Drugs for Pregnant and Lactating Women

Drugs
for
Pregnant
and
Lactating Women

Carl P. Weiner, MD
Professor of Obstetrics, Gynecology, and Reproductive Sciences
Professor of Physiology
University of Maryland School of Medicine
Baltimore, Maryland

Catalin Buhimschi, MD
Clinical Instructor
Yale University School of Medicine
Department of Obstetrics and Gynecology
New Haven, Connecticut

CHURCHILL LIVINGSTONE

An Imprint of Elsevier Science
New York   Edinburgh   London   Philadelphia

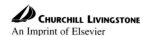
Churchill Livingstone
An Imprint of Elsevier

The Curtis Center
Independence Square West
Philadelphia, PA 19106

Drugs for Pregnant and Lactating Women   ISBN 0-443-06607-8

Notice

Obstetrics/Gynecology is an ever-changing field. Standard safety precautions must be followed, but as new research and clinical experience broaden our knowledge, changes in treatment and drug therapy may become necessary or appropriate. Readers are advised to check the most current product information provided by the manufacturer of each drug to be administered to verify the recommended dose, the method and duration of administration, and contraindications. It is the responsibility of the treating physician, relying on experience and knowledge of the patient, to determine dosages and the best treatment for each individual patient. Neither the Publisher nor the author assumes any liability for any injury and/or damage to persons or property arising from this publication.

The Publisher

Library of Congress Cataloging-in-Publication Data

Weiner, Carl P.
    Drugs for pregnant and lactating women / Carl Weiner.
       p. ; cm
       Includes bibliographical references.
       ISBN 0-443-06607-8
       1. Fetus—Effect of drug on—Handbooks, manuals, etc. 2. Infants (Newborn)—Effect of drugs on—Handbooks, manuals, etc. 3. Obstetrical pharmacology—Handbooks, manuals, etc. 4. Drugs—Side effects—Handbooks, manuals etc. I. Title.
       [DNLM: 1. Pharmaceutical Preparations—contraindications—pregnancy—Handbooks. 2. Breast Feeding—Handbooks. QZ 39 W423d2004]
RG627.6.D79W4562004
618.2'4—dc21   2003053234

Acquisitions Editor: Judith Fletcher/Stephanie Donley
Senior Project Manager: Natalie Ware
Designer: Steven Stave

Printed in China.

Last digit is the print number: 9   8   7   6   5   4   3   2   1

Foreword

This is a dream come true for all of those who care for pregnant and non-pregnant women. There is nothing like this in medical literature. In the past, I have been involved in the publications of several texts on drugs and pregnancy. This new text is on the leading edge of science and knowledge for women and drugs, with more than 720 generic drugs with their 1500 trade names listed in alphabetical order to make identification easy for each drug. Over-the-counter drugs are also included. The information provided in both hard text and electronic versions is very extensive, concise, and user friendly. Its availability as an electronic version for hand-held computer devices, that will be updated for the life of the edition, is particularly exciting. This will not only benefit all health care workers in the field of obstetrics and gynecology, but will also allow instantaneous access to drug related questions.

Included in text and electronic versions are the following headings:

Name
Class
Indications
Dosage with qualifiers
Maternal Considerations
Fetal Considerations
Breastfeeding Safety
References
Summary

Additionally, there are lists of known teratogens, pregnancy drug registries, AHA endocarditis guidelines, FDA category definitions, and the percent of drugs assigned to them also included.

Thanks go to Dr. Weiner for his ingenuity in taking a complicated problem and making it straightforward and simple for those who care for pregnant and non-pregnant women.

This effort is the first to simultaneously embrace text and an electronic version for hand-held computers. The combination of Elsevier—the world's largest health sciences publisher—and Dr. Weiner—an individual who has a long-term interest in female reproduction and especially high-risk obstetrics—assures success of the project.

This is the new frontier in medical publishing and we will look forward to additions and revisions in the electronic format.

Frederick P. Zuspan, MD
Professor and Chairman, Emeritus
The Ohio State University School of Medicine and Public Health, Department of Obstetrics and Gynecology;
Emeritus Editor, American Journal of Obstetrics and Gynecology
Las Vegas, NV

Foreword

The study of medication use in pregnancy is one of the least developed and most neglected areas of clinical pharmacology and drug research. Although pregnancy is widely regarded as a special population due to both the unique maternal physiology and the vulnerability of the developing fetus, researchers and pharmaceutical companies have been reticent to evaluate optimal modalities of treatment in this group. The issue is compounded by the enormous number of medications women are exposed to during pregnancy. Epidemiological surveys indicate nearly two thirds of all pregnant women use four to five drugs during pregnancy, labor and delivery. Women with medical conditions such as epilepsy, diabetes, and hypertension must continue therapy during pregnancy. In some cases, due to a justified or unjustified concern for the developing fetus, the medication prescribed is either withheld, or not adequate to treat the maternal condition, or not monitored closely enough as pregnancy progresses for the needed adjustments in dosing. The result is a double negative, that of fetal exposure without maternal or fetal benefit. The lack of Food and Drug Administration obstetric labeling and the near universal off-label use of drugs are the direct result of the paucity of research and clinical trials in this special population. The public concern stems from the use of drugs in pregnancy based on an empiric approach rather than a scientific basis and does not take into account the many alterations in pregnancy.

There are profound physiologic changes in pregnancy involving the mother, placenta and fetus that may alter absorption, distribution and elimination of drugs. For example, there is a decrease in gastric emptying and an increase in intestinal transit time, both of which may alter gastrointestinal absorption of drugs. Similarly, the physiologic increase in pulmonary blood flow, hyperventilation, or increased tidal volume during pregnancy may increase the absorption of inhalants. The dramatic increase in blood volume with subsequent dilutional hypoalbuminemia, especially in the third trimester, can be associated with a decreased drug binding capacity and may profoundly affect the distribution of many drugs during pregnancy. These are but a few of the many examples of the complex changes in pregnancy that affect the type, dosing, and effectiveness of medications in this special population.

Daily advances in therapeutics dramatically increase the number and types of medications available more rapidly than textbooks can be updated. This new text by Weiner and Buhimschi, Drugs for Pregnant and Lactating Women, helps fill the void. It is a comprehensive resource addressing the unique needs of this special population. Each drug entry includes the generic and trade names, drug class, indication(s) (on and off label), mechanism(s) of action, dosage, maternal and fetal considerations, breastfeeding safety, references, FDA pregnancy and lactation categories, and a summary. Wherever possible, evidence-based recommendations are made. This unique reference combines the printed word with an electronic version updated quarterly to allow for the incorporation of the new therapeutics. This design is user friendly for the busy clinician and includes prescribing information as well as a review of the published experience with the drug in pregnancy and lactation. As the first of its type, Drugs for Pregnant and Lactating Women will simplify the clinician's ability to maintain updated information on medications in pregnancy and facilitate the incorporation of more rigorous study into the use of medications in the pregnant and lactating populations.

Catherine Y. Spong, MD
Chief, Pregnancy and Perinatology Branch
PPB CRMC NICHD NIH
Bethesda, Maryland

Preface

Thousands of pregnant and breast-feeding women take a prescription or over-the-counter drug each day. Though for the most part safe, a small percentage of these actions will have unintended adverse consequences for either mother or child. An additional percentage proves ineffective, due in part to the unique physiology of pregnancy or breastfeeding. And while an unnecessary drug should never be given to the pregnant or breast-feeding woman, an important therapy should never be withheld because of her status. Health care givers are now accustomed to routinely checking the FDA classification of a drug before prescribing it. Unfortunately, this classification system, though simple in concept, is dated, rarely revised as new information becomes available, and too simplistic to account for the physiology and health care needs of pregnant and breast-feeding women. Few drugs are approved by the FDA for use during pregnancy, and even oxytocin is a Category X agent. The important information provided by the manufacturer is often couched in protective legalese and never focuses on the needs of the obstetrical health care provider. Prior attempts to provide the caregiver the needed information have proven dense and filled with descriptions of studies, but not their implications. As a result, they are used in practice as a source of the FDA pregnancy category.

The purpose of this new text is to provide a user friendly, pregnancy-lactation–focused reference for the use of the concerned health care provider. Though we recommend consulting a more complete reference before prescribing an unfamiliar agent, the information provided will aid the safe prescribing of drugs familiar to the physician. The number of new drugs released over the last decade is great, and their known impact on pregnancy and lactation, and vice versa often limited to absent. The authors intend this to be a living text. We have coupled it with a convenient, user-friendly hand-held electronic version that will be updated and expanded on a regular basis. Conflicts in FDA class with existing knowledge are pointed out, and recommendations made wherever possible based on medical evidence. We encourage readers to contact us at Technical.support@elsevier.com with any requests, errors, or conflicts.

Acknowledgment

The production of DRUGS FOR PREGNANT AND LACTATING WOMEN was a long journey that could not have ended successfully without the support of several key people. The authors thank Judy Fletcher who, on behalf of the Publisher, believed in and endorsed a very new concept. We thank Dr. Andrew Malinow, Vice Chair, Department of Anesthesiology, University of Maryland School of Medicine for his meticulous effort to assure the pharmaceutical doses listed in the text were safe and accurate. Lastly, I want to recognize and thank Carol, who spent many evenings alone while I worked on the text. Your support is central. Thank you.

Carl Weiner

Introduction

Frustrated by the absence of a comprehensive resource that recognizes the uniqueness of medical needs during pregnancy and lactation, we created DRUGS FOR PREGNANT AND LACTATING WOMEN as an easy-to-use, reader friendly resource containing the key information required by caregivers to make prescribing decisions. Too often, we check only the FDA Pregnancy Category before making a decision to prescribe or discontinue a medication. Unfortunately, few of us have read these definitions (TABLE 1), understand their limitations, and realize the assigned category is essentially stagnant, based predominantly on information available when the drug was approved in the United States, and only occasionally officially updated to reflect advancing knowledge. Two-thirds of all drugs sold in the U.S. are classified Category C, and less than 1% Category A. With the benefit of added experience, we learn that many Category X drugs are not absolutely contraindicated during pregnancy, and several Category C or D drugs are either clear human teratogens or have frequent and serious adverse fetal effects. These facts are highlighted by a study comparing the categorization of same drugs by the appropriate agencies in the U.S., Australia, and Sweden (Addis A, Sharabi S, Bonati M. Drug Saf 2000; 23:245-53). Only 25% of the 236 drugs common to all 3 systems were placed into the same risk factor category. Nor does the categorization inform the provider how either pregnancy or lactation may alter the patient's response to therapy compared to the nonpregnant state. The FDA is well aware of these limitations and is actively considering revision. Lastly, increasingly busy health care providers are often dependent on either the advertisements in trade journals or the pharmaceutical house detail people for up-to-date information on new drugs. Yet, a recent study observed that promotional claims are frequently misleading and the cited studies were either unretrievable or failed to back-up the particular claim (Villanueva P, Peiro S, Libero J, Pereiro I. Lancet 2003; 361:27-32). This is not a new problem (Wilkes MS, Doblin B, Shapiro M. Ann Intern Med 1992; 116:912-19).

This text seeks to reduce the aforenoted limitations by using brief descriptions to summarize the current level of knowledge. The information on each drug is divided into 10 sections. Those who purchase the electronic version can search by subgroups or names in each of these sections.

The first section of the text lists the generic Name followed by trade names used in the United States. Some drugs have a half dozen or more trade names, and are difficult to remember if you do not use them regularly. While we steadfastly sought to make the text useful to physicians internationally, the sheer number of names used globally proved prohibitive to include at this time.

The second section is the drug Class, such as antibiotic (type), nonsteroidal antiinflammatory (NSAID), anticonvulsant, antihypertensive, etc. This makes it easier to sort drugs in search of alternative or complementary agents when necessary.

The third section lists the Indications for the drug. In most, though not all instances, this list is confined to FDA approved indications. Popular off-label uses are typically reviewed in a subsequent section.

The fourth section is the known or presumed Mechanism of Action. This is frequently either unknown, or while several activities of the drug are known, it is unclear whether they are responsible for the disease-directed action of the drug. Knowledge of the mechanism of action is important for the selection of complementary drugs and the prediction of adverse effects.

The fifth section contains the <u>Dose</u> by specific indication. Also included in this section are most relevant *Contraindications* and *Cautions*. This information is mostly derived from manufacturer-provided material, but tailored for women. You will not find erectile dysfunction or benign prostatic hypertrophy as either an indication or a contraindication for a particular drug, though they certainly might be listed in a general drug text. Also frequently removed from the list are typical corporate liability comments on pregnancy that are not substantiated by either animal or human experience. The dose advice provided has been checked multiple times by at least 3 individuals. However, the very design of this text assumes the prescriber has previously familiarized him or herself with the contents of the package insert. The details provided under <u>Dose</u> are a suitable refresher, but not a substitute. We strongly recommend you confirm the dose when using an unfamiliar drug. Further, we have adopted the approach of simply noting when a dose modification must be considered, rather than trying to be all things for all situations. The standard 'NOTE' mentions the need for either renal or hepatic dosing. This means that, in the face of compromised renal or hepatic function, the physician must take into account altered clearance of the drug. The formulas are usually contained in the package insert or may be discussed with the dispensing pharmacist.

The sixth and seventh sections form the unique core of the text. In the sixth, titled <u>Maternal Considerations</u>, we review how the drug impacts pregnancy and vice versa. We summarize the published experience during pregnancy, highlighting any known problems. Off-label uses are detailed, as is the evidence for efficacy if it exists. We also note applications that have proved unsuccessful. The sad reality is that many drugs used during pregnancy are either ineffective or poorly effective for their most common uses—the tocolytic agents being prime examples. Specific evidence-based recommendations are made wherever possible. It is in this section we also detail the known drug *Side Effects*, again focusing on mother and child. Priapism and impotence may be important side effects in some populations, but not in the one our envisioned reader provides care.

The seventh section is titled <u>Fetal Considerations</u>. Here, the impact of the drug on the human fetus is reviewed, information on placental transfer presented (e.g., the fetal umbilical vein: maternal vein ratio), and any adverse effects summarized. The possible applications of a drug for fetal therapy and an appraisal of its efficacy will also be found here. Animal data are presented when human experience is missing. Rodent teratogenicity studies are summarized, where available, recognizing there are well-known human teratogens, which were not teratogens in rodents (e.g. thalidomide). Of potential relevance is the dose at which the adverse effects are seen in rodents (in terms of multiples of the maximum recommended human dose), and the presence or absence of maternal toxicity that may be the proximate cause of the noted effect. Much of this information is published in peer-reviewed articles, but in some instances, the only source of this information is the manufacturer. It is frightening to us, as practitioners, to find how little is known about many commonly used drugs during pregnancy and lactation. It is our hope readers will be encouraged when confronted with the facts to try and fill in the missing information with quality studies. It is of at least equal concern the number of drugs withheld from women during pregnancy or lactation because of unsubstantiated or, at times, past but refuted theories.

The eighth section is <u>Breastfeeding</u>. We note whether the drug enters human breast milk, and the kinetics of its excretion, if known. The ideal information includes the weight-corrected percent of the maternal dose ingested by the unsupplemented 3kg-newborn and the resulting neonatal blood levels. The number of times the ideal is achieved can be counted on the hands of a single individual. When this information is not known, a milk:plasma (M:P) ratio or concentration is given. This information provides limited information, and may indeed mislead the reader. When no human data are available, animal (typically rodent) is proffered, wherever available. Some of this information is published in peer-reviewed articles, and some by the manufacturer. Occasional conflicts are noted, and wherever possible, specific evidence-based recommendations made. For example, many drugs are used for a limited period or even one-time use. When the patient wishes to continue breastfeeding, but there is reasonable doubt of safety, we will recommend the patient pump her breasts for a period of time before resuming breastfeeding. In other instances, the drug may be safe, but the mother not, for example, the woman with HIV.

Section nine contains salient <u>References</u>. Most are directed at source material, but some are reviews. This information is rarely in packaged inserts (which comprise, for example, the PHYSICIANS DESK REFERENCE) and, cover maternal, fetal, and lactational issues.

The final section is entitled <u>Summary</u>. In this section, the reader will find the FDA category as published in the package insert and a code assigned by the editors for breast-feeding safety (S, safe; NS, not safe; and U, unknown). Often there is some but not enough information for a particular conclusion. In these situations, we have placed a question mark next to the selected code (e.g., S?). The final comments always reflect the need to balance risk. This is a patient-specific process and not given to absolutes. In many instances, the reader is informed there are other alternatives for which there are more experience in pregnancy and lactation. We strongly suggest that wherever possible, the reader seek and use those agents. Pregnancy is not the occasion to be a pioneer, if unnecessary. If there is a post-marketing registry, the telephone number is listed. These registries have the potential to identify important but unusual outcomes.

This text has been prepared to be a living resource. New print editions will be frequent, and those readers with the electronic version will receive periodic updates when they re-synchronize their hand-held computers. Updates will include a growing number of popular herbal remedies with which the obstetrical caregiver will be confronted during the normal course of practice. Readers are encouraged to contact the editors with comments, concerns, and criticisms.

Contents

Acarbose (Precose)

■ **Class**	Oral *hypoglycemic*
■ **Indications**	Diabetes mellitus, type II
■ **Mechanism**	An oral pancreatic α-amylase and intestinal α-glucoside hydrolase inhibitor that delays bowel carbohydrate metabolism, slowing the postprandial rise in glucose

■ **Dosage with Qualifiers**

Diabetes mellitus, type II—begin 25mg (50mg if >60kg); thereafter, 50-100mg PO ac tid based on glucose levels
* **Contraindications**—hypersensitivity to drug or class, DKA, cirrhosis, intestinal obstruction or malabsorbtion syndromes
* **Caution**—renal dysfunction

■ **Maternal Considerations**

Acarbose is the subject of a large ongoing trial to determine whether its use can reduce or delay the onset of type II diabetes in patients with impaired glucose intolerance. There are no adequate reports or well-controlled studies of **acarbose** in pregnant women. There is a single report of 6 pregnant women with impaired glucose tolerance treated with **acarbose**. Glucose levels returned to normal, and the pregnancies were reportedly uncomplicated.
Side effects include intestinal discomfort consisting of pain, diarrhea, flatulence, elevated LFTs, and jaundice.

■ **Fetal Considerations**

There are no adequate reports or well-controlled studies in human fetuses. Only 2% of the oral dose is absorbed. Rodent studies are reassuring, revealing no evidence of teratogenicity or IUGR despite the use of doses almost 10 times higher than those used clinically.

■ **Breastfeeding Safety**

There is no published experience in nursing women. It is unknown whether **acarbose** enters human breast milk. A single rat study suggests **acarbose** might alter the composition of breast milk by inhibiting lipogenesis.

■ **References**

Mercer SW, Williamson DH. Biochem J 1987; 242:235-43.
Product information. Precose, Bayer Corp., 1997.
Zarate A, Ochoa R, Hernandez M, Basurto L. Ginecol Obstet Mex 2000; 68:42-5.

■ **Summary**

* **Pregnancy Category B**
* **Lactation Category U**
* Insulin and diet regulation remain the standard treatments for glucose intolerance during pregnancy.
* There is a growing interest in the use of oral hypoglycemic agents during pregnancy, and **acarbose** is a candidate for future study in this area.

Acebutolol (ACB; Alol; Beloc; Diasectral; Espesil; Lupar; Neptal; Rhotral; Sectral; Sectral LP; Wesfalin)

■ **Class** .... *Antihypertensive; antiarrhythmic, ventricular; hypertension, essential*

■ **Indications** .... Chronic hypertension, ventricular arrhythmias

■ **Mechanism** .... Cardioselective partial β-adrenoceptor antagonist

■ **Dosage with Qualifiers** .... Hypertension—begin 400-800mg PO qd; max 1200mg/d
Ventricular arrhythmia—begin 200-400mg/d; typical dose, 600-1200mg/d
- **Contraindications**—hypersensitivity, CHF, heart block, hypotension, pulmonary disease
- **Caution**—diabetes mellitus, hepatic or renal dysfunction

■ **Maternal Considerations** .... There are no adequate reports or well-controlled studies of **acebutolol** in pregnant women. **Acebutolol** was significantly less successful than either **labetalol** or α-**methyldopa** in controlling chronic arterial hypertension >90mmHg in one small randomized trial. The rates of pregnancy complications among the 3 groups of women were similar.
Side effects include CHF, bronchospasm, fatigue, dizziness, headache, constipation, and diarrhea.

■ **Fetal Considerations** .... There are no adequate reports or well-controlled studies in human fetuses. **Acebutolol** and its main metabolite, N-acetylacebutolol, cross the placenta with a 0.6:0.8 maternal-fetal ratio. A prospective study of **acebutolol's** hemodynamic and renal impact on neonates after chronic *in utero* exposure found hemodynamic failure in 5 of 11 children delivered of treated mothers. Exposed neonates had significantly less early neonatal diuresis, absence of a significant rise in the glomerular filtration rates, and reduced sodium and calcium balances. The direct effect of the drug on the glomerular and tubular functions and/or the renal arteriolar vasomotricity could explain these effects.

■ **Breastfeeding Safety** .... **Acebutolol** and N-acetylacebutolol are concentrated in breast milk (milk-plasma ratios 7:12, respectively) and symptoms of neonatal β-blockade are rarely reported. A neonate might receive pharmacologically active amounts of **acebutolol** if the daily maternal dosage exceeds 400mg/d and/or renal function in the mother is impaired. However, the American Academy of Pediatrics considers **acebutolol** permissible with breastfeeding.

■ **References** .... Yassen H, Boutroy MJ, Monin P, Vert P. Arch Fr Pediatr 1992; 49:351-5.
Committee on Drugs, American Academy of Pediatrics. Pediatrics 1994; 93:137-50.

Lardoux H, Blazquez G, Leperlier E, Gerard J. Arch Mal Coeur Vaiss 1988; 81(Spec No):137-40.
Boutroy MJ, Bianchetti G, Dubruc C, et al. Eur J Clin Pharmacol 1986; 30:737-9.

■ Summary	• **Pregnancy Category B (1st trimester), D (2nd and 3rd trimesters)**
	• **Lactation Category S**
	• There are alternative agents for which there is more experience during pregnancy and lactation.
	• Consider withholding oral **acebutolol** therapy for 12h prior to the anticipated delivery to minimize the risk to the neonate.

Acetaminophen (APAP; Acephen; Aceta; Acetaminophen Uniserts; Anapark; Apacet; Asidon; Calip; Dapacin; Ed-Apap; Feverall; Genapap; Genebs; Mapap; Maranox; Neopap; Oraphen-PD; Panadol; Redutemp; Ridenol; Silapap; Tapanol; Tempra; Tylenol; Uni-Ace)

■ **Class**	Analgesic; antipyretic
■ **Indications**	Mild pain, fever
■ **Mechanism**	Nonspecific cyclooxygenase inhibitor
■ **Dosage with Qualifiers**	Pain and/or fever—650-1000mg PO/PR q4-6h; max 4g/d
	NOTE—included in many combinations
	• **Contraindications**—hypersensitivity to drug or class
	• **Caution**—hepatic or renal dysfunction, chronic alcohol use, G6PD deficiency, PKU
■ **Maternal Considerations**	**Acetaminophen** is metabolized in the liver and excreted by the kidneys. During the 1st trimester, the mean half-life is significantly lower and oral clearance is significantly higher compared to nonpregnant control subjects. Only during pregnancy is weight related to clearance, suggesting the dose may need to be adjusted in obese women. In contrast, there are no obvious differences in clearance at term. Chronic abuse and overdose are the most common problems. The damage appears secondary to free radical toxicity with consumption of glutathione during metabolism. **N-acetylcysteine** is the treatment of choice for an acute overdose.
	Side effects include hepatotoxicity, nephrotoxicity, agranulocytosis, pancytopenia, hemolytic anemia, pancreatitis, rash, angioedema and urticaria.

■ Fetal Considerations ·············· There are no adequate reports or well-controlled studies in human fetuses. **Acetaminophen** crosses the human placenta, reaching steady state in the isolated perfused model within 1h. The F:M ratio for **acetaminophen** approximated 0.12 in the pregnant ewe, and neither sulfate or glucuronide metabolites crossed. **Acetaminophen** use during labor to treat the fever of chorioamnionitis is associated with improved fetal umbilical blood gases, presumably by reducing fetal oxygen demand as the maternal core temperature declines. Although it was previously suggested that exposure to **acetaminophen** was associated with clubfoot and digital abnormalities, these reports are not sustained in large series. However, there appears to be a link between it and gastroschisis and small bowel atresia. Unlike aspirin, **acetaminophen** has no antiplatelet activity and does not pose a hemorrhagic risk to the fetus.

■ Breastfeeding Safety ·············· **Acetaminophen** is excreted in low concentrations into breast milk. The amount of the drug administered to the mother estimated to be available to the neonate ranges from 0.04-0.23%, and it is generally considered compatible with breastfeeding.

■ References ·············· Beaulac-Baillargeon L, Rocheleau S. Eur J Clin Pharmacol 1994; 46:451-4.
Rayburn W, Shukla U, Stetson P, Piehl E. Am J Obstet Gynecol 1986; 155:1353-6.
Kirshon B, Moise KJ Jr, Wasserstrum N. J Reprod Med 1989; 34:955-9.
Weigand UW, Chou RC, Maulik D, Levy G. Pediatr Pharmacol (New York) 1984; 4(3):145-53.
Wang LH, Rudolph AM, Benet LZ. J Pharmacol Exp Ther 1986; 238:198-205.
Committee on Drugs, American Academy of Pediatrics. Pediatrics 1994; 93:137-50.
Werler MM, Sheehan JE, Mitchell AA. Am J Epidemiol 2002; 155:26-31.

■ Summary ·············· • **Pregnancy Category B**
• **Lactation Category S**
• **Acetaminophen** is used throughout pregnancy for analgesia and to reduce fever.
• Like most drugs, it should be used during the 1st trimester only when clearly necessary.

Acetazolamide (Acetadiazol; Acetamide; Azomid; Dehydratin; Diamox; Diamox Sequels; Diamox Sodium; Ederen; Glauconox; Inidrase; Nephramid; Oratrol)

■ **Class**	*Diuretic*
■ **Indications**	Glaucoma, open and closed angle; altitude sickness, prevention and treatment; epilepsy; CHF; drug-induced edema; urinary alkalinization
■ **Mechanism**	Carbonic anhydrase inhibitor

■ **Dosage with Qualifiers**

Glaucoma—125-250mg PO/IV bid to qid
Altitude sickness—250-500mg PO bid beginning 48h before ascent
Epilepsy—375-1000mg (8-30mg/kg/d) PO qd if sole agent; begin 250mg qd if with other agents
Congestive heart failure—250-375mg PO/IV qd (for best results, take on alternate days)
Drug-induced edema—250-375mg PO/IV qd (for best results, take on alternate days)
Urinary alkalinization—5mg/kg PO/IV bid or tid to maintain alkaline urine pH

- **Contraindications**—hypersensitivity to drug or class, hyponatremia, hypokalemia, depressed respiratory function, cirrhosis, hyperchloride acidosis, adrenocortical insufficiency
- **Caution**—hepatic and/or renal dysfunction

■ **Maternal Considerations**

There are no adequate reports or well-controlled studies of **acetazolamide** in pregnant women. Pregnancy is not known to alter the impact, efficacy, and dosing of **acetazolamide**.
Side effects include aplastic anemia, Stevens-Johnson syndrome, toxic epidermal necrolysis, fulminant hepatitis, paresthesias, loss of appetite, taste changes, dyspepsia, and polyuria.

■ **Fetal Considerations**

There are no adequate reports or well-controlled studies in human fetuses. It is unknown whether **acetazolamide** crosses the human placenta. There is no suggestion of teratogenicity in humans despite a long clinical experience. In some rodents, **acetazolamide** is teratogenic (skeletal abnormalities consisting variably of ossification defects or some form of postaxial forelimb ectrodactyly in rats, urinary malformations in mice when combined with **amiloride**).

■ **Breastfeeding Safety**

Acetazolamide is not concentrated in the milk and the neonatal exposure is considered to be less than 1% of the maternal dose. It is generally considered compatible with breastfeeding.

■ **References** ········· Nakatsuka T, Komatsu T, Fujii T. Teratology 1992; 45:629-36.
Academy of Pediatrics. Pediatrics 1994; 93:137-50.

■ **Summary** ·········
- **Pregnancy Category C**
- **Lactation Category S**
- **Acetazolamide** should be used during pregnancy and lactation only if the benefit justifies the potential perinatal risk.

Acetohexamide (Dimelin; Dimelor; Dymelor; Gamadiabet; Ordimel; Toyobexin)

■ **Class** ········· *Oral hypoglycemic; sulfonylurea*

■ **Indications** ········· Diabetes mellitus, type II

■ **Mechanism** ········· A sulfonylurea that acutely stimulates the release of pancreatic insulin and thus requires islet activity

■ **Dosage with Qualifiers** ········· Diabetes mellitus, type II—begin 250mg/d before breakfast in women not receiving another hypoglycemic agent; increase by 250-500mg every 5-7d until desired control
- **Contraindications**—hypersensitivity to drug or class, ketoacidosis, type I diabetes mellitus
- **Caution**—pregnancy

■ **Maternal Considerations** ········· There are no adequate reports or well-controlled studies of **acetohexamide** in pregnant women, and no publications within the last 3 decades. Some oral hypoglycemic drugs are associated with an increased risk of cardiovascular death compared to diet and insulin control of glucose. *Side effects* include hypoglycemia, cholestatic jaundice, gastrointestinal upset, allergic skin reactions, SIADH, hemolytic anemia, various cytopenias, and hepatic porphyria.

■ **Fetal Considerations** ········· There are no adequate reports or well-controlled studies in human fetuses. Although **acetohexamide** apparently crosses the placenta, there are no reports of teratogenicity in humans. Prolonged neonatal hypoglycemia associated with hyperinsulinism is reported. Differences in the extent of the placental transport of various sulfonylureas are reported. Embryotoxicity is noted in rodent studies.

■ **Breastfeeding Safety** ········· There is no published experience in nursing women. It is unknown whether **acetohexamide** enters human breast milk as other sulfonylureas do.

■ **References** ———————————— Kemball ML, McIver C, Milner RD, et al. Arch Dis Child 1970; 45:696-701.

■ **Summary** ————————————
- **Pregnancy Category C**
- **Lactation Category U**
- Insulin and diet regulation remain the standard treatments for glucose intolerance during pregnancy.
- Oral hypoglycemic agents are generally considered contraindicated during pregnancy. However, there is growing interest in the use of these agents during pregnancy, and acetohexamide might be a candidate for future study. If a patient is maintained on **acetohexamide** during pregnancy, she should be switched to insulin 1-2w prior to delivery in hopes of reducing the risk of neonatal hypoglycemia secondary to hyperinsulinism.

Acetylcysteine (Acetyst; Alveolux; Bromuc; Mucomyst; Mucosil; Mucosol; Mukosil; Respaire)

■ **Class** ———————————— *Antidote; mucolytic; antioxidant*

■ **Indications** ———————————— Treatment of acetaminophen or *Amanita phalloides* toxicity; mucolytic in patients with cystic fibrosis

■ **Mechanism** ———————————— A glutathione precursor that breaks disulfide bonds caused by oxidation

■ **Dosage with Qualifiers** ————————————
Acetaminophen toxicity—begin 140mg/kg PO by NG tube; thereafter, 70mg/kg PO q4h ×15-20 doses
Mucolytic—1 nebulizer ampule q6-8h; alternatively 2-5ml of 10% solution or 600mg in 3 divided doses
- **Contraindications**—hypersensitivity to drug or class
- **Caution**—severe respiratory failure, asthma

■ **Maternal Considerations** ————————————
N-acetylcysteine is a prototype antioxidant presently used nearly exclusively during pregnancy for the treatment of maternal drug toxicity associated with free radical excess such as that occurring with **acetaminophen**. There are no adequate and well-controlled studies of **N-acetylcysteine** in pregnant women. It has been used for the treatment of **acetaminophen** toxicity during pregnancy.
Side effects include bronchospasm, anaphylaxis, nausea, vomiting, stomatitis, rhinorrhea, urticaria, and rash.

■ **Fetal Considerations** ————————————
N-acetylcysteine crosses the placenta, reaching equilibrium with maternal sera. In laboratory studies, it reduces embryo toxicity associated with hyperglycemia, hypoxia, and sepsis.

- **Breastfeeding Safety** ⸺ There is no published experience in nursing women. It is unknown whether **N-acetylcysteine** enters human breast milk. It is unlikely short-term administration for an acute problem would pose a risk to the nursing infant.

- **References** ⸺ Boyer JC, Hernandez F, Estorc J, et al. Clin Chem 2001; 47:971-4.
McElhatton PR, Sullivan FM, Volans GN. Reprod Toxicol 1997; 11:85-94.
Horowitz RS, Dart RC, Jarvie DR, et al. J Toxicol Clin Toxicol 1997; 35:447-51.
Buhimschi IA, Buhimschi CS, Weiner CP. Am J Obstet Gynecol 2003; 188:203-8.

- **Summary** ⸺
  - **Pregnancy Category B**
  - **Lactation Category S?**
  - Future investigation may demonstrate a role for **N-acetylcysteine** in the treatment of the fetus for a myriad of pathologic conditions that share excess free radical generation.

Acyclovir (Acivir Cream; Acivir Eye; Avirax; Avorax; Clovicin; Clovix; Entir; Supra-Vir; Zovirax)

- **Class** ⸺ *Antiviral*

- **Indications** ⸺ Primary or secondary herpes infection; treatment or prevention of *Varicella* pneumonia

- **Mechanism** ⸺ A synthetic, acyclic purine nucleoside that inhibits DNA polymerase by direct incorporation

- **Dosage with Qualifiers** ⸺ Genital herpes, recurrent—200mg PO 5x/d ×10d
Genital herpes, suppressive—400mg PO bid for up to a year, or during pregnancy, from 36w onward; with HIV, 400-800mg PO 2-3x/d, or IV 5-10mg/kg q8h ×5-10d
Herpes zoster—800mg PO 5x/d ×7-10d
Varicella, acute—800mg PO qid ×5d
Ocular herpes—3% ointment 5x/d ×7-10d
  - **Contraindications**—hypersensitivity to drug or class
  - **Caution**—renal dysfunction or concurrent nephrotoxic drug

- **Maternal Considerations** ⸺ Treatment is not curative, but rather intended to reduce the duration of symptoms and viral shedding. There is a long clinical experience free of obvious adverse effects. Suppression therapy is both effective and cost-effective whether or not the primary infection occurred during the current pregnancy. Because **acyclovir** is excreted via the kidneys, its half-life may be reduced during pregnancy, but this has not been studied specifically. Its combination with **zidovudine** alters the clearance of both in pregnant rats. *Side effects* include seizures, coma, leukopenia, thrombocytopenia, renal dysfunction, nausea, vomiting, diarrhea, headache, dizziness, lethargy, rash, and confusion.

■ **Fetal Considerations** ·············· There are no adequate reports or well-controlled studies in human fetuses. It is unknown whether **acyclovir** crosses the human placenta. Post-marketing surveillance by Glaxo-Wellcome has not revealed any increase in or pattern of malformations after **acyclovir** exposure during the 1st trimester (756 pregnancies). Rodent studies are reassuring, revealing no evidence of teratogenicity or IUGR despite the use of doses higher than those used clinically.

■ **Breastfeeding Safety** ·············· Though **acyclovir** is passively secreted and achieves concentrations in breast milk higher than maternal serum, it is used to treat neonatal herpetic infection and is generally considered compatible with breastfeeding.

■ **References** ···························· Brown SD, Bartlett MG, White CA. Antimicrob Agents Chemother 2003; 47:991-6.
Scott LL, Hollier LM, McIntire D, et al. Infect Dis Obstet Gynecol 2001; 9:75-80.
Braig S, Luton D, Sibony O, et al. Eur J Obstet Gynecol Reprod Biol 2001; 96:55-8.
Heuchan AM, Isaacs D. Med J Aust 2001; 174:288-92.
Leung DT, Sacks SL. Drugs 2000; 60:1329-52.
Eldridge RR, Ephross SA, Heffner CR, et al. Prim Care Update Obstet Gynecol 1998; 5:190-1.
Scott LL, Alexander J. Am J Perinatol 1998; 15:57-62.
Bork K, Kaiser T, Benes P. Arzneimittelforschung 2000; 50:656-8.
Academy of Pediatrics. Pediatrics 1994; 93:137-50.

■ **Summary** ·····························
- **Pregnancy Category B**
- **Lactation Category S**
- **Acyclovir** significantly reduces the duration of shedding and the number of recurrent HSV outbreaks during pregnancy.

Adapalene (Differin; Differine)

■ **Class** — *Dermatologic, retinoid*

■ **Indications** — Acne vulgaris

■ **Mechanism** — Binds retinoid nuclear receptors to interfere with cellular differentiation, keratinization, and inflammatory processes

■ **Dosage with Qualifiers** — Acne vulgaris—apply (0.1%) cream or gel to the affected area once daily at night
● **Contraindications**—hypersensitivity to drug or class

■ **Maternal Considerations** — Systemic absorption of **adapalene** across human skin is low, with none being detected in the plasma of 6 patients treated for acne in a standardized fashion for 5d with 2g. There are no adequate and well-controlled studies of **adapalene** in pregnant women.
Side effects include erythema, dryness, burning, scaling, and photosensitivity.

■ **Fetal Considerations** — There are no adequate studies of **adapalene** in human pregnancy. It is unknown whether **adapalene** crosses the human placenta. Though the pharmacology is encouraging, there are several reports in humans associating **adapalene** with fetal malformation after cutaneous exposure. The available information is insufficient to conclude cause and effect. Oral administration to rodents at 100-200 times the maximum dose increased the risk of malformation.
No abnormalities were seen in pregnancies exposed to lower concentrations.

■ **Breastfeeding Safety** — There is no published experience in nursing women. It is unknown whether **adapalene** enters human breast milk. Considering the dose and route, it is unlikely to pose a significant risk to the breast-feeding neonate.

■ **References** — No authors. Prescrire Int 1998; 7:148-9.
Autret E, Berjot M, Jonville-Bera AP, et al. Lancet 1997; 350:339.

■ **Summary** — ● **Pregnancy Category C**
● **Lactation Category U**
● **Adapalene** should be used during pregnancy and lactation only if the benefit justifies the potential perinatal risk.
● There are alternative agents for which there is more experience during pregnancy and lactation.

Adenosine (Adenic; Adeno-Jec; Adenocar; Adenocard; Adenoscan; Adenosine Phosphate; ATP)

■ **Class**

Antiarrhythmic, diagnostic

■ **Indications**

Paroxysmal supraventricular tachycardia

■ **Mechanism**

Interrupts reentry pathways by slowing AV node conduction

■ **Dosage with Qualifiers**

Paroxysmal supraventricular tachycardia conversion—
3-6mg IV over 1-2sec; may double to 6mg and then 12mg if
no response after 1-2min
- **Contraindications**—hypersensitivity to drug or class,
  2nd or 3rd degree heart block or sick sinus syndrome
- **Caution**—asthma, chronic obstructive pulmonary disease

■ **Maternal Considerations**

An endogenous purine-based nucleoside, IV **adenosine** is
the first choice for short-term management of paroxysmal
supraventricular arrhythmia after a vagal maneuver fails.
Co-administration of **midazolam** safely reduces the recall
of the unpleasant adverse effects of **adenosine**. For long-
term therapy, β-blocking agents with β-1 selectivity are
first-line drugs; class Ic agents and the class III drug
sotalol are effective therapeutic alternatives.
Adenosine has been used on multiple occasions during
pregnancy to treat paroxysmal supraventricular tachycardia.
Side effects include arrhythmia (bradycardia, ventricular
fibrillation or tachycardia, asystole, complete heart block),
bronchospasm, flushing, chest or groin pressure, dizziness,
nausea, vomiting, apprehension, palpitations, and headache.

■ **Fetal Considerations**

There are no adequate reports or well-controlled studies
in human fetuses. **Adenosine** crosses the human placenta.
And though the kinetics remain to be detailed, it enhances
placental perfusion. Rodent studies are reassuring,
revealing no evidence of teratogenicity. **Adenosine** has
been administered successfully on a number of occasions
directly into the umbilical vein to achieve control of a
fetal supraventricular tachycardia.

■ **Breastfeeding Safety**

There are no adequate reports or well-controlled studies
in nursing women. **Adenosine** is a normal constituent of
human breast milk, though the short half-life suggests
little, if any, of the exogenously administered **adenosine**
will enter the milk.

■ **References**

Chow T, Galvin J, McGovern B. Am J Cardiol 1998; 82:581-621.
Hourigan C, Safih S, Rogers I, et al. Emerg Med
(Fremantle) 2001; 13:51-6.
Acevedo CG, Huambachano A, Perez E, et al. Placenta
1997; 18:387-92.
Trappe HJ, Pfitzner P. Z Kardiol 2001; 90:36-44.
Tan HL, Lie KI. Eur Heart J 2001; 22:458-64.

■ **Summary**
- **Pregnancy Category B**
- **Lactation Category U**
- Useful for the short-term treatment of either maternal or fetal tachycardia.

Albuterol (Airet; Albuterol Sulfate; Asmalin; Asmanil; Asmavent; Butamol; Buventol; Proventil; Salbusian; Salbutamol; Theosal; Ventolin; Ventolin Rotacaps; Volmax)

■ **Class**

Adrenergic agonist; bronchodilator

■ **Indications**

Bronchospasm; exercise-induced asthma

■ **Mechanism**

A selective β-2 agonist

■ **Dosage with Qualifiers**

Bronchospasm—1-2 puffs metered dose inhaler q4-6h, max 12 puffs/d or 2-4mg PO tid/qid
Exercise-induced asthma—2 puffs metered dose inhaler ×1 given 15-30min before exercise
NOTE—numerous drug interactions are known. The reader should consult a detailed text if the patient is or has recently been on an MAO inhibitor or tricyclic antidepressant, a β-adrenoceptor antagonist, a diuretic, or digoxin.
- **Contraindications**—hypersensitivity to drug or class
- **Caution**—hyperthyroidism, cardiovascular disease, diabetes mellitus, seizure disorder.

■ **Maternal Considerations**

In some countries, **albuterol** has been used as a tocolytic agent given IV, SC, or PO (also see **terbutaline** or **ritodrine** whose efficacy it compares to). There is no evidence it will stop preterm or term labor. The maximum delay (compared to placebo), though, of 48h should permit maternal administration of corticosteroids. Betamimetic tocolysis is associated with pulmonary edema, especially with multiple gestation, or in women concurrently receiving glucocorticoid therapy to hasten fetal lung maturation, or in association with infection. The mechanism is unclear. Treatment consists of oxygen supplementation and diuresis. Maternal serum glucose and plasma insulin levels peak soon after cessation of therapy and return to preinfusion levels within 2-3h. The decline in potassium is gradual and plateaus after 2h. Once the **albuterol** infusion is stopped, the potassium returns to normal by 2h. Total WBC counts increase within an hour of initiating therapy. There is no need to administer insulin for hyperglycemia and/or potassium for hypokalemia unless the patient is a known diabetic or is severely affected and requires immediate surgery.

Side effects include bronchospasm with inhaler form, arrhythmia, tremor, nervousness, tachycardia, dizziness, headache, hypertension, nausea, hyperactivity, hypokalemia, and hyperglycemia.

■ **Fetal Considerations**

There are no adequate reports or well-controlled studies in human fetuses. **Albuterol** appears to cross the human placenta, though the kinetics remain to be elucidated. There is no convincing evidence of teratogenicity after 1st trimester exposure. In general, long-term follow-up studies of infants exposed to betamimetic tocolysis are reassuring. **Albuterol,** like other β-adrenoceptor agonists, is associated with a reduction in the incidence of RDS. A single abstract suggests an increased risk of newborn retinopathy. **Albuterol** is teratogenic in mice at doses lower than those used in humans.

■ **Breastfeeding Safety**

There is no published experience in nursing women. It is unknown whether **albuterol** enters human breast milk. Other β-adrenoceptor agonists such as **ritodrine** and **terbutaline** are considered safe for breastfeeding.

■ **References**

Ann Allergy Asthma Immunol 2000; 84:475-80.
Milliez JM, Flouvat B, Delhotal B, Jannet D. Obstet Gynecol 1992; 80:182-5.
Chua S, Razvi K, Wong MT, et al. J Obstet Gynaecol Res 1997; 23:381-7.
Ashworth MF, Spooner SF, Verkuyl DA, et al. Br J Obstet Gynaecol 1990; 97:878-82.
The Worldwide Atosiban versus Beta-agonists Study Group. BJOG 2001; 108:133-42.
Michie CA, Braithwaite S, Schulenberg E, Harvey D. Arch Dis Child 1994; 71:F149.

■ **Summary**

- **Pregnancy Category C**
- **Lactation Category S**
- **Albuterol** should be used during pregnancy and lactation only if the benefit justifies the potential perinatal risk.
- As a tocolytic, **albuterol** has no advantage over any other β-adrenoceptor agonist prolonging pregnancy on average 48h over placebo.
- It is ineffective like all β-adrenoceptor agonists used for preterm prophylaxis.
- β-adrenoceptor agonists should be avoided in diabetic women. If unavoidable, the patient should be aggressively covered with a short-acting insulin.

Alendronate sodium (Fosamax)

■ **Class**	*Bisphosphonates, calcium metabolism*
■ **Indications**	Osteoporosis
■ **Mechanism**	Inhibits osteoclast resorption

■ **Dosage with Qualifiers**

Osteoporosis, postmenopausal treatment—10mg PO qd, or 70mg PO once a week taken with meals
Osteoporosis, postmenopausal prevention—5mg PO qd, or 35mg PO once per week taken with meals
Osteoporosis, steroid-induced—5mg PO qd taken with meals
NOTE—avoid supine position

- **Contraindications**—hypersensitivity to drug or class, hypocalcemia, severe renal dysfunction
- **Caution**—upper GI disease

■ **Maternal Considerations**

There are no adequate reports or well-controlled studies of **alendronate** in pregnant women. There appears only one case report of its use during pregnancy; the woman did respond.
Side effects include esophagitis, gastritis, dysphagia, esophageal ulcer, nausea, vomiting, abdominal pain, arthralgia, myalgias, back pain, constipation, diarrhea, headache, chest pain, flu-like syndrome, and peripheral edema.

■ **Fetal Considerations**

There are no adequate reports or well-controlled studies in human fetuses. **Alendronate** crosses the placenta and in rodents, decreases bone density and delays delivery. Both the total and ionized calcium are reduced in mother and fetus. Its toxic effects are reversed by calcium administration.

■ **Breastfeeding Safety**

There is no published experience in nursing women. It is unknown whether **alendronate** enters human breast milk.

■ **References**

Samdani A, Lachmann E, Nagler W. Am J Phys Med Rehabil 1998; 77:153-6.
Minsker DH, Manson JM, Peter CP. Toxicol Appl Pharmacol 1993; 121:217-23.
Patlas N, Golomb G, Yaffe P, et al. Teratology 1999; 60:68-73.

■ **Summary**

- **Pregnancy Category C**
- **Lactation Category U**
- **Alendronate** should be used during pregnancy and lactation only if the benefit justifies the potential perinatal risk.

Alfentanil (Alfenta; Alfentanyl; Rapifen)

■ **Class** ———————————— *Narcotic*

■ **Indications** ———————— Analgesia either alone or in combination for labor or gynecologic pain

■ **Mechanism** ———————— A short-acting lipophilic opioid

■ **Dosage with Qualifiers** ——— <u>Anesthesia, induction</u>—130-245mcg/kg IV (primarily with underlying cardiac disease undergoing a prolonged surgical procedure; more commonly 8-50mcg/kg at induction to blunt the pressor response to tracheal intubation
<u>Anesthesia, maintenance</u>—3-15mcg/kg IV prn, or 0.5-1mcg/kg/min continuous infusion
NOTE—chest wall rigidity is common and neuromuscular blockers are usually given to enable mask ventilation before tracheal intubation
<u>Conscious sedation</u>—3-8mcg/kg IV ×1
- **Contraindications**—hypersensitivity to drug or class
- **Caution**—chest wall rigidity, N/V, bradycardia, hepatic, renal, or pulmonary dysfunction, head injury, bowel obstruction

■ **Maternal Considerations** ——— **Alfentanil** is a short-acting narcotic with rapid onset. As with other lipophilic opioids, **alfentanil** reduces the total dose of local anesthetic analgesic needed to provide comfort when combined with bupivacaine for epidural analgesia while diminishing the likelihood of an undesired motor blockade. Intravenous **alfentanil** given just prior to intubation reduces the associated pressor response in women with preeclampsia.
Side effects include respiratory arrest or depression, arrhythmia, seizure, coma, abuse or dependency, muscle rigidity, nausea, vomiting, dizziness, hypertension, hypotension, tachycardia, bradycardia, confusion, sweating, dry mouth, constipation, and urinary retention.

■ **Fetal Considerations** ——— **Alfentanil** crosses the placenta when given intravenously, though its transfer rate is lower than **fentanyl** (which approximates antipyrine). Neither human embryo toxicity nor teratogenicity is reported, though 1st trimester human data is limited. **Alfentanil** is embryotoxic in rodents when given for 10-30d at doses 2-3 times the human dose. One limited monkey study concluded offspring had impaired ability to do simple cognitive tasks at 2-3 months of age after exposure at 14w gestation. Lipophilic and hydrophilic characteristics of the drug influence placental transfer, as do fluctuations in maternal flow. Neonatal depression characterized by reduced active and passive tone is reported when **alfentanil** is given shortly before delivery. Occasionally, a narcotic antagonist is necessary. There are no reported fetal or neonatal effects after its use for conduction anesthesia.

■ **Breastfeeding Safety** ⸻ **Alfentanil** is excreted into human the breast milk, though the amount excreted is too small to have any significant effect on the newborn.

■ **References** ⸻

Ashton WB, James MF, Janicki P, Uys PC. Br J Anaesth 1991; 67:741-7.
Cooper RA, Devlin E, Boyd TH, Bali IM. Eur J Anaesthesiol 1993; 10:183-7.
Giroux M, Teixera MG, Dumas JC, et al. Biol Neonate 1997; 72:133-41.
Golub MS, Eisele JH Jr, Donald JM. Am J Obstet Gynecol 1988; 159:1280-6.
Rout CC, Rocke DA. Br J Anaesth 1990; 65:468-74.
Scherer R, Holzgreve W. Eur J Obstet Gynecol Reprod Biol 1995; 59:S17-S29.
Zakowski MI, Ham AA, Grant GJ. Anesth Analg 1994; 79:1089-93.

■ **Summary** ⸻
- **Pregnancy Category C**
- **Lactation Category S**
- **Alfentanil** should be used during pregnancy and lactation only if the benefit justifies the potential perinatal risk.

Allopurinol (Aipico; Alloremed; Alloscan; Alonol; Aloral; Aluline; Aluprin; Apurol; Isanol; Lopurin; Lysuron; Unizuric; Uricemil; Uriconorm-E; Zyloprim; Zyroric)

■ **Class** ⸻ *Miscellaneous, antigout, antioxidant*

■ **Indications** ⸻ Gout, nephrolithiasis secondary to urate or calcium oxalate stones

■ **Mechanism** ⸻ A xanthine oxidase inhibitor that interferes with the conversion of xanthine and hypoxanthine to uric acid

■ **Dosage with Qualifiers** ⸻ Gout prophylaxis—100-800mg PO qd; titrate dose until uric acid <6mg/dl
Urate nephrolithiasis prophylaxis—100-800mg PO qd
Calcium oxalate calculi—200-300mg PO qd
- **Contraindications**—hypersensitivity to drug or class
- **Caution**—renal dysfunction

■ **Maternal Considerations** ⸻ There are no adequate reports or well-controlled studies of **allopurinol** in pregnant women. It is rarely indicated for its traditional indications in pregnant or lactating women. There is a single report of a woman treated during pregnancy for primary gout with **allopurinol.**

She delivered a healthy child at 35w. More often, **allopurinol** has been used during pregnancy for women undergoing treatment of acute leukemia. Of future interest is its potential as an antioxidant. **Allopurinol** was used unsuccessfully in one trial for the treatment of established preeclampsia.

Side effects include agranulocytosis, aplastic anemia, thrombocytopenia, hepatic dysfunction, urticaria, Stevens-Johnson syndrome, toxic epidermal necrolysis, rash, diarrhea, pruritus, nausea, and gout flare.

- **Fetal Considerations** — There are no adequate reports or well-controlled studies in human fetuses. There is no evidence that **allopurinol** is teratogenic in humans. Cleft palate and skeletal defects are reported in some rodents.

- **Breastfeeding Safety** — **Allopurinol** and its metabolite oxypurinol are excreted into breast milk to a limited degree and is considered compatible with breastfeeding.

- **References** — Coddington CC, Albrecht RC, Cefalo RC. Am J Obstet Gynecol 1979; 133:107-8.
  Committee on Drugs. Pediatrics 1994; 93:137-50.
  Fujii T, Nishimura H. Jpn J Pharmacol 1972; 22:201-6.
  Gulmezoglu AM, Hofmeyr GJ, Oosthuisen MM. Br J Obstet Gynaecol 1997; 104:689-96.
  Kamilli I, Gresser U. Clin Investig 1993; 71:161-4.

- **Summary** —
  - **Pregnancy Category C**
  - **Lactation Category S**
  - **Allopurinol** should be used during pregnancy and lactation only if the benefit justifies the potential perinatal risk.

Alosetron hydrochloride (Lotronex)

- **Class** — *Gastrointestinal, antidiarrheal, serotonin receptor antagonist*

- **Indications** — Diarrhea-predominant irritable bowel syndrome

- **Mechanism** — A selective and potent antagonist of the serotonin 5-HT3 receptor

- **Dosage with Qualifiers** — Diarrhea associated with irritable bowel syndrome—1mg PO bid
  - **Contraindications**—hypersensitivity to drug or class, constipation

- **Maternal Considerations** .... There are no published reports of **alosetron** use during pregnancy.
  Side effects include ischemic colitis, constipation, hypertension, allergic rhinitis, dyspepsia, and depressive disorders.

- **Fetal Considerations** .... There are no adequate reports or well-controlled studies in human fetuses. It is unknown whether **alosetron** crosses the human placenta. Rodent studies are generally reassuring, revealing no evidence of teratogenicity or IUGR despite the use of doses higher than those used clinically, with the exception of the mouse, where cleft palate and skeletal defects were reported.

- **Breastfeeding Safety** .... There is no published experience in nursing women. It is unknown whether **alosetron** enters human breast milk. **Alosetron** is excreted into the milk of lactating rats.

- **References** .... There is no published experience in pregnancy or during lactation.

- **Summary** .... • **Pregnancy Category B**
  • **Lactation Category U**
  • **Alosetron** is rarely indicated during pregnancy and should be used only when the benefits outweigh any theoretic risks.

Alprazolam (Alpralid; Alprazolam Intensol; Altraxic; Apo-Alpraz; Xanax; Xanax TS; Xanolam; Zoldac; Zolam; Zopax)

- **Class** .... *Antianxietal, sedative/hypnotic*

- **Indications** .... Acute anxiety

- **Mechanism** .... A short-acting benzodiazepine that reduces anxiety by enhancing GABA effects

- **Dosage with Qualifiers** .... Antianxietal—0.25-0.5mg PO tid, max 4mg/d
  Panic disorder—0.5mg PO tid, up to 1mg after 3-4d
  • **Contraindications**—hypersensitivity to drug or class, glaucoma, pregnancy, CNS depression
  • **Caution**—hepatic or renal dysfunction

- **Maternal Considerations** .... **Alprazolam** is rarely indicated during pregnancy. There are no published reports of **Alprazolam** use during pregnancy. Abrupt cessation of therapy is associated with a discontinuation-emergent syndrome that includes neuropsychiatric, gastrointestinal, dermatologic, cardiovascular, and visual symptoms.

Side effects include physical dependence, syncope, tachycardia, seizures, respiratory depression, coma, drowsiness, light-headedness, dry mouth, depression, headache, constipation, diarrhea, nausea, vomiting, insomnia, blurred vision, hypotension, increased salivation, and dermatitis.

■ **Fetal Considerations**

There are no adequate reports or well-controlled studies in human fetuses. While there is no evidence that **alprazolam** is a human teratogen by either case reports or post-marketing surveillance, **diazepam** has been associated with fetal malformations. There is also concern based on studies with other benzodiazepines that postnatal behavior might be altered by antenatal exposure. Neonatal withdrawal has been reported. Treatment with **phenobarbital** is beneficial.

■ **Breastfeeding Safety**

Alprazolam enters breast milk by passive diffusion. Because of the potential **alprazolam** might alter neurodevelopment, and because of the documented risks of withdrawal, **alprazolam** should be avoided during lactation.

■ **References**

Oo CY, Kuhn RJ, Desai N, et al. Br J Clin Pharmacol 1995; 40:231-6.
St Clair SM, Schirmer RG. Obstet Gynecol 1992; 80:843-6.

■ **Summary**

- **Pregnancy Category D**
- **Lactation Category NS**
- **Alprazolam** should be avoided during pregnancy and lactation unless there are no other safer options.
- There are alternative agents for which there is more experience during pregnancy and lactation.

Alteplase (Actilyse; Activase; Activacin; TPA)

■ **Class**

Thrombolytic

■ **Indications**

Acute MI, acute ischemic stroke, pulmonary embolus

■ **Mechanism**

Human recombinant tissue plasminogen activator is a serine protease that converts plasminogen to plasmin in the presence of fibrin.

■ **Dosage with Qualifiers**

Acute MI—within 4h of symptom onset and based on weight: <67kg, 15mg bolus IV, followed by 0.75mg/kg IV over the next 30min (not to exceed 50mg), then 0.50mg/kg over the next 60min (not to exceed 35mg); >66kg, 15mg bolus IV, followed by 50mg IV over 30min, then 35mg over the next 60min

Pulmonary embolus—100mg IV over 120min; initiate **heparin** therapy near the end or immediately following the **alteplase** when either the PTT or TT returns to less than twice normal

Acute ischemic stroke—given within 4h of symptom onset: 0.9mg/kg IV over 60min; begin with 10% of dose as an IV bolus over 1min (max total dose 90mg)

- **Contraindications**—hypersensitivity to drug or class, intracranial hemorrhage, seizure at onset of stroke, internal bleeding, intracranial neoplasm, aneurysm, hypertension (>185mmHg systolic, 110mmHg diastolic)

■ **Maternal Considerations** — There are no adequate reports or well-controlled studies of **alteplase** in pregnant women. There are case reports of its use during pregnancy for the treatment of PE, MI, and peripheral thrombosis without an apparent increase in risk for hemorrhage, abruption, and PROM or preterm labor. *Side effects* include cerebral hemorrhage, arrhythmias, severe bleeding, anaphylaxis, hypotension, nausea, vomiting, and fever.

■ **Fetal Considerations** — There are no adequate reports or well-controlled studies in human fetuses. It is unknown whether **alteplase** crosses the human placenta. It could theoretically interfere with implantation. In light of its high molecular weight, **alteplase** is unlikely to cross the placenta. Rodent teratogenicity studies have not been conducted.

■ **Breastfeeding Safety** — There is no published experience in nursing women. And while tissue plasminogen activator is a normal constituent of human breast milk, it is unknown whether **alteplase** increases that level.

■ **References** — Huang WH, Kirz DS, Gallee RC, Gordey K. Obstet Gynecol 2000; 96:838.
Baudo F, Caimi TM, Redaelli R, et al. Am J Obstet Gynecol 1990; 163:1274-5.
Grand A, Ghadban W, Perret SP, et al. Ann Cardiol Angeiol 1996; 45:517-22.
Schumacher B, Belfort MA, Card RJ. Am J Obstet Gynecol 1997; 176:716-9.

■ **Summary** —
- **Pregnancy Category C**
- **Lactation Category U**
- **Alteplase** should be used during pregnancy and lactation only if the benefit justifies the potential perinatal risk.
- It is effective for acute thrombotic events that place the patient's survival in question.

Amantadine (Contenton; Endantadine; Infectoflu; Mantandan; Shikitan; Symmetrel; Topharmin)

- **Class** — *Antiviral, extrapyramidal movement disorders*

- **Indications** — Treatment or prevention of influenza, treatment of extrapyramidal reactions or parkinsonism

- **Mechanism** — Unknown; appears to interfere with release of viral nucleic material into the host cell

- **Dosage with Qualifiers** — Influenza—Treatment, 200mg PO qd until 24-48h after symptoms resolve; prophylaxis, 200mg PO qd beginning immediately after exposure and continuing at least 10d
Extrapyramidal reactions—100mg PO qd to tid (max 300mg/d)
Parkinsonism—begin 100mg PO qd, increase to bid after 1w, max 400 mg/d; reduce to 100mg/d if taking other antiparkinsonism drugs
NOTE—renal dosing
  - **Contraindications**—hypersensitivity to drug or class
  - **Caution**—seizure disorder, heart failure, liver disease, cardiovascular disease, geriatric population

- **Maternal Considerations** — The published experience with **amantadine** during pregnancy consists of isolated case reports.
Side effects include CHF, nausea, dizziness, insomnia, anxiety, depression, hallucinations, constipation, ataxia, somnolence, and agitation.

- **Fetal Considerations** — There are no adequate reports or well-controlled studies in human fetuses. It is unknown whether **amantadine** crosses the human placenta. The human experience is of concern. There are several case reports of cardiovascular abnormalities in exposed fetuses. Rats exposed to 7 times the human dose show embryotoxicity and a variety of malformations, while there was no effect at doses 5-6 times the human dose.

- **Breastfeeding Safety** — There is no published experience in nursing women.
Amantadine is excreted into human milk, though the kinetics and safety are unknown.

- **References** — Rosa F. Reprod Toxicol 1994; 8:89-92.
Hagell P, Odin P, Vinge E. Mov Disord 1998; 13:34-8.
Pandit PB, Chitayat D, Jefferies AL, et al. Reprod Toxicol 1994; 8:89-92.
Levy M, Pastuszak A, Koren G. Reprod Toxicol 1991; 5:79-81.

■ **Summary**
- **Pregnancy Category C**
- **Lactation Category U**
- **Amantadine** should be used during pregnancy and lactation only if the benefit justifies the potential perinatal risk.
- There are alternative agents for which there is more experience during pregnancy and lactation.

Ambenonium chloride (Mytelase)

■ **Class** — *Cholinesterase inhibitor*

■ **Indications** — Myasthenia gravis

■ **Mechanism** — Cholinesterase inhibitor with all the pharmacologic actions of acetylcholine

■ **Dosage with Qualifiers** — Myasthenia gravis—begin 5-25mg PO tid; max 200mg/d
NOTE—individualization is the norm; there is a narrow therapeutic margin
- **Contraindications**—hypersensitivity to drug or class, atropine use
- **Caution**—asthma, bradycardia, epilepsy, hyperthyroidism, mechanical gastrointestinal or urinary obstruction

■ **Maternal Considerations** — There are no adequate reports or well-controlled studies of **ambenonium** in pregnant women. The published experience consists of small series and case reports. **Ambenonium** is similar in action to **neostigmine**, but longer acting and with a lower incidence of gastrointestinal side effects.
Side effects include cardiac arrest, bronchospasm, cholinergic crisis, salivation, fasciculation, headache, drowsiness, and gastrointestinal abnormalities such as diarrhea, abdominal pain.

■ **Fetal Considerations** — There are no adequate reports or well-controlled studies in human fetuses. **Ambenonium** is not likely to cross the placenta because it is ionized at physiologic pH. However, other cholinesterase inhibitors have been associated with transient muscular weakness in the neonate.

■ **Breastfeeding Safety** — There is no published experience in nursing women. **Ambenonium** is not likely to be excreted into breast milk because it is ionized at physiologic pH.

■ **References** — Chambers DC, Hall JE, Boyce J. Obstet Gynecol 1967; 29:597-603.

■ **Summary** • **Pregnancy Category C**
 • **Lactation Category U**
 • **Ambenonium** should be used during pregnancy and lactation only if the benefit justifies the potential perinatal risk.

Amikacin (Amikin)

■ **Class** — Antibiotic, aminoglycoside

■ **Indications** — Short-term treatment of serious bacterial infections

■ **Mechanism** — A semisynthetic kanamycin derivative that inhibits protein synthesis by binding to the 30S ribosomal subunit

■ **Dosage with Qualifiers** — Bacterial infection—15mg/kg/d IM/IV divided q8-24h; max 1.5g/d
Urinary tract infection—250mg IM bid
NOTE—renal dosing
 • **Contraindications**—hypersensitivity to drug or class
 • **Caution**—renal dysfunction

■ **Maternal Considerations** — There are no adequate reports or well-controlled studies of **amikacin** in pregnant women. Pregnancy increases the maternal clearance of aminoglycosides in general. Women with normal renal function should receive a dose of **amikacin** that reflects the increased clearance.
Side effects include neuromuscular blockade, renal toxicity, auditory toxicity, rash, fever, headache, paresthesias, vomiting, eosinophilia, anemia, hypotension, and arthralgia.

■ **Fetal Considerations** — There are no adequate reports or well-controlled studies in human fetuses. Placental transfer of **amikacin** may be slightly higher than the β-lactams. Aminoglycosides can damage the fetal kidney presumably because of delayed clearance, and irreversible failure has been reported after some aminoglycosides, but not **amikacin**. **Amikacin** may have less fetal renal toxicity than **gentamicin**. There is no evidence of teratogenicity or interference with fertility. Rodent studies are reassuring, revealing no evidence of teratogenicity or IUGR despite the use of doses higher than those used clinically.

■ **Breastfeeding Safety** — **Amikacin** is excreted into breast milk, but at low concentrations. Oral absorption is poor, suggesting little systemic risk to the neonate.

- **References** ···· Zhang Y, Zhang Q, Xu Z. Zhonghua Fu Chan Ke Za Zhi 1997; 32:288-92.
  Mallie JP, Coulon G, Billerey C, et al. Kidney Int 1988; 33:36-44.
  Bernard B, Abate M, Thielen PF, et al. J Infect Dis 1977; 135:925-32.

- **Summary** ····
  - **Pregnancy Category D**
  - **Lactation Category S**
  - Aminoglycosides are indicated during pregnancy when the benefit outweighs the risk.

Amiloride (Amilospare; Arumil; Midamor)

- **Class** ···· *Antihypertensive, potassium-conserving diuretic*

- **Indications** ···· Adjunct treatment of either hypertension or CHF

- **Mechanism** ···· Inhibits sodium resorption at the distal convoluted tubule, cortical collecting tubule, and collecting duct

- **Dosage with Qualifiers** ····
  Hypertension—5-10mg PO qd; max 20mg
  CHF—5-10mg PO qd; max 20mg
  Lithium induced polyuria—5-10mg PO bid
  NOTE—may be combined with **hydrochlorothiazide**
  - **Contraindications**—hypersensitivity to drug or class, hyperkalemia, renal insufficiency, anuria, potassium-sparing diuretic use
  - **Caution**—diabetes mellitus (increases risk of hyperkalemia)

- **Maternal Considerations** ···· There are no adequate and well-controlled studies of **amiloride** in pregnant women.
  Side effects include aplastic anemia, hyperkalemia, neutropenia, headache, nausea, vomiting, diarrhea, muscle cramps, weakness, and cough.

- **Fetal Considerations** ···· There are no adequate reports or well-controlled studies in human fetuses. **Amiloride** crosses the placenta in modest amounts. Rodent studies are reassuring, revealing no evidence of teratogenicity or IUGR despite the use of doses 20-25 times higher than maximum human dose.

- **Breastfeeding Safety** ···· **Amiloride** is concentrated in breast milk and should probably be avoided while breastfeeding.

- **References** ···· Hall DR, Odendaal HJ. Int J Gynaecol Obstet 1998; 60:63-4.

Aminocaproic acid (Amicar; Capracid; Epsikapron)

■ **Class** ━━━━━━━━━━━━ Hemostatic

■ **Indications** ━━━━━━━━ Hemorrhage associated with excess fibrinolysis (protamine test negative, euglobulin lysis test positive, and platelet count normal)—e.g., placental abruption, missed abortion, cardiac surgery or cirrhosis, treatment of a megakaryocytosis, ITP, agranulocytosis, and hereditary hemorrhagic telangiectasia

■ **Mechanism** ━━━━━━━━ Inhibition of plasminogen activators

■ **Dosage with Qualifiers** ━━ Hemorrhage—typically 4-5g IV or PO over 1st hour, followed by 1g/h IV; max 30g/d
• **Contraindications**—hypersensitivity to drug or class, DIC unassociated with primary fibrinolysis, hemorrhage of unknown etiology
• **Caution**—renal or hepatic dysfunction, coronary artery disease

■ **Maternal Considerations** ━━ There are no adequate reports or well-controlled studies of **aminocaproic acid** in pregnant women. It has been used in a variety of hemorrhagic circumstances. The literature consists predominantly of case reports. *Side effects* include seizures, acute renal failure, cardiac arrhythmias, dizziness, myopathy, myositis, rhabdomyolysis, confusion, and clotting disorders.

■ **Fetal Considerations** ━━━ There are no adequate reports or well-controlled studies in human fetuses. It is unknown whether **aminocaproic acid** crosses the human placenta. **Aminocaproic acid** decreases implantation in a variety of animal models. Rodent teratogenicity studies have not been reported.

■ **Breastfeeding Safety** ━━━ There are no adequate reports or well-controlled studies in nursing women. It is unknown whether **aminocaproic acid** enters human breast milk.

■ **References** ━━━━━━━━ Neubert AG, Golden MA, Rose NC. Obstet Gynecol 1995; 85:831-3.

25

Peng TC, Kickler TS, Bell WR, Haller E. Am J Obstet Gynecol 1991; 165:425-6.
Landers DF, Newland M, Penney LL. J Reprod Med 1989; 34:988-93.

■ **Summary**

- **Pregnancy Category C**
- **Lactation Category U**
- **Aminocaproic acid** should be used during pregnancy and lactation only if the benefit justifies the potential perinatal risk.
- Consideration should be given to the availability of alternative therapies when possible.

Aminoglutethimide (Cytadren)

■ **Class**

Adrenal corticosteroid inhibitor

■ **Indications**

Suppression of adrenal function in women with Cushing's disease until definitive treatment can be undertaken

■ **Mechanism**

Inhibits multiple steps in steroid synthesis including the C-11-, C-18-, and C-21-hydroxylases, thus diminishing the conversion of cholesterol to δ^5-pregnenolone

■ **Dosage with Qualifiers**

Cushing's disease—begin 250mg PO qid under hospitalized supervision; adjust until the desired cortisol level is reached (>2g/d not recommended)
- **Contraindications**—hypersensitivity to drug or class
- **Caution**—may suppress aldosterone leading to hypotension (orthostatic or persistent)

■ **Maternal Considerations**

There are no adequate reports or well-controlled studies of **aminoglutethimide** in pregnant women.
Aminoglutethimide may cause adrenocortical hypofunction, especially under stressful conditions. Patients should be treated with **hydrocortisone** (not **dexamethasone**) and a mineralocorticoid.
Side effects include all manifestations of adrenal insufficiency, neutropenia, agranulocytosis, headache, vomiting, and rash.

■ **Fetal Considerations**

There are no adequate reports or well-controlled studies in human fetuses. Pseudohermaphroditism is observed in about 2/5000 pregnancies treated with **aminoglutethimide**. Rodent studies revealed embryotoxicity and teratogenicity at doses smaller than those usually recommended for humans.

- **Breastfeeding Safety** .... There is no published experience in nursing women. It is unknown whether **aminoglutethimide** enters human breast milk.

- **References** .... No current relevant references.

- **Summary** ....
  - **Pregnancy Category D**
  - **Lactation Category U**
  - **Aminoglutethimide** should be used during pregnancy and lactation only if the benefit justifies the potential perinatal risk.

Aminophylline (Aminophylline; Drafilyn "Z"; Inophyline; Norphyl; Novphyllin; Somophylin; Synthophyllin; Theourin; Truphylline)

- **Class** .... *Antiasthmatic; bronchodilator; xanthine derivative*

- **Indications** .... Relief and prevention of symptoms of asthma and/or reversible bronchospasm

- **Mechanism** .... Unknown; phosphodiesterase inhibitor that increases cAMP

- **Dosage with Qualifiers** ...... Bronchospasm—0.3-0.8mg/kg/h IV preceded by a variety of recommended loading doses (0.3-6mg/kg over 12h IV); alternatively 10-16mg/kg/d PO
  NOTE—See a pharmacologic reference for specific guidance. Serum levels should be periodically monitored and maintained between 10-20mcg/ml.
  - **Contraindications**—hypersensitivity, seizure disorder, peptic ulcer disease, cardiac arrhythmia
  - **Caution**—renal or hepatic dysfunction, CHF

- **Maternal Considerations** ...... **Aminophylline** is a mixture of theophylline and theophylline base. Approximately a third of pregnant women with asthma get worse, a third better, and a third remain clinically unchanged. Well-controlled asthma does not affect pregnancy outcome; uncontrolled asthma may increase the risk of IUGR and preterm delivery. There are no adequate reports or well-controlled studies of **aminophylline** in pregnant women, but there is a long clinical experience. Clearance and the volume of distribution appear increased by pregnancy. IV **aminophylline** is not recommended unless the patient requires hospitalization. Even then, randomized trials suggest it provides no benefit over inhaled steroids. Uterine blood flow, as reflected by Doppler flow, is unaffected. Drug interactions are common and should be sought before prescribing. Commonly used drugs of concern include **ciprofloxacin**, **propranolol**, **lithium,** and **erythromycin** that increase serum levels and **phenytoin** that reduces serum levels.

Side effects include seizures, respiratory arrest, arrhythmias, nausea, vomiting, insomnia, headache, fever, agitation, tremor, and tachycardia.

■ **Fetal Considerations**

There are no adequate reports or well-controlled studies in human fetuses. **Aminophylline** crosses the human placenta rapidly, reaching an F:M ratio approaching unity. While there is no substantive evidence in humans, teratogenicity and embryotoxicity are reported in rats and rabbits at doses that exceed the recommended human dose by 20-50 times. This effect is dose dependent. The proconvulsant effect of **aminophylline** on cortical epileptic after-discharges varies during ontogeny.

■ **Breastfeeding Safety**

Aminophylline is excreted into breast milk and may cause irritability or other signs of toxicity in nursing neonates. However, it is generally considered compatible with breastfeeding.

■ **References**

Wendel PJ, Ramin SM, Barnett-Hamm C, et al. Am J Obstet Gynecol 1996; 175:150-4.
Bernaskova K, Mares P. Epilepsy Res 2000; 39:183-90.
Schatz M. Drug Saf 1997; 16:342-50.
Romero R, Kadar N, Gonzales Govea F, Hobbins JC. Am J Perinatol 1983; 1:31-5.
Shibata M, Wachi M, Kawaguchi M, et al. Methods Find Exp Clin Pharmacol 2000; 22:101-7.
Cosmi EV, Luzi G, Fusaro P, et al. Eur J Obstet Gynecol Reprod Biol 1992; 46:7-11.
Schatz M, Harden K, Forsythe A, et al. J Allergy Clin Immunol 1988; 81:509-17.

■ **Summary**

- **Pregnancy Category C**
- **Lactation Category S**
- **Aminophylline** should be used during pregnancy and lactation only if the benefit justifies the potential perinatal risk.
- Mild asthma during pregnancy is best managed with inhaled β-2 agonists, as necessary; multistep therapy for moderate asthma includes inhaled sodium cromolyn sodium, inhaled beclomethasone dipropionate, and oral theophylline.

Amiodarone (Amiodarex; Amiohexal; Amiorone; Cardarone; Cordarone; Cordarone I.V.; Rythmarone)

- ■ **Class** — Antiarrythmic (*class* III)

- ■ **Indications** — Prevention and suppression of malignant ventricular and supraventricular arrhythmias, atrial fibrillation, and hypertrophic cardiomyopathy

- ■ **Mechanism** — Prolongs phase 3 of the action potential and noncompetitively inhibits α- and β-adrenoceptors

- ■ **Dosage with Qualifiers** — Supraventricular arrhythmia—load 800-1600mg PO qd ×1-3w until response, then 200-600mg PO qd
Ventricular arrhythmia, malignant—load 800-1600mg PO qd ×1-3w until response, then 200-600mg PO qd; alternatively, 150mg IV bolus over 10min, then 1mg/min IV ×6h, then 0.5mg/min IV for 18h
Atrial fibrillation—load 800-1600mg PO qd ×1-3w until response, then 200-600mg PO qd; alternatively, 300mg IV over 1h, then 20mg/kg over 24h, then 600mg PO qd ×1w, then 400 mg/d
Hypertrophic cardiomyopathy—load 800-1600mg PO qd ×1-3w until response, then 200-600mg PO qd
  - • **Contraindications**—hypersensitivity to drug or class, 2nd or 3rd degree block, severe SA node disease, bradycardia
  - • **Caution**—hepatic dysfunction, pulmonary disease, thyroid disease

- ■ **Maternal Considerations** — There are no adequate reports or well-controlled studies of **amiodarone** in pregnant women. The published experience is limited to fewer than 100 pregnancies. There are many alternatives to **amiodarone** during pregnancy. *Side effects* include arrhythmias, heart failure, AV block, hepatic failure, pulmonary toxicity, nausea, vomiting, fatigue, abdominal pain, anorexia, constipation, vision abnormalities, edema, peripheral neuropathy, tremor, ataxia, and dizziness.

- ■ **Fetal Considerations** — There are no adequate reports or well-controlled studies in human fetuses. Placental transport occurs, but the kinetics remains to be detailed. Placental transfer studies suggest low transfer to the fetal compartment especially when the umbilical venous pressure is elevated. Among 64 pregnancies exposed to **amiodarone**, 17% of neonates had hypothyroidism (10 detected at birth, 1 *in utero*), 18% of which had a goiter. Hypothyroidism was transient in all, though 5 were treated short-term. Neurodevelopment assessment of the hypothyroid infants, when carried out, revealed in some instances mild abnormalities often similar to the nonverbal learning disability syndrome. These features were also reported in some **amiodarone**-exposed euthyroid infants, suggesting a direct neurotoxic effect of **amiodarone** during fetal life. Fetal hypothyroidism has been reported in **amiodarone**-resistant fetal arrhythmia.

■ **Breastfeeding Safety** .... **Amiodarone** is excreted in breast milk at concentrations high enough to have a pharmacologic effect. Neonatal hypothyroidism is reported.

■ **References** .... Bartalena L, Bogazzi F, Braverman LE, Martino E. J Endocrinol Invest 2001; 24:116-30.
Vanbesien J, Casteels A, Bougatef A, et al. J. Am J Perinatol 2001; 18:113-6.
Joglar JA, Page RL. Curr Opin Cardiol 2001; 16:40-5.
Schmolling J, Renke K, Richter O, et al. Ther Drug Monit 2000; 22:582-8.
Magee LA, Nulman I, Rovet JF, Koren G. Neurotoxicol Teratol 1999; 21:261-5.
Plomp TA, Vulsma T, de Vijlder JJ. Eur J Obstet Gynecol Reprod Biol 1992; 43:201-7.

■ **Summary** .... • **Pregnancy Category D**
• **Lactation Category NS**
• **Amiodarone** should be avoided during pregnancy and lactation unless no other medical option exists.
• There are alternative agents for which there is more experience during pregnancy and lactation.

Amitriptyline (Amicen; Amilent; Amyzol; Elavil; Larozyl; Pinsanu; Vanatrip)

■ **Class** .... *Antidepressant, tricyclic*

■ **Indications** .... Depression, chronic pain

■ **Mechanism** .... Unknown; inhibits norepinephrine and serotonin reuptake

■ **Dosage with Qualifiers** .... Depression—begin 50-75mg (or 75-100mg if observed in the hospital) PO qhs, max 300mg PO qhs; alternatively, 20-30mg IM q6h
Chronic pain—begin 0.1mg/kg/d, titrate slowly over 2-3w; max 150mg
NOTE—may be combined with **chlordiazepoxide** or **perphenazine**
• **Contraindications**—hypersensitivity to drug or class, use of a MAO inhibitor within 14d
• **Caution**—urinary retention, seizure history, glaucoma, thyroid disease, hepatic dysfunction, suicide risk

■ **Maternal Considerations** ···· Depression is common during and after pregnancy, but typically goes unrecognized. Pregnancy is not a reason a priori to discontinue psychotropic drugs. There are no well-controlled studies of **amitriptyline** during pregnancy. About 7-10% of Caucasians are poor metabolizers, and serum levels should be monitored during pregnancy. Although **amitriptyline** has no effect on placental blood flow in gravid sheep, the pressor response to norepinephrine, but not phenylephrine, is enhanced. *Side effects* include MI, seizures, stroke, agranulocytosis, thrombocytopenia, dry mouth, drowsiness, constipation, urinary retention, blurred vision, increased appetite, and confusion.

■ **Fetal Considerations** ···· Both **amitriptyline** and its sib, nortriptyline, cross the human placenta. Though there is no causal evidence, case reports link CNS/limb abnormalities and developmental delay. And while rodent studies are generally reassuring at doses below 10 times the maximum recommended human dose, studies 10-33 times the maximum recommended dose reveal CNS and facial abnormalities. Long-term effects on serotonergic receptors are postulated but not confirmed.

■ **Breastfeeding Safety** ···· Multiple studies reveal that while **amitriptyline** is excreted into the breast milk, the neonatal concentrations are extremely low.

■ **References** ···· Heikkinen T, Ekblad U, Laine K. Psychopharmacology (Berl) 2001; 153:450-4.
Wisner KL, Perel JM, Findling RL. Am J Psychiatry 1996; 153:1132-7.
Mason BD, Van Petten GR. Am J Obstet Gynecol 1978; 131:868-71.
Kornstein SG. J Clin Psychiatry 2001; 62(Suppl)24:11-7.

■ **Summary** ····
- **Pregnancy Category D**
- **Lactation Category S?**
- **Amitriptyline** should be used during pregnancy only if the benefit justifies the potential perinatal risk.
- As for most psychotropic drugs, using monotherapy and the lowest effective quantity given in divided doses to minimize the peaks may minimize the risks to the perinate.
- **Amitriptyline** is probably a drug of choice for breast-feeding women.

Amlodipine (Norvasc)

Class — Calcium-channel blocker, dihydropyridine

Indications — Chronic hypertension, angina (chronic stable and variant)

Mechanism — Inhibits calcium ion influx into smooth muscle and myocardium

Dosage with Qualifiers — Chronic hypertension—5-10mg PO qd
Angina (chronic stable and variant)—5-10mg PO qd
NOTE—may be combined with **benazepril**, an ACE inhibitor
- **Contraindications**—hypersensitivity to drug or class

Maternal Considerations — There are no well-controlled studies in women of **amlodipine** during pregnancy. Other calcium-channel antagonists are used as inhibitors of myometrial contraction and **amlodipine** has similar properties. There are no reports of its use as a tocolytic agent.
Side effects include arrhythmias, headache, dizziness, fatigue, nausea, palpitations, abdominal pain, muscle cramps, and syncope.

Fetal Considerations — There are no adequate reports or well-controlled studies in human fetuses. It is unknown whether **amlodipine** crosses the human placenta. Rodent studies are reassuring, revealing no evidence of teratogenicity or IUGR despite the use of doses 8 to 23 times the maximum recommended human dose.

Breastfeeding Safety — There is no published experience in nursing women. It is unknown whether **amlodipine** enters human breast milk.

References — Lechner W, Bergant A, Solder E, Kolle D. Wien Med Wochenschr 1996; 146:466-8.

Summary —
- **Pregnancy Category C**
- **Lactation Category U**
- **Amlodipine** should be used during pregnancy and lactation only if the benefit justifies the potential perinatal risk.
- There are alternative agents for which there is more experience during pregnancy and lactation.

Amobarbital (Amybal; Amycal; Amytal Sodium; Isobec; Placidel; Sumital)

- **Class** — Anxiolytic, *hypnotic*

- **Indications** — Anxiety, sedative, hypnotic

- **Mechanism** — Barbiturate

- **Dosage with Qualifiers** — Anxiety—1 tab PO qhs (see Note)
  Sedative—30-50mg PO/IM/IV bid/tid
  Hypnotic—65-200mg PO/IM/IV qhs (IV rate <50 mg/min)
  NOTE—renal and hepatic dosing; often combined with **secobarbital** (50mg/50mg or 100mg/100mg tabs)
  - **Contraindications**—hypersensitivity to drug or class, hepatic dysfunction, porphyria
  - **Caution**—renal dysfunction, respiratory disease

- **Maternal Considerations** — There are no adequate reports or well-controlled studies of **amobarbital** in pregnant women.
  Side effects include respiratory depression, apnea, dyspnea, hepatotoxicity, nausea, vomiting, somnolence, agitation, confusion, ataxia, nervousness, hallucinations, nightmares, constipation, CNS depression, and insomnia.

- **Fetal Considerations** — There are no adequate reports or well-controlled studies in human fetuses. **Amobarbital** crosses the human placenta, achieving an F:M ratio near unity. Though there was some suggestion of a nonspecific risk of malformation in exposed offspring, subsequent studies were reassuring.

- **Breastfeeding Safety** — There is no published experience in nursing women. It is unknown whether **amobarbital** enters human breast milk, though similar agents do.

- **References** — Draffan GH, Dollery CT, Davies DS, et al. Clin Pharmacol Ther 1976; 19:271-5.

- **Summary** —
  - **Pregnancy Category D**
  - **Lactation Category U**
  - While the evidence of **amobarbital** safety during pregnancy is conflicting, alternative agents are available for all indications.

Amoxapine (Asendin)

■ **Class** — Antidepressant (class IV); tricyclic

■ **Indications** — Depression

■ **Mechanism** — Unknown; inhibits norepinephrine and serotonin reuptake

■ **Dosage with Qualifiers** — Depression—begin 50mg PO bid; max 600mg qd
  ● **Contraindications**—hypersensitivity to drug or class, MAO-inhibitor use within 14d, acute MI

■ **Maternal Considerations** — Depression is common during and after pregnancy, but typically goes unrecognized. Pregnancy is not a reason a priori to discontinue psychotropic drugs. There are no adequate and well-controlled studies of **amoxapine** use in pregnant women. There are only scattered case reports to draw upon. **Amoxapine** is similar in efficacy to **imipramine**.
Side effects include seizures, neuroleptic malignant syndrome, tardive dyskinesia, drowsiness, blurred vision, constipation, dry mouth, anxiety, palpitations, insomnia, nightmares, headache, fatigue, profuse sweating, rash, edema, galactorrhea, increased prolactin, and excessive appetite.

■ **Fetal Considerations** — There are no adequate reports or well-controlled studies in human fetuses. Rodent studies are generally reassuring revealing no evidence of teratogenicity. Embryotoxicity was seen at human dose levels, and fetotoxicity at multiples of the recommended human dose.

■ **Breastfeeding Safety** — **Amoxapine** is excreted in the breast milk, though the kinetics and its effect on the newborn have not been studied.

■ **References** — Gelenberg AJ, Wojcik JD, Lydiard RB, et al. J Clin Psychiatry 1984; 45:54-9.
Gelenberg AJ. J Nerv Ment Dis 1979;167:635-6.

■ **Summary** — ● **Pregnancy Category C**
  ● **Lactation Category U**
  ● There are other agents of equal efficacy, such as **imipramine**, for the treatment of depression for which there is more experience during pregnancy.

Amoxicillin (Amoflux; Amoxiden; Amoxil; Amoxin; Amoxipenil; Amoxycillin; Anemol; Apitart; Aspenil; Audumic; Biomox; Bridopen; Excillin; Gemox; Imoxil; Jerramcil; Larotid; Limox; Pensyn; Polymox; Protexillin; Reloxyl; Ronemox; Samosillin; Samthongcillin; Senox; Sigmopen; Suprapen; Trilaxin; Trimox; Twicyl; Unicillin; Virgoxillin; Wymox; Yisulon; Zamocillin)

■ **Class** — Antibiotic, penicillin

■ **Indications** — Gram-positive and -negative infection (systemic, venereal, endocarditis)

■ **Mechanism** — Bactericidal; inhibits biosynthesis of cell wall mucopeptide

■ **Dosage with Qualifiers** — Bacterial infection—250-500mg PO tid, or 500-750mg PO bid
Gonorrhea, uncomplicated—3g PO ×1
Chlamydia trachomatis—500mg PO tid ×7d
Endocarditis prophylaxis—2g PO ×1, 0.5-1h prior to the procedure
H. pylori infection—1g PO bid ×10-14d (combined with either **clarithromycin** and **lansoprazole/omeprazole**).
NOTE—adjust for CrCl: if 10-30ml, administer q12h; if <10ml, administer q24h
- **Contraindications**—hypersensitivity to drug or class
- **Caution**—CMV or EBV infection, renal dysfunction, cephalosporin allergy, PKU

■ **Maternal Considerations** — Similar to **ampicillin**, **amoxicillin** is generally considered safe during pregnancy. It provides a greater than 90% cure rate for Chlamydia. **Amoxicillin** is the most cost-effective treatment of Chlamydia, followed by a single 1g dose of **azithromycin** for nonresponders.
Side effects include thrombocytopenia, agranulocytosis, anaphylaxis, leukopenia, anemia, Stevens-Johnson syndrome, seizures, hepatotoxicity, nausea, vomiting, diarrhea, rash, urticaria, and eosinophilia.

■ **Fetal Considerations** — **Amoxicillin** crosses the placenta but is generally considered safe for the fetus. There are no reports of associated defects, and rodent studies are reassuring.

■ **Breastfeeding Safety** — **Amoxicillin** is excreted into the breast milk in low concentrations, but is generally considered safe during lactation.

■ **References** — Jacobson GF, Autry AM, Kirby RS, et al. Am J Obstet Gynecol 2001; 184:1352-4.
Miller JM, Martin DH. Drugs 2000; 60:597-605.
Edwards RK, Locksmith GJ, Duff P. Obstet Gynecol 2000; 96:60-4.
Hueston WJ, Lenhart JG. Arch Fam Med 1997; 6:551-5.

■ **Summary** ....
- **Pregnancy Category B**
- **Lactation Category S**
- There are no current concerns with **amoxicillin** use in appropriately selected pregnant women.

Amoxicillin/clavulanate potassium
(Amoclan; Amoclav; Augmentin)

■ **Class** .... Antibiotic, penicillin; beta-lactamase inhibitor

■ **Indications** .... Gram-positive and -negative infection (systemic, venereal, endocarditis) with sensitive bacteria

■ **Mechanism** .... Bactericidal; inhibits biosynthesis of cell wall mucopeptide. **Clavulanate** extends the antibiotic spectrum to include bacteria normally resistant to it.

■ **Dosage with Qualifiers** .... Bacterial infection—-250-500mg PO tid, or 500-875mg PO bid
Gonorrhea, uncomplicated—3g PO ×1
Chlamydia trachomatis—500mg PO tid ×7d
Endocarditis prophylaxis—2g PO ×1, 0.5-1h prior to the procedure
H. pylori infection—1g PO bid ×10-14d (combined with **clarithromycin** and **lansoprazole** or **omeprazole**)
NOTE—adjust for CrCl: if 10-30ml, administer q12h; if <10ml, administer q24h
- **Contraindications**—hypersensitivity to drug or class, Augmentin-associated hepatic dysfunction
- **Caution**—CMV or EBV infection, hepatic or renal dysfunction, cephalosporin allergy, PKU

■ **Maternal Considerations** .... Oral **ampicillin** is generally poorly absorbed during labor. **Amoxicillin/clavulanate** was used without success for the treatment of preterm labor and intact membranes. While **amoxicillin/clavulanate** is associated with prolongation of the latency interval after PPROM, there is a greater risk of necrotizing enterocolitis compared to either placebo or **erythromycin**. Macrolides, such as **erythromycin**, are superior for this indication. The incidence of maternal infectious complications is reduced by most antibiotic regimens.
Side effects include thrombocytopenia, agranulocystosis, anaphylaxis, leukopenia, anemia, Stevens-Johnson syndrome, seizures, hepatotoxicity, nausea, vomiting, diarrhea, rash, urticaria, and eosinophilia.

- ■ **Fetal Considerations** .... **Amoxicillin/clavulanate** is not associated with an increased risk of malformation in animal and human studies. However, the numbers of human studies are limited. **Amoxicillin/clavulanate** use may increase the risk of necrotizing enterocolitis when used for prophylaxis in women with preterm PROM.

- ■ **Breastfeeding Safety** .... This class of drug is excreted in milk, but no adverse effects are reported.

- ■ **References** .... Kenyon SL, Taylor DJ, Tarnow-Mordi W, ORACLE Collaborative Group. Lancet 2001; 357:979-94. Czeizel AE, Rockenbauer M, Sorensen HT, Olsen J.Eur J Obstet Gynecol Reprod Biol 2001; 97:188-92.

- ■ **Summary** ....
  - • **Pregnancy Category B**
  - • **Lactation Category S**
  - • **Amoxicillin/clavulanate** does not increase the rate of successful tocolysis in women with preterm labor and intact membranes.
  - • While **amoxicillin/clavulanate** prolongs the latency interval after PPROM, it may be associated with an increased risk of necrotizing enterocolitis. **Erythromycin** is preferred for this indication.

Amphetamine/Dextroamphetamine
(Adderall)

- ■ **Class** .... *Anorexiant, stimulant*

- ■ **Indications** .... Narcolepsy, attention deficit disorder

- ■ **Mechanism** .... Unknown

- ■ **Dosage with Qualifiers** .... ADD—2.5mg PO qam; increase by 2.5mg qw until satisfactory effect; alternatively, 10mg time release PO qam, or 5mg PO immediate release qam up to bid
  Narcolepsy—5-60mg PO qam
  Obesity—5mg PO qam
  - • **Contraindications**—hypersensitivity to drug or class, moderate to severe hypertension, hyperthyroidism, substance abuse, glaucoma, MAO inhibitor use <14d, symptomatic cardiovascular disease
  - • **Caution**—psychosis, mild, hypertension, tics

- **Maternal Considerations** ········· **Amphetamines** are noncatecholamine, sympathomimetic amines with both peripheral and CNS activities. There are no adequate and well-controlled studies of **amphetamine/dextroamphetamine** in pregnant women. **Amphetamine** dependency is associated with preterm delivery. With perhaps the exception of narcolepsy, **amphetamines** should rarely be used during pregnancy. *Side effects* include cardiomyopathy, tachycardia, tremor, psychosis, dependency, headache, hypertension, dizziness, dry mouth, dyspepsia, constipation, abdominal pain, anorexia, weight loss, mood lability, asthenia, diarrhea, and urticaria.

- **Fetal Considerations** ············· There are no adequate reports or well-controlled studies in human fetuses. Infants born to **amphetamine**-dependent women show signs of withdrawal, demonstrating placental transfer. **Amphetamine** is embryotoxic and teratogenic in some rodents when given at high doses. Case controlled studies do not reveal a pattern of teratogenicity, though scattered case reports list various defects associated with 1st trimester usage. Antenatal **amphetamine** exposure is associated with aggressive behavior and delayed development in children under 14 years of age.

- **Breastfeeding Safety** ············· **Amphetamine** is concentrated in human breast milk and generally considered incompatible with breastfeeding.

- **References** ························· Eriksson M, Jonsson B, Steneroth G, Zetterstrom R. Scand J Publ Health 2000; 28:154-7.
Steiner E, Villen T, Hallberg M, Rane A. Eur J Clin Pharmacol 1984; 27:123-4.

- **Summary** ··························· • **Pregnancy Category C**
  • **Lactation Category NS**
  • This schedule II drug is rarely indicated in reproductive-age women and should be avoided.
  • Dependent women should be counseled and enrolled in detoxification programs.

Amphotericin B (Abelcet; AmBisome; Amphocin; Amphotec; Fungilin; Fungizone IV; Fungizone Topical)

- **Class** ····························· *Antifungal*

- **Indications** ······················ Systemic fungal infection

- **Mechanism** ························· Binds to cell wall sterols, changing membrane permeability

- **Dosage with Qualifiers** ········ <u>Systemic fungal infection</u>—aspergillosis, 3-4mg/kg/d IV, max 7.5mg/kg/d; systemic candidiasis, 3.9-6mg/kg/d IV
  NOTE—also available coupled to liposomes (AmBisome) or cholesteryl (Amphotec)
  - **Contraindications**—hypersensitivity to drug or class
  - **Caution**—renal dysfunction

- **Maternal Considerations** ········ There are no adequate reports or well-controlled studies of **amphotericin** in pregnant women. **Amphotericin** has been used during pregnancy without increased risk of complications. It remains the drug of choice for systemic, invasive mycotic infections, whether life-threatening or less severe. Unfortunately little if any information is available regarding the safety of the newer lipid formulations.
  Side effects include seizures, ventricular arrhythmias, asystole, hemorrhagic gastroenteritis, renal failure, thrombocytopenia, agranulocytopenia, hepatic dysfunction, chills, fever, hypertension, nausea, vomiting, headache, anorexia, diarrhea, and rash.

- **Fetal Considerations** ········ There are no adequate reports or well-controlled studies in human fetuses. **Amphotericin** crosses the human placenta and is deposited in the fetal tissues. Therapeutic levels may be found in fetal tissues weeks after cessation. There have been no reports of teratogenicity. Rodent studies are reassuring, revealing no evidence of teratogenicity or IUGR despite the use of doses higher than those used clinically.

- **Breastfeeding Safety** ········ There is no published experience in nursing women. It is unknown whether **amphotericin** enters human breast milk.

- **References** ········ Sobel JD. Drug Saf 2000; 23:77-85.
  Dean JL, Wolf JE, Ranzini AC, Laughlin MA. Clin Infect Dis 1994; 18:364-8.
  Ellinoy BR. Am J Obstet Gynecol 1973; 115:285-6.

- **Summary** ········
  - **Pregnancy Category B**
  - **Lactation Category U**
  - A body of case reports indicates that **amphotericin B** remains the drug of choice for systemic, invasive mycotic infections, whether life-threatening or less severe.

Ampicillin (Adumic; Amblosin; Ampen; Ampesid; Ampibel; Ampicillin; Ampiclox; Ampikel; Ampil; Ampisol; Austrapen; Bionacillin; Cinpillin; Copharcilin; Cryocil; Doktacillin; Fortapen; Herpen; Ingacillin; Isocillin; Marcillin; Nelpicil; Pentrex; Pfizerpen; Principen; Protexillin; Resan; Statcillin; Tampicillin; Tokiocillin; Totacillin; Trilaxan; Ukapen; Vialicina)

- **Class** — *Antibiotic, penicillin*

- **Indications** — GBS and endocarditis prophylaxis, treatment of susceptible gram-positive and -negative organisms

- **Mechanism** — Bactericidal by the inhibition of cell wall mucopeptide synthesis

- **Dosage with Qualifiers** — GBS prophylaxis—2g IV load, then 1-2g IV q4h at least 4h prior to delivery
  Endocarditis prophylaxis—2g IV/IM ×1 (give 30min prior to procedure)
  Endocarditis treatment—12g IV qd
  Bacterial infection—250-500mg PO q6h (max 14g/d), or 0.5-2g IV/IM q6h
  Bacterial meningitis—2g IV loading dose, then 1-2g IV q4-6h.
  Cesarean section prophylaxis—2g IV after umbilical cord clamping
  Gonorrhea—3.5g PO with 1g **probenecid**
  - **Contraindications**—hypersensitivity to drug or drug class, pseudomembranous colitis
  - **Caution**—EBV and CMV infection, penicillin or cephalosporin allergy, renal dysfunction

- **Maternal Considerations** — Well absorbed orally except during labor, **ampicillin** is one of the most commonly used antibiotics during pregnancy. In addition to the noted indications, **ampicillin** was used without success in combination with tocolytic agents to delay or avoid preterm delivery. Plasma clearance is increased during pregnancy, necessitating in some women a higher dose to obtain adequate drug levels.
  Side effects include seizures, thrombocytopenia, agranulocytosis, Stevens-Johnson syndrome, interstitial nephritis, hemolytic anemia, nausea, vomiting, diarrhea, headache, confusion, eosinophilia, and rash.

- **Fetal Considerations** — There is a wide body of clinical experience with **ampicillin** during pregnancy. There is no evidence of teratogenicity in either humans or rodents. Throughout pregnancy, fetal drug levels reach maternal equilibrium 1-3h after administration; thereafter, fetal drug levels exceed maternal values. Amniotic fluid levels are low during early pregnancy, but rise with advancing gestation and may exceed maternal values 6-8h after drug administration.

- **Breastfeeding Safety** ············ Minimal amounts of **ampicillin** are excreted in breast milk. It is generally considered compatible with breastfeeding.

- **References** ············
Kenyon SL, Taylor DJ, Tarnow-Mordi W, ORACLE Collaborative Group. Lancet 2001; 357:979-94.
Nau H. Dev Pharmacol Ther 1987; 10:174-98.
Spinnato JA, Youkilis B, Cook VD, et al. J Matern Fetal Med 2000; 9:348-50.
Zhang Y, Zhang Q, Xu Z. Zhonghua Fu Chan Ke Za Zhi 1997; 32:288-92.
Czeizel AE, Rockenbauer M, Sorensen HT, Olsen J. Am J Obstet Gynecol 2001; 185:140-7.

- **Summary** ············
  - **Pregnancy Category B**
  - **Lactation Category S**
  - **Ampicillin** appears safe and effective for use during pregnancy and lactation when indicated.
  - **Ampicillin** is as effective for post-cesarean prophylaxis as other, broader spectrum agents.

Ampicillin–sulbactam sodium (Ubacillin; Unasyn)

- **Class** ············ *Antibiotic, penicillin*

- **Indications** ············ Bacterial infection secondary to susceptible gram-positive and -negative organisms

- **Mechanism** ············ Bactericidal by the inhibition of cell wall mucopeptide synthesis. Coupling to the β-lactamase inhibitor, **sulbactam** enhances the spectrum of coverage.

- **Dosage with Qualifiers** ············ Bacterial infection—1.5-3g IV/IM q6h; max 8g/d
  NOTE—renal dosing
  - **Contraindications**—hypersensitivity to drug or drug class
  - **Caution**—EBV and CMV infection, penicillin or cephalosporin allergy, renal dysfunction

- **Maternal Considerations** ············ **Ampicillin–sulbactam** is a reasonable selection for prophylaxis in women undergoing cesarean section. It does not prolong the latency interval after PPROM. Because of increased plasma clearance during pregnancy, a dose increase may be necessary to obtain adequate drug levels. *Side effects* include vaginitis, seizures, thrombocytopenia, agranulocytosis, leukopenia, anemia, Stevens-Johnson syndrome, interstitial nephritis, toxic epidermal necrosis, hemolytic anemia, nausea, vomiting, diarrhea, headache, confusion, eosinophilia, and rash.

■ **Fetal Considerations**

Ampicillin–sulbactam reduces neonatal infectious morbidity after PPROM, but to no greater extent than erythromycin, which also prolongs the latency interval. There is no substantive evidence of teratogenicity. Rodent studies are reassuring, revealing no evidence of teratogenicity or IUGR despite the use of doses higher than those used clinically.

■ **Breastfeeding Safety**

Minimal amounts of **ampicillin–sulbactam** are excreted in breast milk. It is generally considered compatible with breastfeeding.

■ **References**

Noyes N, Berkeley AS, Freedman K, Ledger W. Infect Dis Obstet Gynecol 1998; 6:220-3.
Lovett SM, Weiss JD, Diogo MJ, et al. Am J Obstet Gynecol 1997; 176:1030-8.
Lewis DF, Brody K, Edwards MS, et al. Obstet Gynecol 1996; 88:801-5.

■ **Summary**

- **Pregnancy Category B**
- **Lactation Category S**
- **Ampicillin–sulbactam** appears safe and effective for use during pregnancy and lactation when indicated.

Amprenavir (Agenerase)

■ **Class**

Antiviral; protease inhibitor

■ **Indications**

HIV

■ **Mechanism**

HIV-1 protease inhibitor; potent cytochrome p450 inhibitor

■ **Dosage with Qualifiers**

HIV—1200mg PO bid/tid (take with food); increase dose to 1200mg PO tid if given with **efavirenz**
- **Contraindications**—hypersensitivity to drug or class, and **cisapride**, **astemizole**, or **midazolam** use
- **Caution**—hypersensitivity to sulfonamides, hepatic or renal dysfunction

■ **Maternal Considerations**

There is no published experience with **amprenavir** during pregnancy.
Side effects include Stevens-Johnson syndrome, nausea, vomiting, diarrhea, rash, hyperglycemia, hypertriglyceridemia, headache, fatigue, taste change, perioral tingling, and depression.

■ **Fetal Considerations** ⋯⋯⋯ **Amprenavir** crosses the placenta. In various rodents, doses of **amprenavir** well below the recommended human dose were associated with an increased abortion rate and deficient long bone ossification.

■ **Breastfeeding Safety** ⋯⋯⋯ It is unknown whether **amprenavir** is excreted in human breast milk. Breastfeeding is contraindicated in HIV-infected nursing women where formula is available to reduce the risk of neonatal transmission.

■ **References** ⋯⋯⋯ Bawdon RE. Infect Dis Obstet Gynecol 1998; 6:244-6.

■ **Summary** ⋯⋯⋯
- **Pregnancy Category C**
- **Lactation Category NS**
- **Amprenavir** should be used during pregnancy only when the potential benefit justifies the risk to the fetus.
- Physicians are encouraged to register pregnant women under the Antiretroviral Pregnancy Registry (1-800-258-4263) for a better follow-up of the outcome while under treatment with **amprenavir**.

Anagrelide hydrochloride (Agrylin)

■ **Class** ⋯⋯⋯ *Thrombocythemia*

■ **Indications** ⋯⋯⋯ Essential thrombocythemia

■ **Mechanism** ⋯⋯⋯ Unknown

■ **Dosage with Qualifiers** ⋯⋯⋯ Essential thrombocythemia—begin 0.5mg PO qid; increase as necessary to a max of 10mg/d
- **Contraindications**—hypersensitivity to drug or class
- **Caution**—cardiovascular disease, hepatic or renal dysfunction

■ **Maternal Considerations** ⋯⋯⋯ Pregnant women with essential thrombocythemia have an increased risk of 1st trimester loss that is not predictable by the prepregnancy platelet count or reducible by **aspirin** therapy. There are no adequate and well-controlled studies of **anagrelide** in pregnant women. There are only scattered case reports of its use during pregnancy.
Side effects include CHF, stroke, MI, chest pain, hemorrhage, thrombocytopenia, tachycardia, headache, diarrhea, asthenia, abdominal pain, rash, dyspepsia, anorexia, malaise, and paresthesias.

■ **Fetal Considerations** ⋯⋯⋯ There are no adequate reports or well-controlled studies in human fetuses. Rodent studies are reassuring, revealing no evidence of teratogenicity. However, very high doses were associated with delayed delivery and its sequelae.

- **Breastfeeding Safety** — There is no published experience in nursing women. It is unknown whether **anagrelide** enters human breast milk.

- **References** — Wright CA, Tefferi A. Eur J Haematol 2001; 66:152-9.

- **Summary** —
  - **Pregnancy Category C**
  - **Lactation Category U**
  - **Anagrelide** should be used during pregnancy and lactation only if the benefit justifies the potential perinatal risk.

Anakinra (Kineret)

- **Class** — *Antirheumatic*

- **Indications** — Essential thrombocythemia

- **Mechanism** — Inhibits the interleukin-1 type 1 receptor

- **Dosage with Qualifiers** — Rheumatoid arthritis, moderate to severe—100mg SC q24h; check ANC at baseline and q3mo
  - **Contraindications**—hypersensitivity to drug or class, serious infection, concurrent live vaccine
  - **Caution**—renal dysfunction, asthma

- **Maternal Considerations** — There are no published reports of its use during pregnancy. Native interleukin-1 type 1 receptor antagonist has been associated with recurrent pregnancy loss, and is increased in amniotic fluid and umbilical venous blood obtained from pregnancies complicated by preterm PROM. *Side effects* include thrombocytopenia, neutropenia, infection, injection site reaction, sinusitis, URI symptoms, nausea, diarrhea and abdominal pain.

- **Fetal Considerations** — There are no adequate reports or well-controlled studies in human fetuses. It is unknown whether **anakinra** crosses the human placenta. Rodent studies are reassuring, revealing no evidence of teratogenicity or IUGR despite the use of doses higher than those used clinically.

- **Breastfeeding Safety** — There is no published experience in nursing women. It is unknown whether **anakinra** enters human breast milk. Native interleukin-1 type 1 receptor antagonist is present in breast milk, and the concentration increased by mastitis.

- **References** — Fukuda H, Masuzaki H, Ishimaru T. Int J Gynaecol Obstet 2002; 77:123-9.

Unfried G, Tempfer C, Schneeberger C, et al. Fertil Steril 2001; 75:683-7.
Buescher ES, Hair PS. Cell Immunol 2001; 210:87-95.

■ **Summary**
- **Pregnancy Category B**
- **Lactation Category U**
- **Anakinra** should be used during pregnancy and lactation only if the benefit justifies the potential perinatal risk.

Anthralin (Amitase; Anthra-Derm; Anthra-Tex; Anthraderm; Anthraforte; Dithranol; Dritho-Scalp; Drithocreme; Lasan)

■ **Class**
Dermatologic; psoriasis

■ **Indications**
Psoriasis, pustular

■ **Mechanism**
Unknown; inhibits T lymphocytes

■ **Dosage with Qualifiers**
Psoriasis—begin at 0.1% topically and cover for 8-24h; may accelerate to 1-3% topically and cover for 5-60min and apply bid
- **Contraindications**—hypersensitivity to drug or class, lesions on the face or genitals
- **Caution**—renal dysfunction, salicylate allergy

■ **Maternal Considerations**
Pregnancy may precipitate pustular psoriasis. There are no adequate and well-controlled studies of **anthralin** in pregnant women. Though it is generally considered safe for use during pregnancy, there is little data to support a conclusion either way.
Side effects include irritation, contact dermatitis, discoloration of hair and nails, and erythema.

■ **Fetal Considerations**
There are no adequate reports or well-controlled studies in human fetuses. Rodent teratogenicity studies have apparently not been conducted.

■ **Breastfeeding Safety**
There is no published experience in nursing women. It is unknown whether **anthralin** enters human breast milk. The route and dosing frequency suggest it unlikely the breast-feeding neonate would ingest a clinically relevant amount.

■ **References**
Tauscher AE, Fleischer AB, Phelps KC, Feldman SR. J Cutan Med Surg 2002; 6:561-70.
Arnold WP, Boelen RE, van de Kerkof PC. Ned Tijdschr Geneeskd 1995; 139:1170-3.

■ **Summary**

- **Pregnancy Category C**
- **Lactation Category U**
- **Anthralin** should be used during pregnancy and lactation only if the benefit justifies the potential perinatal risk.

Antihemophilic factor (Alphanate; Bioclate; Factor VIII; Green Eight; Haemoctin SDH; Helixate; Hemofil-M; Humate-P; Hyate:C; Koate; Koate-Hp; Kogenate; Melate; Nybcen; Omrixate; Profilate)

■ **Class**
Antihemophilic agent, blood clotting factors

■ **Indications**
Congenital factor VIII deficiency

■ **Mechanism**
Replacement

■ **Dosage with Qualifiers**
Congenital factor VIII deficiency—dose highly variable reflecting weight and severity of deficiency and the presence of inhibitors
NOTE—In general, 1 IU/kg will increase circulating factor VIII by 2%
- **Contraindications**—hypersensitivity to drug or class
- **Caution**—hepatic dysfunction

■ **Maternal Considerations**
Not surprisingly, there are no adequate reports or well-controlled studies of **antihemophilic factor** in pregnant women since the factor VIII deficiency is X-linked. Unbalanced lyonization or crossover during meiosis would account for the rare reports in women if accurate. Replacement is of little clinical use in women with an acquired inhibitor.
Side effects include anaphylaxis, HIV, hepatitis, urticaria, wheezing, nausea, fever, chills, and chest tightness.

■ **Fetal Considerations**
There are no adequate reports or well-controlled studies in human fetuses. Animal studies have not been performed explaining the FDA classification as C.

■ **Breastfeeding Safety**
There are no adequate reports or well-controlled studies in nursing women.

■ **References**
There are no current relevant references.

■ **Summary**
- **Pregnancy Category C**
- **Lactation Category S?**

Antithrombin III concentrate (ATnativ; Thrombate III; Thrombate Iii)

■ **Class**	Anticoagulant, *thrombolytic*
■ **Indications**	ATIII deficiency, congenital or acquired
■ **Mechanism**	Replacement
■ **Dosage with Qualifiers**	ATIII deficiency (congenital or acquired)—treatment of thromboembolism, 50-100U/min IV, titrate to ATIII activity levels; prophylaxis, 50-100U/min IV, titrate to ATIII activity levels NOTE—In general, 1 IU/kg increases ATIII levels by 1-2.1%; goal 80-120% • **Contraindications**—hypersensitivity to drug or class
■ **Maternal Considerations**	There are no adequate studies of **antithrombin III concentrate** in pregnant women. ATIII consumption during normal pregnancy is increased to the level associated with sepsis in the nonpregnant patient. Women with congenital ATIII deficiency have dramatically increased risk of thromboembolic disease during pregnancy. Heparin may be ineffective, depending upon the ATIII level. Replacement is effective prophylaxis and treatment of acute thrombosis and must be performed on an ongoing basis. Preeclampsia is a cause of acquired ATIII deficiency secondary to increased consumption. Several studies suggest ATIII replacement may improve maternal outcome in women with preeclampsia. *Side effects* include dizziness, nausea, bitter taste, cramps, and chest tightness.
■ **Fetal Considerations**	There are no adequate reports or well-controlled studies in human fetuses. There are no reports of adverse fetal effects, and the size of the molecule indicates placental transfer is unlikely. Rodent teratogenicity studies have not apparently been conducted. As an endogenous substance, it is unlikely to have any adverse fetal effects.
■ **Breastfeeding Safety**	There are no adequate reports or well-controlled studies in nursing women. It is unknown whether **antithrombin III concentrate** enters human breast milk.
■ **References**	Yamada T, Yamada H, Morikawa M, et al. J Obstet Gynaecol Res 2001; 27:189-97. Paternoster DM, De Fusco D, Tambuscio B. Int J Gynaecol Obstet 2000; 71:175-6. Weiner CP, Herrig JE, Pelzer GD, Heilskov J. Throm Res Suppl 1990; 58:395-401. Brandt P. Thromb Res Suppl 1981; 22:15-24.

■ **Summary**

- **Pregnancy Category C**
- **Lactation Category U**
- **Antithrombin III concentrate** may be used safely during pregnancy and lactation for the treatment of ATIII deficiency.

Arbutamine (GenESA)

■ **Class**

Cardiac testing, chronotrope, inotrope

■ **Indications**

Provokes cardiac stress in lieu of exercise testing

■ **Mechanism**

Sympathomimetic with β-adrenoceptor selectivity; may limit regional subendocardial perfusion

■ **Dosage with Qualifiers**

Cardiac imaging under stress—administered by a computerized system; use only with continuous cardiac monitoring. Max dose 0.8mcg/kg/min, max total dose 10mcg/kg

- **Contraindications**—hypersensitivity to drug or class, IHSS, history of recurrent ventricular tachycardia, implanted pacemaker

■ **Maternal Considerations**

There are no reports of **arbutamine** use during pregnancy. *Side effects* include tremor, angina, arrhythmia, headache, dizziness, anxiety, and palpitations.

■ **Fetal Considerations**

There are no adequate reports or well-controlled studies in human fetuses. Rodent studies are reassuring, revealing no evidence of teratogenicity.

■ **Breastfeeding Safety**

There are no adequate reports or well-controlled studies in nursing women. It is unknown whether **arbutamine** enters human breast milk. However, considering the indication, it is unlikely the breast-fed neonate would ingest clinically relevant amounts after one-time use.

■ **References**

There is no published experience in pregnancy or during lactation.

■ **Summary**

- **Pregnancy Category B**
- **Lactation Category U**
- Indicated when the medical risks to the mother outweigh any theoretic risk to the fetus.

Ardeparin sodium (Normiflo)

■ **Class** — Anticoagulant; *low-molecular-weight heparin*

■ **Indications** — DVT prophylaxis for joint replacement

■ **Mechanism** — Binds to and accelerates antithrombin III activity; also binds heparin cofactor II

■ **Dosage with Qualifiers** — DVT prophylaxis—begin 50 anti-Xa U/kg SC q12h evening before surgery ×14d
- **Contraindications**—hypersensitivity to drug or class or pork products, bleeding, thrombocytopenia, heparin-induced thrombocytopenia
- **Caution**—IM or IV use, neuraxial anesthesia may be contraindicated depending on dosing regimen desired. Anesthesiologist must know of intended dosing regimen before surgery.

■ **Maternal Considerations** — There are no adequate reports or well-controlled studies of **ardeparin** in pregnant women. This class of drugs is being used with increasing frequency during pregnancy for the treatment of thrombophilia.
Side effects include hemorrhage, injection site hematoma, fever, nausea, vomiting, bruising, arthralgia, and chest pain.

■ **Fetal Considerations** — There are no adequate reports or well-controlled studies in human fetuses. Its molecular weight suggests **ardeparin** does not cross the placenta. Rodent studies at up to 3 times the recommended human dose revealed no evidence of impaired fertility or fetal harm. However, when administered at 7 and 11 times the maximal human dose, scoliosis and cardiac defects, respectively, were noted.

■ **Breastfeeding Safety** — There are no adequate reports or well-controlled studies in nursing women. It is unknown whether **ardeparin** enters human breast milk.

■ **References** — There is no published experience in pregnancy or during lactation.

■ **Summary** —
- **Pregnancy Category C**
- **Lactation Category U**
- There are alternative agents for which there is more experience during pregnancy and lactation.

Argatroban (Acova)

■ **Class** — Anticoagulant; *thrombin inhibitor*

■ **Indications** — Either prophylaxis or treatment of thrombosis in women with heparin-induced thrombocytopenia

■ **Mechanism** — Unknown; directly inhibits thrombin

■ **Dosage with Qualifiers** — Heparin-induced thrombocytopenia—2mcg/kg/min IV; adjust dose based on apTT; maximum 10mcg/kg/min
DIC—0.7mcg/kg/min (response desired is a platelet count >120K/mm³, decreased fibrin or FDP <20, or no decrease in ATIII levels); alternatively 100mcg/kg IV over 1min, then 1-3mcg/kg/min for 6-72h
NOTE—hepatic dosing
- **Contraindications**—hypersensitivity to drug or class, major bleeding
- **Caution**—hepatic dysfunction, severe hypertension, conduction anesthesia, surgery, GI lesions

■ **Maternal Considerations** — There are no adequate reports or well-controlled studies of **argatroban** in pregnant women.
Side effects include hemorrhage, GI bleeding, cardiac arrest, hypotension, fever, diarrhea, nausea, vomiting and cough.

■ **Fetal Considerations** — There are no adequate reports or well-controlled studies in human fetuses. It is unknown whether **argatroban** crosses the human placenta. Rodent studies have not revealed evidence of either impaired fertility or teratogenicity, though the doses used were smaller than those employed clinically.

■ **Breastfeeding Safety** — There are no adequate reports or well-controlled studies in nursing women. It is unknown whether **argatroban** enters human breast milk. **Argatroban** is detected in rat breast milk.

■ **References** — McCrae KR, Bussel JB, Mannucci PM, et al. Hematology (Am Soc Hematol Educ Program) 2001; 282-305.

■ **Summary** —
- **Pregnancy Category B**
- **Lactation Category U**
- **Argatroban** is a somewhat unique drug that should be used only when the risk to the mother outweighs the theoretic risk to the fetus.

Aspirin

- **Class** ························· *Antiplatelet, salicylate, other neurologic agent*

- **Indications** ·············· Fever, mild pain, TIAs, MI, arthritis, rheumatic fever

- **Mechanism** ··············· Unknown, likely multiple as it inhibits the synthesis and release of prostaglandins by interfering with transcription factors, irreversibly inhibits cyclooxygenase, while its analgesia appears 2nd to peripheral and central effects.

- **Dosage with Qualifiers** ········ <u>Fever</u>—325-650mg PO/PR q4h prn
  <u>Analgesia</u>—325-650mg PO/PR q4h prn
  <u>Preeclampsia prophylaxis</u>—81mg PO qd
  <u>Antiphospholipid syndrome</u>—81mg PO qd alone if unassociated with fetal demise, otherwise coupled with **heparin** (fractionated or unfractionated)
  <u>TIA</u>—650mg PO bid
  <u>MI</u>—325mg PO qd to prevent recurrence
  <u>Arthritis</u>—3.6-5.4g PO daily in divided doses
  <u>Rheumatic fever</u>—5-8g PO qd in divided doses; treat for 1-2w, then taper over 2-8w
  NOTE—typically enteric-coated to assure release in the upper small intestine, where absorption is optimal. May be combined with **caffeine** and **butalbital** (without or with **codeine** or **hydrocodone**) and sold as Fiorinal, or with **propoxyphene** and sold as Darvon, or with **dipyridamole**.
  - **Contraindications**—hypersensitivity to drug or class, G6PD deficiency, bleeding disorder
  - **Caution**—GI lesions, renal or hepatic dysfunction, TTP, hypoprothrombinemia

- **Maternal Considerations** ········ **Aspirin** is a potent drug with complex and still unclear mechanisms of action. It is ubiquitous in the pharmacopeia, being combined with a multitude of agents. **Aspirin** is recommended by the American Heart Association for women with a 10y risk of coronary heart disease of 10% or higher, and by the U.S. Preventive Services Task Force for women whose 5y risk of coronary heart disease is 3% or higher. Women ingesting large quantities of **aspirin** are at risk for myriad complications. Chronically high salicylate levels are associated with prolonged pregnancy, increased puerperal bleeding, decreased birth weight, and stillbirth. It is generally recommended that high doses of **aspirin** be avoided during the last trimester. Low-dose **aspirin** alone may be as effective for the treatment for antiphospholipid syndrome characterized by recurrent 1st trimester losses as **aspirin** plus **heparin**. Controversy continues regarding the benefit of low-dose **aspirin** for the prevention of preeclampsia, though no complications of treatment have been documented and several meta-analyses suggest a modest reduction in preeclampsia and IUGR.

Side effects include GI bleeding, thrombocytopenia, anaphylaxis, angioedema, Reye's syndrome, hepatitis, dyspepsia, tinnitus, rash, abnormal LFTs, bruising, and bleeding.

■ **Fetal Considerations**

Aspirin does cross the placenta. Maternal **aspirin** ingestion has been linked to gastroschisis and small intestine atresia independent of fever or cold symptoms. Low-dose **aspirin** doses alter fetal cyclooxygenase activity, but no sequelae are known.

■ **Breastfeeding Safety**

The use of **aspirin** in single doses should not pose any risk to the breast-feeding newborn. In contrast, women on high doses of **aspirin** such as that for arthritis or rheumatic fever might best avoid breastfeeding, as the neonatal salicylate level may reach therapeutic levels.

■ **References**

Pearson TA, Blair SN, Daniels SR, et al. Circulation 2002; 106:388-91.
USPSTF. Ann Intern Med 2002; 136:157-160.
Farquharson R, Quenby S, Greaves M. Obstet Gynecol 2002; 100:408-15.
Duley L, Henderson-Smart D, Knight M, King J. BMJ 2001; 322:329-33.
Empson M, Lassere M, Craig JC, Scott JR. Obstet Gynecol 2002; 99:135-44.
Werler MM, Sheehan JE, Mitchell AA. Am J Epidemiol 2002; 155:26-31.
Coomarasamy A, Papaioannou S, Gee H, Khan KS. Obstet Gynecol 2001; 98:861-6.
Tegeder I, Pfeilschifter J, Geisslinger G. FASEB J 2001; 15:2057-72.
Spigset O, Hagg S. Paediatr Drugs 2000; 2:223-38.
Unsworth J, d'Assis-Fonseca A, Beswick DT, Blake DR. Ann Rheum Dis 1987; 46:638-9.

■ **Summary**

- **Pregnancy Category D**
- **Lactation Category S?**
- **Aspirin** should be used during pregnancy and lactation only if the benefit justifies the potential perinatal risk.
- **Aspirin** may be associated with fetal abnormalities when taken in the 1st trimester.

Atenolol (Alinor; Atolmin; Blotex; B-Vasc; Seles; Tenolin; Tenormin; Tensig)

■ **Class**	Antiadrenergic; *β-1 blocker*
■ **Indications**	Hypertension, MI, and angina pectoris
■ **Mechanism**	Selectively antagonizes the β-1 adrenoceptor
■ **Dosage with Qualifiers**	Hypertension—50mg PO qd; increase to 100mg qd after 7d MI—begin 5mg IV over 5min ×2 (10min apart), then 50mg PO q12h ×7d, then 100mg qd Angina—50mg PO qd, max 200mg qd • **Contraindications**—hypersensitivity to drug or class, 2nd-3rd degree heart block, sinus bradycardia, cardiac insufficiency • **Caution**—renal dysfunction
■ **Maternal Considerations**	Hypertension complicates 5-10% of pregnancies and is a leading cause of maternal and perinatal death and morbidity. Severe hypertension (systolic BP ≥170mmHg and/or diastolic BP ≥110mmHg) should be treated immediately. Mild, chronic hypertension is associated with increased maternal and fetal risks, but there is no consensus as to whether mild to moderate hypertension should be treated during pregnancy. The incidence of transient severe hypertension, antenatal hospitalization, proteinuria and neonatal RDS may be decreased by therapy, but fetal growth may be impaired. Of all β-blockers, the evidence that **atenolol** is associated with IUGR is the strongest. In one small trial, **atenolol** reduced the incidence of preeclampsia in women selected for increased cardiac output. It appears that IUGR reflects excess maternal β-blockade, causing a decrease in cardiac output. *Side effects* include CHF, bronchospasm, bradycardia, cold extremities, fatigue, nausea, rash, and hypotension.
■ **Fetal Considerations**	There are no adequate reports or well-controlled studies in human fetuses. **Atenolol** crosses the placenta. There is no substantive evidence for teratogenicity. As a group, β-blockers are associated with IUGR, though controversy continues as to whether this is drug or disease related. **Atenolol** reduces cardiac output, and failure to reduce the dose to prevent an excessive decline in output is associated with IUGR. Some rodent studies reveal a dose-dependent increase in embryo/fetal resorption.
■ **Breastfeeding Safety**	**Atenolol** is concentrated in breast milk, and significant bradycardia may occur in newborns nursed by women on **atenolol**. It should probably be avoided.

■ **References** — Magee LA. Best Pract Res Clin Obstet Gynaecol 2001; 15:827-45.
Easterling TR, Carr DB, Brateng D, et al. Obstet Gynecol 2001; 98:427-33.
Briggs GG, Nageotte MP. Ann Pharmacother 2001; 35:859-61.
Easterling TR, Brateng D, Schmucker B, et al. Obstet Gynecol 1999; 93:725-33.
Lip GY, Beevers M, Churchill D, et al. Am J Cardiol 1997; 79:1436-8.
Hurst AK, Shotan A, Hoffman K, et al. Pharmacotherapy 1998; 18:840-6.

■ **Summary**
- **Pregnancy Category D**
- **Lactation Category NS**
- **Atenolol** is associated with IUGR unless maternal cardiac output is monitored.
- There are other alternatives with a greater margin of safety.

Atorvastatin calcium (Lipitor)

■ **Class** — Antihyperlipidemia; HMG-CoA reductase inhibitor

■ **Indications** — Hypercholesterolemia, hypertriglyceridemia, dysbetalipoproteinemia, and familial hypercholesterolemia

■ **Mechanism** — Inhibits HMG-CoA reductase

■ **Dosage with Qualifiers** — Hypercholesterolemia, hypertriglyceridemia, dysbetalipoproteinemia, familial hypercholesterolemia—begin 10mg PO qd; monitor response every 8-12w, increasing to a max of 80mg qd
NOTE—monitor LFTs periodically beginning 12w after initiating therapy and with escalation
- **Contraindications**—hypersensitivity to drug or class, active hepatic disease, unexplained elevated LFTs, pregnancy, lactation
- **Caution**—history of liver disease or alcohol abuse

■ **Maternal Considerations** — There is no published experience with **atorvastatin** during pregnancy. The safety of **atorvastatin** during pregnancy has not been established.
Side effects include rhabdomyolysis, hepatotoxicity, dyspepsia, constipation, diarrhea, rash, myalgias, elevated LFTs, or CPK.

■ **Fetal Considerations** — There are no adequate reports or well-controlled studies in human fetuses. It is unknown whether **atorvastatin** crosses the human placenta. **Atorvastatin** does cross the rat placenta and reaches fetal hepatic concentrations similar to maternal plasma. While there is no evidence of teratogenicity in rodents even at high doses, there is a dose-dependent increase in IUGR, a decrease in survival, and behavioral abnormalities that were gender-dependent. These findings are the basis of its category X classification. Rare structural defects have occasionally been reported in association with other HMG-CoA inhibitors.

■ **Breastfeeding Safety** — There are no adequate reports or well-controlled studies in nursing women. It is unknown whether **atorvastatin** enters human breast milk. **Atorvastatin** is excreted into the breast milk of rats. There are no relevant human studies.

■ **References** — Henck JW, Craft WR, Black A, et al. Toxicol Sci 1998; 41:88-99. Dostal LA, Schardein JL, Anderson JA. Teratology 1994; 50:387-94.

■ **Summary**
- **Pregnancy Category X**
- **Lactation Category U**
- Hyperlipidemia is a chronic problem. Cessation of therapy during pregnancy should not significantly impact the long-term course of the disease.
- **Atorvastatin** should be used during pregnancy and lactation only if the benefit justifies the potential perinatal risk.

Atovaquone (Mepron)

■ **Class** — Antiprotozoal

■ **Indications** — Pneumocystis carinii pneumonia in patients intolerant of **trimethoprim-sulfoxisole**

■ **Mechanism** — Unknown

■ **Dosage with Qualifiers** — Pneumocystis carinii pneumonia for patients who cannot tolerate **trimethoprim-sulfoxisole**—750mg PO bid ×21d
Malaria—1000mg PO (with 400mg **proguanil** ×3d)
NOTE—not for prophylaxis; may be combined with **proguanil**
- **Contraindications**—hypersensitivity to drug or class

■ **Maternal Considerations** — There are no adequate reports or well-controlled studies of **atovaquone** during pregnancy. Several studies suggest the combination of **atovaquone** and **proguanil** is effective malaria prophylaxis.
Side effects include rash, fever, nausea, diarrhea, headache, insomnia, hyperglycemia, and elevated amylase.

- **Fetal Considerations** ·········· There are no adequate reports or well-controlled studies in human fetuses. Rodent studies are reassuring revealing no evidence of teratogenicity or IUGR despite the use of doses higher than those used clinically.

- **Breastfeeding Safety** ·········· There are no adequate reports or well-controlled studies in nursing women. It is unknown whether **atovaquone** enters human breast milk. In rats, the milk-plasma ratio approximates 1:3.

- **References** ·········· There is no published experience in pregnancy or during lactation.

- **Summary** ··········
  - **Pregnancy Category C**
  - **Lactation Category U**
  - **Atovaquone** should be used during pregnancy and lactation only if the benefit justifies the potential perinatal risk.

Atracurium (Tracrium)

- **Class** ·········· *Anesthesia, adjunct; musculoskeletal agent, nondepolarizing skeletal muscle relaxant*

- **Indications** ·········· Surgical paralysis

- **Mechanism** ·········· Antagonizes ACh motor endplate receptors; nondepolarizing

- **Dosage with Qualifiers** ·········· Surgical paralysis—0.4-0.5mg/kg IV; may supplement with 0.08-0.10mg/kg q15-25min
  - **Contraindications**—hypersensitivity to drug or class
  - **Caution**—hepatic or renal dysfunction, hypotension, cardiovascular disease, electrolyte abnormalities

- **Maternal Considerations** ·········· **Atracurium** is an intermediate-duration curare derivative producing effective surgical paralysis. There are no adequate reports or well-controlled studies of **atracurium** in pregnant women. The clearance of **atracurium** and clinical duration of **atracurium** are unaltered during pregnancy. In contrast, the clearance of **pancuronium** is increased 27% during cesarean section, and the mean onset time and clinical duration of **cisatracurium** are significantly reduced. *Side effects* include cardiovascular collapse, tachycardia, hypotension, rash, flushing, and urticaria, all due to histamine release and hypertension.

- **Fetal Considerations** ·········· There are no adequate reports or well-controlled studies in human fetuses. **Atracurium** has been used in lieu of **pancuronium** to facilitate fetal procedures. While small amounts are shown to cross the human placenta, its use during cesarean section is not associated with neonatal sequelae. In theory, if used for long-term paralysis of a critically ill pregnant woman, fetal toxicity could be a risk.

■ **Breastfeeding Safety**
There are no adequate reports or well-controlled studies in nursing women. It is unknown whether **atracurium** enters human breast milk. Considering its application, **atracurium** is unlikely to affect the breast-feeding newborn. While some rodent studies report an increase in malformations, they are confounded by the profound respiratory depression associated with the drug.

■ **References**
Pan PH, Moore C. J Clin Anesth 2001; 13:112-7.
Mouw RJ, Klumper F, Hermans J, et al. Acta Obstet Gynecol Scand 1999; 78:763-7.
Atherton DP, Hunter JM. Clin Pharmacokinet 1999; 36:169-89.
Guay J, Grenier Y, Varin F. Clin Pharmacokinet 1998; 34:483.

■ **Summary**
- **Pregnancy Category C**
- **Lactation Category U**
- **Atracurium** should be used during pregnancy and lactation only if the benefit justifies the potential perinatal risk.

Atropine (Atro Ofteno; Atropair; Atropen; Atropinol; Atropisol; Borotropin; Dosatropine; I-Tropine; Isopto Atropine; Isotic cycloma; Liotropina; Minims-Atropine; Ocu-Tropine; Sal-Tropine; Spectro-Atropine)

■ **Class**
Antiarrhythmics, anesthesia

■ **Indications**
Symptomatic bradycardia, organophosphate poisoning, adjunct to anesthesia to reduce secretions

■ **Mechanism**
Antagonizes ACh receptors

■ **Dosage with Qualifiers**
Symptomatic bradycardia—0.5-1mg IV q3-5min prn, max 2mg
Organophosphate poisoning—1-2mg IM/IV q20-30min until muscarinic symptoms resolve
Adjunct to anesthesia—0.4mg IM/SC 30-60min preoperatively to dry oral secretions before expected difficult airway management. Also given with anticholinesterase (**atropine** plus **neostigmine** when reversing neuromuscular paralysis at the end of surgery). NOTE—may be combined with either **difenoxin**, **diphenoxylate**, or **hyoscyamine**, **scopolamine** and **phenobarbital** (Donnatal)

- **Contraindications**—hypersensitivity to drug or class, narrow angle glaucoma, paralytic ileus, asthma, myasthenia gravis

■ **Maternal Considerations** — There are no adequate reports or well-controlled studies of **atropine** in pregnant women.
Side effects include paradoxical bradycardia (usually doses <0.3mg), tachycardia, palpitations, blurred vision, headache, nausea, vomiting, dizziness, dry mouth, restlessness, delirium, tremor, and hot dry skin.

■ **Fetal Considerations** — There are no adequate reports or well-controlled studies in human fetuses. **Atropine** rapidly crosses the human placenta and the fetus will respond to the direct administration of **atropine**.

■ **Breastfeeding Safety** — There are no adequate reports or well-controlled studies in nursing women. It is unknown whether **atropine** enters human breast milk.

■ **References** — Graf JL, Paek BW, Albanese CT, et al. J Pediatr Surg 2000; 35:1388-9.
Kanto J, Lindberg R, Pihlajamaki K, Scheinin M. Pharmacol Toxicol 1987; 60:108-9.

■ **Summary** —
- **Pregnancy Category C**
- **Lactation Category U**
- **Atropine** should be used during pregnancy and lactation only if the benefit justifies the potential perinatal risk.

Attapulgite (Kaopectate)

■ **Class** — Antidiarrheal

■ **Indications** — Diarrhea

■ **Mechanism** — Unknown

■ **Dosage with Qualifiers** — Diarrhea—30ml PO prn, max 6×/d, alternatively 1.2-1.5g after each bowel movement (refer to each manufacturer's dosing formulations)
- **Contraindications**—hypersensitivity to drug or class, bowel obstruction
- **Caution**—fever, volume depletion

■ **Maternal Considerations** — There are no adequate reports or well-controlled studies of **attapulgite** in pregnant women.
Side effects include constipation, dyspepsia, flatulence, nausea, vomiting.

- **Fetal Considerations** ·········· There are no adequate reports or well-controlled studies in human fetuses. It is unknown whether **attapulgite** crosses the human placenta.

- **Breastfeeding Safety** ·········· There is no published experience in nursing women. It is unknown whether **attapulgite** will alter breast milk.

- **References** ·········· There are no relevant publications.

- **Summary** ··········
  - **Pregnancy Category B**
  - **Lactation Category U**
  - There is no published experience in pregnant women, but a long clinical experience supports its occasional use during pregnancy.

Auranofin (Ridaura)

- **Class** ·········· Antiarthritic; *gold compound*

- **Indications** ·········· Rheumatoid arthritis

- **Mechanism** ·········· Unknown

- **Dosage with Qualifiers** ·········· Rheumatoid arthritis—3mg PO bid; may increase to 9mg stepwise after 4-6mo
  - **Contraindications**—hypersensitivity to drug or class, gold toxicity, pulmonary fibrosis, dermatitis, bone marrow aplasia, necrotizing enterocolitis
  - **Caution**—hepatic or renal dysfunction

- **Maternal Considerations** ·········· There is no published experience with **auranofin** during pregnancy.
  Side effects include seizures, nephritic syndrome, renal failure, thrombocytopenia, ulcerative colitis, aplastic anemia, pneumonitis, pulmonary fibrosis, diarrhea, rash, itching, nausea, abdominal pain, conjunctivitis, hematuria, anemia, and anorexia.

- **Fetal Considerations** ·········· There are no adequate reports or well-controlled studies in human fetuses. It is unknown whether **auranofin** crosses the human placenta. Rodent studies reveal an increased risk of embryo and fetal toxicity, gastroschisis and umbilical hernia.

- **Breastfeeding Safety** ·········· There are no adequate reports or well-controlled studies in nursing women. It is unknown whether **auranofin** enters human breast milk. Gold is excreted into rodent milk.

■ **Summary** ·········· • **Pregnancy Category C**
• **Lactation Category U**
• **Auranofin** should be used during pregnancy and lactation only if the benefit justifies the potential perinatal risk.
• There are usually alternative agents for which there is more experience during pregnancy and lactation.

Azatadine maleate (Optimine)

■ **Class** ·········· *Antihistamine*

■ **Indications** ·········· Allergic rhinitis, urticaria

■ **Mechanism** ·········· Unknown

■ **Dosage with Qualifiers** ·········· Allergic rhinitis—1-2mg PO bid
Urticaria—1-2mg PO bid
• **Contraindications**—hypersensitivity, MAO inhibitor within 14d, urinary retention, prostatic hypertrophy
• **Caution**—asthma, glaucoma

■ **Maternal Considerations** ·········· **Azatadine** is an antihistamine with antiserotonergic, anticholinergic, and sedative effects. There is no published experience during pregnancy.
Side effects include agranulocytosis, thrombocytopenia, anaphylaxis, dry mouth, nausea, abdominal pain, urinary retention, headache, constipation, and weight gain.

■ **Fetal Considerations** ·········· There are no adequate reports or well-controlled studies in human fetuses. Rodent studies are reassuring, revealing no evidence of teratogenicity or IUGR despite the use of doses higher than those used clinically.

■ **Breastfeeding Safety** ·········· There are no adequate reports or well-controlled studies in nursing women. It is unknown whether **azatadine** enters human breast milk.

■ **References** ·········· There is no published experience in pregnancy or during lactation.

■ **Summary** ·········· • **Pregnancy Category B**
• **Lactation Category U**
• There are alternative agents for which there is more experience during pregnancy and lactation.

Azathioprine (Imuran)

■ **Class** .... *Immunosuppressant*

■ **Indications** .... Transplant rejection prophylaxis, immune disorders such as SLE, inflammatory bowel disease, and rheumatoid arthritis

■ **Mechanism** .... A purine analog that inhibits T-cell activity

■ **Dosage with Qualifiers** .... <u>Transplant rejection</u>—begin 3-5mg/kg/d PO/IV qd; maintenance 1-3mg/kg/d transplant protocols vary
<u>Crohn's disease and ulcerative colitis</u>—begin 50mg PO qd increasing to 150-250mg PO qd; max 2.5mg/kg/d
<u>Rheumatoid arthritis</u>—begin 1mg/kg PO qd; increase 0.5mg/kg/d after 6-8w; max 2.5mg/kg/d
NOTE—monitor CBC weekly; renal dosing if CrCl <50ml/h
● **Contraindications**—hypersensitivity to drug or class
● **Caution**—pregnancy, lactation

■ **Maternal Considerations** .... There are no adequate reports or well-controlled studies of **azathioprine** in pregnant women. Immune-related disorders are fairly common in reproductive-age women. Women with quiescent inflammatory bowel disease are likely to have an uncomplicated pregnancy, whereas women with active disease are more likely to have complications such as spontaneous abortions, miscarriages, stillbirths, and exacerbation of the disease. Most pregnancies treated with **azathioprine** end successfully, even in transplant patients. It has been used successfully for the treatment of autoimmune hepatitis during pregnancy.
Side effects include pancreatitis, fever, leukopenia, bone marrow suppression, immunosuppression, hepatotoxicity, risk of neoplasm, nausea, vomiting, diarrhea, abdominal pain, rash, increased LFTs, myalgias, and arthralgia.

■ **Fetal Considerations** .... There are no adequate reports or well-controlled studies in human fetuses. **Azathioprine** crosses the human placenta, though the kinetics is unclear. And while no clear pattern of malformation is detectable in the large number of pregnant women exposed, isolated skeletal defects are reported. All immunosuppressants cross the placenta, and their long-term impact on the child later in life is unknown. There are also reports in neonates of reduced IgG and IgM, and leukopenia. It is unclear whether the reported increase in IUGR reflects disease or drug. Heightened immune responses were reported during the pregnancy of a woman whose mother had been treated with **azathioprine** throughout pregnancy.
Azathioprine is teratogenic in rodents treated with human equivalent doses, producing a constellation of malformations that are both skeletal and visceral.

Breastfeeding Safety

Azathioprine is excreted into breast milk, but the pharmacokinetics remains to be elucidated. There are no well-documented instances of neonatal effect.

References

Sgro MD, Barozzino T, Mirghani HM, et al. Teratology 2002; 65:5-9.
Armenti VT, Moritz MJ, Davison JM. Drug Saf 1998; 19:219-32.
Heneghan MA, Norris SM, O'Grady JG, et al. Gut 2001; 48:97-102.
Williamson RA, Karp LE. Obstet Gynecol 1981; 58:247-50.
Scott JR, Branch DW, Holman J. Transplantation 2002; 73:815-6.

Summary

- **Pregnancy Category D**
- **Lactation Category U**
- **Azathioprine** should be used during pregnancy and lactation only if the benefit justifies the potential perinatal risk.
- Consideration should be given to either switching to a different agent with a more reassuring safety profile, or reducing the dose to the minimum required for the control of symptoms.

Azithromycin dihydrate (Aruzilina; Zithromax)

Class

Antibiotic, macrolide

Indications

PID, *Chlamydia*, chancroid, uncomplicated gonorrhea, and community-acquired pneumonia

Mechanism

Inhibits microbial protein synthesis by binding to the P site of the 50S ribosomal subunit

Dosage with Qualifiers

Bacterial infection—500mg PO load ×1, then 250mg PO qd ×6d
Chlamydia or chancroid—1g PO ×1
Uncomplicated gonorrhea—2g PO ×1 (or 1g PO ×1 plus **fluoroquinolone** or **ceftriaxone** or **cefixime**)
PID—500mg IV qd ×2d, then 250mg PO qd ×6d
Community-acquired pneumonia—500mg IV qd ×2-5d, then 500mg PO qd for a total 7-10d
- **Contraindications**—hypersensitivity to drug or class
- **Caution**—hepatic dysfunction, **astemizole** or **terfenadine** use

Maternal Considerations

Azithromycin has a short serum half-life in term pregnant women. Prolonged half-life and high tissular levels were noted in myometrium, placenta, and adipose tissue. Considering its efficacy against other STDs and convenient dosing regimen, **azithromycin** is probably the treatment of choice for *Chlamydia*. Partner pharmacotherapy is cost-effective. **Azithromycin** has been used in combination with **artesunate** as malaria prophylaxis. It was ineffective treatment to reduce lower genital tract colonization with *Ureaplasma urealyticum* in women with preterm labor.

Side effects include angioedema, anaphylaxis, cholestatic jaundice, Stevens-Johnson syndrome, pseudomembranous colitis, diarrhea, nausea, vaginitis, rash, anorexia, and itching.

■ **Fetal Considerations**

There are no adequate reports or well-controlled studies in human fetuses. Less than 3% of maternally administered **azithromycin** crosses the placenta. Not surprisingly, there have been no adverse effects reported in humans. Rodent studies are reassuring, revealing no evidence of teratogenicity or IUGR despite the use of doses higher than those used clinically.

■ **Breastfeeding Safety**

Azithromycin is excreted in breast milk in a dose-dependent fashion. No neonatal effects have been reported.

■ **References**

Kelsey JJ, Moser LR, Jennings JC, Munger MA. Am J Obstet Gynecol 1994; 170:1375-6.
Postma MJ, Welte R, van den Hoek JA, et al. Value Health 2001; 4:266-75.
Ogasawara KK, Goodwin TM. J Matern Fetal Med 1999; 8:12-6.
Ramsey PS, Vaules MB, Vasdev GM, et al. Am J Obstet Gynecol 2003; 188:714-8.
Jacobson GF, Autry AM, Kirby RS, et al. Am J Obstet Gynecol 2001; 184:1352-4.
Heikkinen T, Laine K, Neuvonen PJ, Ekblad U. BJOG 2000; 107:770-5.

■ **Summary**

- **Pregnancy Category B**
- **Lactation Category U**
- **Azithromycin** is an effective antimicrobial agent for a variety of disorders complicating pregnancy.

Aztreonam (Azactam)

■ **Class**

Antibiotic, monobactam

■ **Indications**

Susceptible bacterial infections, including gonorrhea

■ **Mechanism**

Inhibits bacterial cell wall synthesis by binding with high affinity to the penicillin-binding protein 3

- **Dosage with Qualifiers** ········ Bacterial infection—0.5-2g IV/IM q8-12h; max 8g/d
Gonorrhea—1g IM ×1
NOTE—renal dosing
  - **Contraindications**—hypersensitivity to drug or class
  - **Caution**—renal dysfunction

- **Maternal Considerations** ········ There are no adequate reports or well-controlled studies of **aztreonam** in pregnant women. It is one of many antibiotics of potential for use during pregnancy. **Aztreonam** is as effective as **gentamicin** plus **clindamycin** for the treatment of puerperal endomyometritis. *Side effects* include seizures, anaphylaxis, eosinophilia, pseudomembranous colitis, phlebitis, diarrhea, nausea, rash, and elevated LFTs.

- **Fetal Considerations** ········ There are no adequate reports or well-controlled studies in human fetuses. **Aztreonam** crosses the human placenta in therapeutic concentrations, suggesting it might be useful for antepartal chorioamnionitis. Rodent studies are reassuring, revealing no evidence of teratogenicity or IUGR despite the use of doses higher than those used clinically.

- **Breastfeeding Safety** ········ There are no adequate reports or well-controlled studies in human fetuses. It is excreted into the breast milk at trace levels.

- **References** ········ Itakura A, Kurauchi O, Mizutani S, et al. Jpn J Antibiot 1995; 48:749-53.
Clark P. Obstet Gynecol Clin North Am 1992; 19:519-28.
Greenberg RN, Reilly PM, Weinandt WJ, et al. Clin Ther 1987; 10:36-9.
Matsuda S, Oh K, Hirayama H. Jpn J Antibiot 1990; 43:700-5.
Fleiss PM, Richwald GA, Gordon J, et al. Br J Clin Pharmacol 1985; 19:509-11.

- **Summary** ········
  - **Pregnancy Category B**
  - **Lactation Category S**
  - A good agent whose selection may be based more on the cost and availability rather than any particular advantage.
  - Achieves therapeutic levels in the fetal compartment.

Bacampicillin (Ambacomp; Amplibac; Spectrobid)

■ **Class** — Antibiotic (*semisynthetic penicillin*)

■ **Indications** — UTI (E. *coli*, *Proteus mirabilis*, *Streptococcus fecalis* [enterococci], upper and lower respiratory tract [β-hemolytic streptococci, *Streptococcus pyogenes*, *Streptococcus pneumoniae*], urogenital [gonorrhea] and skin [streptococci, staphylococci]) infections

■ **Mechanism** — Rapidly hydrolyzed to **ampicillin** on absorption from the GI tract; inhibits cell wall mucopeptide synthesis

■ **Dosage with Qualifiers** — Bacterial infection—800mg PO q12h
- **Contraindications**—hypersensitivity to drug or drug class, pseudomembranous colitis
- **Caution**—EBV and CMV infection, penicillin or cephalosporin allergy, renal dysfunction

■ **Maternal Considerations** — See **ampicillin**.
Side effects—see **ampicillin**.

■ **Fetal Considerations** — See **ampicillin**.

■ **Breastfeeding Safety** — See **ampicillin**.

■ **References** — Catizone F, Pirillo P, Carlisi T. Minerva Ginecol 1979; 31(9):699-701.

■ **Summary** —
- **Pregnancy Category B**
- **Lactation Category S**
- **Bacampicillin** owes its *in vivo* activity to **ampicillin**.

Bacitracin (Ak-Tracin; Baci-Rx; Baci-IM; Bacticin; Ocutricin; Spectro-Bacitracin)

■ **Class** — Antibiotic, *ophthalmologic, dermatologic*

■ **Indications** — Gram-positive and -negative bacterial infection.

■ **Mechanism** — Bactericidal, cyclic polypeptide that inhibits bacterial cell wall synthesis

- **Dosage with Qualifiers** ⸱⸱⸱⸱⸱ Skin or wound infection—apply cream topically qd to tid
  NOTE—use no longer than 1w; often combined with
  neosporin and **polymixin B**
  - **Contraindications**—hypersensitivity to drug or class
  - **Caution**—myasthenia gravis

- **Maternal Considerations** ⸱⸱⸱⸱⸱ There is no published experience during pregnancy.
  Bacitracin enhances wound healing in nonpregnant surgical
  patients and reduces scarring compared to placebo.
  Side effects include contact dermatitis.

- **Fetal Considerations** ⸱⸱⸱⸱⸱ There are no adequate and well-controlled studies in
  human fetuses. It is unknown whether **bacitracin** crosses
  the human placenta. Considering the dose and route, it is
  unlikely the maternal systemic concentration will reach a
  clinically relevant level. Rodent teratogenicity studies
  have not been performed.

- **Breastfeeding Safety** ⸱⸱⸱⸱⸱ There are no adequate reports or well-controlled studies
  in nursing women. It is unknown whether **bacitracin**
  enters human breast milk. However, considering the dose
  and route, it is unlikely the breast-fed neonate would
  ingest clinically relevant amounts.

- **References** ⸱⸱⸱⸱⸱ Smack DP, Harrington AC, Dunn C, et al. JAMA
  1996; 276:972-7.
  Watcher MA, Wheeland RG. J Dermatol Surg Oncol
  1989; 11:1188-95.

- **Summary** ⸱⸱⸱⸱⸱
  - **Pregnancy Category C**
  - **Lactation Category S**
  - **Bacitracin** promotes wound healing and reduces
    scarring.
  - The long clinical experience with topical administration
    is reassuring.

Baclofen (Lioresal)

- **Class** ⸱⸱⸱⸱⸱ *Muscle relaxant*

- **Indications** ⸱⸱⸱⸱⸱ Control of the spasticity secondary to MS and other spinal
  cord diseases

- **Mechanism** ⸱⸱⸱⸱⸱ Exact mechanism unknown (central-acting muscle relaxant)

- **Dosage with Qualifiers** ⸱⸱⸱⸱⸱ Muscle spasm—begin 5mg PO tid; increase by 15mg qd
  q3d based on response; max 80mg/d
  - **Contraindications**—hypersensitivity to drug or class
  - **Caution**—renal dysfunction, seizure disorder

■ **Maternal Considerations** ⋯⋯⋯ There are no adequate reports or well-controlled studies in pregnant women. The published experience is mostly limited to case reports, mostly of intrathecal use. For example, one documents successful intrathecal use for the treatment of severe tetanus, and another the long-term treatment of severe spasticity after a C5 fracture. **Baclofen** proved superior to placebo for the relief of abortal pain. *Side effects* include CNS depression, seizures, cardiovascular collapse, drowsiness, headache, dizziness, blurred vision and slurred speech, constipation, pruritus, urinary frequency, constipation, and rash.

■ **Fetal Considerations** ⋯⋯⋯ There are no adequate and well-controlled studies in human fetuses. It is unknown whether **baclofen** crosses the human placenta. There is a single case report of neonatal convulsions at 7d of age. Rodent studies reveal an increased prevalence of omphalocele, incomplete ossification of the sternum, vertebral arch widening, and neural tube defects when given at 10 times the recommended dose.

■ **Breastfeeding Safety** ⋯⋯⋯ There are no adequate reports or well-controlled studies in nursing women. **Baclofen** reduces sucking-induced prolactin release, but milk ejection is unchanged. Only about 0.1% of the maternal dose is excreted into human breast milk.

■ **References** ⋯⋯⋯
Engrand N, Van De Perre P, Vilain G, Benhamou D. Eur J Anaesthesiol 2001; 18:261-3.
Munoz FC, Marco DG, Perez AV, Camacho M. Ann Pharmacother 2000; 34:956.
Corli O, Roma G, Bacchini M, et al. Clin Ther 1984; 6:800-7.
Eriksson G, Swahn CG. Scand J Clin Lab Invest 1981; 41:185-7.
Committee on Drugs, American Academy of Pediatrics. Pediatrics 1994; 93:137-50.
Ratnayaka DM, Dhaliwal H, Watkin S. BMJ 2001; 323:85.

■ **Summary** ⋯⋯⋯
• **Pregnancy Category C**
• **Lactation Category S**
• **Baclofen** is rarely necessary during pregnancy and should be given only when the benefits exceed the potential risks.

Balsalazide (Colazal)

■ **Class** ⋯⋯⋯ *Gastrointestinal, inflammatory bowel disease, salicylate*

■ **Indications** ⋯⋯⋯ Ulcerative colitis, acute

■ **Mechanism** ⋯⋯⋯ Exact mechanism unknown (central acting muscle relaxant)

- ■ **Dosage with Qualifiers** ·········· <u>Ulcerative colitis</u>—2.25g PO tid; max use 8w
  - **Contraindications**—hypersensitivity to drug or class
  - **Caution**—renal dysfunction, seizure disorder, antibiotic treatment, pyloric stenosis

- ■ **Maternal Considerations** ········ **Balsalazide** is enzymatically cleaved in the colon to produce **melsalamine**. There are no adequate reports or well-controlled studies in pregnant women.
  Side effects include angioedema, bradycardia, bronchospasm, colitis, nausea, vomiting, diarrhea, abdominal pain, anemia, epistaxis, anxiety, depression, nephritis, arthralgia, alopecia, and dermatitis.

- ■ **Fetal Considerations** ················ There are no adequate and well-controlled studies in human fetuses. It is unknown whether **balsalazide** crosses the human placenta. Rodent studies are reassuring, revealing no evidence of teratogenicity or IUGR despite the use of doses higher than those used clinically.

- ■ **Breastfeeding Safety** ············· There is no published experience in nursing women. It is unknown whether **balsalazide** enters human breast milk.

- ■ **References** ··································· Klotz U. Clin Pharmacokinet 1985; 10:285-302.

- ■ **Summary** ··································· • **Pregnancy Category B**
  - **Lactation Category U**
  - **Balsalazide** should be used during pregnancy and lactation only if the benefit justifies the potential perinatal risk.

Basiliximab (Simulect)

- ■ **Class** ··· *Transplant*

- ■ **Indications** ······························· Renal transplant immunoprophylaxis

- ■ **Mechanism** ······························· IL-2 receptor antagonist

- ■ **Dosage with Qualifiers** ·········· <u>Kidney transplant</u>—20mg IV single dose
  NOTE—**basiliximab** should be given only when it is determined the patient will receive a graft; a second dose should be administered with great caution
  - **Contraindications**—hypersensitivity to drug or class
  - **Caution**—unknown

- ■ **Maternal Considerations** ········ There is no published experience with **basiliximab** during pregnancy.
  Side effects include constipation, diarrhea, nausea, hyperkalemia, hypokalemia, acne, insomnia, angina

pectoris, headache, tremor, hypertension, dysuria, urinary tract infection, edema, fever, asthenia, and hypercholesterolemia.

■ **Fetal Considerations** ⋯⋯⋯ There are no adequate and well-controlled studies in human fetuses. It is unknown whether **basiliximab** crosses the human placenta. Rodent studies are reassuring, revealing no evidence of teratogenicity or IUGR despite the use of doses higher than those used clinically.

■ **Breastfeeding Safety** ⋯⋯⋯ There is no published experience in nursing women. It is unknown whether **basiliximab** enters human breast milk. However, considering the indication and dosing, one time **basiliximab** use is unlikely to pose a clinically significant risk to the breast-feeding neonate.

■ **References** ⋯⋯⋯ No publications of use in pregnancy.

■ **Summary** ⋯⋯⋯
- **Pregnancy Category B**
- **Lactation Category U**
- **Basiliximab** should be given to pregnant women only when the benefits outweigh the potential risks.

Beclomethasone (Beclovent; Beconase; Vanceril; Vanceril DS)

■ **Class** ⋯⋯⋯ *Corticosteroid*

■ **Indications** ⋯⋯⋯ Treatment of asthma, rhinitis, nasal polyp prophylaxis

■ **Mechanism** ⋯⋯⋯ Anti-inflammatory mechanism unknown

■ **Dosage with Qualifiers** ⋯⋯⋯ Asthma—4-16 inhalations/d
Rhinitis—1-2 inhalations in each nostril qd; max 336mcg/d
Nasal polyp prophylaxis—1-2 inhalations in each nostril qd; max 336mcg/d
NOTE—each metered inhalation delivers 42mcg of aerosolized drug
- **Contraindications**—hypersensitivity to drug or class
- **Caution**—local infection

■ **Maternal Considerations** ⋯⋯⋯ **Beclomethasone** has been used during pregnancy without apparent complication, but there are no well-controlled studies involving pregnant women. Its effectiveness requires regular use.
Side effects include irritation of nasal mucous membranes, urticaria, edema, bronchospasm, headache, and nausea.

- **Fetal Considerations** ········· There are no well-controlled studies of **beclomethasone** in human fetuses. It is unknown whether **beclomethasone** specifically crosses the human placenta. Hypoadrenalism may occur in newborns of women using **beclomethasone**, suggesting placental transfer. Rodent studies using up to 10 times the maximum human dose revealed increased frequencies of fetal resorption, cleft palate, delayed ossification, agnathia, and embryocidal effect.

- **Breastfeeding Safety** ········· There are no adequate reports or well-controlled studies in nursing women. It is unknown whether **beclomethasone** enters human breast milk. Other steroids are excreted in low amounts.

- **References** ········· Beck SA. Allergy Asthma Proc 2001; 22:1-4.
Karinski DA, Balkundi D, Rubin LP, Padbury JF. Neonatal Netw 2000; 19:27-32.
Mazzotta P, Loebstein R, Koren G. Drug Saf 1999; 20:361-75.
Brown HM, Storey G. Postgrad Med J 1975; 51:59-64.
Dombrowski MP, Brown CL, Berry SM. J Matern Fetal Med 1996; 5:310-3.
Wendel PJ, Ramin SM, Barnett-Hamm C, et al. Am J Obstet Gynecol 1996; 175:150-4.
Stenius-Aarniala B, Piirila P, Teramo K. Thorax 1988; 43:12-8.

- **Summary** ·········
  - **Pregnancy Category C**
  - **Lactation Category U**
  - **Beclomethasone** should be used during pregnancy and lactation only if the benefit justifies the potential perinatal risk.
  - Fetal adrenal suppression may occur after prolonged maternal systemic steroid administration.

Belladonna (Donnatal; Lomotil; Atropine Sulfate)

- **Class** ········· *Parasympatholytic*

- **Indications** ········· Adjunctive therapy for irritable bowel syndrome, acute enterocolitis, duodenal ulcer, cesarean section (to decrease secretions), fetal bradycardia

- **Mechanism** ········· Anticholinergic; atropine is the active agent

- **Dosage with Qualifiers** ········· Donnatal—0.0194mg/tab, 5ml/elixir (23% alcohol)
Lomotil—0.025mg/tab, 5ml
Atropine sulfate—0.1mg/ml

NOTE—individualize the dose; may be combined with either **opium**, **ergotamine**, **phenobarbital**, or **butabarbital**
- **Contraindications**—hypersensitivity to drug or class
- **Caution**—neuropathy, glaucoma, hepatic diseases, hyperthyroidism, coronary heart diseases, chronic lung diseases

■ **Maternal Considerations**
There are no well-controlled studies in pregnant women. *Side effects* include xerostomia, taste change, blurred vision, bradycardia, palpitation, drowsiness, headache, and anaphylaxis.

■ **Fetal Considerations**
There are no adequate and well-controlled studies in human fetuses. **Belladonna** rapidly crosses the placenta producing a pharmacologic fetal vagotomy with subsequent tachycardia. It decreases fetal breathing. However, no adverse acute or chronic fetal effects are documented in women taking **atropine**. No association with malformations has been documented.

■ **Breastfeeding Safety**
No adequate well-controlled studies determined the passage of **belladonna** in the breast milk; it is generally considered safe for breastfeeding.

■ **References**
Freeman JJ, Altieri RH, Baptiste HJ, et al. J Natl Med Assoc 1994; 86:704-8.
Abboud T, Raya J, Sadry S, et al. Anesth Analg 1983; 62:426-30.
Hellman LM, Filisti LP. Am J Obstet Gynecol 1965; 91:797-805.

■ **Summary**
- **Pregnancy Category C**
- **Lactation Category S**
- **Belladonna** is useful adjuvant therapy for GI symptoms related to irritable bowel syndrome, acute enterocolitis, and duodenal ulcer.
- **Belladonna** decreases fetal breathing.

Benazepril (Lotensin)

■ **Class**
Antihypertensive, ACE-1/A2R antagonist

■ **Indications**
Hypertension, congestive heart failure

■ **Mechanism**
Angiotensin-converting enzyme inhibitor

■ **Dosage with Qualifiers**
<u>Hypertension</u>—begin 10mg qd, max 80mg/d
<u>Congestive heart failure</u>—begin 5mg qd; lower doses when used with a diuretic

NOTE—renal dosing
May be combined with **hydrochlorothiazide.**
- **Contraindications**—hypersensitivity to drug or class, renal artery stenosis, pregnancy
- **Caution**—renal dysfunction, hypovolemia, collagen vascular disease, severe CHF

■ **Maternal Considerations** ····· There is no published experience during pregnancy. However, this class of agents is associated with severe fetal renal toxicity and is considered contraindicated after the 1st trimester.
Side effects include angioedema, hypotension, renal failure, hyperkalemia, elevated BUN/Cr, pancreatitis, liver toxicity, agranulocytosis, dizziness, headache, dyspepsia, cough, rash, urticaria, fatigue, myalgia, diarrhea, and taste changes.

■ **Fetal Considerations** ········· **Benazepril** may cause fetal and neonatal morbidity and death. ACE-inhibitors during the 2nd and 3rd trimesters of pregnancy are associated with hypotension, neonatal skull hypoplasia, renal failure, and oligohydramnios. No such complications are associated with **benazepril** exposure in the 1st trimester. Limited placental transfer is noted in the rat.

■ **Breastfeeding Safety** ········· There is no published experience in nursing women. Minimal amounts of **benazepril** enter the breast milk.

■ **References** ········· Yamamoto S, Takemori E, Hasegawa Y, et al. Arzneimittelforschung 1991; 41:913-23.
Chisholm CA, Chescheir NC, Kennedy M. Am J Perinatol 1997; 14:511-3.
Waldmeier F, Schmid K. Arzneimittelforschung 1989; 39:62-7.

■ **Summary** ·········
- **Pregnancy Category C (1st trimester), D (2nd and 3rd trimesters)**
- **Lactation Category S?**
- **Benazepril** is an ACE inhibitor, which may cause severe fetal and neonatal harm when given after the 1st trimester.
- There are alternative agents with a higher safety profile for which there is more experience during pregnancy and lactation.

Bendroflumethiazide (Bendrofluazide; Benzide; Corzide; Esberizid; Naturetin; Salural)

■ **Class** — Diuretic (*thiazide*)

■ **Indications** — Hypertension

■ **Mechanism** — Mechanism unknown; interferes with electrolyte resorption in the distal renal tubule

■ **Dosage with Qualifiers** — Diuretic—5mg PO qam
Hypertension—5-20mg PO qd
Hypertension (Corzide)—1 tab PO qd
NOTE—Corzide: each tablet contains 5mg of **bendroflumethiazide** plus **nadolol** (40 or 80mg)

- **Contraindications**—hypersensitivity to drug or class, AV block, sinus bradycardia, cardiogenic shock, bradycardia, hypotension, bronchospasm, dizziness, nausea, vomiting, confusion, rash, photosensitivity, and electrolyte abnormalities
- **Caution**—renal dysfunction

■ **Maternal Considerations** — There is no published experience during pregnancy. **Thiazide** diuretics should be avoided during pregnancy except for the treatment of congestive heart disease. It has been suggested but not shown that diuretics in general may hinder placental perfusion by preventing normal plasma expansion. **Thiazide** diuretics are diabetogenic in some women. There are several reports of severe electrolyte imbalance in both mothers and newborns. Hemorrhagic pancreatitis has also been reported after **thiazide** exposure.
Side effects include CHF, thrombocytopenia, agranulocytosis, exfoliative dermatitis.

■ **Fetal Considerations** — There are no adequate and well-controlled studies in human fetuses. It is unknown whether **bendroflumethiazide** crosses the human placenta. Other **thiazide** agents readily cross. Fetal bradycardia associated with fetal hypokalemia has also been reported after maternal **thiazide** use. And while they are not associated with congenital defects, neonatal thrombocytopenia and hypoglycemia are reported.

■ **Breastfeeding Safety** — There is no published experience in nursing women. Many **thiazide** diuretics are excreted into breast milk, but in low concentrations. They are generally considered safe for breast-feeding women.

■ **References** — Finnerty FA, Buchholz JH, Tuckman J. JAMA 1958; 166:1414.
Assoli NS. Clin Pharmacol Ther 1960; 1:48-52.

Flowers CE, Grizzle JE, Easterling WE, Bonner OB. Am J Obstet Gynecol 1962; 84:919-29.
Sibai BM, Grossman RA, Grossman HG. Am J Obstet Gynecol 1984; 150:831-5.
Beermann B, Fahraeus L, Groschisky-Grind M, Lindstrom B. Gynecol Obstet Invest 1980; 11:45-8.
Goldman JA, Neri A, Ovadia J, et al. Am J Obstet Gynecol 1969; 105:556-60.
Rodriguez SU, Leikin SL, Hiller MC. N Engl J Med 1964; 270:881-4.
Pritchard JA, Waley PJ. Am J Obstet Gynecol 1961; 81:1241-4.
Minkowitz S, Soloway HB, Hall JE, Yermakov V. Obstet Gynecol 1964; 24:337-42.
Drug Ther Bull 2001; 39(5):37-40.

■ **Summary**

- **Pregnancy Category D**
- **Lactation Category S**
- **Thiazide** diuretics are contraindicated during pregnancy except for the treatment of congestive heart disease.
- There are alternative agents with a higher safety profile during pregnancy for almost all indications.

Benzocaine (Americaine; Anacaine; Otocain)

■ **Class** — Anesthetic

■ **Indications** — Topical anesthetic, lubricant, relief of pain in acute congestive and serous otitis, acute swimmer's ear, production of anesthesia of mucous membrane

■ **Mechanism** — Stabilizes the neuronal membrane and alters its permeability to sodium ions

■ **Dosage with Qualifiers** — Topical anesthetic (e.g., episiotomy pain)—apply to affected area as needed
Anesthetic lubricant—apply over the intratracheal catheters and pharyngeal and nasal airways with the purpose of attenuating local reflexes
Congestive and serous otitis and acute swimmer's ear—supplied as ear drops
Anesthesia of mucous membrane—supplied as topical gel or local spray; max 20mg
NOTE—combined with **antipyrine** for otic uses
- **Contraindications**—hypersensitivity to drug or class, perforated tympanic membrane
- **Caution**—not known

- ■ **Maternal Considerations** ⋯⋯⋯ There are no well-controlled studies of **benzocaine** during pregnancy. It provides relief from perineal pain associated with episiotomy especially when associated with a corticosteroid. Some practitioners use it as an alternative to **lidocaine** for the symptomatic relief of perineal herpetic lesions.
  Side effects include contact dermatitis, burning, and pruritus.

- ■ **Fetal Considerations** ⋯⋯⋯ There are no well-controlled studies of **benzocaine** in human fetuses. It is unknown whether **benzocaine** crosses the human placenta. Considering the dose and route, it is unlikely the maternal systemic concentration will reach clinically relevant level.

- ■ **Breastfeeding Safety** ⋯⋯⋯ There is no published experience in nursing women. However, considering the dose and route, it is unlikely the breast-fed neonate would ingest clinically relevant amounts.

- ■ **References** ⋯⋯⋯ Goldstein PJ, Lipman M, Luebehusen J. South Med J 1977; 70:806-8.

- ■ **Summary** ⋯⋯⋯
  - **Pregnancy Category C**
  - **Lactation Category U**
  - Postepisiotomy pain can be an annoying complication relieved by local anesthetic.
  - Although frequently used to relieve the pain secondary to genital herpetic lesion, there are no well-controlled trials in this clinical context.

Benzoyl peroxide (Benzac; Brevoxyl; Desquam-E; Desquam-X10; Desquam-X 5)

- ■ **Class** ⋯⋯⋯ Dermatologic

- ■ **Indications** ⋯⋯⋯ Acne vulgaris

- ■ **Mechanism** ⋯⋯⋯ Drying agent

- ■ **Dosage with Qualifiers** ⋯⋯⋯ Acne vulgaris—apply to affected areas qd or bid
  NOTE—also packaged with **clindamycin** or **erythromycin**.
  - **Contraindications**—hypersensitivity to drug or class
  - **Caution**—not known

- ■ **Maternal Considerations** ⋯⋯⋯ **Benzoyl peroxide** is for external use only. There are no well-controlled studies in pregnant women.
  Side effects include dryness, irritation, and pruritus.

- ■ **Fetal Considerations** ············ There are no adequate and well-controlled studies in human fetuses. It is unknown whether **benzoyl peroxide** crosses the human placenta. Rodent teratogen studies have apparently not been conducted. Considering the dose and route, it is unlikely the maternal systemic concentration will reach clinically relevant level.

- ■ **Breastfeeding Safety** ············ There is no published experience in nursing women. It is unknown whether **benzoyl peroxide** enters human breast milk.

- ■ **References** ············ Auffret N. Presse Med 2000; 29:1091-7.
Ives TJ. Am Pharm 1992; NS32:33-8.
Reeves JR. Med Times 1980; 108:82-6.

- ■ **Summary** ············ • **Pregnancy Category C**
  • **Lactation Category U**
  • It is unlikely this drying agent poses a significant risk to the perinate.

Benztropine (Bensylate; Cogentin; Glycopyrrolate)

- ■ **Class** ············ *Antihistamine, parasympatholytic (anticholinergic), antiparkinsonian*

- ■ **Indications** ············ Adjunct therapy for parkinsonism or for the treatment of extrapyramidal reactions

- ■ **Mechanism** ············ Antagonize acetylcholine and histamine receptors

- ■ **Dosage with Qualifiers** ············ Parkinsonism—begin 0.5-1mg qd, increase by 0.5 q5d; max 6mg PO qd
  Extrapyramidal reactions—1-4mg PO qd or bid
  • **Contraindications**—hypersensitivity to drug or class, narrow-angle glaucoma, tardive dyskinesia, ileus
  • **Caution**—CV disease

- ■ **Maternal Considerations** ············ There are no adequate and well-controlled studies of **benztropine** in pregnant women. The published experience is limited to isolated case reports.
  Side effects include tachycardia, anticholinergic psychosis, dry mouth, constipation, tachycardia, sedation, nausea, vomiting, flatulence, anorexia, rash, dizziness, headache, nervousness, tinnitus, edema, and blurred vision.

- ■ **Fetal Considerations** ············ There are no adequate and well-controlled studies in human fetuses. It is unknown whether **benztropine** crosses the human placenta. Exposure to **benztropine** during 1st trimester might be associated with cardiovascular defects. Neonatal paralytic ileus has been reported after **benztropine** use.

- **Breastfeeding Safety** — There is no published experience in nursing women. It is unknown whether **benztropine** enters human breast milk. No adverse neonatal effects are reported with other parasympatholytics such as **atropine**.

- **References** —
Thornburg JE, Moore KE. Res Commun Chem Pathol Pharmacol 1973; 6:313-20.
Falterman CG, Richardson CJ. J Pediatr 1980; 97:308-10.
Committee on Drugs, American Academy of Pediatrics. Pediatrics 1994; 93:137-50.

- **Summary** —
  - **Pregnancy Category C**
  - **Lactation Category U**
  - **Benztropine** should be used during pregnancy and lactation only if the benefit justifies the potential perinatal risk.

Bepridil (Vascor)

- **Class** — *Calcium-channel blocker*

- **Indications** — Chronic stable angina

- **Mechanism** — Inhibits calcium influx into myocardial and vascular smooth muscle

- **Dosage with Qualifiers** — <u>Chronic stable angina</u>—begin 200mg PO qd; max 400mg qd
  - **Contraindications**—hypersensitivity to drug or class, cardiac insufficiency, sick sinus syndrome, 2nd or 3rd degree heart block, hypotension, arrhythmia, prolonged QT interval
  - **Caution**—electrolyte abnormalities, bradycardia, recent MI, hepatic or renal dysfunction

- **Maternal Considerations** — There is no published experience with **bepridil** during human pregnancy.
  Side effects include ventricular arrhythmia, prolonged QT interval, CHF, agranulocytosis, interstitial pulmonary disease, weakness, dizziness, headache, dyspepsia, nausea, tremor, anxiety, drowsiness, dyspnea, dry mouth, paresthesias, insomnia, syncope, flu-like syndrome.

- **Fetal Considerations** — There are no well-controlled studies during pregnancy. Decreased fetal weight and survival were reported in animals exposed to doses more than 30 times the maximal recommended human dose. No teratogenic effects noted in laboratory animals at the same dosages.

■ **Breastfeeding Safety** ⋯⋯⋯ There is no published experience in nursing women. **Bepridil** is excreted into human breast milk, but the kinetics remain to be clarified.

■ **References** ⋯⋯⋯ No publications of use in human pregnancy.

■ **Summary** ⋯⋯⋯
- **Pregnancy Category C**
- **Lactation Category U**
- **Bepridil** should be used during pregnancy and lactation only if the benefit justifies the potential perinatal risk.
- There are alternative agents for which there is more experience during pregnancy and lactation.

Betamethasone (Benoson; Betaderm; Betason; Celestone; Rinderon; Unicort)

■ **Class** ⋯⋯⋯ Corticosteroid

■ **Indications** ⋯⋯⋯ Prevention of RDS in preterm neonates, joint inflammation, arthritis

■ **Mechanism** ⋯⋯⋯ Maturation of type II pneumocytes, enhanced pulmonary compliance, anti-inflammatory

■ **Dosage with Qualifiers** ⋯⋯⋯
Prevention of RDS in preterm neonates in women with preterm labor <34w—12.5mg IM ×2 doses 24h apart
Bursitis/tendonitis—1ml into the tendon sheath or joint combined with a local anesthetic agent
Rheumatoid arthritis or osteoarthritis—0.5-2ml into the joint
- **Contraindications**—hypersensitivity to drug or class, sepsis, uncontrolled diabetes mellitus
- **Caution**—diabetes mellitus, concomitant tocolysis

■ **Maternal Considerations** ⋯⋯⋯ **Betamethasone** may increase the risk of maternal infection in women with PPROM, though most large studies reveal no increase. It can transiently cause an abnormal glucose tolerance test, will worsen existing diabetes mellitus, and is associated with pulmonary edema especially when given with a tocolytic agent in the setting of an underlying infection.
Side effects include adrenal insufficiency and pulmonary edema.

■ **Fetal Considerations** ⋯⋯⋯ **Betamethasone** crosses the human placenta and is one of the few drugs proven to improve perinatal outcome. About half is metabolized to inactive 11-ketosteroid derivatives. An increased risk of neonatal sepsis was suggested but not confirmed. Multiple courses of **betamethasone** are not recommended. Adverse effects noted in animal and human studies are magnified by repeated courses of steroids. They include a profound suppression of fetal breathing, movement, impaired myelination, IUGR, and microcephaly. The fetal heart rate pattern may become transiently nonreactive. Intellectual and motor development, and school achievement are not adversely influenced by steroid treatment. Some suggest emotional stress during organogenesis might cause congenital defects by increasing the level of endogenous **cortisone**. Epidemiologic studies report an association between oral clefting and exposure to corticosteroids during organogenesis. After controlling for 4 confounding factors, it was concluded prenatal exposure increased the risk for cleft lip with or without cleft palate 6-fold. IUGR, shortening of the head and mandible are also suggested as sequelae of chronic steroid use during pregnancy, though it is difficult to separate drug from disease impact. The Collaborative Perinatal Project followed women treated during the 1st trimester. While the number of exposures was limited, no increase in congenital malformations was detected. There was no increase in risk of anomalies when steroids were initiated after organogenesis. Women exposed to topical **cortisone** during pregnancy have no significant increase in birth defects. Female rats exposed to **cortisone** *in utero* exhibit premature vaginal opening. **Cortisone** accelerates fetal rat intestinal maturation, perhaps explaining why corticosteroids decrease the incidence of NEC. In sum, the evidence that **cortisone** is a human teratogen is weak.

■ **Breastfeeding Safety** — There are no adequate reports or well-controlled studies in breast-feeding women. **Cortisone** is present in human milk, but it is unclear whether maternal treatment with **betamethasone** increases the concentration.

■ **References** — Johnson JW, Mitzner W, London WT, et al. Am J Obstet Gynecol 1979; 133:677-84.
Huang WL, Harper CG, Evans SF, et al. Int J Dev Neurosci 2001; 19:415-25.
Sloboda DM, Newnham JP, Challis JR. J Endocrinol 2000; 165:79-91.
Rotmensch S, Liberati M, Celentano C, et al. Acta Obstet Gynecol Scand 1999; 78:768-73.
Rotmensch S, Liberati M, Vishne TH, et al. Acta Obstet Gynecol Scand 1999; 78:493-500.
NIH Consensus Statement 1994; 12:1-24.

■ **Summary** —
- **Pregnancy Category C**
- **Lactation Category U**
- **Betamethasone** reduces the incidence of RDS, intraventricular hemorrhage, and neonatal death.
- There is no convincing scientific evidence that **betamethasone** increases the incidence of maternal or neonatal infection.
- Multiple, repeat courses may incur adverse neonatal effects without additional benefit and should be avoided.

Betamethasone topical (Valisone; Diprolene AF; Diprosone)

■ **Class**	Corticosteroid
■ **Indications**	Steroid responsive dermatitis
■ **Mechanism**	Anti-inflammatory through an unknown mechanism
■ **Dosage with Qualifiers**	Dermatitis—apply to affected area qd or bid (0.05 to 0.01% cream or ointment) NOTE—may be combined with **clotrimazole** • **Contraindications**—hypersensitivity to drug or class
■ **Maternal Considerations**	The absorption level is unlikely to have significant systemic effect when applied topically in small amounts. *Side effects* include adrenal insufficiency, burning, itching, dryness, folliculitis, hypertrichosis, acne, dermatitis, skin atrophy, telangiectasia and hypopigmentation.
■ **Fetal Considerations**	There are no adequate and well-controlled studies in human fetuses. Considering the dose and route, it is unlikely the maternal systemic concentration will reach clinically relevant level.
■ **Breastfeeding Safety**	There is no published experience in pregnancy. However, considering the dose and route, it is unlikely the breast-fed neonate would ingest clinically relevant amounts.
■ **References**	Perucca E, Franchi P, Dezerega V, et al. Rev Chil Obstet Ginecol 1995; 60:125-7.
■ **Summary**	• **Pregnancy Category C** • **Lactation Category U** • Administration of topical **betamethasone** likely poses little additional risk to mother or fetus.

Betaxolol (Betoptic; Kerlone)

■ **Class**	Antihypertensive
■ **Indications**	Hypertension, glaucoma
■ **Mechanism**	β-1 adrenergic receptor antagonist
■ **Dosage with Qualifiers**	Hypertension—10-20mg PO qd; renal disease, begin 5mg PO qd

—1 drop in the affected eye bid; therapy is individualized
- **Contraindications**—hypersensitivity to drug or class, sinus bradycardia, 2nd or 3rd degree AV block, CHF

■ **Maternal Considerations** ...... **Betaxolol** is a cardioselective β-1 adrenergic blocker. There are no adequate reports or well-controlled studies in pregnant women. Clearance is not affected by pregnancy.
Side effects include CHF, bronchospasm, bradycardia, headache, arthralgia, dyspepsia, fatigue, chest pain, edema, pharyngitis, rhinitis, and insomnia.

■ **Fetal Considerations** ...... There are no adequate and well-controlled studies in human fetuses. **Betaxolol** crosses the human placenta rapidly achieving an F:M approaching unity. A similar concentration is found in the amniotic fluid. There is a negative correlation between gestational age and **betaxolol** clearance. In rats, **betaxolol** is associated with miscarriage, IUGR, skeletal and visceral abnormalities, and incomplete descent of the testes.

■ **Breastfeeding Safety** ...... **Betaxolol** is excreted in the breast milk, though the kinetics remain to be elucidated. Caution should be exercised when is administered in nursing mothers.

■ **References** ...... Morselli PL, Boutroy MJ, Bianchetti G, et al. Eur J Clin Pharmacol 1990; 38:477-83.
Boutroy MJ, Morselli PL, Bianchetti G, et al. Eur J Clin Pharmacol 1990; 38:535-9.
Morselli PL, Boutroy MJ, Bianchetti G, Thenot JP. Dev Pharmacol Ther 1989; 13:190-8.

■ **Summary** ......
- **Pregnancy Category C**
- **Lactation Category U**
- **Betaxolol** should be used during pregnancy and lactation only if the benefit justifies the potential perinatal risk.
- There are alternative agents for which there is more experience during pregnancy and lactation.

Bethanechol (Duvoid; Myocholine; Myotonachol; Myotonine; Urecholine)

■ **Class** ...... *Genitourinary*

■ **Indications** ...... Acute, nonobstructive, postoperative or postpartum urinary retention; neurogenic atony of the bladder

■ **Mechanism** ...... Stimulates cholinergic receptors

- **Dosage with Qualifiers** ···· Urinary retention—10-50mg PO tid or qid
  - **Contraindications**—hypersensitivity to drug or class, cystitis, mechanical obstruction, hyperthyroidism, peptic ulcer disease, asthma, parkinsonism, seizures

- **Maternal Considerations** ···· There are no adequate reports or well-controlled studies in pregnant women. It has been used for decades for the treatment of postpartum urinary retention.
  Side effects include bronchospasm, chest pain, diarrhea, headache, flushing, nausea, vomiting, hypotension, urgency, tachycardia, sweating, and miosis.

- **Fetal Considerations** ···· There are no adequate and well-controlled studies in human fetuses. It is unknown whether **bethanechol** crosses the human placenta.

- **Breastfeeding Safety** ···· There is no published experience in nursing women. It is unknown whether **bethanechol** enters human breast milk.

- **References** ···· Gentili A, Migliorini P. Minerva Ginecol 1979; 31:689-92.

- **Summary** ····
  - **Pregnancy Category C**
  - **Lactation Category U**
  - **Bethanechol** should be used during pregnancy and lactation only if the benefit justifies the potential perinatal risk.

Biperiden (Akineton; Bicamol; Tasmolin)

- **Class** ···· Antiparkinsonian, anticholinergic

- **Indications** ···· Adjunct therapy for parkinsonism; control of extrapyramidal disorders secondary to neuroleptic drugs

- **Mechanism** ···· Antagonizes acetylcholine receptors

- **Dosage with Qualifiers** ···· Parkinsonism—2mg PO tid/qid; max 16mg qd
  Extrapyramidal disorder—2mg IM/IV q30min; max 4 doses/d
  - **Contraindications**—hypersensitivity to drug or class, narrow-angle glaucoma, bowel obstruction
  - **Caution**—epilepsy, arrhythmia

- **Maternal Considerations** ···· There are no adequate reports or well-controlled studies in pregnant women.
  Side effects include dry mouth, blurred vision, dizziness, urinary retention, constipation, hematuria, drowsiness, dyspepsia, agitation, and orthostatic hypotension.

- **Fetal Considerations** — There are no adequate reports or well-controlled studies in animal or human fetuses. **Biperiden** apparently crosses the human placenta, though the kinetics remain to be elucidated.

- **Breastfeeding Safety** — There is no published experience in nursing women. It is unknown whether **biperiden** enters human breast milk.

- **References** — Kuniyoshi M, Inanaga K. Kurume Med J 1985; 32:199-202.

- **Summary** —
  - **Pregnancy Category C**
  - **Lactation Category U**
  - **Biperiden** should be used during pregnancy and lactation only if the benefit justifies the potential perinatal risk.

Bismuth subsalicylate (Pepto-Bismol)

- **Class** — *Antidiarrheal*

- **Indications** — Diarrhea, heartburn, nausea

- **Mechanism** — Works topically on the gastric mucosa to inhibit secretion, bind bacterial toxins, and direct antimicrobial activity

- **Dosage with Qualifiers** — Diarrhea—30ml or 2 tab q30min to 1h; max 8 doses in 24h
  - **Contraindications**—hypersensitivity to drug or class
  - **Caution**—hepatic or renal dysfunction, oral anticoagulant or hypoglycemic agents

- **Maternal Considerations** — There are no adequate reports or well-controlled studies in pregnant women. Stool darkening should not be confused with melena. The long clinical experience with this over-the-counter agent is reassuring.
  Side effects include anxiety, loss of hearing, confusion, severe constipation, diarrhea (severe or continuing), difficulty in speaking or slurred speech, dizziness or lightheadedness, drowsiness, and fast or deep breathing.

- **Fetal Considerations** — **Bismuth subsalicylate** is minimally absorbed across the gastric mucosa. Bismuth ion is not transported across the placenta. No reports of adverse fetal outcome have been reported.

- **Breastfeeding Safety** — Bismuth ion is not excreted into milk to any significant degree. Excretion of large amounts of **bismuth subsalicylate** is unlikely considering the lack of systemic absorption.

■ **References** ⸻ Travelers' diarrhea. NIH Consensus Development
Conference. JAMA 1985; 253:2700-4.
Krachler M, Rossipal E, Micetic-Turk D. Eur J Clin Nutr
1999; 53:486-94.

■ **Summary** ⸻
- **Pregnancy Category C**
- **Lactation Category S?**
- The long clinical experience with this over-the-counter agent is reassuring.

Bisoprolol fumarate (Biconor; Concor Plus; Lodoz; Ziak)

■ **Class** ⸻ Antihypertensive, β-blocker

■ **Indications** ⸻ Hypertension

■ **Mechanism** ⸻ β-1 selective adrenoceptor antagonist

■ **Dosage with Qualifiers** ⸻ Hypertension—2.5-40mg PO qd
NOTE—additive effect with thiazide diuretics
- **Contraindications**—hypersensitivity to drug or class, cardiogenic shock, AV block, sinus bradycardia, anuria
- **Caution**—cardiac failure, arterial insufficiency, asthma, thyrotoxicosis, hepatic or renal dysfunction

■ **Maternal Considerations** ⸻ There is no published experience with **bisoprolol** during pregnancy.
Side effects include bradycardia, diarrhea, asthenia, and fatigue.

■ **Fetal Considerations** ⸻ There are no adequate and well-controlled studies in human fetuses. It is unknown whether **bisoprolol** crosses the human placenta. Rodent studies are reassuring, revealing no evidence of teratogenicity or IUGR despite the use of doses higher than those used clinically.

■ **Breastfeeding Safety** ⸻ There is no published experience in nursing women. It is unknown whether **bisoprolol** enters human breast milk.

■ **References** ⸻ Soucek M, Prasek J, Spinarova L. Vnitr Lek 1993; 39:541-8.

■ **Summary** ⸻
- **Pregnancy Category C**
- **Lactation Category U**
- **Bisoprolol** should be used during pregnancy and lactation only if the benefit justifies the potential perinatal risk.
- There are alternative agents for which there is more experience during pregnancy and lactation.

Bleomycin (Blenoxane)

- **Class** — Antineoplastic

- **Indications** — Palliative treatment of squamous cell carcinoma (neck, tongue, cervix, vulva), lymphoma, and associated pleural effusion

- **Mechanism** — Inhibition of DNA, RNA, and protein synthesis

- **Dosage with Qualifiers** — Cancer—varies based on type of neoplasm; most regimens recommend 0.25-0.50U/kg (10-20U/m^2)
  - **Contraindications**—hypersensitivity to drug or class
  - **Caution**—hepatic or renal dysfunction

- **Maternal Considerations** — There are no adequate reports or well-controlled studies in pregnant women. Neutropenia is an important risk. Long-term effects of **bleomycin** on reproductive function are insufficiently studied.
  Side effects include impairment of the pulmonary function (pulmonary fibrosis), rash, urticaria, alopecia, and stomatitis.

- **Fetal Considerations** — There are no adequate reports or well-controlled studies in the human fetus. It is unknown whether **bleomycin** crosses the human placenta. Neonatal leukopenia has been reported shortly after delivery. Long-term follow-up of children exposed *in utero* have not revealed abnormalities. **Bleomycin** is teratogenic in rodents (skeletal malformations, hydroureter, vascular disruptions).

- **Breastfeeding Safety** — There is no published experience in nursing women. It is unknown whether **bleomycin** enters human breast milk. For that reason, it is usually recommended the drug be discontinued in nursing women.

- **References** — Yoshinaka A, Fukasawa I, Sakamoto T, et al. Arch Gynecol Obstet 2000; 264:124-7.
  Rajendran S, Hollingworth J, Scudamore I. Eur J Gynaecol Oncol 1999; 20:272-4.
  Horbelt D, Delmore J, Meisel R, et al. Obstet Gynecol 1994; 84:662-4.
  Aviles A, Neri N. Clin Lymphoma 2001; 2:173-7.

- **Summary** —
  - **Pregnancy Category D**
  - **Lactation Category U**
  - **Bleomycin** should be used during pregnancy and lactation only if the benefit justifies the potential perinatal risk.
  - No teratogenic human fetal effects are reported.

Bretylium (Bretylol)

- **Class** — Antiarrhythmic class III

- **Indications** — Ventricular arrhythmia

- **Mechanism** — Prolongs action potential

- **Dosage with Qualifiers** — Ventricular arrhythmia—5-10mg/kg IM/IV ×1; repeat 1-2h prn until control, then q6h or infusion of 1-2mg/min
  Malignant ventricular arrhythmia—5mg/kg IV ×3; may increase to 10mg/kg and repeat prn, or infusion 1-2/mg/min
  - **Contraindications**—hypersensitivity to drug or class
  - **Caution**—rapid infusion, hepatic, or renal dysfunction

- **Maternal Considerations** — There are no adequate reports or well-controlled studies in pregnant women. The one case report chronicled an uncomplicated course after chronic treatment of prolonged QT syndrome.
  Side effects include hypotension, nausea, vomiting, diarrhea, hiccups, anxiety, and shortness of breath.

- **Fetal Considerations** — There are no adequate and well-controlled studies in human fetuses. It is unknown whether **bretylium** crosses the human placenta.

- **Breastfeeding Safety** — There are no adequate reports or well-controlled studies in nursing women. It is unknown whether **bretylium** enters human breast milk. The one case report noted no neonatal difficulties.

- **References** — Gutgesell M, Overholt E, Boyle R. Am J Perinatol 1990; 7:144-5.

- **Summary**
  - **Pregnancy Category C**
  - **Lactation Category U**
  - **Bretylium** should be used during pregnancy and lactation only if the benefit justifies the potential perinatal risk.
  - There are alternative agents for which there is more experience during pregnancy and lactation.

Bromides—sodium, potassium salts

■ **Class** — Anticonvulsants

■ **Indications** — Epilepsy, seborrheic dermatitis

■ **Mechanism** — Unknown

■ **Dosage with Qualifiers** — Epilepsy—loading dose 450mg/kg; maintenance dose 20-40mg/kg
NOTE—divide the 450mg/kg dose over 5d (90mg/kg/d) and add it to a maintenance dose of 20-40mg/kg (average of 30mg/kg) qd. Thus, a new patient will receive 120mg/kg of potassium bromide each day for 5d, and then return to 30mg/kg qd.
Seborrheic dermatitis—homeopathic doses
• **Contraindications**—hypersensitivity to drug or class

■ **Maternal Considerations** — Oral or topical combinations of potassium and sodium bromide significantly improve seborrheic dermatitis and dandruff after 10 weeks. There are no adequate reports or well-controlled studies in pregnant women.
Side effects include sedation, ataxia, increased urination and rare skin disorders.

■ **Fetal Considerations** — There are no adequate reports or well-controlled studies in human fetuses. IUGR, microcephaly, neonatal bromide intoxication (poor suck, weak cry, diminished Moro reflex, lethargy, hypotonia), rash and sedation are reported after oral use. It is unlikely the maternal systemic concentration will reach clinically relevant level after topical application.

■ **Breastfeeding Safety** — **Bromides** enter human breast milk. It is unlikely the breast-fed neonate would ingest clinically relevant amounts after topical application. The Academy of Pediatrics considers bromides compatible with breastfeeding.

■ **References** — Smith SA, Baker AE, Williams JH Jr. Altern Med Rev 2002; 7:59-67.
Ryan M, Baumann RJ. Pediatr Neurol 1999; 21:523-8.
Miller ME, Cosgriff JM, Roghmann KJ. Am J Obstet Gynecol 1987; 157:826-30.

■ **Summary** — • **Pregnancy Category D**
• **Lactation Category S**
• It is unlikely topically applied **bromides** pose a significant clinical risk to the perinate.

Bromocriptine (Parlodel; Volbro)

■ **Class**	Antiparkinsonian
■ **Indications**	Parkinson's disease, amenorrhea, acromegaly
■ **Mechanism**	Dopamine agonist; stimulator of the dopaminergic receptors

■ **Dosage with Qualifiers**
Parkinson's disease—10-40mg PO qd
Amenorrhea—5-7.5mg PO qhs
Acromegaly—20-30mg PO qd
- **Contraindications**—hypersensitivity to drug or class, uncontrolled hypertension, coronary artery disease
- **Caution**—hypertension, hepatic or renal dysfunction

■ **Maternal Considerations**
Most information regarding **bromocriptine** during pregnancy comes from women treated for infertility with an average duration of exposure of 28d. No special maternal considerations are reported. **Bromocriptine** is used in many countries for the suppression of breast engorgement after delivery. However, rebound engorgement is common after cessation. In 1994, the FDA withdrew approval for that indication after a series of reports describing severe vasospastic events including stroke, MI, cerebral edema, convulsions, and puerperal psychosis.
Side effects include seizures, stroke, MI, headache, dizziness, nausea, hypotension, cramps, fatigue, and constipation.

■ **Fetal Considerations**
There are no adequate reports or well-controlled studies in human fetuses. It is unknown whether **bromocriptine** crosses the human placenta. There are no reports of associated malformations after 1st trimester exposure. Rodent studies are reassuring, revealing no evidence of teratogenicity or IUGR despite the use of doses higher than those used clinically.

■ **Breastfeeding Safety**
Bromocriptine reduces lactation, and its use is generally considered contraindicated during breastfeeding.

■ **References**
Russell CS, Lang C, McCambridge M, Calhoun B. Obstet Gynecol 2001; 98:906-8.
Ionescu O, Vulpoi C, Ungureanu MC, et al. Rev Med Chir Soc Med Nat Iasi 2001; 105:806-9.
Ricci G, Giolo E, Nucera G, et al. Gynecol Obstet Invest 2001; 51:266-70.
Stefos T, Sotiriadis A, Tsirkas P, et al. Acta Obstet Gynecol Scand 2001; 80:34-8.
Turkalj I, Braun P, Krupp P. JAMA 1982; 247:1589-91.
Randall S, Laing J, Chapman AJ, et al. Br J Obstet Gynaecol 1982; 89:20-33.

■ **Summary**
- **Pregnancy Category B**
- **Lactation Category NS**
- **Bromocriptine** is contraindicated during breastfeeding and is not approved in the U.S. for the suppression of breast engorgement postpartum.

Bromodiphenhydramine (Ambenyl; Ambophen; Bromanyl; Bromotuss w/Codeine; Mybanil; Myphetane DC)

■ **Class**

Antihistamine, nonselective

■ **Indications**

Antiallergic, anaphylaxis, dystonic reactions, antitussive, sedation, insomnia

■ **Mechanism**

Central and peripheral H_1 receptor antagonist

■ **Dosage with Qualifiers**

Antiallergic—1-2tsp PO q4-6h
Antitussive, sedation—1-2tsp PO q4-6h
NOTE—combined with **codeine**
- **Contraindications**—hypersensitivity to drug or class, newborns, lactation
- **Caution**—asthma, hyperthyroidism, cardiovascular disease

■ **Maternal Considerations**

Bromodiphenhydramine is a diphenhydramine derivative. There are no adequate reports or well-controlled studies in pregnant women. When combined with **droperidol**, **bromodiphenhydramine** has been advocated as effective in hospital treatment of severe hyperemesis. Overdose is associated with uterine contractions. It is inferior to **nalbuphine** for the relief of pruritus associated with intrathecal **morphine**.
Side effects include somnolence, dry mouth, headache, dizziness, nausea, and vomiting.

■ **Fetal Considerations**

There are no adequate and well-controlled studies in human fetuses. **Bromodiphenhydramine** crosses the human placenta, but the kinetics remain to be detailed. In sheep, transfer is rapid and directly dependent on gestational age. Maternal drug ingestion during rodent pregnancy may alter physical and reflex development. Rodent teratogenicity studies are reassuring, revealing no evidence of teratogenicity or IUGR despite the use of doses higher than those used clinically.

■ **Breastfeeding Safety**

There are no adequate reports or well-controlled studies in nursing women. **Bromodiphenhydramine** is probably excreted into human breast milk.

■ **References** ──────────── Brost BC, Scardo JA, Newman RB. Am J Obstet Gynecol 1996; 175:1376-7.
Nageotte MP, Briggs GG, Towers CV, Asrat T. Am J Obstet Gynecol 174:1801-5.
Yoo GD, Axelson JE, Taylor SM, Rurak DW. J Pharm Sci 1986; 75:685-7.
Kumar S, Tonn GR, Riggs KW, Rurak DW. Drug Metab Dispos 2000; 28:279-85.

■ **Summary** ────────────
- **Pregnancy Category B**
- **Lactation Category U**
- **Bromodiphenhydramine** should be used during pregnancy and lactation only if the benefit justifies the potential perinatal risk.

Budesonide (Budecort; Budeflam; Pulmicort; Rhinocort; Rhinocort Aqua)

■ **Class** ──────────── *Corticosteroid*

■ **Indications** ──────────── Asthma, rhinitis

■ **Mechanism** ──────────── Anti-inflammatory by an unknown mechanism; potent glucocorticoid, weak mineralocorticoid

■ **Dosage with Qualifiers** ──────────
Asthma—0.5-1mg/d inhalation
Rhinitis—metered dose 50mcg/puff inhalation
- **Contraindications**—hypersensitivity to drug or class, primary treatment of status asthmaticus
- **Caution**—infection, systemic steroids

■ **Maternal Considerations** ──────── Asthma can be a serious problem during pregnancy. There are no adequate reports or well-controlled studies of **budesonide** during pregnancy.
Side effects include allergic reaction, stridor, eczema, purpura, back pain, fracture, and myalgia.

■ **Fetal Considerations** ──────────── There are no adequate and well-controlled studies in human fetuses. It is unknown whether **budesonide** crosses the human placenta. Epidemiological study suggests **budesonide** is not a clinically significant teratogen. It appears though to cross the mouse placenta, where **budesonide** increases fetal loss, IUGR, and malformations. Rodents as a group are more susceptible to steroids than humans.

■ **Breastfeeding Safety** ──────────── There is no published experience in nursing women. It is unknown whether **budesonide** enters human breast milk.

■ References — The American College of Obstetricians and Gynecologists (ACOG) and The American College of Allergy, Asthma and Immunology (ACAAI). Ann Allergy Asthma Immunol 2000; 84:475-80.
Mazzotta P, Loebstein R, Koren G. Drug Saf 1999; 20:361-75.
Kallen B, Rydhstroem H, Aberg A. Obstet Gynecol 1999; 93:392-5.
Andersson P, Appelgren LE, Ryrfeldt A. Acta Pharmacol Toxicol 1986; 59:392-402.
Kihlstrom I, Lundberg C. Arzneimittelforschung 1987; 37:43-6.

■ **Summary**
- **Pregnancy Category C**
- **Lactation Category U**
- **Budesonide** should be used during pregnancy and lactation only if the benefit justifies the potential perinatal risk.

Bumetanide (Bumex; Pendock; Segurex)

■ **Class** — Diuretic

■ **Indications** — Heart failure

■ **Mechanism** — Inhibits chloride resorption in the loop of Henle, and in the distal and proximal convoluted tubule

■ **Dosage with Qualifiers** — Heart failure—0.5-2mg/d PO; alternatively, 0.5-1mg IM/IV ×1
- **Contraindications**—hypersensitivity to drug or class, volume and electrolyte depletion, hypokalemia, ototoxicity
- **Caution**—electrolyte abnormalities, hepatic coma, hyperuricemia, anuria

■ **Maternal Considerations** — There is no published experience with **bumetanide** during pregnancy.
Side effects include renal failure, muscle cramps, impaired hearing, ECG changes, dry mouth, upset stomach, thrombocytopenia, vertigo, chest pain, ototoxicity.

■ **Fetal Considerations** — There are no adequate reports or well-controlled studies in human fetuses. It is unknown whether **bumetanide** crosses the human placenta. No teratogenic effects were noted in rodent studies. **Bumetanide** alters *in vitro* Na^{2+} and Cl^- transport across placental membranes.

■ **Breastfeeding Safety** — There is no published experience in nursing women. It is unknown whether **bumetanide** enters human breast milk.

- **References** .... Prieve BA, Yanz JL. Acta Otolaryngol 1984; 98:428-38.
  McClain RM, Dammers KD. J Clin Pharmacol 1981; 21:543-54.

- **Summary** ....
  - **Pregnancy Category D**
  - **Lactation Category U**
  - **Bumetanide** should be used during pregnancy and lactation only if the benefit justifies the potential perinatal risk.

Bupivacaine (Bupivacaine HCl; Marcaine; Sensorcaine)

- **Class** .... *Local anesthetic*

- **Indications** .... Conduction and local anesthesia

- **Mechanism** .... Inhibits nerve impulses by stabilizing neuronal membranes

- **Dosage with Qualifiers** .... Local anesthesia—varies, max 2mg/kg, 400mg/d; onset 2-10min, duration 3-6h
  Conduction anesthesia—varies, recommend consulting a specialty text
  NOTE—available with epinephrine and in a preservative-free solution
  - **Contraindications**—hypersensitivity to drug or class
  - **Caution**—acutely ill patients, hepatic or renal dysfunction, heart block, hypovolemia, hypotension

- **Maternal Considerations** .... **Bupivacaine** is a very popular agent used for neuraxial anesthesia (epidural or spinal) during labor and delivery alone or in combination with either local anesthetic or narcotic agents. Because of its long duration, it is contraindicated for paracervical block.
  Side effects include CNS toxicity, myocardial depression, heart block, bradycardia, ventricular arrhythmias, cardiac arrest, convulsions, respiratory arrest, unconsciousness, hypotension, nausea, vomiting, paresthesias, fever, chills, pruritus, dizziness, restlessness, anxiety, tremor.

- **Fetal Considerations** .... There are no adequate and well-controlled studies in human fetuses. **Bupivacaine** crosses the human placenta, with transfer ratios (agent/antipyrine) *in vitro* approximating 0.4%. Transfer rate increases as the fetal pH declines. It does cross the rodent placenta (F:M ratio approximating 0.3), and decreased pup survival was reported after treatment with high concentrations.

- **Breastfeeding Safety** .... **Bupivacaine** and its major metabolite are found at clinically irrelevant levels after epidural administration. Though it has not been studied after local infiltration, one time use is unlikely to pose a clinically significant risk to the breast-feeding neonate.

- **References** .... Ortega D, Viviand X, Lorec AM, et al. Acta Anaesthesiol Scand 1999; 43:394-7.
Morishima HO, Ishizaki A, Zhang Y, et al. Anesthesiology 2000; 93:1069-74.
Johnson RF, Cahana A, Olenick M, et al. Anesth Analg 1999; 89:703-8.

- **Summary** ....
  - **Pregnancy Category C**
  - **Lactation Category S**
  - **Bupivacaine** is a popular agent for conduction anesthesia during labor.
  - It is contraindicated for paracervical block.

Bupropion (Zyban; Wellbutrin)

- **Class** .... *Antidepressant*, SSRI

- **Indications** .... Depression, smoking cessation

- **Mechanism** .... Unknown mechanism of action; weak blocker of serotonin uptake.

- **Dosage with Qualifiers** .... Depression—100mg PO tid; max dose 150mg PO tid
  Smoking cessation—150-300mg PO bid; patient quits smoking after 5-7d of treatment; 2nd dose should not be later than 6pm and at least 8h after 1st dose
  - **Contraindications**—hypersensitivity to drug or class, seizure disorder, use of MAO inhibitors within 14d, bulimia, anorexia nervosa
  - **Caution**—agitation, insomnia, psychosis, confusion, altered appetite, weight

- **Maternal Considerations** .... There are no adequate reports or well-controlled studies in pregnant women. **Bupropion** is an effective adjunct for smoking cessation therapy. Glaxo-Wellcome maintains an international registry to follow women treated during pregnancy and caregivers are encouraged to register treated patients.
  Side effects include arrhythmias, 3rd degree heart block, Stevens-Johnson syndrome, depression, rash, rhabdomyolysis, dysphagia, vaginal irritation, mania/hypomania, nausea, vomiting, anorexia, sedation, weight loss, weight gain, bronchitis, stomatitis, ataxia, seizure, constipation, and confusion.

- **Fetal Considerations** .... There are no adequate reports or well-controlled studies in human fetuses. It is unknown whether **bupropion** crosses the human placenta. Rodent studies are reassuring, revealing no evidence of teratogenicity or IUGR despite the use of doses higher than those used clinically.

- **Breastfeeding Safety** .... **Bupropion** is excreted into human breast milk achieving M:P ratios of 2.5-8.6. However, the neonatal concentration was below the level of detection in the 3 newborns studied. Confirmatory studies are needed.

- **References** .... Kotlyar M, Hatsukami DK. J Dent Educ 2002; 66:1061-73.
West R, McNeill A, Raw M. Thorax 2000; 55:987-99.
Briggs GG, Samson JH, Ambrose PJ, Shroder DH. Ann Pharmacother 1993; 27:431-3.
Weintraub M, Evan P. Hosp Form 1989; 24:254-9.
Baab SW, Peindl KS, Piontek CM, Wisner KL. J Clin Psychiatry 2002; 63:910-1.

- **Summary** ....
  - **Pregnancy Category B**
  - **Lactation Category S?**
  - **Bupropion** is an adjuvant agent for smoking cessation.
  - Caregivers are encouraged to register treated women with the Glaxo-Wellcome Bupropion International Registry.
  - **Bupropion** should be used during pregnancy and lactation only when the potential benefit justifies the potential perinatal risks.

Buspirone (Ansiced; BuSpar)

- **Class** .... *Sedative*

- **Indications** .... Anxiety

- **Mechanism** .... Mechanism of action is currently unknown

- **Dosage with Qualifiers** .... Anxiety—begin 7.5mg PO bid; increase by 5mg/d q3d until max 60mg/d
  - **Contraindications**—hypersensitivity to drug or class
  - **Caution**—use of MAO inhibitors, hepatic or renal dysfunction

- **Maternal Considerations** .... There is no published experience with **buspirone** during pregnancy.
  Side effects include dizziness, nausea, vomiting, insomnia, rash, headache, fatigue, dry mouth, diarrhea, decreased concentration, hostility, depression, blurred vision, diarrhea, abdominal pain, numbness, and weakness.

- **Fetal Considerations** .... There are no adequate and well-controlled studies in human fetuses. It is unknown whether **buspirone** crosses the human placenta. Rodent studies are reassuring, revealing no evidence of teratogenicity or IUGR despite the use of doses higher than those used clinically.

- **Breastfeeding Safety** .... There is no published experience in nursing women. It is unknown whether **buspirone** enters human breast milk. **Buspirone** is excreted into rodent breast milk.

- **References** .... Kim JA, Druse MJ. Brain Res Dev Brain Res 1996; 92:190-8.

- **Summary** ....
  - **Pregnancy Category B**
  - **Lactation Category U**
  - **Buspirone** should be used during pregnancy and lactation only if the benefit justifies the potential perinatal risk.

Busulfan (Citosulfan; Leukosulfan; Misulban; Myleran)

- **Class** .... *Antineoplastic*

- **Indications** .... Leukemia, myelofibrosis

- **Mechanism** .... Alkylates and cross links DNA

- **Dosage with Qualifiers** .... Leukemia—varies based on the type of neoplasm
  Myelofibrosis—2-4mg PO 2-3×/w
  - **Contraindications**—hypersensitivity to drug or class, resistance to prior treatment, blast crisis, acute lymphocytic leukemia
  - **Caution**—bone marrow depression, seizures

- **Maternal Considerations** .... There are no adequate reports or well-controlled studies in pregnant women. **Busulfan** has been used successfully to treat leukemia and essential polycythemia during pregnancy.
  Side effects include myelosuppression, pulmonary fibrosis, pericardial fibrosis, seizures, and hyperpigmentation.

- **Fetal Considerations** .... There are no adequate and well-controlled studies in human fetuses. It is unknown whether **busulfan** crosses the human placenta. No pattern of anomalies can be discerned. There are reports of IUGR fetuses born to women who were treated with **busulfan** during pregnancy. In rodents, there is a high incidence of carpal and tarsal bone anomalies after small doses of antiproliferatives such as **cytosine arabinoside**, **mitomycin C**, or **busulfan.** Further, infertility may be increased in the offspring of treated rats.

··········· There is no published experience in nursing women. It is unknown whether **busulfan** enters human breast milk.

■ **References** ··········· Ozumba BC, Obi GO. Int J Gynaecol Obstet 1992; 38:49-50.
Wright CA, Tefferi A. Eur J Haematol 2001; 66:152-9.
Diamond I, Anderson MM, McCreadie SR. Pediatrics 1960; 25:85-90.
Dobbing J. Lancet 1977; 1:1155.
Rahman ME, Ishikawa H, Watanabe Y, Endo A. Reprod Toxicol 1996; 10:485-9.

■ **Summary** ···········
- **Pregnancy Category D**
- **Lactation Category U**
- Limited reports indicate busulfan can be used during pregnancy without apparent, adverse fetal effects.
- **Busulfan** should be used during pregnancy and lactation only if the benefit justifies the potential perinatal risk.

Butalbital (Butal compound; Farbital; Fioricet; Fiorinal; Fiormor; Fiortal; Fortabs; Idenal; Isollyl; Laniroif; Lanorinal; Tecnal; Trianal)

■ **Class** ··········· *Anxiolytic, hypnotic*

■ **Indications** ··········· Sedation, insomnia, preoperative sedation, tension headache

■ **Mechanism** ··········· Alters sensory cortex, cerebellar and motor activities

■ **Dosage with Qualifiers** ··········· Sedation—15-30mg PO tid/qid
Insomnia—50-100mg PO qhs (short term)
Preoperative sedation—50-100mg PO 30-60min preoperatively
Tension headache—1-2 tabs Fioricet PO q4h
NOTE—each Fioricet tab contains **butalbital** 50mg, **acetaminophen** 325mg, **caffeine** 40mg; max 6 tabs/d
- **Contraindications**—hypersensitivity to drug or class, porphyria, bronchopneumonia, pulmonary insufficiency
- **Caution**—hepatic or renal dysfunction, history of drug abuse

■ **Maternal Considerations** ··········· There are no adequate reports or well-controlled studies in pregnant women.
Side effects include thrombocytopenia, Stevens-Johnson syndrome, drowsiness, sedation, constipation, dyspnea, nausea, vomiting, SOB, and abdominal pain.

■ **Fetal Considerations** ··········· There are no adequate reports or well-controlled studies in animal and human fetuses. It is unknown whether

butalbital crosses the human placenta. Other barbiturates do cross. Withdrawal seizures have been reported in neonates whose mothers used **butalbital** during pregnancy.

■ **Breastfeeding Safety** .... There is no published experience in nursing women. It is unknown whether **butalbital** enters human breast milk. Other barbiturates enter human breast milk but the kinetics are poorly described.

■ **References** .... Ostrea EM Jr. Am J Obstet Gynecol 1982; 143:597-8.

■ **Summary** ....
- **Pregnancy Category C**
- **Lactation Category U**
- **Butalbital** should be used during pregnancy and lactation only if the benefit justifies the potential perinatal risk.

Butorphanol (Stadol)

■ **Class** .... *Narcotic, analgesic*

■ **Indications** .... Labor pain management, anesthesia

■ **Mechanism** .... Binds to opiate receptors producing agonist antagonist effects

■ **Dosage with Qualifiers** .... Pain—0.5-2mg IV q3-4h prn pain; begin 1mg IV or 2mg IM
Preoperative sedation—2mg IV before induction
Epidural anesthesia—consult a specialty text
- **Contraindications**—hypersensitivity to drug or class, acute MI, coronary insufficiency
- **Caution**—hepatic or renal dysfunction, CNS depression, biliary surgery, substance abuse, impaired pulmonary function, head injury

■ **Maternal Considerations** .... There are no adequate reports or well-controlled studies in pregnant women prior to 37 weeks. **Butorphanol** provides better initial analgesia than **fentanyl** during labor with fewer patient requests for more medication or epidural analgesia. Acute psychosis has been reported after usage. *Side effects* include drowsiness, hypotension, respiratory depression, sedation, dizziness, nausea, vomiting, sweating, headache, euphoria, confusion, nervousness, anorexia, and constipation.

■ **Fetal Considerations** .... There are no adequate and well-controlled studies in human fetuses. **Butorphanol** crosses the human placenta achieving an F:M ratio approximating unity. Its use during labor is associated with a transient (90-120min) sinusoidal fetal heart rhythm. The addition of **butorphanol**, **fentanyl**, or **sufentanil** to epidural **bupivacaine** (0.25%) does not alter FHR short- or long-term variability. Neonatal respiratory depression may occur after parenteral maternal administration. No teratogenic effects are identified in rodents.

■ **Breastfeeding Safety** ⸱⸱⸱⸱⸱⸱⸱⸱⸱ There are no adequate reports or well-controlled studies in nursing women. **Butorphanol** is excreted into human breast milk, but it is estimated the unsupplemented neonate would ingest 4μg per day if the woman is receiving an analgesic dose (2mg IM or 8mg PO) 4 times a day.

■ **References** ⸱⸱⸱⸱⸱⸱⸱⸱⸱⸱⸱⸱⸱⸱⸱⸱⸱ Pittman KA, Smyth RD, Losada M, et al. Am J Obstet Gynecol 1980; 138:797-800.
St Amant MS, Koffel B, Malinow AM. Am J Perinatol 1998; 15:351-6.
Davis A, Yudofsky B, Quidwai S. J Neuropsychiatry Clin Neurosci 1998; 10:236-7.
Atkinson BD, Truitt LJ, Rayburn WF, et al. Am J Obstet Gynecol 1994; 171:993-8.

■ **Summary** ⸱⸱⸱⸱⸱⸱⸱⸱⸱⸱⸱⸱⸱⸱⸱⸱⸱⸱⸱⸱⸱
- **Pregnancy Category C**
- **Lactation Category S**
- **Butorphanol** is a popular agent for labor analgesia given either parenterally or as part of conduction anesthesia.
- **Butorphanol** should be used during pregnancy and lactation only if the benefit justifies the potential perinatal risk.

Cabergoline (Dostinex)

■ **Class** .... *Other, endocrine*

■ **Indications** .... Hyperprolactinemia

■ **Mechanism** .... Stimulates D_2 dopamine receptors

■ **Dosage with Qualifiers** .... Hyperprolactinemia—begin 0.25mg 2×/w then increase 0.25mg/w every month; max 1mg 2×/w; monitor prolactin level
- **Contraindications**—hypersensitivity to drug or class, uncontrolled hypertension
- **Caution**—hepatic dysfunction

■ **Maternal Considerations** .... There are no adequate and well-controlled studies in pregnant women taking **cabergoline**. **Cabergoline** is better tolerated and more effective in inducing a complete biochemical response than **bromocriptine**. Women became pregnant in 1-37mo (mean 12.4mo) with **cabergoline** therapy. It has been used successfully throughout pregnancy to treat a macroprolactinoma. Most tumors associated with macroprolactinoma disappear with therapy. **Cabergoline** is also effective in women resistant or poorly responsive to **bromocriptine**. Prolactin typically trends lower after delivery or 3mo after breastfeeding. *Side effects* include nausea, vomiting, headache, dizziness, constipation, fatigue, abdominal pain, vertigo, hot flashes, dry mouth, depression, and hypotension.

■ **Fetal Considerations** .... There are no adequate and well-controlled studies in human fetuses. It is unknown whether **cabergoline** crosses the human placenta. First trimester exposure is not associated with adverse perinatal outcome. Rodent studies are reassuring, revealing no evidence of teratogenicity or IUGR despite the use of doses higher than those used clinically.

■ **Breastfeeding Safety** .... There is no published experience in nursing women. It is unknown whether **cabergoline** enters human breast milk. **Cabergoline** effectively suppressed lactation in some studies, with less rebound than **bromocriptine**. It should be avoided if breastfeeding is desired.

■ **References** .... Colao A, Sarno AD, Pivonello R, et al. Expert Opin Investig Drugs 2002; 11:787-800.
Liu C, Tyrrell JB. Pituitary 2001; 4:179-85.
Bozhinova S, Porozhanova V, Penkov V. Akush Ginekol 2001; 40:11-4.
Ricci E, Parazzini F, Motta T, et al. Reprod Toxicol 2002; 16:791-3.
Molitch ME. J Reprod Med 1999; 44:1121-6.

Ciccarelli E, Grottoli S, Razzore P, et al. Endocrinol Invest 1997; 20:547-51.
Delgrange E, Maiter D, Donckier J. Eur J Endocrinol 1996; 134: 454-6.
Webster J. Drug Saf 1996; 14:228-38.

■ **Summary**

- **Pregnancy Category B**
- **Lactation Category U**
- Preliminary data suggests no increase in adverse fetal outcomes secondary to **cabergoline** use during pregnancy.
- **Cabergoline** should be avoided if breastfeeding is desired.

Caffeine plus ergotamine (Cafatine; Cafergot; Cafermine; Cafetrate; Ercaf; Ercatab; Ergo-Caff; Gotamine; Micomp-Pb; Migergot; Secadol; Wigraine)

■ **Class**
Combination, central stimulant, antiadrenergic, ergot alkaloid, xanthine derivative

■ **Indications**
Migraine, tension headache, cluster headache

■ **Mechanism**
Combination—see individual drugs

■ **Dosage with Qualifiers**
Headache—1-2 tabs/suppositories PO/PR q30min prn; max 6mg **ergotamine** qd
NOTE—available in tablet or rectal suppository (100mg **caffeine** + 1mg **ergotamine** per tablet, 100/2 suppository)
- **Contraindications**—hypersensitivity, pregnancy, peptic ulcer disease, porphyria
- **Caution**—elderly patients, pediatric patients, history of abuse

■ **Maternal Considerations**
There are only scattered case reports of Cafergot use during pregnancy. This combination is contraindicated in pregnancy due to the oxytocic effects of **ergotamine**. See **caffeine** and **ergotamine** individually.
Side effects include tachycardia, anxiety. In combination with other drugs, Cafergot may cause anaphylaxis, toxic epidermal necrolysis, bone marrow suppression, GI bleeding, and Stevens-Johnson syndrome.

■ **Fetal Considerations**
See **caffeine** and **ergotamine** individually. Jejunal atresia was reported in the child of a woman who ingested Cafergot in 5 consecutive pregnancies. The other 4 ended in spontaneous abortion.

- **Breastfeeding Safety** .... There is no published experience in nursing women. See **caffeine** and **ergotamine** individually.

- **References** .... Graham JM, Marin-Padilla M, Hoefnagel D. Clin Pediatr 1983; 22:226-8.

- **Summary** ....
  - **Pregnancy Category X**
  - **Lactation Category NS**
  - Contraindicated during pregnancy due to the oxytocic effects of **ergotamine**.
  - There are alternative agents with a higher safety profile for which there is more experience during pregnancy and lactation.

Caffeine

- **Class** .... CNS *stimulant, xanthine derivative*

- **Indications** .... Migraine, tension headache, cluster headache, prematurity apnea

- **Mechanism** .... Most of the effects reflect antagonism of A1 and A2 adenosine receptors.

- **Dosage with Qualifiers** .... NOTE—may be combined with **ergotamine** (Cafergot), or other analgesics such as **ASA** or **acetaminophen**
  - **Contraindications**—hypersensitivity to drug or class, peptic ulcer disease, porphyria
  - **Caution**—history of abuse

- **Maternal Considerations** .... There is no clear evidence **caffeine** at moderate levels of ingestion has an adverse effect on pregnancy. Toxicity occurs only in very high dosages (e.g., 25 tablets of Fiorinal [**ASA, butalbital, caffeine**]).
  Side effects include tachycardia, anxiety. In combination with other drugs it may cause anaphylaxis, toxic epidermal necrolysis, bone marrow suppression, GI bleeding, and Stevens-Johnson syndrome.

- **Fetal Considerations** .... There are no adequate and well-controlled studies in human fetuses. **Caffeine** crosses the placenta achieving an F:M ratio near unity. Cardiac arrhythmias are associated with maternal **caffeine** use in excess of 500mg/d. There is no substantive evidence that **caffeine** is either a teratogen or causes IUGR in humans. In rodents, high and sustained doses are associated with a small increase in the prevalence of cleft palate.

■ **Breastfeeding Safety** ⸱⸱⸱⸱⸱⸱⸱⸱⸱⸱⸱⸱⸱⸱⸱ Though it enters human breast milk in small amounts, **caffeine** is generally considered safe for breast-feeding women.

■ **References** ⸱⸱⸱⸱⸱⸱⸱⸱⸱⸱⸱⸱⸱⸱⸱⸱⸱⸱⸱⸱⸱⸱⸱⸱⸱⸱⸱⸱ Clausson B, Granath F, Ekbom A, et al. Am J Epidemiol 2002; 155:429-36.
Signorello LB, Nordmark A, Granath F, et al. Obstet Gynecol 2001; 98:1059-66.
Pollard I, Locquet O, Solvar A, Magre S. Reprod Fertil Dev 2001; 13:435-41.
Grosso LM, Rosenberg KD, Belanger K, et al. Epidemiology 2001; 12:447-55.
Cnattingius S, Signorello LB, Anneren G, et al. N Engl J Med 2000; 343:1839-45.
Koren G. Can Fam Physician. 2000; 46:801-3.

■ **Summary** ⸱⸱⸱⸱⸱⸱⸱⸱⸱⸱⸱⸱⸱⸱⸱⸱⸱⸱⸱⸱⸱⸱⸱⸱⸱⸱⸱⸱⸱
- **Pregnancy Category C**
- **Lactation Category S**
- **Caffeine** is one of the most frequently used drugs during pregnancy, often in combination with products containing **aspirin, acetominophen**, and **codeine**.
- No teratogenic, carcinogenic, or mutagenic effects are known in humans.

Calcifediol (Dical-D; Calcijex)

■ **Class** ⸱⸱⸱⸱⸱⸱⸱⸱⸱⸱⸱⸱⸱⸱⸱⸱⸱⸱⸱⸱⸱⸱⸱⸱⸱⸱⸱⸱⸱⸱⸱⸱ *Vitamin*

■ **Indications** ⸱⸱⸱⸱⸱⸱⸱⸱⸱⸱⸱⸱⸱⸱⸱⸱⸱⸱⸱⸱⸱⸱⸱⸱ Vitamin D deficiency, hypoparathyroidism, osteoporosis, hypocalcemia

■ **Mechanism** ⸱⸱⸱⸱⸱⸱⸱⸱⸱⸱⸱⸱⸱⸱⸱⸱⸱⸱⸱⸱⸱⸱⸱ This active form of vitamin D stimulates intestinal absorption of calcium and phosphorus.

■ **Dosage with Qualifiers** ⸱⸱⸱⸱⸱⸱⸱⸱ Vitamin deficiency—50-100mcg PO qd
Hypoparathyroidism—0.2-1mg PO qd
Osteoporosis—0.6mg PO qd
- **Contraindications**—hypersensitivity to drug or class, hypercalcemia, hypervitaminosis D
- **Caution**—renal failure, renal stones, hyperphosphatemia

■ **Maternal Considerations** ⸱⸱⸱⸱⸱⸱ Vitamin D supplementation is recommended during pregnancy. **Calcifediol** is converted in the kidney to an active form of vitamin D, **calcitriol**. There are no adequate and well-controlled studies in pregnant women. Veiled or dark-skinned pregnant women have an increased risk of vitamin D deficiency, which is associated with disease. *Side effects* include hypercalcemia, elevated creatinine, polydipsia, nausea, and convulsion.

- **Fetal Considerations** .... There are no adequate and well-controlled studies in human fetuses. It is unknown whether **calcifediol** crosses the human placenta, though the placenta synthesizes active vitamin D. **Calcifediol** is reportedly teratogenic in some rodents.

- **Breastfeeding Safety** .... There is no published experience in nursing women. It is unknown whether **calcifediol** enters human breast milk, but supplementation has little effect on milk vitamin D levels.

- **References** .... Grover SR, Morley R. Med J Aust 2001; 175:251-2.
  Brunvand L, Quigstad E, Urdal P, Haug E. Early Hum Dev 1996; 45:27-33.
  Mallet E, Gugi B, Brunelle P, et al. Obstet Gynecol 1986; 68:300-4.
  Cancela L, Le Boulch N, Miravet L. J Endocrinol 1986; 110:43-50.
  Kuoppala T, Tuimala R, Parviainen M, et al. Hum Nutr Clin Nutr 1986; 40:287-93.

- **Summary** ....
  - **Pregnancy Category B**
  - **Lactation Category S**
  - Vitamin D supplementation is generally recommended during pregnancy.
  - Most multivitamin supplements contain adequate quantities of vitamin D in one form or another.

Calcitonin (Calcimar; Miacalcin)

- **Class** .... *Hormone*

- **Indications** .... Osteoporosis, Paget's disease, hypercalcemia

- **Mechanism** .... Unknown

- **Dosage with Qualifiers** .... Osteoporosis—100IU SC or IM qod or 200IU NAS qd
  Paget's disease—begin 100IU SC or IM qd, then 50IU qod
  Hypercalcemia—4IU/kg SC or IM q12h
  - **Contraindications**—hypersensitivity to drug or class
  - **Caution**—renal failure or stones, hyperphosphatemia

- **Maternal Considerations** .... **Calcitonin** regulates calcium homeostatis. There are no adequate reports or well-controlled studies in pregnant women.
  Side effects include rhinitis, back pain, epistaxis, nasal irritation, and headache.

- ■ **Fetal Considerations** ⋯⋯⋯ There are no adequate and well-controlled studies in pregnant women. **Calcitonin** does not cross the placenta. The mechanism by which high doses of **calcitonin** produce IUGR in rabbits is unknown.

- ■ **Breastfeeding Safety** ⋯⋯ There is no published experience in nursing women. It is uknown whether **calcitonin** enters human breast milk. Procalcitonin is a normal constituent of human breast milk. **Calcitonin** inhibits lactation in animals.

- ■ **References** ⋯⋯⋯⋯⋯⋯ Lafond J, Goyer-O'Reilly I, Laramee M, Simoneau L. Endocrine 2001; 14:285-94.
Seki K, Makimura N, Mitsui C, et al. Am J Obstet Gynecol 1991; 164:1248-52.
Woloszczuk W, Kovarik J, Pavelka P. Gynecol Obstet Invest 1981; 12:272-6.
Kovarik J, Woloszczuk W, Linkesch W, Pavelka R. Lancet 1980; 1:199-200.

- ■ **Summary** ⋯⋯⋯⋯⋯⋯⋯
  - **Pregnancy Category C**
  - **Lactation Category U**
  - **Calcitonin** should be used during pregnancy and lactation only if the benefit justifies the potential perinatal risk.

Calcitriol (Rocaltrol)

- ■ **Class** ⋯⋯⋯⋯⋯⋯⋯⋯ *Vitamin*

- ■ **Indications** ⋯⋯⋯⋯⋯⋯ Hypoparathyroidism, osteoporosis, hypocalcemia, supplementation during pregnancy

- ■ **Mechanism** ⋯⋯⋯⋯⋯⋯ Active form of vitamin D; stimulates intestinal absorption of calcium and phosphorus

- ■ **Dosage with Qualifiers** ⋯⋯ Hypocalcemia—0.25mcg-1mcg PO qd
Hypoparathyroidism—0.25-2mcg/d IV; increase the dose every 2-4w as needed
Supplementation during pregnancy—10mcg/d PO
  - **Contraindications**—hypersensitivity to drug or class, hypercalcemia, hypervitaminosis D
  - **Caution**—renal failure or stones, hyperphosphatemia

- ■ **Maternal Considerations** ⋯⋯ **Calcitriol** is an active form of vitamin D. There are no adequate reports or well-controlled studies in pregnant women. **Vitamin D** supplementation is recommended during pregnancy. **Calcitriol** combined with calcium supplementation helps lower systolic blood pressure in older women.

Side effects include nausea, vomiting, anorexia, convulsion, dry mouth, bone pain, polydipsia, irritability, weight loss, increased LFTs, and conjunctivitis.

■ **Fetal Considerations**

There are no adequate and well-controlled studies of the effect of **calcitriol** in human fetuses. It is unknown whether **calcitriol** crosses the human placenta, though the placenta synthesizes active vitamin D. **Calcitriol** has been reported to be teratogenic in rabbits but not rats.

■ **Breastfeeding Safety**

There are no adequate reports or well-controlled studies in nursing women. It is unknown whether **calcitriol** enters human breast milk, but supplementation has little effect on milk vitamin D levels.

■ **References**

Brunvand L, Quigstad E, Urdal P, Haug E. Early Hum Dev 1996; 45:27-33.
Pfeifer M, Begerow B, Minne HW, et al. J Clin Endocrinol Metab 2001; 86:1633-7.
Mallet E, Gugi B, Brunelle P, et al. Obstet Gynecol 1986; 68:300-4.
Cancela L, Le Boulch N, Miravet L. J Endocrinol 1986; 110:43-50.
Kuoppala T, Tuimala R, Parviainen M, et al. Hum Nutr Clin Nutr 1986; 40:287-93.

■ **Summary**

- **Pregnancy Category B**
- **Lactation Category U**
- **Calcitriol** should be used during pregnancy and lactation only if the benefit justifies the potential perinatal risk.
- Most multivitamin supplements contain adequate quantities of vitamin D in one form or another.

Calcium chloride

■ **Class**

Mineral

■ **Indications**

Hypocalcemia, hypermagnesemia

■ **Mechanism**

Modulator of cellular events (e.g., contraction, signaling) via specific membrane channels

■ **Dosage with Qualifiers**

Hypocalcemia—500-1000mg IV slow infusion; do not exceed 1000mg ×1
Hypermagnesemia—500mg IV slow; follow the patient for clinical signs of hypermagnesemia

105

- **Contraindications**—ventricular fibrillation, hypercalcemia, digitalis toxicity, liver dysfunction
- **Caution**—cardiovascular defects, impaired respiratory function, acidosis

■ **Maternal Considerations** ⋯⋯ **Calcium chloride** is lifesaving in women with hypermagnesemia. It provides approximately 3 times more calcium than calcium gluconate. **Calcium chloride** reduces the incidence of parturient paresis in cows and transiently increases cardiac output in gravid ewes during hemorrhagic hypotension.
Side effects include tissue destruction after extravasation, and hyperkalemia-related ECG disturbances.

■ **Fetal Considerations** ⋯⋯ It is unlikely calcium administration increases the fetal concentration. **Calcium chloride** decreases the **aspirin** toxicity in pregnant rats.

■ **Breastfeeding Safety** ⋯⋯ It is unknown whether **calcium chloride** supplementation increases calcium concentration in breast milk.

■ **References** ⋯⋯ Oetzel GR. J Am Vet Med Assoc 1996; 209:958-61.
Vincent RD Jr, Chestnut DH, Sipes SL, et al. Anesth Analg 1992; 74:670-6.
Bohman VR, Cotton DB. Obstet Gynecol 1990; 76:984-6.
Ueno K, Shimoto Y, Yokoyama A, et al. Res Commun Chem Pathol Pharmacol 1983; 39:179-88.

■ **Summary** ⋯⋯
- **Pregnancy Category C**
- **Lactation Category U**
- **Calcium chloride** may be lifesaving in preeclamptic or preterm laboring women with hypermagnesemia secondary to magnesium sulfate infusion.

Camphor (found in Absorbine Arthritic Pain Lotion 10%; Act-On Rub Lotion 1.5%; Anabalm Lotion 3%; Aveeno Anti-Itch Conc. Lotion 0.3%; Avalgesic; Banalg Muscle Pain Reliever 2%; Ben Gay Children's Vaporizing Rub 5%; Campho-Phenique First Aid Gel 10.8%)

■ **Class** ⋯⋯ *Antipruritic/local anesthetic*

■ **Indications** ⋯⋯ Cold relief symptoms, muscle strain

■ **Mechanism** ⋯⋯ Unknown

■ **Dosage with Qualifiers** ⋯⋯⋯ Found in multiple topical preparations
- **Contraindications**—hypersensitivity to drug or class
- **Cautions**—seizures

■ **Maternal Considerations** ⋯⋯⋯ The FDA states over-the-counter drug products may not exceed **camphor** concentrations of 11%. There are no adequate and well-controlled studies in pregnant women. *Side effects* include local irritation and burning sensation.

■ **Fetal Considerations** ⋯⋯⋯ There are no adequate and well-controlled studies in human fetuses. **Camphor** crosses the placenta, but there is no evidence of embryo toxicity or teratogenicity.

■ **Breastfeeding Safety** ⋯⋯⋯ There is no published experience in nursing women. It is unknown whether **camphor** enters human breast milk. Considering the route and dose, it is unlikely the breast-feeding neonate would ingest a clinically significant amount.

■ **References** ⋯⋯⋯ Uc A, Bishop WP, Sanders KD. South Med J 2000; 93:596-8.
American Academy of Pediatrics. Committee on Drugs. Pediatrics 1978; 62:404-6.
Weiss J, Catalano P. Pediatrics 1973; 52:713-4.

■ **Summary** ⋯⋯⋯
- **Pregnancy Category C**
- **Lactation Category S**
- **Camphor** should be used during pregnancy and lactation only if the benefit justifies the potential perinatal risk.

Candesartan (Atacand)

■ **Class** ⋯⋯⋯ *Antihypertensive, ACE-1/A2R-antagonist*

■ **Indications** ⋯⋯⋯ Hypertension

■ **Mechanism** ⋯⋯⋯ AT-1 receptor antagonist

■ **Dosage with Qualifiers** ⋯⋯⋯ Hypertension—begin 16mg PO qd and increase gradually; max 32mg qd
- **Contraindications**—hypersensitivity to drug or class, history of angioedema
- **Caution**—renal artery stenosis, hepatic or renal dysfunction, hyponatremia, heart failure

■ **Maternal Considerations** ⋯⋯⋯ There is no published experience with **candesartan** during pregnancy. It is assumed the effects of **candesartan** are similar to the ACE class of agents. The lowest dose effective should be used when **candesartan** is required for pressure control during pregnancy.

Side effects include fetal and neonatal morbidity/death (see Fetal Considerations), hypovolemia, asthenia, fever, paraesthesia, vertigo, dyspepsia, gastroenteritis, tachycardia, palpitation, leukopenia, hepatotoxicity, neutropenia, hyperkalemia, edema, diarrhea, chest pain, cough, increased LFTs, pruritus, and rash.

■ **Fetal Considerations**
There are no adequate and well-controlled studies in human fetuses. It is unknown whether **candesartan** crosses the human placenta. AT-1 receptors are expressed on many organs of the human fetus. Other ACE inhibitors cross the placenta. And while no adverse fetal effects are reported after 1st trimester exposure, later exposure to agents that interfere with angiotensin is associated with cranial hypoplasia, anuria, reversible or irreversible renal failure, death, oligohydramnios, prematurity, IUGR, and patent ductus arteriosus.

■ **Breastfeeding Safety**
There is no published experience in nursing women. It is unknown whether **candesartan** enters human breast milk.

■ **References**
Hinsberger A, Wingen AM, Hoyer PF. Lancet 2001 19; 357:1620.

■ **Summary**
- **Pregnancy Category C (1st trimester), D (2nd and 3rd trimesters)**
- **Lactation Category U**
- **Candesartan** and other inhibitors of angiotensin's effects should be avoided during pregnancy if possible.
- There are alternative agents for which there is more experience during pregnancy and lactation.
- When the mother's disease requires treatment with **candesartan**, the lowest dose should be used followed by close monitoring of the fetus.

Captopril (Capoten; Tenofax)

■ **Class**
Antihypertensive, ACE-1/A2R-antagonist

■ **Indications**
Hypertension, congestive heart surgery, diabetes, myocardial infarction (acute)

■ **Mechanism**
Angiotensin-converting enzyme inhibitor

■ **Dosage with Qualifiers**
Hypertension—25-50mg PO tid
Congestive heart failure—12.5-50mg PO tid
Diabetic nephropathy—25mg PO tid
NOTE—may be combined with **hydrochlorothiazide**

- **Contraindications**—hypersensitivity to drug or class, renal artery stenosis
- **Caution**—collagen vascular diseases, CHF, renal artery stenosis, hepatic or renal dysfunction, hyponatremia

■ **Maternal Considerations**

There are no adequate and well-controlled studies of **captopril** in pregnant women. Improved pregnancy outcome was noted in mothers treated prenatally with low doses of **captopril**. The lowest dose effective should be used when **captopril** is required during pregnancy. Close monitoring of amniotic fluid and fetal well-being is recommended.

Side effects include angioedema, hypotension, renal failure, hepatic toxicity, pancreatitis, proteinuria, neutropenia, rash, pruritus, hypotension, angioedema, cough, abdominal pain, nausea, vomiting, diarrhea, anorexia, constipation, peptic ulcer, dizziness, headache, malaise, fatigue, insomnia, dry mouth, dyspnea, alopecia, and paresthesias.

■ **Fetal Considerations**

There are no adequate and well-controlled studies in human fetuses. **Captopril** apparently crosses the human placenta, though the kinetics remain to be elucidated. In humans, exposure during the 1st trimester appears reasonably safe. Similar to other ACE inhibitors, fetal exposure during the 2nd and 3rd trimesters is associated with skull hypoplasia, renal failure, limb contractions, craniofacial malformations, hypoplastic lungs, and IUGR. **Captopril** is embryocidal and causes stillbirths in a variety of animals (sheep, rabbits, rats).

■ **Breastfeeding Safety**

Captopril is excreted in breast milk at a very low concentration and is generally considered compatible with breastfeeding.

■ **References**

Easterling TR, Carr DB, Davis C, et al. Obstet Gynecol 2000; 96:956-61.
Bar J, Chen R, Schoenfeld A, et al. J Pediatr Endocrinol Metab 1999; 12:659-65.
Burrows RF, Burrows EA. Aust NZ J Obstet Gynaecol 1998; 38:306-11.
August P, Mueller FB, Sealey JE, Edersheim TG. Lancet 1995; 345:896-7.

■ **Summary**

- **Pregnancy Category C (1st trimester), D (2nd and 3rd trimesters)**
- **Lactation Category S**
- **Captopril** and other inhibitors of angiotensin's effects should be avoided during pregnancy if possible.
- There are alternative agents for which there is more experience during pregnancy and lactation.
- Should the mother's disease require treatment with **captopril**, the lowest dose should be used followed by close monitoring of the fetus.

109

Carbachol (Carbastat; Carboptic; Isopto; Miostat)

■ **Class** .... Parasympathomimetic

■ **Indications** .... Glaucoma

■ **Mechanism** .... Cholinergic receptor agonist; partial cholinesterase inhibitor

■ **Dosage with Qualifiers** .... Glaucoma—2 gtt each eye tid
NOTE—no more than 0.5ml should be administered for satisfactory miosis
  • **Contraindications**—hypersensitivity to drug or class, acute iritis
  • **Caution**—cardiac failure, asthma, hyperthyroidism, gastrointestinal spasm, parkinsonism, recent MI, hypertension

■ **Maternal Considerations** ...... There are no adequate and well-controlled studies of the effect of **carbachol** in pregnant women. **Carbachol** is a potent stimulator of myometrial contractility in rodents. Considering the dose and route, it is unlikely the maternal systemic concentration will reach clinically relevant level. *Side effects* include stinging, burning, flushing, sweating, epigastric distress, abdominal cramps, tightness in urinary bladder, and headache.

■ **Fetal Considerations** .... There are no adequate reports or well-controlled studies in human fetuses. It is unknown whether **carbachol** crosses the human placenta. Considering the dose and route, it is unlikely the maternal systemic concentration reaches a clinically relevant level.

■ **Breastfeeding Safety** .... There is no published experience in pregnancy. It is unknown whether **carbachol** enters human breast milk. However, considering the dose and route, it is unlikely the breast-fed neonate would ingest a clinically relevant amount.

■ **References** .... Garfield RE, Bytautiene E, Vedernikov YP, et al. Am J Obstet Gynecol 2000; 183:118-25.
Boxall DK, Ford AP, Choppin A, et al. Br J Pharmacol 1998; 124:1615-22.
Luckas MJ, Taggart MJ, Wray S. Am J Obstet Gynecol 1999; 181:468-76.

■ **Summary** .... • **Pregnancy Category C**
  • **Lactation Category U**
  • **Carbachol** should be used during pregnancy and lactation only if the benefit justifies the potential perinatal risk.

Carbamazepine (Atretol; Convuline; Epitol; Macrepan; Tegretol)

■ **Class** .... Anticonvulsant

■ **Indications** .... Seizure disorder, trigeminal neuralgia

■ **Mechanism** .... Unknown

■ **Dosage with Qualifiers** .... Seizure disorder—400-600mg PO bid (or 12-25mg/kg/d); max 600mg PO bid
Trigeminal neuralgia—200-400mg PO bid
- **Contraindications**—hypersensitivity, MAO inhibitors in the past 2w
- **Caution**—hepatic or renal failure, bone marrow depression, history of blood dyscrasia, cardiac disease

■ **Maternal Considerations** .... Anticonvulsant drugs should not be discontinued abruptly during pregnancy if used to prevent seizures, as there is a significant possibility of precipitating status epilepticus. There are no adequate and well-controlled studies of **carbamazepine** in pregnant women.
Side effects include seizures, Stevens-Johnson syndrome, arrhythmias, agranulocytosis, thrombocytopenia, and hepatitis.

■ **Fetal Considerations** .... There are no adequate reports or well-controlled studies in human fetuses. **Carbamazepine** rapidly crosses the human placenta, and accumulates in fetal organs including the brain. Epidemiologic study suggests **carbamazepine** is a teratogen causing facial dysmorphism, spina bifida, distal phalange hypoplasia, and developmental delay. In prospective studies involving 1255 exposures, **carbamazepine** increased the rate of neural tube, cardiovascular, urinary tract, and cleft palate anomalies. The combination of **carbamazepine** with other antiepileptic drugs has a synergistic effect on the prevalence of birth defects. Rodent studies reveal an increased prevalence of talipes, cleft palate, and anophthalmos.

■ **Breastfeeding Safety** .... **Carbamazepine** is excreted in human breast milk. Although it is generally considered safe for breast-feeding women, neonatal sequelae reported include cholestatic hepatitis. The infant should be monitored for possible adverse effects, the drug given at the lowest effective dose, and breastfeeding avoided at times of peak drug levels.

■ **References** .... Kaaja E, Kaaja R, Hiilesmaa V. Neurology 2003; 60:575-9.
Iqbal MM, Sohhan T, Mahmud SZ. J Toxicol Clin Toxicol 2001; 39:381-92.
Matalon S, Schechtman S, Goldzweig G, Ornoy A. Reprod Toxicol 2002; 16:9-17.

Diav-Citrin O, Shechtman S, Arnon J, Ornoy A. Neurology 2001(24); 57:321-4.
Holmes LB, Harvey EA, Coull BA, et al. N Engl J Med 2001(12); 344:1132-8.
Bar-Oz B, Nulman I, Koren G, Ito S. Paediatr Drugs 2000; 2:113-26.
Samren EB, van Duijn CM, Christiaens GC, et al. Ann Neurol 1999; 46:739-46.
Frey B, Braegger CP, Ghelfi D. Ann Pharmacother. 2002; 36:644-7.

■ **Summary**

- **Pregnancy Category C**
- **Lactation Category S?**
- **Carbamazepine** should be used during pregnancy and lactation only if the benefit justifies the potential perinatal risk; other anticonvulsants are preferable.
- Monotherapy with the lowest effective quantity given in divided doses to minimize the peaks can minimize the risks.

Carbenicillin (Geocillin)

■ **Class**

Antibiotic

■ **Indications**

Infections with *Escherichia coli*, *Proteus mirabilis*, *Streptococcus fecalis* (enterococci), *Staphylococcus*, *Streptococcus*

■ **Mechanism**

Inhibits synthesis of cell wall mucopeptide

■ **Dosage with Qualifiers**

Adult infection—2-4 tab qd (1 tab = 382mg **carbenicillin**)
- **Contraindications**—hypersensitivity to drug or class
- **Caution**—cephalosporin allergy, seizure disorder, renal dysfunction

■ **Maternal Considerations**

Carbenicillin is indicated for the treatment of acute and chronic infections of the upper and lower urinary tract. There are no adequate reports or well-controlled studies in pregnant women.
Side effects include seizures, anaphylaxis, Stevens-Johnson syndrome, hemolytic anemia, neutropenia, nausea, urticaria, diarrhea, rash, and fever.

■ **Fetal Considerations**

There are no adequate and well-controlled studies in human fetuses. It is unknown whether **carbenicillin** crosses the human placenta. Other penicillins do cross with varying degrees. Rodent studies are reassuring, revealing no evidence of teratogenicity or IUGR despite the use of doses higher than those used clinically.

- **Breastfeeding Safety** ···· There is no published experience in nursing women. **Carbenicillin** is excreted into breast milk in low concentrations, but is generally considered safe during breastfeeding.

- **References** ···· Davies BI, Mummery RV, Brumfitt W. Br J Urol 1975; 47:335-41.
Elek E, Ivan E, Arr M. Int J Clin Pharmacol 1972; 6:223-8.

- **Summary** ····
  - **Pregnancy Category B**
  - **Lactation Category S**
  - **Penicillin**-class drugs are generally considered safe during pregnancy.

Carbidopa (Lodosyn)

- **Class** ···· *Antiparkinsonian*

- **Indications** ···· Parkinson's disease

- **Mechanism** ···· Inhibits peripheral dopamine decarboxylation, crosses blood-brain barrier and can serve as a dopamine precursor

- **Dosage with Qualifiers** ···· Parkinson's disease—the optimal dose is determined by careful titration whether given alone or in combination with **levodopa**. Most patients respond to a 1:10 proportion of **carbidopa** and **levodopa**, provided the daily dosage of **carbidopa** is 70mg or more/d; max 200mg PO qd
NOTE—may be combined with **levodopa** (Sinemet)
  - **Contraindications**—hypersensitivity, glaucoma, melanoma
  - **Caution**—psychosis, asthma, gastric ulcer, renal failure

- **Maternal Considerations** ···· There are no adequate reports or well-controlled studies in pregnant women. Pregnancy may exacerbate Parkinson's disease and have a long-term negative impact on the course of the illness.
Side effects include suicidal ideation, hemolytic anemia, leukopenia, hepatic failure, agitation, headache, and anxiety.

- **Fetal Considerations** ···· There are no adequate reports or well-controlled studies in human fetuses. **Carbidopa** crosses the rat and human placenta, and the fetal blood-brain barrier. Rodent studies are reassuring, revealing no evidence of teratogenicity or IUGR despite the use of doses higher than those used clinically. Its use with **levodopa** is associated with visceral and skeletal malformations in rabbits.

■ **Breastfeeding Safety** .... There are no adequate reports or well-controlled studies in nursing women. It is unknown whether **carbidopa** enters human breast milk.

■ **References** .... Shulman LM, Minagar A, Weiner WJ. Mov Disord 2000; 15:132-5.
Merchant CA, Cohen G, Mytilineou C, et al. J Neural Transm Park Dis Dement Sect 1995; 9:239-42.
Vickers S, Stuart EK, Bianchine JR, et al. Drug Metab Dispos 1974; 2:9-22.

■ **Summary** .... • **Pregnancy Category C**
• **Lactation Category U**
• **Carbidopa** should be used during pregnancy and lactation only if the benefit justifies the potential perinatal risk.

Carbinoxamine (Rondec: carbinoxamine/
dextromethorphan/pseudoephedrine)

■ **Class** .... *Antihistamine*

■ **Indications** .... Cold symptoms

■ **Mechanism** .... Nonselectively antagonizes central and peripheral H_1 receptors

■ **Dosage with Qualifiers** ...... Cold symptoms—5ml PO qid
• **Contraindications**—hypersensitivity to drug or class, MAO inhibitor usage
• **Caution**—glaucoma, hypertension, diabetes, asthma, COPD

■ **Maternal Considerations** ...... There is no published experience with **carbinoxamine** during pregnancy.
Side effects include arrhythmia, hypertension, coronary vasospasm, drowsiness, thickened secretions, and dry mouth.

■ **Fetal Considerations** .... There are no adequate and well-controlled studies in human fetuses. It is unknown whether **carbinoxamine** crosses the human placenta.

■ **Breastfeeding Safety** .... There is no published experience in nursing women. It is unknown whether **carbinoxamine** enters human breast milk.

- **References** — There is no published experience in pregnancy or during lactation.

- **Summary**
  - **Pregnancy Category C**
  - **Lactation Category U**
  - **Carbinoxamine** should be used during pregnancy and lactation only if the benefit justifies the potential perinatal risk.
  - There are alternative agents for which there is more experience during pregnancy and lactation.

Carboprost tromethamine (Hemabate)

- **Class** — *Abortifacient, oxytocic*

- **Indications** — Pregnancy termination, uterine atony

- **Mechanism** — Stimulates prostaglandin F receptors

- **Dosage with Qualifiers** — Pregnancy termination—begin 100mcg IM test dose, then 250mcg IM q90-120min; max 12mg total or use no longer than 2d
  Uterine atony—250mcg IM ×1, may repeat q15-90min; max 2mg
  - **Contraindications**—hypersensitivity to drug or class, acute PID, acute renal, hepatic or pulmonary insufficiency, symptomatic coronary artery disease
  - **Caution**—hypertension, diabetes mellitus, asthma, hepatic or renal dysfunction, anemia, seizure disorder, uterine scar, chorioamnionitis

- **Maternal Considerations** — **Carboprost** is an analog of 15-methylprostaglandin $PGF_2\alpha$. It is a second-line agent for the treatment of uterine atony refractive to **oxytocin** or **methergine/ergotrate** because of the high incidence of GI complaints (21% vs <1%). Some suggest that it is more effective if given directly into the myometrium, but there are no trial data to support the practice. **Carboprost** has also been given both IM and intra-amniotically for pregnancy termination, though PGE_2 is a superior agent for this indication. It can speed cervical ripening (200mcg IM), but once administered may be difficult to control.
  Side effects include pulmonary edema, respiratory distress, hematemesis, uterine rupture, diarrhea, nausea, vomiting, fever, flushing, hypertension, cough, headache, pain, and bronchospasm.

- **Fetal Considerations** — There are no adequate reports or well-controlled studies in human fetuses. It is unknown whether **carboprost**

115

crosses the human placenta. The principal risk reflects that of hypoxia associated with uterine tachysystole.

■ **Breastfeeding Safety** — There is no published experience in nursing women. It is unknown whether **carboprost** enters human breast milk.

■ **References** — Dildy GA 3rd. Clin Obstet Gynecol 2002; 45:330-44. Lamont RF, Morgan DJ, Logue M, Gordon H. Prostaglandins Other Lipid Mediat 2001; 66:203-10. Perry KG Jr, Rinehart BK, Terrone DA, et al. Am J Obstet Gynecol 1999; 181:1057-61.

■ **Summary** —
- **Pregnancy Category C**
- **Lactation Category U**
- **Carboprost** should be used during pregnancy and lactation only if the benefit justifies the potential perinatal risk.

Carisoprodol (Caridolin; Chinchen; Flexartal; Mus-Lax; Neotica; Rela; Rotalin; Scutamil-C; Soma)

■ **Class** — *Muscle relaxant*

■ **Indications** — Muscle spasm

■ **Mechanism** — Blocks interneuronal activity in the descending reticular formation and spinal cord

■ **Dosage with Qualifiers** — Muscle spasm—350mg PO tid and at bedtime or qid
- **Contraindications**—hypersensitivity to drug or class, porphyria
- **Caution**—hepatic or renal dysfunction

■ **Maternal Considerations** — The major metabolite of **carisoprodol** is **meprobamate**. There are no adequate reports or well-controlled studies in pregnant women.
Side effects include anaphylaxis, erythematic multiforme, drowsiness, orthostatic hypotension, vertigo, ataxia, vomiting, tremor, rash, angioedema, and headache.

■ **Fetal Considerations** — There are no adequate reports or well-controlled studies in human fetuses. It is unknown whether **carisoprodol** crosses the human placenta. Rodent teratogenicity studies have not been performed.

■ **Breastfeeding Safety** — **Carisoprodol** is concentrated in breast milk. The absolute dose ingested by an exclusively breast-fed infant was estimated at 1.9mg/kg/d, and the relative dose 4.1% of the weight-adjusted maternal dose. No adverse effects are reported.

■ **References**

Grizzle TB, George JD, Fail PA, Heindel JJ. Fundam Appl Toxicol 1995; 24:132-9.
Nordeng H, Zahlsen K, Spigset O. Ther Drug Monit 2001; 23:298-300.

■ **Summary**

- **Pregnancy Category C**
- **Lactation Category NS?**
- **Carisoprodol** should be used during pregnancy and lactation only if the benefit justifies the potential perinatal risk.

β-Carotene (Vitamin A)

■ **Class**

Vitamin

■ **Indications**

Nutritional supplementation

■ **Mechanism**

Antioxidant

■ **Dosage with Qualifiers**

Supplementation—8000-25000IU PO qd
- **Contraindications**—malabsorption syndrome
- **Caution**—unknown

■ **Maternal Considerations**

Carotene is an antioxidant, and consuming foods rich in β-carotene may help protect from free radicals damage. Some studies suggest the dietary intake of **carotene** may reduce the risk of heart disease and cancer. There are no adequate reports or well-controlled studies in pregnant women. The safety of doses exceeding 6000 USP units during pregnancy is not established.
Side effects include acute toxicity (fatigue, malaise, lethargy, abdominal discomfort), skeletal malformations (cortical thickening, short bones), arthralgia, alopecia, and cracking of the lips.

■ **Fetal Considerations**

There are no adequate reports or well-controlled studies in human fetuses. High doses of **carotene** are teratogenic (bone, heart). There is no evidence of teratogenicity in women consuming 8000-25,000IU.

■ **Breastfeeding Safety**

There is no published experience in nursing women. **Carotene** enters human breast milk and raises its vitamin A level.

■ **References** ···· Fairfield KM, Fletcher RH. JAMA 2002(19); 287:3116-26.
Yamini S, West KP Jr, Wu L, et al. Eur J Clin Nutr 2001;
55:252-9.
Mills JL, Simpson JL, Cunningham GC, et al. Am J Obstet
Gynecol 1997; 177:31-6.
Bahl R, Bhandari N, Wahed MA, et al. J Nutr
2002; 132:3243-8.

■ **Summary** ····
- **Pregnancy Category C**
- **Lactation Category U**
- **Carotene** should be used during pregnancy only if the benefit justifies the potential fetal risk.
- Supplementation is commonplace during pregnancy.

Carteolol (Arteoptik; Cartrol; Ocupress; Optipress)

■ **Class** ···· *Antiadrenergic, glaucoma*

■ **Indications** ···· Hypertension, glaucoma

■ **Mechanism** ···· Antagonizes β-1 and β-2 adrenergic receptors

■ **Dosage with Qualifiers** ···· Hypertension—2.5-10mg PO qd
Chronic open-angle glaucoma and intraocular hypertension—1 gtt of 1% solution bid
NOTE—renal dosing
- **Contraindications**—hypersensitivity to drug or class, asthma, COPD, bradycardia, atrioventricular block, CHF
- **Caution**—diabetes mellitus, hyperthyroidism

■ **Maternal Considerations** ···· There is no published experience with **carteolol** during pregnancy.
Side effects include bronchospasm, asthenia, paresthesia, edema, and back pain.

■ **Fetal Considerations** ···· There are no adequate and well-controlled studies in human fetuses. Rodent studies are reassuring, revealing no evidence of teratogenicity despite the use of doses dramatically higher than those used clinically. There was, however, evidence of fetotoxicity and IUGR at these high doses.

■ **Breastfeeding Safety** ···· There is no published experience in nursing women. It is unknown whether **carteolol** enters human breast milk. It does enter rat milk.

■ **References** ···· Tanaka N, Shingai F, Tamagawa M, Nakatsu I. J Toxicol Sci
1979; 4:47-58.
Tamagawa M, Numoto T, Tanaka N, Nishino H. J Toxicol
Sci 1979; 4:59-77.

■ **Summary**
- **Pregnancy Category C**
- **Lactation Category U**
- **Carteolol** should be used during pregnancy and lactation only if the benefit justifies the potential perinatal risk.
- There are many alternative agents for the treatment of hypertension for which there is more experience during pregnancy and lactation.

Carvedilol (Coreg)

■ **Class** — Antihypertensive

■ **Indications** — Hypertension, CHF

■ **Mechanism** — Selective α-1 and nonselective β-adrenergic receptor antagonists

■ **Dosage with Qualifiers** — Hypertension—6.25-12.5mg PO bid, reevaluate in 2w; max 25mg bid
CHF—3.125-50mg PO bid; max 25-50mg PO bid
- **Contraindications**—hypersensitivity to drug or class, asthma, AV block, bradycardia, CHF (class IV)
- **Caution**—hepatic or renal dysfunction

■ **Maternal Considerations** — There are no adequate reports or well-controlled studies in pregnant women. There are reports of its use for the treatment of peripartal cardiomyopathy.
Side effects include atrioventricular block, bradycardia, thrombocytopenia, sudden death, bronchospasm, fatigue, nausea, vomiting, orthostatic hypotension, bradycardia, headache, gout, and abdominal pain.

■ **Fetal Considerations** — There are no adequate and well-controlled studies in human fetuses. It is unknown whether **carvedilol** crosses the human placenta. **Carvedilol** crosses the rodent placenta, and produces fetotoxicity and IUGR when given in doses that are multiples of the maximum recommended human dose.

■ **Breastfeeding Safety** — There are no adequate reports or well-controlled studies in nursing women. It is unknown whether **carvedilol** enters human breast milk. It does enter the milk of some rodent species.

■ **References** — Sliwa K, Skudicky D, Candy G, et al. Eur J Heart Fail 2002; 4:305-9.

■ **Summary**
- **Pregnancy Category C**
- **Lactation Category U**
- **Carvedilol** should be used during pregnancy and lactation only if the benefit justifies the potential perinatal risk.
- There are alternative agents for which there is more experience during pregnancy and lactation.

Casanthranol (Peri-Colace = casanthranol + dousate sodium)

■ **Class** — Purgative/anthraquinone

■ **Indications** — Constipation

■ **Mechanism** — Stimulates peristalsis

■ **Dosage with Qualifiers** — Constipation—1-2 tab PO qd
- **Contraindications**—hypersensitivity to drug or class, constipation, appendicitis, acute abdomen
- **Caution**—nausea, vomiting

■ **Maternal Considerations** — There are no adequate reports or well-controlled studies in pregnant women.
Side effects include bowel obstruction, abdominal cramps, rash, and electrolyte disorders.

■ **Fetal Considerations** — There are no adequate and well-controlled studies in human fetuses. It is unknown whether **casanthranol** crosses the human placenta. It is not associated with an increased incidence of fetal malformations. Rodent teratogenicity studies have apparently not been performed.

■ **Breastfeeding Safety** — There is no published experience during pregnancy. It is unknown whether **casanthranol** enters human breast milk. A metabolite, anthraquinone is excreted into breast milk and may increase the incidence of diarrhea in infants of nursing mothers. However, it is generally considered safe during breastfeeding.

■ **References** — Heinonen OP, Slone D, Shapiro B. Birth defects and drugs in pregnancy. Littleton MA: Publishing Sciences Group, 1977.
Greenleaf JO, Leonard HSD. Practitioner 1973; 210:259-63.

■ **Summary**
- **Pregnancy Category C**
- **Lactation Category S**
- **Casanthranol** should be used during pregnancy and lactation only if the benefit justifies the potential perinatal risk.

Cefaclor (Ceclor; Ceclor CD; Cefaclor)

■ **Class** — Antibiotic (*2nd-generation cephalosporin*)

■ **Indications** — Bacterial infections (<u>gram-positive aerobes</u>: *Staphylococcus aureus, Streptococcus pneumoniae, Streptococcus pyogenes;* <u>gram-negative anaerobes</u>: *Haemophilus influenzae*)

■ **Mechanism** — Bactericidal—inhibits cell wall synthesis

■ **Dosage with Qualifiers** — <u>Bacterial infection</u>—375-500mg extended release PO bid within 1h of eating, or 250-500mg tid
NOTE—renal dosing
- **Contraindications**—hypersensitivity to drug or class
- **Caution**—penicillin allergy, renal dysfunction, antibiotic-associated colitis, seizure disorder, concomitant use of nephrotoxic drugs

■ **Maternal Considerations** — Because of its antimicrobial spectrum **cefaclor** is used to treat acute bronchitis, pharyngitis, and skin infections. It has poor activity against the anaerobes associated with bacterial vaginosis. There are no adequate reports or well-controlled studies in pregnant women. However, cephalosporins are usually considered safe during pregnancy.
Side effects include anaphylaxis, seizures, pseudomembranous colitis, nephrotoxicity, leukopenia, thrombocytopenia, erythema multiforme, exfoliative dermatitis, and cholestatic jaundice.

■ **Fetal Considerations** — There are no adequate reports or well-controlled studies in human fetuses. It is unknown whether **cefaclor** crosses the human placenta. Rodent studies are reassuring revealing no evidence of teratogenicity or IUGR despite the use of doses higher than those used clinically.

■ **Breastfeeding Safety** — Most cephalosporins are excreted into breast milk. While there are no adequate reports or well-controlled studies in nursing women, **cefaclor** is generally considered compatible with breastfeeding.

■ **References** — Committee on Drugs, American Academy of Pediatrics. Pediatrics 1994; 93:137-50.
Puapermpoonsiri S, Watanabe K, Kato N, Ueno K. Antimicrob Agents Chemother 1997; 41:2297-9.

■ **Summary** —
- **Pregnancy Category B**
- **Lactation Category S**
- **Cefaclor** is used for the treatment of acute bronchitis, pharyngitis, and skin infections.

Cefadroxil (Cedroxim; Droxicef; Duricef; Kefroxil; Nor-Dacef; Ultracef; Wincef)

■ Class — Antibiotic (*1st-generation cephalosporin*)

■ Indications — Bacterial infections (<u>gram-positive aerobes:</u> *Staphylococcus aureus*, β-1 hemolytic streptococci; <u>gram-negative aerobes:</u> *Escherichia coli*, *Proteus mirabilis*, *Klebsiella* species, *Moraxella catarrhalis*)

■ Mechanism — Bactericidal—inhibits cell wall synthesis

■ Dosage with Qualifiers — <u>Bacterial infection</u>—500-1000mg PO qd
NOTE—renal dosing
- **Contraindications**—hypersensitivity to drug or class
- **Caution**—penicillin allergy, renal dysfunction, antibiotic-associated colitis, seizure disorder, concomitant use of nephrotoxic drugs

■ Maternal Considerations — Because of its antimicrobial spectrum, **cefadroxil** is used to treat urinary tract infections and pharyngitis. There are no adequate reports or well-controlled studies in pregnant women. However, cephalosporins are usually considered safe during pregnancy.
Side effects include anaphylaxis, seizures, pseudomembranous colitis, nephrotoxicity, leukopenia, thrombocytopenia, erythema multiforme, exfoliative dermatitis, cholestatic jaundice, diarrhea, nausea, dyspepsia, urticaria, pruritus, and vaginal candidiasis.

■ Fetal Considerations — There are no adequate reports or well-controlled studies in human fetuses. It is unknown whether **cefadroxil** crosses the human placenta. Rodent studies are reassuring, revealing no evidence of teratogenicity or IUGR despite the use of doses higher than those used clinically.

■ Breastfeeding Safety — **Cefadroxil** is excreted into breast milk in low concentrations; it is generally considered compatible with breastfeeding.

■ References — Committee on Drugs, American Academy of Pediatrics. Pediatrics 1994; 93:137-50.
Shetty N, Shulman RI, Scott GM. J Hosp Infect 1999; 41:229-32.

■ Summary —
- **Pregnancy Category B**
- **Lactation Category S**
- **Cefadroxil** is used for the treatment of acute bronchitis, pharyngitis, and skin infections.

Cefamandole (Mandol)

■ **Class** — Antibiotic (2nd-generation cephalosporin)

■ **Indications** — Bacterial infections (<u>gram-positive aerobes</u>: *Staphylococcus aureus, Staphylococcus epidermidis, Streptococcus pneumoniae, Streptococcus pyogenes*; <u>gram-negative aerobes</u>: *Escherichia coli, Klebsiella, Enterobacter, Proteus mirabilis, Morganella morganii*; <u>anaerobic organisms</u>: *Peptococcus, Peptostreptococcus, Clostridium, Bacteroides, Fusobacterium*)

■ **Mechanism** — Bactericidal—inhibits cell wall synthesis

■ **Dosage with Qualifiers** — <u>Bacterial infection</u>—500mg-1.0g IV q4-8h
<u>Cesarean section prophylaxis</u>—1g IV at umbilical cord clamping
- **Contraindications**—hypersensitivity to drug or class
- **Caution**—penicillin allergy, renal dysfunction, antibiotic-associated colitis, seizure disorder, concomitant use of nephrotoxic drugs

■ **Maternal Considerations** — Because of its antimicrobial spectrum, **cefamandole** is used to treat lower respiratory tract infections, urinary tract infections, peritonitis, septicemia, and for post-cesarean section prophylaxis. For the latter, it has no advantage over any other cephalosporin. Cephalosporins are usually considered safe during pregnancy.
Side effects include anaphylaxis, seizures, pseudomembranous colitis, nephrotoxicity, leukopenia, thrombocytopenia, erythema multiforme, exfoliative dermatitis, and cholestatic jaundice.

■ **Fetal Considerations** — There are no adequate reports or well-controlled studies in human fetuses. It is unknown whether **cefamandole** crosses the human placenta. Rodent studies are reassuring, revealing no evidence of teratogenicity or IUGR despite the use of doses higher than those used clinically.

■ **Breastfeeding Safety** — **Cefamandole** is excreted into breast milk in low concentrations; it is generally considered safe during breastfeeding.

■ **References** — Peterson CM, Medchill M, Gordon DS, Chard HL. Obstet Gynecol 1990; 75:179-82.
Ling FW, McNeeley SG Jr, Anderson GD, et al. Clin Ther 1984; 6:669-76.
Duff P, Gibbs RS, Jorgensen JH, Alexander G. Obstet Gynecol 1982; 60:409-12.
Committee on Drugs, American Academy of Pediatrics. Pediatrics 1994; 93:137-50.

■ **Summary** ⸻ • **Pregnancy Category B**
• **Lactation Category S**
• **Cefamandole** is used for the treatment of acute bronchitis, pharyngitis, and skin infections.

Cefazolin (Ancef; Cefazolin; Kefzol; Zolicef)

■ **Class** ⸻ Antibiotic (1st-generation cephalosporin)

■ **Indications** ⸻ Bacterial infections (gram-positive aerobes: Staphylococcus aureus, Staphylococcus epidermidis, Streptococcus pneumoniae; gram-negative aerobes: Escherichia coli, Klebsiella, Enterobacter, Proteus mirabilis)

■ **Mechanism** ⸻ Bactericidal—inhibits cell wall synthesis

■ **Dosage with Qualifiers** ⸻ Acute infection—25-100mg/kg/d IV/IM q8h
Cesarean section prophylaxis—1g IV at umbilical cord clamping
Bacterial endocarditis—1g IV/IM 30min before procedure
NOTE—renal dosing
• **Contraindications**—hypersensitivity to drug or class
• **Caution**—penicillin allergy, renal dysfunction, antibiotic-associated colitis, seizure disorder, concomitant use of nephrotoxic drugs

■ **Maternal Considerations** ⸻ Because of its antimicrobial spectrum, **cefazolin** is used to treat lower respiratory tract infections, genitourinary tract infections, skin infections, peritonitis, septicemia, endocarditis, for post-cesarean section prophylaxis, and intrapartum for group B streptococcus. **Cefazolin** is superior to **clindamycin** and **erythromycin** for group B streptococcus prophylaxis in patients with a nonanaphylactic penicillin allergy. The prophylactic administration of **cefazolin** preoperatively, intraoperatively, or postoperatively reduces the incidence of post-cesarean section infection. For this indication, it has no clinical advantage over any other cephalosporin, and cost is often the deciding factor. Prophylaxis is usually discontinued within 24h of the surgical procedure. Cephalosporins are usually considered safe during pregnancy.
Side effects include seizures, pseudomembranous colitis, nephrotoxicity, leukopenia, thrombocytopenia, erythema multiforme, and Stevens-Johnson syndrome.

■ **Fetal Considerations** ⸻ There are no adequate reports or well-controlled studies in human fetuses. **Cefazolin** rapidly crosses the human placenta, achieving concentrations greater than or equal to the MIC(90) for group B streptococcus maternal, fetal, and AF samples. Rodent studies are reassuring, revealing no evidence of teratogenicity or IUGR despite the use of doses higher than those used clinically.

■ **Breastfeeding Safety** ⋯⋯⋯⋯ While there are no adequate reports or well-controlled studies in nursing women, **cefazolin** is apparently excreted into human breast milk. And though the kinetics remain to be elucidated, it is generally considered compatible with breastfeeding.

■ **References** ⋯⋯⋯⋯⋯⋯ Fiore Mitchell T, Pearlman MD, Chapman RL, et al. Obstet Gynecol 2001; 98:1075-9.
Wing DA, Hendershott CM, Debuque L, Millar LK. Obstet Gynecol 1998; 92:249-53.
Millar LK, Wing DA, Paul RH, Grimes DA. Obstet Gynecol 1995; 86:560-4.
Philipson A, Stiernstedt G, Ehrnebo M. Clin Pharmacokinet 1987; 12:136-44.

■ **Summary** ⋯⋯⋯⋯⋯⋯⋯
- **Pregnancy Category B**
- **Lactation Category S**
- **Cefazolin** is superior to both **clindamycin** and **erythromycin** for group B streptococcus prophylaxis in patients with a nonanaphylactic penicillin allergy.

Cefdinir (Omnicef)

■ **Class** ⋯⋯⋯⋯⋯⋯⋯⋯⋯ Antibiotic (*1st-generation cephalosporin*)

■ **Indications** ⋯⋯⋯⋯⋯⋯ Bacterial infections (gram-positive aerobes: *Staphylococcus aureus, Staphylococcus epidermidis, Streptococcus pneumoniae*; gram-negative aerobes: *Escherichia coli, Klebsiella, Enterobacter, Proteus mirabilis*)

■ **Mechanism** ⋯⋯⋯⋯⋯⋯ Bactericidal—inhibits cell wall synthesis

■ **Dosage with Qualifiers** ⋯⋯ Acute infection—600mg PO qd for 10d, or 300mg PO bid ×10d
- **Contraindications**—hypersensitivity to drug or class
- **Caution**—penicillin allergy, renal dysfunction, antibiotic-associated colitis, seizure disorder, concomitant use of nephrotoxic drugs

■ **Maternal Considerations** ⋯⋯ There are no adequate reports or well-controlled studies in pregnant women. It appears effective and safe during pregnancy for the treatment of acute infections, but has no unique advantage over other cephalosporins for most indications. Cost is often a key decision factor.

Side effects include diarrhea, vaginal moniliasis, vaginitis, rash, nausea, headache, abdominal pain, dyspepsia, flatulence, vomiting, anorexia, constipation, abnormal stools, asthenia, dizziness, insomnia, leukorrhea, pruritus, and somnolence.

■ **Fetal Considerations** — There are no adequate reports or well-controlled studies in human fetuses. It is unknown whether **cefdinir** crosses the human placenta. Rodent studies are reassuring, revealing no evidence of teratogenicity or IUGR despite the use of doses higher than those used clinically.

■ **Breastfeeding Safety** — Most cephalosporins are excreted into breast milk. While there is no published experience in nursing women, **cefdinir** is generally considered compatible with breastfeeding.

■ **References** — Guay DR. Rel Clin Ther 2002; 24:473-89.

■ **Summary** —
- **Pregnancy Category B**
- **Lactation Category S**
- **Cefdinir** is used for the treatment of community-acquired pneumonia, acute bronchitis, maxillary sinusitis, and otitis media.
- There are other cephalosporins for which there is more experience regarding use during pregnancy and lactation.

Cefditoren (Spectracef)

■ **Class** — Antibiotic (*1st-generation cephalosporin*)

■ **Indications** — Bacterial infections, hospital-acquired pneumonia

■ **Mechanism** — Bactericidal—inhibits cell wall synthesis

■ **Dosage with Qualifiers** — Acute infection—200-400mg PO with food bid for 10d
Hospital-acquired pneumonia—400mg PO with food bid ×14d
NOTE—renal dosing
- **Contraindications**—hypersensitivity to drug or class, hypersensitivity to milk proteins, carnitine deficiency
- **Caution**—penicillin allergy, renal dysfunction, antibiotic-associated colitis, concomitant use of nephrotoxic drugs, seizures

■ **Maternal Considerations** — There is no published experience with **cefditoren** during pregnancy. Cephalosporins are generally considered safe during pregnancy.

Side effects include seizures, nausea, diarrhea, pseudomembranous colitis, abdominal pain, dyspepsia, flatulence, vomiting, anorexia, constipation, abnormal stools, Stevens-Johnson syndrome, vaginal moniliasis, vaginitis, headache, asthenia, dizziness, insomnia, rash, leukorrhea, pruritus, and somnolence.

■ **Fetal Considerations** — There are no adequate reports or well-controlled studies in human fetuses. It is unknown whether **cefditoren** crosses the human placenta. Rodent studies are reassuring, revealing no evidence of teratogenicity or IUGR despite the use of doses higher than those used clinically.

■ **Breastfeeding Safety** — Most cephalosporins are excreted into breast milk. While there is no published experience in nursing women, **cefditoren** is generally considered compatible with breastfeeding.

■ **References** — Guay DR. Rel Clin Ther 2002; 24:473-89.

■ **Summary**
- **Pregnancy Category B**
- **Lactation Category S**
- **Cefditoren** is used for the treatment of community-acquired pneumonia, acute bronchitis, maxillary sinusitis, and otitis media.
- There are other cephalosporins for which there is more experience regarding use during pregnancy and lactation.

Cefepime (Maxipime)

■ **Class** — Antibiotic (*4th-generation cephalosporin*)

■ **Indications** — Bacterial infections (<u>gram-positive aerobes</u>: *Staphylococcus aureus* (methicillin resistant), *Staphylococcus epidermidis*, *Streptococcus pneumoniae*; <u>gram-negative aerobes</u>: *Escherichia coli*, *Klebsiella*, *Enterobacter*, *Proteus mirabilis*, *Pseudomonas aeruginosa*)

■ **Mechanism** — Bactericidal—inhibits cell wall synthesis

■ **Dosage with Qualifiers** — <u>Bacterial infection</u>—1-2g IV or IM q12h
<u>Uncomplicated UTI</u>—0.5-1g IV/IM q12h
NOTE—renal dosing
- **Contraindications**—hypersensitivity to drug or class
- **Caution**—penicillin allergy, renal dysfunction, antibiotic-associated colitis, seizure disorder, concomitant use of nephrotoxic drugs

- **Maternal Considerations** ⋯⋯ **Cefepime** is used to treat lower respiratory tract infections, genitourinary tract infections, skin infections, and neutropenic patients because of its antimicrobial spectrum. Limited study suggests it is effective as **cefotaxime** for the treatment of acute obstetric and gynecologic infections. Third and 4th-generation cephalosporins, such as **cefotaxime, cefoperazone, ceftriaxone, ceftazidime** or **ceftizoxime** are generally not recommended for surgical prophylaxis. Despite these recommendations, they have been accepted by the medical community for prophylaxis and are today commonly misused. Cephalosporins are usually considered safe during pregnancy.
  Side effects include anaphylaxis, seizures, pseudomembranous colitis, nephrotoxicity, leukopenia, thrombocytopenia, erythema multiforme, exfoliative dermatitis, Stevens-Johnson syndrome, and cholestatic jaundice.

- **Fetal Considerations** ⋯⋯ There are no adequate reports or well-controlled studies in human fetuses. It is unknown whether **cefepime** crosses the human placenta. Rodent studies are reassuring, revealing no evidence of teratogenicity or IUGR despite the use of doses higher than those used clinically.

- **Breastfeeding Safety** ⋯⋯ Most cephalosporins are excreted into breast milk. While there is no published experience in nursing women, **cefepime** is generally considered compatible with breastfeeding.

- **References** ⋯⋯ Newton ER, Yeomans ER, Pastorek JG, et al. J Antimicrob Chemother 1993; 32(Suppl B):195-204.
  Kai S, Kohmura H, Ishikawa K, et al. Jpn J Antibiot 1992; 45:642-60.

- **Summary** ⋯⋯
  - **Pregnancy Category B**
  - **Lactation Category S**
  - Third and 4th-generation cephalosporins are generally not recommended for surgical prophylaxis.
  - There are alternative agents for which there is more experience during pregnancy and lactation.

Cefixime (Suprax; Ultraxime)

- **Class** ⋯⋯ Antibiotic (*3rd-generation cephalosporin*)

- **Indications** ⋯⋯ Bacterial infections (<u>gram-positive aerobes</u>: *Staphylococcus pyogenes, Streptococcus pneumoniae*; <u>gram-negative aerobes</u>: *Escherichia coli, Proteus, Haemophilus influenzae, Moraxella catarrhalis, Neisseria gonorrhoeae*)

■ **Mechanism** ⋯⋯⋯⋯⋯⋯⋯⋯ Bactericidal—inhibits cell wall synthesis

■ **Dosage with Qualifiers** ⋯⋯ Bacterial infection—400mg PO qd
Gonorrhea (uncomplicated)—400mg PO ×1
NOTE—renal dosing
- **Contraindications**—hypersensitivity to drug or class
- **Caution**—penicillin allergy, renal dysfunction, antibiotic-associated colitis, seizure disorder, concomitant use of nephrotoxic drugs

■ **Maternal Considerations** ⋯⋯ **Cefixime** has been discontinued in the U.S. It is used to treat lower respiratory tract infections, otitis media, pharyngitis, acute bronchitis, acute exacerbation of chronic bronchitis, gonorrhea, genitourinary tract infections, skin infections, and neutropenic patients because of its antimicrobial spectrum. **Cefixime** is an effective and safe oral medication during pregnancy for the treatment of acute obstetric and sexually transmitted diseases such as gonorrhea. Third and 4th generation cephalosporins, such as **cefotaxime**, **cefoperazone**, **ceftriaxone**, **ceftazidime,** and **ceftizoxime,** are generally not recommended for surgical prophylaxis. Despite these recommendations, they have been accepted by the medical community for prophylaxis and are today commonly misused. Cephalosporins are usually considered safe during pregnancy.
Side effects include anaphylaxis, seizures, pseudomembranous colitis, neutropenia, thrombocytopenia, erythema multiforme, exfoliative dermatitis, and cholestatic jaundice.

■ **Fetal Considerations** ⋯⋯⋯⋯ There are no adequate reports or well-controlled studies in human fetuses. It is unknown whether **cefixime** crosses the human placenta. Transfer across the rodent placenta is poor. Rodent studies are reassuring, revealing no evidence of teratogenicity or IUGR despite the use of doses higher than those used clinically.

■ **Breastfeeding Safety** ⋯⋯⋯⋯ Most cephalosporins are excreted into breast milk. While there is no published experience in nursing women, **cefixime** is generally considered compatible with breastfeeding. Transfer into rodent milk occurs at low levels.

■ **References** ⋯⋯⋯⋯⋯⋯⋯⋯⋯ Mahon BE, Rosenman MB, Graham MF, Fortenberry JD. Am J Obstet Gynecol 2002; 186:1320-5.
Gray RH, Wabwire-Mangen F, Kigozi G, et al. Am J Obstet Gynecol 2001; 185:1209-17.
Donders GG. Drugs 2000; 59:477-85.
Ramus RM, Sheffield JS, Mayfield JA, Wendel GD Jr. Am J Obstet Gynecol 2001; 185:629-32.
Wilton LV, Pearce GL, Mann RD. Br J Clin Pharmacol 1996; 41:277-84.
Halperin-Walega E, Batra VK, Tonelli AP, Barr A, Yacobi A. Drug Metab Dispos 1988; 16:130-4.

■ **Summary** ──────── • **Pregnancy Category B**
• **Lactation Category S**
• Third and 4th-generation cephalosporins are generally not recommended for surgical prophylaxis.
• There are alternative agents for which there is more experience during pregnancy and lactation.

Cefmetazole (Zefazone)

■ **Class** ──────── Antibiotic (2nd-generation cephalosporin)

■ **Indications** ──────── Bacterial infection (<u>gram-positive aerobes</u>: Staphylococcus aureus, Staphylococcus epidermidis, Streptococcus pneumoniae, Streptococcus pyogenes; <u>gram-negative aerobes</u>: Escherichia coli, Klebsiella, Enterobacter, Proteus mirabilis, Morganella morganii; <u>anaerobic organisms</u>: Peptococcus, Peptostreptococcus, Clostridium, Bacteroides, Fusobacterium)

■ **Mechanism** ──────── Bactericidal—inhibits cell wall synthesis

■ **Dosage with Qualifiers** ──────── <u>Bacterial infection</u>—2gm IV q6-12h for 5-14d
<u>Perioperative prophylaxis</u>—1-2g IV 30-90min prior to procedure; may be repeated in 8-16h
• **Contraindications**—hypersensitivity to drug or class
• **Caution**—penicillin allergy, renal dysfunction, antibiotic-associated colitis, seizure disorder, concomitant use of nephrotoxic drugs

■ **Maternal Considerations** ──────── There are no adequate reports or well-controlled studies in pregnant women. **Cefmetazole** is highly effective against most causes of bacterial vaginosis during pregnancy. **Cefmetazole** appears equivalent to **cefoxitin** in reducing post-cesarean section endometritis. Cephalosporins are usually considered safe during pregnancy.
Side effects include anaphylaxis, Stevens-Johnson syndrome, renal failure, diarrhea, headache, hypotension, nausea, rash, pruritus, fever, epigastric pain, vaginitis, pleural effusion, dyspnea, and erythema.

■ **Fetal Considerations** ──────── There are no adequate reports or well-controlled studies in human fetuses. **Cefmetazole** rapidly crosses the human placenta, yielding fetal levels in excess of the typical MIC. Rodent studies are reassuring, revealing no evidence of teratogenicity or IUGR despite the use of doses higher than those used clinically.

■ **Breastfeeding Safety** ··············· Only a scant amount of **cefmetazole** is excreted into human breast milk, and it is generally considered compatible with breastfeeding.

■ **References** ····························· Crombleholme WR, Green JR, Ohm-Smith M, et al. J Antimicrob Chemother 1989; 23(Suppl D): 97-104.
Puapermpoonsiri S, Watanabe K, Kato N, Ueno K. Antimicrob Agents Chemother 1997; 41:2297-9.
Ninomiya K, Yoshimoto T, Hasegawa Y. Jpn J Antibiot 1984; 37:14-7.
Cho N, Fukunaga K, Kunii K. Jpn J Antibiot 1981; 34:915-24.

■ **Summary** ····························· • **Pregnancy Category B**
• **Lactation Category S**
• **Cefmetazole** is an effective agent for the treatment of bacterial vaginosis and postpartum endometritis.
• Selection is often based on cost.

Cefonicid (Monocid)

■ **Class**··································· Antibiotic (2nd-generation cephalosporin)

■ **Indications** ····························· Bacterial infections (gram-positive aerobes: Staphylococcus aureus, Staphylococcus epidermidis, Streptococcus pneumoniae; gram-negative aerobes: Escherichia coli, Klebsiella, Enterobacter, Proteus mirabilis, Pseudomonas aeruginosa, Neisseria gonorrhoeae; gram-positive anaerobes: Clostridium perfringens, Peptostreptococcus, Peptococcus, Propionibacterium acnes; gram-negative anaerobes: Fusobacterium nucleatum)

■ **Mechanism**······························ Bactericidal—inhibits cell wall synthesis

■ **Dosage with Qualifiers** ········· Bacterial infection—10-25mg/kg (or 1g) IV q24h
Cesarean section prophylaxis—1g IV 30min prior to procedure
• **Contraindications**—hypersensitivity to drug or class
• **Caution**—penicillin allergy, renal dysfunction, antibiotic-associated colitis, seizure disorder, concomitant use of nephrotoxic drugs

■ **Maternal Considerations** ········ Because of its antimicrobial spectrum, **cefonicid** is used to treat lower respiratory tract infections, genitourinary tract infections, skin infections, septicemia, and for surgical prophylaxis. It appears effective and safe during pregnancy for the treatment of acute infections and post-cesarean section prophylaxis, but has no unique advantage over other cephalosporins for most indications. Cost is often a key decision factor. Cephalosporins are usually considered safe during pregnancy.

Side effects include anaphylaxis, seizures, neutropenia, pseudomembranous colitis, thrombocytopenia, erythema multiforme, exfoliative dermatitis, cholestatic jaundice, and positive Coombs' test.

■ **Fetal Considerations**

There are no adequate reports or well-controlled studies in human fetuses. It is unknown whether **cefonicid** crosses the human placenta. Rodent studies are reassuring, revealing no evidence of teratogenicity or IUGR despite the use of doses higher than those used clinically.

■ **Breastfeeding Safety**

Cefonicid is excreted at low concentrations into human breast milk, but is generally considered compatible with breastfeeding.

■ **References**

Fejgin MD, Markov S, Goshen S, et al. Int J Gynaecol Obstet 1993; 43:257-61.
Faro S, Martens MG, Hammill HA, et al. Am J Obstet Gynecol 1990; 162:900-10.
Duff P, Robertson AW, Read JA. Obstet Gynecol 1987; 70:718-21.
Lou MA, Wu YH, Jacob LS, Pitkin DH. Infect Dis 1984; 6(Suppl 4):S816-20.

■ **Summary**

- **Pregnancy Category B**
- **Lactation Category S**
- **Cefonicid** is effective and safe during pregnancy for the treatment of acute obstetric infection and surgical prophylaxis.
- A favorable cost profile is a key factor in its selection.

Cefoperazone (Cefobid)

■ **Class**

Antibiotic (*3rd-generation cephalosporin*)

■ **Indications**

Bacterial infections (<u>gram-positive aerobes</u>: *Staphylococcus aureus, Staphylococcus epidermidis, Streptococcus pneumoniae, Streptococcus pyogenes, Enterococcus*; <u>gram-negative aerobes</u>: *Escherichia coli, Klebsiella, Enterobacter, Citrobacter, Proteus mirabilis, Pseudomonas aeruginosa, Neisseria gonorrhoeae*; <u>gram-positive anaerobes</u>: *Clostridium perfringens, Peptostreptococcus, Peptococcus, Propionibacterium acnes*)

■ **Mechanism**

Bactericidal—inhibits cell wall synthesis

■ **Dosage with Qualifiers**

<u>Bacterial infection</u>—1-2g IV or IM q12h
<u>Cesarean section prophylaxis</u>—1-2g IV
NOTE—may be combined with **Sulbactam**

- **Contraindications**—hypersensitivity to drug or class
- **Caution**—penicillin allergy, renal dysfunction, antibiotic-associated colitis, seizure disorder, concomitant use of nephrotoxic drugs, altered hepatic function

■ **Maternal Considerations** ⋯⋯ Because of its antimicrobial spectrum, **cefoperazone** is used to treat lower respiratory tract infections, genitourinary tract infections, skin infections, septicemia, and for surgical prophylaxis. **Cefoperazone** appears effective and safe during pregnancy for the treatment of acute infections. Clearance is only modestly affected by pregnancy. Third and 4th generation cephalosporins, such as **cefotaxime, cefoperazone, ceftriaxone, ceftazidime,** and **ceftizoxime,** are generally not recommended for surgical prophylaxis. Despite these recommendations, they have been accepted by the medical community for prophylaxis and are today commonly misused.
Side effects include anaphylaxis, serum sickness, pseudomembranous colitis, neutropenia, rash, urticaria, thrombocytopenia, and nausea.

■ **Fetal Considerations** ⋯⋯ There are no adequate reports or well-controlled studies in human fetuses. **Cefoperazone** crosses the human placenta, but to a lower degree than **ceftizoxime**. Rodent studies are reassuring, revealing no evidence of teratogenicity or IUGR despite the use of doses higher than those used clinically.

■ **Breastfeeding Safety** ⋯⋯ **Cefoperazone** is excreted in small amounts into human breast milk, and is generally considered compatible with breastfeeding.

■ **References** ⋯⋯ Geroulanos S, Marathias K, Kriaras J, Kadas B. J Chemother 2001; (13)1:23-6.
Ng NK, Sivalingam N. Med J Malaysia 1992; 47:273-9.
Ogita S, Imanaka M, Matsumoto M, et al. Am J Obstet Gynecol 1988; 158:23-7.
Fortunato SJ, Bawdon RE, Maberry MC, Swan KF. Obstet Gynecol 1990; 75:830-3.
Gonik B, Feldman S, Pickering LK, Doughtie CG. Antimicrob Agents Chemother 1986; 30:874-6.
Gilstrap LC 3rd, St Clair PJ, Gibbs RS, Maier RC. Antimicrob Agents Chemother 1986; 30:808-9.
Matsuda S, Kashiwagura T, Hirayama H. Jpn J Antibiot 1985; 38:223-9.

■ **Summary** ⋯⋯
- **Pregnancy Category B**
- **Lactation Category S**
- **Cefoperazone** appears effective and safe during pregnancy for the treatment of acute obstetric infection.
- Third and 4th generation cephalosporins are generally not recommended for surgical prophylaxis.

Ceforanide

■ **Class** — Antibiotic (2nd-generation cephalosporin)

■ **Indications** — Bacterial infection, surgical prophylaxis

■ **Mechanism** — Bactericidal—inhibits cell wall synthesis

■ **Dosage with Qualifiers** — Bacterial infection—500mg-1g IV bid
Surgical prophylaxis—500mg-1g IV ×1
- **Contraindications**—hypersensitivity to drug or class
- **Caution**—penicillin allergy, renal dysfunction, antibiotic-associated colitis, seizure disorder, concomitant use of nephrotoxic drugs

■ **Maternal Considerations** — There are no adequate and well-controlled studies of **ceforanide** in pregnant women. It appears to have no unique advantage over other cephalosporins for most indications. Cephalosporins are usually considered safe during pregnancy.
Side effects include anaphylaxis, serum sickness, pseudomembranous colitis, diarrhea, nausea, vomiting, constipation, headache, and fever.

■ **Fetal Considerations** — There are no adequate and well-controlled studies in human fetuses. It is unknown whether **ceforanide** crosses the human placenta. Rodent studies are reassuring, revealing no evidence of teratogenicity or IUGR despite the use of doses higher than those used clinically.

■ **Breastfeeding Safety** — Most cephalosporins are excreted into breast milk. While there is no published experience in nursing women, **ceforanide** is generally considered compatible with breastfeeding.

■ **References** — Saravolatz LD, Lee C, Drukker B. Obstet Gynecol 1985; 66:513-6.

■ **Summary** —
- **Pregnancy Category B**
- **Lactation Category S**
- **Ceforanide** appears safe during pregnancy for the treatment of acute obstetric infections such as chorioamnionitis.

Cefotaxime (Claforan; Zetaxim)

- **Class** — Antibiotic (3rd-generation cephalosporin)

- **Indications** — Bacterial infections (<u>gram-positive aerobes</u>: *Staphylococcus aureus, Staphylococcus epidermidis, Streptococcus pneumoniae, Streptococcus pyogenes, Enterococcus*; <u>gram-negative aerobes</u>: *Escherichia coli, Klebsiella, Enterobacter, Citrobacter, Proteus mirabilis, Pseudomonas aeruginosa, Neisseria gonorrhoeae*; <u>gram-positive anaerobes</u>: *Clostridium perfringens, Peptostreptococcus, Peptococcus, Propionibacterium acnes*)

- **Mechanism** — Bactericidal—inhibits cell wall synthesis

- **Dosage with Qualifiers** — <u>Bacterial infection</u>—1-2g IM or IV q8h
  <u>Gonorrhea</u>—1g IM ×1
  <u>Surgical prophylaxis</u>—1g IV/IM 30-90min preoperatively
  NOTE—renal dosing
  - **Contraindications**—hypersensitivity to drug or class
  - **Caution**—penicillin allergy, renal dysfunction, antibiotic-associated colitis, seizure disorder, concomitant use of nephrotoxic drugs

- **Maternal Considerations** — **Cefotaxime** is used to treat lower respiratory tract infections, genitourinary tract infections, skin infections, septicemia, and for surgical prophylaxis because of its antimicrobial spectrum. **Cefotaxime** appears effective and safe during pregnancy for the treatment of acute infections. High amniotic fluid concentrations suggest it may be advantageous for the treatment of chorioamnionitis. Third and 4th generation cephalosporins, such as **cefotaxime, cefoperazone, ceftriaxone, ceftazidime,** and **ceftizoxime,** are generally not recommended for surgical prophylaxis. Despite these recommendations, they have been accepted by the medical community for prophylaxis and are today commonly misused.
  Side effects include anaphylaxis, serum sickness, pseudomembranous colitis, diarrhea, nausea, vomiting, constipation, headache, fever, neutropenia, thrombocytopenia, rash, and urticaria.

- **Fetal Considerations** — There are no adequate reports or well-controlled studies in human fetuses. **Cefotaxime** crosses the human placenta. And though the kinetics remain to be elucidated, it achieves amniotic fluid concentrations that exceed the MIC90 for most strains of *E. coli*. Rodent studies are reassuring, revealing no evidence of teratogenicity or IUGR despite the use of doses higher than those used clinically.

- **Breastfeeding Safety** — Scant quantities of **cefotaxime** are excreted into human breast milk, and it is generally considered compatible with breastfeeding.

- **References** .... Geroulanos S, Marathias K, Kriaras J, Kadas B. J Chemother 2001; (13)1:23-6.

  Kafetzis DA, Siafas CA, Georgakopoulos PA, Papadatos CJ. Acta Paediatr Scand 1981; 70:285-8.

  Kafetzis DA, Lazarides CV, Siafas CA, et al. J Antimicrob Chemother 1980; 6(Suppl A):135-41.

  Ninomiya K, Hasegawa Y, Kanamoto T, et al. Jpn J Antibiot 1982; 35:1882-92.

  Yasuda J, Yamamoto T, Ito M, et al. Jpn J Antibiot 1982; 35:1877-81.

- **Summary** ....
  - **Pregnancy Category B**
  - **Lactation Category S**
  - **Cefotaxime** appears effective and safe during pregnancy for the treatment of acute obstetric infection and surgical prophylaxis.
  - Third and 4th generation cephalosporins are generally not recommended for surgical prophylaxis.

Cefotetan (Apatef; Cefotan)

- **Class** .... Antibiotic (2nd-generation cephalosporin)

- **Indications** .... Bacterial infections (gram-positive aerobes: *Staphylococcus aureus, Staphylococcus epidermidis, Streptococcus pneumoniae, Streptococcus pyogenes, Enterococcus*; gram-negative aerobes: *Escherichia coli, Klebsiella, Enterobacter, Citrobacter, Proteus mirabilis, Pseudomonas aeruginosa, Neisseria gonorrhoeae*; gram-positive anaerobes: *Clostridium perfringens, Peptostreptococcus, Peptococcus, Propionibacterium acnes*)

- **Mechanism** .... Bactericidal—inhibits cell wall synthesis

- **Dosage with Qualifiers** .... Bacterial infection—1-3g IM or IV q12h
  Preoperative prophylaxis—1-2g IV 30-60 min prior to surgery
  Cesarean section surgical prophylaxis—1-2g IV after umbilical cord clamping
  NOTE—renal dosing
  - **Contraindications**—hypersensitivity to drug or class
  - **Caution**—penicillin allergy, renal dysfunction, antibiotic-associated colitis, seizure disorder, concomitant use of nephrotoxic drugs

- **Maternal Considerations** .... Because of its antimicrobial spectrum, **cefotetan** is used to treat lower respiratory tract infections, genitourinary tract infections, skin infections, septicemia, and surgical prophylaxis. **Cefotetan** appears effective and safe during pregnancy for the treatment of acute infections. However, it has no activity against *Chlamydia trachomatis*. When used for the treatment of pelvic inflammatory disease, appropriate antichlamydial coverage should be added. Single dose **cefotetan** can replace the multidose **cefoxitin** regimen for post-cesarean section prophylaxis with considerable cost savings. Case reports describe maternal hemolysis associated with **cefotetan** for post-cesarean section prophylaxis.

Side effects include anaphylaxis, agranulocytosis, prolonged INR, pseudomembranous colitis, neutropenia, thrombocytopenia, rash, urticaria, and hemolysis.

■ **Fetal Considerations**
There are no adequate reports or well-controlled studies in human fetuses. **Cefotetan** crosses both rodent and human placentas, though the kinetics remain to be elucidated. Rodent studies are reassuring, revealing no evidence of teratogenicity or IUGR despite the use of doses higher than those used clinically.

■ **Breastfeeding Safety**
While there are no adequate reports or well-controlled studies in nursing women, **cefotetan** is excreted in scant quantities into human breast milk and is generally considered compatible with breastfeeding.

■ **References**
Spinnato JA, Youkilis B, Cook VD, et al. J Matern Fetal Med 2000; 9:348-50.
Naylor CS, Steele L, Hsi R, et al. Am J Obstet Gynecol 2000; 182:1427-8.
Todd MW, Benrubi G. Hosp Formul 1990; 25:446-8,450.
Noyes N, Berkeley AS, Freedman K, Ledger W. Infect Dis Obstet Gynecol 1998; 6:220-3.
Suzuki H, Imamura K, Yoshida T, et al. J Antimicrob Chemother 1983; 11:179-83.
Martin C, Thomachot L, Albanese J. Clin Pharmacokinet 1994; 26:248-58.

■ **Summary**
• **Pregnancy Category B**
• **Lactation Category S**
• **Cefotetan** appears effective and safe during pregnancy for the treatment of acute obstetric infection and for surgical prophylaxis.

Cefoxitin (Cefxitin; Mefoxin)

■ **Class** — Antibiotic (2nd-generation cephalosporin)

■ **Indications** — Bacterial infections (<u>gram-positive aerobes</u>: *Staphylococcus aureus, Staphylococcus epidermidis, Streptococcus pneumoniae, Streptococcus pyogenes*, Enterococcus; <u>gram-negative aerobes</u>: *Escherichia coli*, Klebsiella, Enterobacter, Citrobacter, *Proteus mirabilis, Pseudomonas aeruginosa, Neisseria gonorrhoeae*; <u>gram-positive anaerobes</u>: *Clostridium perfringens*, Peptostreptococcus, Peptococcus, *Propionibacterium acnes*)

■ **Mechanism** — Bactericidal—inhibits cell wall synthesis

■ **Dosage with Qualifiers** — <u>Bacterial infection</u>—1-2g IV q6-q8h; alternatively for severe infection, 2g q4h or 3g q6h
<u>Perioperative prophylaxis</u>—2g IV, 30-60min preoperatively
NOTE—renal dosing
- **Contraindications**—hypersensitivity to drug or class
- **Caution**—penicillin allergy, renal dysfunction, antibiotic-associated colitis, seizure disorder, concomitant use of nephrotoxic drugs

■ **Maternal Considerations** — **Cefoxitin** is used to treat lower respiratory tract infections, genitourinary tract infections, skin infections, septicemia, and for surgical prophylaxis because of its antimicrobial spectrum. It is a preferred agent for the treatment of PID where inpatient and outpatient therapy (combined with **doxycycline**) yield similar results. **Cefoxitin** appears effective and safe during pregnancy for the treatment of acute infection, though there are more cost-effective regimens for post-cesarean section prophylaxis. It is not beneficial for elective cesarean delivery.
Side effects include anaphylaxis, agranulocytosis, serum sickness, pseudomembranous colitis, neutropenia, thrombocytopenia, acute renal failure, and hemolytic anemia.

■ **Fetal Considerations** — There are no adequate and well-controlled studies in human fetuses. **Cefoxitin** crosses the human placenta achieving an F:M ratio approximating 0.6 45min after maternal injection. Rodent studies are reassuring, revealing no evidence of teratogenicity or IUGR despite the use of doses higher than those used clinically.

■ **Breastfeeding Safety** — Most cephalosporins are excreted into breast milk. There is little detectable **cefoxitin** in human breast milk after post-cesarean section prophylaxis. It is generally considered compatible with breastfeeding.

■ **References** — Amstey MS, Casian-Colon AE. Obstet Gynecol 1997; 90:667-8.
Todd MW, Benrubi G. Hosp Formul 1990; 25:446-8,450.

Bagratee JS, Moodley J, Kleinschmidt I, Zawilski W. BJOG 2001; 108:143-8.

Ness RB, Soper DE, Holley RL, et al. Am J Obstet Gynecol 2002; 186:929-37.

Noyes N, Berkeley AS, Freedman K, Ledger W. Infect Dis Obstet Gynecol 1998; 6:220-3.

Dubois M, Delapierre D, Chanteux L, et al. J Clin Pharmacol 1981; 21:477-83.

Roex AJ, van Loenen AC, Puyenbroek JI, Arts NF. Eur J Obstet Gynecol Reprod Biol 1987; 25:299-302.

Ness RB, Soper DE, Holley RL, et al. Am J Obstet Gynecol 2002; 186:929-37.

■ **Summary**
- **Pregnancy Category B**
- **Lactation Category S**
- **Cefoxitin** appears effective and safe during pregnancy for the treatment of acute obstetric infection.
- There are more cost-effective regimens for post-cesarean section prophylaxis.

Cefpodoxime (Banan; Cepodem; Vantin)

■ **Class** Antibiotic (3rd-generation cephalosporin)

■ **Indications** Bacterial infections (gram-positive aerobes: Staphylococcus aureus, Staphylococcus epidermidis, Streptococcus pneumoniae, Streptococcus pyogenes, Enterococcus; gram-negative aerobes: Escherichia coli, Klebsiella, Enterobacter, Citrobacter, Proteus mirabilis, Pseudomonas aeruginosa, Neisseria gonorrhoeae; gram-positive anaerobes: Clostridium perfringens, Peptostreptococcus, Peptococcus, Propionibacterium acnes)

■ **Mechanism** Bactericidal—inhibits cell wall synthesis

■ **Dosage with Qualifiers** Bacterial infection—100-400mg PO bid, max 800mg qd
Surgical prophylaxis—100mg PO bid ×3d
- **Contraindications**—hypersensitivity to drug or class
- **Caution**—penicillin allergy, renal dysfunction, antibiotic-associated colitis, seizure disorder, concomitant use of nephrotoxic drugs

■ **Maternal Considerations** There is little published experience with **cefpodoxime** during pregnancy. Third and 4th generation cephalosporins are generally not recommended for surgical prophylaxis. Despite these recommendations, they have been accepted by the medical community for prophylaxis and are commonly misused. Cephalosporins are usually considered safe during pregnancy.

Side effects include anaphylaxis, seizure, diarrhea, pseudomembranous colitis, leukopenia, anemia, thrombocytopenia, Stevens-Johnson syndrome, nausea, dyspepsia, rash, and pruritus.

■ **Fetal Considerations** — There are no adequate and well-controlled studies in human fetuses. It is unknown whether **cefpodoxime** crosses the human placenta. Rodent studies are reassuring, revealing no evidence of teratogenicity or IUGR despite the use of doses higher than those used clinically.

■ **Breastfeeding Safety** — Most cephalosporins are excreted into breast milk. While there is no published experience in nursing women, **cefpodoxime** reportedly is excreted in breast milk at modest levels. The kinetics remain to be detailed.

■ **References** — Hayashi H, Yaginuma Y, Yamashita T, et al. Chemotherapy 2000; 46:213-8.
Escande F, Borde M, Pateyron F. Arch Pediatr 1997; 4:1116-8.
Mikamo H, Izumi K, Ito K, et al. Jpn J Antibiot 1993; 46:269-73.

■ **Summary** —
● **Pregnancy Category B**
● **Lactation Category U**
● **Cefpodoxime** appears effective and safe during pregnancy for the treatment of acute obstetric infection.
● There are alternative agents for which there is more experience during pregnancy and lactation.
● Third and 4th generation cephalosporins are generally not recommended for surgical prophylaxis.

Cefprozil (Cefzil; Procef)

■ **Class** — Antibiotic (2nd-generation cephalosporin)

■ **Indications** — Bacterial infections (<u>gram-positive aerobes</u>: *Staphylococcus aureus, Staphylococcus epidermidis, Streptococcus pneumoniae, Streptococcus pyogenes, Enterococcus*; <u>gram-negative aerobes</u>: *Escherichia coli, Klebsiella, Enterobacter, Citrobacter, Proteus mirabilis, Pseudomonas aeruginosa, Neisseria gonorrhoeae*; <u>gram-positive anaerobes</u>: *Clostridium perfringens, Peptostreptococcus, Peptococcus, Propionibacterium acnes*)

■ **Mechanism** — Bactericidal—inhibits cell wall synthesis

■ **Dosage with Qualifiers** — Bacterial infection—250-500mg PO qd or bid
NOTE—renal dosing
● **Contraindications**—hypersensitivity to drug or class

- **Caution**—penicillin allergy, renal dysfunction, antibiotic-associated colitis, seizure disorder, concomitant use of nephrotoxic drugs

■ **Maternal Considerations** There is no published experience with **cefprozil** during pregnancy. Cephalosporins are usually considered safe during pregnancy.
Side effects include anaphylaxis, seizures, pseudomembranous colitis, nephrotoxicity, leukopenia, thrombocytopenia, and erythema multiforme.

■ **Fetal Considerations** There are no adequate and well-controlled studies in human fetuses. It is unknown whether **cefprozil** crosses the human placenta. Small quantities cross the rodent placenta. Rodent studies are reassuring, revealing no evidence of teratogenicity or IUGR despite the use of doses higher than those used clinically.

■ **Breastfeeding Safety** **Cefprozil** is excreted into human breast milk in very small quantities, but even if one assumes the concentration in milk remains constant at the highest observed, a neonate ingesting an average of 800ml of milk per day would ingest a maximum of about 3mg of **cefprozil** per day.

■ **References** Shyu WC, Shah VR, Campbell DA, et al. Antimicrob Agents Chemother 1992; 36:938-41.
Nakanomyo H, Ishikawa K, Esumi Y, et al. Jpn J Antibiot 1990(l); 43:1325-34.

■ **Summary**
- **Pregnancy Category B**
- **Lactation Category S**
- There are alternative agents for which there is more experience during pregnancy and lactation.

Ceftazidime (Ceptaz; Fortaz; Tazicef; Tazidime)

■ **Class** Antibiotic (*3rd-generation cephalosporin*)

■ **Indications** Bacterial infections (gram-positive aerobes: *Staphylococcus aureus, Staphylococcus epidermidis, Streptococcus pneumoniae, Streptococcus pyogenes, Enterococcus*; gram-negative aerobes: *Escherichia coli, Klebsiella, Enterobacter, Citrobacter, Proteus mirabilis, Pseudomonas aeruginosa, Neisseria gonorrhoeae*; gram-positive anaerobes: *Clostridium perfringens, Peptostreptococcus, Peptococcus, Propionibacterium acnes*)

■ **Mechanism** Bactericidal—inhibits cell wall synthesis

- **Dosage with Qualifiers** ⋯⋯ <u>Bacterial infection</u>—1g IV or IM q8-12h (2g IV or IM q8h for meningitis)
NOTE—renal dosing
  - **Contraindications**—hypersensitivity to drug or class
  - **Caution**—penicillin allergy, impaired renal function, antibiotic-associated colitis, seizure disorder, concomitant use of nephrotoxic drugs

- **Maternal Considerations** ⋯⋯ **Ceftazidime** is a 3rd generation cephalosporin that retains a broad spectrum of *in vitro* antimicrobial activity and clinical utility in serious infections, particularly those due to major nosocomial pathogens, and respiratory infections in patients with cystic fibrosis. **Ceftazidime**-containing regimens are important for febrile episodes in neutropenic patients. There are no adequate and well-controlled studies of **ceftazidime** in pregnant women. Maternal renal elimination is increased during pregnancy. Third and 4th generation cephalosporins are not generally recommended for surgical prophylaxis. Despite these recommendations, they have been accepted by the medical community for prophylaxis and are today commonly misused.
Side effects include seizures, agranulocytosis, thrombocytopenia, and anaphylaxis.

- **Fetal Considerations** ⋯⋯ There are no adequate and well-controlled studies in human fetuses. **Ceftazidime** crosses the human placenta achieving an F:M ratio in the 2nd trimester approximating 0.15 and the M:AF ratio approximates 0.19. Rodent studies are reassuring, revealing no evidence of teratogenicity or IUGR despite the use of doses higher than those used clinically.

- **Breastfeeding Safety** ⋯⋯ **Ceftazidime** is excreted into human breast milk in very small quantities, but even if one assumes the concentration in milk remains constant at the highest observed, a neonate ingesting an average of 800ml of milk per day would ingest a maximum of about 4mg of **ceftazidime** per day.

- **References** ⋯⋯
Geroulanos S, Marathias K, Kriaras J, Kadas B. J Chemother 2001; (13)1:23-6.
Rains CP, Bryson HM, Peters DH. Drugs 1995; 49:577-617.
Nathorst-Boos J, Philipson A, Hedman A, Arvisson A. Am J Obstet Gynecol 1995; 172:163-6.
Kuzemko J, Crawford C. Lancet 1989; 2:385.
Tassi PG, Tarantini M, Cadenelli GP, et al. Int J Clin Pharmacol Ther Toxicol 1987; 25:582-8.
Jorgensen NP, Walstad RA, Molne K. Acta Obstet Gynecol Scand 1987; 66:29-33.
Kulakov VI, Voropaeva SD, Kasabulatov NM. Akush Ginekol (Mosk) 1995; 2:17-9.
Blanco JD, Jorgensen JH, Castaneda YS, Crawford SA. Antimicrob Agents Chemother 1983; 23:479-80.

■ **Summary** • **Pregnancy Category B**
• **Lactation Category S**
• Third and 4th generation **cephalosporins** are generally not recommended for surgical prophylaxis. There are alternative agents for which there is more experience during pregnancy and lactation.

Ceftibuten (Cedax)

■ **Class** — Antibiotic (3rd-generation cephalosporin)

■ **Indications** — Bacterial infections (<u>gram-positive aerobes</u>: Staphylococcus aureus, Staphylococcus epidermidis, Streptococcus pneumoniae, Streptococcus pyogenes, Enterococcus; <u>gram-negative aerobes</u>: Escherichia coli, Klebsiella, Enterobacter, Citrobacter, Proteus mirabilis, Pseudomonas aeruginosa, Neisseria gonorrhoeae; <u>gram-positive anaerobes</u>: Clostridium perfringens, Peptostreptococcus, Peptococcus, Propionibacterium acnes)

■ **Mechanism** — Bactericidal—inhibits cell wall synthesis

■ **Dosage with Qualifiers** — <u>Bacterial infection</u>—400mg PO qd 1-2h after meals
NOTE—renal dosing
• **Contraindications**—hypersensitivity to drug or class
• **Caution**—penicillin allergy, renal dysfunction, antibiotic-associated colitis, seizure disorder, concomitant use of nephrotoxic drugs

■ **Maternal Considerations** — **Ceftibuten** is effective treatment for acute UTI during pregnancy. There is little experience during pregnancy with other indications. Third and 4th generation cephalosporins are not generally recommended for surgical prophylaxis. Despite these recommendations, they have been accepted by the medical community for prophylaxis and are today commonly misused. Cephalosporins are usually considered safe during pregnancy.
Side effects include seizures, agranulocytosis, thrombocytopenia, and anaphylaxis.

■ **Fetal Considerations** — There are no adequate reports or well-controlled studies in human fetuses. It is unknown whether **ceftibuten** crosses the human placenta. Rodent studies are reassuring, revealing no evidence of teratogenicity or IUGR despite the use of doses higher than those used clinically.

■ **Breastfeeding Safety** — Most cephalosporins are excreted into breast milk. However, the concentration of **ceftibuten** in breast milk is minimal and considered compatible with breastfeeding.

■ References ·········· Krcmery S, Hromec J, Demesova D. Int J Antimicrob
Agents 2001; 17:279-82.
Barr WH, Lin CC, Radwanski E, et al. Diagn Microbiol
Infect Dis 1991; 14:93-100.

■ Summary ············
- **Pregnancy Category B**
- **Lactation Category S**
- Third and 4th generation cephalosporins are generally
  not recommended for surgical prophylaxis. There are
  alternative agents for which there is more experience
  during pregnancy and lactation.

Ceftizoxime (Cefizox)

■ **Class** ············· *Antibiotic (3rd-generation cephalosporin)*

■ **Indications** ············· Bacterial infections (gram-positive aerobes: *Staphylococcus
aureus, Staphylococcus epidermidis, Streptococcus pneumoniae,
Streptococcus pyogenes, Enterococcus;* gram-negative aerobes:
*Escherichia coli, Klebsiella, Enterobacter, Citrobacter, Proteus
mirabilis, Pseudomonas aeruginosa, Neisseria gonorrhoeae;* gram-
positive anaerobes: *Clostridium perfringens, Peptostreptococcus,
Peptococcus, Propionibacterium acnes*)

■ **Mechanism** ············· Bactericidal—inhibits cell wall synthesis

■ **Dosage with Qualifiers** ············· Bacterial infection—1-2g IV or IM q8-12h; alternatively for
severe infection, 3-4g IV or IM q8h
Gonorrhea—1g IM
NOTE—renal dosing
- **Contraindications**—hypersensitivity to drug or class
- **Caution**—penicillin allergy, renal dysfunction,
  antibiotic-associated colitis, seizure disorder,
  concomitant use of nephrotoxic drugs

■ **Maternal Considerations** ············· **Ceftizoxime** appears effective and safe for the treatment
of acute infections during pregnancy. It has no effect on
the interval to delivery, or the duration of pregnancy in
women treated for preterm labor with intact membranes.
Third and 4th generation cephalosporins are not generally
recommended for surgical prophylaxis. Despite these
recommendations, they have been accepted by the
medical community for prophylaxis and are today
commonly misused. Cephalosporins are usually
considered safe during pregnancy.
Side effects include rash, anaphylaxis, pruritus, eosinophilia,
and hepatic enzyme elevation.

- **Fetal Considerations** ···· There are no adequate reports or well-controlled studies in human fetuses. **Ceftizoxime** concentrations are higher in cord blood and amniotic fluid than in maternal blood, perhaps because of more avid binding to fetal serum proteins. Rodent studies are reassuring, revealing no evidence of teratogenicity or IUGR despite the use of doses higher than those used clinically.

- **Breastfeeding Safety** ···· Most cephalosporins are excreted into breast milk, but the amount of **ceftizoxime** excreted is minimal and generally considered compatible with breastfeeding.

- **References** ···· Mercer BM, Arheart KL. Lancet 1995; 346:1271-9.
  Gordon M, Samuels P, Shubert P, et al. Am J Obstet Gynecol 1995; 172:1546-52.
  Fortunato SJ, Welt SI, Stewart JT. Am J Obstet Gynecol 1993; 168:914-5.
  Fortunato SJ, Welt SI, Eggleston M, et al. J Perinatol 1990; 10:252-6.
  Yamamoto T, Yasuda J, Kanao M, Okada H. Jpn J Antibiot 1988; 41:1164-71.
  Cho N, Fukunaga K, Kunii K, Tezuka K, Kobayashi I. Jpn J Antibiot 1988; 41:1142-54.

- **Summary** ····
  - **Pregnancy Category B**
  - **Lactation Category S**
  - Third and 4th generation cephalosporins are generally not recommended for surgical prophylaxis. There are alternative agents for which there is more experience during pregnancy and lactation.

Ceftriaxone (Cef-3; Rocephin; Rowecef)

- **Class** ···· Antibiotic (3rd-generation cephalosporin)

- **Indications** ···· Bacterial infections (gram-positive aerobes: *Staphylococcus aureus, Staphylococcus epidermidis, Streptococcus pneumoniae, Streptococcus pyogenes, Enterococcus;* gram-negative aerobes: *Escherichia coli, Klebsiella, Enterobacter, Citrobacter, Proteus mirabilis, Pseudomonas aeruginosa, Neisseria gonorrhoeae;* gram-positive anaerobes: *Clostridium perfringens, Peptostreptococcus, Peptococcus, Propionibacterium acnes*)

- **Mechanism** ···· Bactericidal—inhibits cell wall synthesis

- **Dosage with Qualifiers** ···· Gonorrhea—250mg IM ×1 (see CDC STD guidelines)
  Bacterial infection—1-2g IV qd
  Preoperative prophylaxis—1g IV

- **Contraindications**—hypersensitivity to drug or class
- **Caution**—penicillin allergy, renal dysfunction, antibiotic-associated colitis, seizure disorder, concomitant use of nephrotoxic drugs

■ **Maternal Considerations**

Ceftriaxone appears effective and safe during pregnancy for the treatment of acute infections. **Ceftriaxone** (single dose given IM) is a drug of choice for the treatment of gonorrhea in pregnancy. Third and 4th generation cephalosporins are not generally recommended for surgical prophylaxis. Despite these recommendations, they have been accepted by the medical community for prophylaxis and are today commonly misused. Cephalosporins are usually considered safe during pregnancy.
Side effects include thrombocytopenia, anaphylaxis, diarrhea, pseudomembranous colitis, eosinophilia, and vomiting.

■ **Fetal Considerations**

There are no adequate reports or well-controlled studies in human fetuses. **Ceftriaxone** rapidly crosses the human placenta reaching therapeutic concentrations in the fetal compartments. Some studies suggest that intrapartum prophylaxis with **ceftriaxone** decreases the rates of bacterial colonization and early-onset infection in newborns. Rodent studies are reassuring, revealing no evidence of teratogenicity or IUGR despite the use of doses higher than those used clinically. However, **ceftriaxone** weakly impairs *in vitro* rat nephrogenesis at all doses studied except 1000ug/ml, which blocked kidney development completely.

■ **Breastfeeding Safety**

Most cephalosporins are excreted into breast milk, but the amount of **ceftriaxone** excreted is <5% of a 2g maternal dose. It is generally considered compatible with breastfeeding.

■ **References**

Hercogova J, Brzonova I. Curr Opin Infect Dis 2001; 14:133-7.
Ramus RM, Sheffield JS, Mayfield JA, Wendel GD Jr. Am J Obstet Gynecol 2001; 185:629-32.
Shaffer EA. Curr Gastroenterol Rep 2001; 3:166-73.
Roberts JA. Urol Clin North Am 1999; 26:753-63.
Nathanson S, Moreau E, Merlet-Benichou C, Gilbert T. J Am Soc Nephrol 2000; 11:874-84.
Wing DA, Hendershott CM, Debuque L, Millar LK. Obstet Gynecol 1999; 94:683-8.
Saez-Llorens X, Ah-Chu MS, Castano E, et al. Clin Infect Dis 1995; 21:876-80.
Temmerman M, Njagi E, Nagelkerke N, et al. J Reprod Med 1995; 40:176-80.
Bourget P, Quinquis-Desmaris V, Fernandez H. Ann Pharmacother 1993; 27:294-7.

■ **Summary**
- **Pregnancy Category B**
- **Lactation Category S**
- **Ceftriaxone** appears effective and safe during pregnancy for the treatment of acute obstetric infections.
- Third and 4th generation cephalosporins are generally not recommended for surgical prophylaxis.

Cefuroxime (Ceftin; Kefurox; Zinacef)

■ **Class** — Antibiotic (*2nd-generation cephalosporin*)

■ **Indications** — Bacterial infections (<u>gram-positive aerobes</u>: *Staphylococcus aureus, Staphylococcus epidermidis, Streptococcus pneumoniae, Streptococcus pyogenes, Enterococcus*; <u>gram-negative aerobes</u>: *Escherichia coli, Klebsiella, Enterobacter, Citrobacter, Proteus mirabilis, Pseudomonas aeruginosa, Neisseria gonorrhoeae*; <u>gram-positive anaerobes</u>: *Clostridium perfringens, Peptostreptococcus, Peptococcus, Propionibacterium acnes*)

■ **Mechanism** — Bactericidal—inhibits cell wall synthesis

■ **Dosage with Qualifiers** — <u>Bacterial infection</u>—0.75-1.5g IM/IV q6-8h; max 3.0g q8h for bacterial meningitis
<u>Surgical prophylaxis</u>—1.5g IV ×1
NOTE—renal dosing
- **Contraindications**—hypersensitivity to drug or class
- **Caution**—penicillin allergy, renal dysfunction, antibiotic-associated colitis, seizure disorder, concomitant use of nephrotoxic drugs

■ **Maternal Considerations** — There are no adequate reports or well-controlled studies of **cefuroxime** in pregnant women. It appears to be safe and effective during pregnancy for the treatment of acute infections, especially pyelonephritis. One investigator suggested it was a first choice option for the treatment of acute pyelonephritis during pregnancy due to its tolerance, microbiological activity and superior clinical effect compared to **cephradine**. Cephalosporins are usually considered safe during pregnancy.
Side effects include thrombocytopenia, anaphylaxis, pseudomembranous colitis, eosinophilia, diarrhea, vomiting, interstitial nephritis, neutropenia, and elevated hepatic enzyme.

■ **Fetal Considerations** — There are no adequate reports or well-controlled studies in human fetuses. **Cefuroxime** crosses the human placenta, is unaffected by gestational age and anemia, but requires a dose of at least 1500mg to achieve the typical MIC in the fetus. There is no evidence of teratogenicity after 1st trimester exposure, and children of women treated with **cefuroxime** are normal at 18m. Rodent studies are reassuring, revealing no evidence of teratogenicity or IUGR despite the use of doses higher than those used clinically.

■ **Breastfeeding Safety**

Most cephalosporins are excreted into breast milk. While there are no adequate reports or well-controlled studies in nursing women, **cefuroxime** is generally considered compatible with breastfeeding.

■ **References**

Ovalle A, Martinez MA, Wolff M, et al. Rev Med Chil 2000; 128:749-57.
Berkovitch M, Segal-Socher I, Greenberg R, et al. Br J Clin Pharmacol 2000; 50:161-5.
Ovalle A, Martinez MA, Wolff M, et al. Rev Med Chil 2000; 128:749-57.
Manka W, Solowiow R, Okrzeja D. Drug Saf 2000; 22:83-8.
Holt DE, Fisk NM, Spencer JA, et al. Arch Dis Child 1993; 68:54-7.
De Leeuw JW, Roumen FJ, Bouckaert PX, et al. Obstet Gynecol 1993; 81:255-60.
Kristensen GB, Beiter EC, Mather O. Acta Obstet Gynecol Scand 1990; 69:497-500.

■ **Summary**
- **Pregnancy Category B**
- **Lactation Category S**
- A reasonable candidate for the noted indications.

Celecoxib (Celebrex)

■ **Class**

NSAID

■ **Indications**

Osteoarthritis, rheumatoid arthritis, familial adenomatous polyposis, acute pain

■ **Mechanism**

Cyclooxygenase-2 (COX-2) inhibitor

■ **Dosage with Qualifiers**

Osteoarthritis—200mg PO qd
Rheumatoid arthritis—100-200mg PO bid
Familial adenomatous polyposis—200mg PO bid; begin with 100mg PO qd
Pain, acute—200mg PO bid
- **Contraindications**—hypersensitivity to drug or class, nonsteroidal drug-induced asthma, nonsteroidal drug-induced urticaria, aspirin triad, hepatic and renal failure

- **Caution**—nasal polyps, GI bleeding, renal or hepatic dysfunction, CHF, hypertension, dehydration, fluid retention, asthma

■ **Maternal Considerations**

Celecoxib is the prototype COX-2 inhibitor. There are no adequate reports or well-controlled studies in pregnant women. *In vitro* studies reveal inhibition of uterine contractions by COX-2 inhibition. In one small trial, **celecoxib** was employed as a tocolytic agent. The authors concluded it was similar to indomethacin but with a lower frequency of adverse fetal effects. **Celecoxib** (80 and 160mg/kg/d) significantly reduces fertility, prolongs pregnancy, and inhibits normal cervical ripening in rats. *Side effects* include GI bleeding, GI ulceration, esophagitis, hypersensitivity reaction, bronchospasm, heart failure, hepatic toxicity, renal papillary necrosis, diarrhea, abdominal pain, flatulence, dizziness, and pharyngitis.

■ **Fetal Considerations**

There are no adequate reports or well-controlled studies in human fetuses. **Celecoxib** presumably crosses the human placenta, as do other NSAIDs, and can cause ductus arteriosus constriction late in pregnancy. It reduces renal blood and urine flows in the ovine fetus. **Celecoxib** increases the incidence of VSD and other fetal alterations such as fused ribs and misshapen sternum in rabbits treated during organogenesis. There is a dose-dependent increase in the frequency of diaphragmatic hernia in rats.

■ **Breastfeeding Safety**

There are no adequate reports or well-controlled studies in nursing women. A single case report found a concentration of 133ng/ml approximately 5h after a 100mg dose and an elimination half-life of 4.0-6.5h. If this level were sustained, the amount ingested by a 3.5kg newborn in 24h should be subclinical.

■ **References**

Sookvanichsilp N, Pulbutr P. Contraception 2002; 65:373-8.
Stika CS, Gross GA, Leguizamon G, et al. Am J Obstet Gynecol 2002; 187:653-60.
Slattery MM, Friel AM, Healy DG, Morrison JJ. Obstet Gynecol 2001; 98:563-9.
Davies NM, McLachlan AJ, Day RO, Williams KM. Clin Pharmacokinet 2000; 38:225-42.
Kajino H, Roman C, Clyman RI. Biol Neonate 2002; 82:257-62.
Bukowski R, Mackay L, Fittkow C, et al. Am J Obstet Gynecol 2001; 184:1374-8.
Knoppert DC, Stempak D, Baruchel S, Koren G. Pharmacotherapy 2003; 23:97-100.

■ **Summary**

- **Pregnancy Category C**
- **Lactation Category U**
- **Celecoxib** should be used during pregnancy and lactation only if the benefit justifies the potential perinatal risk.

Cephalexin (Alsporin; Biocef; Carnosporin; Cefaseptin; Cephin; Ceporexin-E; Check; Ed A-Ceph; Keflet; Keflex; Lopilexin; Mamlexin; Synecl; Winlex)

■ **Class** — Antibiotic (*1st-generation cephalosporin*)

■ **Indications** — Bacterial infections (<u>gram-positive aerobes</u>: *Staphylococcus aureus*, β-1 hemolytic streptococci; <u>gram-negative aerobes</u>: *Escherichia coli*, *Proteus mirabilis*, *Klebsiella* species, *Moraxella catarrhalis*)

■ **Mechanism** — Bactericidal—inhibits cell wall synthesis

■ **Dosage with Qualifiers** — <u>Bacterial infection</u>—250mg-1g PO q6h
  - **Contraindications**—hypersensitivity to drug or class
  - **Caution**—penicillin allergy, renal dysfunction, antibiotic associated colitis

■ **Maternal Considerations** — **Cephalexin** is used for the treatment of urinary tract infections, acute obstetric infections, and pharyngitis because of its antimicrobial spectrum. **Cephalexin** appears effective and safe during pregnancy for the treatment of acute bacterial infection. It is extensively used for the oral phase of treatment for pyelonephritis. *Side effects* include neutropenia, thrombocytopenia, anaphylaxis, pseudomembranous colitis, diarrhea, nausea, and elevated hepatic enzymes.

■ **Fetal Considerations** — There are no adequate reports or well-controlled studies in human fetuses. **Cephalexin** crosses the human placenta in a carrier-mediated fashion. The magnitude of transfer is greater than **cephapirin**, and produces a fetal concentration above the MIC for most sensitive pathogens. There is no evidence of teratogenicity. Rodent studies are also reassuring, revealing no evidence of teratogenicity or IUGR despite the use of doses higher than those used clinically.

■ **Breastfeeding Safety** — Most cephalosporins are excreted into breast milk, but the amount of **cephalexin** excreted is small and generally considered compatible with breastfeeding.

■ **References** — Czeizel AE, Rockenbauer M, Sorensen HT, Olsen J. Am J Obstet Gynecol 2001; 184:1289-96.
Wing DA, Hendershott CM, Debuque L, Millar LK. Obstet Gynecol 1998; 92:249-53.
Pfau A, Sacks TG. Clin Infect Dis 1992; 14:810-4.
Kudo Y, Urabe T, Fujiwara A, Yamada K, Kawasaki T. Biochim Biophys Acta 1989; 978:313-8.
Creatsas G, Pavlatos M, Lolis D, Kaskarelis D. Curr Med Res Opin 1980; 7:43-6.

Campbell-Brown M, McFadyen. Br J Obstet Gynaecol 1983; 90:1054-9.
Griffith RS. Postgrad Med J 1983; 59(Suppl 5):16-27.
Stage AH, Glover DD, Vaughan JE. J Reprod Med 1982; 27:113-9.
Kafetzis DA, Siafas CA, Georgakopoulos PA, Papadatos CJ. Acta Paediatr Scand 1981; 70:285-8.

■ **Summary**

- **Pregnancy Category B**
- **Lactation Category S**
- A popular cephalosporin for which there is a broad and reassuring experience during pregnancy.

Cephalothin (Keflin; Seffin)

■ **Class**
Antibiotic (*1st-generation cephalosporin*)

■ **Indications**
Bacterial infections (<u>gram-positive aerobes</u>: *Staphylococcus aureus*, β-1 hemolytic streptococci; <u>gram-negative aerobes</u>: *Escherichia coli*, *Proteus mirabilis*, *Klebsiella* species, *Moraxella catarrhalis*)

■ **Mechanism**
Bactericidal—inhibits cell wall synthesis

■ **Dosage with Qualifiers**
<u>Bacterial infection</u>—500mg-2gm IM/IV q4-6h
<u>Surgical prophylaxis</u>—1-2g IV 30-60min preoperatively
- **Contraindications**—hypersensitivity to drug or class
- **Caution**—penicillin allergy, renal dysfunction, antibiotic-associated colitis, seizure disorder, concomitant use of nephrotoxic drugs

■ **Maternal Considerations**
The elimination half-life of this 1st generation cephalosporin is reduced by 1/3 during pregnancy. Primary treatment of UTIs with a 1st generation cephalosporin during pregnancy may no longer be appropriate because a significant number of isolates (11%) are resistant to **cephalothin**. Prophylactic **cephalothin** decreases the incidence of endometritis in women undergoing midtrimester abortion.
Side effects include anemia, thrombocytopenia, anaphylaxis, pseudomembranous colitis, diarrhea, nausea, and elevated hepatic enzymes.

■ **Fetal Considerations**
There are no adequate reports or well-controlled studies in human fetuses. Rodent studies are reassuring, revealing no evidence of teratogenicity or IUGR despite the use of doses higher than those used clinically.

■ **Breastfeeding Safety** .... Most cephalosporins are excreted into breast milk, but the amount of **cephalothin** excreted is small and generally considered compatible with breastfeeding.

■ **References** .... Philipson A, Stiernstedt G, Ehrnebo M. Clin Pharmacokinet 1987; 12:136-44.
Angel JL, O'Brien WF, Finan MA, et al. Obstet Gynecol 1990; 76:28-32.
Fan YD, Pastorek JG 2nd, Miller JM Jr, Mulvey J. Am J Perinatol 1987; 4:324-6.
Spence MR, King TM, Burkman RT, Atienza MF. Obstet Gynecol 1982; 60:502-5.
Noschel H, Peiker G, Voigt R, et al. Arch Toxicol Suppl 1980; 4:380-4.
Kafetzis DA, Siafas CA, Georgakopoulos PA, Papadatos CJ. Acta Paediatr Scand 1981; 70:285-8.

■ **Summary** ....
- **Pregnancy Category B**
- **Lactation Category S**
- A popular cephalosporin for which there is a broad and reassuring experience with use during pregnancy.

Cephapirin (Cefadyl)

■ **Class** .... Antibiotic (*1st-generation cephalosporin*)

■ **Indications** .... Bacterial infections (<u>gram-positive aerobes</u>: *Staphylococcus aureus*, β-1 hemolytic streptococci; <u>gram-negative aerobes</u>: *Escherichia coli*, *Proteus mirabilis*, *Klebsiella* species, *Moraxella catarrhalis*)

■ **Mechanism** .... Bactericidal—inhibits cell wall synthesis

■ **Dosage with Qualifiers** .... <u>Bacterial infection</u>—1-2g IV/IM q4-6h; max 12g qd
- **Contraindications**—hypersensitivity to drug or class
- **Caution**—penicillin allergy, renal dysfunction, antibiotic-associated colitis, seizure disorder, concomitant use of nephrotoxic drugs

■ **Maternal Considerations** .... **Cephapirin** appears effective and safe for the treatment of acute infection during pregnancy.
Side effects include anemia, thrombocytopenia, anaphylaxis, pseudomembranous colitis, diarrhea, nausea, and elevated hepatic enzymes.

■ **Fetal Considerations** .... There are no adequate reports or well-controlled studies in human fetuses. **Cephapirin** crosses the human placenta, and though the magnitude of transfer is less than **cephalexin**, it does produce a fetal concentration above the MIC for most sensitive pathogens. Rodent studies are reassuring, revealing no evidence of teratogenicity or IUGR despite the use of doses higher than those used clinically.

■ **Breastfeeding Safety** — Most cephalosporins are excreted into breast milk, but the amount of **cephapirin** excreted is small and generally considered compatible with breastfeeding.

■ **References** — Dashow EE, Read JA, Coleman FH. Obstet Gynecol 1986; 68:473-8.
Prades M, Brown MP, Gronwall R, Miles NS. Am J Vet Res 1988; 49:1888-90.
Levin DK, Gorchels C, Andersen R. Am J Obstet Gynecol 1983; 147:273-7.
Creatsas G, Pavlatos M, Lolis D, Kaskarelis D. Curr Med Res Opin 1980; 7:43-6.
Kafetzis DA, Siafas CA, Georgakopoulos PA, Papadatos CJ. Acta Paediatr Scand 1981; 70:285-8.

■ **Summary** —
- **Pregnancy Category B**
- **Lactation Category S**
- A fairly large clinical experience with **cephapirin** during pregnancy is reassuring.

Cephradine (Anspor; Cefamid; Cefradina; Eskefrin; Nobitina; Velosef)

■ **Class** — Antibiotic (1st-generation cephalosporin)

■ **Indications** — Bacterial infections (<u>gram-positive aerobes</u>: Staphylococcus aureus, β-1 hemolytic streptococci; <u>gram-negative aerobes</u>: Escherichia coli, Proteus mirabilis, Klebsiella species, Moraxella catarrhalis)

■ **Mechanism** — Bactericidal—inhibits cell wall synthesis

■ **Dosage with Qualifiers** — <u>Bacterial infection</u>—250-500mg PO q6h
<u>UTI</u>—up to 1g PO q6h
- **Contraindications**—hypersensitivity to drug or class
- **Caution**—penicillin allergy, renal dysfunction, antibiotic-associated colitis, seizure disorder, concomitant use of nephrotoxic drugs

■ **Maternal Considerations** — **Cephradine** has been used for the treatment of UTI and pharyngitis because of its antimicrobial spectrum. However, its elimination half-life is decreased by 25% during pregnancy, which might in part explain why

cefuroxime proved superior in one randomized trial for the treatment of UTI.

Side effects include anemia, thrombocytopenia, anaphylaxis, pseudomembranous colitis, diarrhea, nausea, and elevated hepatic enzymes.

■ **Fetal Considerations**

There are no adequate reports or well-controlled studies in human fetuses. **Cephradine** rapidly crosses the human placenta and is found in the amniotic fluid within hours of maternal administration. Rodent studies are reassuring, revealing no evidence of teratogenicity or IUGR despite the use of doses higher than those used clinically.

■ **Breastfeeding Safety**

Cephradine is excreted into human breast milk. Its M:P ratio approximates 0.2, suggesting **cephradine** should be compatible with breastfeeding.

■ **References**

Ovalle A, Martinez MA, Wolff M, et al. Rev Med Chil 2000; 128:749-57.
Lange IR, Rodeck C, Cosgrove R. Br J Obstet Gynaecol 1984; 91:551-4.
Philipson A, Stiernstedt G, Ehrnebo M. Clin Pharmacokinet 1987; 12:136-44.
Mischler TW, Corson SL, Larranaga A, et al. J Reprod Med 1978; 21:130-6.

■ **Summary**

- **Pregnancy Category B**
- **Lactation Category S**
- A fairly large experience with **cephradine** during pregnancy is reassuring, though there are alternative agents which may be superior for use during pregnancy.

Cetirizine (Alltec; Zyrtec)

■ **Class**

Antihistamine, 2nd-generation

■ **Indications**

Allergic rhinitis, urticaria

■ **Mechanism**

Inhibition of peripheral H_1 receptors

■ **Dosage with Qualifiers**

Allergic rhinitis—5-10mg PO qd; max 10mg qd
Urticaria—5-10mg PO qd; max 10mg qd
NOTE—may be combined with **pseudoephedrine**
- **Contraindications**—hypersensitivity to drug or class
- **Caution**—hepatic or renal dysfunction, CNS depressant use

■ **Maternal Considerations** ⋯⋯⋯ There are no adequate reports or well-controlled studies in pregnant women. The product labels state medications for allergic rhinitis should be avoided during pregnancy owing to lack of fetal safety, though the majority of agents have human data that refute this position.
Side effects include bronchospasm, hepatitis, hypersensitivity, somnolence, fatigue, dry mouth, pharyngitis, dizziness, abdominal pain, and diarrhea.

■ **Fetal Considerations** ⋯⋯⋯ There are no adequate reports or well-controlled studies in human fetuses. It is unknown whether **cetirizine** crosses the human placenta. Neither 1st- (e.g., **chlorpheniramine**) nor 2nd-generation (e.g., **cetirizine**) antihistamines are incriminated as human teratogens. However, 1st-generation antihistamines are preferred as there is more conclusive evidence of safety. Rodent studies are reassuring, revealing no evidence of teratogenicity or IUGR despite the use of doses higher than those used clinically.

■ **Breastfeeding Safety** ⋯⋯⋯ There are no adequate reports or well-controlled studies in nursing women. **Cetirizine** enters human breast milk, though the kinetics remain to be elucidated.

■ **References** ⋯⋯⋯ Paris-Kohler A, Megret-Gabeaud ML, Fabre C, et al. Allerg Immunol (Paris) 2001; 33:399-403.
Mazzotta P, Loebstein R, Koren G. Drug Saf 1999; 20:361-75.
Einarson A, Bailey B, Jung G, et al. Ann Allergy Asthma Immunol 1997; 78:183-6.

■ **Summary** ⋯⋯⋯ • **Pregnancy Category B**
• **Lactation Category U**
• A reasonable selection for the listed indications, though there are alternative agents for which there is more experience during pregnancy and lactation.

Chenodiol (Chelobil; Chendal; Chenix; Chenocol; Chino; Chebil; Chenodex; Soluston)

■ **Class** ⋯⋯⋯ *Gallstone solubilizer*

■ **Indications** ⋯⋯⋯ Gallstones (cholesterol)

■ **Mechanism** ⋯⋯⋯ Reduces hepatic synthesis of cholesterol

■ **Dosage with Qualifiers** ⋯⋯⋯ <u>Gallstones</u>—250mg PO bid × 2w, increase by 250mg/w until the max tolerated or recommended dose is reached (13-16mg/kg/d) in 2 divided doses

- **Contraindications**—hypersensitivity to drug or class, acute cholecystitis, cholangitis, gallstone pancreatitis, intrahepatic cholestasis, primary biliary cirrhosis or sclerosing cholangeitis
- **Caution**—gallstones

■ **Maternal Considerations** — Because of potential hepatotoxicity, poor response rates in some subgroups of **chenodiol**-treated patients, and an increased cholecystectomy rate in other treated subgroups, **chenodiol** is not appropriate treatment for many patients with gallstones. There are no adequate reports or well-controlled studies of **chenodiol** in pregnant women. Maternal pregnancy outcome may be improved in pregnancies complicated by intrahepatic cholestasis by treatment with **urso-deoxicholic acid**.
Side effects include diarrhea, dyspepsia, nausea, vomiting, constipation, and dizziness.

■ **Fetal Considerations** — There are no adequate reports or well-controlled studies in human fetuses. It is unknown if **chenodiol** crosses the placenta. Bile acid levels are lower in both amniotic fluid and umbilical blood samples from pregnancies treated for intrahepatic cholestasis with **urso-deoxicholic acid**, suggesting placental transfer. Serious hepatic, renal and adrenal lesions occurred in rhesus fetuses given 60-90mg/kg/d (4-6 × MRHD) from day 21 to day 45 of pregnancy. Hepatic lesions occurred in neonatal baboons whose mothers received 18-38mg/kg (1-2 × MRHD) throughout pregnancy. Fetal malformations were not observed. Neither fetal liver damage nor fetal abnormalities occurred in reproduction studies in rats and hamsters.

■ **Breastfeeding Safety** — There are no adequate reports or well-controlled studies in nursing women. It is unknown whether **chenodiol** enters human breast milk.

■ **References** — Mazzela G, Nicola R, Francesco A, et al. Hepatology 2001; 33:504-8.
Palmer AK, Heywood R. Toxicology 1974; 2:239-46.
Carey WD, Tangedahl TN. Postgrad Med 1982; 71:163-72.

■ **Summary** —
- **Pregnancy Category X**
- **Lactation Category U**
- **Chenodiol** is generally considered contraindicated in women who are or may become pregnant, though there is no human data to support it.
- **Chenodiol** should be used during pregnancy and lactation only if the benefit justifies the potential perinatal risk.

Chloral Hydrate (Aquachloral; Chloralhydrat; Chloralix; Dormel; Kloral; Noctec)

■ **Class**	*Sedative, hypnotic*
■ **Indications**	Insomnia, anxiety, alcohol withdrawal
■ **Mechanism**	Unknown
■ **Dosage with Qualifiers**	Insomnia, anxiety—500mg-1g PO prn qhs Alcohol withdrawal—500mg-1g PO q6h NOTE—also available in suppository form • **Contraindications**—hypersensitivity to drug or class, cardiac disease, hepatic failure • **Caution**—depression, drug abuse, porphyria
■ **Maternal Considerations**	**Chloral hydrate** is an anxiolytic hypnotic. There are no adequate reports or well-controlled studies in pregnant women. There is a case report of successful hemodialysis during pregnancy for the treatment of a **chloral hydrate** overdose. *Side effects* include hypersensitivity, leukopenia, dependence, respiratory depression, hyperbilirubinemia, and angioedema.
■ **Fetal Considerations**	There are no adequate reports or well-controlled studies in human fetuses. Chronic use during pregnancy may result in neonatal withdrawal, suggesting placental transfer. Rodent teratogenicity studies have apparently not been performed. Equine studies suggest a higher frequency of miscarriage after **chloral hydrate**.
■ **Breastfeeding Safety**	There are no adequate reports or well-controlled studies in nursing women. **Chloral hydrate** is excreted into human breast milk and may cause neonatal sedation.
■ **References**	Akpokodje JU, Akusu MO, Osuagwu AI. Vet Rec 1986; 118:306. Vaziri ND, Kumar KP, Mirahmadi K, Rosen SM. South Med J 1977; 70:377-8.
■ **Summary**	• **Pregnancy Category C** • **Lactation Category NS?** • **Chloral hydrate** should be used during pregnancy and lactation only if the benefit justifies the potential perinatal risk.

Chlorambucil (Leukeran; Linfolysin)

■ **Class** ⋯⋯⋯⋯ *Antineoplastic, alkylating agent*

■ **Indications** ⋯⋯⋯ Palliative therapy for a variety of cancers including leukemia, lymphomas, trophoblastic disease

■ **Mechanism** ⋯⋯⋯ Alkylating agent (crosslinks DNA and RNA and inhibits protein synthesis)

■ **Dosage with Qualifiers** ⋯ Cancer—varies based on the type of neoplasm. Most regimens recommend 0.1-0.2mg/kg/d × 3-6w
- **Contraindications**—hypersensitivity to drug or class, resistance to drug
- **Caution**—neutropenia, thrombocytopenia, seizures, fever, hepatotoxicity, epilepsy

■ **Maternal Considerations** ⋯ **Chlorambucil** is an alkylating agent. There are no adequate reports or well-controlled studies in pregnant women. There are many case reports of a successful outcome in women treated with **chlorambucil** throughout pregnancy.
Side effects include bone marrow suppression, nausea, vomiting, confusion, anxiety, seizures, skin hypersensitivity, and pulmonary fibrosis.

■ **Fetal Considerations** ⋯ There are no adequate reports or well-controlled studies in animal and human fetuses. It is unknown whether **chlorambucil** crosses the human placenta. The sole report of a **chlorambucil**-associated birth defect is unilateral renal agenesis in one fetus of a set of twins. The lack of reports suggests **chlorambucil** is not a major human teratogen, and fetal tolerance later in gestation is quite high. **Chlorambucil** is a teratogen in rodents, causing postclosure exencephaly and axial skeletal abnormalities.

■ **Breastfeeding Safety** ⋯ There are no adequate reports or well-controlled studies in nursing women. It is unknown whether **chlorambucil** enters human breast milk.

■ **References** ⋯⋯⋯ Padmanabhan R, Samad PA. Reprod Toxicol 1999; 13:189-201.
Evans AC Jr, Soper JT, Clarke-Pearson DL, et al. Gynecol Oncol 1995; 59:226-30.
Curry SL, Blessing JA, DiSaia PJ, et al. Obstet Gynecol 1989; 73:357-62.

■ **Summary** ⋯⋯⋯
- **Pregnancy Category D**
- **Lactation Category U**
- **Chlorambucil** should be used during pregnancy and lactation only if the benefit justifies the potential perinatal risk.

158

Chloramphenicol (Amphicol; Archifen; Aromycetin; Bekamycetin; Biomycetin; Chlomin; Chloradrops; Chlornitromycin; Chlorocort; Chlorofair; Chloromycetin; Chloromyxin; Chloronitrin; Chloroptic; Cloramfeni; Cloramplast; Cloromicetin; Danmycetin; Denicol; Econochlor; Heminevrin; I-Chlor; Infa-Chlor; Isopto; Kemicetina; Leukomycin; Mychel; Newlolly; Ocu-Chlor; Ophthochlor; Optomycin; Spectro-Chlor; Sunchlormycin; Troymycetin; Vernacetin)

■ **Class** .... *Antibiotic*

■ **Indications** .... Bacterial infections (<u>gram-positive and -negative bacteria</u>: *Rickettsia*, lymphogranuloma psittacosis, *Vibrio cholerae*, *Salmonella typhi*, *Haemophilus influenzae*)

■ **Mechanism** .... Bacteriostatic—interferes with protein synthesis

■ **Dosage with Qualifiers** .... <u>Bacterial infections</u>—50-100mg/kg IV qd; max 100mg/kg/d
<u>Rickettsial infections</u>—50-100mg/kg IV qd; max 100mg/kg/d
<u>Ophthalmic</u>—1-2 gtts/eye q4-6×/d ×72h then adjust to response
NOTE—**chloramphenicol** is not considered a first-line therapy
  ● **Contraindications**—hypersensitivity to drug or class, pregnancy, infancy, mild infectious process
  ● **Caution**—hepatic failure, G6PD deficiency, bone marrow suppression

■ **Maternal Considerations** .... There are no adequate reports or well-controlled studies in pregnant women.
Side effects include bone marrow suppression, nausea, fever, rash, urticaria, pruritus, neuropathy, optic neuritis, blurred vision, vomiting, confusion, headache, mental confusion, "gray baby syndrome," thrombocytopenia, aplastic anemia, agranulocytosis, and pseudomembranous colitis.

■ **Fetal Considerations** .... There are no adequate reports or well-controlled studies in human fetuses. It is unknown whether **chloramphenicol** crosses the human placenta. Thiamphenicol does cross the rodent placenta. **Chloramphenicol** is not teratogenic in either humans or rodents. It does cause neonatal "gray baby syndrome." Case reports document successful treatment of meningoencephalitis in neonates caused by maternal *Mycoplasma hominis*.

■ **Breastfeeding Safety** .... There are no adequate reports or well-controlled studies in nursing women. It is not known whether **chloramphenicol** enters human breast milk. Caution is advised in nursing mothers due to the danger of developing "gray baby syndrome" in neonates.

■ **References** ⋯⋯⋯⋯⋯⋯⋯⋯⋯⋯⋯ Knausz M, Niederland T, Dosa E, Rozgonyi F. J Med
Microbiol 2002; 51:187-8.
Stallings SP. Obstet Gynecol Surv 2001; 56:37-42.
Czeizel AE, Rockenbauer M, Sorensen HT, Olsen J. Eur J
Epidemiol 2000; 16:323-7.
Amstey MS. Clin Infect Dis 2000; 30:237.

■ **Summary** ⋯⋯⋯⋯⋯⋯⋯⋯⋯⋯⋯⋯⋯
- **Pregnancy Category C**
- **Lactation Category U**
- The risk of neonatal "gray baby syndrome" is a major negative factor for the use of **chloramphenicol**.
- **Chloramphenicol** should be used during pregnancy and lactation only if the benefit justifies the potential perinatal risk.

Chlordiazepoxide (Benzodiapin; Chlordiazachel; Chuichin; Kalbrium; Karmoplex; Libnum; Libritabs; Librium; Medilium; Poxi; Reposans; Restocalm; Ripolin; Vapine; Zenecin)

■ **Class** ⋯⋯⋯⋯⋯⋯⋯⋯⋯⋯⋯⋯⋯⋯ Benzodiazepine (long-acting)

■ **Indications** ⋯⋯⋯⋯⋯⋯⋯⋯⋯⋯⋯ Anxiety, severe alcohol dependence

■ **Mechanism** ⋯⋯⋯⋯⋯⋯⋯⋯⋯⋯⋯ Enhances GABA effects and acts through benzodiazepine receptors

■ **Dosage with Qualifiers** ⋯⋯⋯⋯ Anxiety—5-10mg PO tid or qid
Severe anxiety—20-25mg PO tid or qid
Alcohol withdrawal—50-100mg PO IM /IV; max 300mg qd
- **Contraindications**—hypersensitivity to drug or class
- **Caution**—alcohol, hepatic or renal failure

■ **Maternal Considerations** ⋯⋯⋯ There are no adequate reports or well-controlled studies in pregnant women. The available information is insufficient to determine whether the potential benefits of benzodiazepines to the mother outweigh the risks to the fetus. High peak concentrations are avoided by dividing the daily dosage into 2 or 3 doses.
Side effects include agranulocytosis, drowsiness, ataxia, confusion, rash, edema, menstrual irregularities, decreased libido, and extrapyramidal effects.

■ **Fetal Considerations** ⋯⋯⋯⋯⋯ Benzodiazepines are rapidly transferred across the placenta during early and late pregnancy, and 1st trimester exposure to this class of drugs has been linked to an increased risk of anomalies. While there are no well-controlled studies in human fetuses, the overall experience has been reassuring. In some 550 children followed up to 4 years, there was no increase in either malformations or adverse effects on neurobehavioral development and IQ. Some infants exposed in the 3rd trimester exhibit either the floppy infant syndrome, or marked neonatal withdrawal symptoms. Symptoms vary from mild sedation, hypotonia, and reluctance to suck, to apneic spells, cyanosis, and impaired metabolic responses to cold stress, and may persist for hours to months after birth. This correlates with the pharmacokinetic and placental transfer of the benzodiazepines and their disposition in the neonate. **Chlordiazepoxide** retards motor development and physical maturation in mice. Rodent studies reveal no increased risk of congenital anomalies, IUGR, or adverse effects on lactation.

■ **Breastfeeding Safety** — There are no adequate reports or well-controlled studies in nursing women. The drug enters human breast milk in low concentrations such that only high clinical doses might be expected to exert an effect on the nursing newborn.

■ **References** — Iqbal MM, Sobhan T, Ryals T. Psychiatr Serv 2002; 53:39-49.
McElhatton PR. Reprod Toxicol 1994; 8:461-75.
Kanto JH. Drugs 1982; 23:354-80.

■ **Summary** —
- **Pregnancy Category D**
- **Lactation Category S?**
- **Chlordiazepoxide** should be used during pregnancy and lactation only if the benefit justifies the potential perinatal risk.
- **Benzodiazepines** should be used as monotherapy at the lowest effective dose for the shortest possible duration.
- High peak concentrations are avoided by dividing the daily dosage into 2 or 3 doses.

Chlorhexidine (Peridex; PerioGard; Plakicide; Savacol)

■ **Class** — *Miscellaneous*

■ **Indications** — Gingivitis, cleansing of the birth canal to prevent infection

■ **Mechanism** — Antibacterial

■ **Dosage with Qualifiers** — Gingivitis, infection prevention—15ml PO, swish/spit bid
- **Contraindications**—hypersensitivity to drug or class

■ **Maternal Considerations** — While there are no adequate reports or well-controlled studies in pregnant women, **chlorhexidine** is considered safe for cleansing of the birth canal, and may be as effective as **ampicillin** for the prevention of neonatal group B streptococcus. Its use during labor may also decrease HIV transmission. It does not, however, reduce the incidence of postpartum endometritis.

Side effects include staining of teeth, taste change, and salivary gland inflammation.

■ **Fetal Considerations** ⋯⋯⋯⋯ There are no adequate reports or well-controlled studies in human fetuses. It is unknown whether **chlorhexidine** crosses the human placenta. Exposure to **chlorhexidine** during birth is not associated with any increase in neonatal mortality rate due to sepsis, fever, poor feeding, apnea or dyspnea in newborns.

■ **Breastfeeding Safety** ⋯⋯⋯⋯ It is not known whether **chlorhexidine** enters human milk. While there are no adequate reports or well-controlled studies in nursing women, the quantity of drug absorbed systemically during a brief encounter is likely minimal.

■ **References** ⋯⋯⋯⋯⋯⋯⋯⋯ Gaillard P, Mwanyumba F, Verhofstede C, et al. AIDS 2001(16); 15:389-96.
Sweeten KM, Eriksen NL, Blanco JD. Am J Obstet Gynecol 1997; 176:426-30.
Facchinetti F, Piccinini F, Mordini B, Volpe A. J Matern Fetal Neonatal Med 2002; 11:84-8.
Kaihura CT, Ricci L, Bedocchi L, et al. Acta Biomed Ateneo Parmense 2000; 71(Suppl 1):567-71.
Stray-Pedersen B, Bergan T, Hafstad A, et al. Int J Antimicrob Agents 1999; 12:245-51.

■ **Summary** ⋯⋯⋯⋯⋯⋯⋯⋯⋯ • **Pregnancy Category B**
• **Lactation Category S?**
• **Chlorhexidine** is safe to use for cleansing of the birth canal; its use during labor may decrease group B streptococcus and HIV transmission.

Chloroquine (Aralen; Aralen Injection; Chlorofoz; Dichinalex; Lariago; Quinalan)

■ **Class** ⋯⋯⋯⋯⋯⋯⋯⋯⋯⋯ *Antiprotozoal*

■ **Indications** ⋯⋯⋯⋯⋯⋯⋯⋯ Malaria prophylaxis and treatment, amebiasis

■ **Mechanism** ⋯⋯⋯⋯⋯⋯⋯⋯ Unknown

■ **Dosage with Qualifiers** ⋯⋯⋯ Malaria prophylaxis—500mg PO qw; begin 2w before travel and continue until 8w post exposure (500mg phosphate = 300mg base)

Malaria treatment—begin 1g PO ×1, then 500mg PO 6-8h later, then 500mg PO qd ×2
Amebiasis—begin 1g qd ×2, then 500mg PO qd ×2-3w

- **Contraindications**—hypersensitivity to drug or class, porphyria, retinal field changes
- **Caution**—gastrointestinal disorder, neurologic disease, hepatic failure

■ **Maternal Considerations**

Chloroquine is closely related to hydroxychloroquine and has similar uses. While there are no adequate reports or well-controlled studies in pregnant women, a body of clinical experience suggests **chloroquine** is safe during pregnancy. **Chloroquine** is also used as an adjunct for the treatment of SLE in women who have failed to respond to first-line agents. Recent studies suggest it may have a role in the treatment of HIV, and thus may have a role in HIV-infected breast-feeding women. While prolonged treatment with quinine-type drugs is associated with pigmentary retinopathy, the risk is not increased during pregnancy. *Side effects* include agranulocytosis, thrombocytopenia, aplastic anemia, dermatitis, ototoxicity, vomiting, dizziness, diarrhea, and pruritus.

■ **Fetal Considerations**

Chloroquine crosses the placenta achieving an F:M ratio approximating 0.7-0.8. Fetal retinopathy was noted in some animal studies but more recent investigation casts doubt on the association and suggests it is safe during the 1st trimester. No increase in spontaneous abortion or major birth defects is reported in humans.

■ **Breastfeeding Safety**

Chloroquine enters human breast milk achieving an M:P ratio ranging from 0.268 to 0.462. Some studies suggest it may actually be concentrated. However, it is generally considered compatible with breastfeeding.

■ **References**

Klinger G, Morad Y, Westall CA, et al. Lancet 2001(8); 358:813-4.
McGready R, Thwai KL, Cho T, et al. Trans R Soc Trop Med Hyg 2002; 96:180-4.
Motta M, Tincani A, Faden D, et al. Lancet 2002; 359:524-5.
Koren G. Can Fam Physician 1999; 45:2869-70.
Boelaert JR, Piette J, Sperber K. J Clin Virol 2001; 20:137-40.
Akintonwa A, Gbajumo SA, Mabadeje AF. Ther Drug Monit 1988; 10:147-9.

■ **Summary**

- **Pregnancy Category C**
- **Lactation Category S**
- **Chloroquine** should be used during pregnancy and lactation only if the benefit justifies the potential perinatal risk.

Chlorothiazide (Azide; Chlothin; Diurazide; Diuret; Diuril; Saluretil)

■ **Class** — *Diuretic*

■ **Indications** — Hypertension, peripheral edema

■ **Mechanism** — Inhibits resorption of sodium and chloride

■ **Dosage with Qualifiers** — Edema—500-1000mg PO qd or bid
Hypertension—250-500mg PO qd or bid
NOTE—may be combined with **methyldopa** or **reserpine**
- **Contraindications**—hypersensitivity to drug or class, electrolyte imbalances

■ **Maternal Considerations** — Though popular among obstetricians for the treatment of edema and weight gain in the 1970s, there are no adequate reports or well-controlled studies in pregnant women. Physiologic edema should not be treated. Thiazide diuretics may be diabetogenic. Severe electrolyte imbalances in both mother and newborn are reported. Hemorrhagic pancreatitis is also reported after thiazide exposure.
Side effects include renal failure, hyponatremia, hypochloremia, hypomagnesemia, glucose intolerance, hyperlipidemia, and photosensitivity.

■ **Fetal Considerations** — There are no adequate reports or well-controlled studies in human fetuses. Thiazide diuretics readily cross the placenta. There is no clear evidence **chlorothiazide** increases the risk of malformation. However, older studies suggest thiazide diuretics may decrease placental perfusion by preventing normal plasma expansion and increase the risk of IUGR. Thrombocytopenia and hypoglycemia are major risks. The mechanism for the thrombocytopenia is unknown. Fetal bradycardia following exposure is the result of electrolyte imbalance (hypokalemia).

■ **Breastfeeding Safety** — Thiazide diuretics enter human breast milk in low concentrations. And while there are no adequate reports or well-controlled studies in nursing women, they are generally considered compatible with breastfeeding.

■ **References** — Finnerty FA, Buchholz JH, Tuckman J. JAMA 1958; 166:1414.
Sibai BM, Grossman RA, Grossman HG. Am J Obstet Gynecol 1984; 150:831-5.
Beermann B, Fahraeus L, Groschisky-Grind M, Lindstrom B. Gynecol Obstet Invest 1980; 11:45-8.
Goldman JA, Neri A, Ovadia J, et al. Am J Obstet Gynecol 1969; 105:556-60.
Rodriguez SU, Leikin SL, Hiller MC. N Engl J Med 1964; 270:881-4.

Pritchard JA, Waley PJ. Am J Obstet Gynecol 1961; 81:1241-4.
Hall DR, Odendaal HJ. Int J Gynaecol Obstet 1998; 60:63-4.
George JD, Price CJ, Tyl RW, et al. Fundam Appl Toxicol 1995; 26:174-80.

■ **Summary**
- **Pregnancy Category D**
- **Lactation Category S**
- **Chlorothiazide,** like other thiazides, poses a risk to the perinate and is generally contraindicated during pregnancy except for the treatment of CHF.

Chlorotrianisene (Estregur; Tace)

■ **Class**
Antineoplastics, hormones/hormone modifiers

■ **Indications**
Severe vasomotor symptoms, atrophic vaginitis

■ **Mechanism**
Estrogen receptor agonist

■ **Dosage with Qualifiers**
Severe vasomotor symptoms—12-25mg PO qd; treat for 30d
Atrophic vaginitis—12-25mg PO qd; treat for 30d
- **Contraindications**—hypersensitivity to drug or class, pregnancy, breast carcinoma, hepatic carcinoma, thromboembolic disorder, smoker over 35 years old
- **Caution**—hypertension, diabetes mellitus, hepatic dysfunction, hyperlipidemia, depression

■ **Maternal Considerations**
Chlorotrianisene is an estrogen analog that was and may still be used in some countries for the suppression of lactation. It is ineffective. **Chlorotrianisene** increases the risk of thromboembolism during pregnancy and postpartum. It is generally considered contraindicated during pregnancy.
Side effects include deep venous thrombosis.

■ **Fetal Considerations**
There are no adequate reports or well-controlled studies in pregnant women. It is unknown whether **chlorotrianisene** crosses the human placenta. There is suboptimal data linking oral contraceptive use with the VACTREL syndrome (vertebral, anal, cardiac, tracheoesophageal, renal, limb malformations).

■ **Breastfeeding Safety**
There is no published experience in nursing women. It is unknown whether **chlorotrianisene** enters human breast milk. The use of estrogen analogs for lactation suppression has been discontinued due to poor efficacy and the risk of thrombosis.

165

■ **References** .... Niebyl JR, Bell WR, Schaaf ME, et al. Am J Obstet Gynecol 1979; 134:518-22.
Phillips WP. J Ark Med Soc 1975; 72:163-7.

■ **Summary** ....
- **Pregnancy Category D**
- **Lactation Category NS**
- **Chlorotrianisene** is generally considered contraindicated during pregnancy and lactation.
- Treated nonpregnant women with an intact uterus should be monitored closely for signs of endometrial, ovarian, and breast cancers, and appropriate diagnostic measures taken to rule out malignancy.

Chlorpheniramine (Allerkyn; Chlor-Trimeton; Cloroetano; Clorten; Comin; Cophene-B; Corometon; Evenin; Histacort; Histex; Kelargine; Methyrit; Polaramine; Polaronil; Reston)

■ **Class** .... Antihistamine, 1st-generation

■ **Indications** .... Allergic rhinitis, anaphylaxis

■ **Mechanism** .... Antagonizes cholinergic receptors

■ **Dosage with Qualifiers** .... Allergic rhinitis—4mg PO q4-6h
Anaphylaxis—5-20mg SC/IM q6-12h prn
NOTE—often combined with **hydrocodone, phenylephrine, phenylpropanolamine**, or **pseudoephedrine**
- **Contraindications**—hypersensitivity to drug or class
- **Caution**—gastrointestinal obstruction, sedative

■ **Maternal Considerations** .... There are no adequate reports or well-controlled studies in pregnant women, and its safety during pregnancy is not established. However, **chlorpheniramine** is widely available in over-the-counter preparations and has not to date been implicated with adverse effects during pregnancy. In general, 1st-generation antihistamines are preferred to later generations because of the longer use experience.
Side effects include hypotension, dry mouth, nausea, vomiting, and constipation.

■ **Fetal Considerations** .... Though there are no adequate reports or well-controlled studies in human fetuses, epidemiological study indicates **chlorpheniramine** is not a human teratogen. It is unknown whether **chlorpheniramine** crosses the human placenta. Rodent studies are reassuring, revealing no evidence of teratogenicity or IUGR despite the use of doses higher than those used clinically. In rodents,

chlorpheniramine stimulates glycosaminoglycan alterations leading to palatal mesenchyme and cleft palate malformation.

■ **Breastfeeding Safety** — There is no published experience with **chlorpheniramine** in nursing women. Because preterm and term neonates can have adverse reactions to antihistamines, it should probably be avoided in the 3rd trimester.

■ **References** — The American College of Obstetricians and Gynecologists (ACOG) and The American College of Allergy, Asthma and Immunology (ACAAI). Ann Allergy Asthma Immunol 2000; 84:475-80.
Mazzotta P, Loebstein R, Koren G. Drug Saf 1999; 20:361-75.
Young GL, Jewell D. Cochrane Database Syst Rev 2000; CD000027.
Brinkley LL, Morris-Wiman J. Am J Anat 1986; 176:379-89.
Wilk AL, King CT, Pratt RM. Teratology 1978; 18:199-209.

■ **Summary**
- **Pregnancy Category B**
- **Lactation Category NS?**
- **Chlorpheniramine** should be used during pregnancy and lactation only if the benefit justifies the potential perinatal risk.

Chlorpromazine (Artomin; Fenactil; Klorazin; Megaphen; Promacid; Protran; Romazine; Sonazine; Thorazine)

■ **Class** — *Tranquilizer*

■ **Indications** — Psychosis, nausea, vomiting, hiccups, tetanus, porphyria (acute)

■ **Mechanism** — Unknown; believed to antagonize the D_2 dopamine receptors

■ **Dosage with Qualifiers** — Psychosis—200-800mg IM qd; divide dose tid or qid
Nausea—10-25mg PO q4-6h
Hiccups—25-50mg PO tid or qid; if no response PO, may be given IM/IV
Tetanus—25-50mg IM/IV q6-8h
Porphyria (acute)—25-50mg IM tid or qid
- **Contraindications**—hypersensitivity to drug or class, sedation, bone marrow depression, Parkinson's disease
- **Caution**—hepatic failure, hypotension

- **Maternal Considerations** ⸺ There are no adequate reports or well-controlled studies in pregnant women. **Chlorpromazine** seems safe and effective when used for the preceding indications during pregnancy.
  Side effects include seizure, thrombocytopenia, agranulocytosis, and neuroleptic malignant syndrome.

- **Fetal Considerations** ⸺ There are no adequate reports or well-controlled studies in human fetuses. **Chlorpromazine** rapidly crosses the placenta, and an extrapyramidal syndrome can occur in newborns of women given **chlorpromazine** during labor. There is no evidence **chlorpromazine** is a human teratogen. Rodent studies are also reassuring, though learning and behavioral abnormalities are reported in some studies. The injection of **chlorpromazine** into each rat uterine horn significantly reduces the number of implantation sites.

- **Breastfeeding Safety** ⸺ There are no adequate reports or well-controlled studies in nursing women. **Chlorpromazine** is excreted into human breast milk, though the kinetics remain to be elucidated. The occasional dose of **chlorpromazine** is probably compatible with breastfeeding.

- **References** ⸺ Yang RZ, Xie XY, Sun HY, et al. Contraception 1998; 58:315-20.
  Yoshida K, Smith B, Craggs M, Kumar R. Psychol Med 1998; 28:81-91.
  Finnerty M, Levin Z, Miller LJ. Am J Psychiatry 1996; 153:261-3.
  Hammond JE, Toseland PA. Arch Dis Child 1970; 45:139-40.
  Hill RM, Desmond MM, Kay JL. J Pediatr 1966; 69:589-95.

- **Summary** ⸺
  - **Pregnancy Category C**
  - **Lactation Category S?**
  - **Chlorpromazine** should be used during pregnancy and lactation only if the benefit justifies the potential perinatal risk.

Chlorpropamide (Arodoc; Chlordiabet; Chlorprosil; Diabenil; Diabinese; Diamide; Diatanpin; Dibetes; Gliconorm; Glycermin; Glymese; Insilange; Meldian; Mellitos; Milligon; Norgluc; Normoglic; Orodiabin; Promide; Tanpinin)

- **Class** ⸺ *Antidiabetic; 1st-generation sulfonylurea*

- **Indications** ⸺ Diabetus mellitus type II, diabetes insipidus

■ **Mechanism** ⸺ Stimulates release of insulin from pancreatic islet β cell

■ **Dosage with Qualifiers** ⸺ Diabetes—100-500mg PO qd
Diabetes insipidus—200-500mg PO qd
- **Contraindications**—hypersensitivity to drug or class, diabetic ketoacidosis, sulfonamides allergy
- **Caution**—hepatic or renal dysfunction

■ **Maternal Considerations** ⸺ There are no adequate reports or well-controlled studies in pregnant women. Current study suggests that some modern oral hypoglycemic drugs are safe and useful, not only later in pregnancy but also in the 1st trimester, providing excellent control of blood glucose. The treatment of women with gestational diabetes after delivery does not alter the timing or reduce the ultimate frequency of type II diabetes. **Chlorpropamide** and other sulfonylureas may provoke an **Antabuse**-like reaction if the patient consumes alcohol. There are alternative agents with minimal placental transport that are better candidates for maternal therapy. Older reports note its use for diabetes insipidus. Presently, DDAVP is preferred for this indication.
Side effects include hypoglycemia, agranulocytosis, anemia, thrombocytopenia, cholestatic jaundice, hepatic dysfunction, blurred vision, nausea, vomiting, weight gain, pruritus, and photosensitivity.

■ **Fetal Considerations** ⸺ **Chlorpropamide** crosses the placenta and has a long half-life. It significantly reduces birthweight and perinatal mortality in the offspring of diabetic women without increasing the incidence of birth defects. More recent studies suggest that some oral hypoglycemic agents are relatively safe during pregnancy with no increased risk of macrosomia, hypoglycemia, and lung immaturity, though there are alternative agents with less placental transfer. Rodent teratogenicity studies have not been conducted.

■ **Breastfeeding Safety** ⸺ While there are no adequate studies in nursing mothers, **chlorpropamide** enters the breast milk, achieving an M:P ratio of 0.2, and neonatal hypoglycemia has been reported.

■ **References** ⸺
Langer O, Conway DL, Berkus MD, et al. N Engl J Med 2000; 343:1134-8.
Elliott BD, Schenker S, Langer O, Johnson R, Prihoda T. Am J Obstet Gynecol 1994; 171:653-60.
Robinson AG, Verbalis JG. Curr Ther Endocrinol Metab 1994; 5:1-6.
Stowers JM, Sutherland HW, Kerridge DF. Diabetes 1985; 34(Suppl 2):106-10.
Coetzee EJ, Jackson WP. S Afr Med J 1984(21); 65:635-7.
Onegova RF. Probl Endokrinol (Mosk) 1978; 24:67-70.

■ **Summary**

- **Pregnancy Category C**
- **Lactation Category NS**
- **Chlorpropamide** should be used during pregnancy and lactation only if the benefit justifies the potential perinatal risk.
- There are alternative agents with less placental transport that are better candidates for maternal therapy.

Chlorthalidone (Hydro; Hygroton; Servidone; Thalidone; Thalitone; Urolin)

■ **Class** — Diuretic, thiazide

■ **Indications** — Hypertension, peripheral edema

■ **Mechanism** — Inhibits sodium and chloride reabsorption in the distal convoluted tubules

■ **Dosage with Qualifiers** — Hypertension—25-100mg PO qd
Edema—begin 30-60mg PO qd; max 120mg/d
NOTE—may also be combined with **clonidine** or **reserpine**
- **Contraindications**—hypersensitivity to drug or class, anuria, sensitivity to sulfonamides
- **Caution**—hepatic or renal dysfunction, and bronchial asthma

■ **Maternal Considerations** — **Chlorthalidone** is an oral diuretic with a prolonged action (48-72h). There are no adequate reports or well-controlled studies in pregnant women. Physiologic edema should not be treated.
Side effects include aplastic anemia, agranulocytosis, thrombocytopenia, exfoliative dermatitis, anorexia, nausea, vomiting, hypokalemia, constipation, vertigo, dizziness, purpura, photosensitivity, leukopenia, rash, hyperglycemia, pancreatitis, and orthostatic hypotension.

■ **Fetal Considerations** — There are no adequate reports or well-controlled studies in human fetuses. **Chlorthalidone** crosses the placenta, achieving an F:M ratio approximating 0.15. Rodent studies are reassuring, revealing no evidence of teratogenicity or IUGR despite the use of doses higher than those used clinically.

■ **Breastfeeding Safety** — While **chlorthalidone** is excreted into human breast milk, the pharmacokinetics remain to be clarified. It is generally considered compatible with breastfeeding.

■ **References** ⋯⋯⋯⋯⋯ Mulley BA, Parr GD, Pau WK, et al. Eur J Clin Pharmacol 1978; 13:129-31.

■ **Summary** ⋯⋯⋯⋯⋯⋯
- **Pregnancy Category B**
- **Lactation Category S?**
- **Thiazide** diuretics are rarely indicated during pregnancy and lactation.
- **Chlorthalidone** should be given during pregnancy and lactation only if the potential benefit outweighs the potential risks to the perinate.

Chlorzoxazone (Biomioran; Eze D.S.; Myoforte; Paraflex; Parafon Forte DSC; Relax-ds; Relaxazone; Remular; Strifon Forte DSC)

■ **Class** ⋯⋯⋯⋯⋯⋯⋯⋯ *Muscle relaxant*

■ **Indications** ⋯⋯⋯⋯⋯⋯ Muscle spasms

■ **Mechanism** ⋯⋯⋯⋯⋯ Depresses CNS activity

■ **Dosage with Qualifiers** ⋯⋯ Muscle spasm—250-750mg PO tid or qid
NOTE—should be prescribed in conjunction with other treatment modalities, such as physical therapy
- **Contraindications**—hypersensitivity to drug or class, alcohol consumption
- **Caution**—hepatic or renal failure

■ **Maternal Considerations** ⋯⋯ There are no adequate reports or well-controlled studies in pregnant women. **Chlorzoxazone** should not be taken if there is an allergy to any skeletal muscle relaxant.
Side effects include nausea, vomiting, diarrhea, loss of appetite, headache, severe weakness, unusual increase in sweating, fainting, breathing difficulties, irritability, convulsions, feeling of paralysis, and loss of consciousness.

■ **Fetal Considerations** ⋯⋯⋯ There are no adequate reports or well-controlled studies in human fetuses. It is unknown whether **chlorzoxazone** crosses the human placenta. Rodent teratogenicity studies have not been performed.

■ **Breastfeeding Safety** ⋯⋯⋯ There is no published experience in nursing women. It is unknown whether **chlorzoxazone** enters human breast milk.

■ **References** ⋯⋯⋯⋯⋯⋯ There is no published experience in pregnancy or during lactation.

■ **Summary**
- **Pregnancy Category C**
- **Lactation Category U**
- **Chlorzoxazone** should be used during pregnancy and lactation only if the benefit justifies the potential perinatal risk.
- It should be combined with other measures to relieve discomfort.

Cholera vaccine

■ **Class** — Vaccine

■ **Indications** — Travel to a cholera endemic area

■ **Mechanism** — Active immunity

■ **Dosage with Qualifiers** — Cholera susceptibility—0.5ml intradermal q1w ×2 doses, then q1m ×2 doses; boosters 0.3-0.5ml after 5y
- **Contraindications**—hypersensitivity to drug or class, any acute illness
- **Caution**—avoid intravenous injection

■ **Maternal Considerations** — **Cholera vaccine** is a sterile suspension of killed *Vibrio cholerae*. There are no adequate reports or well-controlled studies of **cholera vaccine** in pregnant women.
Side effects include erythema, induration, pain, and tenderness at the site of injection; malaise, headache, and mild-to-moderate temperature elevations that may persist for 1-2 days.

■ **Fetal Considerations** — There are no adequate and well-controlled studies in human fetuses. It is likely **cholera vaccine**-induced IgG crosses the human placenta. There is no evidence of fetal harm. Rodent studies have not been performed.

■ **Breastfeeding Safety** — There are no adequate reports or well-controlled studies in nursing women. **Cholera vaccine**-induced antibodies enter human breast milk.

■ **References** — Hahn-Zoric M, Carlsson B, Jalil F, et al. Scand J Infect Dis 1989; 21:421-6.

■ **Summary**
- **Pregnancy Category C**
- **Lactation Category S**
- **Cholera vaccine** should be used during pregnancy and lactation only if the benefit justifies the potential perinatal risk.

Cholestyramine (Choles; Cholybar; Cuemid; Questran; Questran Light)

■ **Class** .... *Cholesterol lowering*

■ **Indications** .... Hypercholesterolemia

■ **Mechanism** .... Binds intestinal bile acids in a nonabsorbable complex

■ **Dosage with Qualifiers** .... Hypercholesterolemia—begin 4g PO 1-6x/d; maintenance 4-8g in 2 divided doses
NOTE—take before meals and always mix with water
- **Contraindications**—hypersensitivity to drug or class, biliary obstruction
- **Caution**—constipation

■ **Maternal Considerations** .... **Cholestyramine** is the chloride salt of a basic anion exchange resin. There are no adequate reports or well-controlled studies in pregnant women. **Cholestyramine** is not systemically absorbed, but could interfere with the uptake of fat-soluble vitamins. While **cholestyramine** is used by some for the treatment of cholestasis of pregnancy, its efficacy is in doubt. **Cholestyramine** failed to lower cholesterol levels in rats, but did so in rabbits. *Side effects* include severe constipation, flatulence, gastric pain, anorexia, dyspepsia, headache, rash, fatigue, and weight loss.

■ **Fetal Considerations** .... There are no adequate reports or well-controlled studies in human fetuses. **Cholestyramine** is not systemically absorbed, but could interfere with the uptake of fat-soluble vitamins. Rodent studies are reassuring, revealing no evidence of infertility, increased pregnancy loss, teratogenicity, or IUGR despite the use of doses higher than those used clinically.

■ **Breastfeeding Safety** .... There is no published experience in nursing women. It is unknown whether **cholestyramine** enters human breast milk.

■ **References** .... Lammert F, Marschall HU, Matern S. Curr Treat Options Gastroenterol 2003; 6:123-132.
Palinski W, D'Armiento FP, Witztum JL, et al. Circ Res 2001; 89:991-6.
Haave NC, Innis SM. J Dev Physiol 1989; 12:11-4.
Olsson R, Tysk C, Aldenborg F, Holm B. Gastroenterology 1993; 105:267-71.
Hassan AS, Hackley JJ, Johnson LL. Atherosclerosis 1985; 57:139-48.
Innis SM. Am J Obstet Gynecol 1983; 146:13-6.

■ **Summary** • **Pregnancy Category C**
• **Lactation Category U**
• **Cholestyramine** should be used during pregnancy and lactation only if the benefit justifies the potential perinatal risk.

Ciclopirox olamine (Brumixol; Batrafen; Loprox Laca)

■ **Class** Antifungal

■ **Indications** Yeast infection

■ **Mechanism** Chelates polyvalent cations (Fe^{3+} or Al^{3+}) inhibiting metal-dependent enzymes responsible for degradation of peroxides within fungal cell

■ **Dosage with Qualifiers** Yeast infection—apply cream 1% or lotion 1% onto the affected and surrounding skin bid
• **Contraindications**—hypersensitivity to drug or class
• **Caution**—hepatic or renal failure

■ **Maternal Considerations** There are no adequate reports or well-controlled studies in pregnant women. Treatment of mycotic cervical inflammation during pregnancy is followed by a significant reduction in symptoms and the number of active colonies. *Side effects* include itching at the site of application, worsening of the condition being treated, and mild to severe burning.

■ **Fetal Considerations** There are no adequate reports or well-controlled studies in human fetuses. It is unknown whether **ciclopirox olamine** crosses the human placenta. Though well absorbed by the female rodent, placental transfer is low, and the fetal tissue concentration is always lower than in maternal blood. Rodent studies are reassuring, revealing no evidence of teratogenicity or IUGR despite the use of doses higher than those used clinically.

■ **Breastfeeding Safety** There is no published experience in nursing women. It is unknown whether **ciclopirox olamine** enters human breast milk.

■ **References** Novachkov V, Damianov L, Tsankova M, Ivanov S. Akush Ginekol 1999; 38:54-5.
Kellner HM, Arnold C, Christ OE, et al. Arzneimittelforschung 1981; 31:1337-53.

■ **Summary**

- **Pregnancy Category B**
- **Lactation Category U**
- **Ciclopirox olamine** should be used during pregnancy and lactation only if the benefit justifies the potential perinatal risk.
- There are alternative agents for which there is more experience during pregnancy and lactation.

Cidofovir (Vistide)

■ **Class** — *Antiviral*

■ **Indications** — Cytomegalovirus retinitis in AIDS patients

■ **Mechanism** — Inhibits viral DNA synthesis

■ **Dosage with Qualifiers** — CMV retinitis—5mg/kg IV qw administered over 1h; drink copious amounts of water to avoid renal failure
NOTE—administer with **probenecid**; renal dosing
- **Contraindications**—hypersensitivity to drug or class, direct intraocular injection
- **Caution**—renal failure

■ **Maternal Considerations** — There is no published experience with **cidofovir** during pregnancy. Its use was associated with breast adenocarcinoma in female rats.
Side effects include neutropenia, renal failure, uveitis, nausea, vomiting, anorexia, and anemia.

■ **Fetal Considerations** — There are no adequate reports or well-controlled studies in human fetuses. It is unknown whether **cidofovir** crosses the human placenta. Rodent studies conducted at doses below the MRHD revealed maternal and embryotoxicity associated with skeletal malformations.

■ **Breastfeeding Safety** — There is no published experience in nursing women. It is unknown whether **cidofovir** enters human breast milk. Breastfeeding is contraindicated in HIV-infected nursing women where formula is available to reduce the risk of neonatal transmission.

■ **References** — McNicholl IR, Palmer SM, Ziska DS, Cleary JD. Ann Pharmacother 1999; 33:607-14.
Awan AR, Field HJ. Antimicrob Agents Chemother 1993; 37:2478-82.

■ **Summary**
- **Pregnancy Category C**
- **Lactation Category U**
- **Cidofovir** should be used during pregnancy and lactation only if the benefit justifies the potential perinatal risk.
- Physicians are encouraged to register pregnant women under the Antiretroviral Pregnancy Registry (1-800-258-4263) for a better follow-up of the outcome while under treatment with **cidofovir**.

Cimetidine (Beamat; Cimebec; Cimetegal; Cimetidine In Sodium Chloride; Cimewet; Ciwidine; Edalene; Gerucim; Paoweian; Procimeti; Proctospre; Tagagel; Tagamed; Tagamet; Tagamin; Tratol; Ulcinfan; Ulpax; Valmagen; Wergen)

■ **Class**

Antihistamine, antiulcer

■ **Indications**

Peptic ulcer disease, GERD, Zollinger-Ellison syndrome

■ **Mechanism**

Antagonizes histamine H_2 receptors

■ **Dosage with Qualifiers**

Gastric ulcer—300mg PO/IM/IV qid; max 2.5g/d
GERD—400mg PO qac or qhs or 800mg PO bid ×12w
Zollinger-Ellison syndrome—300-600mg PO/IM/IV qid
NOTE—renal dosing
- **Contraindications**—hypersensitivity to drug or class

■ **Maternal Considerations**

There are no adequate reports or well-controlled studies in pregnant women, and evidence documenting the safety of acid-suppressing drugs during pregnancy is very limited. Antacids and antacid/alginic acid combinations or **sucralfate** constitute first-line medical therapy. If the symptoms are not adequately relieved or if complications develop, treatment with **cimetidine** or **ranitidine** may be considered. The treatment of the "heartburn" with **cimetidine** is not followed by significant maternal adverse reactions. Drugs that inhibit hepatic microsomal enzymes, such as **cimetidine**, may promote the accumulation of unexpectedly high (possibly toxic) blood concentrations of **lidocaine**. **Cimetidine** has some antiandrogenic effect. *Side effects* include neutropenia, thrombocytopenia, agranulocytosis, headache, diarrhea, vomiting, rash, and hepatic failure.

■ **Fetal Considerations** ⋯⋯⋯⋯ There are no adequate reports or well-controlled studies in human fetuses. Studies conducted in pregnant subjects found no relation between drug exposure and either preterm delivery or IUGR. Rodent studies reveal inhibition of both testicular descent and genital differentiation and causes cryptorchidism postnatally. These events might occur in human fetuses when high doses of **cimetidine** are administered to pregnant women around the end of the 1st trimester.

■ **Breastfeeding Safety** ⋯⋯⋯ There are no adequate reports or well-controlled studies in nursing women. **Cimetidine** enters human breast milk. The percentage of the maternal dose ingested based on neonatal body weight is <10%, which should be safe under normal conditions.

■ **References** ⋯⋯⋯⋯⋯⋯⋯⋯ Ruigomez A, Garcia Rodriguez LA, Cattaruzzi C, et al. Am J Epidemiol 1999; 150:476-81.
Broussard CN, Richter JE. Drug Saf 1998; 19:325-37.
Katz PO, Castell DO. Gastroenterol Clin North Am 1998; 27:153-67.
Takeshi S, Kai H, Suita S. Surgery 2002; 131(1 Suppl):S301-5.
Oo CY, Kuhn RJ, Desai N, McNamara PJ. Clin Pharmacol Ther 1995; 58:548-55.

■ **Summary** ⋯⋯⋯⋯⋯⋯⋯⋯⋯ • **Pregnancy Category B**
• **Lactation Category S**
• Antacids and antacid/alginic acid combinations or sucralfate constitute first-line medical therapy.
• If symptoms are not adequately relieved or if complications develop, treatment with **cimetidine** or **ranitidine** may be considered.

Cinoxacin (Cinobac)

■ **Class** ⋯⋯⋯⋯⋯⋯⋯⋯⋯⋯⋯ *Antibiotic, quinolone*

■ **Indications** ⋯⋯⋯⋯⋯⋯⋯⋯ Urinary tract infection from E. *coli*, P. *mirabilis*, P. *vulgaris*, *Klebsiella,* and E*nterobacter* species

■ **Mechanism** ⋯⋯⋯⋯⋯⋯⋯ Bactericidal; inhibits DNA synthesis (activity of DNA gyrase and topoisomerase)

■ **Dosage with Qualifiers** ⋯⋯ UTI (prophylaxis)—250mg PO qhs ×5mo
UTI (treatment)—250mg PO q6h or 500mg PO q12h ×7-12d
NOTE—renal dosing
• **Contraindications**—hypersensitivity to drug or class
• **Caution**—not known

■ **Maternal Considerations** ⋯⋯ There is no published experience with **cinoxacin** during pregnancy.
Side effects include skin rash, urticaria, pruritus, edema, angioedema, eosinophilia, itching, redness, swelling, dizziness, headache, increased sensitivity of skin to sunlight, and thrombocytopenia.

■ **Fetal Considerations** ⋯⋯ There are no adequate reports or well-controlled studies in human fetuses. The use of the new quinolones during the 1st trimester of pregnancy is not associated with an increased prevalence of malformations or musculoskeletal problems; however, longer follow-up and MRI of the joints may be warranted to exclude subtle cartilage and bone damage. While rodent studies did not reveal evidence of teratogenicity, **cinoxacin** was associated with bone development abnormalities in young animals.

■ **Breastfeeding Safety** ⋯⋯ There is no published experience in nursing women. It is unknown whether **cinoxacin** enters human breast milk.

■ **References** ⋯⋯ Peters HJ. Z Arztl Fortbild 1995; 89:279-86.
Cristiano P, Morelli G, Simioli F, et al. Minerva Med 1989; 80:393-5.
Bardi M, Manzoni A. Clin Ter 1988; 127:185-8.

■ **Summary** ⋯⋯
- **Pregnancy Category C**
- **Lactation Category U**
- **Cinoxacin** should be used during pregnancy and lactation only if the benefit justifies the potential perinatal risk.
- There are alternative agents for which there is more experience during pregnancy and lactation.

Ciprofloxacin (Ciloxan; Cipro; Cyprobay)

■ **Class** ⋯⋯ Antibiotic, *quinolone*

■ **Indications** ⋯⋯ Anthrax, cystitis (gram-negative infection), enteric fever

■ **Mechanism** ⋯⋯ Bactericidal—inhibits DNA gyrase and topoisomerase

■ **Dosage with Qualifiers** ⋯⋯ UTI, uncomplicated cystitis—250-750mg PO bid
UTI, severe—200-400mg IV bid
Anthrax—400mg IV bid (or 500mg PO bid) ×60d
Gonorrhea—500mg PO ×1
- **Contraindications**—hypersensitivity
- **Caution**—renal or hepatic failure, dehydration, diabetes, seizure disorder, sun exposure

■ **Maternal Considerations** ⋯⋯ Fluoroquinolone therapy is widely used as a treatment for gonorrhea because it is a relatively inexpensive, oral, and single-dose therapy. However, fluoroquinolone-resistant disease is being identified more frequently. A test for cure is essential. There are no adequate reports or well-controlled studies in pregnant women. **Ciprofloxacin** is also usually selected when penicillin-class agents have no effect on gram-negative rods. **Ciprofloxacin** has the best safety profile of second-line drugs for drug-resistant tuberculosis. It is the drug of choice for prophylaxis among asymptomatic pregnant women exposed to B*acillus anthracis*. In instances where the strain is penicillin-sensitive, prophylaxis with **amoxicillin**, 500mg tid ×60d, may be considered. Isolates of B. *anthracis* implicated in the recent bioterrorist attacks are susceptible to **penicillin** in laboratory tests, but may contain penicillinase activity. Penicillins are not recommended for treatment of anthrax. **Ciprofloxacin** has also been used to treat Q fever during pregnancy.

Side effects include seizures, pseudomembranous colitis, psychosis, hypersensitivity, nausea, vomiting, dizziness, rash, increased CK levels, arthropathy (animal), photosensitivity, pruritus, agitation, confusion, tendonitis, arthralgia, and elevated hepatic enzymes.

■ **Fetal Considerations** ⋯⋯ There are no adequate reports or well-controlled studies in human fetuses. **Ciprofloxacin** crosses the human placenta, and can be found in amniotic fluid in low quantities. Short-duration treatment with **ciprofloxacin** appears free of adverse fetal responses. As a class, the new quinolones do not appear associated with an increased risk of malformation or musculoskeletal problems in humans. The effect of prolonged exposure such as that required for Crohn's disease or anthrax prophylaxis remains unknown. Longer follow-up and MRI of the joints may be warranted to exclude subtle cartilage and bone damage. There are no clinically significant musculoskeletal dysfunctions reported in children exposed to fluoroquinolones *in utero*. Treatment of fetal mice, dogs, and rabbits with other quinolones is associated with an acute arthropathy of the weight-bearing joints.

■ **Breastfeeding Safety** ⋯⋯ There are no adequate reports or well-controlled studies in lactating human mothers. **Ciprofloxacin** enters human breast milk, and oral doses of this drug are concentrated in breast milk at levels higher than serum. C. *difficile* pseudomembranous colitis has been reported in a breast-fed neonate whose mother was taking **ciprofloxacin**. In some animals, slow **ciprofloxacin** elimination results in blood levels out of proportion to that ingested. Because of the potential for some quinolones to cause arthropathy in juvenile animals, they should be avoided in pregnant and lactating women.

■ **References** .... Centers for Disease Control and Prevention. JAMA
2001; 286:2396-7.
MMWR Morb Mortal Wkly Rep 2001; 50:960.
Connell W, Miller A. Drug Saf 1999; 21:311-23.
Loebstein R, Addis A, Ho E, et al. Antimicrob Agents
Chemother 1998; 42:1336-9.
Koul PA, Wani JI, Wahid A. Lancet 1995; 346:307-8.
Berkovitch M, Pastuszak A, Gazarian M, et al. Obstet
Gynecol 1994; 84:535-8.
Siefert HM, Maruhn D, Maul W, et al.
Arzneimittelforschung 1986; 36:1496-502.
Harmon T, Burkhart G, Applebaum H. J Pediatr Surg
1992; 7:744-6.
Gardner DK, Gabbe SG, Harter C. Clin Pharm 1992; 11:352-4.

■ **Summary** ....
- **Pregnancy Category C**
- **Lactation Category NS**
- **Ciprofloxacin** should be used during pregnancy only if the benefit justifies the potential perinatal risk.
- It should be avoided while breastfeeding.
- There are alternative agents for which there is more experience during pregnancy and lactation.

Cisapride (Propulsid; Viprasen)

■ **Class** .... *Gastrointestinal drug*

■ **Indications** .... GERD

■ **Mechanism** .... Stimulates gastric motility by triggering the release of acetylcholine by the myenteric plexus

■ **Dosage with Qualifiers** .... GERD—10-20mg PO qac 15min before meals and hs; max 20mg PO qid
NOTE—check serum electrolytes and ECG before initiating
- **Contraindications**—hypersensitivity, arrhythmia, sinus node dysfunction, atrioventricular block, CHF, ventricular arrhythmia, bradyarrhythmia
- **Caution**—electrolyte imbalances, prolongs QT interval on ECG

■ **Maternal Considerations** .... There are no adequate reports or well-controlled studies in pregnant women. Antacids and antacid/alginic acid combinations or sucralfate constitute first-line medical therapy. **Cisapride** is reserved for patients with severe symptoms. Rodent studies suggest decreased fertility after exposure to **cisapride**.
Side effects include severe arrhythmias (torsades de pointes), pancytopenia, thrombocytopenia, anemia, hepatic failure, headache, nausea, vomiting, fatigue, and depression.

- **Fetal Considerations** ···· There are no adequate reports or well-controlled studies in human fetuses. It is unknown whether **cisapride** crosses the human placenta. There were no differences in maternal history, birthweight, gestational age at delivery, and rates of live births, spontaneous or therapeutic abortions, fetal distress, and major or minor malformations among the group of pregnant women exposed to **cisapride**; 3/4 of exposures occurred during organogenesis. **Cisapride** rapidly crosses the ovine placenta with an average F:M ratio of 0.71. Rodent studies are reassuring, revealing no evidence of teratogenicity. Embryotoxicity was noted at doses that were multiples of the MRHD.

- **Breastfeeding Safety** ···· **Cisapride** enters human breast milk, but at low concentrations of 6ng/ml. Thus, the amount ingested by the neonate is likely without clinical effect.

- **References** ···· Marshall JK, Thompson AB, Armstrong D. Can J Gastroenterol 1998; 12:225-7.
  Broussard CN, Richter JE. Drug Saf 1998; 19:325-37.
  Bailey B, Addis A, Lee A, et al. G Dig Dis Sci 1997; 42:1848-52.
  Veereman-Wauters G, Monbaliu J, Meuldermans W, et al. Drug Metab Dispos 1991; 19:168-72.
  Hofmeyr GJ, Sonnendecker EW. Eur J Clin Pharmacol 1986; 30:735-6.

- **Summary** ····
  - **Pregnancy Category C**
  - **Lactation Category S?**
  - **Cisapride** should be used during pregnancy and lactation only if the benefit justifies the potential perinatal risk.
  - There is considerably more experience with metoclopramide during pregnancy and lactation.
  - **Cisapride** should be reserved for patients with severe symptoms unresponsive to other agents.

Cisplatin (Asiplatin; Platinol)

- **Class** ···· Antineoplastic

- **Indications** ···· Chemotherapy (cancer: ovary, bladder, lung, esophageal, cervical, breast, gastric, lymphoma, myeloma, sarcoma)

- **Mechanism** ···· Binds and crosslinks DNA

- **Dosage with Qualifiers** — Cancer—Varies with the tumor. Most regimens recommend 100mg/m²/cycle and require 3-4 cycles. NOTE—Prehydration and maintenance of an adequate urinary output are absolute requirements
  - **Contraindications**—hypersensitivity to drug or class, myelosuppresion, pregnancy, lactation
  - **Caution**—renal or hepatic failure, neuropathy, hearing impairment, myelosuppression

- **Maternal Considerations** — There are no adequate reports or well-controlled studies in pregnant women. Patients should be advised to avoid pregnancy during treatment. The published literature consists mostly of case reports. **Cisplatin** has been used during pregnancy for women discovered to have ovarian or other malignancies. Good outcomes are possible. Pregnancy and fetal age impact on cisplatin protein binding because of lower albumin levels. The resulting higher levels of free drug in the mother and fetus may increase the risk of toxicity in both. **Cisplatin** causes severe mitochondrial toxicity in the maternal rat kidney. *Side effects* include nephrotoxity, ototoxicity, neuropathy, optic neuritis, papilledema, seizures, anemia, hypokalemia, hypoglycemia, blurred vision, paresthesia, ataxia, elevated hepatic enzymes, rash, urticaria, muscle weakness, and loss of taste.

- **Fetal Considerations** — There are no adequate reports or well-controlled studies in human fetuses. **Cisplatin** crosses the human placenta. Low fetal protein concentration increases the percentage of free drug. Malformations in offspring of women treated with **cisplatin** are rare. **Cisplatin** is embryotoxic and teratogenic in mice. Damage to the fetal renal and hepatic mitochondria as a result of transplacental drug exposure appears mild.

- **Breastfeeding Safety** — **Cisplatin** enters human breast milk at concentrations at or below the level of detection, and is generally considered compatible with breastfeeding.

- **References** —
Gerschenson M, Paik CY, Gaukler EL, et al. Reprod Toxicol 2001; 15:525-31.
Zemlickis D, Klein J, Moselhy G, Koren G. Med Pediatr Oncol 1994; 23:476-9.
Otton G, Higgins S, Phillips KA, Quinn M. Int J Gynecol Cancer 2001; 11:413-7.
Marana HR, de Andrade JM, da Silva Mathes AC, et al. Gynecol Oncol 2001; 80:272-4.
Yoshinaka A, Fukasawa I, Sakamoto T, et al. Arch Gynecol Obstet 2000; 264:124-7.
Ben-Baruch G, Menczer J, Goshen R, et al. J Natl Cancer Inst 1992; 84:451-2.
de Vries EG, van der Zee AG, Uges DR, Sleijfer DT. Lancet 1989; 1:497.
Kopf-Maier P, Erkenswick P, Merker HJ. Toxicology 1985; 34:321-31.

■ **Summary**

- **Pregnancy Category D**
- **Lactation Category S**
- Patients should be advised to avoid pregnancy during treatment.
- However, should pregnancy occur or the neoplasm be discovered during pregnancy, there is increasing evidence for the relative safety of **cisplatin** during gestation.

Citalopram hydrobromide (Celexa)

■ **Class**
Antidepressant

■ **Indications**
Depression

■ **Mechanism**
Serotonin reuptake inhibition

■ **Dosage with Qualifiers**
Depression—20-60mg PO qd
- **Contraindications**—hypersensitivity to drug or class, MAO inhibitor use, abrupt withdrawal
- **Caution**—seizure disorder, mania, hepatic or renal dysfunction, suicidal ideation

■ **Maternal Considerations**
Depression is an important and often unrecognized problem during pregnancy and the puerperium. Pregnancy is not a reason to discontinue therapy. There are no adequate reports or well-controlled studies in pregnant women, despite the fact the drug appears to be growing in popularity.
Side effects include nephrotoxity, ototoxicity, neuropathy, optic neuritis, seizures, anemia, hypokalemia, and hypoglycemia.

■ **Fetal Considerations**
There are no adequate reports or well-controlled studies in human fetuses. **Citalopram** crosses the human placenta, achieving an F:M ratio approximating 0.66. The use of antidepressants in early pregnancy does not seem to carry significant risk for the human infant during the newborn period. While the clinical reports are generally reassuring, neonatal withdrawal syndrome has been reported after 3rd trimester exposure. Rodent studies reveal cardiovascular and skeletal defects.

■ **Breastfeeding Safety**
Citalopram enters human breast milk, but the neonatal concentration is very low and likely poses no threat to breast-feeding neonates.

■ **References**
Doehaerd S. Related Rev Med Brux 2001; 22:A264-6.
Ericson A, Kallen B, Wiholm B. Eur J Clin Pharmacol 1999; 55:503-8.

Nordeng H, Lindemann R, Perminov KV, Reikvam A. Acta Paediatr 2001; 90:288-91.
Heikkinen T, Ekblad U, Kero P, et al. Clin Pharmacol Ther 2002; 72:184-91.

■ **Summary**

- **Pregnancy Category C**
- **Lactation Category S?**
- **Citalopram** should be used during pregnancy and lactation only if the benefit justifies the potential perinatal risk.
- There are alternative agents for which there is more experience during pregnancy and lactation.

Clarithromycin (Biaxin; Biaxin XL; Klacid XL)

■ **Class** — Antibiotic, macrolide

■ **Indications** — Infections (<u>gram-positive aerobes</u>: Staphylococcus aureus [methicillin-resistant], Staphylococcus pyogenes, Streptococcus pneumoniae; <u>gram-negative aerobes</u>: Haemophilus influenzae, Moraxella catarrhalis; <u>other microorganisms</u>: Mycoplasma pneumoniae, Chlamydia pneumoniae, Mycobacterium avium complex, Mycobacterium intracellulare, Helicobacter pylori)

■ **Mechanism** — Inhibits bacterial protein synthesis by binding to the 50S ribosomal subunit

■ **Dosage with Qualifiers** — <u>Bacterial infection</u>—250-500mg PO bid
<u>Mycoplasma avium cellulare infection</u>—15mg/kg PO qd; dose divided q12h
<u>Coxiella burnetii (Q fever) during pregnancy</u>—250-500mg PO bid

- **Contraindications**—hypersensitivity to drug or class
- **Caution**—hepatic dysfunction or renal failure

■ **Maternal Considerations** — **Clarithromycin** is used for the treatment of lower respiratory tract infections, genitourinary tract infections, skin infections, neutropenic patients, AIDS-related infections, acute maxillary sinusitis, and active duodenal ulcer. There are no adequate reports or well-controlled studies in pregnant women. It was suggested that Helicobacter pylori infection might be a cause of persistent hyperemesis gravidarum. **Clarithromycin** has also been used successfully for the treatment of Q fever during pregnancy. Studies in rats, rabbits, and monkeys indicate **clarithromycin** does not impair fertility.
Side effects include anaphylaxis, Stevens-Johnson syndrome, arrhythmia, pseudomembranous colitis, diarrhea, nausea, abdominal pain, dyspepsia, headache, and rash.

■ **Fetal Considerations** ···················· There are no adequate reports or well-controlled studies in human fetuses. **Clarithromycin** crosses the human placenta to a greater degree than other macrolides (6% maternal dose), making it a candidate in treatment trials of genital mycoplasma and ureaplasma infections during pregnancy. Post-marketing studies are reassuring. No teratogenic effects are noted in most studies of rats, rabbits, and monkeys. However, there are reports of a modest increase in cardiovascular malformations and cleft palate in certain rodent strains.

■ **Breastfeeding Safety** ················ There are no adequate reports or well-controlled studies in nursing women. **Clarithromycin** enters human breast milk reaching levels as high as 75% of the maternal concentration.

■ **References** ································· Witt A, Sommer EM, Cichna M, et al. Am J Obstet Gynecol 2003; 188:816-9.
Rouveix B, Levacher M, Giroud JP. Rev Pneumol Clin 1999; 55:338-43.
Jover-Diaz F, Robert-Gates J, Andreu-Gimenez L, Merino-Sanchez J. Infect Dis Obstet Gynecol 2001; 9:47-9.
Gilljam M, Berning SE, Peloquin CA, et al. Eur Respir J 1999; 14:347-51.
Einarson A, Phillips E, Mawji F, et al. Am J Perinatol 1998; 15:523-5.
Drinkard CR, Shatin D, Clouse J. Pharmacoepidemiol Drug Saf 2000; 9:549-56.
Jacoby EB, Porter KB. Am J Perinatol 1999; 16:85-8.
Amsden GW. Clin Ther 1996; 18:56-72.
Sedlmayr T, Peters F, Raasch W, Kees F. Geburtshilfe Frauenheilkd 1993; 53:488-91.

■ **Summary** ······························
- **Pregnancy Category C**
- **Lactation Category U**
- **Clarithromycin** should be used during pregnancy and lactation only if the benefit justifies the potential perinatal risk.
- High placental transfer during the 1st trimester makes it an attractive agent for the treatment of mycoplasma and ureaplasma infections.

Clavulanate potassium

■ **Class** — Anti-infective

■ **Indications** — Combined with **penicillin**, **amoxicillin**, and **ticarcillin** to broaden their antibacterial spectrum to cover certain gram-negative bacteria

■ **Mechanism** — β-lactamase inhibitor

■ **Dosage with Qualifiers** — See **penicillin**, **amoxicillin**, and **ticarcillin**.
- **Contraindications**—hypersensitivity to drug or class
- **Caution**—see antibiotics (**penicillin**, **ticarcillin**, **amoxicillin**)

■ **Maternal Considerations** — See **penicillin**, **amoxicillin**, and **ticarcillin**.
Side effects include nausea, vomiting, diarrhea, abdominal pain, colitis, anorexia,and pseudomembranous colitis; at high doses, seizures, platelet dysfunction, hemolytic anemia, encephalitis, and nephritis.

■ **Fetal Considerations** — There are no well-controlled studies in human fetuses. **Clavulanate** crosses the human placenta, appearing in umbilical blood within 1h after administration, reaching a peak at 2-3h. Rodent studies are reassuring when **clavulanate** is administered concomitantly with **penicillin** or **amoxicillin**, revealing no evidence of teratogenicity or IUGR despite the use of doses higher than those used clinically.

■ **Breastfeeding Safety** — While there are no reports specifically addressing the passage of **clavulanate** into the breast milk, it is generally considered compatible with breastfeeding.

■ **References** — See **penicillin**, **amoxicillin**, and **ticarcillin**.

■ **Summary** —
- **Pregnancy Category B**
- **Lactation Category S**
- **Clavulanate** is combined with **penicillin, amoxicillin, and ticarcillin** to broaden their antibacterial spectrum to include certain gram-negative bacteria.

Clemastine fumarate (Allerhist-1; Contac 12 Hour Allergy; Tavist; Tavist-1)

- **Class** — *Antihistamine*

- **Indications** — Rhinitis, urticaria

- **Mechanism** — Antagonizes central and peripheral H_1 receptors

- **Dosage with Qualifiers** — Allergic rhinitis—1.34-2.68mg PO bid or tid prn
  Urticaria—1.34-2.68mg PO bid or tid prn; max 8.04mg qd
  - **Contraindications**—hypersensitivity to drug or class, asthma, hypersensitivity, acute attacks of asthma, known alcohol intolerance
  - **Caution**—glaucoma

- **Maternal Considerations** — There are no adequate reports or well-controlled studies in pregnant women. MAO inhibitors such as **isocarboxazid** (Marplan), **phenelzine** (Nardil), or **tranylcypromine** (Parnate) prolong the anticholinergic effects of antihistamines. See **chlorpheniramine**.
  Side effects include seizures, anaphylaxis, sedation, drowsiness, dizziness, agranulocytosis, dry mouth, extreme sleepiness, confusion, weakness, ringing in the ears, blurred vision, large pupils, flushing, fever, shaking, insomnia, hallucinations, and possibly seizures.

- **Fetal Considerations** — There are no adequate reports or well-controlled studies in human fetuses. It is unknown whether **clemastine** crosses the human placenta. Symptoms of toxicity in neonates include excitement, hyperreflexia, tremors, ataxia, fever, seizures, fixed dilated pupils, dry mouth, and facial flushing. The dose that causes seizures approximates the lethal dose. See **chlorpheniramine**.

- **Breastfeeding Safety** — There is no published experience in nursing women. It is unknown whether **clemastine** enters breast milk.

- **References** — There is no published experience in pregnancy or lactation.

- **Summary** —
  - **Pregnancy Category B**
  - **Lactation Category U**
  - There are alternative agents for which there is more experience during pregnancy and lactation.

Clindamycin (Cleocin; Cleocin T; Cleocin Phosphate; Clinda-Derm; Euroclin; Turimycin)

■ **Class** — Antibiotic (*other antimicrobials*)

■ **Indications** — Infections (gram-positive aerobes: *Staphylococcus aureus, Staphylococcus epidermidis*, streptococci, pneumococci; gram-negative aerobes: *Bacteroides fragilis, Fusobacterium* species; gram-positive anaerobes: *Propionibacterium, Eubacterium, Actinomyces* species; gram-positive anaerobes: peptostreptococci, *Peptococcus, Clostridia*; group B streptococcus prophylaxis in **penicillin**-allergic women, bacterial vaginosis, acne vulgaris)

■ **Mechanism** — Bactericidal; inhibits bacterial protein synthesis

■ **Dosage with Qualifiers** — Bacterial infections—150-450mg PO qid ×7-14d; max 4.8g/d; alternatively, 300-900mg IV q6-12h
Bacterial vaginosis—1 applicator PV qhs ×3-7d
Acne vulgaris—apply 1% gel topically bid
NOTE—available in oral, parenteral, topical and vaginal gel formats
- **Contraindications**—hypersensitivity to drug or class, colitis
- **Caution**—hepatic or renal failure

■ **Maternal Considerations** — Because of its antimicrobial spectrum, **clindamycin** is used for the treatment of serious infections caused by anaerobes, respiratory tract infections, postpartum endometritis, pneumonitis, and soft tissue infections caused by streptococci and staphylococci. **Clindamycin** is a popular drug for the treatment of acne in reproductive-age women. There are no adequate reports or well-controlled studies in pregnant women. Higher doses of **clindamycin** should be used during pregnancy, as its half-life in maternal serum appears shorter during pregnancy. When combined with **gentamicin** in patients with PPROM, there is a significant reduction in the incidence of histological chorioamnionitis, but not the frequency of funisitis. **Clindamycin** vaginal gel does not reduce the incidence of preterm delivery in women with bacterial vaginosis. It is the antibiotic of choice for prophylaxis for neonatal group B sepsis in patients allergic to penicillin, though there is growing resistance.
Side effects include diarrhea, thrombocytopenia, anaphylaxis, esophagitis, pseudomembranous colitis, nausea, vomiting, rash, and jaundice.

■ **Fetal Considerations** — There are no adequate reports or well-controlled studies in human fetuses. **Clindamycin** crosses the human placenta, achieving fetal levels above the typical MICs. There are no reports linking **clindamycin** with fetal malformations. Rodent studies are reassuring, revealing no evidence of teratogenicity or IUGR despite the use of doses higher than those used clinically.

■ **Breastfeeding Safety** **Clindamycin** enters human breast milk. While case reports describe bloody stools in nursing newborns whose mothers were treated with **clindamycin**, it is usually considered compatible with breastfeeding.

■ **References** Bland ML, Vermillion ST, Soper DE, Austin M. Am J Obstet Gynecol 2001; 184:1125-6.
Kekki M, Kurki T, Pelkonen J, et al. Obstet Gynecol 2001; 97:643-8.
Ovalle A, Martinez MA, Kakarieka E, et al. J Matern Fetal Neonatal Med 2002; 12:35-41.
Brumfield CG, Hauth JC, Andrews WW. Am J Obstet Gynecol 2000; 182:1147-51.
Steen B, Rane A. Br J Clin Pharmacol 1982; 13:661-4.
Philipson A. Clin Pharmacokinet 1979; 4:297-309.

■ **Summary** • **Pregnancy Category B**
• **Lactation Category S**
• An effective drug, either alone or combined with **gentamicin** for a variety of pregnancy-related infections.

Clofazimine (Lamprene)

■ **Class** Antimycobacterials

■ **Indications** Lepromatous leprosy

■ **Mechanism** Bactericidal; preferentially binding to mycobacterial DNA

■ **Dosage with Qualifiers** Lepromatous leprosy—100mg PO bid for 10d, then 2×/w ×4mo
• **Contraindications**—hypersensitivity to drug or class.
• **Caution**—abdominal pain, diarrhea, skin discoloration, depression or suicide, skin dryness and ichthyosis, stains soft contact lenses

■ **Maternal Considerations** Uneven distribution and prolonged retention in the tissues are special features of **clofazimine** metabolism. There are no adequate reports or well-controlled studies in pregnant women.

Side effects include hyperpigmentation of the skin and conjunctiva and abdominal pain. These effects resolve upon cessation of therapy.

■ **Fetal Considerations** ⋯⋯⋯⋯ There are no adequate reports or well-controlled studies in human fetuses. **Clofazimine** crosses the placenta, though the kinetics remain to be elucidated. Hyperpigmentation of the neonate that resolves gradually is reported in humans. Rodent studies are generally reassuring, revealing no evidence of teratogenicity despite the use of doses higher than those used clinically. However, embryotoxicity and IUGR were noted.

■ **Breastfeeding Safety** ⋯⋯⋯ **Clofazimine** is excreted in the breast milk, though the kinetics remain to be elucidated. Hyperpigmentation of the newborn resolving over 5mo was reported.

■ **References** ⋯⋯⋯⋯⋯⋯⋯ Lopes VG, Sarno EN. Rev Assoc Med Bras 1994; 40:195-201.
Holdiness MR. Clin Pharmacokinet 1989; 16:74-85.
Farb H, West DP, Pedvis-Leftick A. Obstet Gynecol 1982; 59:122-3.

■ **Summary** ⋯⋯⋯⋯⋯⋯⋯⋯
- **Pregnancy Category C**
- **Lactation Category U**
- **Clofazimine** should be used during pregnancy and lactation only if the benefit justifies the potential perinatal risk.
- There are alternative agents for which there is more experience during pregnancy and lactation.

Clofibrate (Apoterin; Atromid-S; Cartagyl; Clofibral; Clofibrato; Clofipront; Coles)

■ **Class** ⋯⋯⋯⋯⋯⋯⋯⋯⋯⋯ *Antihyperlipemic*

■ **Indications** ⋯⋯⋯⋯⋯⋯⋯ Hypercholesterolemia

■ **Mechanism** ⋯⋯⋯⋯⋯⋯ Fibrates act through the nuclear PPAR system which regulates lipid metabolism

■ **Dosage with Qualifiers** ⋯⋯⋯ Hypercholesterolemia—2g PO qd, in divided doses
NOTE—success is defined as triglyceride level reduced 20-70%, HDL increased by 10-25%, or LDL decreased
- **Contraindications**—severe renal or hepatic dysfunction, gallbladder disease, primary biliary cirrhosis
- **Caution**—significant hepatic or renal dysfunction, rhabdomyolysis and severe hyperkalemia (with preexisting renal insufficiency)

■ **Maternal Considerations** ⋯⋯⋯ There are no adequate reports or well-controlled studies of **clofibrate** in pregnant women. **Clofibrate** typically reduces serum cholesterol a modest amount and serum triglycerides somewhat more. Substantial reductions in cholesterol and triglycerides can occur in type III hyperlipidemia. No study has shown a convincing reduction in fatal MI. There is little information on the effect of **clofibrate** on cholesterol metabolism during human pregnancy. For that reason, women of childbearing potential taking **clofibrate** should use effective contraception. In patients who plan to become pregnant, **clofibrate** should be withdrawn several months before conception.

Side effects include mild abdominal and bowel irritation, myalgia, increased CPK, gallstones, increased serum transaminase, water retention, and breast enlargement.

■ **Fetal Considerations** ⋯⋯⋯⋯ There are no adequate and well-controlled studies in human fetuses. It is unknown whether **clofibrate** crosses the human placenta. It does cross the rodent placenta and alters fetal cholesterol metabolism. While teratogenic studies have not demonstrated any effect attributable to **clofibrate**, it is known that serum of the rabbit fetus accumulates a higher concentration of **clofibrate** than that in the mother.

■ **Breastfeeding Safety** ⋯⋯⋯⋯ There is no published experience in nursing women. It is unknown whether **clofibrate** enters human breast milk. Animal studies revealed increase in neonatal and pup mortality rates during lactation.

■ **References** ⋯⋯⋯⋯⋯⋯⋯⋯⋯⋯⋯⋯ Wilson GN, King T, Argyle JC, Garcia RF. Pediatr Res 1991; 29:256-62.
Ujhazy E, Onderova E, Horakova M, et al. Pharmacol Toxicol 1989; 64:286-90.
Nyitray M, Szaszovsky E, Druga A. Arch Toxicol Suppl 1980; 4:463-5.
Muller DP, Pavlou C, Whitelaw AG, McLintock D. Br J Obstet Gynaecol 1978; 85:127-33.

■ **Summary** ⋯⋯⋯⋯⋯⋯⋯⋯⋯⋯⋯⋯⋯⋯ • **Pregnancy Category C**
• **Lactation Category U**
• **Clofibrate** should be used during pregnancy and lactation only if the benefit justifies the potential perinatal risk and there are no other reasonable options.

Clomiphene (Clomid; Clomifene; Milophene; Serophene)

■ **Class** — *Infertility, hormone, hormone modifier*

■ **Indications** — Ovulation induction

■ **Mechanism** — Binds to estrogen receptors with both stimulatory and inhibitory effects

■ **Dosage with Qualifiers** — Ovulation induction—50mg PO qd for 5d (menstrual cycle day 5-10); max 100mg PO qd
- **Contraindications**—hypersensitivity to drug or class, pregnancy, abnormal uterine bleeding, adrenal gland dysfunction, thyroid disease, pituitary tumor, endometrial cancer
- **Caution**—polycystic ovary syndrome, hepatic failure

■ **Maternal Considerations** — There are no indications for **clomiphene** during pregnancy. Ovarian hyperstimulation may occur even when used as directed. There is an increased incidence of multiple pregnancy, including bilateral tubal pregnancy and coexisting tubal and intrauterine pregnancy. *Side effects* include thromboembolism, ovarian hyperstimulation syndrome, multiple pregnancy, ovarian enlargement, nausea, vomiting, hot flashes, abdominal distension, breast tenderness, blurred vision, headache, and abnormal uterine bleeding.

■ **Fetal Considerations** — There are no adequate reports or well-controlled studies in human fetuses. It is unknown whether **clomiphene** crosses the human placenta. Although a myriad of fetal abnormalities are reported in pregnancies after **clomiphene**-induced ovulation, no discernable pattern has emerged. Rare ocular abnormalities (persistent hyperplastic primary vitreous and retinal aplasia) have been reported in several children of women taking high doses during pregnancy. Rodent studies revealed hydramnios, and weak, edematous fetuses with wavy ribs and bone changes.

■ **Breastfeeding Safety** — There is no published experience in nursing women. It is not known whether **clomiphene** is excreted in human milk.

■ **References** — Lynch A, McDuffie R Jr, Murphy J, et al. Obstet Gynecol 2002; 99:445-51.
Nagao T, Yoshimura S. Teratog Carcinog Mutagen 2001; 21:213-21.
Clark JH, Guthrie SC, McCormack SA. Adv Exp Med Biol 1981; 138:87-98.
Canales ES, Lasso P, Soria J, Zarate A. Br J Obstet Gynaecol 1977; 84:758-9.
Bishai R, Arbour L, Lyons C, Koren G. Teratology 1999; 60:143-5.

■ **Summary**
- **Pregnancy Category X**
- **Lactation Category U**
- **Clomiphene** is contraindicated during pregnancy.
- There is no indication for its use during lactation.
- Patient should be evaluated carefully to exclude pregnancy prior to beginning ovulation induction.

Clomipramine (Anafranil)

■ **Class** — *Antidepressant, tricyclic*

■ **Indications** — Obsessive compulsive disorder, depression

■ **Mechanism** — Exact mechanism unknown; inhibits norepinephrine and serotonin reuptake

■ **Dosage with Qualifiers** — Obsessive-compulsive disorder—begin 25mg PO qhs, then increase 75mg qhs; max 250mg qhs
Depression—100-250mg PO qd in 3 divided doses
- **Contraindications**—hypersensitivity to drug or class, myocardial infarction, glaucoma, pheochromocytoma, prior usage of MAO inhibitors, suicidal ideation
- **Caution**—hepatic or renal dysfunction, seizure disorder

■ **Maternal Considerations** — There are no adequate reports or well-controlled studies in pregnant women. A variety of withdrawal symptoms may occur with abrupt discontinuation of **clomipramine**. *Side effects* include dry mouth, sedation, headache, constipation, and seizures.

■ **Fetal Considerations** — There are no adequate reports or well-controlled studies in human fetuses. It is unknown whether **clomipramine** crosses the human placenta. Withdrawal symptoms, including jitteriness, tremor, and seizures, have been reported in neonates whose mothers had taken **clomipramine** until delivery. Rodent studies are reassuring, revealing no evidence of teratogenicity or IUGR despite the use of doses higher than those used clinically. Neonatal **clomipramine** on days 8-21 produced behavioral and physiologic abnormalities in the adult resembling those found in human depression.

■ **Breastfeeding Safety** — Since only trace amounts of **clomipramine** are found in human breast milk, it is likely compatible with breastfeeding.

■ **References** — Feng P, Ma Y, Vogel GW. Brain Res Dev Brain Res 2001; 129:107-10.

Wisner KL, Perel JM, Foglia JP. J Clin Psychiatry
1995; 56:17-20.
Rodriguez Echandia EL, Foscolo MR, Gonzalez A. Ann NY
Acad Sci 1988; 525:80-8.
Schimmell MS, Katz EZ, Shaag Y, et al. J Toxicol Clin
Toxicol 1991; 29:479-84.

■ **Summary**

- **Pregnancy Category C**
- **Lactation Category S?**
- **Clomipramine** should be used during pregnancy only if the benefit justifies the potential perinatal risk.

Clonazepam (Klonopin)

■ **Class**

Anxiolytics, *benzodiazepine*

■ **Indications**

Absence seizures, anxiety, periodic leg movement, neuralgia

■ **Mechanism**

Binds to benzodiazepine receptors

■ **Dosage with Qualifiers**

Absence seizures—0.5-5mg PO tid
Anxiety—0.25-0.5mg PO bid or tid
Panic disorder—0.5-1mg PO bid or tid
Periodic leg movement—0.5-2mg PO tid
Neuralgia—2-4mg PO qd
NOTE—treatment should not be withdrawn abruptly

- **Contraindications**—hypersensitivity to drug or class
- **Caution**—hepatic failure

■ **Maternal Considerations**

There are no adequate reports or well-controlled studies in pregnant women. In case reports, **clonazepam** was unrelated to complications of pregnancy, labor, or delivery. Several investigators have used **clonazepam** for seizure prophylaxis in severe preeclampsia.
Side effects include respiratory depression, neutropenia, hepatic failure, ataxia, confusion, visual changes, drowsiness, and behavioral changes.

■ **Fetal Considerations**

There are no adequate reports or well-controlled studies in human fetuses. **Clonazepam** crosses the human placenta, achieving an F:M ratio approximating 0.60. While congenital anomalies are reported in 13% of infants whose mothers took **clonazepam** during pregnancy in combination with other anti-epileptic drugs, there is no pattern of anomalies. The majority of exposed infants are normal at birth and have normal postnatal development. Exposure in the late 3rd trimester and during labor seems to carry greater risks to the perinate. While the neonatal withdrawal syndrome is rare, children born to treated women may have symptoms varying from mild sedation, hypotonia, and reluctance to suck, to apnea spells, cyanosis, and impaired metabolic responses to cold stress. These symptoms can persist from hours to months after birth.

■ **Breastfeeding Safety**

There are no adequate reports or well-controlled studies in nursing mothers. **Clonazepam** enters human breast milk. Limited study suggests the breast-feeding neonate could ingest a clinically relevant amount. Breast-fed newborns should be observed closely for side effects.

■ **References**

Eros E, Czeizel AE, Rockenbauer M, et al. Eur J Obstet Gynecol Reprod Biol 2002; 101:147-54.
McElhatton PR. Reprod Toxicol 1994; 8:461-75.
Soderman P, Matheson I. Eur J Pediatr 1988; 147:212-3.
Fisher JB, Edgren BE, Mammel MC, Coleman JM. Obstet Gynecol 1985; 66(3 Suppl):34S-35S.

■ **Summary**

- **Pregnancy Category D**
- **Lactation Category NS?**
- There is no substantive evidence that **clonazepam** alone is a teratogen in humans.
- Exposure in the late 3rd trimester and during labor seems to carry greater risks to the perinate.
- **Clonazepam** should be used during pregnancy and lactation only if the benefit justifies the potential perinatal risk.

Clonidine (Catapres; Catapres-TTS; Duraclon)

■ **Class**

Antihypertensive

■ **Indications**

Hypertension

■ **Mechanism**

α_2-adrenergic receptor agonists (centrally acting)

■ **Dosage with Qualifiers**

Hypertension—0.1-0.3mg PO bid; max 1.2mg PO bid
Also used for analgesia or as an adjunctive anesthetic-neuraxial given IV or PO
NOTE—caution should be used due to potential rebound hypertension
- **Contraindications**—hypersensitivity
- **Caution**—cardiovascular disease, hepatic and renal failure

■ **Maternal Considerations** ········ **Clonidine** is popular for treatment-seeking opiate abusers, particularly those with concurrent cocaine use. The abuse potential of the drug warrants further study in this high-risk population. There are no adequate reports or well-controlled studies in pregnant women. Women withdrawing from a variety of illicit narcotics may benefit from **clonidine** initially and then **methadone** if symptoms persist. The combination of epidural **clonidine** with **bupivacaine/fentanyl** for pain control during labor improves analgesia, and reduces the supplementation rate and frequency of shivering. Though hypotension and bradycardia are drug dependent, no adverse maternal hemodynamic effects are noted if used in low doses mixed with opioids and local anesthetic. However, troublesome maternal sedation has been reported.

Side effects include drowsiness, dry mouth, constipation, headache, rash, nausea, edema, and dry eyes.

■ **Fetal Considerations** ··············· There are no adequate reports or well-controlled studies in human fetuses. **Clonidine** readily crosses the placenta achieving an F:M ratio of 1. Amniotic fluid concentrations are up to 4 times those in serum. Neonates of women receiving **clonidine** during labor are not sedated, but may experience some hypotension. **Clonidine** does not negatively affect the fetal heart rate pattern. Rodent studies are reassuring, revealing no evidence of teratogenicity or IUGR despite the use of doses higher than those used clinically. However, there is an increase in the rate of embryo absorption.

■ **Breastfeeding Safety** ··············· **Clonidine** is concentrated in human breast milk reaching an M:P ratio approximating 2. Caution is advised.

■ **References** ···················· Paech MJ, Pavy TJ, Orlikowski CE, Evans SF. Reg Anesth Pain Med 2000; 25:34-40.
Tremlett MR, Kelly PJ, Parkins J, et al. Br J Anaesth 1999; 83:257-61.
Aveline C, El Metaoua S, Masmoudi A, Boelle PY, Bonnet F. Anesth Analg 2002; 95:735-40.
Anderson F, Paluzzi P, Lee J, et al. Obstet Gynecol 1997; 90:790-4.
Dashe JS, Jackson GL, Olscher DA, et al. Obstet Gynecol 1998; 92:854-8.
Hartikainen-Sorri AL, Heikkinen JE, Koivisto M. Obstet Gynecol 1987; 69:598-600.

■ **Summary** ······························ • **Pregnancy Category C**
• **Lactation Category NS?**
• **Clonidine** should be used during pregnancy and lactation only if the benefit justifies the potential perinatal risk.

Clorazepate (Gen-Xene; Mendon; Nevracten; Tranxene)

■ **Class** — *Sedative, anxiolytic; benzodiazepine*

■ **Indications** — Anxiety, alcohol withdrawal

■ **Mechanism** — Enhances GABA effects by binding to benzodiazepine receptors

■ **Dosage with Qualifiers** — Anxiety—15-60mg PO qd in divided doses
Alcohol withdrawal—30mg ×1, then 30-60mg/d in divided doses
- **Contraindications**—hypersensitivity to drug or class, substance abuse, glaucoma, acute angina, suicidal ideation
- **Caution**—none

■ **Maternal Considerations** — There are no adequate reports or well-controlled studies in pregnant women. All benzodiazepine derivatives are lipophilic, undissociated agents, which readily penetrate membranes. **Clorazepate** is rapidly absorbed with peak concentrations reached within 2h. The absorption half-life approximates 0.77h and elimination half-life is 1.3h in pregnant women.
Side effects include hepatic failure, drowsiness, headache, hypotension, and dry mouth.

■ **Fetal Considerations** — There are no adequate reports or well-controlled studies in pregnant women. **Clorazepate** appears to cross the placenta more slowly than other benzodiazepines. An increased risk of malformations is reported in some studies for some benzodiazepines. The lowest effective dose of **clorazepate** should be used during delivery, because high doses are associated with floppy infant syndrome. Rodent teratogenicity studies have not apparently been performed.

■ **Breastfeeding Safety** — There is no published experience in nursing mothers. **Clorazepate** is excreted into human breast milk at low concentrations, though the kinetics remain to be detailed. As with other benzodiazepines in breast milk, caution is advised.

■ **References** — McElhatton PR. Reprod Toxicol 1994; 8:461-75.
Patel DA, Patel AR. JAMA 1980; 244:135-6.
Rey E, d'Athis P, Giraux P, et al. Eur J Clin Pharmacol 1979; 15:175-80.

■ **Summary** • **Pregnancy Category D**
• **Lactation Category U**
• **Clorazepate** should be used during pregnancy and lactation only if the benefit justifies the potential perinatal risk.
• There are usually other options available for which there is more experience during pregnancy and lactation.

Clotrimazole (Canastene; Clomaz; Clomine; Fungicide; Gyne-Lotrimin; Lotrimin; Mycelex; Mycelex-G)

■ **Class** — *Antifungal, dermatologic*

■ **Indications** — *Tinea pedis, cruris, versicolor, corporis*; cutaneous and vulvovaginal candidiasis

■ **Mechanism** — Alters membrane permeability

■ **Dosage with Qualifiers** — Yeast infection—1% lotion bid 2-4w for cutaneous candidiasis
Vaginal candidiasis—vaginal cream should be inserted qhs ×7d
• **Contraindications**—hypersensitivity to drug or class
• **Caution**—none

■ **Maternal Considerations** — There are no adequate reports or well-controlled studies in pregnant women. Vaginal candidiasis (moniliasis or thrush) is a common and frequently distressing infection for many women. Treatments for 7d may be necessary during pregnancy rather than the shorter courses more commonly used for nonpregnant women. Topical **clotrimazole** appears to be more effective than **nystatin** for treating symptomatic vaginal candidiasis in pregnancy. Candida sepsis should be considered in the differential diagnosis of sepsis following CVS.
Side effects include erythema, burning, edema, pruritus, and vaginal irritation.

■ **Fetal Considerations** — There are no adequate reports or well-controlled studies in human fetuses. It is unknown whether **clotrimazole** crosses the human placenta. There is little maternal, systemic absorption after dermal application. Thus, considering the dose and route, it is unlikely the maternal systemic concentration will reach clinically relevant level. One case report describes fetal death at 18 weeks' gestation in association with a retained IUD and asymptomatic intraamniotic and fetal infection by *Candida albicans*. Rodent studies are reassuring, revealing no evidence of teratogenicity or IUGR despite the use of doses higher than those used clinically.

■ **Breastfeeding Safety** .... There are no adequate reports or well-controlled studies in nursing mothers. It is unknown whether **clotrimazole** enters human breast milk. However, considering the route and level of maternal systemic absorption, it is unlikely the breast-feeding neonate would ingest a clinically significant amount.

■ **References** ....
Young GL, Jewell D. Cochrane Database Syst Rev 2000; CD000225.
Czeizel AE, Toth M, Rockenbauer M. Epidemiology 1999; 10:437-40.
Weisberg M. Clin Ther 1986; 8:563-7.
Guaschino S, Michelone G, Stola E, et al. Biol Res Pregnancy Perinatol 1986; 7:20-2.
Fleury F, Hughes D, Floyd R. Am J Obstet Gynecol 1985; 152:968-70.
Segal D, Gohar J, Huleihel M, Mazor M. Scand J Infect Dis 2001; 33:77-8.

■ **Summary** ....
- **Pregnancy Category B**
- **Lactation Category S?**
- There is no evidence that either thrush or **clotrimazole** in pregnancy is harmful to the baby.
- Treatments ×7d for vaginitis may be necessary during pregnancy in contrast to the shorter courses used in nonpregnant women.

Cloxacillin (Amplium; Austrastaph; Bactopen; Chuckin; Cloxapen; Methocillin; Prostafilina; Prostaphlin; Tegopen)

■ **Class** .... *Antimicrobial*

■ **Indications** .... Bacterial infection, treatment of staphylococcal mastitis

■ **Mechanism** .... Bactericidal; inhibits bacterial wall mucopeptide synthesis

■ **Dosage with Qualifiers** .... Bacterial infection—250-500mg PO q6h; take 1h before or after meals
NOTE—discontinued in the U.S. **Cloxacilin** loses potency when used with **erythromycin**, **gentamicin**, and **kanamycin**. It should not be added to blood products and IV lipids.
- **Contraindications**—hypersensitivity to drug or class
- **Caution**—hepatic or renal failure

199

■ **Maternal Considerations** .... **Cloxacillin sodium** is a broad-spectrum antibiotic effective against penicillinase-producing *Staphylococcus* and is usually combined with **ampicillin**. There are no adequate reports or well-controlled studies in pregnant women. Before its withdrawal in the U.S., **cloxacillin** was used for the treatment of mastitis. There is a significant increase in the free plasma fraction of the **cloxacillin** during pregnancy beginning in the 2nd trimester and peaking at delivery. A similarly increased free-of-fraction **cloxacillin** is found in cord blood, which increases further during the 1st postnatal week. **Cloxacillin** is highly concentrated in the kidneys.
Side effects include seizures, thrombocytopenia, agranulocytosis, and renal failure.

■ **Fetal Considerations** .... There are no adequate reports or well-controlled studies in human fetuses. **Cloxacillin** crosses the human placenta. Fetal drug levels rise slowly to equilibrium with the maternal circulation 1-3h after drug administration. Thereafter, fetal drug levels exceed maternal values. Amniotic fluid levels are low during early gestation, rising progressively near term until they exceed maternal values 6-8h after drug administration. Rodent studies are reassuring, revealing no evidence of teratogenicity or IUGR despite the use of doses higher than those used clinically.

■ **Breastfeeding Safety** .... There is no published experience in nursing mothers. **Cloxacillin** is excreted in the breast milk of both humans and cows.

■ **References** .... Herngren L, Ehrnebo M, Boreus LO. Dev Pharmacol Ther 1983; 6:110-24.
Anderson JC. J Comp Pathol 1977; 87:611-21.
Brander GC, Watkins JH, Gard RP. Vet Rec 1975; 97:300-4.

■ **Summary** .... • **Pregnancy Category B**
• **Lactation Category U**
• There are other options for which there is more experience during pregnancy and lactation.

Clozapine (Clozaril; Entumin; Etumine)

■ **Class** .... *Antipsychotic*

■ **Indications** .... Atypical psychosis, schizophrenia

■ **Mechanism** .... Unknown; may antagonize D2 dopamine receptors

■ **Dosage with Qualifiers** ········ Psychosis (schizophrenia)—begin 12.5mg PO qd or bid, increasing up to 25-50mg in 3-7d; titer to symptoms to 150-300mg PO bid; max 900mg/d
NOTE—check CBC count q2w for agranulocytosis
- **Contraindications**—hypersensitivity to drug or class, myocarditis, myeloproliferative disorder, glaucoma, CNS depression
- **Caution**—renal or hepatic failure, seizure and cardiac disease, bone marrow suppression

■ **Maternal Considerations** ······· There are no adequate reports or well-controlled studies in pregnant women. **Clozapine** is a relatively new medication for treatment-resistant schizophrenia. It is effective in responsive patients experiencing positive (hallucinations, delusions, bizarre behavior, hostility) and negative (withdrawal, blunted emotions, lack of motivation, and inability to experience pleasure or enjoyment) symptoms. Negative symptoms seem to respond better to **clozapine** compared to traditional antipsychotics. Studies in rats revealed a rapid increase in the level of serum prolactin with peak values at 15 and 60min. Clinical experience suggests most current psychotropic drugs are relatively safe for use in pregnancy. *Side effects* include agranulocytosis, leukopenia, neuroleptic malignant syndrome, thrombosis, constipation, arrhythmias, and cardiac arrest.

■ **Fetal Considerations** ·············· There are no adequate reports or well-controlled studies in the human fetus. It is unknown whether **clozapine** crosses the human placenta. Rodent studies are reassuring, revealing no evidence of teratogenicity or IUGR despite the use of doses higher than those used clinically.

■ **Breastfeeding Safety** ············ There are no adequate reports or well-controlled studies in nursing women. It is unknown whether **clozapine** enters human breast milk. Animal studies suggest **clozapine** enters breast milk and can affect neonatal behavior. Other antipsychotic medications are excreted into human breast milk. If breastfeeding continues, the infant should be monitored for possible adverse effects, the drug given at the lowest effective dose, and breastfeeding avoided at times of peak drug levels.

■ **References** ·············· Dickson RA, Hogg L. Psychiatr Serv 1998; 49:1081-3.
Kaplan B, Modai I, Stoler M, et al. J Am Board Fam Pract 1995; 8:239-41.
Barnas C, Bergant A, Hummer M, et al. Am J Psychiatry 1994; 151:945.

■ **Summary** ··············
- **Pregnancy Category B**
- **Lactation Category U**
- As for most psychotropic drugs, using monotherapy and the lowest effective quantity given in divided doses to minimize the peaks can minimize the risks.

Cocaine

■ **Class** — *Sympatomimetic; topical anesthesia*

■ **Indications** — Topical anesthetic for mucosa

■ **Mechanism** — Inhibits norepinephrine reuptake in the human peripheral circulation

■ **Dosage with Qualifiers** — Topical <u>anesthesia</u>—dose varies with the area to be anesthetized, vascularity of the tissues, individual tolerance, and the technique of anesthesia.
NOTE—highly restricted access in the U.S.; no indication during pregnancy; for use as a topical anesthetic of mucosa only
NOTE—the lowest dosage needed to provide effective anesthesia should be administered
- **Contraindications**—hypersensitivity
- **Caution**—cardiovascular disease, hypertension

■ **Maternal Considerations** — Cocaine is a highly addictive drug and is abused widely. There are no adequate reports or well-controlled studies in pregnant women. Maternal cocaine use is a significant public health problem, particularly in urban areas and among women of low socioeconomic status. Cocaine stimulates isolated myometrial contractile activity, and several clinical studies report an association between cocaine and preterm labor. Although cocaine inhibits uterine neuronal and extraneuronal uptake of catecholamines, and increases circulating levels of catecholamines in experimental animals, it is unlikely that facilitation of the α-adrenergic pathway is the sole mechanism of action. Cocaine-exposed women have a higher risk of medical complications including syphilis, gonorrhea, and hepatitis; psychiatric, nervous, emotional disorders; PROM, abruptio placentae, and domestic violence.

■ **Fetal Considerations** — There are no adequate reports or well-controlled studies in the human fetus. **Cocaine** crosses the human placenta and is associated with placental abruption, free radical production and fetal encephalopathy. **Cocaine**-exposed children are at increased risk of significant cognitive deficits, and a doubling of the rate of developmental delay during the first 2 years of life. **Cocaine** has teratogenic or adverse effects on the developing brain. **Cocaine**-exposed infants require medical attention for central nervous system irritation, cardiac anomalies, apnea, and feeding difficulties. It is estimated $500 million (U.S.) in additional health expenditures result from the direct hospital costs of **cocaine**-exposed neonates. Ongoing maternal drug use is associated with worse developmental outcomes among a group of drug-exposed infants.

- **Breastfeeding Safety** .... There are no adequate reports or well-controlled studies in nursing mothers. **Cocaine** freely enters human breast milk and is stable.

- **References** .... Bauer CR, Shankaran S, Bada HS, et al. Am J Obstet Gynecol 2002; 186:487-95.
Refuerzo JS, Sokol RJ, Blackwell SC, et al. Am J Obstet Gynecol 2002; 186:1150-4.
Nassogne MC, Evrard P, Courtoy PJ. Ann NY Acad Sci 1998; 846:51-68.
Chasnoff IJ, Lewis DE, Squires L. Pediatrics 1987; 80:836-8.
Bailey DN. Am J Clin Pathol 1998; 110:491-4.
Delaney DB, Larrabee KD, Monga M. Am J Perinatol 1997; 14:285-8.
Schuler ME, Nair P, Kettinger L. Arch Pediatr Adolesc Med 2003; 157:133-8.

- **Summary** ....
  - **Pregnancy Category C**
  - **Lactation Category NS**
  - There are no indications for **cocaine** use during pregnancy and lactation.

Codeine

- **Class** .... *Analgesic, narcotic*

- **Indications** .... Antitussive, expectorant

- **Mechanism** .... Opiate receptor stimulant

- **Dosage with Qualifiers** .... Pain management—15-60mg PO/IM qid
Antitussive—10-20mg PO q4-6h
NOTE—also combined with **aspirin**, **acetaminophen**, **ibuprofen**, **propoxyphene**, and others
  - **Contraindications**—hypersensitivity to drug or class
  - **Caution**—hepatic or renal dysfunction, increased intracranial pressure, hypothyroidism, acute alcoholism, chronic lung disease

- **Maternal Considerations** .... **Codeine** is metabolized to **morphine**. There are no adequate reports or well-controlled studies in pregnant women. **Codeine** is contained in many tablets prescribed for the relief of headaches. It is commonly used alone and in combination to relieve episiotomy pain during the puerperium. Combining **codeine** with a NSAID significantly enhances pain relief. **Codeine** is not effective for the relief of uterine cramps. **Codeine** overdose may be reversed with **naloxone**.

Side effects include dizziness, euphoria, nausea, vomiting, constipation, dry mouth, urinary retention, and itching.

■ **Fetal Considerations**
There are no adequate reports or well-controlled studies in human fetuses. Rodent studies are reassuring, revealing no evidence of teratogenicity, though IUGR is seen at doses below those producing maternal toxicity.

■ **Breastfeeding Safety**
There are no adequate reports or well-controlled studies in nursing mothers. **Codeine** and its metabolite **morphine** are excreted in human breast milk. Breast-feeding neonates have low plasma levels during the first few days of life in part secondary to the low concentration in milk, and in part due to the small amount of milk produced. Thus, moderate **codeine** use (up to 60mg) is probably compatible with breastfeeding.

■ **References**
Meny RG, Naumburg EG, Alger LS, et al. J Hum Lact 1993; 9:237-40.
Williams J, Price CJ, Sleet RB, et al. Fundam Appl Toxicol 1991; 16:401-13.
Bloomfield SS, Mitchell J, Cissell G, Barden TP. Am J Med 1986; 80:65-70.
Jacobson J, Bertilson SO. J Int Med Res 1987; 15:89-95.

■ **Summary**
- **Pregnancy Category C**
- **Lactation Category S**
- **Codeine** should be used during pregnancy and lactation only if the benefit justifies the potential perinatal risk.

Colchicine (Colsalide Improved; Coluric)

■ **Class**
Antigout

■ **Indications**
Gout (acute), chronic familial Mediterranean fever (prophylaxis)

■ **Mechanism**
Unknown; interferes with microtubule growth affecting mitosis and other, microtubule-dependent functions

■ **Dosage with Qualifiers**
Gout (acute)—1-1.2mg PO ×1, then 0.5-0.6mg PO q1-2h; max 4-8mg PO/24h; allow 2-3d between courses; alternatively, administered 1-2mg IV load, then 0.5mg IV q6h; max 4mg; allow 7d between courses
Gout (prophylaxis)—0.6mg PO 1-4×/w
Familial Mediterranean fever (prophylaxis)—1-2mg PO div dose bid or tid

- **Contraindications**—hypersensitivity to drug or class, cardiovascular diseases, diarrhea, nausea, vomiting, or stomach pain, blood dyscrasia
- **Caution**—hepatic or renal failure, impaired GI function

■ **Maternal Considerations** Gout is extremely rare in pregnancy. There are no adequate reports or well-controlled studies in pregnant women. **Colchicine** is found in some herbs such as **ginkgo biloba**. **Colchicine**-induced myopathy and neuropathy appear more common than previously recognized. Patients receiving long-term therapy should be monitored carefully.
Side effects include loss of hair, gastrointestinal symptoms, and loss of appetite.

■ **Fetal Considerations** There are no adequate reports or well-controlled studies in human fetuses. **Colchicine** crosses the human placenta. And while the kinetics remain to be elucidated, it is detectable after maternal ingestion of herbal remedies where the concentration is high enough to affect neutrophil adherence. It does cross the rodent placenta, and is teratogenic at doses of 1.25 and 1.5mg/kg in mice and 10mg/kg in hamsters. Because of its mechanism of action, it is suggested women who take **colchicine** during fertilization have an increased likelihood of an aneuploid fetus. As a result, some authors do not advise discontinuation of **colchicine** before pregnancy but recommend amniocentesis for karyotyping. The evidence supporting this recommendation is scant.

■ **Breastfeeding Safety** There is no published experience in nursing women. **Colchicine** is excreted into human breast milk in low quantities. It usually considered compatible with breastfeeding.

■ **References** Guillonneau M, Aigrain EJ, Galliot M, et al. Eur J Obstet Gynecol Reprod Biol 1995; 61:177-8.
Ditkoff EC, Sauer. J Assist Reprod Genet 1996; 13:684-5.
Petty HR, Fernando M, Kindzelskii AL, et al. Chem Res Toxicol 2001; 14:1254-8.
Ehrenfeld M, Brzezinski A, Levy M, Eliakim M. Br J Obstet Gynaecol 1987; 94:1186-91.
Ben-Chetrit E, Scherrmann JM, Levy M. Arthritis Rheum 1996; 39:1213-7.

■ **Summary**
- **Pregnancy Category D**
- **Lactation Category S**
- **Colchicine** should be used during pregnancy and lactation only if the benefit justifies the potential perinatal risk.
- Patients should be warned against using herbal products known to contain **colchicine**.

Colesevelam (Welchol)

■ **Class** — Cholesterol lowering

■ **Indications** — Hypercholesterolemia

■ **Mechanism** — High capacity bile acid binding molecule

■ **Dosage with Qualifiers** — Hypercholesterolemia—4-6 tab PO qd (1 tab = 625mg **colesevelam**)
NOTE—medication should be taken with food
- **Contraindications**—hypersensitivity to drug or class
- **Caution**—constipation, triglycerides elevated (>300mg/dl), dysphagia, major GI surgery

■ **Maternal Considerations** — There is no published experience with **colesevelam** during pregnancy. Malabsorption of fat-soluble vitamins might occur during use.
Side effects include nausea, bloating, belching, flatulence, and weight loss.

■ **Fetal Considerations** — There are no adequate reports or well-controlled studies in human fetuses. It is unknown whether **colesevelam** crosses the human placenta. Rodent studies are reassuring, revealing no evidence of teratogenicity or IUGR despite the use of doses higher than those used clinically.

■ **Breastfeeding Safety** — There are no adequate reports or well-controlled studies in pregnant women. It is unknown whether **colesevelam** enters human breast milk.

■ **References** — Shepherd J, Packard CJ, Bicker S, et al. N Engl J Med 1980; 302:1219-22.

■ **Summary** —
- **Pregnancy Category B**
- **Lactation Category U**
- **Colesevelam** should be used during pregnancy and lactation only if the benefit justifies the potential perinatal risk.
- There are other agents for which there is more experience during pregnancy and lactation.

Colestipol (Colestid)

■ **Class** ⸱⸱⸱⸱⸱⸱⸱⸱⸱⸱⸱⸱ Antihyperlipemic; bile acid sequestrant

■ **Indications** ⸱⸱⸱⸱⸱⸱⸱⸱⸱⸱ Hypercholesterolemia, digitoxin overdose

■ **Mechanism** ⸱⸱⸱⸱⸱⸱⸱⸱⸱ Binds bile acids in the intestine creating a nonabsorbable complex

■ **Dosage with Qualifiers** ⸱⸱⸱⸱ Hypercholesterolemia—2-16g qd; begin at 2g qd or bid, increase in 2g increments at 1 or 2mo intervals
Digitoxin overdose—10g PO ×1, then 5g PO q6-8h
- **Contraindications**—hypersensitivity to drug or class
- **Caution**—constipation, vitamin absorption interference

■ **Maternal Considerations** ⸱⸱⸱ There are no adequate reports or well-controlled studies in pregnant women. **Colestipol** is an adjunctive therapy for the reduction of elevated serum total and LDL-C in patients with primary hypercholesterolemia (elevated LDL-C) who do not respond adequately to diet. Chronic use of **colestipol** may lead to increased bleeding secondary to the hypoprothrombinemia of vitamin K deficiency.
Side effects include nausea, bloating, belching, flatulence, and weight loss.

■ **Fetal Considerations** ⸱⸱⸱⸱⸱⸱ There are no adequate reports or well-controlled studies in human fetuses. It is unknown whether **colestipol** crosses the human placenta. However, it is not absorbed systemically (less than 0.17% of the dose), and thus should not directly cause fetal harm at the recommended dosages. Rodent studies are reassuring, revealing no evidence of teratogenicity or IUGR despite the use of doses higher than those used clinically.

■ **Breastfeeding Safety** ⸱⸱⸱⸱⸱⸱ There are no adequate reports or well-controlled studies in breastfeeding women. **Colestipol** is not absorbed into the systemic circulation, which suggests a direct effect on breastfeeding is not possible. However, prolonged use could induce malabsorption and decrease the milk concentration of vitamins A, D, and K.

■ **References** ⸱⸱⸱⸱⸱⸱⸱⸱⸱⸱ Webster HD, Bollert JA. Toxicol Appl Pharmacol 1974; 28:57-65.

■ **Summary** ⸱⸱⸱⸱⸱⸱⸱⸱⸱⸱
- **Pregnancy Category B**
- **Lactation Category S?**
- **Colestipol** should be used during pregnancy and lactation only if the benefit justifies the potential perinatal risk.

Cortisone (Cortisyl; Cortone)

■ **Class** .... Corticosteroid

■ **Indications** .... Adrenal insufficiency, inflammation

■ **Mechanism** .... Unknown

■ **Dosage with Qualifiers** .... Adrenal insufficiency—25-300mg PO qd
Inflammation suppression—25-300mg PO qd
NOTE—Chronic treatment may cause adrenal
suppression; use the lowest dose for shortest time.
Patients with systemic infection or surgical stress require
supplemental therapy.
- **Contraindications**—hypersensitivity to drug or class,
  CHF, active untreated infections (however, may be used
  in patients under treatment for tuberculous meningitis)
- **Caution**—seizure disorder, diabetes, hypertension,
  osteoporosis, hepatic dysfunction

■ **Maternal Considerations** .... There are no adequate reports or well-controlled studies
in pregnant women. **Cortisone** circulates both bound and
unbound, the latter active representing a small
percentage. Hepatic synthesis of the steroid-binding
protein increases under the influence of estrogen during
early pregnancy. Women with Cushing's disease may
require additional **cortisone** to saturate the newly formed
binding protein and prevent the free **cortisone** level from
falling during the first 2 or 3mo of pregnancy. It is
suggested but poorly documented that chronic steroid
administration increases the incidence of maternal
infection. Women who receive a short-term burst of
steroids, such as those with PPROM, have no increased
incidence of chorioamnionitis. The potent fluorinated
steroids, **betamethasone** and **dexamethasone**, are
more effective at accelerating fetal lung maturity than
the less potent corticosteroids, **cortisol**, **cortisone**, and
prednisone.
Side effects include adrenal insufficiency, psychosis,
immunosuppression, peptic ulcer, CHF, osteoporosis,
pseudotumor cerebri, pancreatitis, hypokalemia,
hypertension, Cushing features, ecchymosis, acne, and
impaired wound healing.

■ **Fetal Considerations** .... There are no adequate reports or well-controlled studies in
human fetuses. Primate studies suggest almost complete
conversion of **cortisol** to **cortisone** by the placenta. Some
suggest emotional stress during organogenesis may cause
congenital malformations by increasing the level of
cortisone. Retrospective epidemiologic studies have sought
an association between oral clefting and exposure to
corticosteroids. After controlling for confounding factors, it
was concluded that prenatal exposure to corticosteroids
increase the risk of cleft lip with or without cleft palate

6 fold. IUGR, shortening of the head and mandible are also suggested sequelae. Yet, the Collaborative Perinatal Project followed women treated during the 1st trimester. And while the number of exposures was limited, no increase in congenital malformations was detected. There was no increase in risk of anomalies after organogenesis. Women exposed to topical **cortisone** during pregnancy have no significant increase in birth defects. Female rats exposed to **cortisone** *in utero* exhibit premature vaginal opening. **Cortisone** accelerates fetal rat intestinal maturation, perhaps explaining why corticosteroids decrease the incidence of NEC. In sum, the evidence that **cortisone** is a human teratogen is weak.

■ **Breastfeeding Safety**

There are no adequate reports or well-controlled studies in breastfeeding women. **Cortisone** is present in human milk, but it is unclear whether maternal treatment increases the concentration.

■ **References**

Avci S, Yilmaz C, Sayli U. J Hand Surg [Am] 2002; 27:322-4.
Hansen D, Lou HC, Olsen J. Ugeskr Laeger 2001; 163:1051-7.
McCoy SJ, Shirley BA. Life Sci 1992; 50:621-8.
Dombrowski MP. Maternal Fetal Med 1996; 5:310-3.
Israel EJ, Schiffrin EJ, Carter EA, et al. Gastroenterology 1990; 99:1333-8.
Slikker W Jr, Althaus ZR, Rowland JM, et al. J Pharmacol Exp Ther 1982; 223:368-74.
Cziezel A, Rockenbauer M. Teratology 1997; 56:335-340.
Collaborative Group on Antenatal Therapy. J Pediatr 1984; 104:259-67.
Vermillion ST, Soper DE, Bland ML, Newman RB. Am J Obstet Gynecol 2000; 183:925-9.

■ **Summary**

- **Pregnancy Category C**
- **Lactation Category U**
- **Cortisone** should be used during pregnancy and lacation only if the benefit justifies the potential perinatal risk.

Cromolyn (Cromoglicic Acid; Cromogloz; Gastrocrom; Inostral; Intal; NasalCrom; Opticrom)

■ **Class**

Antiasthmatic; *mast cell stabilizer; opthalmics*

■ **Indications**

Chronic and exercise-induced asthma, allergic conjunctivitis, mastocytosis, food allergies, inflammatory bowel disease

■ **Mechanism**

Inhibits mast cell degranulation

- **Dosage with Qualifiers** .... Mastocytosis—200mg PO qid
  Food allergy—200mg PO qid
  Inflammatory bowel disease—200mg PO qid
  Asthma and exercise-induced asthma (chronic treatment)—20mg NEB qid
  Allergic rhinitis—1 puff per nostril bid or tid (5.2mg/spray)
  Allergic conjunctivitis, vernal keratitis—1 gtt OS/OD 4-6x/d
  - **Contraindications**—hypersensitivity to drug or class
  - **Caution**—arrhythmia

- **Maternal Considerations** .... **Cromolyn** is a relatively short-acting NSAID taken daily to prevent symptoms. It is available in a metered-dose inhaler or a nebulizer solution. There are no adequate reports or well-controlled studies in pregnant women. There is an increase in adverse outcomes during pregnancy in women whose asthma is poorly controlled. Rodent studies using parenterally administered drug were not associated with adverse effects.
  Side effects include bronchospasm, anaphylaxis, throat irritation, dry throat, bitter taste, cough, wheezing, and dizziness.

- **Fetal Considerations** .... There are no adequate reports or well-controlled studies in human fetuses. It is unknown whether **cromolyn** crosses the human placenta. Rodent studies are reassuring, revealing no evidence of teratogenicity despite the use of doses higher than those used clinically. Adverse fetal effects (increased resorptions and decreased fetal weight) were noted only at very high parenterally administered doses that produced maternal toxicity.

- **Breastfeeding Safety** .... There are no adequate reports or well-controlled studies in breast-feeding women. It is unknown whether **cromolyn** enters human breast milk. Early prophylaxis against food allergies appears to be best achieved by breastfeeding. Exclusive breastfeeding should be encouraged for as long as possible when there is a family history of allergy.

- **References** .... Schatz M. Semin Perinatol 2001; 25:145-52.
  Mazzotta P, Loebstein R, Koren G. Drug Saf 1999; 20:361-75.
  Popescu IG, Comanescu C, Murariu D, Stancu C. Med Interne 1981; 19:185-9.
  Gerrard JW, Shenassa M. Ann Allergy 1983; 51:300-2.
  Ashton MJ, Clark B, Jones KM, et al. Toxicol Appl Pharmacol 1973; 26:319-28.

- **Summary** ....
  - **Pregnancy Category B**
  - **Lactation Category S?**
  - **Cromolyn** should be used during pregnancy and lactation only if the benefit justifies the potential perinatal risk.
  - Virtually none of the commonly used asthma medications are contraindicated during pregnancy if their use is justified by the severity of the asthma in pregnancy.

Cyanocobalamin (Antipernicin; B-12-1000; Berubigen; Betalin 12; Betlovex; Blu-12; Cobal; Cobalparen; Cobavite; Cobex; Cobolin-M; Compensal; Corubeen; Corubin; Cpc-Carpenters; Crystamine; Crysti-12; Cyano-Plex; Cyanocob; Cyanoject; Cyomin; Cytacon; Cytaman; Depinar; Depo-Cobolin; Docemine; Dodecamin; La-12; Lifaton; Nascobal; Neurin-12; Neurodex; Neuroforte-R; Norivite; Ottovit; Pan B-12; Primabalt; Rubesol-1000; Rubisol; Rubivite; Rubramin Pc; Ruvite; Shovite; Sytobex; Vibal; Vibisone; Vita Liver; Vita-Plus B-12; Vitabee 12; Vitamin B-12; Yobramin)

■ **Class** — Vitamin; *hematinic*

■ **Indications** — Vitamin B_{12} deficiency, pernicious anemia

■ **Mechanism** — Coenzyme involved in major biochemical reactions

■ **Dosage with Qualifiers** — Vitamin B_{12} deficiency—30mcg qd ×5-10d, then 100-1000mcg SC/IM qmo; PO route can be used for maintenance
Pernicious anemia—100mcg qd ×6-7d, then 100-1000mcg SC/IM qmo
Recommended daily allowance—6mcg PO qd
  ● **Contraindications**—hypersensibility to drug or class
  ● **Caution**—pruritus, diarrhea, urticaria

■ **Maternal Considerations** — "Intrinsic factor" is essential for the adequate alimentary absorption of **cyanocobalamin**. The recommended daily intake is 4µg. **Cyanocobalamin** deficiency and the compensatory rise in homocysteine are significant risk factors for cardiovascular disease. There are no adequate reports or well-controlled studies in pregnant women. **Cyanocobalamin** deficiency has been linked to early pregnancy loss.
Side effects include anaphylaxis, thrombosis, pruritus, diarrhea, and urticaria.

■ **Fetal Considerations** — There are no adequate reports or well-controlled studies in human fetuses. There is efficient transfer of **cyanocobalamin** against a concentration gradient from mother to fetus by 16 weeks' gestation. IUGR fetuses have impaired hepatic **cyanocobalamin** storage ability. In one study, amniotic fluid **cyanocobalamin** levels were lower when the fetus had a NTD. Increased **folate** intake reduces the risk of neural tube defects and possibly other malformations. Evidence suggests the beneficial effect of **folate** is related to improved function of methionine synthase, a **cyanocobalamin**-dependent enzyme converting homocysteine to methionine. Rodent teratogenicity studies have not been performed.

- **Breastfeeding Safety** — While there are no adequate reports or well-controlled studies in breastfeeding women, **cyanocobalamin** is generally considered safe for breastfeeding women in therapeutic doses. The recommended daily intake is 4 µg.

- **References** —
Fairfield KM, Fletcher RH. JAMA 2002; 287:3116-26.
Reznikoff-Etievant MF, Zittoun J, Vaylet C, Pernet P, Milliez J. Eur J Obstet Gynecol Reprod Biol 2002; 104:156-9.
Berg MJ, Van Dyke DC, Chenard C, et al. J Am Diet Assoc 2001; 101:242-5.
Walker MC, Smith GN, Perkins SL, et al. Am J Obstet Gynecol 1999; 180:660-4.
Abbas A, Snijders RJ, Nicolaides KH. Br J Obstet Gynaecol 1994; 101:215-9.
Abbas A, Snijders RJ, Sadullah S, Nicolaides KH. Fetal Diagn Ther 1994; 9:14-8.
Economides DL, Ferguson J, Mackenzie IZ, et al. Br J Obstet Gynaecol 1992; 99:23-5.

- **Summary** —
  - **Pregnancy Category C**
  - **Lactation Category S**
  - **Cyanocobalamin** is contained in most prenatal vitamin tablets, though the evidence it improves pregnancy outcome overall is weak.

Cyclamate

- **Class** — *Artificial sweetener*

- **Indications** — Food sweetener

- **Mechanism** — Stimulation of the sweet receptors

- **Dosage with Qualifiers** — Food sweetener—max 1.5g qd
  - **Contraindications**—hypersensibility
  - **Caution**—unknown

- **Maternal Considerations** — **Cyclamate** is 30 times sweeter than sucrose and has been used in foods since the 1950s. It was removed from food products in the U.S. and Canada in the 1970s after several animal studies suggested it posed an increased risk of papillary carcinoma of the bladders in rats fed the maximum dietary level. However, there are no adequate well-controlled studies in human subjects, and epidemiologic study does not suggest an increased incidence of cancer in humans. While still banned in the U.S., it is available in Canada and Europe. The scientific community is reviewing current data that may support **cyclamate** approval again.

- **Fetal Considerations** .... No adequate or well-controlled studies have been performed in human fetuses. **Cyclamate** crosses the human placenta. Rodent teratogenicity studies reveal no increase in adverse outcomes.

- **Breastfeeding Safety** .... There is no published experience in nursing women. It is unknown whether **cyclamate** enters human breast milk.

- **References** .... Schmahl D, Habs M. Arzneimittelforschung 1980; 30:1905-6.
Oser BL, Carson S, Cox GE, et al. Toxicology 1975; 4:315-30.
Ward VL, Zeman FJ. J Nutr 1971; 101:1635-46.
Massobrio M, Coppo F, Rappelli F. Minerva Ginecol 1971; 23:507-35.
Pitkin RM, Reynolds WA, Filer LJ Jr. Am J Obstet Gynecol 1970; 108:1043-50.

- **Summary** ....
  - **Pregnancy Category D**
  - **Lactation Category U**
  - Artificial sweetener of unclear risk during pregnancy and lactation.

Cyclobenzaprine (Flexeril)

- **Class** .... *Muscle relaxant*

- **Indications** .... Muscle spasm

- **Mechanism** .... Believed to act centrally

- **Dosage with Qualifiers** ...... Muscle spasm—10mg PO tid; max 40-60mg/d
  - **Contraindications**—hypersensitivity to drug or class, prior use of MAO inhibitors in the last 14d, hyperthyroidism, recent MI, arrhythmias
  - **Caution**—glaucoma

- **Maternal Considerations** ...... **Cyclobenzaprine** relieves skeletal muscle spasm of local origin without interfering with muscle function. It is ineffective in muscle spasm due to CNS disease. There is no published experience with **cyclobenzaprine** during pregnancy.
Side effects include arrhythmias, seizures, myocardial infarction, hepatitis, nausea, vomiting, dry mouth, dizziness, asthenia, dyspepsia, blurred vision, and nervousness.

- **Fetal Considerations** .... There are no adequate reports or well-controlled studies in human fetuses. It is unknown whether **cyclobenzaprine** crosses the human placenta. Rodent studies are reassuring, revealing no evidence of teratogenicity or IUGR despite the use of doses higher than those used clinically.

- **Breastfeeding Safety** — There is no published experience in nursing women. It is unknown whether **cyclobenzaprine** enters human breast milk.

- **References** — Harwood MI, Chang SI. J Fam Pract 2002; 51:118.
  Stein WM, Read S. J Pain Symptom Manage 1997; 14:255-8.
  Kobayashi H, Hasegawa Y, Ono H. Eur J Pharmacol 1996; 311:29-35.

- **Summary** —
  - **Pregnancy Category B**
  - **Lactation Category U**
  - There is no published experience during pregnancy.

Cyclophosphamide (Cytokan; Cytoxan; Endoxon; Neosar; Neosar for Injection)

- **Class** — *Antineoplastic; alkylating agent; antirheumatic*

- **Indications** — Chemotherapy (cancer: ovary, bladder, lung, esophageal, cervical, breast, gastric, lymphoma, myeloma, sarcoma, gestational trophoblastic disease), mycosis fungoides, immune disorders such as rheumatoid arthritis

- **Mechanism** — Alkylates and crosslinks DNA (nitrogen mustard)

- **Dosage with Qualifiers** — Chemotherapy—varies depending on tumor and protocol
  Mycosis fungoides—2-3mg/kg PO qd
  Rheumatoid arthritis—1.5-3mg/kg PO qd
  NOTE—hydration is essential
  - **Contraindications**—hypersensitivity to drug or class, bone marrow depression
  - **Caution**—renal or hepatic failure, leukopenia, thrombocytopenia, recent radiation, recent chemotherapy

- **Maternal Considerations** — **Cyclophosphamide** is an alkylating agent used to treat cancer of the ovary, breast, and blood and lymph systems. Transient sterility is common after **cyclophosphamide**, and there is a risk of secondary malignancy. There are no adequate reports or well-controlled studies in pregnant women. There are multiple case reports suggesting it can be used with a good pregnancy outcome.
  Side effects include infertility, CHF, malignancy, anaphylaxis, leukopenia, thrombocytopenia, cardiomyopathy, alopecia, rash, headache, nausea, vomiting, dizziness, and stomatitis.

- **Fetal Considerations** — There are no adequate reports or well-controlled studies in human fetuses. **Cyclophosphamide** crosses the human placenta, though the kinetics remain to be detailed. Population studies have not convincingly demonstrated teratogenicity in humans, though neonatal hematologic suppression and secondary malignancies in the offspring are reported. Studies conducted in rodents suggest an increased incidence of fetal malformations and decreased implantation.

■ **Breastfeeding Safety** — **Cyclophosphamide** enters human breast milk in high concentration and is generally considered not compatible with breastfeeding. Neonatal neutropenia has been reported.

■ **References** — Kart Koseoglu H, Yucel AE, Kunefeci G, et al. Lupus 2001; 10:818-20.
Ozalp SS, Yalcin OT, Tanir HM. Eur J Gynaecol Oncol 2001; 22:221-2.
Altintas A, Vardar MA. Eur J Gynaecol Oncol 2001; 22:154-6.
Ben-Arie A, Piura B, Biran H, et al. Acta Obstet Gynecol Scand 2001; 80:672-3.
Zemlickis D, Lishner M, Erlich R, Koren G. Teratog Carcinog Mutagen 1993; 13:139-43.
Sharon N, Neumann Y, Kenet G, et al. Pediatr Hematol Oncol 2001; 18:247-52.
Peters BG, Bray JJ, Masidonski P, Mahon SM. Oncol Nurs Forum 2001; 28:639-42.
Amato D, Niblett JS. Med J Aust 1977; 1:383-4.
Meirow D, Epstein M, Lewis H, et al. Hum Reprod 2001; 16:632-7.
Enns GM, Roeder E, Chan RT, et al. Am J Med Genet 1999; 86:237-41.

■ **Summary** — • **Pregnancy Category D**
• **Lactation Category NS**
• **Cyclophosphamide** should be used during pregnancy and lactation only if the benefit justifies the potential perinatal risk.
• Breastfeeding should be avoided during therapy.

Cycloserine (Cicloserina; Cyclorin; Seromycin)

■ **Class** — *Antituberculosis*

■ **Indications** — Active pulmonary and extrapulmonary tuberculosis

■ **Mechanism** — Interferes with the synthesis of the bacterial cellular wall

■ **Dosage with Qualifiers** — TB—250mg PO q12h ×2w; continue 0.5-1g/d in divided doses based on blood levels (max 1g/d)

- **Contraindications**—epilepsy, depression, severe anxiety, psychosis, severe renal insufficiency, alcoholism
- **Caution**—drowsiness, headache, mental confusion, tremors, vertigo, loss of memory, psychoses

■ **Maternal Considerations** ⸺ There are no adequate reports or well-controlled studies in pregnant women. The published experience is limited to case reports with no obvious pregnancy-related adverse effects.

■ **Fetal Considerations** ⸺ There are no adequate reports or well-controlled studies in human fetuses. It is unknown whether **cycloserine** crosses the human placenta. No teratogenic effects have been described in human fetuses.

■ **Breastfeeding Safety** ⸺ **Cycloserine** is excreted into human breast milk in small quantities, though the kinetics remain to be detailed. No adverse effects have been reported. It is generally considered compatible with breastfeeding.

■ **References** ⸺ Lessnau KD, Qarah S. Chest 2003; 123:953-6.
Sanguigno N. Scand J Respir Dis Suppl 1970; 71:178-9.
Tran JH, Montakantikul P. J Hum Lact 1998; 14:337-40.

■ **Summary** ⸺
- **Pregnancy Category C**
- **Lactation Category S**
- **Cycloserine** should be used during pregnancy and lactation only if the benefit justifies the potential perinatal risk.

Cyclosporine (Ciclosporin; Neoral, Sandimmune, SangCya)

■ **Class** ⸺ *Immunosuppression*

■ **Indications** ⸺ Prevention of transplant organ rejection

■ **Mechanism** ⸺ Believed to act through inhibition of T-lymphocytes

■ **Dosage with Qualifiers** ⸺ Prevention of transplant rejection—5-10mg/kg/d PO in 2 divided doses; 5-6mg/kg IV 4-12h before surgery
- **Contraindications**—hypersensitivity to drug or class, hypertension
- **Caution**—hepatic or renal failure

■ **Maternal Considerations** ⸺ There are no adequate reports or well-controlled studies in pregnant women. **Cyclosporine** promotes growth of 1st trimester human cytotrophoblasts by apparently increasing their invasive ability. Successful pregnancy after solid organ transplantation is common. Preconception criteria for the optimal transplant recipient include good transplant graft function, no evidence of rejection, a minimum of 1 to 2 years post-transplant and either no or well-controlled hypertension. For these women, pregnancy is generally without significant adverse effect. Because preeclampsia develops in 30% of pregnant renal transplant patients, especially those with pretransplant arterial hypertension, blood pressure, renal function, proteinuria, and weight should be monitored every 2-4 weeks until the 3rd trimester, and then every week. Antihypertensive agents should be changed to those tolerated during pregnancy. **Cyclosporine** alters placental endothelin-1/nitric oxide vasoactive balance. Yet newborns of transplant recipient mothers are typically AGA and normotensive.

Side effects include seizures, thrombocytopenia, anaphylaxis, leukopenia, infection, hyperglycemia, hyperkalemia, and hyperuricemia.

■ **Fetal Considerations**
There are no adequate reports or well-controlled studies in human fetuses. Transfer of **cyclosporine** across the isolated perfused placenta is poor, <5% of the maternal load. This is consistent with a case report. Most pregnancies and their offspring have normal postnatal growth and development after maternal immunosuppressive therapy. Some studies suggest a higher risk of stillbirth, preterm delivery and IUGR in transplant patients treated with **cyclosporine**. Whether this is due to the disease or **cyclosporine** is unknown. Children born to transplanted women taking **cyclosporine** have normal renal function despite prolonged exposure *in utero.*

■ **Breastfeeding Safety**
There are no adequate reports or well-controlled studies in nursing mothers. **Cyclosporine** is excreted into human breast milk at low quantities. However, breast-fed infants of treated mothers ingest less than 300ug per day and absorb undetectable amounts. In rats, neonatal exposure to **cyclosporine** in breast milk causes significant alterations in T-cell maturation and inhibition of lymphoproliferative responsiveness to mitogen activation.

■ **References**
Sgro MD, Barozzino T, Mirghani HM, et al. Teratology 2002; 65:5-9.
Giudice PL, Dubourg L, Hadj-Aissa A, et al. Nephrol Dial Transplant 2000; 15:1575-9.
Di Paolo S, Monno R, Stallone G, et al. Am J Kidney Dis 2002; 39:776-83.
Yan F, Li D, Sun X, Zhu Y, et al. Zhonghua Fu Chan Ke Za Zhi 2002; 37:74-6.
Nandakumaran M, Eldeen AS. Dev Pharmacol Ther 1990; 15:101-5.
Raddadi AA, Baker Damanhoury Z. Br J Dermatol 1999; 140:1197-8.
Wu A, Nashan B, Messner U, et al. Clin Transplant 1998; 12:454-64.
Padgett EL, Seelig LL Jr. Transplantation 2002; 73:867-74.

Nyberg G, Haljamae U, Frisenette-Fich C, Wennergren M, Kjellmer I. Transplantation 1998; 65:253-5.
Munoz-Flores-Thiagarajan KD, Easterling T, Davis C, Bond EF. Obstet Gynecol 2001; 97:816-8.

■ **Summary**
- **Pregnancy Category C**
- **Lactation Category S?**
- **Cyclosporine** should be used during pregnancy and lactation only if the benefit justifies the potential perinatal risk.

Cyproheptadine (Actinal; Aptide; Cyheptin; Huavine; Ioukmin; Nekomin; Oractine; Periactin; Setomin)

■ **Class**

Antihistamines, sedating

■ **Indications**

Allergic rhinitis

■ **Mechanism**

Central and peripheric H_1 receptor antagonist, serotonin receptor antagonist

■ **Dosage with Qualifiers**

Allergic rhinitis—4mg PO tid
- **Contraindications**—hypersensitivity to drug or class, gastric ulcer, glaucoma, MAO inhibitors used up to 14d prior, bladder neck obstruction
- **Caution**—none

■ **Maternal Considerations**

There are no adequate reports or well-controlled studies in pregnant women. **Cyproheptadine** is used to prevent or relieve symptoms of rhinitis (inflammation of the mucous membranes of the nasal passages, often associated with hayfever and other seasonal allergies); skin itching and hives; and tissue swelling (angioedema). It is also used to stimulate appetite in women with anorexia nervosa (8mg PO qid).
Side effects include agranulocytosis, dry mouth, nausea, vomiting, urinary retention, dizziness, headache, rash, diarrhea, weight gain, and glucose intolerance.

■ **Fetal Considerations**

There are no adequate reports or well-controlled studies in human fetuses. It is unknown whether **cyproheptadine** crosses the human placenta. Rodent studies are reassuring, revealing no evidence of teratogenicity or IUGR despite the use of doses higher than those used clinically. **Cyproheptadine** alters insulin-secreting B cell function in the fetal rat pancreas when given to pregnant rats at a dose that has no apparent effects on the maternal pancreas.

Breastfeeding Safety .... There is no published experience in nursing women. It is unknown whether **cyproheptadine** enters human breast milk.

References .... Chow SA, Fischer LJ. Drug Metab Dispos 1987; 15:740-8.
Chow SA, Fischer LJ. Toxicol Appl Pharmacol 1986; 84:264-77.
Rodriguez Gonzalez MD, Lima Perez MT, Sanabria Negrin JG. Teratog Carcinog Mutagen 1983; 3:439-46.
Kasperlik-Zaluska A, Migdalska B, Hartwig W, et al. Br J Obstet Gynaecol 1980; 87:1171-3.

Summary ....
- **Pregnancy Category B**
- **Lactation Category U**
- There are alternative, selective agents for which there is more experience during pregnancy and lactation.

Cytarabine (Cytosar-U; Tarabine PFS)

Class .... *Antineoplastic; antimetabolite*

Indications .... Leukemia

Mechanism .... Interferes with RNA and DNA chain elongation after incorporation

Dosage with Qualifiers .... Cancer—varies with protocol; most recommend 100mg/m²/d by continuous IV infusion (days 1 to 7) or 100mg/m² IV q12h (days 1 to 7)
Meningeal leukemia—30mg/m² q4d until CSF findings were normal (intrathecal administration)
- **Contraindications**—hypersensitivity to drug or class, pregnancy, infertility
- **Caution**—renal or hepatic failure

Maternal Considerations .... There are no adequate reports or well-controlled studies in pregnant women. The coexistence of leukemia and pregnancy is extremely rare. **Cytarabine** is used during pregnancy to achieve remission of the acute episodes. It is an essential component of the drug regimen used for the treatment of acute myelogenic leukemia. Once remission is achieved the dose should be readjusted. *Side effects* include anemia, bruising, nausea, vomiting, hair loss, leukopenia, bone marrow suppression, and pancreatitis.

Fetal Considerations .... There are no adequate reports or well-controlled studies in human fetuses. **Cytarabine** does appear to cross the human placenta, though the kinetics remain to be detailed. In humans, **cytarabine** is associated with fetal brachycephaly, hypoplasia of the anterior cranial base and the midface, cranial synostoses, IUGR and neonatal leukopenia and elevation of neonatal hepatic transaminases. Unaffected neonates appear to mature normally. In rodents, **cytarabine** causes microcephalia and joint anomalies.

■ **Breastfeeding Safety** ·········· There are no adequate reports or well-controlled studies in nursing women. It is unknown whether **cytarabine** enters human breast milk.

■ **References** ············· Ono-Yagi K, Ohno M, Iwami M, et al. Acta Neuropathol 2000; 403-8.
Requena A, Velasco JG, Pinilla J, Gonzalez-Gonzalez A. Eur J Obstet Gynecol Reprod Biol 1995; 63:139-41.
Caligiuri MA, Mayer RJ. Semin Oncol 1989; 16:388-96.
Cantini E, Yanes B. South Med J 1984; 77:1050-2.
Fassas A, Kartalis G, Klearchou N, et al. Nouv Rev Fr Hematol 1984; 26:19-24.

■ **Summary** ·············
- **Pregnancy Category D**
- **Lactation Category U**
- **Cytarabine** should be used during pregnancy and lactation only if the benefit justifies the potential perinatal risk.
- **Cytarabine** would appear to be a modest human teratogen.

Dacarbazine (DTIC-Dome)

■ **Class**	*Antineoplastic; alkylating agent*
■ **Indications**	Melanoma, Hodgkin's disease
■ **Mechanism**	Primary action appears alkylation of nucleic acids
■ **Dosage with Qualifiers**	<u>Melanoma, Hodgkin's disease</u>—numerous dosing schedules depend on disease, response, and concomitant therapy: 375mg/m²; 850mg/m²; 250mg/m²/d ×5d; 2-4.5mg/kg/d ×10d; 650-1450mg/m² are the most frequent regimens; intra-arterial administration is no longer recommended • **Contraindications**—hypersensitivity to drug or class • **Caution**—hepatic or renal dysfunction
■ **Maternal Considerations**	There are no adequate reports or well-controlled studies in pregnant women. There are multiple case reports of **dacarbazine** use during pregnancy with a good outcome. *Side effects* include leukopenia, alopecia, thrombocytopenia, anorexia, nausea, vomiting, hepatotoxicity, diarrhea, fever, myalgias, hepatic or renal dysfunction, and photosensitivity.
■ **Fetal Considerations**	There are no adequate reports or well-controlled studies in human fetuses. It is unknown whether **dacarbazine** crosses the human placenta. No teratogenic effects are described in human fetuses, and long-term follow-up studies of children exposed *in utero* in the 1st trimester are reassuring. **Dacarbazine** is both teratogenic and embryotoxic in rodents when given at multiples of the maximum recommended human dose.
■ **Breastfeeding Safety**	There are no adequate reports or well-controlled studies in nursing women. It is unknown whether **dacarbazine** enters human breast milk.
■ **References**	Aviles A, Neri N. Clin Lymphoma 2001; 2:173-7. Aviles A, Diaz-Maqueo JC, Talavera A, et al. Am J Hematol 1991; 36:243-8. Green DM, Zevon MA, Lowries G, et al. N Engl J Med 1991; 325:141-6.
■ **Summary**	• **Pregnancy Category C** • **Lactation Category U** • **Dacarbazine** should be used during pregnancy and lactation only if the benefit justifies the potential risk. • Women of childbearing potential should use contraception during therapy and for at least 4 months after completion of therapy.

Daclizumab (Zenapax)

■ **Class** — *Immunosuppressive*

■ **Indications** — Transplant, kidney

■ **Mechanism** — IL-2 receptor antagonist

■ **Dosage with Qualifiers** — Transplant—1.0mg/kg IV q14d ×5 doses
NOTE—begin within 24h pretransplant; interacts with echinacea
- **Contraindications**—hypersensitivity to drug or class
- **Caution**—unknown

■ **Maternal Considerations** — There are no adequate reports or well-controlled studies in pregnant women. It is recommended that women of childbearing potential use contraception before and during therapy, and for 4 months after completion of therapy with **daclizumab**.
Side effects include pulmonary edema, renal tubular necrosis, nausea, vomiting, diarrhea, constipation, abdominal or chest pain, dyspepsia, tremor, headache, edema, dizziness, dysuria, dyspnea, fever, acne, and cough.

■ **Fetal Considerations** — There are no adequate reports or well-controlled studies in human fetuses. It is unknown whether **daclizumab** crosses the human placenta. No teratogenic effects are described in human fetuses. Animal teratogenicity studies have not been conducted.

■ **Breastfeeding Safety** — There are no published reports in nursing mothers. It is unknown whether **daclizumab** enters human breast milk.

■ **References** — There is no published experience in pregnancy or during lactation.

■ **Summary** —
- **Pregnancy Category C**
- **Lactation Category U**
- **Daclizumab** should be used during pregnancy and lactation only if the benefit justifies the potential risk.

Dactinomycin (Cosmegen)

■ **Class** .... *Antineoplastics, antibiotics*

■ **Indications** .... Gestational trophoblastic tumors, Wilms' tumor, Ewing's sarcoma, uterine carcinoma

■ **Mechanism** .... Inhibits RNA and protein synthesis

■ **Dosage with Qualifiers** .... Gestational trophoblastic tumors—12mcg/kg IV ×5d
Wilms' tumor—15mcg/kg IV ×5d
Rhabdomyosarcoma—15mcg/kg IV ×5d
Ewing's sarcoma—protocols vary; most recommend dose should not exceed 15mcg/kg or 400-600mcg/m^2 qd IV ×5d
- **Contraindications**—hypersensitivity to drug or class, herpes zoster, varicella infection
- **Caution**—hepatic or renal dysfunction may enhance radiation injury to tissues

■ **Maternal Considerations** .... **Dactinomycin** is a derivative of *Streptomyces parvulus* and extensively used for the treatment of gestational trophoblastic tumors. No deleterious, long-term effects are described in women treated with combination regimens that include **dactinomycin** for germ cell ovarian cancer. There are no adequate and well-controlled studies of **dactinomycin** in pregnant women.
Side effects include aplastic anemia, thrombocytopenia, leukopenia, pancytopenia, flushing, alopecia, acute folliculitis, nausea, vomiting, fever, lethargy, abdominal pain, myalgias, anorexia, increased LFTs, hepatotoxicity, GI ulceration, pharyngitis, and stomatitis. Tissue necrosis after extravasation may manifest days to weeks after treatment.

■ **Fetal Considerations** .... There are no adequate reports or well-controlled studies in human fetuses. It is unknown whether **dactinomycin** crosses the human placenta. No teratogenic effects are described in humans. In rodents, it is both embryotoxic and teratogenic when given at multiples of the maximum recommended human dose.

■ **Breastfeeding Safety** .... There is no published experience in nursing women. It is unknown whether **dactinomycin** enters human breast milk. It is generally considered incompatible with breastfeeding.

■ **References** .... Kendall A, Gillmore R, Newlands E. Curr Opin Obstet Gynecol 2002; 14:33-8.
Nagai K, Ikenoue T, Mori N. J Matern Fetal Med 2001; 10:136-40.
Suzuka K, Matsui H, Iitsuka Y, et al. Obstet Gynecol 2001; 97:431-4.
Matsui H, Suzuka K, Iitsuka Y, et al. Gynecol Oncol 2000; 78:28-31.
Goldstein DP. Surg Forum 1967; 18:426-8.

Dalteparin (Fragmin)

- **Class** ································· Anticoagulant, *low-molecular-weight heparin*

- **Indications** ····························· Prophylaxis and treatment for DVT, unstable angina

- **Mechanism** ······························· Binds to antithrombin III and accelerates its inhibition of thrombin and factor Xa.

- **Dosage with Qualifiers** ··········· DVT prophylaxis—begin 2500U SC or IV 1-2h preoperatively, then qd ×5-14d; increase dose to 5000U SC in high-risk women or during pregnancy
  DVT treatment—200U/kg/d SC in divided doses; max 18,000U/dose, overlap with oral anticoagulation 2-3d
  Unstable angina—120U/kg; max 10,000U SC q12h
  NOTE—2500U SC once daily is of similar antithrombotic efficacy to 5000U of unfractionated heparin bid
  - **Contraindications**—hypersensitivity to drug or class, active bleeding, thrombocytopenia, epidural catheters, antibodies to drug, prosthetic heart valve, spinal puncture
  - **Caution**—diabetic retinopathy, hepatic or renal dysfunction, recent surgery or stroke, pregnancy, GI bleeding

- **Maternal Considerations** ·········· **Dalteparin** is a low-molecular-weight heparin (5000MW) (LMWH) with improved bioavailability, increased plasma elimination half-life, and greater factor Xa inhibitory activity compared to unfractionated **heparin**. **Dalteparin** given once or twice daily (IV or SC) is as effective as unfractionated **heparin** for the initial treatment of acute deep vein thrombosis. LMWHs are increasingly popular during pregnancy for the treatment of various thrombophilias and the antiphospholipid syndrome. LMWHs differ in pharmacologic profiles. The mean retention time of anti-Xa activity varies from 5.2h (**dalteparin**) to 7h (**enoxaparin**, **nadroparin**). The bioavailability of a prophylactic dose of LMWHs range from 86% (**dalteparin**) to 98% (**enoxaparin**, **nadroparin**). Though equal in efficacy and amenable to once a day dosing for prophylaxis in the nonpregnant patient, they are more expensive than unfractionated **heparin** and have the same risks. **Heparin** and heparin products are not treatments for preeclampsia. The therapeutic dose of

dalteparin during pregnancy is based on maternal weight. At least during pregnancy, the interpatient variability is wide. Clearance is enhanced significantly by pregnancy. The initial prophylactic dose for most pregnant women in the 1st trimester is 5000U daily. Anti-Xa activity is measured after initiating therapy, and again periodically (at least each trimester) to confirm the adequacy of the prophylactic or therapeutic dose. 5000U SC should produce an anti-Xa activity of 0.20-0.40U/ml (0.4-0.7U/mL for full anticoagulation) 3h after injection. Women treated with LMWHs for prevention of thromboembolic complications are at risk of developing an epidural or spinal hematoma after neuraxial anesthesia. LMWHs are best replaced with unfractionated **heparin** at 36w because of their long half-lives, and inability to measure residual activity (anti-Xa levels). One prospective study of bone density in women receiving LMWH found no significant change in mean bone density between baseline and 6 weeks' postpartum.

Side effects include bleeding, thrombocytopenia, fever, pruritus, osteoporosis, easy bruising, epistaxis, injection site reaction, and elevated LFTs.

■ **Fetal Considerations** — **Dalteparin**, similar to other LMWHs and unfractionated heparin, does not cross the placenta. It is generally safe and effective for the noted indications during pregnancy. Rodent studies are reassuring revealing no evidence of teratogenicity despite the use of doses higher than those used clinically.

■ **Breastfeeding Safety** — Only trace amounts of **dalteparin** (2500U × 1 IU, and measured as anti-Xa activity) enter human breast milk. It is highly unlikely that puerperal treatment will have any clinically relevant effect on the nursing infant.

■ **References** —
Farquharson RG, Sephton V, Quenby SM. J Soc Gyn Invest 2003; 10(Suppl):308A.
Ulander V, Stenqvist P, Kaaja R. Thromb Res 2002; 106:13.
Laurent P, Dussarat GV, Bonal J, et al. Drugs 2002; 62:463-77.
Richter C, Sitzmann J, Lang P, et al. Br J Clin Pharmacol 2001; 52:708-10.
O'Shaughnessy DF. Hematology 2000; 4:373-80.
Rey E, Rivard GE. Int J Gynaecol Obstet 2000; 71:19-24.
Samama MM, Gerotziafas GT. Semin Thromb Hemost 2000; 26(Suppl 1):31-8.
Dunn CJ, Jarvis B. Drugs 2000; 60:203-37.
Blomback M, Bremme K, Hellgren M, Lindberg H. Blood Coagul Fibrinolysis 1998; 9:343-50.

■ **Summary** —
- **Pregnancy Category B**
- **Lactation Category S**
- **Dalteparin** should be used during pregnancy only if the benefit justifies the potential perinatal risk.
- The possibility of once daily administration and the reduced need for laboratory monitoring may in some

instances translate into a cost advantage compared to unfractionated heparin or warfarin. Unfortunately, this is not true during pregnancy where the increased clearance generally necessitates twice a day dosing and measurement of anti-Xa activity.

- LMWHs are best replaced with unfractionated heparin at around 36w because of their long half-lives, possible need for surgical delivery and/or neuraxial anesthesia, and inability to easily obtain anti-Xa levels.
- LMWHs may have lower frequencies of thrombocytopenia and osteoporosis compared to unfractionated heparin.

Danazol (Danocrine; Danatrol; Danokrin; Danogen; Ectopal; Zoldan-A)

■ **Class** — Hormone, other gynecologic action

■ **Indications** — Endometriosis, fibrocystic breast disease, hereditary angioedema

■ **Mechanism** — Suppression of the pituitary-ovarian axis

■ **Dosage with Qualifiers** — Endometriosis—begin 200-400mg PO bid depending on severity; continue for 3-6mo trial
Fibrocystic breast disease—50-200mg PO bid for 2-6mo, then adjust dose
Hereditary angioedema—200mg PO tid until response, then half dose for 1-3mo
NOTE—begin during menstruation
- **Contraindications**—hypersensitivity to drug or class, undiagnosed genital bleeding, pregnancy, breastfeeding, porphyria
- **Caution**—hepatic, renal or cardiac dysfunction, epilepsy, migraine

■ **Maternal Considerations** — There are no indications during pregnancy for **danazol**. It should be discontinued if the patient becomes pregnant. **Danazol** is not an effective contraceptive. It decreases the maternal progesterone level if taken during the 1st trimester.
Side effects include alteration of the lipid profile (low HDL), contraceptive failure, pseudotumor cerebri, weight gain, acne and seborrhea, mild hirsutism, virilization, edema, hair loss, hoarseness, menstrual irregularities, flushing, sweating, vaginal dryness, reduction in breast size, hypertension, anxiety, and thromboembolism.

■ **Fetal Considerations** ⋯⋯⋯⋯ There are no adequate and well-controlled studies in human fetuses. It is unknown whether **danazol** crosses the human placenta. Though the FDA classifies **danazol** as category X, there is no reason *a priori* to terminate an exposed pregnancy. **Danazol** can have an androgenic effect on female fetuses (vaginal atresia, clitoral hypertrophy, labial fusion, ambiguous genitalia). Thus, exposed fetuses should undergo a detailed ultrasound examination. Rodent studies are reassuring, revealing no evidence of teratogenicity or IUGR despite the use of doses higher than that used clinically. **Danazol** is associated with inhibition of fetal development in rabbits.

■ **Breastfeeding Safety** ⋯⋯⋯⋯ There is no published experience in nursing women. It is unknown whether **danazol** enters human breast milk. It is generally considered contraindicated during breastfeeding.

■ **References** ⋯⋯⋯⋯⋯⋯⋯⋯⋯⋯

Bianchi S, Busacca M, Agnoli B, et al. Hum Reprod 1999; 14:1335-7.
Zayed F, Abu-Heija A. Obstet Gynecol Surv 1999; 54:121-30.
Rabe T, Kiesel L, Franke C, et al. Biol Res Pregnancy Perinatol 1984; 5:149-52.
Igarashi M, Iizuka M, Abe Y, Ibuki Y. Hum Reprod 1998; 13:1952-6.
Kingsbury AC. Med J Aust 1985; 143:410-1.
Brunskill PJ. Br J Obstet Gynaecol 1992; 99:212-5.
Schwartz R. Am J Dis Child 1982; 136:474.

■ **Summary** ⋯⋯⋯⋯⋯⋯⋯⋯⋯⋯
- **Pregnancy Category X**
- **Lactation Category NS?**
- There are no indications for **danazol** during pregnancy; it is considered contraindicated.
- A pregnancy test is recommended immediately prior to initiating therapy.
- **Danazol** may virilize a female fetus (vaginal atresia, clitoral hypertrophy, labial fusion, urogenital sinus defect, ambiguous genitalia), but these abnormalities have not been reported if discontinued by 8w.

Dantrolene (Danlene; Dantralen; Dantrium; Dantrium IV)

■ **Class** ⋯⋯⋯⋯⋯⋯⋯⋯⋯⋯⋯⋯ *Muscle relaxant*

■ **Indications** ⋯⋯⋯⋯⋯⋯⋯⋯ Chronic spasticity, malignant hyperthermia

■ **Mechanism** ⋯⋯⋯⋯⋯⋯⋯⋯ Interferes with the release of the calcium from sarcoplasmic reticulum

■ **Dosage with Qualifiers** ⋯⋯ Chronic spasticity—begin 25mg PO qd; max 400mg/d
Malignant hyperthermia prevention—4-8mg/kg/d PO q6-8h
1-2d preoperatively with last dose 3-4h prior to surgery;
same dose post crisis
Malignant hyperthermia crisis—1-2.5mg/kg IV ×1,
may repeat q5min until patient improves; max 10mg/kg
Neuroleptic malignant syndrome—1mg/kg IV ×1, repeat
until symptoms improve; max 10mg/kg
NOTE—monitor LFTs

- **Contraindications**—hypersensitivity to drug or class, cirrhosis
- **Caution**—age >35y, pulmonary disease, cardiomyopathy

■ **Maternal Considerations** ⋯⋯ There are no adequate reports or well-controlled studies of **dantrolene** in pregnant women, though it has been used for both the prevention and treatment of acute malignant hyperthermia and neuroleptic malignant syndrome where it may be lifesaving. However, prevention of malignant hypertension is not usually recommended. Instead, a non-triggering anesthetic should be selected. *Side effects* include hepatic dysfunction, pleural effusion, pericarditis, constipation, bowel obstruction, abdominal pain, diarrhea, dizziness, pruritus, vomiting, tachycardia, depression, seizure, headache, aplastic anemia, and myalgia.

■ **Fetal Considerations** ⋯⋯ There are no adequate reports or well-controlled studies in human fetuses. It readily crosses the placenta, achieving equal maternal and fetal whole blood levels by delivery. No adverse neonatal effects are reported. **Dantrolene** is embryocidal in rodents when administered at a multiple of the maximum recommended human dose.

■ **Breastfeeding Safety** ⋯⋯ **Dantrolene** is excreted in human breast milk. Though the kinetics remain to be detailed, it is generally considered incompatible with breastfeeding. Breastfeeding may resume after therapy.

■ **References** ⋯⋯ Russell CS, Lang C, McCambridge M, Calhoun B. Obstet Gynecol 2001; 98:906-8.
Fricker RM, Hoerauf KH, Drewe J, Kress HG. Anesthesiology 1998; 89:1023-5.
Ben Abraham R, Cahana A, Krivosic-Horber RM, Perel A. QJM 1997; 90:13-8.
Shime J, Gare D, Andrews J, Britt B. Am J Obstet Gynecol 1988; 159:831-4.

■ **Summary** ⋯⋯
- **Pregnancy Category C**
- **Lactation Category NS**
- **Dantrolene** should be used during pregnancy and lactation only if the benefit justifies the potential perinatal risk.

Dapsone (Avlosulfon; Dapson; Dapsoderm-X)

■ **Class** — Antimycobacterial

■ **Indications** — Pneumocystis carinii pneumonia, dermatitis herpetiformis, malaria suppression, leprosy

■ **Mechanism** — Bactericidal/bacteriostatic by some unknown mechanism

■ **Dosage with Qualifiers** — Pneumocystis carinii pneumonia—100mg PO qd; usually given with trimethropim (20mg/kg qd ×3w)
Dermatitis herpetiformis—begin 50mg PO qd, increase to 300mg qd as needed
Malaria suppression—100mg PO qw, give with **pyrimethamine** 12.5mg PO qw
Leprosy prophylaxis—100mg PO qd ×24mo
Leprosy treatment—50mg PO qd
- **Contraindications**—hypersensitivity to drug or class
- **Caution**—cardiac, renal or hepatic dysfunction, G6PD deficiency

■ **Maternal Considerations** — There are no adequate reports or well-controlled studies of **dapsone** in pregnant women. **Dapsone**, alone or in combination with **pyrimethamine**, **trimethoprim-sulfamethoxazole**, **pentamidine**, is the most commonly used drug for PCP prophylaxis. **Dapsone** should be administered in combination with one or more antileprosy drugs to avoid resistance.
Side effects include hemolysis, aplastic anemia, peripheral neuropathy, nausea, vomiting, abdominal pains, pancreatitis, vertigo, blurred vision, tinnitus, insomnia, fever, headache, fatigue, malaise, psychosis, pulmonary eosinophilia, albuminuria, nephrotic syndrome, renal papillary necrosis, exfoliative dermatitis, erythema multiforme, toxic epidermal necrolysis, phototoxicity, drug-induced lupus-like syndrome, and infectious mononucleosis-like syndrome.

■ **Fetal Considerations** — There are no adequate reports or well-controlled studies in human fetuses. Transfer across the human placenta likely occurs, as there are reports of neonatal methemoglobinemia after maternal **dapsone**. **Dapsone** appears unassociated with fetal abnormalities in humans. Rodent teratogenicity studies have not been performed.

■ **Breastfeeding Safety** — **Dapsone** is excreted in breast milk in substantial amounts with the unsupplemented breast-fed infant receiving some 15% of the maternal dose. Hemolytic reactions can occur in newborns. Caution is advised. Breastfeeding is contraindicated in HIV infected nursing women where formula is available to reduce the risk of neonatal transmission.

- **References** — Kabra NS, Nanavati RN, Srinivasan G. Indian Pediatr 1998; 35:553-5.
  Lush R, Iland H, Peat B, Young G. Aust NZ J Med 2000; 30:105-7.
  Bhargava P, Kuldeep CM, Mathur NK. Int J Lepr Other Mycobact Dis 1996; 64:457-8.
  Erstad BL. Clin Pharm 1992; 11:800-5.
  Edstein MD, Veenendaal JR, Newman K, Hyslop R. Br J Clin Pharmacol 1986; 22:733-5.
  Kahn G. J Am Acad Dermatol 1985; 13:838-9.

- **Summary** —
  - **Pregnancy Category C**
  - **Lactation Category S?**
  - **Dapsone** should be used during pregnancy and lactation only if the benefit justifies the potential perinatal risk.
  - Hemolysis in neonates is the most common adverse effect seen in patients with or without G6PD deficiency.

Daunorubicin (Cerubidine; DaunoXome)

- **Class** — *Antineoplastic, antibiotic*

- **Indications** — HIV-associated Kaposi's sarcoma, acute myelogenic leukemia, acute lymphoblastic leukemia

- **Mechanism** — Inhibits topoisomerase and binds DNA

- **Dosage with Qualifiers** — Kaposi's sarcoma—dose varies with protocol; most recommend 40mg/m² IV
  Acute myelogenic leukemia—dose varies with protocol; most recommend 40mg/m² IV
  Acute lymphoblastic leukemia—dose varies with protocol; most recommend 40mg/m² IV
  - **Contraindications**—hypersensitivity to drug or class
  - **Caution**—hepatic, renal or cardiac dysfunction, myelosuppression

- **Maternal Considerations** — **Daunorubicin** is an anthracycline antibiotic. **Daunoxome** is an encapsulated form designed to maximize selectivity for solid tumors such as Kaposi's sarcoma. The specific mechanism by which the **daunorubicin** citrate liposome delivers the drug to solid tumors is not known. There are no adequate and well-controlled studies of **daunorubicin** in pregnant women. There are multiple reports of its use during pregnancy with a successful outcome.
  Side effects include bone marrow suppression, hepatic and cardiac toxicity, alopecia, nausea, vomiting, diarrhea, mucositis, back pain, flushing, chest tightness, fever, and local tissue necrosis at the site of drug extravasation.

- **Fetal Considerations** ········· There are no adequate reports or well-controlled studies in human fetuses. **Daunorubicin** crosses the human placenta, but in the isolated perfused model the global transfer was less than 3%. Not surprisingly, there are multiple reports of its use during pregnancy, including 1st trimester, without evidence of an adverse fetal effect. And though children (and presumably fetuses) have greater sensitivity to the cardiotoxic effects of **daunorubicin** than adults, there are no such reports in exposed fetuses. Rodent studies reveal at doses a fraction of that used in the human an increased prevalence of anophthalmia, microphthalmia, and incomplete ossification when given alone, and esophageal atresia with tracheoesophageal fistula if **daunorubicin** is combined with **adriamycin**.

- **Breastfeeding Safety** ········· There is no published experience in nursing women. **Daunorubicin** is excreted into human breast milk, but in the only case reported, the total amount delivered in the milk (maximum concentration of active antibiotic: 0.24mg/L) was negligible.

- **References** ········· Leslie KK. Clin Obstet Gynecol 2002; 45:153-64.
Dezube BJ. Expert Rev Anticancer Ther 2002; 2:193-200.
Achtari C, Hohlfeld P. Am J Obstet Gynecol 2000; 183:511-2.
Grohard P, Akbaraly JP, Saux MC, et al. J Gynecol Obstet Biol Reprod (Paris) 1989; 18:595-600.
Egan PC, Costanza ME, Dodion P, Egorin MJ, Bachur NR. Cancer Treat Rep 1985; 69:1387-89.
Merei JM, Farmer P, Hasthorpe S, et al. Anat Rec 1997; 249:240-8.

- **Summary** ·········
  - **Pregnancy Category D**
  - **Lactation Category S?**
  - **Daunorubicin** should be used during pregnancy and lactation only if the benefit justifies the potential perinatal risk.

Deferoxamine (Desferal)

- **Class** ········· Antidote; *chelator*

- **Indications** ········· Iron toxicity

- **Mechanism** ········· Chelation

- **Dosage with Qualifiers** ········· Acute iron intoxication—1g IM ×1, then 500mg IM q4h ×2, may repeat; do not exceed 6g/24h

<u>Chronic iron overload</u>— 500-1000mg IM qd, plus 2000mg IV (not to exceed 15 mg/kg/h) with each transfused unit of PRBCs

- **Contraindications**—hypersensitivity to drug or class, severe renal disease or anuria
- **Cautions**—IV route should be used only in instances of cardiovascular collapse or with blood transfusion

■ **Maternal Considerations**

There are no adequate reports or well-controlled studies in pregnant women. There are case reports of its use during pregnancy and lactation in women with transfusion-dependent homozygous β-thalassemia. *Side effects* include ocular disturbances such as blurred vision, cataracts, decreased acuity, color perception and night vision, injection site irritation, pruritus, tachycardia, hypotension, shock, nausea, vomiting, diarrhea, and abdominal pain.

■ **Fetal Considerations**

There are no adequate reports or well-controlled studies in human fetuses. It is unknown whether **deferoxamine** crosses the human placenta. However, there are over 50 published cases without evidence of adverse fetal effects. Rodent studies reveal an increased incidence of delayed ossification and skeletal anomalies when administered at multiples of the recommended human dose.

■ **Breastfeeding Safety**

There are no adequate reports or well-controlled studies in nursing women. It is unknown whether **deferoxamine** enters human breast milk. Case reports suggest **deferoxamine** therapy does not alter the iron content of human breast milk.

■ **References**

Pafumi C, Zizza G, Caruso S, et al. Ann Hematol 2000; 79:571-3.
Surbek DV, Glanzmann R, Nars PW, Holzgreve W. J Perinat Med 1998; 26:240-3.
Singer ST, Vichinsky EP. Am J Hematol 1999; 60:24-6.
Perniola R, Magliari F, Rosatelli MC, De Marzi CA. Gynecol Obstet Invest 2000; 49:137-9.

■ **Summary**

- **Pregnancy Category C**
- **Lactation Category U**
- **Deferoxamine** should be used during pregnancy and lactation only if the benefit justifies the potential perinatal risk.

Delavirdine (Rescriptor)

- **Class** — *Retroviral* (NNRTIs)

- **Indications** — HIV

- **Mechanism** — Non-nucleoside reverse transcriptase inhibitor that induces allosteric changes in HIV-1 reverse transcriptase rendering it incapable of converting viral RNA to DNA

- **Dosage with Qualifiers** — HIV—400mg PO tid
  - **Contraindications**—hypersensitivity to drug or class
  - **Cautions**—unknown

- **Maternal Considerations** — There are no adequate reports or well-controlled studies in pregnant women. Because **delavirdine** increases the plasma concentrations of several protease inhibitors, it may also be beneficial as a component of salvage therapy in combination with protease inhibitors.
  Side effects include skin rash, angioedema, Stevens-Johnson syndrome, anemia, GI bleeding, pancreatitis, thrombocytopenia, neutropenia, pancytopenia, granulocytosis, fatigue, nausea, vomiting, diarrhea, abdominal pain, hematuria, dry skin, elevated LFTs, flu-like symptoms, bradycardia, headache, anxiety, and edema.

- **Fetal Considerations** — There are no adequate reports or well-controlled studies in human fetuses. It is unknown whether **delavirdine** crosses the human placenta. In rodents, **delavirdine** causes embryotoxicity and VSDs at doses that are multiples of the maximum recommended human dosage.

- **Breastfeeding Safety** — There is no published experience in nursing women. It is unknown whether **delavirdine** enters human breast milk. Breastfeeding is contraindicated in HIV infected nursing women where formula is available to reduce the risk of neonatal transmission.

- **References** — There is no published experience in pregnancy or during lactation.

- **Summary** —
  - **Pregnancy Category C**
  - **Lactation Category U**
  - **Delavirdine** should be used during pregnancy and lactation only if the benefit justifies the potential perinatal risk.
  - Physicians are encouraged to register pregnant women under the Antiretroviral Pregnancy Registry (1-800-258-4263) for a better follow-up of the outcome while under treatment with **delavirdine**.

Demecarium (Humorsol; Tosmilen)

- **Class** .... *Cholinesterase inhibitors; miotic; ophthalmic*

- **Indications** .... Open-angle glaucoma

- **Mechanism** .... Cholinesterase inhibitor

- **Dosage with Qualifiers** .... Glaucoma—1-2 drops (0.125% or 0.25%) in the affected eye
  - **Contraindications**—hypersensitivity to drug or class, uveal inflammation, glaucoma associated with iridocyclitis
  - **Caution**—narrow angle-closure glaucoma, bronchial asthma, spastic GI disturbances, peptic ulcer, pronounced bradycardia and hypotension, recent MI, epilepsy, parkinsonism

- **Maternal Considerations** .... **Demecarium** is a cholinesterase inhibitor with sustained activity. It produces miosis and ciliary muscle contraction, and should be used only when shorter-acting miotics have proved inadequate. There is no published experience with **demecarium** during pregnancy.
  Side effects include salivation, urinary incontinence, diarrhea, profuse sweating, muscle weakness, respiratory difficulties, shock, cardiac irregularities, stinging, burning, tearing, lid muscle twitching, and headache.

- **Fetal Considerations** .... There are no adequate reports or well-controlled studies in human fetuses. It is unknown whether **demecarium** crosses the placenta. Considering the dose and route, it is unlikely the maternal systemic concentration will reach clinically relevant level. Rodent teratogenicity studies have apparently not been performed.

- **Breastfeeding Safety** .... There is no published experience in nursing women. It is unknown whether **demecarium** enters human breast milk. However, considering the indication and dosing, **demecarium** use is unlikely to pose a clinically significant risk to the breast-feeding neonate.

- **References** .... There is no published experience in pregnancy or during lactation.

- **Summary** ....
  - **Pregnancy Category X**
  - **Lactation Category U**
  - **Demecarium** should be used during pregnancy only if the benefit justifies the potential risk.
  - There are alternative agents for which there is more experience regarding use during pregnancy and lactation.

Demeclocycline (Bioterciclin; Clortetrin; Declomycin; Ledermycin)

■ **Class** .... Antibiotic (*tetracyclines*)

■ **Indications** .... Bacterial infections (<u>gram-negative microorganisms</u>: *Haemophilus ducreyi* (chancroid), *Yersinia pestis*, *Francisella tularensis*, *Pasteurella pestis*, *Pasteurella tularensis*, *Bartonella*, *Bacteroides* species, *Vibrio* species, *Brucella*, *Escherichia coli*, *Enterobacter aerogenes*, *Shigella*, *Haemophilus influenzae*, *Klebsiella*; <u>gram-positive</u>: *Streptococcus pyogenes*, *Streptococcus faecalis*, *Streptococcus pneumoniae*, *Staphylococcus aureus*, *Neisseria gonorrhoeae*, *Listeria monocytogenes*, *Clostridium*, *Bacillus anthracis*, *Fusobacterium fusiforme* [Vincent's infection], *Rickettsiae*, *Treponema pallidum*, *Actinomyces*, amebiasis)

■ **Mechanism** .... Bacteriostatic; inhibits protein synthesis

■ **Dosage with Qualifiers** .... <u>Bacterial infection, amebiasis, rickettsiae</u>—150mg PO qid or 300mg PO bid
<u>Gonorrhea</u>—600mg PO ×1; follow with 300mg q12h ×4d
NOTE—renal dosing
● **Contraindications**—hypersensitivity to drug or class, diabetes insipidus
● **Caution**—hepatic or renal dysfunction

■ **Maternal Considerations** .... There are no adequate reports or well-controlled studies of **demeclocycline** during pregnancy. Outside pregnancy, **demeclocycline** may cause diabetes insipidus-like syndrome (polyuria, polydipsia, and weakness) that is nephrogenic in origin, dose-dependent and reversible on discontinuation.
Side effects include photosensitization, diabetes insipidus syndrome, pseudotumor cerebri, thrombocytopenia, hemolytic anemia, hepatic or renal dysfunction, increased BUN, glossitis, enterocolitis, acute fatty liver disease, and vaginal candidiasis.

■ **Fetal Considerations** .... There are no adequate reports or well-controlled studies in human fetuses. It is unknown whether **demeclocycline** crosses the human placenta. Other tetracyclines may cause a permanent discoloration of the teeth (yellow-gray-brown teeth) when given during the latter half of pregnancy, or during childhood prior to 8 years of age. In rodents, exposure to **demeclocycline** is associated with tooth discoloration. Exposure to other tetracyclines is associated with delayed bone growth.

■ **Breastfeeding Safety** .... There is no published experience in nursing women. It is unknown whether **demeclocycline** enters human breast milk. It likely enters human breast milk, as do other tetracyclines, and is generally considered incompatible with breastfeeding.

■ **References** Thomas JP, Bradley EL Jr. Ala J Med Sci 1973; 10:89-97.
Iwamoto HK, Brennan WR. Toxicol Appl Pharmacol 1969; 14:33-40.
Zyngier S, Schmuziger P. Rev Farm Bioquim Univ Sao Paulo 1970; 8:173-6.
Jha VK, Jayachandran C, Singh MK. Vet Res Commun 1989; 13:225-30.
Hendeles L, Trask PA. J Am Dent Assoc 1983; 107:12.

■ **Summary**
- **Pregnancy Category D**
- **Lactation Category NS**
- There are alternative agents during pregnancy for almost all indications.

Desipramine (Deprexan; Norpramin; Pertofrane)

■ **Class** — *Antidepressant, tricyclic*

■ **Indications** — Depression

■ **Mechanism** — Unknown; inhibits the norepinephrine and serotonin reuptake

■ **Dosage with Qualifiers** — Depression—Begin 25-75mg PO qam, increase gradually to a maximum of 300mg/d (typical 100-200mg qd)
- **Contraindications**—hypersensitivity to drug or class, usage of MAO inhibitor drugs in the past 14d, coronary artery disease
- **Caution**—heart disease, glaucoma, thyroid disease, seizure disorde

■ **Maternal Considerations** — Depression is a commonly overlooked and undertreated disorder during pregnancy and the puerperium. Pregnancy is not a reason a priori to discontinue psychotropic drugs. Women with a history of depression are at high risk for recurrence during pregnancy and the puerperium. **Desipramine** is a metabolite of **imipramine**. **Desipramine** lowers the threshold for seizures. There are no adequate and well-controlled studies of **desipramine** in pregnant women. There are marked interindividual differences during pregnancy in the metabolism of the tricyclic antidepressants. Tricyclic antidepressants are effective for the treatment of postpartum depression.
Side effects include stroke, MI, arrhythmias, thrombocytopenia, seizures, urinary retention, and glaucoma.

- **Fetal Considerations** — There are no adequate reports or well-controlled studies in human fetuses. It is unknown whether **desipramine** crosses the human placenta. No evidence of teratogenicity is seen in rhesus monkey fetuses exposed to **imipramine** despite a high incidence of maternal toxicity and abortion. A large body of study on the impact of *in utero* exposure to **desipramine** on postnatal neurologic function is inconclusive.

- **Breastfeeding Safety** — **Desipramine** is excreted in small quantities into human breast milk, but is not detectable in the blood of breast-feeding newborns. No adverse effects are reported in breast-feeding neonates.

- **References** — Wisner KL, Parry BL, Piontek CM. N Engl J Med 2002; 347:194-9.
  Yoshida K, Smith B, Craggs M, Kumar RC. J Affect Disord 1997; 43:225-37.
  Ware MR, DeVane CL. J Clin Psychiatry 1990; 51:482-4.
  Gelenberg AJ, Wojcik JD, Lydiard RB, et al. J Clin Psychiatry 1984; 45:54-9.
  Sjoqvist F, Bertilsson L. Adv Biochem Psychopharmacol 1984; 39:359-72.
  Hendrickx. Teratology 1975; 11:219-21.
  Stancer HC, Reed KL. Am J Psychiatry 1986; 143:1597-600.

- **Summary**
  - **Pregnancy Category C**
  - **Lactation Category S**
  - Tricyclic antidepressants are effective second-line therapies (behind serotonin reuptake inhibitors) for postpartum depression.
  - Pregnancy is not a reason a priori to discontinue psychotropic drugs.

Desmopressin (DDAVP Desmopressin; Octim)

- **Class** — *Antidiuretic hormone*

- **Indications** — Diabetes insipidus, nocturnal enuresis, factor VIII deficiency, von Willebrand's disease

- **Mechanism** — Synthetic analog of hormone arginine vasopressin

- **Dosage with Qualifiers** — Diabetes insipidus—10-40mcg NAS qhs; 1-2mcg SC/IV bid also acceptable (10mcg = 40U)
  von Willebrand's disease—0.3mcg/kg IV ×1; alternatively NAS to provide 300mcg
  Factor VIII deficiency—0.3mcg/kg IV ×1; alternatively NAS ×1
  Nocturnal enuresis—10-40mcg NAS qhs

- **Contraindications**—hypersensitivity to drug or class, coronary artery disease, IIB von Willebrand's disease
- **Caution**—hyponatremia, electrolyte imbalance

■ **Maternal Considerations** ⋯⋯ The metabolic clearance rate of **arginine vasopressin** increases 4-fold during human pregnancy. As opposed to natural hormone, **desmopressin** (1-deamino-[8-D-arginine] vasopressin) has no uterotonic action in antidiuretic doses. It is the treatment of choice for most patients with von Willebrand's disease type 1 (vWD). Types 2 and 3 are usually unresponsive, and best treated with either FFP or concentrates containing von Willebrand's factor. There is a high risk of delayed postpartum hemorrhage in vWD type 1, especially during the first week. The risk is independent of the factor VIII level during the 3rd trimester, and reflects the rapid clearance of the various factor VIII components postpartum. The risk of postpartum hemorrhage is especially high in women with type 2 or 3 vWD. Hemorrhage may occur up to 5w postpartum. Administer **desmopressin** at least 30min prior to a surgical procedure to maintain hemostasis during the procedure and immediately postoperatively. Maternal **desmopressin** use reduces and stabilizes plasma osmolality and increases amniotic fluid volume. It has been proposed as a possible treatment of oligohydramnios, and if given intra-amniotically, polyhydramnios.
Side effects include hyponatremia, cerebral edema, rhinitis, flushing, abdominal pain, rhinitis, and thrombotic accidents.

■ **Fetal Considerations** ⋯⋯ There are no adequate reports or well-controlled studies in human fetuses. It is unknown whether **desmopressin** crosses the human placenta. No adverse fetal effects are reported when **desmopressin** is used during human pregnancy. Rodent studies are reassuring revealing no evidence of teratogenicity or IUGR despite the use of doses higher than those used clinically. In sheep, intra-amniotic **desmopressin** inhibits fetal urination without cardiovascular effect or change in fetal swallowing.

■ **Breastfeeding Safety** ⋯⋯ There are no adequate reports or well-controlled studies in nursing women. A single study found minimal **desmopressin** in human breast milk after a single nasal spray. Considering the dose and dosing frequency, it seems unlikely a significant quantity would reach the breast-feeding neonate. It has been used to treat diabetes insipidus during the puerperium.

■ **References** ⋯⋯
Kouides PA. Best Pract Res Clin Haematol 2001; 14:381-99.
Ross MG, Cedars L, Nijland MJ, Ogundipe A. Am J Obstet Gynecol 1996; 174:1608-13.
Kullama LK, Nijland MJ, Ervin MG, Ross MG. Am J Obstet Gynecol 1996; 174:78-84.
Davison JM, Sheills EA, Philips PR, et al. Am J Physiol 1993; 264:F348-53.

Chediak JR, Alban GM, Maxey B. Am J Obstet Gynecol 1986; 155:618-24.
Burrow GN, Wassenaar W, Robertson GL, Sehl H. Acta Endocrinol (Copenh) 1981; 97:23-5.

■ **Summary**
- **Pregnancy Category B**
- **Lactation Category S**
- **Desmopressin** is effective therapy for women with either diabetes insipidus, or type 1 vWD during pregnancy in if necessary, or in the puerperium.

Dexamethasone (Aeroseb-Dex; Corotason; Curson; Decaderm; Decadron; Decarex; Decaspray; Decofluor; Desigdron; Dexone; Dms; Hexadrol; Isopto; Lebedex; Lozusu; Maxidex; Millicorten; Mymethasone; Predni; Taidon)

■ **Class** — Corticosteroid

■ **Indications** — Accelerating fetal lung maturity, adrenal insufficiency, inflammatory states, congenital adrenal hyperplasia, allergic reactions, testing for Cushing's syndrome, cerebral edema, shock

■ **Mechanism** — Unknown

■ **Dosage with Qualifiers** — Prevention of RDS in preterm neonates—6mg IM q12h ×4 doses
Cerebral edema—10mg IV, then 4mg IM q6h
Adrenal insufficiency—0.03-0.15mg/kg PO, IV, IM qd
Inflammatory states—0.75-9mg PO, IV, IM qd
Inflammatory ocular—1-2 gtt q1-6h
Congenital adrenal hyperplasia—0.5mg and 2mg PO qd
Allergic reactions—0.75-9mg PO qd
Shock—1-6mg/kg IV q2-6h prn
Diagnostic test for Cushing's disease—2.0mg of dexamethasone PO q6h for 48h; 24h urine collection required to calculate 17-hydroxycorticosteroid production
Postoperative N/V—4-5mg IV
NOTE—also available in a multitude of preparations for dermatologic and opthalmologic uses;
Inhalation 1 puff = 100mcg; 3 puffs = 3-4 puffs/d
Equivalent doses: dexamethasone 0.75mg = methylprednisolone 4mg = hydrocortisone 20mg
- **Contraindications:** hypersensitivity to drug or class, fungal infections, active untreated infections (however, may be used in patients under treatment for tuberculosis meningitis), and lactation

- **Caution**—seizure disorder, diabetes, hypertension, osteoporosis, hepatic dysfunction

■ **Maternal Considerations** ········ **Dexamethasone** is used widely for the acceleration of fetal lung maturity. Most large studies conclude the risk of maternal infection in women after PPROM is not increased by **dexamethasone**. It may transiently cause an abnormal glucose tolerance test, and will worsen diabetes mellitus. Large doses such as those given to hasten the fetal lung maturation are associated with pulmonary edema, especially when combined with a tocolytic agent in the setting of an underlying infection. **Dexamethasone** does not reduce the maternal perception of fetal movements and short-term variability. It is not contraindicated in women with severe preeclampsia requiring preterm delivery. Women chronically treated must be monitored closely for hypertension or glucose intolerance, and treated with stress replacement doses postoperatively and postpartum. **Dexamethasone** is an effective antiemetic for nausea and vomiting after general anesthesia for pregnancy termination. There are as yet uncorroborated reports that IV **dexamethasone** helps modify the clinical course of the so-called HELLP syndrome both ante and postpartum. It may also reduce itching in women with intrahepatic cholestasis of pregnancy.

Side effects include immunosuppression, pancreatitis, fluid retention, cardiovascular failure, pseudotumor cerebri, suppression of growth and development in children, myositis, Cushing's disease, decreased carbohydrate tolerance, osteoporosis, hepatic dysfunction, thromboembolism, insomnia, and anxiety.

■ **Fetal Considerations** ···················· Antenatal corticosteroid administration is the only therapy conclusively demonstrated to reduce the perinatal morbidity and death associated with preterm delivery. Newborns of treated women have lower incidences of RDS, NEC, IVH, and shorter hospital stays. Corticosteroids should be restricted to a single course. There is little evidence repeat courses provide additional benefit, and there is evidence of potential harm. **Dexamethasone** readily crosses the human placenta, which cannot metabolize it. Infants of women treated chronically should be carefully observed for signs of hypoadrenalism. Complete fetal heart block has been treated with **dexamethasone** during pregnancy with positive result. Some studies suggest that in contrast to **betamethasone**, **dexamethasone** does not alter biophysical parameters of the fetus (i.e., fetal breathing) when administered for the enhancement of lung maturation. However, oligohydramnios is reportedly more common. When initiated by 6-7w, **dexamethasone** can prevent or diminish virilization due to congenital adrenal hyperplasia. It is continued until a definitive diagnosis is established by DNA analysis of chorionic villi at 11-13w. Some suggest emotional stress during organogenesis can cause congenital malformations by increasing the level of **cortisone**. Corticosteroids produce oral clefting in some rodents. Some epidemiological studies conclude after controlling for confounding factors that prenatal exposure to corticosteroids adds a 6-fold increase in the risk for cleft lip with or without cleft palate, IUGR, shortening of the head and mandible. In contrast, the Collaborative Perinatal Project followed women treated during the 1st trimester. While the number of exposures was limited, no increase in congenital malformations was detected. There was no increased risk of anomalies after organogenesis. Antenatal **dexamethasone** for fetal lung maturation is associated with diminished growth (12g at 24-26w, 63g at 27-29w, 161g at 30-32w, and 80g at 33-34w gestation) and decreased myelination in several animal models. The long-term impacts of these effects remain to be established. Corticosteroids (e.g. **cortisone**) accelerate fetal rat intestinal maturation, perhaps explaining why corticosteroids decrease the incidence of NEC.

■ **Breastfeeding Safety** .... There are no adequate reports or well-controlled studies in breast-feeding women. **Dexamethasone** is excreted into human breast milk, but it is unclear whether maternal treatment increases the concentration of **cortisone** in breast milk.

■ **References** ....
Lammert F, Marschall HU, Matern S. Curr Treat Options Gastroenterol 2003; 6:123-132.
Moritz K, Butkus A, Hantzis V, et al. Endocrinology 2002; 143:1159-65.
Fujii Y, Uemura A. Obstet Gynecol 2002; 99:58-62.
New MI. Curr Urol Rep 2001; 2:11-8.
Wong JP, Kwek KY, Tan JY, Yeo GS. Aust NZ J Obstet Gynaecol 2001; 41:339-41.
Ritzen EM. Semin Neonatol 2001; 6:357-62.
Nevagi SA, Kaliwal BB. Indian J Exp Biol 2001; 39:1163-5.
Spiliotis BE. J Pediatr Endocrinol Metab 2001; 14:1299-302.
Guinn DA, Atkinson MW, Sullivan L, et al. JAMA 2001; 286:1581-7.
Mushkat Y, Ascher-Landsberg J, Keidar R, et al. Eur J Obstet Gynecol Reprod Biol 2001; 97:50-2.
Isler CM, Barrilleaux PS, Magann EF, et al. Am J Obstet Gynecol 2001; 184:1332-7.
Bloom SL, Sheffield JS, McIntire DD, Leveno KJ. Obstet Gynecol 2001; 97:485-90.
Goldenberg RL, Wright LL. Obstet Gynecol 2001; 97:316-7.

■ **Summary** ....
- **Pregnancy Category C**
- **Lactation Category U**
- **Dexamethasone** is effective for the reduction of neonatal RDS and other complications of prematurity. The administration of a corticosteroid is standard of care for threatened preterm delivery.
- There is no evidence of increased benefit by serial administration; there is evidence of fetal harm.

Dexchlorpheniramine (Dex-Cpm; Dexchlor; Mylaramine; Polaramine)

■ **Class** — Antihistaminic, *decongestant (nasal)*

■ **Indications** — Allergic rhinitis, anaphylaxis

■ **Mechanism** — Antagonizes central and peripheral H_1 receptors

■ **Dosage with Qualifiers** —
Allergic rhinitis—2-4mg PO q4-6h; max 24mg/24h
Anaphylaxis—5-20mg SC, IM q6-12h prn; max 40mg/24h
  - **Contraindications**—see **Chlorpheniramine**
  - **Caution**—see **Chlorpheniramine**

■ **Maternal Considerations** — **Dexchlorpheniramine** is the active metabolite of **chlorpheniramine**. There are no adequate reports or well-controlled studies in pregnant women, and its safety during pregnancy is not established. However, **chlorpheniramine** is widely available in over-the-counter preparations and has not been implicated with adverse effects during pregnancy.
Side effects include hypotension, dry mouth, nausea, vomiting, and constipation.

■ **Fetal Considerations** — **Dexchlorpheniramine** has not been incriminated as a human teratogen. See **Chlorpheniramine.**

■ **Breastfeeding Safety** — There are no adequate reports or well-controlled studies in nursing women. It is unknown whether **dexchlorpheniramine** enters human breast milk. There are no reports of adverse effects on the breast-feeding neonate despite widespread availability.

■ **References** — See **Chlorpheniramine**.

■ **Summary** —
  - **Pregnancy Category B**
  - **Lactation Category S**
  - **Dexchlorpheniramine** should be used during pregnancy and lactation only if the benefit justifies the potential risk.

Dexmedetomidine (Precedex)

■ **Class**	*Adrenergic agonist; sedative; anesthetic adjunct during induction, maintenance; postoperative analgesia*
■ **Indications**	Sedation of ventilated patients
■ **Mechanism**	Selective α-2 adrenoceptor agonist
■ **Dosage with Qualifiers**	Sedation—begin 1mcg/kg IV over 10min, then 0.2-0.7mcg/kg/h IV Anesthestic adjunct—0.5-0.6mcg/kg iv Postoperative pain—0.4mcg/kg iv NOTE—avoid abrupt withdrawal • **Contraindications**—hypersensitivity to drug or class • **Caution**—cardiovascular disease, bradycardia, 2nd/3rd degree heart block, sick sinus syndrome, hypotension, transient hypertension, hypovolemia, diabetes mellitus, hepatic or renal dysfunction, adrenal insufficiency, tachycardia, anemia, and thirst.
■ **Maternal Considerations**	There are no adequate reports or well-controlled studies of **dexmedetomidine** in pregnant women. It is a potent neuroprotector and has been explored in several perinatal models. *Side effects* include bradycardia, hypotension, atrial fibrillation, pulmonary edema, pleural effusion, bronchospasm, hypokalemia, leukocytosis, adrenal insufficiency, nausea, and vomiting.
■ **Fetal Considerations**	There are no adequate reports or well-controlled studies in human fetuses. **Dexmedetomidine** crosses the human placenta, which also binds a large fraction delaying transfer. Rodent studies are generally reassuring, revealing no evidence of teratogenicity, though embryotoxicity and IUGR occurs in some models. It is a potent neuroprotector that has been explored in perinatal models.
■ **Breastfeeding Safety**	There is no published experience in nursing women. It is unknown whether **dexmedetomidine** enters human breast milk. **Dexmedetomidine** is excreted into rodent milk. Considering its indications, it is unlikely to pose a clinically significant risk to women who choose to breastfeed.
■ **References**	Ala-Kokko TI, Pienimaki P, Lampela E, et al. Acta Anaesthesiol Scand 1997; 41:313-9. Laudenbach V, Mantz J, Lagercrantz H, et al. Anesthesiology 2002; 96:134-41. Hayashi Y, Maze M. Br J Anaesth 1993; 71:108-18. Peden CJ, Prys-Roberts C. Br J Anaesth 1992; 68:123-5.

Dexmethylphenidate (Focalin)

■ **Class** ⋯⋯⋯⋯⋯⋯⋯⋯⋯⋯⋯⋯⋯⋯⋯⋯⋯ CNS *stimulant*

■ **Indications** ⋯⋯⋯⋯⋯⋯⋯⋯⋯⋯ Attention deficit disorder

■ **Mechanism** ⋯⋯⋯⋯⋯⋯⋯⋯⋯⋯ Unknown; stimulates CNS activity

■ **Dosage with Qualifiers** ⋯⋯ Attention deficit disorder—begin 2.5mg PO bid; increase by 5-10mg/d qw, max dose 20mg/d
- **Contraindications**—hypersensitivity to drug or class, history of severe anxiety, glaucoma, motor tics, MAO inhibitor use within 14d
- **Caution**—cardiovascular disease, hypertension, seizure disorder, psychosis, substance abuse, hyperthyroidism

■ **Maternal Considerations** ⋯⋯ There are no published reports of **dexmethylphenidate** use during pregnancy.
Side effects include seizures, dependency, arrhythmia, angina, thrombocytopenia, leukopenia, nervousness, insomnia, abdominal pain, headache, dizziness, palpitations, blurred vision, anorexia, weight loss, dyskinesia, and rash.

■ **Fetal Considerations** ⋯⋯⋯ There are no adequate reports or well-controlled studies in human fetuses. It is unknown whether **dexmethylphenidate** crosses the human placenta. Rodent studies are reassuring, revealing no evidence of teratogenicity, though delayed ossification is seen at the highest dose level.

■ **Breastfeeding Safety** ⋯⋯⋯ There is no published experience in nursing women. It is unknown whether **dexmethylphenidate** enters human breast milk.

■ **References** ⋯⋯⋯⋯⋯⋯⋯⋯⋯ There is no published experience in pregnancy or during lactation.

■ **Summary** ⋯⋯⋯⋯⋯⋯⋯⋯⋯⋯
- **Pregnancy Category C**
- **Lactation Category U**
- **Dexmethylphenidate** should be used during pregnancy and lactation only if the benefit justifies the potential perinatal risk.

Dextroamphetamine (Amphaetex; Das; Dexampex; Dexedrina; Dexedrine; Dextrostat; Ferndex; Oxydess; Spancap No. 1)

■ **Class** .... *Stimulant, CNS; amphetamine; adrenergic agonist*

■ **Indications** .... Attention deficit disorder with hyperactivity, narcolepsy, obesity

■ **Mechanism** .... CNS stimulant

■ **Dosage with Qualifiers** .... <u>Attention deficit disorder</u>—5mg PO qd/bid; increase up to 5mg/wk prn, max 40mg qd
<u>Narcolepsy</u>—10-60mg PO qd; begin 10mg PO qd and increase 10mg/w if necessary
<u>Obesity</u>—5-30mg PO qd 30min before breakfast
- **Contraindications**—hypersensitivity to drug or class, hypertension, glaucoma, hyperthyroidism, Tourette's syndrome
- **Caution**—mild hypertension

■ **Maternal Considerations** .... There are no adequate reports or well-controlled studies of **dextroamphetamine** in pregnant women. There are case reports of its use for the treatment of narcolepsy during pregnancy. Since **amphetamines** are used to decrease appetite and maintain adequate body weight, its usage during pregnancy should be immediately discouraged once pregnancy is diagnosed.
Side effects include arrhythmia, palpitation, insomnia, irritability, dry mouth, diarrhea, tremor, anorexia, and personality changes.

■ **Fetal Considerations** .... There are no adequate reports or well-controlled studies in human fetuses. **Amphetamines** cross the human placenta. One case report describes severe congenital body deformity, tracheoesophageal fistula, and anal atresia in the newborn of a mother who took **dextroamphetamine** throughout the 1st trimester. Epidemiologic study reveals that birth weight is unaffected if discontinued prior to 28w, but is significantly lower if discontinued later. **Dextroamphetamine** is embryotoxic and teratogenic when administered to some but not all rodents.

■ **Breastfeeding Safety** .... **Amphetamines** are excreted in human milk and are generally considered incompatible with breastfeeding.

■ **References** .... Hoover-Stevens S, Kovacevic-Ristanovic R. Clin Neuropharmacol 2000; 23:175-81.
Naeye RL. Pharmacology 1983; 26:117-20.
Briggs GG, Samson JH, Crawford DJ. Am J Dis Child 1975; 129:249-50.

■ Summary

- **Pregnancy Category C**
- **Lactation Category NS**
- **Dextroamphetamine** should be used during pregnancy and lactation only if the benefit justifies the potential perinatal risk.
- There are few indications for **dextroamphetamine** during pregnancy, which would preclude its temporary cessation.

Dextromethorphan (Bio-Tuss Dm; Biophen-Dm; Equi-Tuss Dm; Genophen-Dm Elixir; Io Tuss-Dm; Iodur-Dm; Iogan-Dm; Iophen D-C; Iophen-DM; Iotuss-Dm; Myodine Dm; Oridol Dm; Roganidin-Dm; Sil-O-Tuss Dm; Tosmar Dm; Tri-Onex Dm; Tussi-Organidin DM; Tussi-R-Gen Dm; Tusside; Tussidin Dm; Tusso-DM; Aquabid-Dm; Broncot; Fenex Dm; Gani-Tuss-Dm Nr; Guaibid Dm; Guaifenesin Dm; Guaifenesin W/Dextromethorphan; Guiadrine Dm; Humibid DM; Iofen-Dm Nf; Muco-Fen-Dm; Mucobid Dm; Numobid Dx; Pancof-HC; Q-Mibid-Dm; RobafenDm; Sudal-DM; Tusnel; Tussi-Organidin DM NR; Tussi-Organidin DM-S NR; Tussidin Dm Nr; Tussin Dm; Dectuss DM; Phen-Tuss DM; Phenergan w/Dextromethorphan; Pherazine DM; Promethazine w/DM; Prothazine)

■ **Class** — *Antitussive, expectorant*

■ **Indications** — Cough

■ **Mechanism** — Suppression of the cough center

■ **Dosage with Qualifiers** — Antitussive—10-30mg PO q4h; max 120mg qd (contains alcohol)
NOTE—may be combined with **guaifenesin** or **promethazine**
- **Contraindications**—hypersensitivity to drug or class, usage of MAO inhibitors in the last 14d
- **Caution**—concomitant usage of serotonergic drugs

■ **Maternal Considerations** — There are no adequate reports or well-controlled studies of **dextromethorphan** in pregnant women. It is commonly found in many over-the-counter preparations. No adverse pregnancy outcomes are associated with its use.
Side effects include abuse, serotonin syndrome, sedation, dizziness, and abdominal pain.

- **Fetal Considerations** .... There are no adequate reports or well-controlled studies in human fetuses. It is unknown whether **dextromethorphan** crosses the human placenta. The wide and long-term clinical experience suggests any fetal risk of **dextromethorphan** containing cough preparations is small. Rodent studies are reassuring, revealing no evidence of teratogenicity or IUGR despite the use of doses higher than that used clinically. **Dextromethorphan** is a teratogen in the chick embryo, a poor model for such studies.

- **Breastfeeding Safety** .... There are no adequate reports or well-controlled studies in nursing women. It is unknown whether **dextromethorphan** enters human breast milk. However, the wide and long-term clinical experience suggests any risk to the breast-feeding neonate is small.

- **References** .... Debus O, Kurlemann G, Gehrmann J, Krasemann T. Chest 2001; 120:1038-40.
Einarson A, Lyszkiewicz D, Koren G. Chest 2001; 119:466-9.
Martinez-Frias ML, Rodriguez-Pinilla E. Teratology 2001; 63:38-41.

- **Summary** ....
  - **Pregnancy Category C**
  - **Lactation Category S**
  - **Dextromethorphan** should be used during pregnancy and lactation only if the benefit justifies the potential perinatal risk.

Dextrothyroxine (Choloxin)

- **Class** .... Antihyperlipidemic

- **Indications** .... Hypercholesterolemia

- **Mechanism** .... Stimulates hepatic catabolism and excretion of cholesterol

- **Dosage with Qualifiers** .... Hypercholesterolemia—begin 1-2mg PO qd; increase to max 4-8mg/d
  - **Contraindications**—hypersensitivity to drug or class, cardiac arrhythmia, tachycardia, CHF
  - **Caution**—hepatic or renal dysfunction

- **Maternal Considerations** .... **Dextrothyroxine** is the dextrorotatory isomer of **thyroxine**. There are no adequate and well-controlled studies of **dextrothyroxine** in pregnant women.
Side effects include angina, arrhythmia, MI, insomnia, nervousness, palpitations, tremors, loss of weight, changes in libido, and gallstones.

- **Fetal Considerations** ⋯⋯ There are no adequate reports or well-controlled studies in human fetuses. It is unknown whether **dextrothyroxine** crosses the human placenta. Rodent studies are reassuring, revealing no evidence of teratogenicity or IUGR despite the use of doses higher than those used clinically.

- **Breastfeeding Safety** ⋯⋯ There is no published experience in nursing women. It is unknown whether **dextrothyroxine** enters human breast milk.

- **References** ⋯⋯ There is no published experience in pregnancy or during lactation.

- **Summary** ⋯⋯
  - **Pregnancy Category C**
  - **Lactation Category U**
  - **Dextrothyroxine** should be used during pregnancy and lactation only if the benefit justifies the potential perinatal risk.

Dezocine (Dalgan)

- **Class** ⋯⋯ *Narcotic*

- **Indications** ⋯⋯ Moderate to severe pain

- **Mechanism** ⋯⋯ Binds to various opiate receptors

- **Dosage with Qualifiers** ⋯⋯ Pain, moderate to severe—begin 5mg IV q2-4h or 10mg IM q3-6h; max dose 10mg IV and 20mg IM
  - **Contraindications**—hypersensitivity to drug or class
  - **Caution**—head injury, hepatic or renal dysfunction, sulfite allergy, drug dependency, biliary surgery, impaired lung function

- **Maternal Considerations** ⋯⋯ **Dezocine** is a synthetic opioid agonist-antagonist. There is no published experience with **dezocine** during pregnancy.
  Side effects include respiratory depression or arrest, hypotension, nausea, vomiting, dizziness, headache, pruritus, euphoria, and anxiety.

- **Fetal Considerations** ⋯⋯ There are no adequate and well-controlled studies in human fetuses. It is unknown whether **dezocine** crosses the human placenta. Evidence of rodent teratogenicity is noted in the manufacturer's information, but not detailed.

- **Breastfeeding Safety** ⋯⋯ There is no published experience in nursing women. It is unknown whether **dezocine** enters human breast milk.

■ **References** .... There is no published experience in pregnancy or during lactation.

■ **Summary** ....
- **Pregnancy Category C**
- **Lactation Category U**
- **Dezocine** should be used during pregnancy and lactation only if the benefit justifies the potential perinatal risk.
- There are alternative agents for which there is more experience during pregnancy and lactation.

Diatrizoate (Amidotrizoate; Angiovist 282; Berlex; Bolus Infusion Set; Burron Infusion Set; Cystografin; Cystografin Dilute; Cystografin Dilute w/Set; Hypaque; Hypaque Meglumine; Hypaque-Cysto; Hypaque-Cysto 100Ml/300Ml; Hypaque-Cysto 250Ml/500Ml; Reno-M-30; Reno-M-60; Reno-M-Dip; Urovist Cysto; Urovist Cysto 100Ml in 300Ml; Urovist Cysto 300Ml in 500Ml; Urovist Cysto Pediatric; Urovist Meglumine; Urovist Meglumine DIU/CT)

■ **Class** .... *Diagnostic, nonradioactive*

■ **Indications** .... Retrograde cystourethrography

■ **Mechanism** .... Radiographic contrast agent

■ **Dosage with Qualifiers** .... Retrograde cystourethrography—25-300ml instilled within the urinary bladder
NOTE—also used for IV contrast
- **Contraindications**—hypersensitivity to drug or class
- **Caution**—sensitivity to iodine, urinary tract infection

■ **Maternal Considerations** .... There are no adequate reports or well-controlled studies of **diatrizoate** in pregnant women. **Diatrizoate** is a contrast agent frequently used to study bladder structure or function, fallopian tube patency and in the past for a variety of fetal imaging studies.
Side effects include hematuria, retrograde infection, renal failure, hypersensitivity, and anaphylactic reaction.

■ **Fetal Considerations** .... There are no adequate reports or well-controlled studies in human fetuses. It is unknown whether **diatrizoate** crosses the human placenta. Postnatally, **diatrizoate** is used diagnostically to distinguish NEC from microcolon of prematurity. Rodent teratogenicity studies have not been performed.

- ■ **Breastfeeding Safety** — There is no published experience in nursing women. It is unknown whether **diatrizoate** enters human breast milk. However, considering the indication and dosing, one-time **diatrizoate** use is unlikely to pose a clinically significant risk to the breast-feeding neonate.

- ■ **References** — Krasna IH, Rosenfeld D, Salerno P. J Pediatr Surg 1996; 31:855-8.
  Harman CR, Menticoglou SM, Bowman JM, Manning FA. Fetal Ther 1989; 4:78-82.
  Samuel N, Dicker D, Landman J, et al. J Ultrasound Med 1986; 5:425-8.

- ■ **Summary**
  - **Pregnancy Category C**
  - **Lactation Category U**
  - **Diatrizoate** should be used during pregnancy and lactation only if the benefit justifies the potential perinatal risk.

Diazepam (Alupram; Anlin; Baogin; Britazepam; Centrazepam; Chuansuan; Desloneg; Diastat; Diatran; Dizac; Euphorin; Evacalm; Jinpanfan; Mandro; Meval; Nellium; Nerozen; Nixtensyn; Notense; Parzam; Pomin; Rival; Tensium; Tranquil; Valitran; Valium; Valrelease; Winii; Zepaxid)

- ■ **Class** — *Anxiolytic, benzodiazepine, muscle relaxant*

- ■ **Indications** — Anxiety, alcohol withdrawal, seizure disorder, status epilepticus, muscle spasm

- ■ **Mechanism** — Binds benzodiazepine and possibly GABA receptors centrally

- ■ **Dosage with Qualifiers** — Anxiety—2-10mg IV, IM tid/qid
  Alcohol withdrawal—5mg PO tid/qid prn
  Seizure disorder—2-10mg PO bid/qid
  Status epilepticus—5-10mg IV q10-15min
  Muscle spasm—2-10mg PO bid/qid
  - **Contraindications**—hypersensitivity to drug or class, glaucoma, CNS depression, shock, coma, and barbiturate and alcohol use
  - **Caution**—renal or hepatic dysfunction, psychosis, pulmonary dysfunction

- ■ **Maternal Considerations** — There are no adequate reports or well-controlled studies of **diazepam** in pregnant women. It is a beneficial adjunct to IV fluids and vitamins for the treatment of 1st trimester hyperemesis. **Diazepam** was previously used for prophylaxis and treatment of eclamptic convulsions, but proved less effective than **magnesium sulfate**. Pregnancy may unmask a preexisting potential for chorea (chorea gravidarum), and benzodiazepines may aid chorea control. **Diazepam** is a useful antianxietal in women undergoing fetal therapy procedures such as cordocentesis. After surgery, patients should be cautioned against operating machinery or driving. **Flumazenil** (a specific benzodiazepine-receptor antagonist) is indicated for complete or partial reversal of the sedative effects, or treatment of **benzodiazepine** overdose.

Side effects include severe burning and vascular irritation, withdrawal syndrome, hepatic toxicity, pancytopenia, neutropenia, hypotension, nausea, vomiting, vertigo, blurred vision, and rash.

■ **Fetal Considerations**

There are no adequate reports or well-controlled studies in human fetuses. **Diazepam** rapidly crosses the human placenta, with the F:M ratio approaching unity within 15min of maternal injection. Several studies suggest an increased risk of fetal malformation when **diazepam** is used during the 1st trimester. These have not been confirmed subsequently. Postnatal follow-up until age 4y is likewise reassuring, revealing no adverse effects on neurodevelopment. Decreased fetal movement frequently accompanies IV administration. Prolonged CNS depression may occur in neonates, apparently due to their inability to metabolize **diazepam**. The shortest course and the lowest dose should be used when indicated during pregnancy. Some newborns exposed antenatally exhibit either the floppy infant syndrome, or marked neonatal withdrawal symptoms. Symptoms vary from mild sedation, hypotonia, reluctance to suck, apneic spells, cyanosis, and impaired metabolic responses to cold stress. Such symptoms may persist for hours to months after birth. Rodent studies suggest an increased incidence of fetal malformations (skeletal defects) when administered at much higher doses than ones used clinically. Further, a large body of rodent behavioral studies reveals behavioral alterations that persist into adulthood.

■ **Breastfeeding Safety**

Diazepam is excreted into human breast milk. The maximum neonatal exposure is estimated at 3% of the maternal dose. Problems may arise if the neonate is premature, or the maternal dose particularly high. Neonatal lethargy, sedation, and weight loss have been reported.

■ **References**

Iqbal MM, Sobhan T, Aftab SR, Mahmud SZ. Del Med J 2002; 74:127-35.
Iqbal MM, Sobhan T, Ryals T. Psychiatr Serv 2002; 53:39-49.
Duley L, Henderson-Smart D. Cochrane Database Syst Rev 2000; CD000127.
Ditto A, Morgante G, la Marca A, De Leo V. Gynecol Obstet Invest 1999; 48:232-6.

Suita S, Taguchi T, Yamanouchi T, et al. J Pediatr Surg 1999; 34:1652-7.

Belfort MA, Anthony J, Saade GR. Semin Perinatol 1999; 23:65-78.

Gulmezoglu AM, Duley L. BMJ 1998; 316:975-6.

Chatterjee A, Mukheree J. J Obstet Gynaecol Res 1997; 23:289-93.

Chien PF, Khan KS, Arnott N. Br J Obstet Gynaecol 1996; 103:1085-91.

Jauniaux E, Jurkovic D, Lees C, et al. Hum Reprod 1996; 11:889-92.

Lancet 1995; 345:1455-63.

McElhatton PR. Reprod Toxicol 1994; 8:461-75.

Golbe LI. Neurol Clin 1994; 12:497-508.

Levy M, Spino M. Pharmacotherapy 1993; 13:202-11.

Stahl MM, Saldeen P, Vinge E. Br J Obstet Gynaecol 1993; 100:185-8.

Borgatta L, Jenny RW, Gruss L, Ong C, Barad D. J Clin Pharmacol 1997; 37:186-92.

Brandt R. Arzneimittelforschung 1976; 26:454-7.

■ **Summary**

- **Pregnancy Category D**
- **Lactation Category S?**
- **Diazepam** should be used during pregnancy and lactation only if the benefit justifies the potential perinatal risk.
- Many indications for **diazepam** have other alternative agents considered to have a higher safety margin during pregnancy and lactation.

Diazoxide (Hyperstat; Proglycem)

■ **Class** — *Antihypertensive, antihypoglycemic*

■ **Indications** — Hypertension

■ **Mechanism** — Directly relaxes peripheral arteriole smooth muscle

■ **Dosage with Qualifiers** — Hypertension—1-3mg/kg IV q5-15min; max 150mg IV
- **Contraindications**—hypersensitivity to drug or class, sulfonamides or thiazide diuretics
- **Caution**—coronary artery disease

■ **Maternal Considerations** — The choice of antihypertensive depends in part on physician experience, and in part on what is known about adverse maternal and fetal side effects. **Diazoxide** has been used for the treatment of severe hypertension during pregnancy, but is associated with a high risk of hypotension and its attendent fetal distress. Smaller but more frequent dosing protocols reputedly reduce that risk. There are many alternatives including **labetalol, ketanserin, hydralazine, nitroprusside, nicardipine** (in low doses), and **nifedipine** of seemingly equal efficacy with much lower complication rates.

Side effects include arrhythmias, seizures, MI, hyperglycemia, hypotension, nausea, vomiting, weakness, and CHF.

■ **Fetal Considerations** .... There are no adequate reports or well-controlled studies in human fetuses. **Diazoxide** crosses the human placenta, though the kinetics remain to be elucidated. Rodent studies are generally reassuring, revealing no evidence of teratogenicity, though IUGR is seen at the highest doses.

■ **Breastfeeding Safety** .... There is no published experience in nursing women. It is unknown whether **diazoxide** enters human breast milk.

■ **References** .... Duley L, Henderson-Smart DJ. Cochrane Database Syst Rev 2000; CD001449.
Lowe SA, Rubin PC. J Hypertens 1992; 10:201-7.
Michael CA. Aust NZ J Obstet Gynaecol 1986; 26:26-9.

■ **Summary** ....
- **Pregnancy Category C**
- **Lactation Category U**
- **Diazoxide** is indicated outside pregnancy for the rapid reduction of blood pressure.
- There are many other alternatives (e.g. **labetalol, ketanserin**, and **nifedipine**) during pregnancy of seemingly equal efficacy with much lower complication rates.

Dichlorphenamide (Daranide; Defenamida)

■ **Class** .... *Carbonic anhydrase inhibitor*

■ **Indications** .... Glaucoma (open-angle)

■ **Mechanism** .... Carbonic anhydrase inhibitors decrease intraocular pressure by reducing aqueous humor inflow

■ **Dosage with Qualifiers** .... Glaucoma—100-200mg PO q12h until response then maintain 25-50mg 1-3/d
- **Contraindications**—hypersensitivity to drug or class
- **Caution**—hypokalemia

- **Maternal Considerations** ········· There is no published experience with **dichlorphenamide** during pregnancy. **Dichlorphenamide** should be used with caution because it could produce brisk diuresis followed by hypokalemia.
  Side effects include constipation, anorexia, nausea, vomiting, weight loss, urinary frequency, renal colic, renal calculi, skin rash, headache, weakness, pruritus, leukopenia, agranulocytosis, thrombocytopenia, nervousness, sedation, depression, confusion, dizziness, and paresthesias of the hands, feet, and tongue.

- **Fetal Considerations** ············· There are no adequate reports or well-controlled studies in human fetuses. It is unknown whether **dichlorphenamide** crosses the human placenta. Rodent studies reveal teratogenic effects (skeletal anomalies) at high doses.

- **Breastfeeding Safety** ············· There is no published experience in nursing women. It is unknown whether **dichlorphenamide** enters human breast milk.

- **References** ··········· Purichia N, Erway LC. Dev Biol 1972; 27:395-405.
  Hallesy DW, Layton WM Jr. Riv Patol Nerv Ment 1966; 87:6-8.

- **Summary** ···········
  - **Pregnancy Category B**
  - **Lactation Category U**
  - **Dichlorphenamide** should be used during pregnancy and lactation only if the benefit justifies the potential perinatal risk.

Diclofenac (Berifen Gel; Blesin; Cataflam; Clofen; Diclofenac Sodium; Oritaren; Silino; Voltaren)

- **Class** ········· NSAID; *analgesic*

- **Indications** ········· Dysmenorrhea, mild to moderate pain, rheumatoid arthritis or osteoarthritis, ankylosing spondylitis

- **Mechanism** ········· Inhibits cyclooxygenase and lipoxygenase leading to reduced prostaglandin synthesis

- **Dosage with Qualifiers** ········· Dysmenorrhea—begin 100mg PO, then 50mg PO tid
  Mild to moderate pain—begin 50mg PO bid to tid
  Rheumatoid arthritis or osteoarthritis—50mg PO bid to tid; max 225mg qd
  Ankylosing spondylitis—25mg PO qid
  - **Contraindications**—hypersensitivity to drug or class, NSAID-induced asthma, nasal polyps, GI bleeding, liver
  - **Caution**—hypertension, nasal polyps, CHF, GI bleeding history

■ Maternal Considerations ⋯⋯⋯ There are no adequate reports or well-controlled studies in pregnant women. **Diclofenac** is a short-acting NSAID with antipyretic, anti-inflammatory, and analgesic properties. It is useful for the relief of ureteral colic or postsurgical pain during pregnancy. In several studies, **diclofenac** had a morphine sparing effect. While rodent studies reveal very high doses of some NSAIDs are associated with dystocia and prolongation of pregnancy, similar studies in humans are missing for **diclofenac**. Cyclooxygenase inhibitors like **diclofenac** may modulate the quantity and degradation of collagen in the rat cervix. **Diclofenac** does not interfere with cervical ripening induced by **misoprostol**. Like other NSAIDs, **diclofenac** alters renal function to decrease free water clearance and increases the toxicity of certain drugs such as **digoxin**. NOTE—with caution, may be combined with **misoprostol** (Arthrotec)

Side effects include anaphylaxis, bleeding, bronchospasm, thrombocytopenia, Stevens-Johnson syndrome, interstitial nephritis, impairment of the liver and kidney function, abdominal pain, urticaria, drowsiness, and tinnitus.

■ Fetal Considerations ⋯⋯⋯ There are no adequate reports or well-controlled studies in human fetuses. **Diclofenac** rapidly crosses the human placenta even in the 1st trimester yielding an F:M ratio approximating unity. Premature closure of the ductus arteriosus is reported. Rodent studies are generally reassuring, revealing no evidence of teratogenicity or IUGR despite the use of doses higher than those used clinically. High doses were associated with fetal toxicity.

■ Breastfeeding Safety ⋯⋯⋯ There are no adequate reports or well-controlled studies in nursing women. Most NSAIDs enter human milk to some extent. The chemical structure and preliminary study suggest passage should be low and occasional use without clinically significant risk. **Ibuprofen** is generally preferred for breast-feeding women.

■ References ⋯⋯⋯

Ivy LC, Grace WC, Ben CC, Chung HP. Contraception 2003; 67:101-5.

Ergene U, Pekdemir M, Canda E, et al. Int Urol Nephrol 2001; 33:315-9.

Hohlagschwandtner M, Ruecklinger E, Husslein P, Joura EA. Obstet Gynecol 2001; 98:1089-92.

Siddik SM, Aouad MT, Jalbout MI, et al. Reg Anesth Pain Med 2001; 26:310-5.

Al-Waili NS. Arch Med Res 2001; 32:148-54.

Siu SS, Yeung JH, Lau TK. Hum Reprod 2000; 15:2423-5.

Bogdanenko EV, Sviridov IuV, Sadovnikov VB, Zhdanov RI. Eksp Klin Farmakol 1999; 62:55-7.

Zenker M, Klinge J, Kruger C, et al. J Perinat Med 1998; 26:231-4.

Mas C, Menahem S. Aust NZ J Obstet Gynaecol 1999; 39:106-7.

Bienkiewicz A. Horm Metab Res 1995; 27:79-82.

Montenegro MA, Palomino H. J Craniofac Genet Dev Biol 1990; 10:83-94.

Needs CJ, Brooks PM. Br J Rheumatol 1985; 24:291-7.

■ **Summary** —
- **Pregnancy Category B**
- **Lactation Category S?**
- There are alternative agents for which there is more experience during pregnancy and lactation.

Dicloxacillin (Dacocillin; Dycill; Dynapen; Maclicine; Orbenin; Pathocil; Staphcillin)

■ **Class** — Antibiotics (*penicillin*)

■ **Indications** — Bacterial infections (gram-positive aerobes: penicillin-resistant *Staphylococcus*), osteomyelitis, mastitis

■ **Mechanism** — Bactericidal; inhibits cell wall synthesis

■ **Dosage with Qualifiers** — Skin infection—125-500mg PO q6h 1h before or after a meal
Osteomyelitis—250-500mg PO q6h before or after a meal
Mastitis—250-500mg PO q6h before or after a meal
NOTE—renal dosing; GI absorption of **dicloxacillin** is delayed if taken after a meal
- **Contraindications**—hypersensitivity to drug or class
- **Caution**—cephalosporin allergy, neonates, renal or hepatic dysfunction, and Epstein-Barr virus or cytomegalovirus infections

■ **Maternal Considerations** — There are no adequate reports or well-controlled studies of **dicloxacillin** in pregnant women. **Dicloxacillin** is a penicillinase-resistant, acid-resistant semisynthetic broad-spectrum penicillin. It is an excellent drug for the treatment of postpartum mastitis.
Side effects—seizures, pseudomembranous colitis, agranulocytosis, anemia, thrombocytopenia, leukopenia, epigastric or abdominal pain, nausea, vomiting, diarrhea, dizziness, fatigue, fever, increased LFTs, and eosinophilia

■ **Fetal Considerations** — There are no adequate reports or well-controlled studies in human fetuses. **Dicloxacillin** crosses the human placenta. The fetal concentrations are relatively low, perhaps because of the high degree of protein binding in the mother. Rodent studies are reassuring, revealing no evidence of teratogenicity or IUGR despite the use of doses higher than those used clinically.

■ **Breastfeeding Safety** — There is no published experience in nursing women. It is unknown whether **dicloxacillin** enters human breast milk. The extensive clinical experience with its use for mastitis is reassuring. Other penicillin agents are excreted into human breast milk, but are generally considered safe.

■ **References** ⋯⋯⋯⋯⋯⋯⋯ Herngren L, Ehrnebo M, Boreus LO. Dev Pharmacol Ther 1983; 6:110-24.
Anderson JC. J Comp Pathol 1977; 87:611-21.
Nau H. Dev Pharmacol Ther 1987; 10:174-98.
Depp R, Kind AC, Kirby WM, Johnson WL. Am J Obstet Gynecol 1970; 107:1054-7.
MacAulay MA, Berg SR, Charles, D. Am J Obstet Gynecol 1968; 102:1162-8.
Brander GC, Watkins JH, Gard RP. Vet Rec 1975; 97:300-4.

■ **Summary** ⋯⋯⋯⋯⋯⋯⋯⋯⋯
- **Pregnancy Category B**
- **Lactation Category S**
- A drug of choice for the treatment of postpartum mastitis.

Dicyclomine (A-Spas; Antispas; Bentyl; Bo-Cyclomine; Coochil; Dedoxia; Diciclomina; Dicyclocot; Magesan; Medispaz-Im; Protylol)

■ **Class** ⋯⋯⋯⋯⋯⋯⋯⋯⋯⋯⋯ *Anticholinergic; gastrointestinal*

■ **Indications** ⋯⋯⋯⋯⋯⋯⋯⋯ Irritable bowel syndrome

■ **Mechanism** ⋯⋯⋯⋯⋯⋯⋯⋯ Decreases GI motility by inhibiting smooth muscle contractility

■ **Dosage with Qualifiers** ⋯⋯ <u>Irritable bowel syndrome</u>—20mg PO qid; max 40mg PO qid
- **Contraindications**—hypersensitivity to drug or class, ulcerative colitis, paralytic ileus, toxic megacolon, myasthenia gravis, reflux esophagitis, glaucoma
- **Caution**—cardiovascular disease, hyperthyroidism

■ **Maternal Considerations** ⋯⋯ There are no adequate reports or well-controlled studies of **dicyclomine** in pregnant women.
Side effects include drowsiness, blurred vision, respiratory distress, tachycardia, urticaria, confusion, constipation, mydriasis, nausea, vomiting, palpitations, tachycardia, fever, psychosis, and photophobia

■ **Fetal Considerations** ⋯⋯⋯ There are no adequate reports or well-controlled studies in human fetuses. It is unknown whether **dicyclomine** crosses the human placenta. Epidemiologic studies are reassuring. **Dicyclomine** was a component of **Bendectin**, a popular but no longer marketed drug used to treat nausea and vomiting during pregnancy. Initially consisting of **doxylamine**, **dicyclomine**, and **pyridoxine**, **dicyclomine** was dropped from the formulation in 1976. **Bendectin** was ultimately discontinued in 1983 after an

257

onslaught of lawsuits suggesting it caused congenital malformations. Subsequent studies revealed no difference in the prevalence of birth defects between mothers who had taken **Bendectin** during the 1st trimester and those who had not. Rodent studies are reassuring, revealing no evidence of teratogenicity or IUGR despite the use of doses higher than those used clinically.

■ **Breastfeeding Safety**
There is no published experience in nursing women. **Dicyclomine** is excreted in human milk. As there are case reports noting severe respiratory symptoms in neonates directly receiving **dicyclomine**, it is considered incompatible with breastfeeding.

■ **References**
Magee LA, Mazzotta P, Koren G. Am J Obstet Gynecol 2002; 185:S256-61.
Boneva RS, Moore CA, Botto L, et al. Am J Epidemiol 1999; 149:717-25.
McKeigue PM, Lamm SH, Linn S, Kutcher JS. Teratology 1994; 50:27-37.

■ **Summary**
- **Pregnancy Category B**
- **Lactation Category NS?**
- **Dicyclomine** should be used during pregnancy only if the benefit justifies the potential perinatal risk.
- There are alternative agents for which there is more experience during pregnancy and lactation.

Didanosine (DDI; Videx; Videx EC)

■ **Class**
Antiviral

■ **Indications**
HIV infection

■ **Mechanism**
Reverse transcriptase inhibitor

■ **Dosage with Qualifiers**
HIV infection—200mg PO q12h
NOTE—if weight <60kg, 125mg PO q12h
- **Contraindications**—hypersensitivity to drug or class, history of pancreatitis, neuropathy
- **Caution**—gout, neuropathy, renal or hepatic dysfunction, concomitant use of neurotoxic agents

■ **Maternal Considerations**
There are no adequate reports or well-controlled studies of **didanosine** in pregnant women. Human pharmacokinetic studies suggest that maternal plasma clearance is significantly greater antepartum than postpartum after IV administration. Clearance during pregnancy is unaltered after PO administration. **Didanosine** is no more

effective than **zidovudine** as a monotherapy. HIV patients with <400 viral copies/ml respond faster (2 consecutive viral loads <400 copies/ml) and maintain it for 4 years when treated with a multiregimen treatment that includes **didanosine**, **stavudine**, and **nelfinavir** compared to **lamivudine**, **zidovudine,** and **nelfinavir**. Resistant strains are known. **Didanosine** is a cause of diabetes mellitus. Blood glucose levels should be monitored frequently especially when **didanosine** is combined with other drugs such as **pentamidine** and **dapsone** that cause hyperglycemia. **Didanosine** does not cure HIV, nor does it reduce the risk of HIV transmission by sexual contact or blood contamination. Fatal lactic acidosis has been reported in pregnant women who have received a combination of **didanosine** and **stavudine**. The long-term effects of **didanosine** on both treated women and neonates are presently unknown.

Side effects include pancreatitis, neuropathy, hepatotoxicity, optic neuritis, thrombocytopenia, diabetes mellitus, nausea, vomiting, diarrhea, rhabdomyolysis, rash, abdominal pain, arthralgia, and anorexia.

■ Fetal Considerations

There are no adequate reports or well-controlled studies in human fetuses. **Didanosine** rapidly crosses the isolated human placenta, and it efficiently crosses *in vivo* the macaque placenta. It is estimated the fetal levels would be therapeutic. Rodent studies are reassuring revealing no evidence of teratogenicity or IUGR despite the use of doses higher than those used clinically. **Didanosine** does cross the rodent placenta.

■ Breastfeeding Safety

There is no published experience in nursing women. It is unknown whether **didanosine** enters human breast milk. It is generally recommended that wherever possible, HIV-infected women not breastfeed to avoid the risk of HIV transmission to the neonate.

■ References

Bardsley-Elliot A, Perry CM. Paediatr Drugs 2000; 2:373-407.
Wang Y, Livingston E, Patil S, et al. J Infect Dis 1999; 180:1536-41.
Bawdon RE, Sobhi S, Dax J. Am J Obstet Gynecol 1992; 167:1570-4.
Tuntland T, Odinecs A, Pereira CM, Nosbisch C, Unadkat JD. Am J Obstet Gynecol 1999; 180:198-206.
Munshi MN, Martin RE, Fonseca VA. Diabetes Care 1994; 17:316-7.

■ Summary

- **Pregnancy Category B**
- **Lactation Category U**
- **Didanosine** should be used during pregnancy and lactation only if the benefit justifies the potential perinatal risk.
- Physicians are encouraged to register pregnant women under the Antiretroviral Pregnancy Registry (1-800-258-4263) for a better follow-up of the outcome while under treatment with **didanosine**.

Dienestrol (DV; Estraguard; Ortho Dienoestrol)

■ **Class** — *Hormone, estrogen*

■ **Indications** — Atrophic vaginitis

■ **Mechanism** — Stimulates estrogen receptors

■ **Dosage with Qualifiers** — Atrophic vaginitis—1 intravaginal application 3×/w
- **Contraindications**—hypersensitivity to drug or class, history thromboembolic disease, cancer (ovarian, uterine, breast), unexplained vaginal bleeding
- **Caution**—hepatic or renal dysfunction, history of depression

■ **Maternal Considerations** — **Dienestrol** is a synthetic, nonsteroidal estrogen suitable for intravaginal use. It is also an oxidative metabolic product of **diethylstilbestrol**. Estrogen compounds are contraindicated during pregnancy.
Side effects include depression, thromboembolic events (stroke, MI), endometrial carcinoma, gallbladder disease, pancreatitis, hypertension, nausea, vomiting, abnormal uterine bleeding, migraine, libido change, increase in size of uterine fibromyomas, vaginal candidiasis, breast tenderness, and erythema nodosum.

■ **Fetal Considerations** — There are no adequate reports or well-controlled studies in human fetuses. It is unknown whether **dienestrol** crosses the human placenta. The genital tract has the ability to metabolize **dienestrol**. **Estrogens** are contraindicated during pregnancy.

■ **Breastfeeding Safety** — There is no published experience in nursing women. It is unknown whether **dienestrol** enters human breast milk. Estrogens are usually considered incompatible with breastfeeding.

■ **References** — Miller RK, Heckmann ME, McKenzie RC. J Pharmacol Exp Ther 1982; 220:358-65.
Korach KS, McLachlan JA. Arch Toxicol Suppl 1985; 8:33-42.
Harper MJ. Anat Rec 1968; 162:433-52.

■ **Summary** —
- **Pregnancy Category X**
- **Lactation Category NS?**
- **Dienestrol** is contraindicated during pregnancy and lactation.

Diethylpropion (Depletite; Diethylpropion HCl; Dietil; Dipro; Durad; M-Orexic; Radtue; Tenuate; Tenuate Dospan; Tepanil)

■ **Class** — Anorexiant, CNS *stimulant*

■ **Indications** — Obesity

■ **Mechanism** — The mechanism of appetite suppression is unknown (possible inhibitor of norepinephrine and dopamine reuptake).

■ **Dosage with Qualifiers** — Obesity—25mg PO tid before meals, or extended release tab qd
- **Contraindications**—hypersensitivity to drug or class, use of MAO inhibitor drugs within the last 14d, cardiovascular disease, glaucoma, hyperthyroidism

■ **Maternal Considerations** — There are no adequate reports or well-controlled studies of **diethylpropion** in pregnant women. The published experience consists of isolated case reports.
Side effects include pulmonary hypertension, arrhythmias, psychosis, dry mouth, constipation, and restlessness.

■ **Fetal Considerations** — There are no adequate reports or well-controlled studies in human fetuses. It is unknown whether **diethylpropion** crosses the human placenta. Neonatal withdrawal has been described in neonates delivered of women who used **diethylpropion** during pregnancy. There is a single case report of sacral agenesis associated with multiple anomalies of the lower limb in a woman taking **diethylpropion** during the first month of pregnancy. Rodent studies are reassuring, revealing no evidence of teratogenicity or IUGR despite the use of doses higher than those used clinically.

■ **Breastfeeding Safety** — There are no adequate reports or well-controlled studies in nursing women. **Diethylpropion** is excreted into human breast milk, though the kinetics remain to be elucidated.

■ **References** — Abraham E. Clin Orthop 1979; 145:168-71.
Silverman M, Okun R. Curr Ther Res Clin Exp 1971; 13:648-53.
Boileau PA. Appl Ther 1968; 10:763-5.

■ **Summary**
- **Pregnancy Category B**
- **Lactation Category U**
- There is no strong clinical indication for **diethylpropion** during pregnancy.

Diethylstilbestrol (Stilphostrol)

■ **Class** .... *Hormone, estrogen, antineoplastics*

■ **Indications** .... Metastatic breast cancer

■ **Mechanism** .... Binds and stimulates estrogen receptors

■ **Dosage with Qualifiers** .... Metastatic breast cancer—15mg PO qd
- **Contraindications**—hypersensitivity, male with breast carcinoma, estrogen dependent carcinoma, pregnancy, active thrombophlebitis or thromboembolic disorders
- **Caution**—cardiovascular disease, coronary artery disease, seizure disorder, hepatic adenoma, hypercalcemia, glucose tolerance

■ **Maternal Considerations** .... **Diethylstilbestrol** was administered to approximately 3 million pregnant women in the U.S. and in the Netherlands between 1947 and 1975. There was an increased risk of mammary carcinomas in exposed women. Pregnancy does not appear to influence adversely the tumor characteristics or prognosis of patients who have developed these malignancies.
Side effects include depression, nervousness, dizziness, chest pain, shortness of breath, nausea, vomiting, leg edema, erythema nodosum, decreased libido, fatigue, and increased coagulation factors II, VII, VIII, IX and X.

■ **Fetal Considerations** .... There are no adequate reports or well-controlled studies in human fetuses. It or a metabolite presumably crosses the human placenta. **Diethylstilbestrol**-exposed daughters frequently have developmental disorders of the cervix and corpus uteri (hypoplasia of the uterine cavity, uterine corpus, and cervix; T-shaped uterine cavity, constrictions of the uterine cavity, and bilateral hydrosalpinges). They have an increased risk of spontaneous abortion, ectopic pregnancy and infertility, and possibly an increased risk of cervical incompetence. Spontaneous uterine rupture at term has also been described. An increased risk of hypospadias in the sons exposed to DES *in utero* was reported. Rodent experiments reveal that **diethylstilbestrol** increases the incidence of genital tumors in not only 2nd generation but also 3rd generation animals. However, recent studies report no increased risk of lower genital tract abnormalities in 3rd generation women.

■ **Breastfeeding Safety** .... Estrogens are contraindicated for lactation suppression. **Diethylstilbestrol** does not effectively suppress lactation.

■ **References** .... Klip H, Verloop J, van Gool JD, et al. Lancet 2002; 359:1102-7.

Hernandez-Diaz S. Lancet 2002; 359:1081-2.
Kaufman RH, Adam E. Obstet Gynecol 2002; 99:197-200.
Althuisius SM, Dekker GA, Hummel P, et al. Am J Obstet Gynecol 2001; 185:1106-12.
Hatch EE, Herbst AL, Hoover RN, et al. Cancer Causes Control 2001; 12:837-45.
Treffers PE, Hanselaar AG, Helmerhorst TJ, et al. Ned Tijdschr Geneeskd 2001; 145:675-80.
Palmer JR, Hatch EE, Rao RS, et al. Am J Epidemiol 2001; 154:316-21.
Keller C, Nanda R, Shannon RL, et al. Int J Gynecol Cancer 2001; 11:247-50.
Hanselaar A, van Loosbroek M, Schuurbiers O, et al. Cancer 1997; 79:2229-36.
Herbst AL, Anderson D. Semin Surg Oncol 1990; 6:343-6.
van Gils AP, Tham RT, Falke TH, Peters AA. AJR Am J Roentgenol 1989; 153:1235-8.
Adams DM, Druzin ML, Cederqvist LL. Obstet Gynecol 1989; 73:471-3.
Brown DD. Br Med J 1969; 1:51.

■ **Summary**
- **Pregnancy Category X**
- **Lactation Category NS**
- **Diethylstilbestrol** is contraindicated during pregnancy and lactation.

Diflunisal (Dolobid; Dopanone; Fluodonil; Noaldol)

■ **Class** — *Analgesic*, NSAID; *salicylates*

■ **Indications** — Mild to moderate pain, osteoarthritis, rheumatoid arthritis

■ **Mechanism** — Inhibits cyclooxygenase and lipoxygenase leading to reduced prostaglandin synthesis

■ **Dosage with Qualifiers** — Pain—begin 1000mg PO ×1; then 500mg PO q12h
Osteoarthritis—250-500mg PO q12h
Rheumatoid arthritis—250-500mg PO q12h
- **Contraindications**—hypersensitivity to drug or class, asthmatic attacks, urticaria, aspirin-precipitated rhinitis
- **Caution**—nasal polyps, GI bleeding, hypertension, cardiac failure, hepatic or renal dysfunction

■ **Maternal Considerations** — **Diflunisal** is an NSAID with anti-inflammatory, antipyretic, and analgesic properties. Similar to many NSAIDs, **diflunisal** inhibits platelet aggregation. There are no adequate reports or well-controlled studies of **diflunisal** in pregnant women. **Diflunisal** is superior to **aspirin** for postepisiotomy pain.

Side effects include peptic ulceration, GI bleeding, anaphylaxis, thrombocytopenia, Stevens-Johnson syndrome, nephritis, hepatic or renal failure

■ **Fetal Considerations**

There are no adequate reports or well-controlled studies in human fetuses. It is unknown whether **diflunisal** crosses the human placenta. Treated *Cynomolgus* monkeys experience no increased rates of abortion, IUGR, or malformation. Rodent studies reveal embryotoxicity and teratogenicity (skeletal malformations) in doses 1-8 times the recommended human dose. In the human fetus, other NSAIDs can cause in the 3rd trimester constriction of the ductus arteriosus, followed by tricuspid incompetence and pulmonary hypertension. Platelet dysfunction, intracranial bleeding, or renal dysfunction may result in permanent renal failure, oligohydramnios, or necrotizing enterocolitis.

■ **Breastfeeding Safety**

There is no published experience in nursing women. **Diflunisal** is excreted into human milk achieving an M:P ratio less than 0.07. Considering the indications and dosing, occasional **diflunisal** use is unlikely to pose a clinically significant risk to the breast-feeding neonate.

■ **References**

Rowland JM, Robertson RT, Cukierski M, et al. Fundam Appl Toxicol 1987; 8:51-8.
Kollenberg LO, Hudyma EO, Robbins JM. J Am Podiatr Med Assoc 1985; 75:517-22.
Clark RL, Robertson RT, Minsker DH, et al. Teratology 1984; 30:319-32.
De Vroey P. Curr Med Res Opin 1978; 5:544-7.

■ **Summary**

- **Pregnancy Category C**
- **Lactation Category S?**
- **Diflunisal** and other NSAIDs are probably safe if used occasionally for the noted indications during pregnancy and lactation.

Digitoxin (Coramedan; Crystodigin)

■ **Class**

Antiarrhythmic, inotrope, cardiac glycoside

■ **Indications**

Heart failure, atrial flutter, atrial fibrillation, supraventricular tachycardia

■ **Mechanism**

Inhibits Na^+-K^+ transmembrane ATPase

- **Dosage with Qualifiers** ⋯⋯ Heart failure—0.2mg PO qd ×4d; maintenance dose varies between 0.05-0.3mg qd
Atrial flutter—0.2-0.3mg PO qd
Atrial fibrillation—0.2-0.3mg PO qd
Supraventricular tachycardia—0.3mg PO qd
Rapid digitalization—0.6mg, then 0.4mg in 4-6h, then 0.2mg q4-6h until drug level therapeutic
  - **Contraindications**—hypersensitivity to drug or class, ventricular tachycardia, cardiac disease, and hypersensitive carotid sinus syndrome
  - **Caution**—hypokalemia, hepatic and renal failure

- **Maternal Considerations** ⋯⋯ There are no adequate reports or well-controlled studies of **digitoxin** in pregnant women. **Digitoxin** is a crystalline-pure cardiac glycoside obtained from D*igitalis purpurea* and is identical to the pharmacologic action of digitalis. Excretion is slow (14-21d). Serum levels should be monitored periodically during pregnancy. Pregnant women receiving the usual dose of 0.25mg tend to have subnormal levels and may require a small increase during the last trimester.
Side effects include digitalis intoxication that includes nausea, vomiting, visual disturbance, electrolyte abnormalities (hypo/hyperkalemia), and bradycardia.

- **Fetal Considerations** ⋯⋯ There are no adequate reports or well-controlled studies in human fetuses. **Digoxin** and presumably **digitoxin** cross the healthy human placenta reaching F:M ratios approximating 0.8. However, the human placenta is rich in digoxin receptors, and transfer is greatly reduced when there is hydrops. Fetal bradycardia is reported. Studies are compromised by tests, which failed to differentiate between **digoxin** and endogenous digoxin-like substances. Rodent teratogenicity studies have not been performed.

- **Breastfeeding Safety** ⋯⋯ There is no published experience in nursing women. It is unknown whether **digitoxin** enters human breast milk. Endogenous digoxin-like substances are normal components of breast milk.

- **References** ⋯⋯ Van Gundy JC, Bolam DL, Swigart SA, Nelson RM Jr. Nebr Med J 1986; 71:300-2.
Soyka LF. Clin Perinatol 1975; 2:23-35.

- **Summary** ⋯⋯
  - **Pregnancy Category C**
  - **Lactation Category U**
  - **Digitoxin** should be used during pregnancy and lactation only if the benefit justifies the potential perinatal risk.
  - There are alternative digoxin-type agents with shorter elimination times.

Digoxin (Digacin; Digitek; Lanicor; Lanoxicaps; Lanoxin)

■ **Class** .... Antiarrhythmic, inotrope, cardiac glycoside

■ **Indications** .... Congestive heart failure, atrial fibrillation/flutter, paroxysmal atrial tachycardia

■ **Mechanism** .... Inhibits Na$^+$-K$^+$ transmembrane ATPase

■ **Dosage with Qualifiers** .... Congestive heart failure—begin with a loading dose of 0.75-1.25mg PO, or 0.5-1mg IV/IM followed by a maintenance dose 0.125-0.5mg PO qd
NOTE—**digoxin** levels should be maintained between 0.8-2ng/ml
Atrial fibrillation/flutter—0.125-0.5mg PO qd
Paroxysmal atrial tachycardia—0.125-0.5mg PO qd
Fetal arrhythmia—1mg IV to load, 0.25-1mg PO bid
Rapid digitalization—0.4-0.6mg IV/PO, then 0.1-0.3mg q6-8h guided by the **digoxin** level
- **Contraindications**—hypersensitivity to drug or class, ventricular fibrillation, ventricular tachycardia, atrioventricular accessory pathway, sick sinus syndrome
- **Caution**—bradycardia, atrioventricular block, MI, cardiomyopathy, constrictive pericarditis, renal or hepatic dysfunction

■ **Maternal Considerations** .... There is a long clinical experience during pregnancy and the puerperium with **digoxin** for the treatment of benign arrhythmias and cardiomyopathy. A full cardiovascular evaluation is recommended prior to its initiation. Potential stimulants, such as smoking, **caffeine**, and **alcohol** should be eliminated. Although no antiarrhythmic drug is completely safe during pregnancy, most are well tolerated and add relatively little risk. Drug therapy should be avoided during the 1st trimester and drugs with the best safety record used as first-line therapy. Women with peripartal cardiomyopathy who have persistently abnormal ventricular function must be continuously treated with **digoxin**, diuretics, anticoagulation, and have the same relatively poor prognosis as patients with dilated cardiomyopathy. Heart transplantation may be necessary for survival.
Side effects include hallucinations, blurred vision, thrombocytopenia, arrhythmia, bradycardia, delirium, and electrolyte abnormalities (hypo/hyperkalemia).

■ **Fetal Considerations** .... There are no adequate reports or well-controlled studies in human fetuses. **Digoxin** crosses the placenta with a typical F:M ratio ranging from 0.6-0.8. **Digoxin** is generally considered first-line therapy for the treatment of fetal SVT in the absence of hydrops. Treatment is aimed initially at slowing the ventricular response rate and ultimately conversion to sinus rhythm. However, there are no trails confirming that conversion reflects therapeutic efficacy or disease natural history. After adequate maternal digitalization, conversion to normal sinus rhythm should occur within 72h, reported successes often occur after weeks. Certainly, the addition of a second agent would be desirable if there is no response. The fetal response is worse if tricuspid regurgitation is already present. Placental transport is dramatically reduced when there is hydrops, and this appears inversely proportional to the umbilical venous pressure. Certainly in this instance, many fetal medicine specialists consider **flecainide** the drug of choice. Direct fetal **digoxin** administration (IM) can be successful after more traditional intensive trials of transplacental therapy with **digoxin**, **verapamil**, and **procainamide**, either separately or in combination, fail. Transplacental **digoxin** therapy has also been used to improve ionotropy in fetuses with complete heart block. Despite adequate therapy and many times improvement in the fetal status *in utero*, many fetuses require postnatal pacemaker implantation or heart transplant. Rodent teratogenicity studies have not been performed.

■ Breastfeeding Safety

There are no adequate reports or well-controlled studies in nursing women. **Digoxin** enters human breast milk in low concentration, achieving an M:P ratio approximating 0.7. As a result, the **digoxin** level of the breast-fed neonate would be subtherapeutic. Endogenous digoxin-like substances are a normal component of breast milk.

■ References

Ebenroth ES, Cordes TM, Darragh RK. Pediatr Cardiol 2001; 22:483-7.
Krapp M, Baschat AA, Gembruch U, et al. Ultrasound Obstet Gynecol 2002; 19:158-64.
Jouannic JM, Le Bidois J, Fermont L, et al. Fetal Diagn Ther 2002; 17:120-3.
Jones LM, Garmel SH. Obstet Gynecol 2001; 98:921-3.
Baughman KL. Curr Treat Options Cardiovasc Med 2001; 3:469-480.
Facchini M, Bauersfeld U, Fasnacht M, Candinas R. Schweiz Med Wochenschr 2000; 130:1962-9.
Oudijk MA, Ambachtsheer EB, Stoutenbeek P, Meijboom EJ. Ned Tijdschr Geneeskd 2001(23); 145:1218-9.
Brackley KJ, Ismail KM, Wright JG, Kilby MD. Fetal Diagn Ther 2000; 15:355-8.
Schmolling J, Renke K, Richter O, et al. Ther Drug Moni 2000; 22:582-8.
Lisowski LA, Verheijen PM, Benatar AA, et al. J Am Coll Cardiol 2000; 35:771-7.
Joglar JA, Page RL. Drug Saf 1999; 20:85-94.
Mozas J, Miranda JA, Barranco M. Int J Gynaecol Obstet 1995; 50:293-4.
Chao RC, Ho ES, Hsieh KS. Am Heart J 1992; 124:1095-8.
Cameron AD, Walker JJ, Nimrod CA. BMJ 1988; 297:623.
Weiner CP, Thompson MI. Am J Obstet Gynecol 1988; 158:570-3.

Weiner CP, Landas S, Persoon TJ. Am J Obstet Gynecol 1987; 157:368-71.
Kleinman CS, Copel JA, Weinstein EM, et al. J Clin Ultrasound 1985; 13:265-73.
Reinhardt D, Richter O, Genz T, Pottoff S. Eur J Pediatr 1982; 138:49-52.

■ **Summary**

- **Pregnancy Category C**
- **Lactation Category S**
- **Digoxin** is indicated for the treatment of mild to moderate heart failure. Concomitant ACE-inhibitor agents should be discontinued during the 1st trimester if possible.
- **Digoxin** has a long clinical track record of treating both maternal and fetal arrhythmias; it is one of the safest antiarrhythmics to use during pregnancy.

Dihydroergotamine (D.H.E. 45; Migranal)

■ **Class**

Ergot alkaloids; migraine

■ **Indications**

Migraine and cluster headache

■ **Mechanism**

Constricts cranial and peripheral vessels

■ **Dosage with Qualifiers**

Migraine—1mg IM/IV, may repeat qh ×2; max 2mg IV, or 3mg/attack or 6mg/w; alternatively, 1 spray (0.5mg) NAS each nostril, may repeat in 15min; max 4 sprays/attack, 8 sprays/w

Cluster headache—1mg IM/IV, may repeat q1h ×2; max 2mg IV, or 3mg/attack or 6mg/w

NOTE—prime pump with 4 sprays, discard unused portion after 8h

- **Contraindications**—hypersensitivity to drug or class, coronary artery disease, uncontrolled hypertension, basilar migraine, peripheral vascular disease, cerebrovascular disease, 5HT1 agonist within 24h, severe hepatic or renal dysfunction, concurrent vasoconstrictors, sepsis, potent CYP3A4 inhibitor use
- **Caution**—cardiac risk factors

■ **Maternal Considerations**

There are no adequate reports or well-controlled studies of **dihydroergotamine** in pregnant women. It possesses oxytocic properties and was used in several older trials to assist the induction of labor. It was used occasionally in the past during pregnancy for the treatment of "low" blood pressure. Neither of the last two are indications. **Dihydroergotamine** is effective for the treatment of menstrual migraine.

Side effects include hypertension, peripheral or bowel ischemia, coronary spasm, MI, chest pain, tachycardia, bradycardia, nausea, vomiting, numbness in fingers and toes, leg weakness, and itching.

■ **Fetal Considerations** ⋯⋯⋯ There are no adequate reports or well-controlled studies in human fetuses. It is unknown whether **dihydroergotamine** crosses the human placenta. In one series, women with "low" blood pressure were treated for 1w and the fetal umbilical artery S/D ratio increased 22%, thus suggesting placental transfer. In guinea pigs, chronic administration of **dihydroergotamine** is associated with IUGR.

■ **Breastfeeding Safety** ⋯⋯ There is no published experience in nursing women. It is unknown whether **dihydroergotamine** enters human breast milk. It is known that ergots inhibit prolactin, and that ergotamine is excreted into human breast milk and can have adverse effects on the breast-fed neonate. It would be reasonable to stop breastfeeding until the headache has resolved.

■ **References** ⋯⋯⋯⋯⋯⋯⋯ Silberstein SD. J Womens Health Gend Based Med 1999; 8:919-31.
Goeschen K, Behrens O, Muhlhaus K, et al. Z Geburtshilfe Perinatol 1989; 193:264-7.

■ **Summary** ⋯⋯⋯⋯⋯⋯⋯⋯ ● **Pregnancy Category X**
● **Lactation Category NS**
● Contraindicated during pregnancy and lactation.
● There are alternative agents for which there is more experience during pregnancy and lactation.

Dihydrotachysterol (DHT; Hytakerol; Tachyrol)

■ **Class** ⋯⋯⋯⋯⋯⋯⋯⋯⋯ *Vitamin, mineral*

■ **Indications** ⋯⋯⋯⋯⋯⋯⋯ Osteoporosis, hypocalcemia, renal osteodystrophy

■ **Mechanism** ⋯⋯⋯⋯⋯⋯⋯ Stimulates bone mineralization as well as intestinal calcium and phosphorus absorption

■ **Dosage with Qualifiers** ⋯⋯ Osteoporosis—0.6mg PO qd; give with calcium and fluoride
Hypocalcemia—begin 0.8-2.4mg PO qd for several days, then 0.2-1mg PO qd
Renal osteodystrophy—0.1-0.6mg PO qd
● **Contraindications**—hypersensitivity to drug or class, hypercalcemia, hypervitaminosis D
● **Caution**—renal stones, hyperphosphatemia, hypervitaminosis D

- **Maternal Considerations** .... There are no adequate reports or well-controlled studies of **dihydrotachysterol** (**vitamin D**) in pregnant women, though it is part of most prenatal vitamin preparations. **Dihydrotachysterol** and **calcitriol** are both effective for the management of hypoparathyroidism during pregnancy. The dose required typically needs to be readjusted during the latter half of gestation. The dose of **calcitriol** should be reduced during lactation.
  Side effects include hypercalcemia, renal dysfunction, hypercalciuria, convulsion, polydipsia, nausea, vomiting, anorexia, anemia, weakness, and metastatic calcifications.

- **Fetal Considerations** .... There are no adequate reports or well-controlled studies in human fetuses. It is unknown whether **dihydrotachysterol** crosses the human placenta. Nor is it known whether **dihydrotachysterol** increases fetal calcium. However, fetal supravalvular aortic stenosis may be associated with hypercalcemia secondarily to hypervitaminosis D, and hypercalcemia can occur during treatment with **dihydrotachysterol**. Rodent teratogenicity studies reveal similar abnormalities.

- **Breastfeeding Safety** .... There are no adequate reports or well-controlled studies in nursing women. While **dihydrotachysterol** increases the amount of calcium in breast milk, hypercalcemia is not seen in breast-fed neonates. It is considered unlikely to have a clinically significant effect on the breast-feeding neonate.

- **References** .... Caplan RH, Beguin EA. Obstet Gynecol 1990; 76:485-9.
  Klotz HP. Sem Ther 1963; 39:559-60.

- **Summary** ....
  - **Pregnancy Category C**
  - **Lactation Category S?**
  - **Dihydrotachysterol** should be used during pregnancy and lactation only if the benefit justifies the potential perinatal risk.
  - Both mother and infant should be monitored to detect hypercalcemia during breastfeeding.

Diltiazem (Cardizem; Clarute; Dilacor XR; Lacerol; Tiazac)

- **Class** .... *Antiarrhythmic* (*class* IV)

- **Indications** .... Angina, atrial fibrillation, atrial flutter

- **Mechanism** .... Calcium-channel blocker

- **Dosage with Qualifiers** ···· <u>Angina</u>—begin 30mg PO qid; max 360mg/d
<u>Atrial flutter/fibrillation</u>—20mg (0.25 mg/kg) IV, over 2min; if inadequate response, 0.35mg/kg IV over 2min, then continue infusion with 10(5-15)mg/h for 24h
NOTE—may be packaged with **enalapril**
  - **Contraindications**—hypersensitivity to drug or class, AV block, hypotension, bradycardia, sick sinus syndrome, MI
  - **Caution**—hepatic or renal dysfunction

- **Maternal Considerations** ···· There are no adequate reports or well-controlled studies of **diltiazem** in pregnant women. Clearance is unaltered by pregnancy in the rabbit. **Diltiazem** is used for the treatment of acute cardiac rhythm emergencies. In vitro and in vivo studies demonstrated effective inhibition of myometrial contractions and vasodilatation of arteries collected from normal and preeclamptic women. Oral **diltiazem** has no advantage over **nifedipine** as a tocolytic agent. The cardiovascular alterations following either drug appear minimal in normotensive, pregnant women. Case reports during pregnancy document successful treatment of maternal angina secondary to coronary spasm.
Side effects include edema, headache, nausea, vomiting, dizziness, asthenia, rush, flushing, first-degree AV block, pulmonary congestion, photosensitivity, urticaria, dry mouth, dyspnea, hyperuricemia, osteoarticular pain, sexual difficulties, tinnitus, and erythema multiforme (Stevens-Johnson syndrome, toxic epidermal necrolysis).

- **Fetal Considerations** ···· There are no adequate reports or well-controlled studies in human fetuses. It is unknown whether **diltiazem** crosses the human placenta. It does rapidly cross the rabbit placenta. Rodent studies suggest an increased incidence of skeletal and aortic arch malformations in some species at doses of **diltiazem** administered in multiples of the recommended human dose. Another study of rabbits concluded that chronic in utero exposure altered postnatal metabolism.

- **Breastfeeding Safety** ···· There are no adequate reports or well-controlled studies in nursing women. **Diltiazem** enters human milk and may reach maternal serum levels. Though generally considered safe for breast-feeding women, it may be wise to consider another calcium-channel blocker.

- **References** ····
Bregante MA, Aramayona JJ, Fraile LJ, et al. Xenobiotica 2000; 30:831-41.
El-Sayed YY, Holbrook RH Jr, Gibson R, et al. J Matern Fetal Med 1998; 7:217-21.
Scott WJ Jr, Resnick E, Hummler H, et al. Reprod Toxicol 1997; 11:207-14.
Maekawa K, Ohnishi H, Hirase T, et al. J Intern Med 1994; 235:489-92.
Ivorra MD, Chulia S, Noguera MA, D'Ocon MP. Pharmacology 1994; 49:33-41.

Kook H, Yoon YD, Baik YH. J Korean Med Sci 1996; 11:250-7.
Reviriego J, Fernandez-Alfonso MS, Guerra P, Marin J.
J Cardiovasc Pharmacol 1990; 16:128-38.
Fraile LJ, Bregante MA, Garcia MA, Solans C. Xenobiotica
2001; 31:177-85.
Poli E, Merialdi A, Coruzzi G. Pharmacol Res 1990;
22:115-24.
Lubbe WF. NZ Med J 1987; 100:121.

■ **Summary**

- **Pregnancy Category C**
- **Lactation Category S?**
- **Diltiazem** should be used during pregnancy and lactation only if the benefit justifies the potential perinatal risk.

Dimenhydrinate (Amosyt; Biodramina; Di-Men; Dimeno; Dimetabs; Dinate; Dommanate; Dramamine injection; Dramanate; Dramavance; Dramocen; Dramoject; Dymenate; Hydrate; Marmine; Or-Dram; Shodram; T-Circ; Travelgum; Wehamine)

■ **Class** — *Anticholinergic, antiemetic, antivertigo*

■ **Indications** — Motion sickness, migraine headache

■ **Mechanism** — Exact mechanism of action is unknown

■ **Dosage with Qualifiers** — Motion sickness—50-100mg PO, IM, IV q4-6h; begin at least 30min before anticipated activity, max 400mg/d
Migraine—50-100mg PO

- **Contraindications**—hypersensitivity to drug or class
- **Caution**—neonates, seizure disorder, glaucoma, concomitant use of ototoxic medication

■ **Maternal Considerations** — There are no adequate reports or well-controlled studies of **dimenhydrinate** in pregnant women. It is popular agent in many locales for the relief of nausea and vomiting during pregnancy, though the practice is unsupported by a single clinical trial. Both **dimenhydrinate** and **diphenhydramine** are considered treatment options for severe migraine headache during pregnancy. **Caution** is warranted since several investigators report an increase in uterine activity associated with **dimenhydrinate**.
Side effects include drowsiness, headache, fatigue, increase appetite, abdominal pain, nausea, vomiting, diarrhea, increased bronchial secretion, anorexia, and nervousness.

■ **Fetal Considerations** ···········   There are no adequate reports or well-controlled studies in human fetuses. It is unknown whether **dimenhydrinate** crosses the human placenta. There is no indication that **dimenhydrinate** increases the risk of fetal abnormalities when given at any stage of pregnancy. Rodent studies are reassuring, revealing no evidence of teratogenicity or IUGR despite the use of doses higher than those used clinically.

■ **Breastfeeding Safety** ·········   There is no published experience in nursing women. **Dimenhydrinate** is excreted in small quantities into human breast milk, though the kinetics remain to be elucidated. A long clinical experience is reassuring.

■ **References** ···········   Aube M. Neurology 1999; 53:S26-8.
Lemay M, Samaan M, St Michel P, Granger L, Pigeon R. Can Med Assoc J 1982; 127:606-7.

■ **Summary** ···········
  • **Pregnancy Category B**
  • **Lactation Category S?**
  • **Dimenhydrinate** should be used during pregnancy and lactation only if the benefit justifies the potential perinatal risk.

Dinoprostone (Cervidil; Prepidil; Prostin E2; Prostin E2 Vaginal Suppository)

■ **Class** ···········   *Labor induction; prostaglandin; oxytocic*

■ **Indications** ···········   Cervical ripening

■ **Mechanism** ···········   Unknown

■ **Dosage with Qualifiers** ·········   Cervical ripening—0.5mg gel PV endocervical, may repeat q6h ×2; alternatively, 10mg insert PV into the posterior fornix (remain supine 2h), remove with onset of labor or uterine tachysystole
NOTE—available in either gel or tablet-like insert formats
  • **Contraindications**—hypersensitivity to drug or class, other oxytocics, vaginal delivery itself contraindicated, undiagnosed vaginal bleeding, uterine hypertonicity, uterine tachysystole, fetal distress, imminent delivery, CPD, prior cesarean section or other major uterine surgery, grand multiparity
  • **Caution**—ROM, asthma, glaucoma, increased intraocular pressure, hepatic or renal dysfunction

■ Maternal Considerations

Dinoprostone is the naturally occurring PGE_2. It is effective when administered by oral, vaginal or intracervical routes for cervical ripening preceding either vaginal delivery or pregnancy termination. Efficacy is maintained after membrane rupture. Complications include tachysystole and uterine rupture. Outpatient use has been advocated, but there is no dose that assures the absence of tachysystole. The risk of the latter is especially great in women with a prior cesarean section. **Dinoprostone** reduces the risk of postpartum hemorrhage in high-risk patients. It has also been used to treat atony. Hypertension has been reported on occasion. The safety profile of **dinoprostone** is good; it has been used successfully in women with a wide range of medical complications.

Side effects include bronchospasm, bradycardia, hypertension, arrhythmias, uterine rupture, fetal acidosis, PROM, nausea, vomiting, diarrhea, headache, uterine contractions, dizziness, flushing, fever, cough, chills, and dyspnea.

■ Fetal Considerations

There are no adequate reports or well-controlled studies in human fetuses. It is unknown whether **dinoprostone** crosses the human placenta. Its effects on the fetus appear to reflect complications of uterine activity. Rodent studies reveal embryotoxicity and an increased prevalence of skeletal anomalies when given during organogenesis.

■ Breastfeeding Safety

There is no published experience in nursing women. It is unknown whether **dinoprostone** enters human breast milk. However, considering the indication and dosing, **dinoprostone** use is unlikely to pose a clinically significant risk to the breast-feeding neonate. PGE_2 is naturally excreted into breast milk and has been reported as a cause of neonatal diarrhea.

■ References

Stitely ML, Satin AJ. Clin Obstet Gynecol 2002; 45:114-24.
Biem SR, Turnell RW, Olatunbosun O, Tauh M, Biem HJ. J Obstet Gynaecol Can 2003; 25:23-31.
Van Selm M, Kanhai HH, Keirse MJ. Acta Obstet Gynecol Scand 1995; 74:270-4.
Kelly AJ, Kavanagh J, Thomas J. Cochrane Database Syst Rev 2001; (2):CD003101.
Voss DH, Cumminsky KC, Cook VD, et al. J Matern Fetal Med 1996; 5:186-93.

■ Summary

- **Pregnancy Category C**
- **Lactation Category S**
- **Dinoprostone** should be used during pregnancy only if the benefit justifies the potential perinatal risk.
- Other prostaglandin compounds, such as **misoprostol**, have similar efficacy, the same degree of safety but lower cost.

Diphenhydramine (Allerdryl 50; Allergia-C; Allergina; Amidryl; Banophen; Beldin; Belix; Ben-A-Vance; Ben-Rex; Bena-D10; Benadryl; Benadryl Steri-Dose; Benahist; Benapon; Bendramine; Benoject; Bydramine; Dibenil; Dimidril; Diphen; Diphenacen-50; Diphenhist; Dytuss; Fynex; Genahist; Hydramine; Hydril; Hyrexin; Noradryl; Norafed; Nordryl; Pharm-A-Dry; Restamin; Shodryl; Tega Dryl; Truxadryl; Tusstat; Uad Dryl; Wehdryl)

- **Class** .... *Antihistamine*

- **Indications** .... Antihistamine, motion sickness, anaphylaxis, sedation, insomnia, dystonic reactions

- **Mechanism** .... Nonselective central and peripheral H_1 receptor antagonist

- **Dosage with Qualifiers** .... Antihistaminic—25-50mg PO/IV/IM q6h prn
  Anaphylaxis—1-1.25mg/kg PO/IV/IM q4-6h; max 300mg/d
  Dystonic reactions—25-50mg PO tid/qid; max 300mg/d
  Sedation—25-50mg PO qid prn
  Insomnia—50mg PO qhs
  Motion sickness—25-50mg PO q4-6h prn; max 300mg/d
  - **Contraindications**—hypersensitivity to drug or class, concomitant use of alcohol
  - **Caution**—glaucoma, asthma, hyperthyroidism, cardiovascular disease, glaucoma, peptic ulcer

- **Maternal Considerations** .... There are no adequate reports or well-controlled studies of **diphenhydramine** in pregnant women. It has a long history of use in obstetrics. **Diphenhydramine** is a useful adjunct for women who have allergic reactions to local anesthesia, laminaria, and serum albumin, or for the treatment of severe migraine headaches.
  Side effects include drowsiness, somnolence, dry mouth, nausea, vomiting, headache, abdominal pain, fever, and diarrhea.

- **Fetal Considerations** .... There are no adequate reports or well-controlled studies in human fetuses. Though **diphenhydramine** crosses the human placenta, the kinetics remain to be elucidated. There is no evidence of increased fetal risk if administered during any stage of pregnancy. **Diphenhydramine** may cause neonatal depression if administered during labor. Rodent studies are reassuring, revealing no evidence of teratogenicity or IUGR despite the use of doses higher than those used clinically.

- **Breastfeeding Safety** .... There is no published experience in nursing women. It is unknown whether **diphenhydramine** enters human breast milk. Irritability is the most common adverse reaction reported in the newborns of women using antihistamines while breastfeeding.

■ **References** .... Miller AA. J Perinatol 2000; 20:390-1.
Aube M. Neurology 1999; 53:S26-8.
Garfield RE, Bytautiene E, Vedernikov YP, et al. Am J
Obstet Gynecol 2000; 183:118-25.
Brost BC, Scardo JA, Newman RB. Am J Obstet Gynecol
1996; 175:1376-7.
Ito S, Blajchman A, Stephenson M, et al. Am J Obstet
Gynecol 1993; 168:1393-9.
Yoo SD, Rurak DW, Taylor SM, Axelson JE. J Pharm Sci
1993; 82:145-9.
Leathem AM. Clin Pharm 1986; 5:660-8.
Woods JR Jr, Brinkman CR III, Assali NS. Obstet Gynecol
1976; 48:195-202.
Schardein JL, Hentz DL, Petrere JA, Kurtz SM. Toxicol Appl
Pharmacol 1971; 18:971-6.

■ **Summary** ....
- **Pregnancy Category B**
- **Lactation Category S**
- **Diphenhydramine** appears safe and effective for use during pregnancy.

Dipyridamole (Persantine)

■ **Class** .... *Platelet inhibitors*

■ **Indications** .... Thrombus prophylaxis—DVT, angina, valvulopathy

■ **Mechanism** .... A phosphodiesterase inhibitor that blocks platelet adhesion and stimulates coronary artery dilatation

■ **Dosage with Qualifiers** .... Thromboembolism—150-400mg PO qd (usually given in combination with either **coumadin** or **aspirin**)
Angina—50mg PO tid
Valvulopathy—75-100mg PO qid
- **Contraindications**—hypersensitivity to drug or class
- **Caution**—hypotension

■ **Maternal Considerations** .... Thromboembolus is a major complication of mechanical heart valves. The risk is greatly reduced but not eliminated by regimens of anticoagulation with **coumadin** or therapeutic **heparin** in addition to an antiplatelet agent. **Coumadin** is relatively contraindicated during pregnancy. The regimen of **dipyridamole**, **aspirin** and **ticlopidine** also appears to be effective prophylaxis. Because preeclampsia is associated with a subclinical DIC state, and IUGR with placental thrombosis, a number of studies have examined the role of **dipyridamole** to reduce their incidence. For the most part, **dipyridamole** adds little to the beneficial effects of 81mg of **aspirin** for these indications. **Dipyridamole** has also been used for the treatment of essential thrombocythemia during pregnancy.

Side effects include hypotension, MI, arrhythmias, bronchospasm, rash, dyspnea, nausea, vomiting, tachycardia, flushing, and diarrhea.

■ Fetal Considerations

There are no adequate reports or well-controlled studies in human fetuses. It is unknown whether **dipyridamole** crosses the human placenta. The addition of **dipyridamole** to **aspirin** does not enhance the beneficial effect of **aspirin** on preventing IUGR. **Dipyridamole** use is associated with decreased Doppler measured flow resistance in the umbilical artery. Rodent studies are reassuring, revealing no evidence of teratogenicity or IUGR despite the use of doses higher than those used clinically.

■ Breastfeeding Safety

There is no published experience in nursing women. **Dipyridamole** enters human milk, though the kinetics remain to be elucidated. There is no evidence to suggest a neonatal effect that would preclude breastfeeding. It has been used to treat respiratory difficulties in newborns with congenital diaphragmatic hernia.

■ References

Ueno M, Masuda H, Nakamura K, Sakata R. Surg Today 2001; 31:1002-4.
Hassouna A, Allam H. Cardiovasc Surg 2001; 9:478-81.
Knight M, Duley L, Henderson-Smart DJ, King JF. Cochrane Database Syst Rev 2000; CD000492.
North RA, Ferrier C, Gamble G, Fairley KF, Kincaid-Smith P. Aust N Z J Obstet Gynaecol 1995; 35:357-62.
Kincaid-Smith P. Blood Press 1994; 3:18-23.
Griesshammer M, Heimpel H, Pearson TC. Leuk Lymphoma 1996; 22 (Suppl 1):57-63.
Menashe Y, Ben-Baruch G, Greenspoon JS, et al. J Reprod Med 1993; 38:625-9.
Hirose S, Yamada A, Kasugai M, Ishizuka T, Tomoda Y. Asia Oceania J Obstet Gynaecol 1992; 18:187-93.
Uzan S, Beaufils M, Breart G, Bazin B, Capitant C, Paris J. Lancet 1991; 337:1427-31.
Wallenburg HC, Rotmans N. Lancet 1988; 1:939.
Wallenburg HC, Rotmans N. Am J Obstet Gynecol 1987; 157:1230-5.

■ Summary

- **Pregnancy Category B**
- **Lactation Category S?**
- **Dipyridamole** appears safe for the noted indications during pregnancy and lactation.

Dirithromycin (Dynabac; Norton)

■ **Class** — Antibiotic, macrolide

■ **Indications** — Bacterial infections (<u>gram positive aerobes</u>: Staphylococcus aureus (methicillin-susceptible only), Streptococcus pneumoniae, Streptococcus pyogenes; <u>gram-negative aerobes</u>: Legionella pneumophila, Moraxella catarrhalis, Bordetella pertussis; <u>other bacteria</u>: Mycoplasma pneumoniae)

■ **Mechanism** — Bactericidal; inhibits protein synthesis by binding to the P site of the 50S ribosomal subunit

■ **Dosage with Qualifiers** — <u>Bacterial infection</u>—500mg PO qd
- **Contraindications**—hypersensitivity to drug or class, bacteremia
- **Caution**—renal or hepatic dysfunction

■ **Maternal Considerations** — There is no published experience with **dirithromycin** during pregnancy. **Dirithromycin** is converted in the intestine to the microbiologically active **erythromycylamine**. Both **azithromycin** and **dirithromycin** have a low risk of drug interactions, but they are less well known. **Dirithromycin** is comparable in efficacy to **erythromycin** for the treatment of skin and soft tissue infections with significantly less nausea. Once a day dosing aids compliance.
Side effects include arrhythmias, pseudomembranous colitis, anorexia, anxiety, constipation, depression, dry mouth, dysmenorrhea, edema, epistaxis, fever, flu syndrome, gastritis, gastroenteritis, hemoptysis, hyperventilation, mouth ulceration, myalgia, nervousness, paraesthesia, peripheral edema, somnolence, sweating, syncope, palpitation, taste perversion, tinnitus, tremor, dehydration, urinary frequency, vaginal moniliasis, vaginitis, vasodilatation, and malaise.

■ **Fetal Considerations** — There are no adequate reports or well-controlled studies in human fetuses. It is unknown whether **dirithromycin** crosses the human placenta. Other macrolides cross the placenta. Rodent studies are reassuring, revealing no evidence of teratogenicity despite the use of doses higher than those used clinically. Very high doses were associated with IUGR.

■ **Breastfeeding Safety** — There is no published experience in nursing women. It is unknown whether **dirithromycin** enters human breast milk. It is excreted into rodent milk. Other macrolides are considered compatible with breastfeeding.

■ **References** — There is no published experience in pregnancy or during lactation.

■ **Summary**

- **Pregnancy Category C**
- **Lactation Category U**
- **Dirithromycin** should be used during pregnancy and lactation only if the benefit justifies the potential perinatal risk.
- There are alternative agents for which there is more experience during pregnancy and lactation.

Disopyramide (Norpace)

■ **Class** — Antiarrhythmics (class I A)

■ **Indications** — Ventricular arrhythmia

■ **Mechanism** — Stabilizes cell membrane by modifying the action potential in phase 0

■ **Dosage with Qualifiers** — Ventricular arrhythmia—load 300mg ×1, then 150mg PO q6h; adjust prn
- **Contraindications**—hypersensitivity to drug or class, cardiogenic shock, 2nd or 3rd AV block, CHF, prolongation of the Q-T interval, cardiomyopathy
- **Caution**—hypoglycemia, atrial tachyarrhythmias, renal or hepatic dysfunction

■ **Maternal Considerations** — There are no adequate reports or well-controlled studies of **disopyramide** in pregnant women. Pregnancy alters the percentage of free drug circulating in the plasma. Treatment of a cardiac arrhythmia during pregnancy with **disopyramide** is complicated by reported risks of hemorrhage or hypotension or contractions leading to fetal distress. Patients should be monitored intensively to avoid or detect complications. In point, **disopyramide** is superior to placebo for the induction of labor.
Side effects include CHF, arrhythmia, thrombocytopenia, hypotension, dizziness, blurred vision, nausea, vomiting, diarrhea, abdominal pain, dry mucous membranes, anxiety, urinary retention, pruritus, rash, and constipation.

■ **Fetal Considerations** — There are no adequate reports or well-controlled studies of **disopyramide** in human fetuses. It crosses the human placenta, achieving an F:M ratio approximating 0.26 for **disopyramide**, and 0.43 for its main metabolite, N-monodesalkyl disopyramide. Rodent studies are reassuring revealing no evidence of teratogenicity despite doses higher than those used clinically. The highest doses were associated with embryotoxicity and IUGR.

■ **Breastfeeding Safety** ⋯⋯⋯ There are no adequate reports or well-controlled studies in nursing women. Though **disopyramide** is concentrated in human breast milk over maternal plasma after oral administration, the unsupplemented newborn would ingest <2mg/kg. Not surprisingly, **disopyramide** is at or below the level of detection in the neonate.

■ **References** ⋯⋯⋯⋯⋯⋯

Abbi M, Kriplani A, Singh B. J Reprod Med 1999; 44:653-5.
Grand A. Ann Cardiol Angeiol 1992; 41:549-64.
Tadmor OP, Keren A, Rosenak D, et al. Am J Obstet Gynecol 1990; 162:482-6.
Hoppu K, Neuvonen PJ, Korte T. Br J Clin Pharmacol 1986; 21:553.
MacKintosh D, Buchanan N. Br J Clin Pharmacol 1985; 19:856-7.
Barnett DB, Hudson SA, McBurney A. Br J Clin Pharmacol 1982; 14:310-2.
Ellsworth AJ, Horn JR, Raisys VA, Miyagawa LA, Bell JL. DICP 1989; 23:56-7.

■ **Summary** ⋯⋯⋯⋯⋯

- **Pregnancy Category C**
- **Lactation Category S?**
- **Disopyramide** should be used during pregnancy and lactation only if the benefit justifies the potential perinatal risk.

Disulfiram (Antabuse; Antadict; Aversan; Disulfiram; Tetmosol)

■ **Class** ⋯⋯⋯⋯⋯⋯⋯ *Drug cessation*

■ **Indications** ⋯⋯⋯⋯⋯ Alcohol dependence

■ **Mechanism** ⋯⋯⋯⋯⋯ Inhibits acetaldehyde dehydrogenase

■ **Dosage with Qualifiers** ⋯⋯⋯ Alcohol dependence—begin 500mg PO qam ×1w; continue 500-125mg PO qam, tapering from high to low slowly
NOTE—must abstain from alcohol >12h before administration

- **Contraindications**—hypersensitivity to drug or class, alcohol use <12 h, metronidazole use, coronary artery disease, psychosis
- **Caution**—diabetes mellitus, seizures, hepatic or renal dysfunction

■ **Maternal Considerations** ⋯⋯ There are no adequate reports or well-controlled studies of **disulfiram** in pregnant women. **Disulfiram** is a deterrant to alcohol consumption in patients with a history of

alcohol abuse. Its use is increasingly more common in reproductive-age women. The safety of **disulfiram** during pregnancy is not established. The published literature consists mostly of case reports and small series.
Side effects include cardiovascular collapse, arrhythmia, seizure, coma, psychosis, optic neuritis, hepatitis, rash, drowsiness, fatigability, headache, allergic dermatitis, and a metallic or garlic-like taste.

■ **Fetal Considerations** ⋯⋯ There are no adequate reports or well-controlled studies in human fetuses. It is unknown whether **disulfiram** crosses the human placenta. There are several case reports of limb abnormalities in alcoholic women treated with **disulfiram** during pregnancy. In *vitro*, **disulfiram** is embryotoxic, affecting both DNA synthesis and morphological development.

■ **Breastfeeding Safety** ⋯⋯ There is no published experience in nursing women. It is unknown whether **disulfiram** enters human breast milk.

■ **References** ⋯⋯ Reitnauer PJ, Callanan NP, Farber RA, Aylsworth AS. Teratology 1997; 56:358-62.
Helmbrecht GD, Hoskins IA. Am J Perinatol 1993; 10:5-7.
Thompson PA, Folb PI. J Appl Toxicol 1985; 5:1-10.
Gardner RJ, Clarkson JE. N Z Med J 1981;93:184-6.
Nora AH, Nora JJ, Blu J. Lancet 1977; 2:664.

■ **Summary** ⋯⋯
- **Pregnancy Category C**
- **Lactation Category U**
- **Disulfiram** should be used during pregnancy and lactation only if the benefit justifies the potential perinatal risk.

Divalproex (Depakote)

■ **Class** ⋯⋯ Anticonvulsant, *migraine*

■ **Indications** ⋯⋯ Seizures, mania, migraine prophylaxis

■ **Mechanism** ⋯⋯ Acetaldehyde dehydrogenase inhibition

■ **Dosage with Qualifiers** ⋯⋯ Seizures—10-15mg/kg/d PO in 1-3 divided doses, increase by 5-10mg/kg/d every week; max 60mg/kg/d; therapeutic trough = 50-100mcg/ml
Mania—250mg tid PO, increase by 5-10mg/kg/d every 2-3 days; max 60mg/kg/d; therapeutic trough = 50-100mcg/ml
Migraine prophylaxis—250-500mg PO bid
NOTE—take with food

- **Contraindications**—hypersensitivity to drug or class, hepatic dysfunction or disease
- **Caution**—renal dysfunction, bone marrow suppression, bleeding tendencies, congenital metabolic disorders

■ **Maternal Considerations**

There are no adequate reports or well-controlled studies of **divalproex** in pregnant women. **Divalproex** is a stabilized form of **valproic acid**. It disassociates into **valproate** in the GI track. While the metabolism of **valproate** is unaltered by pregnancy, clearance is increased primarily because of decreased binding. It is suggested the drug be taken in multiple divided doses to avoid high peaks. (See **valproic acid.**)

Side effects include congenital neural tube defects, nausea, vomiting, diarrhea, abdominal pain, hepatotoxicity, pancreatitis, hyponatremia, SIADH, aplastic anemia, thrombocytopenia, pancytopenia, bleeding, hyperammonemia, psychosis, Stevens-Johnson syndrome, dyspepsia, alopecia, tremor, appetite changes, insomnia, peripheral edema, blurred vision, tinnitus, and respiratory disorders.

■ **Fetal Considerations**

There are no adequate reports or well-controlled studies in human fetuses. **Valproate** and its metabolites cross the placenta by perhaps a proton linked transport system, and is concentrated in fetal plasma at least in part because of increased protein binding. **Valproate** is a human teratogen. **Divalproex** exposure during the 1st trimester increases the risk of a fetal neural tube defect by about 10 times, or to a prevalence of 1-2%. This association likely reflects pharmacogenetics since preconception maternal folate supplementation does not necessarily reduce the risk of recurrence in subsequent pregnancies. Other associated malformations involve the cardiovascular system and the limbs. Its combination with other anticonvulsants increases the risks of malformation. As for most psychotropic drugs, using monotherapy and the lowest effective quantity given in divided doses to minimize the peaks can minimize the risks. (See **valproic acid.**)

■ **Breastfeeding Safety**

There are no adequate reports or well-controlled studies in nursing women. Only small amounts of valproate (1-10%) enter human breast milk, and its serum concentration in breast-fed neonates is subclinical. (See **valproic acid.**)

■ **References**

Nakamura H, Ushigome F, Koyabu N, et al. Pharm Res 2002; 19:154-61.
Duncan S, Mercho L, Lopes-Cendes I, et al. Epilepsia 2001; 42:750-3.
Philbert A, Pedersen B, Dam M. Acta Neurol Scand 1985; 72:460-3.
von Unruh GE, Froescher W, Hoffmann F, Niesen M. Ther Drug Monit 1984; 6:272-6.

■ **Summary**
- **Pregnancy Category D**
- **Lactation Category S**
- **Divalproex** should be used during pregnancy only if the benefit justifies the potential perinatal risk.
- As for most psychotropic drugs, using monotherapy and the lowest effective quantity given in divided doses to minimize the peaks can minimize the risks.
- There are alternatives for migraine prophylaxis during pregnancy.
- Exposed women should undergo a targeted ultrasound examination to search for fetal neural tube defects.

Dobutamine (Dobutrex)

■ **Class**

Adrenergic agonist; inotrope, hypotension, shock

■ **Indications**

Cardiac decompensation

■ **Mechanism**

Stimulates β-1 adrenergic receptors

■ **Dosage with Qualifiers**

Cardiac decompensation—2-10mcg/kg/min IV; max 40mcg/kg/min
- **Contraindications**—hypersensitivity to drug or class, idiopathic hypertrophic subaortic stenosis, hypertension
- **Caution**—history of recent MI, arrhythmia or sulfite allergy

■ **Maternal Considerations**

There are no adequate reports or well-controlled studies of **dobutamine** in pregnant women. **Dobutamine** is a direct acting β-adrenergic ionotropic agent producing a pressor effect with less chronotropy than the β-adrenergic agents, plus some degree of vasodilation (e.g., pulmonary vascular resisitance) but no dopaminergic renal effects. **Dobutamine** is recommended for ionotropic support of women with cardiac decompensation during pregnancy. It is used to improve ventricular function in women with idiopathic dilated cardiomyopathy. **Dobutamine** can also induce a modest but unsustained increase in cardiac output in patients with idiopathic pulmonary hypertension. The diagnosis of peripartal cardiomyopathy is limited to women with CHF and decreased LV systolic function during the last month of pregnancy or within 5mo of delivery. Women whose ventricular function is normal at rest and exercise may have their **dobutamine** tapered and ultimately discontinued after 6-12mo. The **dobutamine** challenge test is used to assess ventricular function in women with a history of peripartal cardiomyopathy who have regained normal resting LV size and performance. **Digoxin** is recommended prior to **dobutamine** when treatment is necessary for atrial fibrillation.

Side effects include tachycardia, arrhythmia, phlebitis, hypotension, nausea, vomiting, headache, angina, palpitations, shortness of breath, hypertension, myocardial ischemia, and ventricular fibrillation.

■ **Fetal Considerations** .... There are no adequate reports or well-controlled studies in human fetuses. **Dobutamine** crosses the human placenta, though the kinetics remain to be elucidated. **Dobutamine** has been used in twin twin transfusion syndrome with possible benefit. Rodent studies are reassuring revealing no evidence of teratogenicity or IUGR despite the use of doses higher than those used clinically.

■ **Breastfeeding Safety** .... There is no published experience in nursing women. It is unknown whether **dobutamine** enters human breast milk.

■ **References** .... Fishburne JI, Meis PJ, Urban RB, et al. Am J Obstet Gynecol 1980; 137:944-52.
Baughman KL. Curr Treat Options Cardiovasc Med 2001; 3:469-480.
Mareschal-Desandes R, Hascoet JM, Bosser G, et al. Arch Pediatr 2002; 9:377-81.
Hibbard JU, Lindheimer M, Lang RM. Obstet Gynecol 1999; 94:311-6.
Lampert MB, Weinert L, Hibbard J, Korcarz C, Lindheimer M, Lang RM. Am J Obstet Gynecol 1997; 176:189-95.
Brown G, O'Leary M, Douglas I, Herkes R. Anaesth Intensive Care 1992; 20:80-3.

■ **Summary** .... • **Pregnancy Category B**
• **Lactation Category U**
• **Dobutamine** should be used during pregnancy and lactation only if the benefit justifies the potential perinatal risk.

Docetaxel (Taxotere)

■ **Class** .... *Antineoplastic; antimitotic*

■ **Indications** .... Breast cancer, lung cancer, gestational choriocarcinoma

■ **Mechanism** .... Mitotic inhibitor

■ **Dosage with Qualifiers** ...... <u>Cancer</u>—dose varies per protocol; most regimens recommend 60-100mg/m^2

- **Contraindications**—hypersensitivity to drug or class, agranulocytosis
- **Caution**—renal or hepatic dysfunction

■ **Maternal Considerations** ······ There are no adequate reports or well-controlled studies of **docetaxel** in pregnant women. There is one case report of its use during pregnancy.
Side effects include thrombocytopenia, leukopenia, anemia, agranulocytosis, myelosuppression, skin rash, edema, stomatitis.

■ **Fetal Considerations** ·············· There are no adequate reports or well-controlled studies in human fetuses. It is unknown whether **docetaxel** crosses the human placenta. While there is no evidence of teratogenicity, rodent studies reveal clear evidence of both embryo and fetal toxicity at doses far below those used in humans.

■ **Breastfeeding Safety** ··········· There is no published experience in nursing women. It is unknown whether **docetaxel** enters human breast milk. However, it is generally considered incompatible with breastfeeding in light of its pharmacologic mechanism.

■ **References** ····························· De Santis M, Lucchese A, De Carolis S, Ferrazani S, Caruso A. Eur J Cancer Care 2000; 9:235-7.
Winquist E, Carey M. Gynecol Oncol 2000; 79:523-4.

■ **Summary** ······························
- **Pregnancy Category D**
- **Lactation Category NS**
- **Docetaxel** should be used during pregnancy and lactation only if the benefit justifies the potential perinatal risk.
- Alternative agents should be sought for which there is more experience during pregnancy and lactation.

Docusate calcium, sodium, potassium
(Colace; Ediclone; Kasof; Laxagel; Prenate-90; Rapilax; Regulax; Surfak; Wasserlax)

■ **Class** ···························· Laxative

■ **Indications** ····················· Constipation

■ **Mechanism** ···················· Retains moisture and fat within the large bowel

■ **Dosage with Qualifiers** ········· Constipation—100mg PO qd, bid
NOTE—may be packaged with **casanthranol**

- **Contraindications**—hypersensitivity to drug or class, fecal impaction, mineral oil use, acute abdomen, colitis, GI obstruction
- **Caution**—nausea, vomiting

■ **Maternal Considerations** .... While there are no adequate reports or well-controlled studies of **docusate** in pregnant women, there is a long clinical experience with virtually no reported complications. **Docusate** is frequently used postpartum to avoid constipation in women who have had a repaired episiotomy. It may rarely potentiate the hepatotoxicity of other drugs.
Side effects include bitter taste, nausea, rash, diarrhea, throat irritation, and intestinal obstruction.

■ **Fetal Considerations** .... **Docusate** is not absorbed systemically and thus does not cross the placenta. A three generational rodent study failed to identify any adverse effects on reproduction. There are reports of neonatal hypomagnesemia after maternal abuse of stool softeners.

■ **Breastfeeding Safety** .... There are no adequate reports or well-controlled studies in nursing women. **Docusate** is not absorbed systemically and thus will not enter human breast milk.

■ **References** .... Gattuso JM, Kamm MA. Drug Saf 1994; 10:47-65.
Schindler AM. Lancet 1984; 2:822.
MacKenzie K, Henwood S, Foster G, et al. Fundam Appl Toxicol 1990; 15:53-62.

■ **Summary** ....
- **Pregnancy Category C**
- **Lactation Category S**
- Most laxatives are relatively safe if used intermittently in the absence of contraindications.

Dofetilide (Tikosyn)

■ **Class** .... *Antiarrhythmic, class* III

■ **Indications** .... Atrial flutter/fibrillation

■ **Mechanism** .... Prolongs the phase 3 action potential

■ **Dosage with Qualifiers** .... Atrial flutter/fibrillation—500mcg PO q12h; adjust dose based on QTc and creatinine clearance
NOTE—renal dosing; restricted access in the U.S.
- **Contraindications**—hypersensitivity to drug or class, QT prolongation (>440-500msec), renal failure, hypokalemia

- **Caution**—bradycardia, electrolyte abnormalities, renal dysfunction, CYP 3A4 inhibitors

■ **Maternal Considerations** ········ There is no published experience with **dofetilide** during pregnancy.
Side effects include ventricular arrhythmias, QT interval prolongation, chest pain, dizziness, headache, nausea, dyspepsia, diarrhea, flu-like symptoms, and rash.

■ **Fetal Considerations** ············ There are no adequate reports or well-controlled studies in human fetuses. It is unknown whether **dofetilide** crosses the human placenta. Rodent studies reveal that **dofetilide** produces a spectrum of defects similar to **phenytoin** including cardiac, digital and oral facial clefting malformations possibly by blocking potassium channels.

■ **Breastfeeding Safety** ············ There is no published experience in nursing women. It is unknown whether **dofetilide** enters human breast milk.

■ **References** ························ Danielsson BR, Skold AC, Azarbayjani F. Curr Pharm Des 2001; 7:787-802.

■ **Summary** ·························
- **Pregnancy Category C**
- **Lactation Category U**
- **Dofetilide** should be used during pregnancy and lactation only if the benefit justifies the potential perinatal risk.
- There are alternative agents for which there is more experience during pregnancy and lactation.

Dolasetron mesylate (Anzemet)

■ **Class** ···························· *Nausea/vomiting*

■ **Indications** ····················· Severe nausea or vomiting secondary to either chemotherapy or anesthesia

■ **Mechanism** ······················ Selective 5-HT3 receptor antagonist

■ **Dosage with Qualifiers** ········· Nausea and vomiting, post-op—typically 12.5mg IV ×1 15min before surgery ends
Nausea and vomiting, chemotherapy—100mg PO ×1 1h pre-chemo, or 1.8mg/kg IV ×1 15min pre-chemo
- **Contraindications**—hypersensitivity to drug or class
- **Caution**—hypomagnesemia, prolonged QT

■ **Maternal Considerations** ········ There is no published experience with **dolasetron** during pregnancy.

Side effects include arrhythmia, headache, diarrhea, abdominal pain, fever, fatigue, dizziness, increased LFTs, leukopenia, hypertension, pain, drowsiness, and urinary retention.

■ **Fetal Considerations** ········· There are no adequate reports or well-controlled studies in human fetuses. It is unknown whether **dolasetron** crosses the placenta. Rodent studies are reassuring revealing no evidence of teratogenicity or IUGR despite the use of doses higher than those used clinically.

■ **Breastfeeding Safety** ········· There is no published experience in nursing women. It is unknown whether **dolasetron** enters human breast milk.

■ **References** ········· There is no published experience in pregnancy or during lactation.

■ **Summary** ·········
- **Pregnancy Category B**
- **Lactation Category U**
- **Dolasetron** should be used during pregnancy and lactation only if the benefit justifies the potential perinatal risk.
- There are many alternative agents for which there is more experience during pregnancy and lactation.

Dopamine (Intropin)

■ **Class** ········· *Inotrope, adrenergic agonist*

■ **Indications** ········· Shock, refractory CHF

■ **Mechanism** ········· Stimulates α and β-1 adrenergic and dopaminergic receptors

■ **Dosage with Qualifiers** ········· <u>Adjunct for shock</u>—1-50mcg/kg/min IV; max 20-50μg/kg/min
2-5mcg/kg/m primarily dopaminergic receptor effects, but may exhibit a pressor effect
5-10mcg/kg/m primarily β-adrenergic effects with inotropy and chronotropy
>10mcg/kg/m primarily α-adrenergic effects with peripheral vasoconstriction
<u>Refractory CHF</u>—1-3μg/kg/min IV
- **Contraindications**—hypersensitivity to drug, class or sulfites, ventricular fibrillation, pheochromocytoma
- **Caution**—diabetes mellitus, occlusive vascular diseases, Raynaud's syndrome, usage of MAO inhibitors

■ **Maternal Considerations** ⋯⋯⋯ There are no adequate reports or well-controlled studies of **dopamine** in pregnant women. **Dopamine** is a natural catecholamine that produces both positive chronotropiuc and ionotropic effects. Several investigators have applied its vasodilating properties to the treatment of preeclamptic hypertension. A low dose infusion of **dopamine** aids the management of acute renal failure caused by preeclampsia. A treatment program of IV fluids, **furosemide** and/or **dopamine** has been suggested for preeclamptic women with anuria (output <100ml/24h). If unsuccessful, early dialysis should be considered. The evidence for the use of prophylactic medical interventions, such as the use of loop diuretics, **mannitol** and low-dose **dopamine** is poor. Studies in monkeys report both increase and decrease in the uterine blood flow depending on dose.
Side effects include anaphylaxis, asthma, gangrene, hypotension, tachycardia, ventricular arrhythmia, ectopic beats, angina, palpitation, widened QRS complex, bradycardia, hypertension, vasoconstriction, dyspnea, azotemia, headache, anxiety, and pilo-erection.

■ **Fetal Considerations** ⋯⋯⋯ There are no adequate reports or well-controlled studies in human fetuses. There are specific **dopamine** receptors on the human placenta. Rodent studies are reassuring, revealing no evidence of teratogenicity or IUGR despite the use of doses higher than those used clinically. Maternal toxicity occurred and was associated with decreased neonatal survival.

■ **Breastfeeding Safety** ⋯⋯⋯ There is no published experience in nursing women. It is unknown whether **dopamine** enters human breast milk.

■ **References** ⋯⋯⋯ Keiseb J, Moodley J, Connolly CA. Hypertens Pregnancy 2002; 21:225-34.
Brown G, O'Leary M, Douglas I, Herkes R. Anaesth Intensive Care 1992; 20:80-3.
Mantel GD. Best Pract Res Clin Obstet Gynaecol 2001; 15:563-81.
Martinez de Ita AL, Garcia Caceres E, Helguera Martinez AM, Cejudo Carranza E. Ginecol Obstet Mex 1998; 66:462-8.
Nasu K, Yoshimatsu J, Anai T, Miyakawa I. Gynecol Obstet Invest 1996; 42:140-1.

■ **Summary** ⋯⋯⋯ • **Pregnancy Category C**
• **Lactation Category NS**
• **Dopamine** should be used during pregnancy and lactation only if the benefit justifies the potential perinatal risk.

Doxazosin (Cardura)

- **Class** — Antihypertensive; antiadrenergic

- **Indications** — Hypertension

- **Mechanism** — Selective antagonist of peripheral α-1 adrenergic receptors

- **Dosage with Qualifiers** — Hypertension—1mg PO qd, increase slowly (dose range 1-8mg qd); max 16mg qd
  - **Contraindications**—hypersensitivity to drug or class
  - **Caution**—hepatic or renal dysfunction

- **Maternal Considerations** — There are no adequate reports or well-controlled studies of **doxazosin** in pregnant women. It is similar to **atenolol**. *Side effects* include arrhythmias, headache, nausea, vomiting, somnolence, edema, dyspnea, asthenia, diarrhea, angina, fatigue, hypotension, back pain, flu-like syndrome, diarrhea, dry mouth, blurred vision, and dyspepsia.

- **Fetal Considerations** — There are no adequate reports or well-controlled studies in human fetuses. It is unknown whether **doxazosin** crosses the human placenta. Rodent studies are reassuring, revealing no evidence of teratogenicity or IUGR despite the use of doses higher than those used clinically.

- **Breastfeeding Safety** — There are no adequate reports or well-controlled studies in nursing women. It is unknown whether **doxazosin** enters human breast milk. It is concentrated in rodent milk. Similar agents are generally considered compatible with breastfeeding.

- **References** — There is no published experience in pregnancy or during lactation.

- **Summary** —
  - **Pregnancy Category B**
  - **Lactation Category U**
  - There are many alternatives for which there is greater experience during pregnancy and lactation.

Doxepin (Sinequan; Zonalon)

■ **Class**	*Antidepressant, tricyclic*
■ **Indications**	Depression, anxiety, pruritus (topical)
■ **Mechanism**	Exact mechanism unknown, but does inhibit norepinephrine and serotonin reuptake
■ **Dosage with Qualifiers**	<u>Depression</u>—begin 25-75mg PO qhs (alternatively 50mg PO tid), increase gradually based on response; max 300mg qd <u>Anxiety</u>—begin 25-75mg PO qhs (alternatively 25mg PO tid), increase gradually based on response; max 300mg qd <u>Pruritus</u>—apply cream qid to affected area (5%C); systemic absorption significant with widespread application • **Contraindications**—hypersensitivity to drug or class, glaucoma, urinary retention • **Caution**—advanced age
■ **Maternal Considerations**	There are no adequate reports or well-controlled studies of **doxepin** in pregnant women. ***Side effects*** include dry mouth, blurred vision, constipation, urinary retention, drowsiness, extrapyramidal symptoms, confusion, disorientation, hallucinations, numbness, paresthesias, ataxia, seizures, eosinophilia, leukopenia, thrombocytopenia, purpura, lowered libido, testicular swelling, gynecomastia, rash, and anorexia.
■ **Fetal Considerations**	There are no adequate reports or well-controlled studies in human fetuses. It is unknown whether **doxepin** crosses the human placenta.
■ **Breastfeeding Safety**	There are no adequate reports or well-controlled studies in nursing women. While only small amounts of **doxepin** and its active metabolite enter breast milk, one report described apnea and drowsiness though the neonatal plasma **doxepin** was just into the detectable range. Caution is suggested.
■ **References**	Frey OR, Scheidt P, von Brenndorff AI. Ann Pharmacother 1999; 33:690-3. Wisner KL, Perel JM, Findling RL. Am J Psychiatry 1996; 153:1132-7.
■ **Summary**	• **Pregnancy Category C** • **Lactation Category NS?** • **Doxepin** should be used during pregnancy and lactation only if the benefit justifies the potential perinatal risk. • There are other agents available for which there is greater experience during pregnancy and lactation.

Doxorubicin (Adriamycin)

- **Class** — Antineoplastic

- **Indications** — Cancer (bladder, breast, bronchogenic, gastric, ovary, thyroid, leukemia, lymphoma, Hodgkin's lymphoma, bone, Wilms' tumor, neuroblastoma, bone)

- **Mechanism** — Interferes with DNA synthesis by binding to it

- **Dosage with Qualifiers** — Cancer—dose varies per protocol; most regimens recommend 60-75mg/m^2 IV q3w
  NOTE—hepatic and renal dosing; use of a cardioprotectant agent (**dexrazoxane**) during treatment recommended. **Doxorubicin** should not be administered IM since severe local tissue necrosis might occur.
  - **Contraindications**—hypersensitivity to drug or class, hyperbilirubinemia, cardiomyopathy, CHF, myelosuppression, previous treatment with complete courses of **doxorubicin, idarubicin, daunorubicin**
  - **Caution**—hepatic dysfunction, concomitant radiation therapy

- **Maternal Considerations** — There are no adequate reports or well-controlled studies of **doxorubicin** in pregnant women. Irreversible myocardial toxicity may occur during or months after therapy. **ACE inhibitors** and **dexrazoxane** offer cardioprotection. Women diagnosed during pregnancy with breast cancer are frequently treated during the 1st trimester of pregnancy with a complex regimen including **fluorouracil, doxorubicin**, and **cyclophosphamide**. *Side effects* include include potentiation of **cyclophosphamide** toxicity, arrhythmia, pericarditis, alopecia, hyperpigmentation, nausea, vomiting, stomatitis, cellulites, tissue necrosis, acute myeloid leukemia, fever, chills and urticaria, and neurotoxicity.

- **Fetal Considerations** — Though there are no adequate reports or well-controlled studies in human fetuses. There are numerous uncontrolled series and case reports whose interpretations are complicated by the fact that **doxorubicin** is often given with other agents. There is no firm evidence of teratogenicity or perinatal myocardial dysfunction in fetuses of women treated with **doxorubicin**. Women treated during the 2nd and 3rd trimesters of pregnancy experience little increase in the rate of complication during labor and delivery. There is essentially no long-term follow-up of exposed fetuses. **Doxorubicin** is associated with a series of anomalies in rats similar to VATER-esophageal atresia, tracheo-esophageal fistula, and cloacal and urogenital anomalies.

- **Breastfeeding Safety** — There are no adequate reports or well-controlled studies in nursing women. **Doxorubicin** is concentrated in human breast milk achieving maximum M:P ratios approximating 4.4. However, the maximum concentration of active drug approximates 0.24mg/L. Thus, the amount ingested by the breast-feeding neonate would be insignificant.

■ **References**

Merei JM. Pediatr Surg Int 2002; 18:36-9.
Merei JM, Hasthorpe S, Hutson JM. Eur J Pediatr Surg 2002; 12:3-7.
Gwyn KM, Theriault RL. Curr Treat Options Oncol 2000; 1:239-43.
Meyer-Wittkopf M, Barth H, Emons G, Schmidt S. Ultrasound Obstet Gynecol 2001; 18:62-6.
Menegola E, Broccia ML, Renzo FD. Teratog Carcinog Mutagen 2001; 21:283-93.
Liu MI, Hutson JM. BJU Int 2000; 86:107-12.
Berry DL, Theriault RL, Holmes FA, et al. J Clin Oncol 1999; 17:855-61.
d'Incalci M, Broggini M, Buscaglia M, Pardi G. Lancet 1983; 1:75.
Egan PC, Costanza ME, Dodion P, Egtorin MJ, Bachur NR. Cancer Treat Rep 1985; 69:1387-9.

■ **Summary**

- **Pregnancy Category D**
- **Lactation Category S?**
- **Doxorubicin** should be used during pregnancy and lactation only if the benefit justifies the potential perinatal risk.
- Successful pregnancies are the norm despite chemotherapy.

Doxycycline (Doxy; Doxy-100; Doxychel; Doxycycline Hyclate; Monodox; Vibramycin; Vibra-Tabs)

■ **Class**

Antibiotic, tetracycline

■ **Indications**

Gonorrhea, *chlamydia*, PID, malaria, Lyme disease, anthrax

■ **Mechanism**

Bacteriostatic; inhibits protein synthesis

■ **Dosage with Qualifiers**

Gonorrhea, uncomplicated—100mg PO bid ×7d; for complicated use in combination with another agent such as **ceftriaxone**, **cefixime**, or **ciprofloxacin** (if not pregnant or breastfeeding)
Chlamydia —100mg PO bid ×7d
PID—100mg PO bid ×10-14d with another agent such as **ceftriaxone** 250mg IM

<u>Malaria</u>—100mg PO qd beginning 1-2d before departure and continuing through 4w after exposure
<u>Lyme disease</u>—100mg PO bid ×14-21d (28d if associated with arthritis)
<u>Anthrax</u>—100mg IV, PO q12h; postexposure, 100mg PO q12h for 60d or until disease excluded
NOTE—**doxycycline** is the 1st choice for pregnant women infected with anthrax
- **Contraindications**—hypersensitivity to drug or class, pregnancy; see **tetracycline**
- **Caution**—hepatic or renal dysfunction; see **tetracycline**

■ **Maternal Considerations** ⋯⋯ **Doxycycline** is synthetically derived from oxytetracycline. See **tetracycline**.
Side effects include neutropenia, thrombocytopenia, hepato-toxicity, pseudo-membranous colitis, anorexia, epigastric distress, nausea, vomiting, diarrhea, stomatitis, glossitis, black hairy tongue, dysphagia, hoarseness, renal toxicity, dizziness, headache, and teeth discoloration; see **tetracycline**.

■ **Fetal Considerations** ⋯⋯ Use of **tetracycline** class during tooth development (3rd trimester, infancy and in children <8y) may cause permanent discoloration of the teeth. See **tetracycline**.

■ **Breastfeeding Safety** ⋯⋯ See **tetracycline**.

■ **References** ⋯⋯ See **tetracycline**.

■ **Summary** ⋯⋯
- **Pregnancy Category D**
- **Lactation Category NS**
- See **tetracycline**.

Dronabinol (Marinol)

■ **Class** ⋯⋯ Antiemetic

■ **Indications** ⋯⋯ Nausea and vomiting associated with chemotherapy, AIDS-related anorexia

■ **Mechanism** ⋯⋯ Activates cannabinoid receptors

■ **Dosage with Qualifiers** ⋯⋯ <u>Nausea/vomiting (chemo)</u>—5mg/m^2 PO ×1 1-3h before first dose of chemotherapy; max 4-6×/d
<u>Anorexia (AIDS)</u>—2.5mg PO bid; max 20mg qd
- **Contraindications**—hypersensitivity to drug or class
- **Caution**—schizophrenia

■ **Maternal Considerations** — There are no adequate reports or well-controlled studies of **dronabinol** in pregnant women. Several publications suggest a relationship between cannabis use and head and neck cancers in a dose-response manner for frequency and duration of use. Interaction was observed with cigarette smoking and alcohol use.

Side effects include anxiety, euphoria, dizziness, dry mouth, mood disturbances, ataxia, paranoia, orthostatic hypotension, tachycardia, hallucinations, palpitations, tachycardia, facial flush, and conjunctivitis.

■ **Fetal Considerations** — There are no adequate reports or well-controlled studies in human fetuses. It is unknown whether **dronabinol** crosses the human placenta. Rodent studies are reassuring revealing no evidence of teratogenicity or IUGR despite the use of doses higher than those used clinically.

■ **Breastfeeding Safety** — There is no published experience in nursing women. It is unknown whether **dronabinol** enters human breast milk. Breastfeeding is contraindicated in HIV-infected nursing women where formula is available to reduce the risk of neonatal transmission.

■ **References** — Carriot F, Sasco AJ. Rev Epidemiol Sante Publique 2000; 48:473-83.
Lee MJ. Obstet Gynecol Clin North Am 1998; 25:65-83.
Reiter GS. AIDS Clin Care 1996; 8:89-91, 93, 96.
Doyle E, Spence AA. Br J Anaesth 1995; 74:359-61.

■ **Summary** —
- **Pregnancy Category B**
- **Lactation Category NS**
- **Dronabinol** should be used during pregnancy and lactation only if the benefit justifies the potential perinatal risk.
- There are alternative agents for which there is more experience during pregnancy and lactation.

Droperidol (Inapsine)

■ **Class** — Antiemetic; antivertigo; anxiolytic; sedative

■ **Indications** — Perioperative nausea and vomiting

■ **Mechanism** — Unknown; antagonizes dopamine and α-adrenergic receptors

■ **Dosage with Qualifiers** — Nausea and vomiting (perioperative)—0.625-1.25mg IM/IV q3-4h prn
- **Contraindications**—hypersensitivity to drug or class, prolonged QT interval

295

- **Caution**—history of reaction to other drugs causing tardive dyskinesia, hypotension, CNS depression, CHF, bradycardia, diuretics, hypokalemia, hypomagnesemia, hepatic or renal dysfunction, and alcohol abuse

■ **Maternal Considerations**

There are no adequate reports or well-controlled studies of **droperidol** in pregnant women. It has been used in emergency rooms for the acute management of migraine headache with success similar to **meperidine**. **Droperidol** reduces nausea and vomiting after epidural **morphine** similar in efficacy to **dexamethasone**. The addition of **metoclopramide** appears to enhance its efficacy. In one study, it was inferior to **granisetron** after cesarean section. There is a black box warning currently issued by the FDA based on reports of prolonged QT associated dysrhythmia. The dozens of cases reported to the FDA were in fact multiple reports of 3 cases.
Side effects include tardive dyskinesia (treat with **diphenhydramine** or **cogentin**), arrhythmia, hypotension, prolonged QT interval, bronchospasm, laryngospasm, delirium, drowsiness, chills, anxiety, nightmares, fever, and hypertension.

■ **Fetal Considerations**

There are no adequate reports or well-controlled studies in human fetuses. It is unknown whether **droperidol** crosses the human placenta. Rodent studies are reassuring, revealing no evidence of teratogenicity or IUGR despite the use of doses higher than those used clinically. Neonatal mortality was increased perhaps because of maternal neglect.

■ **Breastfeeding Safety**

There is no published experience in nursing women. It is unknown whether **droperidol** enters human breast milk. However, considering the indications, its short-term use is unlikely to pose a significant risk to the breast-feeding neonate.

■ **References**

Richman PB, Allegra J, Eskin B, et al. Am J Emerg Med 2002; 20:39-42.
Tzeng JI, Wang JJ, Ho ST, Tang CS, Liu YC, Lee SC. Br J Anaesth 2000; 85:865-8.
Fujii Y, Tanaka H, Toyooka H. Acta Anaesthesiol Scand 1998; 42:921-5.
Bailey P, Norton R, Karan S. Anesthesiology 2002; 97:288-9.
Gan TJ, White PF, Scuderi PE, Watcha MF, Kovac A. Anesthesiology 2002; 97:287.

■ **Summary**

- **Pregnancy Category C**
- **Lactation Category S**
- **Droperidol** should be used during pregnancy and lactation only if the benefit justifies the potential perinatal risk.
- **Droperidol** has long been a cheap and effective antiemetic used for prophylaxis at cesarean section, though rescue therapy may not be as effective as the 5HT3 blockers like **odansetron** or **granisetron**.

Econazole nitrate (Spectazole)

- **Class** — Antifungal; *topical, dermatologic*

- **Indications** — Tinea and cutaneous candidiasis

- **Mechanism** — Unknown

- **Dosage with Qualifiers** — Tinea—apply cream to affected area qd
  Cutaneous candidiasis—apply cream to affected area bid
  - **Contraindications**—hypersensitivity
  - **Cautions**—unknown

- **Maternal Considerations** — **Econazole** has been used for the treatment of *Candida* vaginitis with success somewhat inferior to **clotrimazole**. Systemic absorption of **econazole** is extremely low. There is no published experience with **econazole** during pregnancy. However, it was effective *in vitro* using samples obtained from pregnant women. **Econazole** prolongs pregnancy in rats when given orally.
  Side effects include burning, itching, redness, and rash.

- **Fetal Considerations** — There are no adequate reports or well-controlled studies in human fetuses. It is unknown whether **econazole** crosses the human placenta. Considering the dose and route, it is unlikely the maternal systemic concentration will reach clinically relevant level. Rodent studies are reassuring, revealing no evidence of teratogenicity or IUGR despite the use of doses higher than those used clinically. Embryotoxic effects were noted in rodents after oral administration of 10-40 times the human dose.

- **Breastfeeding Safety** — There is no published experience in nursing women. It is unknown whether **econazole** enters human breast milk. It is present in rodent breast milk after high oral doses. Considering the indication, dosing, and route, it seems unlikely to pose a clinically significant risk to the breast-feeding neonate.

- **References** — Guaschino S, Michelone G, Stola E, et al. Biol Res Pregnancy Perinatol 1986; 7:20-2.

- **Summary** —
  - **Pregnancy Category C**
  - **Lactation Category S?**
  - There are other antifungal agents with higher clinical efficacy and more experience during pregnancy.

Edrophonium (Enlon; Reversol; Tensilon)

■ **Class** .... *Miscellaneous; cholinesterase inhibitor*

■ **Indications** .... Diagnosis of myasthenia gravis, anesthesia adjunct

■ **Mechanism** .... Cholinesterase inhibitor

■ **Dosage with Qualifiers** .... Myasthenia gravis, diagnosis—2mg IV over 15-30sec; if no response after 1min, repeat with 8mg. If a reaction, halt infusion and administer atropine 0.5mg IV
Anesthesia, adjunct—reversal of non-depolarizing neuromuscular blockade, 500mcg/kg IV given 1min after atropine 0.02mg/kg IV push
  • **Contraindications**—hypersensitivity, intestinal obstruction
  • **Caution**—asthma, arrhythmia

■ **Maternal Considerations** .... **Edrophonium** is a short- and rapid-acting cholinergic drug. There are no adequate reports or well-controlled studies of **edrophonium** in pregnant women. While there is no supporting literature in the last 30 years, older literature suggests anticholinesterases may trigger preterm labor. *Side effects* include severe cholinergic reaction, arrhythmias, respiratory paralysis, diplopia, tearing, seizures, dysphagia, dysarthria, dysphonia, hypotension, diarrhea, and abdominal pain.

■ **Fetal Considerations** .... There are no adequate reports or well-controlled studies in human fetuses. It is unknown whether **edrophonium** crosses the human placenta. Chemical structure suggests it will not cross the placenta. There are no reports of either fetal toxicity or teratogenicity. Rodent teratogenicity studies have apparently not been performed.

■ **Breastfeeding Safety** .... There is no published experience in nursing women. It is unknown whether **edrophonium** enters human breast milk. The chemical structure suggests it will not be excreted into the breast milk. Considering the indication, one-time **edrophonium** use is unlikely to pose a clinically significant risk to the breast-feeding neonate.

■ **References** .... Drachman DB. N Engl J Med 1978; 298:186-93.

■ **Summary** ....
  • **Pregnancy Category C**
  • **Lactation Category S**
  • **Edrophonium** should be used during pregnancy and lactation only if the benefit justifies the potential perinatal risk.

Efavirenz (Sustiva)

■ **Class** — Antiviral

■ **Indications** — HIV infection

■ **Mechanism** — Non-nucleoside reverse transcriptase inhibitor

■ **Dosage with Qualifiers** — HIV infection—600mg PO qd
- **Contraindications**—hypersensitivity
- **Caution**—hepatic dysfunction, **cisapride** use, **triazolam** use, **midazolam** use, **astemizole** use

■ **Maternal Considerations** — There are no adequate reports or well-controlled studies of **efavirenz** in pregnant women. Hepatotoxicity may be more common during pregnancy. Perhaps the most relevant consideration when initiating a pregnant woman on a non-nucleoside reverse transcriptase inhibitor is whether normally tolerated side effects will be magnified by pregnancy.
Side effects include Stevens-Johnson syndrome, dermatitis, erythema multiforme, rash, drowsiness, insomnia, abnormal dreams, hyperlipidemia, diarrhea, nausea, vomiting, fever, and hepatic dysfunction.

■ **Fetal Considerations** — There are no adequate reports or well-controlled studies in human fetuses. **Efavirenz** crosses the placenta achieving an F:M ratio approximating unity. Its use has been associated with CNS malformations in monkey fetuses at doses that approximate the human, and with neural tube defects in exposed human fetuses. Rodent studies reveal an increased frequency of reabsorbtions.

■ **Breastfeeding Safety** — There is no published experience in nursing women. It is unknown whether **efavirenz** enters human breast milk. Breastfeeding is contraindicated in HIV-infected women where formula is available to reduce the risk of neonatal transmission. **Efavirenz** is excreted in the breast milk of rats.

■ **References** — Hill JB, Sheffield JS, Zeeman GG, Wendel GD Jr. Obstet Gynecol 2001; 98:909-11.
Taylor GP, Low-Beer N. Drug Saf 2001; 24:683-702.
De Santis M, Carducci B, De Santis L, Cavaliere AF, Straface G. Arch Intern Med 2002; 162:355.
Fundaro C, Genovese O, Rendeli C, Tamburrini E, Salvaggio E. AIDS 2002; 16:299-300.

■ **Summary**
- **Pregnancy Category C**
- **Lactation Category NS**
- The goal of HIV treatment during pregnancy is achievement and maintenance of a zero viral load.

- The early experience with **efavirenz** during pregnancy is concerning; it is likely a human teratogen.
- **Efavirenz** should be used during pregnancy and lactation only if the benefit justifies the potential perinatal risk.
- There are alternative agents for which there is more experience during pregnancy and lactation.
- Physicians are encouraged to register pregnant women under the Antiretroviral Pregnancy Registry (1-800-258-4263) for a better follow-up of the outcome while under treatment with **efavirenz**.

Enalapril (Vasotec)

■ **Class** — ACE-I, A2R-*antagonist*

■ **Indications** — Hypertension, CHF, myocardial infarction, nephropathy

■ **Mechanism** — Angiotensin-converting enzyme inhibitor

■ **Dosage with Qualifiers** — Hypertension—begin 5mg PO qd (max 40mg qd); alternatively 0.625-1.25mg IV, then up to 5mg IV q6h
CHF—begin 2.5mg PO qd (max 40mg qd)
MI—begin 2.5mg PO qd (max 40mg qd), quickly titrate dose up
Nephropathy—5-20mg PO qd
NOTE—also combined with either **hydrochlorothiazide** or **felodipine**
- **Contraindications**—hypersensitivity, renal artery stenosis
- **Caution**—renal dysfunction, hypovolemia, severe CHF, collagen vascular disease

■ **Maternal Considerations** — There are no adequate reports or well-controlled studies of **enalapril** in pregnant women. It is generally well tolerated and pregnancy does not alter dosing.
Side effects include angioedema, hypotension, renal failure, hyperkalemia, hepatotoxicity, neutropenia, pancreatitis, dizziness, nausea, vomiting, fatigue, dyspepsia, rash, urticaria, and myalgia.

■ **Fetal Considerations** — There are no adequate reports or well-controlled studies in human fetuses. **Enalapril** crosses the human placenta, but does not equilibrate, at least in the isolated perfused model, even after 6h. And while no adverse fetal effects are reported after 1st trimester exposure, later exposure to agents which interfere with angiotensin action is associated with cranial hypoplasia, anuria, reversible or irreversible renal failure, death, oligohydramnios, prematurity, IUGR, and patent ductus arteriosus. This "ACEI fetopathy" does not have a counterpart in experimental animals because humans develop these systems prior to calvarial ossification at the end of 1st trimester. **Enalapril** produces fetal hypotension in the rhesus macaques.

■ **Breastfeeding Safety**
There are no adequate reports or well-controlled studies in nursing women. Trace amounts of **enalapril** are detected in breast milk, though the kinetics remain to be elucidated. Until further study, the infant should be monitored for possible adverse effects, the drug given at the lowest effective dose, and breastfeeding avoided at times of peak drug levels if breastfeeding continues.

■ **References**
Tabacova SA, Kimmel CA. Reprod Toxicol 2001; 15:467-78.
Miller RK, Jessee L, Barrish A, Gilbert J, Manson JM. Teratology 1998; 58:76-81.
Ducsay CA, Umezaki H, Kaushal KM, et al. Am J Obstet Gynecol 1996; 175:50-5.
Burrows RF, Burrows EA. Aust NZ J Obstet Gynaecol 1998; 38:306-11.
Redman CW, Kelly JG, Cooper WD. Eur J Clin Pharmacol 1990; 38:99.

■ **Summary**
- **Pregnancy Category C (1st trimester), D (2nd and 3rd trimesters)**
- **Lactation Category S?**
- **Enalapril** and other inhibitors of angiotensin's actions should be avoided during pregnancy if possible.
- There are alternative agents for which there is more experience during pregnancy and lactation.
- When the mother's disease requires treatment with **enalapril**, the lowest doses should be used followed by close monitoring of the fetus.

Encainide

- **Class** — Antiarrhythmic, Class I

- **Indications** — Ventricular arrhythmias

- **Mechanism** — Stabilizes membrane charge by depressing the phase 0 action potential

- **Dosage with Qualifiers** — Ventricular arrhythmia (maternal or fetal)—10-50mg PO qid
  - **Contraindications**—hypersensitivity, cardiogenic shock, AV block (partial or complete)
  - **Caution**—heart failure, hepatic or renal dysfunction, prolonged QT interval

- **Maternal Considerations** — There are no adequate reports or well-controlled studies of **encainide** in pregnant women. There is only a single case report of **encainide** use for a maternal arrhythmia. *Side effects* include cardiac arrest, CHF, arrhythmia, dizziness, blurred vision, headache, tremor, fatigue, palpitations, asthenia, tremor, constipation, edema, and abdominal pain.

- **Fetal Considerations** — There are no adequate reports or well-controlled studies in human fetuses. It is unknown whether **encainide** crosses the human placenta. A related drug, **flecainide**, does cross the human placenta and reaches therapeutic levels in the fetus. Rodent studies are reassuring, revealing no evidence of teratogenicity or IUGR despite the use of doses higher than those used clinically.

- **Breastfeeding Safety** — There is no published experience in nursing women. It is unknown whether **encainide** enters human breast milk. **Flecainide** is excreted at low levels and is generally considered safe during breastfeeding.

- **References** — Fagih B, Sami M. Can J Cardiol 1999; 15:113-7.

- **Summary**
  - **Pregnancy Category C**
  - **Lactation Category U**
  - **Encainide** should be used during pregnancy and lactation only if the benefit justifies the potential perinatal risk.
  - There are other, similar agents for which there is greater experience regarding use during pregnancy

Enoxacin (Penetrex)

- **Class** — Antibiotic, quinolone

- **Indications** — UTI, uncomplicated gonorrhea

- **Mechanism** — Bactericidal by inhibition of DNA gyrase

- **Dosage with Qualifiers** — UTI, uncomplicated—200mg PO bid ×7d (avoid meals)
  UTI, complicated—400mg PO bid ×14d (avoid meals)
  Gonorrhea, uncomplicated—400mg PO ×1
  - **Contraindications**—hypersensitivity
  - **Caution**—pregnancy, lactation, renal or hepatic dysfunction, seizure disorder, diabetes mellitus, sun exposure

- **Maternal Considerations** — There are no published reports of **enoxacin** use during pregnancy. It is a broad-spectrum agent with high oral absorption. It is not effective for the treatment of syphilis.
  Side effects include anaphylaxis, phototoxicity, pseudomembranous colitis, seizures, psychoses, nausea, vomiting, diarrhea, dyspepsia, lightheadedness, pruritus, rash, arthralgia, and tendon rupture.

- **Fetal Considerations** — There are no adequate reports or well-controlled studies in human fetuses. It is unknown whether **enoxacin** crosses the human placenta. Rodent studies are reassuring, revealing no evidence of teratogenicity or IUGR despite the use of doses higher than those used clinically. Adverse effects were associated with maternal toxicity.
  As a class, the new quinolones do not appear associated with an increased risk of malformation or musculoskeletal problems in humans. Longer follow-up and MRI of the joints may be warranted to exclude subtle cartilage and bone damage. There are no clinically significant musculoskeletal dysfunctions reported in children exposed to other fluoroquinolones *in utero.*

- **Breastfeeding Safety** — There is no published experience in nursing women. It is unknown whether **enoxacin** enters human breast milk. It does enter rodent milk, and other quinolone type drugs are excreted into human breast milk. In some animals, slow elimination of a related agent, **ciprofloxacin,** results in blood levels out of proportion to the dose ingested. Because of the potential for some quinolones to cause arthropathy in juvenile animals, they should be avoided in pregnant and lactating women until more information is available.

- **References** — No published experience in pregnancy or during lactation.

■ **Summary**
- **Pregnancy Category C**
- **Lactation Category NS?**
- **Enoxacin** should be used during pregnancy and lactation only if the benefit justifies the potential perinatal risk.
- There are alternative agents for which there is more experience during pregnancy and lactation.

Enoxaparin (Lovenox)

■ **Class**

Anticoagulant, low-molecular-weight heparinoid

■ **Indications**

Prevention and treatment of venous thrombosis in the maternal or placental circulations

■ **Mechanism**

Binds antithrombin III, accelerates inhibition of factor Xa

■ **Dosage with Qualifiers**

Prophylaxis—DVT (episode within 12mo of pregnancy, no thrombophilia), begin at 20-40mg SC qd; DVT (associated with thrombophilia), depends on the thrombophilia and medical history. Consult a specialty text such as *High Risk Pregnancy: Management Options.*
Antiphospholipid syndrome—begin at 20-40mg SC qd
Cesarean section—at least 40mg SC qd until patient is active
Treatment of acute thrombosis—1-1.5mg/kg SC q12h
NOTE—target for anti-Xa activity depends on indication and laboratory test used
NOTE—manufacturer has specifically sought to discourage its use during pregnancy
- **Contraindications**—hypersensitivity, active bleeding, thrombocytopenia
- **Caution**—diabetic retinopathy, renal dysfunction

■ **Maternal Considerations**

The incidence of PE and DVT is higher in pregnant compared to nonpregnant patients, reaching a rate of 0.05 and 1% in all pregnancies, and as high as 3% after cesarean section. Pregnancy increases the clearance of both heparin and low-molecular-weight heparinoids such as **enoxaparin** requiring dose monitoring periodically throughout pregnancy (anti-Xa activity of 0.20-0.40U/ml for prophylaxis, and 0.4-0.7U/ml for full anticoagulation). **Enoxaparin** may have a lower risk of osteoporosis and allergic thrombocytopenia than unfractionated heparin. Acute thrombosis should be treated with therapeutic levels for the remainder of pregnancy and at least 6w postpartum (a minimum of 3mo total). **Enoxaparin** has also been used during pregnancy for prophylaxis in women with thrombophilia or mechanical heart valve or antiphospholipid syndrome. There have been multiple maternal deaths in treated women with a mechanical heart valve. The manufacturer specifically discourages its use for this indication. Unlike unfractionated heparin, **enoxaparin** cannot be predictably reversed with protamine. Women treated with LMWHs for prevention of thromboembolic complications are at risk of developing an epidural or spinal hematoma after neuraxial anesthesia. Therefore, women should be instructed to withhold their next injection once contractions begin, or 12h prior to a planned induction of labor. Preferably, LMWHs are replaced with unfractionated **heparin** at 36w. **Enoxaparin** should be discontinued 12-24h (depending on daily dose) before placement of a neuraxial (epidural or spinal) anesthesia. **Enoxaparin** should not be (re)instituted until at least 2h after removal of an indwelling epidural catheter. One prospective study of bone density in women receiving LMWH found no significant change in mean bone density between baseline and 6 weeks postpartum.

Side effects include epidural/spinal hematoma, thrombocytopenia, paralysis, CHF, pneumonia, anemia, hemorrhage, fever, injection site hematoma or bruising, hematuria, and elevated transaminases.

■ **Fetal Considerations**
Neither unfractionated nor fractionated heparin crosses the human placenta, and thus does not pose a direct risk to the human fetus. Epidemiological studies are reassuring. Rodent studies are reassuring, revealing no evidence of teratogenicity or IUGR despite the use of doses higher than those used clinically.

■ **Breastfeeding Safety**
There are no adequate reports or well-controlled studies in nursing women. One investigation found no anti-Xa activity in the breast milk from a single patient. **Enoxaparin** is unlikely to cross in light of its high molecular weight, and if it does cross and is ingested by the nursing newborn, it is likely to be degraded.

■ **References**
James D, Steer P, Weiner CP, Gonik B (Eds.) High Risk Pregnancy: Management Options, 2nd ed. Philadelphia: WB Saunders, 2000.
Laurent P, Dussarat GV, Bonal J, et al. Drugs 2002; 62:463-77.
Lepercq J, Conard J, Borel-Derlon A, et al. BJOG 2001; 108:1134-40.
Rowan JA, McCowan LM, Raudkivi PJ, North RA. Am J Obstet Gynecol 2001; 185:633-7.
Bar J, Mashiah R, Cohen-Sacher B, et al. Thromb Res 2001; 101:235-41.
Casele HL, Laifer SA, Woelkers DA, Venkataramanan R. Am J Obstet Gynecol 1999; 181:1113-7.
Backos M, Rai R, Baxter N, et al. Br J Obstet Gynaecol 1999; 106:102-7.
Dimitrakakis C, Papageorgiou P, Papageorgiou I, et al. Haemostasis 2000; 30:243-8.

■ **Summary** ⸺ • **Pregnancy Category B**
• **Lactation Category S?**
• **Enoxaparin** is a more costly alternative to
unfractionated **heparin** with likely equal efficacy but a
lower risk of osteoporosis and thrombocytopenia.
• The dose of **enoxaparin** administered *must* be monitored
periodically throughout pregnancy and puerperium
by the measurement of anti-Xa activity to assure
therapeutic levels.

Ephedrine

■ **Class** ⸺ *Sympathomimetic*

■ **Indications** ⸺ Nasal decongestant, pressor support after epidural
analgesia

■ **Mechanism** ⸺ Causes release of epinephrine and norepinephrine from
nerve endings resulting in mainly β-adrenergic
stimulation; also a weak direct-acting vasopressor

■ **Dosage with Qualifiers** ⸺ Decongestant—25-50mg PO q6h (max 150mg/d)
NOTE—may be combined with **theophylline**, **pentobarbital**
or potassium iodide
• **Contraindications**—hypersensitivity, thyroid toxicosis,
porphyria, coronary artery disease, hypertension, use of
a MAO inhibitor within 14d
• **Caution**—glaucoma, arrhythmia, hyperthyroidism

■ **Maternal Considerations** ⸺ There are no adequate reports or well-controlled studies
of **ephedrine** in pregnant women. When abused as a
decongestant, **ephedrine** may exacerbate the
hypertension associated with preeclampsia. There is a
long clinical experience with the use of **ephedrine** during
labor to treat hypotension associated with neuraxial
anesthesia. It is considered the vasopressor of choice
unless contraindicated by maternal condition (e.g.,
coexisting valvular stenosis) and is protective of the
uterine circulation, perhaps through release of nitric oxide
in the placental vessels.
Side effects include arrhythmias, insomnia, nervousness,
dizziness, and tachycardia.

■ **Fetal Considerations** ⸺ There are no adequate reports or well-controlled studies in
human fetuses. **Ephedrine** apparently crosses the placenta,
though the kinetics remain to be elucidated. Rodent
teratogenicity studies have not been conducted. The long
clinical experience with the drug, both in over-the-counter
preparations and in the labor suite, is reassuring.

- **Breastfeeding Safety** ⋯⋯ There are no adequate reports or well-controlled studies in nursing women. **Ephedrine** is excreted and concentrated into breast milk, but less than 1% of the ingested dose is excreted. Thus, it is generally considered safe for breast-feeding women.

- **References** ⋯⋯⋯ Ducros L, Bonnin P, Cholley BP, et al. Anesthesiology 2002; 96:612-6.
Cooper DW, Carpenter M, Mowbray P, et al. Anesthesiology 2002; 97:1582-90.
Emmett RS, Cyna AM, Andrew M, Simmons SW. Cochrane Database Syst Rev 2001; 3:CD002251.
Findlay JW, Butz RF, Sailstad JM, et al. Br J Clin Pharmacol 1984; 18:901-6.
Li P, Tong C, Eisenach JC. Anesth Analg 1996; 82:288-93.

- **Summary** ⋯⋯⋯
  - **Pregnancy Category C**
  - **Lactation Category S**
  - **Ephedrine** is commonly found in many over-the-counter preparations.
  - It is a popular agent for the treatment of hypotension associated with conduction anesthesia.

Epinephrine (Adrenalin Chloride; Ana-Guard; Epifrin; EpiPen; Glaucon; Philip; Racepinephrine; Sus-Phrine)

- **Class** ⋯⋯⋯ *Sympathomimetic/ionotrope/pressor*

- **Indications** ⋯⋯⋯ Severe asthma, anaphylaxis, cardiac arrest

- **Mechanism** ⋯⋯⋯ Potent activator of α- and β-adrenoceptors

- **Dosage with Qualifiers** ⋯⋯ Severe asthma—0.1-0.5mg SC q10-15min
Anaphylaxis—0.1-0.5mg SC q10-15min (or 0.1-0.25mg IV over 5-10min)
Cardiac arrest—0.5-1mg IV q3-5min prn (or 1mg via ET tube, 0.1-1mg intracardiac); may follow with 1-4mcg/min constant infusion
NOTE—usually a 1:10,000 solution; may be combined with a local anesthetic
  - **Contraindications**—hypersensitivity, narrow angle glaucoma, coronary artery disease, cardiovascular disease, sulfite allergy
  - **Caution**—asthma, hyperthyroidism

- **Maternal Considerations** ⋯⋯ **Epinephrine** is commonly used for the relief of severe bronchospasm secondary to allergy. There are no adequate reports or well-controlled studies of **epinephrine** in pregnant women. Theoretically, it could lead to a decrease in uterine blood flow. **Epinephrine** in solution with local anesthetic decreases vascular absorption of local anesthetic, intensifying neural blockade and in some cases prolonging the duration of the block. The maternal response may be potentiated by a variety of drugs and by preeclampsia.

Side effects include stroke, cerebral hemorrhage, arrhythmias, hypertension, tachycardia, tremor, nausea, vomiting, and headache.

■ **Fetal Considerations**

There are no adequate reports or well-controlled studies in human fetuses. **Epinephrine** apparently rapidly crosses the human placenta, which is rich in catecholamine receptors. It is teratogenic in mice at 25 times the maximum human dose.

■ **Breastfeeding Safety**

There is no published experience in nursing women. It is unknown whether **epinephrine** enters human breast milk. However, considering the indication and dosing, one-time **epinephrine** use is unlikely to pose a clinically significant risk to the breast-feeding neonate.

■ **References**

Nguyen TT, Tseng YT, McGonnigal B, et al. Placenta 1999; 20:3-11.

■ **Summary**

- **Pregnancy Category C**
- **Lactation Category U**
- **Epinephrine** should be used during pregnancy and lactation only if the benefit justifies the potential perinatal risk.

Epoetin alfa (EPO; Epogen; Eprex; Erythropoietin; Procrit)

■ **Class**

Hematologic, hematopoietic; hormone

■ **Indications**

Transfusion reduction or severe hyporegenerative anemia secondary to AZT therapy, chronic renal failure, or chemotherapy

■ **Mechanism**

Stimulates RBC production

■ **Dosage with Qualifiers**

Transfusion reduction—300U/kg SC 3×/w beginning 10d preoperative
AZT–related anemia—150U/kg SC/IV 3×/w beginning for 8w; may increase to 300U/kg for 3w if poor response
Renal failure-related anemia—50-100U/kg IV/SC 3×/w
Chemotherapy related anemia—150U/kg SC/IV 3×/w beginning for 8w; may increase to 300U/kg for 3w if poor response

- **Contraindications**—hypersensitivity
- **Caution**—hypertension, iron, folate or vitamin B_{12} deficiency, CHF, coronary artery disease, seizure disorder, sickle cell anemia

■ **Maternal Considerations** ⋯⋯ There are no adequate reports or well-controlled studies of **epoetin** in pregnant women. Adjuvant **epoetin** safely enhances the efficacy of iron sucrose in the treatment of gestational iron deficiency anemia resistant to orally administered iron alone.

Side effects include severe hypertension, CHF, MI, stroke, DVT, seizures, headache, arthralgia, tachycardia, fever, diarrhea, nausea, vomiting, dyspnea, dizziness, rash, paresthesias.

■ **Fetal Considerations** ⋯⋯ There are no adequate reports or well-controlled studies in human fetuses. It is unknown whether **epoetin** crosses the human placenta. In the offspring of rats treated with 500U/kg, a diverse group of abnormalities was observed, including delayed ossification. There were no effects below that dose.

■ **Breastfeeding Safety** ⋯⋯ There is no published experience in nursing women. It is unknown whether **epoetin** enters human breast milk.

■ **References** ⋯⋯ Danko J, Huch R, Huch A. Lancet 1990; 335:737-8.
Sifakis S, Angelakis E, Vardaki E, et al. Gynecol Obstet Invest 2001; 51:150-6.
Breymann C, Visca E, Huch R, Huch A. Am J Obstet Gynecol 2001; 184:662-7.

■ **Summary** ⋯⋯
- **Pregnancy Category C**
- **Lactation Category U**
- **Epoetin** should be used during pregnancy and lactation only if the benefit justifies the potential perinatal risk.
- A growing body of evidence suggests it is advantageous for certain women with iron deficiency.

Epoprostenol (Flolan)

■ **Class** ⋯⋯ *Antihypertensive, platelet inhibitor; prostaglandin; other*

■ **Indications** ⋯⋯ Pulmonary hypertension

■ **Mechanism** ⋯⋯ Prostacyclin is a direct vasodilator.

■ **Dosage with Qualifiers** ⋯⋯ Pulmonary hypertension—2ng/kg/min IV, increase 1-2ng/min q15min; infuse through a central line
- **Contraindications**—hypersensitivity, CHF, pulmonary edema

- **Maternal Considerations** .... **Epoprostenol** is prostacyclin. Primary pulmonary hypertension (PPH) is a rare, progressive condition aggravated by the physiologic changes of pregnancy. **Epoprostenol** has been used to treat women in the immediate postpartum period with apparent success. The maternal mortality rate ranges from 30-50%.
  Side effects include pulmonary edema, rebound pulmonary hypertension, thrombocytopenia, headache, nausea, vomiting, anxiety, tachycardia, hypotension, chest pain, diarrhea, paresthesias, dyspnea.

- **Fetal Considerations** .... There are no adequate reports or well-controlled studies in human fetuses. It is unknown whether **epoprostenol** crosses the human placenta. A small amount of carbacyclin is transferred. The placenta and fetus synthesize large quantities of prostacyclin. There is no reason to suspect toxicity. Rodent studies are reassuring, revealing no evidence of teratogenicity or IUGR despite the use of doses higher than those used clinically.

- **Breastfeeding Safety** .... There is no published experience in nursing women. It is unknown whether **epoprostenol** is excreted into breast milk.

- **References** .... Stewart R, Tuazon D, Olson G, Duarte AG. Chest 2001; 119:973-5.
  Badalian SS, Silverman RK, Aubry RH, Longo J. J Reprod Med 2000; 45:149-52.
  Walenga RW, Kuhn DC, Stuart MJ. Prostaglandins 1989; 37:121-34.

- **Summary** ....
  - **Pregnancy Category B**
  - **Lactation Category U**
  - **Epoprostenol** has been successfully employed in several women with life-threatening pulmonary hypertension.

Eprosartan mesylate (Teveten)

- **Class** .... Antihypertensive, AT1 *antagonist*

- **Indications** .... Hypertension

- **Mechanism** .... Highly specific AT1 receptor antagonist

- **Dosage with Qualifiers** .... Hypertension—600-800mg PO qd
  - **Contraindications**—hypersensitivity, pregnancy
  - **Caution**—renal artery stenosis, volume depletion, CHF

■ **Maternal Considerations** ⋯⋯⋯ There is no published human experience during pregnancy.

Side effects include severe hypertension, CHF, MI, stroke, DVT, seizures, headache, arthralgia, tachycardia, fever, diarrhea, nausea, vomiting, dyspnea, dizziness, rash, and paresthesias.

■ **Fetal Considerations** ⋯⋯⋯ There are no adequate reports or well-controlled studies in human fetuses. It is unknown whether **eprosartan** crosses the human placenta. Similar class drugs are known teratogens. And while no adverse fetal effects are reported after 1st trimester exposure, later exposure to agents which interfere with angiotensin action is associated with cranial hypoplasia, anuria, reversible or irreversible renal failure, death, oligohydramnios, prematurity, IUGR, and patent ductus arteriosus. This "ACEI fetopathy" does not have a counterpart in experimental animals because humans develop these systems prior to calvarial ossification at the end of 1st trimester.

■ **Breastfeeding Safety** ⋯⋯⋯ There is no published experience in nursing women. It is unknown whether **eprosartan** enters human breast milk. **Eprosartan** is excreted into rodent breast milk. Until further study, the infant should be monitored for possible adverse effects, the drug given at the lowest effective dose, and breastfeeding avoided at times of peak drug levels if breastfeeding continues.

■ **References** ⋯⋯⋯ No published experience in pregnancy or during lactation.

■ **Summary** ⋯⋯⋯
- **Pregnancy Category C (1st trimester) D (2nd and 3rd trimesters)**
- **Lactation Category U**
- **Eprosartan** and other inhibitors of angiotensin's actions should be avoided during pregnancy if possible.
- There are alternative agents for which there is more experience during pregnancy and lactation.
- When the mother's disease requires treatment with **eprosartan**, the lowest doses should be used followed by close monitoring of the fetus.

Ergocalciferol (Biocatines D2 masiva; Deltalin; Drisdol; Radiostol; Vitamin D)

■ **Class** .... *Vitamin*

■ **Indications** .... Rickets, hypoparathyroidism, familial hypophosphatemia

■ **Mechanism** .... Vitamin D_2 stimulates intestinal absorption of calcium and phosphorus, and mineralization. It is converted in the liver to 25-hydroxyergocalciferol and then in the kidney to the active 1,25-dihydroxyergocalciferol.

■ **Dosage with Qualifiers** .... Rickets, osteomalacia—12,000 to 500,000U PO qd or 250mcg IM qd
Hypoparathyroidism—50,000 to 200,000U PO qd (supplement with 500mg elemental calcium 6×/d)
Familial hypophosphatemia—12,000 to 80,000U PO qd (supplement with 1-2g elemental phosphorus/d)
NOTE—1 mcg = 40U
- **Contraindications**—hypersensitivity, renal osteodystrophy, hypercalcemia, hypervitaminosis A
- **Caution**—renal dysfunction or stones, CVD

■ **Maternal Considerations** .... **Ergocalciferol** is a synthetic regulator of calcium. There are no adequate reports or well-controlled studies of **ergocalciferol** in pregnant women. There is a long clinical experience of vitamin D supplementation during pregnancy and lactation without complications. The recommended minimal daily requirement is 400U. The safety of larger doses is unknown.
Side effects include hypercalcemia, nausea, vomiting, anorexia, anemia, weakness, and renal dysfunction.

■ **Fetal Considerations** .... There are no adequate reports or well-controlled studies in human fetuses. It is unknown whether **ergocalciferol** crosses the human placenta. Maternal vitamin D supplementation does not significantly increase the neonatal level. **Ergocalciferol** or a metabolite crosses the rodent placenta. Hypervitaminosis D has been associated with a syndrome characterized by supravalvular aortic stenosis, elfin facies, and mental retardation. Rare reports in fetal rats suggesting anomalous bone development when administered in high doses with cortisone.

■ **Breastfeeding Safety** .... There are no adequate reports or well-controlled studies in nursing women. It is unknown whether **ergocalciferol** enters human breast milk. Vitamin D is a normal component of breast milk, and **ergocalciferol** has little effect on vitamin D metabolites in human breast milk. It is likely simple supplementation is safe during lactation. However, there is a single case report of a woman given large doses of vitamin D where 25-hydroxycholecalciferol was identified in her breast milk and the neonate developed hypercalcemia.

■ **References** .... Di Gregorio S, Danilowicz K, Rubin Z, Mautalen C. Nutrition 2000; 16:1052-5.
Takeuchi A, Okano T, Tsugawa N, et al. J Nutr 1989; 119:1639-46.
Clements MR, Fraser DR. J Clin Invest 1988; 81:1768-73.

■ **Summary** ....
- **Pregnancy Category C**
- **Lactation Category S**
- **Ergocalciferol** is considered safe and effective during pregnancy and lactation when used in therapeutic amounts.

Ergotamine (Ergomar; Ergostat; Medihaler-Ergotamine; Wigrettes)

■ **Class** .... *Ergot alkaloid*

■ **Indications** .... Abort or prevent migraine headache

■ **Mechanism** .... Complex and multiple; partial agonist/antagonist against tryptaminergic, dopaminergic and α-adrenergic receptors depending upon site

■ **Dosage with Qualifiers** .... Abort or prevent migraine headache—1 tab SL q30min prn at first sign of attack; max 3 tabs qd, or 5 tabs qwk
NOTE—2mg tablets
- **Contraindications**—hypersensitivity to drug or class, PVD, CAD, hypertension, hepatic or renal dysfunction, severe pruritus, sepsis, and pregnancy
- **Caution**—breastfeeding

■ **Maternal Considerations** .... There are no adequate reports or well-controlled studies in pregnant women. **Ergotamine** is a highly active uterine contractile agonist. Inadvertent use may lead to abortion. **Ergotamine** produces constriction of both arteries and veins. It causes constriction of peripheral and cranial blood vessels and depresses the central vasomotor centers. The pain of a migraine attack is believed secondary to greatly increased amplitude of pulsations in the cranial arteries, especially the meningeal branches of the external carotid artery. **Ergotamine** reduces extracranial blood flow, decreases the amplitude of pulsation in the cranial arteries, and decreases hyperperfusion of the territory of the basilar artery. It is effective in controlling up to 70% of acute migraine attacks, so that it is now considered specific for the treatment of this headache syndrome. **Atropine** or antiemetic compounds of the phenothiazine group may relieve the associated nausea and vomiting. There is a case report of its association with maternal MI following a **ergotamine** associated abortion.

Side effects include nausea, vomiting (up to 10%), leg weakness, myalgia, numbness and paresthesias of the fingers and toes, precordial pain, transient changes in heart rate, edema, and pruritus.

■ **Fetal Considerations**
There are no adequate reports or well-controlled studies in human fetuses. It is unknown whether **ergotamine** crosses the human placenta. While there is no clear evidence it is a teratogen, the severe vasoconstriction associated with toxicity could lead to profound fetal hypoxia and death. It has also been associated with Mobius syndrome.

■ **Breastfeeding Safety**
There are no adequate reports or well-controlled studies in nursing women. **Ergotamine** is excreted into human breast milk. Theoretically, excessive dosing or prolonged administration of **ergotamine** might inhibit lactation. Though generally considered incompatible with breastfeeding, the only published study found no effect on milk production or infant weight gain.

■ **References**
Marti V, Salas E, Torner P, Dominguez de las Rozas JM. Med Clin (Barc) 1999; 113:758-9.
Raymond GV. Teratology 1995; 51:344-7.
de Groot AN, van Dongen PW, van Roosmalen J, Eskes TK. Eur J Obstet Gynecol Reprod Biol 1993; 51:73-7.
Au KL, Woo JS, Wong VC. Eur J Obstet Gynecol Reprod Biol 1985; 19:313-5.
Graf WD, Shepard TH. J Child Neurol 1997; 12:225-7.
Moretti ME, Lee A, Ito S. Can Fam Physician 2000; 46:1753-7.
Jolivet A, Robyn C, Huraux-Rendu C, Gautray JP. J Gynecol Obstet Biol Reprod (Paris) 1978; 7:129-34.

■ **Summary**
• **Pregnancy Category X**
• **Lactation Category NS?**
• **Ergotamine** should be used during pregnancy and lactation only if the benefit justifies the potential perinatal risk.
• There are alternative agents for which there is a higher safety profile and more experience during pregnancy and lactation.

Erythromycin (A/T/S; Akne-Mycin; C-Solve-2; Del-Mycin; Dumotrycin; E-Base; ETS; Emgel; Endoeritrin; Erisone; Eritomicina; Erycette; Erygel; Erythra-Derm; Ilotycin; Mercina; PCE; Proterytrin; Retcin; Romycin; Sansac; Staticin; T-Stat)

■ **Class** — Antibiotic, *macrolide*

■ **Indications** — Bacterial infection, certain STDs, prophylaxis for rheumatic heart disease, bacterial endocarditis and GBS

■ **Mechanism** — Inhibits protein synthesis by binding the P site of the 50S ribosomal subunit

■ **Dosage with Qualifiers** — Bacterial infection—250-500mg PO q6h-12h
NOTE—may be combined with a sulfa agent to improve coverage of H. *influenzae*
- **Contraindications**—hypersensitivity, cisapride use, astemizole use
- **Caution**—myasthenia gravis, hepatic dysfunction

■ **Maternal Considerations** — The routine use of macrolide antibiotics prolongs the latency interval and reduces infectious morbidity in women with PPROM, but offers no benefit in women with preterm labor and intact membranes. **Erythromycin** reduces the frequency of preterm delivery in women with either asymptomatic bacteriuria or symptomatic lower genital tract infections. However, the practice of routine screening for BV in asymptomatic women who are at low risk for preterm delivery cannot be supported based on evidence from the literature. The frequency of group B streptococcus resistance renders it a poor selection for prophylaxis. **Erythromycin** is an effective alternative therapy for the treatment of chlamydial infection. Partner treatment is, overall, cost-effective among women aged 15 to 29. Though an alternative for the treatment of syphilis in penicillin allergic patients, placental transport is low (<5%). Thus, **erythromycin** is not recommended for the treatment of syphilis during pregnancy. **Penicillin**-allergic women should be desensitized.
Side effects include anaphylaxis, hepatotoxicity, thrombophlebitis, ventricular arrhythmia, bradycardia, hypotension, nausea, vomiting, diarrhea, pruritus, anorexia, abdominal pain, jaundice, eosinophilia, and elevated hepatic transaminases.

■ **Fetal Considerations** — There are no adequate reports or well-controlled studies in human fetuses. **Erythromycin** crosses the human placenta achieving an F:M concentration ratio of 0.3.

■ **Breastfeeding Safety** — There are no adequate reports or well-controlled studies in nursing women. **Erythromycin** is excreted into human breast milk, achieving an M:P ratio approximating unity.

Rodent studies are reassuring, revealing no evidence of teratogenicity or IUGR despite the use of doses higher than those used clinically.

■ **References** Kenyon S, Boulvain M, Neilson J. Cochrane Database Syst Rev 2001; 4:CD001058.
Kenyon SL, Taylor DJ, Tarnow-Mordi W; ORACLE Collaborative Group. Lancet 2001; 357:979-94.
Manning SD, Foxman B, Pierson CL, et al. Obstet Gynecol 2003; 101:74-9.
Louik C, Werler MM, Mitchell AA. Am J Obstet Gynecol 2002; 186:288-90.
Gray RH, Wabwire-Mangen F, Kigozi G, et al. Am J Obstet Gynecol 2001; 185:1209-17.
Postma MJ, Welte R, van den Hoek JA, et al. Value Health 2001; 4:266-75.
Mercer BM, Miodovnik M, Thurnau GR, et al. JAMA 1997; 278:989-95.
Sheffield JS, Sanchez PJ, Morris G, et al. Am J Obstet Gynecol 2002; 186:569-73.
Heikkinen T, Laine K, Neuvonen PJ, Ekblad U. BJOG 2000; 107:770-5.
Zhang Y, Zhang Q, Xu Z. Zhonghua Fu Chan Ke Za Zhi 1997; 32:288-92.

■ **Summary**
- **Pregnancy Category B**
- **Lactation Category S**
- **Erythromycin** is one option for the treatment of PPROM to prolong the latency period.
- **Erythromycin** reduces the frequency of preterm delivery in women with either asymptomatic bacteriuria or symptomatic lower genital tract infections.
- **Erythromycin** is an effective alternative therapy for the treatment of *Chlamydia* infection; partner treatment is cost-effective.
- Poor placental transport renders it a poor choice for the treatment of fetal infection.

Esmolol (Brevibloc)

■ **Class** *Antihypertensive, antiarrhythmic class* II

■ **Indications** Hypertension (perioperative), supraventricular tachycardia

■ **Mechanism** β-1 receptor antagonist

■ **Dosage with Qualifiers** <u>Perioperative hypertension/tachycardia</u>—begin 150mcg/kg/min IV; titrate up by 50mcg/kg/min for a max of 300mcg/kg/min

<u>Supraventricular tachycardia</u>—begin 500mcg/kg/min ×1min, then 50mcg/kg/min ×4min; repeat cycle if no effect, titrating infusion up by 50mcg/kg/min after each loading dose

- **Contraindications**—hypersensitivity, sinus bradycardia, AV heart block, cardiogenic shock
- **Caution**—asthma

■ **Maternal Considerations** ········ **Esmolol** is a short acting β-1 blocker employed for the rapid but short-term control of either hypertension or supraventricular arrhythmia. There are no adequate reports or well-controlled studies of **esmolol** in pregnant women. It has been used successfully for blood pressure control in women with preeclampsia or pheochromocytoma before induction of general anesthesia, and in women with terbutaline overdose or hypertrophic obstructive cardiomyopathy.
Side effects include bronchospasm, hypotension, cardiac failure, dizziness, nausea, vomiting, somnolence, fatigue, and phlebitis.

■ **Fetal Considerations** ············· There are no adequate reports or well-controlled studies in human fetuses. **Esmolol** crosses the human placenta, and fetal bradycardia may continue days after delivery despite the short effect in adults. Rodent studies are reassuring, revealing no evidence of teratogenicity or IUGR despite the use of doses higher than those used clinically. Maternal toxicity is associated with embryo lethality.

■ **Breastfeeding Safety** ··············· There is no published experience in nursing women. It is unknown whether **esmolol** is excreted into breast milk.

■ **References** ································· Ostman PL, Chestnut DH, Robillard JE, et al. Anesthesiology 1988; 69:738-41.
Gilson GJ, Knieriem KJ, Smith JF, et al. J Reprod Med 1992; 37:277-9.

■ **Summary** ···································
- **Pregnancy Category C**
- **Lactation Category U**
- **Esmolol** should be used during pregnancy and lactation only if the benefit justifies the potential perinatal risk.

Esomeprazole (Nexium)

■ **Class** — Antiulcer; *proton pump inhibitor; gastrointestinal*

■ **Indications** — GERD, erosive esophagitis, H. *pylori* infection treatment

■ **Mechanism** — A proton pump inhibitor reducing gastric parietal cell release of hydrogen

■ **Dosage with Qualifiers** — GERD—20-40mg PO qd ×4-8w; max 80mg qd
Erosive esophagitis—20-40mg PO qd ×4-8w; max 80mg qd
H. *pylori*—40mg PO qd ×10d taken with **amoxicillin** and **clarithromycin**
- **Contraindications**—hypersensitivity
- **Caution**—hepatic dysfunction, long-term use

■ **Maternal Considerations** — There are no adequate reports or well-controlled studies of **esomeprazole** in pregnant women. **Esomeprazole** is cost-effective compared with **omeprazole** in the acute treatment of reflux esophagitis and GERD without esophagitis. These drugs are being used with increasing frequency during pregnancy, and there is a great need for additional study.
Side effects include hepatic dysfunction, diarrhea, and headache.

■ **Fetal Considerations** — There are no adequate reports or well-controlled studies in human fetuses. It is unknown whether **esomeprazole** crosses the human placenta. One epidemiological study including 600 pregnancies is reassuring. Rodent studies are reassuring, revealing no evidence of teratogenicity or IUGR despite the use of doses higher than those used clinically.

■ **Breastfeeding Safety** — There is no published experience in nursing women. It is unknown whether **esomeprazole** is excreted into breast milk.

■ **References** — Wahlqvist P, Junghard O, Higgins A, Green J. Pharmacoeconomics 2002; 20:279-87.
Nikfar S, Abdollahi M, Moretti ME, Magee LA, Koren G. Dig Dis Sci 2002; 47:1526-9.

■ **Summary** —
- **Pregnancy Category B**
- **Lactation Category U**
- **Esomeprazole** should be used during pregnancy and lactation only if the benefit justifies the potential perinatal risk.
- There are alternative agents for which there is more experience during pregnancy and lactation.

Estazolam (Eurodin; Nuctalon; ProSom; Sedarest)

■ **Class** — Benzodiazepine; sedative/hypnotic

■ **Indications** — Insomnia

■ **Mechanism** — Binds to the benzodiazepine receptor, enhancing GABA effects

■ **Dosage with Qualifiers** — Insomnia—1-2mg PO qhs prn
- **Contraindications**—hypersensitivity, pregnancy, depressed respiratory function, and sleep apnea
- **Caution**—hepatic or renal dysfunction, suicidal ideation, history of substance abuse

■ **Maternal Considerations** — There is no published experience with **estazolam** during pregnancy. Other drugs of this class such as **diazepam** are considered to be contraindicated during pregnancy. *Side effects* include somnolence, headache, asthenia, dizziness, and disorientation.

■ **Fetal Considerations** — There are no adequate reports or well-controlled studies in human fetuses. It is unknown whether **estazolam** crosses the human placenta. Transplacental movement of similar drugs is known to occur and neonatal depression is reported. See **diazepam**.

■ **Breastfeeding Safety** — There is no published experience in nursing women. It is unknown whether **estazolam** enters human breast milk. See **diazepam**.

■ **References** — No published experience in pregnancy or during lactation.

■ **Summary** —
- **Pregnancy Category X**
- **Lactation Category U**
- Benzodiazepines such as **estazolam** are generally contraindicated during pregnancy.
- There are alternative agents for which there is more experience during pregnancy and lactation.

Estradiol (Alora; Climara; Estrace; Estraderm; Estring; Fempatch; Vivelle)

■ **Class** .... *Estrogen, hormone*

■ **Indications** .... Contraception (when used in combination with a progestational agent), vasomotor symptoms, osteoporosis prevention, atrophic vaginitis, primary ovarian failure, breast cancer palliation

■ **Mechanism** .... A natural estrogen that binds to estrogen receptors developing and maintaining female sex characteristics; has both receptor- and nonreceptor-mediated activities

■ **Dosage with Qualifiers** .... Vasomotor symptoms—1-2mg PO qd, cycle 21d on and 7d off, add a progestin days 14-21 if uterus present
Osteoporosis prevention—0.5mg PO qd, cycle 21d on and 7d off, add a progestin days 14-21 if uterus present
Atrophic vaginitis—1-2mg PO qd, cycle 21d on and 7d off, add a progestin days 14-21 if uterus present
Primary ovarian failure—1-2mg PO qd
Breast cancer palliation—10mg PO tid ×3mo
NOTE—also available in a variety of preparations as **ethinyl estradiol,** a more potent synthetic. Delivery systems include oral tablets, vaginal tablets, creams, rings, and subcutaneous and transdermal formulations produced by various manufacturers.
● **Contraindications**—hypersensitivity, undiagnosed vaginal bleeding, thromboembolic disease, estrogen-dependent breast cancer, pregnancy
● **Caution**—hepatic dysfunction

■ **Maternal Considerations** .... **Estradiol** is a naturally occurring **estrogen**, and as such may have a different risk profile than synthetic or phytoestrogens. There are no indications for **estradiol** during pregnancy. Recent studies suggest **estrogen** plus **medroxyprogesterone** for the treatment of menopausal symptoms increases the risk of breast cancer and cardiovascular disease.
Side effects include thromboembolism, stroke, MI, endometrial and breast cancer, gallbladder disease, pancreatitis, hypertension, breast tenderness, hepatic adenoma, bloating, nausea, vomiting, headache, dizziness, depression, weight gain, libido changes, intolerance to contact lenses, migraine, and rash.

■ **Fetal Considerations** .... There are no adequate reports or well-controlled studies in human fetuses. While **diethylstilbestrol** and other synthetic/environmental estrogens are recognized teratogens with the potential for transgenerational effects, few studies support this effect for naturally occurring substances like **estradiol**. There is no clear evidence of fetal harm after inadvertent exposure during the

1st trimester. Some studies have suggested prenatal exposure to **estradiol** might alter immune programming.

■ **Breastfeeding Safety** — Though **estradiol** is excreted into breast milk and has been reported to reduce the amount of milk produced, it is not effective as an inhibitor of lactation. All pharmacokinetic studies have shown that the transfer to breast milk of both **progesterone** and **estrogen** when taking a contraceptive pill is of the same order as natural hormones. Estrogen-containing contraceptives should be initiated after the 6th week of lactation when the lipid profile has returned to normal and the risk of thrombosis is identical to that of the general population.

■ **References** — Karpuzoglu-Sahin E, Hissong BD, Ansar Ahmed S. J Reprod Immunol 2001; 52:113-27.
Herbst AL. Gynecol Oncol 2000; 76:147-56.
Barlow S, Kavlock RJ, Moore JA, et al. Teratology 1999; 60:365-75.
Hook EB. Teratology 1994; 49:162-6.

■ **Summary** —
- **Pregnancy Category X**
- **Lactation Category S**
- There is no indication for **estradiol** during pregnancy.
- There is no clear evidence of fetal harm after inadvertent exposure during the 1st trimester.

Estrogens, conjugated (Azumon; Conjugen; Emopremarin; Mannest; Menopak-E; Ovest; Premarin; Trepova)

■ **Class** — Estrogens, hormone

■ **Indications** — Primary ovarian failure, vasomotor symptoms of menopause, osteoporosis

■ **Mechanism** — Bind to estrogen receptors; has both receptor- and nonreceptor-mediated activities

■ **Dosage with Qualifiers** — Vasomotor symptoms—0.3-1.25mg PO qd for 21d, and then 7d off; add a progestin days 14-21 if uterus present
Osteoporosis—0.625mg PO qd for 21d, and then 7d off; add a progestin days 14-21 if uterus present
Primary ovarian failure—1.25mg PO qd for 21d, and then 7d off; add a progestin days 14-21 if uterus present
NOTE—may be combined with **medroxyprogesterone**, **meprobamate**, or **methyltestosterone**
- **Contraindications**—hypersensitivity, pregnancy, undiagnosed vaginal bleeding, thromboembolic disease, estrogen-dependent breast cancer
- **Caution**—lactation, hepatic dysfunction

- **Maternal Considerations** ⋯⋯ **Conjugated estrogens** is a mixture of estrogens extracted from natural sources, most commonly pregnant mares' urine. They have been long known to increase the risk of endometrial cancer. There are no indications for **conjugated estrogens** during pregnancy. Recent studies suggest **estrogen** plus **medroxyprogesterone** for the treatment of menopausal symptoms increases the risk of breast cancer and cardiovascular disease. See **estradiol**. *Side effects* include thromboembolism, stroke, MI, endometrial and breast cancer, gallbladder disease, pancreatitis, hypertension, breast tenderness, hepatic adenoma, bloating, nausea, vomiting, headache, dizziness, depression, weight gain, libido changes, intolerance to contact lenses, migraine, and rash.

- **Fetal Considerations** ⋯⋯ **Estrogen** has a myriad of effects on the developing embryo/fetus; many are poorly understood. See **estradiol**.

- **Breastfeeding Safety** ⋯⋯ See **estradiol**.

- **References** ⋯⋯ See **estradiol**.

- **Summary** ⋯⋯
  - **Pregnancy Category X**
  - **Lactation Category S**
  - There is no indication for **estradiol** during pregnancy.
  - There is no clear evidence of fetal harm after inadvertent exposure during the 1st trimester.

Estrogens, esterified (Amnestrogen; Estratab; Evex; Femogen; Menest)

- **Class** ⋯⋯ Estrogens, hormone

- **Indications** ⋯⋯ Hormone replacement, primary ovarian failure, vasomotor symptoms of menopause and osteoporosis

- **Mechanism** ⋯⋯ Bind to estrogen receptors; has both receptor- and nonreceptor-mediated activities

- **Dosage with Qualifiers** ⋯⋯ Vasomotor symptoms—1.25mg PO qd, cycle 21d on and 7d off, add a progestin days 14-21 if uterus present
  Osteoporosis prevention—0.3mg PO qd, cycle 21d on and 7d off, add a progestin days 14-21 if uterus present
  Atrophic vaginitis—0.3-1.25mg PO qd, cycle 21d on and 7d off, add a progestin days 14-21 if uterus present
  Primary ovarian failure—1-25mg PO qd
  Breast cancer palliation—10mg PO tid ×3mo
  NOTE—may be combined with **methyltestosterone**

- **Contraindications**—hypersensitivity, pregnancy, undiagnosed vaginal bleeding, thromboembolic disease, **estrogen**-dependent breast cancer
- **Caution**—lactation, hepatic dysfunction

■ **Maternal Considerations**

Esterified estrogens are prepared synthetically from plant sources. There are no indications for **esterified estrogens** during pregnancy. Recent studies suggest **estrogen** plus **medroxyprogesterone** for the treatment of menopausal symptoms increases the risk of breast cancer and cardiovascular disease. It has been long known to increase the risk of endometrial cancer. See **estradiol**.
Side effects include thromboembolism, stroke, MI, endometrial and breast cancer, gallbladder disease, pancreatitis, hypertension, breast tenderness, hepatic adenoma, bloating, nausea, vomiting, headache, dizziness, depression, weight gain, libido changes, intolerance to contact lenses, migraine, and rash.

■ **Fetal Considerations**

Estrogen has a myriad of effects on the developing embryo/fetus; many are poorly understood. See **estradiol**.

■ **Breastfeeding Safety**

See **estradiol**.

■ **References**

See **estradiol**.

■ **Summary**

- **Pregnancy Category X**
- **Lactation Category S**
- There is no indication for **estradiol** during pregnancy.
- There is no clear evidence of fetal harm after inadvertent exposure during the 1st trimester.

Estropipate (Harmonet; Ogen; Ortho-Est)

■ **Class**

Estrogen, hormone

■ **Indications**

Hormone replacement for hypogonadism, vasomotor symptoms of menopause and osteoporosis

■ **Mechanism**

Binds to estrogen receptors developing and maintaining female sex characteristics; it has both receptor- and nonreceptor-mediated activities.

■ **Dosage with Qualifiers**

Vasomotor symptoms—0.625-5mg PO qd, cycle 21d on and 7d off, add a progestin days 14-21 if uterus present
Osteoporosis prevention—0.625mg PO qd, cycle 21d on and 7d off, add a progestin days 14-21 if uterus present
Hypogonadism—1.75-7.5mg PO qd, cycle 21d on and 7d off, add a progestin days 14-21 if uterus present

- **Contraindications**—hypersensitivity, pregnancy, undiagnosed vaginal bleeding, thromboembolic disease, **estrogen**-dependent breast cancer
- **Caution**—lactation, hepatic dysfunction

■ **Maternal Considerations**

Estropipate was formerly known as piperazine estrone sulfate. There are no indications for **estropipate** during pregnancy. Recent studies suggest **estrogen** plus **medroxyprogesterone** for the treatment of menopausal symptoms increases the risk of breast cancer and cardiovascular disease. It has been long known to increase the risk of endometrial cancer. See **estradiol**.
Side effects include thromboembolism, stroke, MI, endometrial and breast cancer, gallbladder disease, pancreatitis, hypertension, breast tenderness, hepatic adenoma, bloating, nausea, vomiting, headache, dizziness, depression, weight gain, libido changes, intolerance to contact lenses, migraine, rash.

■ **Fetal Considerations**

Estrogen has a myriad of effects on the developing embryo/fetus; many are poorly understood. See **estradiol**.

■ **Breastfeeding Safety**

See **estradiol**.

■ **References**

See **estradiol**.

■ **Summary**

- **Pregnancy Category X**
- **Lactation Category S**
- There is no indication for **estropipate** during pregnancy.
- There is no clear evidence of fetal harm after inadvertent exposure during the 1st trimester.

Ethacrynic acid (Edecrin)

■ **Class**

Diuretic type 1; loop diuretic

■ **Indications**

Hypertension, peripheral edema

■ **Mechanism**

Inhibits sodium and chloride resorption in the loop of Henle and proximal/distal tubules

■ **Dosage with Qualifiers**

Hypertension—begin 25mg PO qd; max 100mg/d
Peripheral edema—25mg qd; max 200mg PO bid
- **Contraindications**—hypersensitivity, anuria
- **Caution**—renal or hepatic dysfunction

■ **Maternal Considerations**

There are no adequate reports or well-controlled studies of **ethacrynic acid** in pregnant women. **Ethacrynic acid** is a potent loop diuretic and rarely indicated. It was used in the past for preeclampsia, pulmonary edema, and diabetes insipidus.

Side effects include hepatotoxicity, neutropenia, thrombocytopenia, agranulocytosis, deafness, anorexia, abdominal pain, nausea, vomiting, diarrhea, hyperglycemia, phlebitis, deafness, tinnitus, rash, and weakness.

■ **Fetal Considerations**

There are no adequate reports or well-controlled studies in human fetuses. It is unknown whether **ethacrynic acid** crosses the human placenta. Rodent studies are reassuring, revealing no evidence of teratogenicity or IUGR despite the use of doses higher than those used clinically.

■ **Breastfeeding Safety**

There is no published experience in nursing women. It is unknown whether **ethacrynic acid** enters human breast milk.

■ **References**

Wilson AL, Matzke GR. Drug Intell Clin Pharm 1981; 15:21-6.

■ **Summary**

- **Pregnancy Category B**
- **Lactation Category U**
- Superior agents with fewer side effects for which there is more experience during pregnancy are preferred.

Ethambutol (Afimocil; Carnotol; Cidanbutol; Coxytol; Danbutol; Myambutol)

■ **Class**

Antimycobacterial

■ **Indications**

Mycobacterial infections

■ **Mechanism**

Inhibits growing *Mycobacterium*

■ **Dosage with Qualifiers**

Mycobacterial infections—15-25mg/kg qd, max 1g/dose
Tuberculosis adjuvant therapy—15-25mg/kg qd, max 2.5g/dose; given as part of multidrug therapy
NOTE—renal dosing
- **Contraindications**—hypersensitivity, optic neuritis
- **Caution**—renal dysfunction, ophthalmologic disorders

■ **Maternal Considerations**

There are no adequate reports or well-controlled studies of **ethambutol** in pregnant women. Untreated tuberculosis poses a significant threat to mother, fetus, and family. Adherence to treatment can be difficult because of a general fear of any medication and pregnancy-related nausea. All 4 first-line drugs (**isoniazid**, **rifampin**, **ethambutol,** and **pyrazinamide)** have excellent safety records in pregnancy. The published experience consists of relatively small to moderate series and case reports. **Side effects** include thrombocytopenia, neuropathy (optic, peripheral), anorexia, nausea, vomiting, joint pain, abdominal pain, fever, headache, hallucinations, pruritus, elevated LFTs.

■ **Fetal Considerations** — There are no adequate reports or well-controlled studies in human fetuses. **Ethambutol** reportedly crosses the human placenta achieving an F:M ratio approximating unity. There are no reports suggesting an adverse fetal effect. Rodent studies are reassuring, revealing no evidence of teratogenicity or IUGR despite the use of doses higher than those used clinically.

■ **Breastfeeding Safety** — There are no adequate reports or well-controlled studies in nursing women. Only small quantities of **ethambutol** are excreted into breast milk, and it is generally considered compatible with breastfeeding. The dose ingested by the neonate is inadequate to treat tuberculosis.

■ **References** — Tripathy SN. Int J Gynaecol Obstet 2003; 80:247-53.
Bothamley G. Drug Saf 2001; 24:553-65.
Brost BC, Newman RB. Obstet Gynecol Clin North Am 1997; 24:659-73.
Holdiness MR. Early Hum Dev 1987; 15:61-74.
Tran JH, Montakantikul P. J Hum Lact 1998; 14:337-40.
Shneerson JM, Francis RS. Tubercle 1979; 60:167-9.

■ **Summary** —
- **Pregnancy Category B**
- **Lactation Category S**
- Pregnancy does not alter the importance of treating mycobacterial infection.
- **Ethambutol** is considered safe and effective during pregnancy and lactation.

Ethinyl estradiol (Estinyl; Feminone; Mikrofollin)

■ **Class** — Estrogen, hormone

■ **Indications** — Contraception (used with a progestational agent), vasomotor symptoms, osteoporosis prevention, atrophic vaginitis, primary ovarian failure, breast cancer palliation

■ **Mechanism** — Synthetic estradiol with both receptor- and nonreceptor-mediated activities

- **Dosage with Qualifiers** ⋯⋯⋯ Vasomotor symptoms—1-2mg PO qd, cycle 21d on and 7d off, add a progestin days 14-21 if uterus present
Osteoporosis prevention—0.5mg PO qd, cycle 21d on and 7d off, add a progestin days 14-21 if uterus present
Atrophic vaginitis—1-2mg PO qd, cycle 21d on and 7d off, add a progestin days 14-21 if uterus present
Primary ovarian failure—1-2mg PO qd
Breast cancer palliation—10mg PO tid ×3mo
  - **Contraindications**—hypersensitivity, pregnancy, undiagnosed vaginal bleeding, thromboembolic disease, estrogen-dependent breast cancer
  - **Caution**—lactation, hepatic dysfunction

- **Maternal Considerations** ⋯⋯⋯ There are no indications for **estradiol** during pregnancy. Recent studies suggest **estrogen** plus **medroxyprogesterone** for the treatment of menopausal symptoms increases the risk of breast cancer and cardiovascular disease.
Side effects include thromboembolism, stroke, MI, endometrial and breast cancer, gallbladder disease, pancreatitis, hypertension, breast tenderness, hepatic adenoma, bloating, nausea, vomiting, headache, dizziness, depression, weight gain, libido changes, intolerance to contact lenses, migraine, rash.

- **Fetal Considerations** ⋯⋯⋯ There are no adequate reports or well-controlled studies in human fetuses. While **diethylstilbestrol** and other synthetic/environmental estrogens are recognized teratogens with the potential for transgenerational effects, few studies support this effect for naturally occurring substances like **estradiol**. There is no clear evidence of fetal harm after inadvertent exposure during the 1st trimester. Some studies have suggested prenatal exposure to **estradiol** might alter immune programming.

- **Breastfeeding Safety** ⋯⋯⋯ Though **estradiol** is excreted into breast milk and has been reported to reduce the amount of milk produced, it is not effective as an inhibitor of lactation. All pharmacokinetic studies have shown that the transfer to breast milk of both **progesterone** and **estrogen** when taking a contraceptive pill is of the same order as natural hormones. **Estrogen**-containing contraceptives should be initiated after the 6th week of lactation when the lipid profile has returned to normal and the risk of thrombosis is identical to that of the general population.

- **References** ⋯⋯⋯ See **estradiol**.

- **Summary** ⋯⋯⋯
  - **Pregnancy Category X**
  - **Lactation Category S**
  - There is no indication for **estradiol** during pregnancy.
  - There is no clear evidence of fetal harm after inadvertent exposure during the 1st trimester.

Ethosuximide (Thosutin; Zarontin)

■ **Class** — Anticonvulsant

■ **Indications** — Treatment of absence epilepsy (petit mal)

■ **Mechanism** — Depresses motor cortex and elevates the threshold of the CNS for convulsion

■ **Dosage with Qualifiers** — Absence epilepsy—250mg PO bid; monitor levels, max 1.5g/d
- **Contraindications**—hypersensitivity
- **Caution**—bone marrow depression, hepatic or renal dysfunction, mixed seizures, abrupt withdrawal, porphyria

■ **Maternal Considerations** — There are no adequate reports or well-controlled studies of **ethosuximide** in pregnant women. Metabolism does not appear to be significantly altered by pregnancy, only the volume of distribution. Patients may experience drowsiness. Discontinuation of the drug may be considered during pregnancy if the risk of convulsion does not pose a significant health threat to the mother. There is no interaction between **ethosuximide** and oral contraceptive agents.
Side effects include agranulocytosis, SLE, Stevens-Johnson syndrome, pancytopenia, anorexia, dyspepsia, nausea, vomiting, diarrhea, irritability, headache, dizziness, rash, hirsutism, and gingival hyperplasia.

■ **Fetal Considerations** — There are no adequate reports or well-controlled studies in human fetuses. **Ethosuximide** crosses the human placenta achieving an F:M ratio approximating unity. The associations between **ethosuximide** and either birth defects or behavioral disorders are unclear.

■ **Breastfeeding Safety** — There are no adequate reports or well-controlled studies in nursing women. **Ethosuximide** is excreted into human breast milk achieving M:P ratios approximating 0.8-0.9 with an estimated total exposure of 3.6-11mg/kg. Serum concentrations in breast-fed neonates range from 15-40ng/ml.

■ **References** — Tomson T, Villen T. Ther Drug Monit 1994; 16:621-3.
Tejerizo Lopez LC, de Santiago Obeso J, Henriquez Esquiroz JM, et al. An Esp Pediatr 1987; 27:352-6.
Samren EB, van Duijn CM, Koch S, et al. Epilepsia 1997; 38:981-90.
Kuhnz W, Koch S, Jakob S, et al. Br J Clin Pharmacol 1984; 18:671-7.
Koup JR, Rose JQ, Cohen ME. Epilepsia 1978; 19:535-9.

- **Pregnancy Category C**
- **Lactation Category S**
- **Ethosuximide** should be used during pregnancy and lactation only if the benefit justifies the potential perinatal risk.

Ethyl alcohol (Ethanol)

■ **Class** — *Toxicology*

■ **Indications** — Methanol or ethylene glycol intoxication

■ **Mechanism** — Inhibits alcohol dehydrogenase

■ **Dosage with Qualifiers** — Methanol intoxication—begin 1000mg/kg IV over 1-2h, then 100mg/kg/h IV over 1-2h to keep ethanol level at 100-130mcg/dl
Ethylene glycol intoxication—begin 1000mg/kg IV over 1-2h, then 100mg/kg/h IV over 1-2h to keep ethanol level at 100-130mcg/dl

- **Contraindications**—hypersensitivity, epilepsy, diabetic coma
- **Caution**—hepatic or renal dysfunction, diabetes mellitus, gout

■ **Maternal Considerations** — **Ethyl alcohol** is one of the most commonly abused drugs during pregnancy. The patient may misrepresent **ethyl alcohol** use. Antenatal alcohol interviews have the greatest correlation with postnatal outcome and should be part of each prenatal record.
Side effects include euphoria and intoxication.

■ **Fetal Considerations** — **Ethyl alcohol** is the most common teratogen (prevalence 0.5-2/1000 births) and typically reflects chronic consumption. In addition to the well-described fetal alcohol syndrome (pre- and postnatal IUGR, CNS anomalies, and a wide spectrum of malformations, the most typical being the craniofacial features), recent evidence suggests **ethyl alcohol** may decrease endothelial responses. Tobacco and/or cocaine use are synergistic in their adverse fetal effects. The effects of antenatal exposure on brain development are varied.

■ **Breastfeeding Safety** — **Ethyl alcohol** is excreted into the breast milk, but the quantity ingested by the neonate is too small to have a significant impact.

■ **References** ·············· Turcotte LA, Aberle NS, Norby FL, et al. Alcohol 2002; 26:75-81.
Jacobson SW, Chiodo LM, Sokol RJ, Jacobson JL. Pediatrics 2002; 109:815-25.
Mattson SN, Schoenfeld AM, Riley EP. Alcohol Res Health 2001; 25:185-91.

■ **Summary** ··············
- **Pregnancy Category X**
- **Lactation Category S**
- Each intake interview during pregnancy should include specific questions on maternal **ethyl alcohol** usage.

Etidocaine hydrochloride (Duranest)

■ **Class** ·············· *Anesthetic, local*

■ **Indications** ·············· Anesthesia for minor surgery

■ **Mechanism** ·············· Stabilizes the neuronal membrane by inhibiting ionic fluxes required for initiation and transmission

■ **Dosage with Qualifiers** ·············· Nerve block—max 8mg/kg at a single injection up to 400mg
NOTE—contains **epinephrine**
- **Contraindications**—hypersensitivity
- **Caution**— severe shock, heart block, peripheral vascular disease, hypertension

■ **Maternal Considerations** ·············· **Etidocaine** is a rapid onset (3-5min), long duration (5-10h) local anesthetic agent with more profound motor block than seen after injection of equianalgesic concentrations of **bupivacaine**. It is a popular agent in some locales for use in labor epidural and spinal anesthesia. However, it is not used for labor epidural analgesia due to the motor block. There are no adequate and well-controlled
studies of **etidocaine** in pregnant women. Tachycardia may be a sign of intravascular injection.
Side effects include maternal hypotension, fetal bradycardia (after paracervical block), tachycardia, convulsions, nervousness, and lightheadedness.

■ **Fetal Considerations** ·············· There are no adequate reports or well-controlled studies in human fetuses. **Etidocaine** crosses the human placenta achieving an F:M ratio approximating 0.3. Uterine blood flow is preserved in the absence of maternal hypotension. Local anesthetics cross when used for epidural, paracervical, pudendal or caudal nerve blocks may cause varying degrees of toxicity. Rodent studies are reassuring, revealing no evidence of teratogenicity or IUGR despite the use of doses higher than those used clinically.

■ **Breastfeeding Safety** .... There is no published experience in nursing women. It is unknown whether **etidocaine** enters human breast milk. Considering the indications and dosing, limited **etidocaine** use is unlikely to pose a clinically significant risk to the breast-feeding neonate.

■ **References** .... Nau H. Dev Pharmacol Ther 1985; 8:149-81.
Morgan DJ, Cousins MJ, McQuillan D, Thomas J. Eur J Clin Pharmacol 1977; 12:359-65.
Wilson J Acta Anesth Scand Suppl 1975; 60:97-9.

■ **Summary** ....
- **Pregnancy Category B**
- **Lactation Category S**
- A local anesthetic with a large clinical experience during pregnancy.

Etidronate (Didronel)

■ **Class** .... *Bisphosphonates*

■ **Indications** .... Paget's disease, hypercalcemia

■ **Mechanism** .... Inhibits bone formation, growth and osteoclast reabsorption

■ **Dosage with Qualifiers** .... Paget's disease—5-10mg/kg/d; max 10mg/kg/d for <6m, or 11-20mg/kg/d for <3m
Hypercalcemia—7.5 mg/kg/d IV ×3-7d, then 20mg/kg/d PO ×30-90d
- **Contraindications**—hypersensitivity, renal dysfunction
- **Caution**—long bone fracture, enterocolitis, cardiac failure

■ **Maternal Considerations** .... There is no published experience with **etidronate** during pregnancy.
Side effects include fractures, seizures, nausea, vomiting, diarrhea, and bone pain.

■ **Fetal Considerations** .... There are no adequate reports or well-controlled studies in human fetuses. It is unknown whether **etidronate** crosses the human placenta. Rodent studies are reassuring, revealing no evidence of teratogenicity or IUGR despite the use of doses higher than those used clinically.

■ **Breastfeeding Safety** .... There is no published experience in nursing women. It is unknown whether **etidronate** is excreted into human breast milk.

■ **References** .... Nolen GA, Buehler EV. Toxicol Appl Pharmacol 1971; 18:548-61.

- **Summary** .... • **Pregnancy Category B**
  - **Lactation Category U**
  - There is no published experience during pregnancy.
  - **Etidronate** should be used during pregnancy and lactation only if the benefit justifies the potential perinatal risk.

Etodolac (Lodine)

- **Class** .... NSAID

- **Indications** .... Mild to moderate pain, osteoarthritis, rheumatoid arthritis

- **Mechanism** .... Inhibits cyclooxygenase, lipoxygenase and reduces prostaglandin synthesis

- **Dosage with Qualifiers** .... Pain—200-400mg PO q6-8h prn, max 1.2g qd
  Osteoarthritis—300-500mg PO bid, max 1.2g qd
  Rheumatoid arthritis—300-500mg PO bid, max 1.2g qd
  - **Contraindications**—hypersensitivity to it or other NSAIDs
  - **Caution**—GI bleeding, hypertension, CHF

- **Maternal Considerations** .... **Etodolac** is an NSAID antipyretic analgesic. There is no published experience during human pregnancy. See **indomethacin**.
  Side effects include anaphylaxis, GI bleeding, acute renal failure, thrombocytopenia, agranulocytosis, interstitial nephritis, hepatotoxicity, Stevens-Johnson syndrome, dyspepsia, nausea, constipation, tinnitus, and fluid retention.

- **Fetal Considerations** .... There are no adequate reports or well-controlled studies in human fetuses. It is unknown whether **etodolac** crosses the human placenta. Other NSAIDs do cross. The pharmacologic profile suggests it is likely to have risks similar to those of **indomethacin** including oligohydramnios and ductal constriction. Rodent studies performed at doses approximating the recommended human dose are associated with an increased prevalence of limb abnormalities. Higher doses delayed parturition and increased the perinatal loss rate. See **indomethacin**.

- **Breastfeeding Safety** .... There is no published experience in nursing women. It is not known whether **etodolac** is excreted into human breast milk. See **indomethacin**.

- **References** .... No published experience in pregnancy or during lactation.

■ **Summary**

- **Pregnancy Category C**
- **Lactation Category U**
- The pharmacologic profile suggests it is likely to have risks similar to those of **indomethacin**.
- There are alternative agents for which there is more experience during pregnancy and lactation.

Etomidate (Amidate)

■ **Class**

Anesthetic, general

■ **Indications**

Induction of general anesthesia

■ **Mechanism**

Unknown

■ **Dosage with Qualifiers**

Induction of general anesthesia—0.3mg/kg IV (range 0.2-0.6mg/kg) over 30-60sec
- **Contraindications**—hypersensitivity
- **Caution**—unknown

■ **Maternal Considerations**

Etomidate is a short-acting (3-5min) hypnotic drug without analgesic activity. It has little to no effect on cardiac contractility, and is therefore used to induce general anesthesia for cesarean delivery in women with coexisting cardiac disease.
Side effects include shock, myoclonic movements, nausea, vomiting, apnea, and injection site reactions.

■ **Fetal Considerations**

There are no adequate reports or well-controlled studies in human fetuses. Transfer across the rodent placenta occurs, reaching concentrations roughly equal to maternal plasma. Rodent studies reveal no evidence of teratogenicity, though embryo and fetal toxicity occurs, and IUGR is seen when the mothers are exposed long-term to high concentrations.

■ **Breastfeeding Safety**

There is no published experience in pregnancy. It is unknown whether **etomidate** crosses the human placenta. However, considering the indications, it is unlikely the breast-fed neonate would ingest clinically relevant amounts.

■ **References**

Beltrame D, di Salle E, Giavini E, et al. Reprod Toxicol 2001; 15:195-213.
Downing JW, Buley RJ, Brock-Utne JG, Houlton PC. Br J Anaesth 1979; 51:135-40.
Houlton PJ, Downing JW, Buley RJ, Brock-Utne JG. S Afr Med J 1978; 54:773-5.

■ Summary
- **Pregnancy Category C**
- **Lactation Category S?**
- **Etomidate** should be used during pregnancy and lactation only if the benefit justifies the potential perinatal risk.
- There are alternative agents for which there is more experience during pregnancy and lactation.

Etretinate (Tegison)

■ **Class** — Dermatologic; retinoid

■ **Indications** — Severe psoriasis

■ **Mechanism** — Unknown

■ **Dosage with Qualifiers** — Severe psoriasis—0.75-1mg/kg in 2 to 3 divided doses until response, then maintenance of 0.5-0.75mg/kg/d; max 1.5mg/kg
- **Contraindications**—hypersensitivity
- **Caution**—hepatic dysfunction

■ **Maternal Considerations** — There are no published studies in pregnant women. Drug levels may persist for years after treatment, though the relevance of these levels to subsequent pregnancy outcome is unknown. Psoriasis is not lethal, and the use of **etretinate** is absolutely contraindicated during pregnancy. Women should be tested for pregnancy within 2w of initiating therapy and use effective contraception. *Side effects* include pseudotumor cerebri, hepatotoxicity, corneal opacities, hyperostosis, hyperlipidemia, and elevated hepatic transaminases.

■ **Fetal Considerations** — **Etretinate** is a human and rodent teratogen with the majority of fetuses exposed during organogenesis affected. Multiple organ systems are affected including neural tube defects, facial dysmorphia, limb and digit malformations, microcephaly and skeletal defects. Exposed fetuses should be referred to an appropriate fetal evaluation unit. **Etretinate** has been used to treat harlequin fetuses with improvement in their skin condition but no change in mortality.

■ **Breastfeeding Safety** — There is no published experience in nursing women. It is unknown whether **etretinate** enters human breast milk. It is excreted into rodent milk.

■ **References** — Beltrame D, di Salle E, Giavini E, et al. Reprod Toxicol 2001; 15:195-213.

Reiners J, Lofberg B, Kraft JC, Kochhar DM, Nau H. Reprod Toxicol 1988; 2:19-29.

■ **Summary**
- **Pregnancy Category X**
- **Lactation Category U**
- **Etretinate** is absolutely contraindicated during pregnancy.

Exemestane (Aromasin)

■ **Class**
Antineoplastic; hormone modifier

■ **Indications**
Estrogen-sensitive breast cancer in women who have progressed on **tamoxifen**

■ **Mechanism**
Irreversible, steroid aromatase inhibitor

■ **Dosage with Qualifiers**
Adjuvant therapy for breast cancer—25mg PO qd
- **Contraindications**—hypersensitivity
- **Caution**—hepatic or renal dysfunction

■ **Maternal Considerations**
There is no published experience with **exemestane** during pregnancy.
Side effects include hot flashes, nausea, fatigue, increased sweating, and increased appetite.

■ **Fetal Considerations**
There are no adequate reports or well-controlled studies in human fetuses. It is unknown whether **exemestane** crosses the human placenta. It does cross the rodent placenta, achieving concentrations roughly equal to maternal plasma. While an increase in embryo resorption and IUGR are seen, there is no increase in the incidence of malformations.

■ **Breastfeeding Safety**
There is no published experience in nursing women. It is unknown whether **exemestane** enters human breast milk. It is excreted into rodent milk.

■ **References**
Beltrame D, di Salle E, Giavini E, et al. Reprod Toxicol 2001; 15:195-213.

■ **Summary**
- **Pregnancy Category D**
- **Lactation Category U**
- **Exemestane** should be used during pregnancy and lactation only if the benefit justifies the potential perinatal risk.

Factor IX (Alphanine; Bebulin VH; Immuno; Konyne 80; Mononine; Profilnine SD; Proplex T)

■ **Class** — Blood components/substitute

■ **Indications** — Factor IX deficiency (prevention and control of bleeding), treatment of anticoagulant overdose

■ **Mechanism** — Factor IX replacement

■ **Dosage with Qualifiers** — Bleeding—dose (IU) = kg × % desired increase ×1.2 (1.2 for recombinant otherwise ×1 for concentrate) given slow IV push
Prophylaxis—20-30IU/kg 1-2×/w given slow IV push
Anticoagulant overdose—(kg × % desired increase in Factor IX) given slow IV push
  • **Contraindications**—hypersensitivity to mouse proteins, hepatic dysfunction, DIC, hyperfibrinolytic states
  • **Caution**—thrombophilia

■ **Maternal Considerations** — **Factor IX** is a stabile, lyophilized concentrate either recombinant or made from pooled human plasma. It is purified by immunoaffinity chromatography, which reduces the risk of virus transmission. There are no adequate reports or well-controlled studies in pregnant women. **Factor IX** deficiency is typically an X-linked disorder, and thus symptoms occur only in women with unbalanced lyonization.
Side effects include thromboembolic disease, viral disease, flushing, tingling, fever, chills, nausea, vomiting, urticaria, headache, blood pressure changes, and injection site reaction.

■ **Fetal Considerations** — There are no adequate reports or well-controlled studies in human fetuses. Placental transfer is unlikely. Rodent teratogenicity studies have not been conducted.

■ **Breastfeeding Safety** — There are no adequate reports or well-controlled studies in nursing women. It is unknown whether **factor IX** enters human breast milk. However, any ingested factor would likely be degraded.

■ **References** — Shobeiri SA, West EC, Kahn MJ, Nolan TE. Obstet Gynecol Surv 2000; 55:729-37.

■ **Summary** —
  • **Pregnancy Category C**
  • **Lactation Category S**
  • Rarely indicated in pregnancy or during lactation.

Famciclovir (Famvir)

- **Class** — Antiviral

- **Indications** — Treatment of genital herpes and herpes zoster

- **Mechanism** — Inhibits viral DNA polymerase

- **Dosage with Qualifiers** — Genital herpes (1st episode)—250mg PO tid ×7d
  Genital herpes (recurrent)—125mg PO bid ×5d
  Genital herpes (prophylaxis)—250mg PO bid
  Herpes zoster—500mg PO tid ×7d
  NOTE—renal dosing
  - **Contraindications**—hypersensitivity
  - **Caution**—renal dysfunction

- **Maternal Considerations** — **Famciclovir** is metabolized to the active **penciclovir**. There are no adequate reports or well-controlled studies in pregnant women. With a dosing profile superior to **acyclovir**, drugs in this class decrease both asymptomatic shedding and the number of clinical recurrences. It is likely that the same is true during pregnancy, a supposition supported by randomized trials and cohort studies demonstrating a lower-than-expected asymptomatic shedding rate. Drug clearance is slower in nonpregnant women compared to men.
  Side effects include headache, nausea, vomiting, diarrhea, fatigue, itching, paresthesias, and flatulence.

- **Fetal Considerations** — There are no adequate reports or well-controlled studies in human fetuses. It is unknown whether **famciclovir** crosses the human placenta. Rodent studies are reassuring, revealing no evidence of teratogenicity or IUGR despite the use of doses higher than those used clinically.

- **Breastfeeding Safety** — There is no published experience in nursing women. It is unknown whether **famciclovir** is excreted in human breast milk. **Famciclovir** is excreted in concentrations higher than plasma in lactating rats.

- **References** — Leung DT, Sacks SL. Drugs 2000; 60:1329-52.
  Baker DA. Int J Fertil Womens Med 1998; 43:243-8.
  Scott LL. Clin Obstet Gynecol 1999; 42:134-48.

- **Summary**
  - **Pregnancy Category B**
  - **Lactation Category U**
  - This class of agents has several potential applications during pregnancy.
  - Physicians are encouraged to register pregnant women under the Famciclovir Pregnancy Registry (1-888-669-6682) maintained by the manufacturer for a better follow-up of the outcome while under treatment with **famciclovir**.

Famotidine (Pepcid)

- **Class** — *Antiulcer; antihistamine; anti-GERD*

- **Indications** — Treatment of gastric ulcer disease, GERD, and Zollinger-Ellison syndrome

- **Mechanism** — H_2-receptor antagonist

- **Dosage with Qualifiers** — GERD—20-40mg PO qhs for 12w
  Gastric ulcer—20-40mg PO qhs for 4-6w
  Zollinger-Ellison syndrome—20-60mg PO q6h, max 160mg PO q6h
  NOTE—renal dosing
  - **Contraindications**—hypersensitivity, PKU
  - **Caution**—renal dysfunction

- **Maternal Considerations** — There are no adequate reports or well-controlled studies in pregnant women. There are only rare reports of its use during pregnancy. A single dose of **famotidine** administered to parturients PO 3h before surgery is more effective neutralizing gastric secretion than **omeprazole**. *Side effects* include pancytopenia, leukopenia, thrombocytopenia, jaundice, bronchospasm, headache, taste change, constipation, diarrhea, acne, dizziness, dry skin, periorbital edema, myalgias, elevated LFTs, tinnitus, proteinuria, and elevated BUN/creatinine levels.

- **Fetal Considerations** — There are no adequate reports or well-controlled studies in human fetuses. **Famotidine** crosses the placenta achieving an F:M ratio approximating 0.40. Rodent studies are reassuring, revealing no evidence of teratogenicity or IUGR despite the use of doses higher than those used clinically.

- **Breastfeeding Safety** — There are no adequate reports or well-controlled studies in nursing women. **Famotidine** is excreted into human milk to a lesser extent than **cimetidine** and **ranitidine**, though the kinetics remain to be elucidated.

- **References** — Jacoby EB, Porter KB. Am J Perinatol 1999; 16:85-8.
  Lin CJ, Huang CL, Hsu HW, Chen TL. Acta Anaesthesiol Sin 1996; 34:179-84.
  Dicke JM, Johnson RF, Henderson GI, et al. Am J Med Sci 1988; 295:198-206.

- **Summary** —
  - **Pregnancy Category B**
  - **Lactation Category U**
  - **Famotidine** is effective for the treatment of GERD and peptic ulcer disease, and has a reassuring safety profile in animals.
  - There is little published experience during human pregnancy and lactation.

Felbamate (Felbatol; Taloxa)

■ **Class** — Anticonvulsant

■ **Indications** — Second-line therapy for seizure disorders

■ **Mechanism** — Unknown

■ **Dosage with Qualifiers** — Seizure disorder—400-1200mg PO tid (max 3600mg/d)
NOTE—renal dosing
- **Contraindications**—hypersensitivity
- **Caution**—hepatic or renal dysfunction, history of blood dyscrasias

■ **Maternal Considerations** — Epilepsy is a common neurologic disorder affecting 1 million American reproductive-age women. There are no adequate reports or well-controlled studies of **felbamate** in pregnant women. Drug interactions between enzyme-inducing antiepileptic drugs like **felbamate** and hormonal contraceptives are well documented, increasing the risk of an unplanned pregnancy. Using either a higher hormone content oral contraceptive or a second contraceptive is suggested. Planned pregnancy is highly recommended and counseling before conception is crucial covering folic acid supplementation, optimal control of seizure activity, monotherapy with the lowest effective antiepileptic drug dose, and medication adherence. Drug dose adjustments are often necessary and should be based on clinical symptoms and not solely on serum drug concentrations. *Side effects* include aplastic anemia, hepatic failure, anorexia, nausea, vomiting, headache, insomnia, dizziness, somnolence, constipation, nervousness, tremor, diplopia, depression, abdominal pain, and ataxia.

■ **Fetal Considerations** — There are no adequate reports or well-controlled studies in human fetuses. It is unknown whether **felbamate** crosses the human placenta. It does cross the rodent placenta. Rodent studies are reassuring, revealing no evidence of teratogenicity despite the use of doses higher than those used clinically. IUGR was noted.

■ **Breastfeeding Safety** — There are no adequate reports or well-controlled studies in nursing women. **Felbamate** is excreted into human breast milk, though the kinetics remain to be elucidated. **Felbamate** is excreted into rodent breast milk, and there is a higher neonatal death rate in breast-fed pups. If breastfeeding continues, the infant should be monitored for possible adverse effects, the drug given at the lowest effective dose, and breastfeeding avoided at times of peak drug levels.

■ **References** — Chang SI, McAuley JW. Ann Pharmacother 1998; 32:794-801.
Morrell MJ. Epilepsia 1996; 37(Suppl 6):S34-44.

■ **Summary** .... • **Pregnancy Category C**
• **Lactation Category U**
• **Felbamate** is a second-line treatment for several seizure disorders.
• **Felbamate** should be used during pregnancy and lactation only if the benefit justifies the potential perinatal risk.

Felodipine (Plendil)

■ **Class** .... Antihypertensive; calcium-channel blocker

■ **Indications** .... Treatment of chronic hypertension

■ **Mechanism** .... Dihydropyridine calcium-channel blocker

■ **Dosage with Qualifiers** .... Chronic hypertension—5mg PO qd (max 20mg/d)
• **Contraindications**—hypersensitivity
• **Caution**—hepatic dysfunction, CHF

■ **Maternal Considerations** .... There are no adequate reports or well-controlled studies of **felodipine** in pregnant women. The published experience consists of isolated case reports where **felodipine** was used successfully for the treatment of severe hypertension during pregnancy without adverse effect. Calcium-channel blockers are the most effective tocolytic agents. **Felodipine** decreases placental blood flow and prolongs parturition in rabbits.
Side effects include edema, headache, flushing, dizziness, nausea, abdominal pain, diarrhea, rhinorrhea, chest pain, palpitations, muscle cramps, and weakness.

■ **Fetal Considerations** .... There are no adequate reports or well-controlled studies in human fetuses. It is unknown whether **felodipine** crosses the human placenta. **Felodipine** is associated with an increased prevalence of digital anomalies in rodents possibly secondary to the observed decrease in placental blood flow. Prolonged parturition is associated with an increased perinatal mortality.

■ **Breastfeeding Safety** .... There is no published experience in nursing women. It is unknown whether **felodipine** enters human breast milk. It is excreted into rodent milk.

■ **References** .... Casele HL, Windley KC, Prieto JA, et al. J Reprod Med 1997; 42:378-81.
Danielson MK, Danielsson BR. Arzneimittelforschung 1993; 43:106-9.
Lundgren Y, Thalen P, Nordlander M. Pharmacol Toxicol 1992; 71:361-4.

Danielsson BR, Reiland S, Rundqvist E, Danielson M. Teratology 1989; 40:351-8.

■ **Summary**
- **Pregnancy Category C**
- **Lactation Category U**
- **Felodipine** should be used during pregnancy and lactation only if the benefit justifies the potential perinatal risk.
- There are other agents with a superior safety profile for which there is more experience during pregnancy and lactation.

Fenofibrate (Tricor)

■ **Class** — Antihyperlipidemic, cholesterol-lowering

■ **Indications** — Hyperlipidemia

■ **Mechanism** — Unclear; interferes with triglyceride synthesis

■ **Dosage with Qualifiers** — Hypertriglyceridemia—begin 54mg PO qd with meals adjusting q4-8w; max 160mg qd
Hypercholesterolemia—begin 54mg PO qd with meals adjusting q4-8w; max 160mg qd
Mixed dyslipidemia—begin 54mg PO qd with meals adjusting q4-8w; max 160mg qd
NOTE—54mg tablet = 67mg capsule
- **Contraindications**—hypersensitivity, hepatic or renal dysfunction, gallbladder disease
- **Caution**—oral anticoagulants

■ **Maternal Considerations** — There are no adequate reports or well-controlled studies of **fenofibrate** in pregnant women. One rodent study concludes that pregnant and nonpregnant rats respond differently to **fenofibrate**, and that high maternal doses were associated with delayed delivery. Hyperlipidemia is not acutely life-threatening. Cessation of medication during pregnancy is suggested.
Side effects include hepatitis, pancreatitis, cholelithiasis, myositis, myopathy, elevated LFTs, abdominal pain, headache, constipation, rhinitis, and nausea.

■ **Fetal Considerations** — There are no adequate reports or well-controlled studies in human fetuses. It is unknown whether **fenofibrate** crosses the human placenta. **Fenofibrate** causes IUGR given at doses equivalent to the recommended human dose, and is embryotoxic and teratogenic (predominantly bony abnormalities) at doses 7-10 times the MRHD.

There is no published experience in nursing women. It is unknown whether **fenofibrate** enters human breast milk.

■ **References** Soria A, Bocos C, Herrera E. J Lipid Res 2002; 43:74-81.

■ **Summary**
- **Pregnancy Category C**
- **Lactation Category U**
- **Fenofibrate** should be used during pregnancy and lactation only if the benefit justifies the potential perinatal risk.
- Hyperlipidemia is not acutely life threatening. Cessation of medication during pregnancy is suggested.
- There are alternative agents for which there is more experience during pregnancy and lactation.

Fenoldopam (Corlopam)

■ **Class** *Antihypertensive*

■ **Indications** Acute severe hypertension

■ **Mechanism** Dopamine D_1-like and α-2 adrenergic receptor agonist

■ **Dosage with Qualifiers** Severe hypertension—0.025-0.3mcg/kg/min IV; increase q15min 0.05-0.1mcg/kg/min until reaching max dose of 1.6mcg/kg/min for 48h
- **Contraindications**—hypersensitivity
- **Caution**—glaucoma, acute cerebral vascular disease, hypokalemia, sulfite allergy, asthma, hepatic dysfunction

■ **Maternal Considerations** **Fenoldopam** is an alternative for treatment of a hypertensive crisis if unresponsive to **sodium nitroprusside**. There are no adequate reports or well-controlled studies of **fenoldopam** in pregnant women. In isolated systems, it causes relaxation of the rodent myometrium.
Side effects include reflex tachycardia, MI, CHF, arrhythmias, leukocytosis, hypokalemia, headache, flushing, nausea, vomiting, sweating, back pain, abdominal pain, palpitations, constipation, and nasal congestion.

■ **Fetal Considerations** There are no adequate reports or well-controlled studies in human fetuses. It is unknown whether **fenoldopam** crosses the human placenta. It relaxes thromboxane constricted human umbilical arteries. Rodent studies are reassuring, revealing no evidence of teratogenicity or IUGR despite the use of doses higher than those used clinically. **Fenoldopam** induces a diuresis in fetal sheep.

■ **Breastfeeding Safety** ⋯⋯⋯⋯ There are no adequate reports or well-controlled studies in nursing women. It is unknown whether **fenoldopam** enters human breast milk. It is excreted into rodent milk.

■ **References** ⋯⋯⋯⋯⋯⋯⋯⋯ Sato N, Tanaka KA, Szlam F, et al. Anesth Analg 2003; 96:539-44.
Estan L, Berenguer A, Martinez-Mir I, et al. Gen Pharmacol 1993; 24:397-401.
Segar JL, Smith FG, Guillery EN, et al. Am J Physiol 1992; 263:R868-73.

■ **Summary** ⋯⋯⋯⋯⋯⋯⋯⋯⋯⋯ • **Pregnancy Category B**
• **Lactation Category U**
• **Fenoldopam** is an alternative to **sodium nitroprusside** in women with hypertensive crisis unresponsive to other antihypertensive agents.

Fenoprofen (Nalfon)

■ **Class** ⋯⋯⋯⋯⋯⋯⋯⋯⋯⋯⋯⋯ *Analgesic*; NSAID

■ **Indications** ⋯⋯⋯⋯⋯⋯⋯⋯ Arthritis, mild to moderate pain

■ **Mechanism** ⋯⋯⋯⋯⋯⋯⋯⋯ Inhibits both cyclooxygenase and lipoxygenase; reduces prostaglandin synthesis

■ **Dosage with Qualifiers** ⋯⋯ Osteoarthritis or rheumatoid arthritis—300-600mg PO tid/qid; max 3200mg/d
Pain relief—200mg PO q4-6h prn
NOTE—take with meals
• **Contraindications**—hypersensitivity to drug or class, NSAID asthma
• **Caution**—GI bleeding, hypertension, CHF, nasal polyps

■ **Maternal Considerations** ⋯⋯ **Fenoprofen** is a non-steroidal, anti-inflammatory, antipyretic agent. There are no adequate reports or well-controlled studies of **fenoprofen** in pregnant women. Similar to other NSAIDs, it is effective for the relief of episiotomy pain. In rodents, **fenoprofen** prolongs parturition, and it reduces contractions of isolated myometrium from monkeys and humans.
Side effects include anaphylaxis, GI bleeding, renal failure, bronchospasm, thrombocytopenia, agranulocytosis, hepatic toxicity, dyspepsia, nausea, headache, constipation, abdominal pain, dizziness, rash, fluid retention, and tinnitus.

- **Fetal Considerations** There are no adequate reports or well-controlled studies in human fetuses. It is unknown whether **fenoprofen** crosses the human placenta. **Fenoprofen** prolongs gestation in rodents, as do other NSAIDs. It is otherwise poorly studied during pregnancy.

- **Breastfeeding Safety** There is no published experience in nursing women. It is unknown whether **fenoprofen** enters human breast milk.

- **References** Johnson WL, Harbert GM, Martin CB. Am J Obstet Gynecol 1975; 123:364-75.
Gruber CM, Bauer RO, Bettigole JB, et al. J Med 1979; 10:65-8.

- **Summary**
  - **Pregnancy Category B (D in 3rd trimester)**
  - **Lactation Category U**
  - **Fenoprofen** offers no clear advantage over other NSAIDs for which there is more experience during pregnancy and lactation.

Fentanyl (Fentanyl Oralet; Oralet; Sublimaze)

- **Class** *Analgesic, narcotic; anesthetic, general*

- **Indications** Anesthesia, preoperative analgesia, regional anesthesia, postoperative pain relief

- **Mechanism** Binds to various opiate receptors

- **Dosage with Qualifiers** Preoperative analgesia—50-100mcg IV 30-60min prior to surgery
Anesthesia, adjunct—2-50mcg/kg IV depending on needs
Labor epidural anesthesia—approximately 25mcg intrathecal; 40-50mcg epidural: usually followed by a dose of 20-30mcg/hr mixed in solution of dilute local anesthetics (consult a specialty text)
Labor analgesia (IV)—begin 50mcg IV, thereafter 25mcg q20-30min prn
Postoperative pain relief—50-100mcg IV q1-2h prn
NOTE—also available in oral and transdermal forms
  - **Contraindications**—hypersensitivity to drug or class
  - **Caution**—hepatic, renal, or pulmonary dysfunction, bowel obstruction, CNS depressant use, hypotension, biliary disease, seizure disorder, inflammatory bowel disease

- **Maternal Considerations** **Fentanyl** is a short-acting opiate with considerable risk of abuse. It is often combined during labor with local anesthetics to minimize motor blockade for epidural anesthesia. **Fentanyl** may be used safely in women with severe preeclampsia. It is a useful adjunct to a paracervical block for suction curettage. The chance of a successful external version is increased by its use with spinal blockade.

Side effects include respiratory depression or arrest, dependency, laryngospasm, bronchospasm, arrhythmias, ileus, cardiac arrest, nausea, vomiting, weakness, dry mouth, confusion, sweating euphoria, itching, hypotension, and bradycardia.

■ **Fetal Considerations**

There are no adequate reports or well-controlled studies in human fetuses. **Fentanyl** rapidly crosses the human placenta achieving an F:M ratio approximating unity. It crosses the fetal blood brain barrier and has been used for fetal analgesia where a reduction in endorphin levels is demonstrated. Rodent studies are generally reassuring, revealing no evidence of teratogenicity or IUGR despite the use of doses higher than those used clinically. It is embryotoxic in rodents.

■ **Breastfeeding Safety**

There are no adequate reports or well-controlled studies in nursing women. **Fentanyl** enters human breast milk, but is not likely to pose a risk to the neonate of an alert, breast-feeding woman.

■ **References**

Wong CY, Ng EH, Ngai SW, Ho PC. Hum Reprod 2002; 17:1222-5.
Head BB, Owen J, Vincent RD Jr, et al. Obstet Gynecol 2002; 99:452-7.
Fisk NM, Gitau R, Teixeira JM, et al. Anesthesiology 2001; 95:828-35.
Cooper J, Jauniaux E, Gulbis B, Quick D, Bromley L. Br J Anaesth 1999; 82:929-31.
Cheng CJ, Sia AT, Lim EH, et al. Can J Anaesth 2001; 48:570-4.
Birnbach DJ, Matut J, Stein DJ, et al. Anesth Analg 2001; 93:410-3.
Leuschen MP, Wolf LJ, Rayburn WF. Clin Pharm 1990; 9:336-7.

■ **Summary**

- **Pregnancy Category C**
- **Lactation Category S**
- **Fentanyl** is a short-acting opiate widely used during pregnancy for analgesia of multiple types.

Ferrous gluconate

■ **Class** ⸺ *Mineral*

■ **Indications** ⸺ Iron deficiency and supplementation

■ **Mechanism** ⸺ Essential component in many proteins including hemoglobin

■ **Dosage with Qualifiers** ⸺ Iron deficiency—2-3mg/kg elemental Fe PO qd in divided doses
Iron supplementation—15-30mg elemental Fe qd
NOTE—300mg = 35mg elemental Fe; do not take within 2h of tetracyclines or antacids, which may bind the Fe. Also available in parenteral form.
NOTE—available as ferrous fumarate and ferrous sulfate.
- **Contraindications**—hypersensitivity to drug or class, hemochromatosis, hemolytic anemia, thalassemia, hemosiderosis, peptic ulcer disease, ulcerative colitis.
- **Caution**—chronic therapy

■ **Maternal Considerations** ⸺ Though iron supplementation is widely practiced during pregnancy in the industrialized world, there is no convincing evidence it changes either long- or short-term outcomes. Severe anemia may be an important cause of maternal death, but there is a lack of convincing evidence regarding the risks of mild to moderate maternal anemia. Women anemic due to iron deficiency should first receive a reticulocytic dose followed by supplementation for the duration of pregnancy. Women with disorders of iron utilization (e.g., thalassemia) should not be routinely supplemented.
Side effects include dyspepsia, nausea, vomiting, diarrhea, constipation, and dark stools.

■ **Fetal Considerations** ⸺ There is no evidence that maternal iron supplementation influences the fetal iron status.

■ **Breastfeeding Safety** ⸺ Maternal iron supplementation does not alter the concentration of iron in breast milk.

■ **References** ⸺ Graves BW, Barger MK. J Midwifery Womens Health 2001; 46:159-66.
Rasmussen K. J Nutr 2001; 131:590S-601S.

■ **Summary** ⸺
- **Pregnancy Category A**
- **Lactation Category S**
- Though the risk of routine iron supplementation during pregnancy and lactation is probably minimal, there is no improvement in perinatal outcome or reduction in maternal morbidity in the industrialized world.

Fexofenadine (Allegra)

■ **Class** — Antihistamine

■ **Indications** — Allergic rhinitis, chronic urticaria

■ **Mechanism** — Selective H_1 antagonist

■ **Dosage with Qualifiers** —
Allergic rhinitis—180mg PO qd
Chronic urticaria—60mg PO bid
NOTE—may be combined with **pseudoephedrine**
- **Contraindications**—hypersensitivity to drug or class
- **Caution**—renal dysfunction

■ **Maternal Considerations** — **Fexofenadine** is a 3rd generation antihistamine effective for the symptomatic relief of allergic rhinitis. There are no adequate reports or well-controlled studies of **fexofenadine** in pregnant women. While increasingly preferred for its nonsedating properties, there are no published controlled trials or population studies of **fexofenadine** use during pregnancy.
Side effects include dysmenorrhea, drowsiness, nausea, flu-like symptoms, dyspepsia, and fatigue.

■ **Fetal Considerations** — There are no adequate reports or well-controlled studies in human fetuses. It is unknown whether **fexofenadine** crosses the human placenta. While there is no evidence of teratogenicity in rodents, there is a dose-dependent increase in IUGR and decrease in the survival of pups.

■ **Breastfeeding Safety** — There is no published experience in nursing women. It is unknown whether **fexofenadine** enters human breast milk.

■ **References** — Mazzotta P, Loebstein R, Koren G. Drug Saf 1999; 20:361-75.

■ **Summary** —
- **Pregnancy Category C**
- **Lactation Category U**
- **Fexofenadine** should be used during pregnancy and lactation only if the benefit justifies the potential perinatal risk.
- There are alternative agents, including inhaled steroids and 1st-generation antihistamines such as **chlorpheniramine,** for which there is wide experience during pregnancy and lactation.

Filgrastim (Neupogen)

■ **Class** .... *Hematopoeitic agent; biologic response modifier*

■ **Indications** .... Severe chronic neutropenia, AIDS neutropenia, bone marrow transplantation, chemotherapy-induced neutropenia, progenitor cell donors

■ **Mechanism** .... Human granulocyte colony stimulating factor

■ **Dosage with Qualifiers** .... Severe chronic neutropenia—10mcg/kg SC qd
AIDS neutropenia—1-10mcg/kg SC qd
Neutropenia post bone marrow transplantation—10mcg/kg IV qd >24h after either chemotherapy or transplant
Chemotherapy-induced neutropenia—5mcg/kg SC/IV qd ×2w; may increase by 5mcg/kg per chemo cycle
Progenitor cell donors—10mcg/kg SC qd
- **Contraindications**—hypersensitivity to drug or class, hypersensitivity to E. *coli* proteins
- **Caution**—hepatic or renal dysfunction

■ **Maternal Considerations** .... There are no adequate reports or well-controlled studies of **filgrastim** in pregnant women. It has been used to treat severe chronic neutropenia and chemotherapy-induced neutropenia during pregnancy without obvious adverse effect.
Side effects include anaphylaxis, thrombocytopenia, nausea, vomiting, musculoskeletal, abdominal and bone pain, rash, splenomegaly, hypotension, local swelling and erythema.

■ **Fetal Considerations** .... There are no adequate reports or well-controlled studies in human fetuses. It is unknown whether **filgrastim** crosses the human placenta. There is no evidence to suggest it is a human teratogen. However, rodent studies using high doses reveal evidence of embryotoxicity, IUGR, and delayed external differentiation.

■ **Breastfeeding Safety** .... There are no adequate reports or well-controlled studies in nursing women. It is unknown whether **filgrastim** enters human breast milk.

■ **References** .... Dale DC, Cottle TE, Fier CJ, et al. Am J Hematol 2003; 72:82-93.
Cottle TE, Fier CJ, Donadieu J, Kinsey SE. Semin Hematol 2002; 39:134-40.

■ **Summary** .... - **Pregnancy Category C**
- **Lactation Category U**
- **Filgrastim** should be used during pregnancy and lactation only if the benefit justifies the potential perinatal risk.

Flavoxate (Urispas)

■ **Class** — Anticholinergic; antispasmodic

■ **Indications** — Bladder spasm

■ **Mechanism** — Antagonizes muscarinic receptors

■ **Dosage with Qualifiers** — Bladder spasm—100-200mg PO qid/tid
- **Contraindications**—hypersensitivity to drug or class, intestinal obstruction, GI bleeding, and achalasia
- **Cautions**—unknown

■ **Maternal Considerations** — There is no published experience with **flavoxate** during pregnancy. In nonpregnant women, **flavoxate** first increases then decreases uterine contractions.
Side effects include leukopenia, nausea, vomiting, dry mouth, dizziness, blurred vision, tachycardia, palpitations, headache, drowsiness, dysuria, urticaria, and fever.

■ **Fetal Considerations** — There are no adequate reports or well-controlled studies in human fetuses. It is unknown whether **flavoxate** crosses the placenta. Rodent studies are reassuring, revealing no evidence of teratogenicity or IUGR despite the use of doses higher than those used clinically.

■ **Breastfeeding Safety** — There is no published experience in nursing women. It is unknown whether **flavoxate** enters human breast milk.

■ **References** — Coutinho EM, Darze E, Gesteira SK. Int J Gynaecol Obstet 1980; 17:581-4.

■ **Summary** —
- **Pregnancy Category B**
- **Lactation Category U**
- **Flavoxate** should be used during pregnancy and lactation only if the benefit justifies the potential perinatal risk. There are few if any indications.

Flecainide (Tambocor)

■ **Class** Antiarrhythmic, class 1C

■ **Indications** Ventricular or atrial arrhythmias

■ **Mechanism** Depresses action potential by stabilizing cell membranes

■ **Dosage with Qualifiers** Ventricular arrhythmia—100mg PO q12h (max 400mg qd; increase dose by 50mg/d q4d)
Atrial arrhythmia—50mg PO q12h (max 400mg qd; increase dose by 50mg/d q4d)
- **Contraindications**—hypersensitivity to drug or class, cardiogenic shock, severe AV block, bi- or trifascicular block
- **Caution**—CHF, hepatic or renal dysfunction, prolonged QT interval

■ **Maternal Considerations** There are no adequate reports or well-controlled studies of **flecainide** in pregnant women. **Flecainide** has been used successfully for the treatment of maternal arrhythmias during pregnancy.
Side effects include ventricular arrhythmia, CHF, cardiac arrest, arrhythmia, dizziness, blurred vision, dyspepsia, headache, nausea, vomiting, fatigue, weakness, constipation, and chest pain.

■ **Fetal Considerations** There are no adequate reports or well-controlled studies in human fetuses. **Flecainide** rapidly crosses the placenta, achieving an F:M ratio approximating unity, and like **digoxin,** is concentrated in amniotic fluid. An accepted second-line agent for the treatment of fetal SVT, the popularity of **flecainide** as a first-line agent, especially with hydrops, is growing. An elevated umbilical venous pressure, such as that associated with hydrops fetalis, reduces the placental transport of both **flecainide** and **digoxin.**

■ **Breastfeeding Safety** Though **flecainide** is excreted in human breast milk achieving an M:P ratio approximating 2.5, the quantity consumed would be unlikely to produce a neonatal plasma level above 100ng/ml, a subtherapeutic level.

■ **References**
Fagih B, Sami M. Can J Cardiol 1999; 15:113-7.
Ebenroth ES, Cordes TM, Darragh RK. Pediatr Cardiol 2001; 22:483-7.
Schmolling J, Renke K, Richter O, et al. Ther Drug Monit 2000; 22:582-8.
Krapp M, Baschat AA, Gembruch U, et al. Ultrasound Obstet Gynecol 2002; 19:158-64.
Simpson JM, Sharland GK. Heart 1998; 79:576-81.
Bourget P, Pons JC, Delouis C, et al. Ann Pharmacother 1994; 28:1031-4.
McQuinn RL, Pisani A, Wafa S, et al. Clin Pharmacol Ther 1990; 48:262-7.

Fluconazole (Diflucan)

■ **Class** ··· *Antifungal*

■ **Indications** ····························· Candidiasis, cryptococcal meningitis

■ **Mechanism** ····························· Inhibits cytochrome P450 and C-14 demethylation

■ **Dosage with Qualifiers** ········ Esophageal or oropharyngeal candidiasis—200mg PO/IV ×1, then 100mg PO/IV qd
Vaginal candidiasis—150mg PO ×1
Cryptococcal meningitis—400mg PO/IV ×1, then 200mg PO/IV qd

- **Contraindications**—hypersensitivity to drug or class, use of **astemizole**, **cisapride**, or **terfenidine**
- **Caution**—hepatic or renal dysfunction

■ **Maternal Considerations** ········ There are no adequate reports or well-controlled studies of **fluconazole** in pregnant women. It has been used for the treatment of coccidioidomycosis during pregnancy and *Candida* sepsis postpartum. The systemic antifungal drug with which there has been the most experience is **amphotericin B**.
Side effects include hepatotoxicity, seizures, angioedema, Stevens-Johnson syndrome, agranulocytosis, nausea, vomiting, headache, rash, dizziness, diarrhea, dyspepsia, and taste changes.

■ **Fetal Considerations** ··············· There are no adequate reports or well-controlled studies in human fetuses. It is unknown whether **fluconazole** crosses the human placenta. Four children are described with a similar and rare pattern of anomalies. The features include brachycephaly, abnormal facies, abnormal calvarial development, cleft palate, femoral bowing, thin ribs and long bones, arthrogryposis and congenital heart disease. Each was associated with chronic, parenteral use in the 1st trimester. Limited duration oral therapy is unlikely to pose a teratogenic risk. **Fluconazole** does not appear to increase the risks of IUGR or preterm delivery. It has been used for the treatment of congenital candidiasis. Rodent studies conducted at multiples of the

MRHD revealed a variety of ossification defects considered consistent with inhibition of estrogen synthesis. There was an increased risk of cleft palate in rats when combined with **phenytoin**.

■ **Breastfeeding Safety** ⸻ There are no adequate reports or well-controlled studies in nursing women. **Fluconazole** enters human breast milk at concentrations similar to maternal plasma. It is generally recommended that breastfeeding be avoided.

■ **References** ⸻
Sorensen HT, Nielsen GL, Olesen C, et al. Br J Pharmacol 1999; 48:234-8.
Jick SS. Pharmacotherapy 1999; 19:221-2.
Lee BE, Feinberg M, Abraham JJ, Murthy ARK. Pediatr Infect Dis J 1992; 11:1062-4.
Tiboni GM, Iammarrone E, Giampietro F, et al. Teratology 1999; 59:81-7.

■ **Summary** ⸻
- **Pregnancy Category C**
- **Lactation Category NS?**
- **Fluconazole** should be used during pregnancy and lactation only if the benefit justifies the potential perinatal risk.
- Current evidence suggests it may be a weak teratogen.
- There are alternative agents for which there is more experience during pregnancy and lactation.

Flucytosine (Ancoban)

■ **Class** ⸻ Antifungal

■ **Indications** ⸻ Severe fungal infection

■ **Mechanism** ⸻ Unknown

■ **Dosage with Qualifiers** ⸻ Severe fungal infection—50-150mg/kg PO qd in 4 divided doses
- **Contraindications**—hypersensitivity to drug or class
- **Caution**—hepatic or renal dysfunction, bone marrow depression

■ **Maternal Considerations** ⸻ There are no adequate reports or well-controlled studies of **flucytosine** in pregnant women. It has been used during pregnancy for the treatment of cryptococcal meningitis and pneumonia, and *Candida* septicemia. The systemic antifungal drug with which there has been the most experience is **amphotericin B**.

- **Maternal Considerations** — There are no adequate reports or well-controlled studies of **flumazenil** in pregnant women. It has been used successfully during pregnancy for the treatment of benzodiazepine overdose.
  Side effects include withdrawal syndrome, seizures, arrhythmias, dizziness, nausea, vomiting, sweating, blurred vision, headache, bradycardia or tachycardia, anxiety, fatigue, shivering, and confusion.

- **Fetal Considerations** — There are no adequate reports or well-controlled studies in human fetuses. Since **flumazenil** can apparently reverse maternally administered **diazepam** in the both the fetus and neonate, it likely crosses the human placenta. Rodent studies reveal no evidence of teratogenicity, but embryotoxicity occurs at high doses. Behavioral changes were noted in rat pups after late pregnancy exposure.

- **Breastfeeding Safety** — There is no published experience in nursing women. It is unknown whether **flumazenil** enters human breast milk. Considering the indication, limited or one time **flumazenil** use is unlikely to pose a clinically significant risk to the breast-feeding neonate.

- **References** — Dixon JC, Speidel BD, Dixon JJ. Acta Paediatr 1998; 87:225-6.
  Shibata T, Kubota N, Yokoyama H. Masui 1994; 43:572-4.
  Stahl MM, Saldeen P, Vinge E. Br J Obstet Gynaecol 1993; 100:185-8.

- **Summary** —
  - **Pregnancy Category C**
  - **Lactation Category U**
  - **Flumazenil** should be used during pregnancy and lactation only if the benefit justifies the potential perinatal risk.

Flunisolide (AeroBid; Nasalide; Nasarel)

- **Class** — *Corticosteroid, inhalation*

- **Indications** — Asthma prophylaxis, allergic rhinitis

- **Mechanism** — Unknown

- **Dosage with Qualifiers** — Asthma prophylaxis—2 puffs INH bid (approx 50mcg per puff)
  Allergic rhinitis—2 sprays/nostril bid/tid
  - **Contraindications**—hypersensitivity to drug or class, status asthmaticus, respiratory infection

- **Maternal Considerations** ⋯⋯ There is no published experience with **flunisolide** during pregnancy, though inhaled corticosteroids are a cornerstone of asthma therapy. They are used widely during pregnancy without apparent adverse effects. *Side effects* include adrenal insufficiency, nausea, vomiting, diarrhea, headache, sore throat, nasal congestion, dyspepsia, flu-like symptoms, palpitations, abdominal pain, anorexia, peripheral edema, dizziness, cough, eczema, and hypertension.

- **Fetal Considerations** ⋯⋯ There are no adequate reports or well-controlled studies in human fetuses. It is unknown whether **flunisolide** crosses the human placenta. In rodents, **flunisolide** is both embryotoxic and teratogenic at 100 times the MRHD. Although systemically administered corticosteroids are teratogenic in some rodents, and a weak effect in humans cannot be excluded, the concentration of drug absorbed systemically suggests the risk of a significant fetal effect is low.

- **Breastfeeding Safety** ⋯⋯ There is no published experience in nursing women. It is unknown whether **flunisolide** enters human breast milk. Considering the concentration and quantity absorbed systemically, it is unlikely the plasma level achieved will be clinically relevant to lactation.

- **References** ⋯⋯ There is no published experience in pregnancy or during lactation.

- **Summary** ⋯⋯
  - **Pregnancy Category C**
  - **Lactation Category U**
  - **Flunisolide** should be used during pregnancy and lactation only if the benefit justifies the potential perinatal risk.

Fluocinolone topical (Synalar)

- **Class** ⋯⋯ Corticosteroid

- **Indications** ⋯⋯ Steroid-responsive dermatitis

- **Mechanism** ⋯⋯ Unknown

- **Dosage with Qualifiers** ⋯⋯ Steroid-responsive dermatitis—apply to affected area bid/qid
  NOTE—0.01, or 0.025% cream, ointment or salve
  - **Contraindications**—hypersensitivity to drug or class

■ **Maternal Considerations** ⋯⋯ There is no published experience with **fluocinolone** during pregnancy.
Side effects include adrenal insufficiency, irritation, burning, itching, dryness, folliculitis, hypertrichosis, acne, hypopigmentation, skin atrophy, and striae.

■ **Fetal Considerations** ⋯⋯ There are no adequate reports or well-controlled studies in human fetuses. It is unknown whether **fluocinolone** crosses the human placenta. While systemically administered corticosteroids including **fluocinolone** are teratogenic in some rodents, and a weak effect in humans cannot be excluded, the concentration of drug absorbed systemically suggests the risk of an adverse fetal effect is low.

■ **Breastfeeding Safety** ⋯⋯ There are no adequate reports or well-controlled studies in nursing women. It is unknown whether **fluocinolone** enters human breast milk. However, considering the concentration and quantity absorbed systemically, it is unlikely the plasma level achieved will be clinically relevant to lactation.

■ **References** ⋯⋯ There is no published experience in pregnancy or during lactation.

■ **Summary** ⋯⋯
- **Pregnancy Category C**
- **Lactation Category U**
- **Fluocinolone** should be used during pregnancy and lactation only if the benefit justifies the potential perinatal risk.

Fluorouracil (Adrucil)

■ **Class** ⋯⋯ *Antimetabolite; antineoplastic*

■ **Indications** ⋯⋯ Malignancies including breast, colon, basal cell, and gestational trophoblast

■ **Mechanism** ⋯⋯ Pyrimidine analog that inhibits both DNA and RNA synthesis

■ **Dosage with Qualifiers** ⋯⋯ Malignancy—Depends on tumor and protocol
NOTE—available in a topical preparation for the treatment of basal cell carcinoma
- **Contraindications**—hypersensitivity to drug or class, myelosuppression, serious infection, recent surgery
- **Caution**—hepatic or renal dysfunction, prior use of alkylating agents, coronary artery disease

- ■ **Maternal Considerations** ⸺ There are no adequate reports or well-controlled studies of **fluorouracil** in pregnant women. **Fluorouracil** is most commonly used during pregnancy in the 2nd and 3rd trimesters for the treatment of metastatic breast cancer where it is often combined with **doxorubicin** and **cyclophosphamide**. It should be used only when there is significant risk for the mother's survival.

  Side effects include leukopenia, thrombocytopenia, agranulocytosis, GI bleeding, nausea, vomiting, diarrhea, anorexia, enteritis, alopecia, dermatitis, photosensitivity, erythema, ulceration, stomatitis, lethargy, malaise, headache, and confusion.

- ■ **Fetal Considerations** ⸺ There are no adequate reports or well-controlled studies in human fetuses. **Fluorouracil** apparently crosses the human placenta, since maternal administration is associated with fetal immunosuppression. Although there is little published epidemiologic study, there are multiple case reports of normal pregnancy outcome after early exposure. Little is known about the long-term effects of intrauterine exposure to **fluorouracil**. **Fluorouracil** crosses the rodent placenta and produces a variety of defects involving the skeleton and palate.

- ■ **Breastfeeding Safety** ⸺ There is no published experience in nursing women. It is unknown whether **fluorouracil** enters human breast milk.

- ■ **References** ⸺ Inoue T, Horii I. J Toxicol Sci 2002; 27:79-86.
  Gwyn KM, Theriault RL. Curr Treat Options Oncol 2000; 3:239-43.

- ■ **Summary** ⸺ • **Pregnancy Category D**
  - **Lactation Category NS**
  - **Fluorouracil** should be used during pregnancy and lactation only if the benefit justifies the potential perinatal risk.

Fluoxetine (Prozac; Sarafem)

- ■ **Class** ⸺ *Antidepressant, SSRI*

- ■ **Indications** ⸺ Depression, premenstrual dysphoric syndrome, obsessive-compulsive disorder, bulimia

- ■ **Mechanism** ⸺ Selectively inhibits reuptake of serotonin

- ■ **Dosage with Qualifiers** ⸺ Depression—begin 20mg PO qd (in AM or PM); increase as needed after several weeks to 60mg qd
  Premenstrual dysphoric syndrome—20mg PO qd; max 80mg/d

Obsessive-compulsive disorder—begin 20mg PO qd; increase as needed after several weeks to 80mg
Bulimia—60mg PO qd

- **Contraindications**—hypersensitivity to drug or class, use of an MAO inhibitor within 14d
- **Caution**—hepatic or renal dysfunction, seizure history, suicide threat

■ **Maternal Considerations** ········ Depression is common during and after pregnancy, but typically goes unrecognized. Pregnancy is not a reason a priori to discontinue psychotropic drugs. There are no adequate reports or well-controlled studies of **fluoxetine** in pregnant women. **Fluoxetine** is effective treatment for postpartum depression, and is as effective as a course of cognitive-behavioral counseling in the short term.
Side effects include serotonin syndrome, insomnia, nausea, diarrhea, tremor, headache, anorexia, anxiety, dry mouth, decreased libido, delayed or absent orgasm, abnormal dreams, sedation, sweating, and itching.

■ **Fetal Considerations** ············ There are no adequate reports or well-controlled studies in human fetuses. It is unknown whether **fluoxetine** crosses the human placenta. Prospectively ascertained pregnancy outcomes after SSRIs, mainly **fluoxetine**, reveal no teratogenic effect. Nor are there differences in birth weight and acute neonatal outcome between treated and untreated pregnancies. Exposure throughout gestation does not adversely affect cognition, language development, or the temperament of preschool and early-school-age children. Rodent studies too are reassuring, though the rates of IUGR and stillbirth are higher in rats treated with multiples of the MRHD. Prolonged prenatal SSRI exposure in rats is associated with reduced behavioral pain responses and increased parasympathetic cardiac modulation in recovery following an acute neonatal noxious event. In sheep, **fluoxetine** has transient effects on fetal behavioral and acid base status.

■ **Breastfeeding Safety** ············ Maternal serum and peak breast milk concentrations of **fluoxetine** and its active metabolite, **norfluoxetine** predict nursing infant serum **norfluoxetine** concentrations. Neonatal serum concentrations are typically low in nursing women taking 20mg/d or less. Thus, breastfeeding is not contraindicated.

■ **References** ···································· Hoffbrand S, Howard L, Crawley H. Cochrane Database Syst Rev 2001; (2):CD002018.
Cohen LS, Heller VL, Bailey JW, et al. Biol Psychiatry 2000; 48:996-1000.
Calil HM. J Clin Psychiatry 2001; (Suppl 62)22:24-9.
Addis A, Koren G. Psychol Med 2000; 30:89-94.
Nulman I, Rovet J, Stewart DE, et al. Am J Psychiatry 2002; 159:1889-95.
Oberlander TF, Eckstein Grunau R, Fitzgerald C, et al. Pediatr Res 2002; 51:443-53.
Morrison JL, Chien C, Riggs KW, et al. Pediatr Res 2002; 51:433-42.

Morrison JL, Chien C, Gruber N, et al. Brain Res Dev Brain Res 2001; 131:47-56.
Hendrick V, Stowe ZN, Altshuler LL, et al. Biol Psychiatry 2001; 50:775-82.

■ **Summary**

- **Pregnancy Category C**
- **Lactation Category S, conditionally**
- **Fluoxetine** should be used during pregnancy and lactation only if the benefit justifies the potential perinatal risk.

Fluoxymesterone (Alomon; Android-F; Fluoron; Fuloan; Halotestin; Hysterone; Ora-Testryl; Oratestin)

■ **Class**

Androgen; hormone

■ **Indications**

Postpartum breast engorgement, palliative therapy for breast cancer

■ **Mechanism**

Binds androgen receptors producing multiple androgenic and anabolic effects

■ **Dosage with Qualifiers**

Postpartum breast engorgement—2.5mg PO ×1 shortly after delivery, then 5-10mg PO qd ×4-5d
Breast cancer, palliation—10-40mg PO qd
- **Contraindications**—hypersensitivity to drug or class, breast cancer, hepatic or renal dysfunction, pregnancy

■ **Maternal Considerations**

There is no published experience with **fluoxymesterone** during pregnancy, nor are there any recognized indications for its use during pregnancy.
Side effects include polycythemia, liver tumors, menstrual irregularities, hirsutism, acne, electrolyte imbalance, libido changes, headache, deepened voice, and dyspepsia.

■ **Fetal Considerations**

There are no adequate reports or well-controlled studies in human fetuses. It is unknown whether **fluoxymesterone** specifically or an active metabolite cross the human placenta. Androgens are recognized human teratogens leading to masculinization of the female fetus.

■ **Breastfeeding Safety**

Fluoxymesterone is ineffective for the suppression of lactation and is no longer used. It is unknown whether **fluoxymesterone** enters human breast milk.

■ **References**

No current relevant references

■ **Summary**

- **Pregnancy Category X**
- **Lactation Category U**
- Contraindicated during pregnancy and lactation.

Fluphenazine decanoate (Prolixin)

■ **Class** ·················· *Antipsychotic, class 3; phenothiazines*

■ **Indications** ············ Psychosis (e.g., chronic schizophrenia)

■ **Mechanism** ············ Unclear; dopamine D_2 receptor antagonist

■ **Dosage with Qualifiers** ···· <u>Psychosis</u>—begin 12.5-25mg IM; response within 12-96h, dose q2-4w
NOTE—also available as **fluphenazine enanthate,** which has an even longer duration of action
- **Contraindications**—hypersensitivity to drug or class, CNS depression, bone marrow depression, severe hypotension, pheochromocytoma
- **Caution**—hepatic dysfunction, seizure disorder, myasthenia gravis, Parkinson's disease, severe CV disease

■ **Maternal Considerations** ···· **Fluphenazine** is a long-acting parenteral antipsychotic typically used in institutional settings. There are no adequate reports or well-controlled studies in pregnant women. Consistent with its biochemistry, **fluphenazine** increases maternal prolactin.
Side effects include seizures, neuroleptic malignant syndrome, aplastic anemia, agranulocytosis, cholestatic jaundice, nausea, anorexia, headache, depression, leukopenia, hyperprolactinemia, tardive dyskinesia, sedation, pseudo-parkinsonism, drowsiness, blurred vision, dry mouth, constipation, photosensitivity, and urinary retention.

■ **Fetal Considerations** ········ There are no adequate reports or well-controlled studies in human fetuses. It is unknown whether **fluphenazine** crosses the human placenta. Rodent studies reveal bone and CNS malformations. The incidence of these malformations increases significantly when diphenylhydantoin is administered concurrently. Peroxidative bioactivation of phenothiazines to their cation radical by human placental peroxidase may be one mechanism for their developmental toxicity.

■ **Breastfeeding Safety** ······· There is no published experience in nursing women. It is unknown whether **fluphenazine** enters human breast milk.

■ **References** ··············· Yang X, Kulkarni AP. Teratog Carcinog Mutagen 1997; 17:139-51.
Abdel-Hamid HA, Abdel-Rahman MS, Abdel-Rahman SA. J Appl Toxicol 1996; 16:221-5.

- **Pregnancy Category C**
- **Lactation Category U**
- **Fluphenazine** should be used during pregnancy and lactation only if the benefit justifies the potential perinatal risk.

Flurandrenolide topical (Cordan; Haelan)

■ **Class** — Corticosteroid, topical; dermatologic

■ **Indications** — Steroid-responsive dermatitis

■ **Mechanism** — Anti-inflammatory mechanism unknown

■ **Dosage with Qualifiers** — Steroid-responsive dermatitis—apply to affected area qd/qid
NOTE—available as 0.025 or 0.05% in cream, ointment or lotion; may be combined with **neomycin**
- Contraindications—hypersensitivity to drug or class

■ **Maternal Considerations** — There are no adequate reports or well-controlled studies of **flurandrenolide** in pregnant women.
Side effects include adrenal suppression, burning, itching, dryness, acne, hypopigmentation, hypertrichosis, and contact dermatitis.

■ **Fetal Considerations** — There are no adequate reports or well-controlled studies in human fetuses. Rodent teratogenicity studies have apparently not been performed. While systemically administered corticosteroids are teratogenic in some rodents, and a weak effect in humans cannot be excluded, the concentration of drug absorbed systemically if applied to a small area suggests the risk of a significant fetal effect is low.

■ **Breastfeeding Safety** — There is no published experience in nursing women. It is unknown whether **flurandrenolide** enters human breast milk. It is unlikely the limited systemic concentration achieved after application to a small area is clinically relevant to lactation.

■ **References** — No current relevant references

■ **Summary** —
- **Pregnancy Category C**
- **Lactation Category S?**
- **Flurandrenolide** should be used during pregnancy and lactation only if the benefit justifies the potential perinatal risk.

Flurazepam (Dalmane; Fluleep; Midorm; Niotal; Paxane)

- **Class** — *Benzodiazepine, class 3; sedative/hypnotic*

- **Indications** — Insomnia, short-term relief

- **Mechanism** — Binds to benzodiazepine receptors

- **Dosage with Qualifiers** — Insomnia—15-30mg PO qh
  - **Contraindications**—hypersensitivity to drug or class, pregnancy
  - **Caution**—hepatic or pulmonary dysfunction, sleep apnea

- **Maternal Considerations** — There are no adequate reports or well-controlled studies of **flurazepam** in pregnant women. There are other hypnotics on the market with better pharmacologic and safety profiles such as **zolpidem**. Prolonged use of hypnotics is not advised.
  Side effects include coma, dependence, sedation, dizziness, ataxia, confusion, headache, nausea, and elevated LFTs.

- **Fetal Considerations** — There are no adequate reports or well-controlled studies in human fetuses. **Flurazepam** crosses the human placenta, though the kinetics remain to be elucidated. Benzodiazepines such as **diazepam** and **chlordiazepoxide** may be associated with an increased risk of malformations after 1st trimester exposure. Rodent teratogenicity studies with **flurazepam** specifically have apparently not been performed. Neonatal depression was reported in a neonate of a woman taking **flurazepam** for the 10d preceding delivery. The long-term neurologic effects of *in utero* exposure are unknown.

- **Breastfeeding Safety** — There are no adequate reports or well-controlled studies in nursing women. Older abstracts suggest **flurazepam** enters human breast milk.

- **References** — No current relevant references

- **Summary** —
  - **Pregnancy Category X**
  - **Lactation Category U**
  - There are no indications that require the use of **flurazepam** during pregnancy.
  - There are other hypnotics on the market, such as **zolpidem**, with better pharmacologic and safety profiles.

Flurbiprofen (Ansaid)

- **Class** — *Analgesic*; NSAID

- **Indications** — Dysmenorrhea, osteoarthritis, analgesia (mild to moderate pain), antipyretic

- **Mechanism** — Inhibits cyclooxygenases and lipoxygenase; reduces prostaglandin synthesis

- **Dosage with Qualifiers** — Dysmenorrhea—begin 100mg PO ×1, then 50-100mg PO bid/tid
  Osteoarthritis—50-100mg PO bid/tid
  Analgesia (mild to moderate pain)—begin 100mg PO ×1, then 50-100mg PO bid/tid
  - **Contraindications**—hypersensitivity to drug or class, ASA/NSAID-induced asthma
  - **Caution**—hypertension, history GI bleeding, CHF, nasal polyps

- **Maternal Considerations** — **Flurbiprofen** has analgesic, antipyretic, and anti-inflammatory activities. There are no adequate reports or well-controlled studies of **flurbiprofen** in pregnant women. **Flurbiprofen** is equivalent to **aspirin** and superior to **codeine** as an analgesic for postpartum uterine pain. It is unknown whether **flurbiprofen** offers any advantage over other, similar NSAIDs. **Flurbiprofen** prolongs rat parturition as do most NSAIDs.
  Side effects include GI bleeding, acute renal failure, bronchospasm, thrombocytopenia, interstitial nephritis, hepatotoxicity, agranulocytosis, dyspepsia, nausea, abdominal pain, dizziness, headache, rash, urticaria, increased LFTs, fluid retention, tinnitus, and drowsiness.

- **Fetal Considerations** — There are no adequate reports or well-controlled studies in human fetuses. **Flurbiprofen** crosses the human placenta. Other NSAIDs cause ductus arteriosus constriction and oligohydramnios secondary to fetal oliguria. **Flurbiprofen** is known to do so in rats. Rodent studies are generally reassuring, revealing no evidence of teratogenicity or IUGR despite the use of doses higher than that used clinically. High doses are associated in the rodent with embryotoxicity and increased perinatal mortality secondary to delayed parturition.

- **Breastfeeding Safety** — The elimination half-life of **flurbiprofen** during early lactation is slightly prolonged (mean 4.8h) compared to adult males. The peak plasma concentrations are comparable to those reported for healthy volunteers. In 10 of 12 women (3-5d postpartum), the **flurbiprofen** concentration in breast milk was less than 0.050mcg/ml. The remaining women did not exceed 0.07mcg/ml.

This concentration is insufficient to pose a risk to the breast-feeding neonate.

■ **References** Smith IJ, Hinson JL, Johnson VA, et al. J Clin Pharmacol 1989; 29:174-84.
Bloomfield SS, Mitchell J, Cissell G, Barden TP. Am J Med 1986; 80:65-70.

■ **Summary**
- **Pregnancy Category B (1st and 2nd trimesters), D (3rd trimester)**
- **Lactation Category S**
- An NSAID for which there is little experience regarding use in pregnancy.
- **Flurbiprofen** offers no clear advantage over other NSAIDs for which there is more experience.

Fluticasone (Cutivate; Flonase; Flonase Aq; Flovent; Flunase; Zoflut)

■ **Class** *Corticosteroid, inhalational, topical; dermatologic*

■ **Indications** Asthma prophylaxis

■ **Mechanism** Anti-inflammatory mechanism unknown

■ **Dosage with Qualifiers** Asthma prophylaxis—begin 88mcg bid if on bronchodilator alone; max 880mcg bid, taper to lowest effective dose
NOTE—available as 44-, 110-, 220mcg/puff; also available for intranasal and topical use; may be combined with **salmeterol**, a β-mimetic agent
- **Contraindications**—hypersensitivity to drug or class, acute asthma, status asthmaticus
- **Cautions**—unknown

■ **Maternal Considerations** There are no adequate reports or well-controlled studies of **fluticasone** in pregnant women. **Fluticasone** is a popular agent in women with asthma and commonly encountered during pregnancy. It is not effective for the treatment of pregnancy rhinitis.
Side effects include adrenal suppression, bronchospasm, glaucoma, cataracts, Cushingoid features, headache, nasal congestion, sinusitis, and pharyngitis.

■ **Fetal Considerations** There are no adequate reports or well-controlled studies in human fetuses. It is unknown whether **fluticasone** crosses the human placenta. While systemically administered corticosteroids including **fluticasone** are teratogenic in some rodents and a weak effect in humans cannot be excluded, the concentration of drug absorbed suggests the risk of an adverse fetal effect is low. There are no documented epidemiological studies with intranasal corticosteroids during pregnancy; however, inhaled corticosteroids have not been incriminated as teratogens and are commonly used by pregnant women who have asthma. Less than 0.1% of an inhaled dose crosses the rodent placenta.

■ **Breastfeeding Safety**   There are no adequate reports or well-controlled studies in nursing women. It is unknown whether **fluticasone** enters human breast milk. Measurable but small amounts enter rat breast milk. However, considering the concentration and quantity absorbed systemically, it is unlikely the plasma level achieved will be clinically relevant to lactation.

■ **References**   Mazzotta P, Loebstein R, Koren G. Drug Saf 1999; 20:361-75. Ellegard EK, Hellgren M, Karlsson NG. Clin Otolaryngol 2001; 26:394-400.

■ **Summary**   • **Pregnancy Category C**
• **Lactation Category S**
• **Fluticasone** should be used during pregnancy and lactation only if the benefit justifies the potential perinatal risk.

Fluvastatin (Lescol; Lescol XL)

■ **Class**   *Antihyperlipidemic*

■ **Indications**   Hypercholesterolemia, mixed dyslipidemia, secondary prevention of cardiac events

■ **Mechanism**   HMG-CoA reductase competitive inhibitor

■ **Dosage with Qualifiers**   Hypercholesterolemia—begin 20mg PO qh; max 40mg bid
Mixed dyslipidemia—begin 20mg PO qh; max 40mg bid
Secondary prevention of cardiac events—begin 20mg PO qh; max 40mg bid
NOTE—check LFT after 3mo or upon increasing dose
• **Contraindications**—hypersensitivity to drug or class, active hepatic disease
• **Caution**—hepatic or renal disease, alcohol abuse

■ **Maternal Considerations**   **Fluvastatin** is a competitive inhibitor of the enzyme responsible for the conversion of 3-hydroxy-3-methylglutaryl-coenzyme A (HMG-CoA) to mevalonate, a precursor of cholesterol. There are no adequate reports or well-controlled studies of **fluvastatin** in pregnant women.

Hyperlipidemia is a chronic illness, and discontinuing treatment during pregnancy is unlikely to compromise patient care. Published experience is confined to a case report. However, there is an unexpected high maternal mortality rate in rats during lactation. Supplementation with mevalonic acid completely blocks and/or ameliorates death, cardiac myopathy, and other adverse effects. Thus, the adverse maternal effects result from exaggerated pharmacologic activity at the dose levels administered, i.e., inhibition of the enzyme HMG-CoA reductase, its immediate product mevalonic acid, and cholesterol biosynthesis. It is not known whether pregnancy enhances the toxicity of **fluvastatin** in humans.

Side effects include pancreatitis, hepatic toxicity, rhabdomyolysis, constipation, dyspepsia, flatulence, nausea, diarrhea, abdominal pain, myalgias, muscle weakness, and elevated CPK or LFTs.

■ **Fetal Considerations** — There are no adequate reports or well-controlled studies in human fetuses. It is not known whether **fluvastatin** crosses the placenta. In rodents, **fluvastatin** is associated with delayed and abnormal skeletal development. There is one report of VATER in the child of a woman who took **fluvastatin** during the 1st trimester. Similar class drugs are associated with rare reports of malformations.

■ **Breastfeeding Safety** — There is no published experience in nursing women. It is unknown whether **fluvastatin** enters human breast milk.

■ **References** — Seguin J, Samuels P. Obstet Gynecol 1999; 93:847.
Hrab RV, Hartman HA, Cox RH Jr. Teratology 1994; 50:19-26.

■ **Summary** —
- **Pregnancy Category X**
- **Lactation Category U**
- **Fluvastatin** is presently considered contraindicated during pregnancy.

Fluvoxamine (Floxyfral; Luvox)

■ **Class** — Antidepressant

■ **Indications** — Obsessive-compulsive disorder

■ **Mechanism** — Selectively inhibits serotonin reuptake

■ **Dosage with Qualifiers** — Obsessive-compulsive disorder—begin at 50mg PO qh; increase by 50mg q3-4d; max 300mg/d
NOTE—taper gradually if discontinued

- **Contraindications**—hypersensitivity to drug or class, concurrent or recent use of **astemizole**, **cisapride**, **terfenidine** or an MAO inhibitor within 14d.
- **Caution**—CV disease, suicide risk, seizure disorder

■ **Maternal Considerations** ········ There are no adequate reports or well-controlled studies of **fluvoxamine** in pregnant women. It is chemically unrelated to the other SSRIs. The few published case reports suggest no adverse effects when used at recommended doses.
Side effects include seizures, bradycardia, hepatic toxicity, toxic epidermal necrosis, withdrawal syndrome, nausea, vomiting, constipation, agitation, headache, sweating, flatulence, and palpitations.

■ **Fetal Considerations** ·········· There are no adequate reports or well-controlled studies in human fetuses. Though the kinetics need further clarification, **fluvoxamine** crosses the human placenta and is excreted into the amniotic fluid. There is no evidence of teratogenicity or any other adverse effect in humans after 1st trimester exposure. SSRI antidepressants are not teratogenic in animals. **Fluvoxamine** is associated in rodents with an increase in perinatal mortality that is predominantly attributed to maternal toxicity. Self-resolving neurologic signs were observed in newborns exposed to **fluoxetine** at the end of pregnancy.

■ **Breastfeeding Safety** ·········· There are no adequate reports or well-controlled studies in nursing women. **Fluvoxamine** is excreted in low concentrations into human breast milk, but the resulting neonatal levels are below the limit of detection.

■ **References** ·················· Kulin NA, Pastuszak A, Sage SR, et al. JAMA 1998; 279:609-10.
No author, Prescrire Int 1999; 8:157-9.
Hostetter A, Ritchie JC, Stowe ZN. Biol Psychiatry 2000; 48:1032-4.
Hendrick V, Fukuchi A, Altshuler L, et al. Br J Psychiatry 2001; 179:163-6.
Kristensen JH, Hackett LP, Kohan R, Paech M, Ilett KF. J Hum Lact 2002; 18:139-43.

■ **Summary** ··················
- **Pregnancy Category C**
- **Lactation Category S**
- **Fluvoxamine** should be used during pregnancy only if the benefit justifies the potential perinatal risk.

Folic acid (Acido; Folasic; Folicet; Folico; Folvite; Nifolin; Renal Multivit Form Forte Zinc)

■ **Class** — Hematinic; *vitamin*

■ **Indications** — Pregnancy supplementation, prevention of recurrent NTDs, megaloblastic anemia

■ **Mechanism** — Required for erythropoiesis and DNA synthesis

■ **Dosage with Qualifiers** — Pregnancy supplementation—0.8-1mg PO qd
Prevention of recurrent NTDs—5mg PO qd prior to conception
Megaloblastic anemia—0.4mg PO qd ×4-5d; max 1mg/d
NOTE—available in PO or parenteral forms
- **Contraindications**—undiagnosed anemia
- **Caution**—unknown

■ **Maternal Considerations** — Suboptimal preconception folate and vitamin B_6 reserves, especially when combined, may increase the risk of spontaneous abortion. Women who become pregnant before folate restoration is complete have an increased risk of folate insufficiency during conception and pregnancy. As a consequence, they may be at increased risk of preterm birth.
Side effects include nausea, vomiting, anorexia, flatulence, irritability, altered sleep pattern, erythema, rash, and itching.

■ **Fetal Considerations** — NTDs and other pregnancy complications are linked to impaired MTHFR function. Each doubling of the serum folate concentration roughly halves the risk of an NTD. It is suggested that high levels of folate supplementation might blunt the negative impact of antiepileptic drugs. The high prevalence of mutated MTHFR genotypes in spontaneously aborted embryos supports the potentially protective role of periconceptional folic acid supplementation.

■ **Breastfeeding Safety** — Maternal **folate** stores are depleted during lactation without supplementation. Supplementation minimizes maternal loss and significantly increases the concentration of **folate** in milk.

■ **References** — Ronnenberg AG, Goldman MB, Chen D, et al. Obstet Gynecol 2002; 100:107-13.
Lumley J, Watson L, Watson M, Bower C. Cochrane Database Syst Rev 2001; (3):CD001056.
Wald NJ, Law MR, Morris JK, Wald DS. Lancet 2001; 358:2069-73.
Mackey AD, Picciano MF. Am J Clin Nutr 1999; 69:285-92.
Schwahn B, Rozen R. Am J Pharmacogenomics 2001; 1:189-201.

Zetterberg H, Regland B, Palmer M, et al. Eur J Hum Genet 2002; 10:113-8.

■ **Summary**
- **Pregnancy Category A**
- **Lactation Category S**
- Preconception **folate** supplementation reduces the incidence of NTDs and possibly other birth defects.
- Preconception **folate** supplementation may reduce the incidence of spontaneous abortion in couples that are each carriers of an MTHFR mutation.
- **Folate** should be provided to every pregnant woman.

Fomepizole (Antizol)

■ **Class** — Antidote; toxicology

■ **Indications** — Ethylene glycol or methanol toxicity

■ **Mechanism** — Inhibits alcohol dehydrogenase

■ **Dosage with Qualifiers** — Ethylene glycol toxicity—begin 15mg/kg IV q12h; then 10mg/kg q12h ×4, then 15mg/kg q12h until ethylene glycol level below 20mg/dl and pH normal
Methanol toxicity—begin 15mg/kg IV q12h; then 10mg/kg q12h ×4, then 15mg/kg q12h until ethylene glycol level below 20mg/dl and pH normal
- **Contraindications**—hypersensitivity to drug or class

■ **Maternal Considerations** — There are no adequate reports or well-controlled studies of **fomepizole** in pregnant women. The published experience consists of a single case report. However, the risks of ethylene or methanol toxicity to mother and fetus outweigh any theoretic risk of the drug.
Side effects include seizures, nausea, vomiting, headache, dizziness, metallic taste, abnormal smell, and rash.

■ **Fetal Considerations** — There are no adequate reports or well-controlled studies in human fetuses. It is unknown whether **fomepizole** crosses the placenta. Animal reproduction studies have not been performed.

■ **Breastfeeding Safety** — There are no adequate reports or well-controlled studies in nursing women. It is unknown whether **fomepizole** enters human breast milk. However, it is unlikely a patient requiring treatment will breastfeed during that period.

■ **References** — Velez LI, Kulstad E, Shepherd G, Roth B. Vet Hum Toxicol 2003; 45:28-30.

Fondaparinux (Arixtra)

■ **Class** ⸳⸳⸳⸳⸳⸳⸳⸳⸳⸳⸳⸳⸳⸳⸳⸳⸳⸳⸳⸳⸳⸳⸳⸳⸳⸳⸳⸳⸳⸳⸳⸳⸳⸳⸳⸳⸳⸳⸳ Anticoagulant

■ **Indications** ⸳⸳⸳⸳⸳⸳⸳⸳⸳⸳⸳⸳⸳⸳⸳⸳⸳⸳⸳⸳⸳⸳⸳ DVT prophylaxis for hip or knee replacement, surgery for hip fracture

■ **Mechanism** ⸳⸳⸳⸳⸳⸳⸳⸳⸳⸳⸳⸳⸳⸳⸳⸳⸳⸳⸳⸳⸳⸳⸳ Selectively binds antithrombin III potentiating factor Xa neutralization and inhibiting thrombin formation

■ **Dosage with Qualifiers** ⸳⸳⸳⸳⸳⸳ DVT prophylaxis for hip replacement—2.5mg SC qd for 5-10d beginning 6-8h post surgery
DVT prophylaxis after hip fracture surgery—2.5mg SC qd for 5-10d beginning 6-8h post surgery
DVT prophylaxis for knee replacement—2.5mg SC qd for 5-10d beginning 6-8h post surgery
NOTE—monitor renal function and CBC; avoid regional anesthesia within 24h
- **Contraindications**—hypersensitivity to drug or class, active bleeding, weight <50kg, CrCl<30ml/min, thrombocytopenia associated with antiplatelet antibodies, IM administration, bacterial endocarditis, neuraxial analgesia
- **Caution**—renal dysfunction, history of GI bleeding, hemorrhagic stroke, heparin-induced thrombocytopenia, active or recent peptic ulcer disease, and diabetic retinopathy

■ **Maternal Considerations** ⸳⸳⸳⸳⸳⸳ There is no published experience with **fondaparinux** during pregnancy. **Fondaparinux** is the first in a new class of antithrombotic agents developed for the prevention and treatment of VTE. It inhibits thrombin generation by selectively inhibiting factor Xa. **Fondaparinux** is rapidly absorbed, reaching its maximum concentration in approximately 2h. The terminal half-life of 13-21h permits once-daily dosing. **Fondaparinux's** reproducible linear pharmacokinetic profile suggests individual dose adjustments will not be required for the vast majority of the population and that there will be no need for routine hemostatic monitoring. At therapeutic concentrations (>2mg/L), **fondaparinux** exhibits >94% binding to its target protein, antithrombin.

■ **Fetal Considerations** There are no adequate and well-controlled studies in human fetuses. *In vitro*, **fondaparinux** does not cross the human placenta, suggesting the fetus is not directly at risk.

■ **Breastfeeding Safety** There are no adequate reports or well-controlled studies in nursing women. It is unknown whether **fondaparinux** enters human breast milk.

■ **References** Lagrang F, Vergnes C, Brun JL, et al. Thromb Haemost 2002; 87:831-5.

■ **Summary**
  - **Pregnancy Category B**
  - **Lactation Category U**
  - Though there is no published experience during pregnancy, **fondaparinux** remains an attractive possibility for DVT prophylaxis during pregnancy.
  - There are alternative agents for which there is more experience during pregnancy and lactation.

Formoterol, inhaled (Foradil Aerolizer)

■ **Class** *Adrenergic agonist; bronchodilator*

■ **Indications** Asthma prophylaxis, treatment of exercise-induced asthma; COPD maintenance

■ **Mechanism** β-2 agonist

■ **Dosage with Qualifiers** Asthma prophylaxis—12mcg INH (inhalation) q12h
Treatment of exercise-induced asthma—12mcg INH 15-30min prior to exercise; may repeat q12h prn, max 24mcg/d
COPD maintenance—12mcg INH q12h; max 24mcg/d
  - **Contraindications**—hypersensitivity to drug or class, acute asthma
  - **Caution**—arrhythmia, CV disease, hypertension, diabetes mellitus, hypokalemia, seizure disorder

■ **Maternal Considerations** **Formoterol** is a long-acting betamimetic agent used for asthma prophylaxis. It is not for acute treatment. There are no adequate reports or well-controlled studies of **formoterol** in pregnant women. Only 33 pregnant women were reported to have used **formoterol** in a post-marketing survey. No adverse effects were noted. There is some reduction in rodent myometrial contractility when studied *in vitro*.

Side effects include arrhythmia, paradoxical bronchospasm, hypokalemia, nervousness, tremor, headache, dry mouth, nausea, dizziness, insomnia, chest pain, muscle cramps, dyspepsia, and dysphonia.

■ **Fetal Considerations** — There are no adequate reports or well-controlled studies in human fetuses. Rodent studies are reassuring, revealing only delayed ossification, IUGR and increased perinatal mortality at doses >2000 times the MRHD.

■ **Breastfeeding Safety** — There is no published experience in nursing women. It is unknown whether **formoterol** enters human breast milk. The transfer of similar agents, such as **terbutaline** is very low.

■ **References** — Wilton LV, Shakir SA. Drug Saf 2002; 25:213-23.
Bardou M, Cortijo J, Loustalot C, et al. Naunyn Schmiedebergs Arch Pharmacol 1999; 360:457-63.
Shinkai N, Takayama S. J Pharm Pharmacol 2000; 52:1417-23.

■ **Summary** —
- **Pregnancy Category C**
- **Lactation Category U**
- **Formoterol** should be used during pregnancy and lactation only if the benefit justifies the potential perinatal risk.

Foscarnet (Foscavir)

■ **Class** — Antiviral

■ **Indications** — **Acyclovir**-resistant HSV, CMV retinitis, AIDS

■ **Mechanism** — Selectively inhibits viral DNA polymerase

■ **Dosage with Qualifiers** — Acyclovir-resistant HSV—40mg/kg IV given over 1h q8h for 2-3w
CMV retinitis, AIDS—begin at 60mg/kg IV given over 1h q8h; administer maintenance dose ×2-3w
NOTE—renal dosing
- **Contraindications**—hypersensitivity to drug or class
- **Caution**—renal dysfunction, malnutrition, CNS disorders

■ **Maternal Considerations** — **Foscarnet** exerts its antiviral activity by a selective inhibition at the pyrophosphate-binding site on virus-specific DNA polymerases. There are no adequate reports or well-controlled studies of **foscarnet** in pregnant women, and the indications are limited. **Foscarnet** was used successfully during pregnancy in one woman with

AIDS for the treatment of genital acyclovir-resistant herpes simplex virus type 2, and in another HIV-infected woman with myeloradiculitis.

Side effects include renal failure, anemia, pancreatitis, bone marrow suppression, thrombocytopenia, leukopenia, agranulocytopenia, bronchospasm, seizures, nausea, vomiting, diarrhea, fever, headache, weakness, hypocalcemia, hypophosphatemia, and hypomagnesemia.

■ **Fetal Considerations**
There are no adequate reports or well-controlled studies in human fetuses. It is unknown whether **foscarnet** crosses the human placenta. Rodent studies were for the most part reassuring, revealing a modest increase in minor skeletal abnormalities.

■ **Breastfeeding Safety**
There is no published experience in nursing women. It is unknown whether **foscarnet** enters human breast milk. However, it is concentrated in rat breast milk.

■ **References**
Alvarez-McLeod A, Havlik J, Drew KE. Clin Infect Dis 1999; 29:937-8.
Alla P, de Jaureguiberry JP, Legier HP, et al. Rev Med Interne 1999; 20:514-6.

■ **Summary**
• **Pregnancy Category C**
• **Lactation Category U**
• **Foscarnet** should be used during pregnancy and lactation only if the benefit justifies the potential perinatal risk.

Fosfomycin tromethamine (Monurol)

■ **Class**
Antibiotic

■ **Indications**
Acute cystitis with susceptible strains

■ **Mechanism**
Bactericidal

■ **Dosage with Qualifiers**
Acute cystitis—3g PO ×1
• **Contraindications**—sensitivity to drug or class
• **Caution**—hepatic dysfunction

■ **Maternal Considerations**
Fosfomycin is an orally active, broad-spectrum bactericidal agent that has the advantage of single-dose administration. There are no adequate reports or well-controlled studies of **fosfomycin** in pregnant women. In several controlled trials conducted in pregnant women, it was similar in efficacy to other commonly used agents.

Side effects include diarrhea, vaginitis, nausea, vomiting, headache, weakness, dizziness, and dyspepsia.

■ **Fetal Considerations** ⋯⋯⋯ There are no adequate reports or well-controlled studies in human fetuses. **Fosfomycin** readily crosses the human placenta, though the kinetics remain to be elucidated. Rodent studies are reassuring; fetal toxicity is seen only when the dose used produced maternal toxicity.

■ **Breastfeeding Safety** ⋯⋯ There is no published experience in nursing women. It is unknown whether **fosfomycin** enters human breast milk.

■ **References** ⋯⋯⋯⋯ Krcmery S, Hromec J, Demesova D. Int J Antimicrob Agents 2001; 17:279-82.
Reeves DS. Infection 1992; 20(Suppl 4):S313-6.
Ferreres L, Paz M, Martin G, Gobernado M. Chemotherapy 1977; 23(Suppl 1):175-9.

■ **Summary** ⋯⋯⋯⋯⋯
- **Pregnancy Category B**
- **Lactation Category U**
- **Fosfomycin** should be used during pregnancy and lactation only if the benefit justifies the potential perinatal risk.
- There are other agents available for which there is greater experience during pregnancy and lactation.

Fosinopril (Monopril)

■ **Class** ⋯⋯⋯⋯ ACE-1/A2R-*antagonist*

■ **Indications** ⋯⋯⋯ Hypertension, CHF, acute MI, nephropathy

■ **Mechanism** ⋯⋯⋯ ACE inhibitor

■ **Dosage with Qualifiers** ⋯⋯ Hypertension—begin 10mg PO qd; max 80mg/d; lower dose required with diuretic
CHF—begin 10mg PO qd; max 80mg/d
Acute MI—10-20mg PO qd
Nephropathy—20mg PO qd
NOTE—renal dosing; may also be combined with **hydrochlorothiazide**
- **Contraindications**—hypersensitivity to drug or class, hereditary or ACE-related angioedema, pregnancy
- **Caution**—renal artery stenosis, severe CHF, renal dysfunction, connective tissue disease, volume depletion, hyponatremia

- **Maternal Considerations** ⸱⸱⸱⸱⸱⸱ A long-acting ACE inhibitor, there is no published experience with **fosinopril** during pregnancy. **Fosinopril** is rarely if ever necessary during pregnancy.
Side effects include angioedema, hypotension, acute renal failure, hepatic toxicity, agranulocytosis, pancreatitis, cough, dizziness, fatigue, hyperkalemia, nausea, vomiting, elevated BUN, creatinine, musculoskeletal pain, and URI symptoms.

- **Fetal Considerations** ⸱⸱⸱⸱⸱⸱ There are no adequate reports or well-controlled studies in human fetuses. It is unknown whether **fosinopril** crosses the human placenta. However, this class of drugs is known to have adverse human fetal renal effects leading to disability or death. Similar effects occur with **fosinopril** in rodents.

- **Breastfeeding Safety** ⸱⸱⸱⸱⸱⸱ There is no published experience in nursing women. It is unknown whether **fosinopril** enters human breast milk.

- **References** ⸱⸱⸱⸱⸱⸱ Grove KL, Mayo RJ, Forsyth CS, et al. Toxicol Lett 1995; 80:85-95.

- **Summary** ⸱⸱⸱⸱⸱⸱
  - **Pregnancy Category D, C in 1st trimester**
  - **Lactation Category U**
  - ACE-I and A2R-antagonists should be avoided during pregnancy unless there are no alternatives.
  - Should an ACE-I/A2R-antagonist be required, **fosinopril** is a poor selection during pregnancy because of its long half-life.
  - There are alternative agents for which there is more experience during pregnancy and lactation.

Fosphenytoin (Cerebyx)

- **Class** ⸱⸱⸱⸱⸱⸱ *Anticonvulsant*

- **Indications** ⸱⸱⸱⸱⸱⸱ Status epilepticus, seizure disorder, seizure prevention prior to neurosurgery

- **Mechanism** ⸱⸱⸱⸱⸱⸱ See **phenytoin**

- **Dosage with Qualifiers** ⸱⸱⸱⸱⸱⸱ Status epilepticus—15-20mg phenytoin equivalents/kg IV ×1
Seizure disorder—load 10-20mg phenytoin equivalents/kg IV/IM, then 4-6mg phenytoin equivalents/kg IV/IM
Seizure prophylaxis before neurosurgery—load 10-20mg phenytoin equivalents/kg IV/IM, then 4-6mg phenytoin equivalents/kg IV/IM
NOTE—therapeutic level 10-20mcg/ml

- **Contraindications**—hypersensitivity to drug or class, sinus bradycardia, 2nd or 3rd degree AV block, SA block
- **Caution**—hypotension, hepatic or renal dysfunction, cardiovascular disease, diabetes mellitus, and porphyria

■ **Maternal Considerations** .... **Fosphenytoin** is converted *in vivo* to **phenytoin**. There are no adequate reports or well-controlled studies of **fosphenytoin** in pregnant women, but the risks should be similar to **phenytoin**. The risk of seizure during pregnancy may rise because of increased clearance. Maternal serum levels should be monitored throughout gestation. *Side effects* include cardiovascular collapse, hypotension, bradycardia, arrhythmias, Stevens-Johnson syndrome, toxic delirium, pancytopenia, thrombocytopenia, leukopenia, agranulocytosis, hepatic toxicity, anemia, dizziness, nystagmus, itching, paresthesias, headache, somnolence, nausea, vomiting, ataxia, tremor, dry mouth, blurred vision, fever, constipation, and electrolyte change.

■ **Fetal Considerations** .... There are no adequate reports or well-controlled studies in human fetuses. See **phenytoin**.

■ **Breastfeeding Safety** .... There is no published experience in nursing women. It is unknown whether **fosphenytoin** enters human breast milk. See **phenytoin**.

■ **References** .... There is no published experience in pregnancy or during lactation. See **phenytoin**.

■ **Summary** ....
- **Pregnancy Category D**
- **Lactation Category NS**
- Functionally equivalent to **phenytoin**.
- **Fosphenytoin** should be used during pregnancy and lactation only if the benefit justifies the potential perinatal risk.

Frovatriptan (Froval)

■ **Class** .... *Migraine*

■ **Indications** .... Migraine

■ **Mechanism** .... Selective 5HT-1 agonist

■ **Dosage with Qualifiers** .... <u>Migraine</u>—2.5mg PO ×1, may repeat after 2h; max 7.5mg/24h
- **Contraindications**—hypersensitivity to drug or class, coronary artery disease, CV disease, peripheral vascular disease, ischemic bowel disease, uncontrolled

hypertension, hemiplegic or basilar migraine, use of an ergot or 5H1 agonist within 24h.
- **Caution**—cardiac risk factors

■ **Maternal Considerations** — There is no published experience with **frovatriptan** during pregnancy.
Side effects include acute MI, coronary vasospasm, arrhythmias, subarachnoid hemorrhage, hypertensive crisis, stroke, bowel ischemia, dizziness, fatigue, flushing, paresthesias, dry mouth, bone pain, dyspepsia, neck or jaw tightness, and chest pressure.

■ **Fetal Considerations** — There are no adequate reports or well-controlled studies in human fetuses.

■ **Breastfeeding Safety** — There is no published experience in nursing women. It is unknown whether **frovatriptan** enters human breast milk. Considering the limited dosing regimen and the safety of similar class agents, **frovatriptan** is likely compatible with breastfeeding. If desired, the patient may pump her breasts for 24h and then resume breastfeeding.

■ **References** — There is no published experience in pregnancy or during lactation.

■ **Summary**
- **Pregnancy Category C**
- **Lactation Category ?**
- **Frovatriptan** should be used during pregnancy and lactation only if the benefit justifies the potential perinatal risk.

Furazolidone (Furoxone)

■ **Class** — Antibiotic

■ **Indications** — Bacterial infection

■ **Mechanism** — Interferes with enzyme systems

■ **Dosage with Qualifiers** — Bacterial infection—100mg PO qid ×5-10d
- **Contraindications**—hypersensitivity to drug or class, use of an MAO inhibitor within 2w, alcohol use
- **Caution**—G6PD deficiency

■ **Maternal Considerations** — **Furazolidone** is a metabolite of **nitrofurantoin** and should have a similar degree of safety during pregnancy. It is alternative treatment for giardiasis. There are no adequate reports or well-controlled studies in pregnant women. See **nitrofurantoin**.

Side effects include hypertension, hemolytic anemia, hypoglycemia, nausea, vomiting, abdominal pain, headache, rash, urticaria, fever, and arthralgia.

■ **Fetal Considerations** — There are no adequate reports or well-controlled studies in human fetuses. See **nitrofurantoin.**

■ **Breastfeeding Safety** — There is no published experience in nursing women. **Furazolidone** is excreted into rodent breast milk. See **nitrofurantoin.**

■ **References** — There is no published experience in pregnancy or during lactation.

■ **Summary** —
- **Pregnancy Category C**
- **Lactation Category S**
- **Furazolidone** is a metabolite of **nitrofurantoin** and should have a similar degree of safety during pregnancy.
- **Furazolidone** should be used during pregnancy and lactation only if the benefit justifies the potential perinatal risk.

Furosemide (Lasix)

■ **Class** — *Diuretic*

■ **Indications** — Pulmonary or peripheral edema, hypertension, hypercalcemia

■ **Mechanism** — Inhibits the reabsorption of sodium and chloride in the loop of Henle

■ **Dosage with Qualifiers** — Pulmonary edema—begin at 40mg IV ×1 slowly, assess response; may increase to 80mg IV q1h prn
Peripheral edema—20-80mg PO qd to bid; max 600mg qd
Hypertension—40mg PO bid; max 600mg qd
Hypercalcemia—80-100mg IV q1-2h, or 120mg PO qd
- **Contraindications**—hypersensitivity to drug or class, hypersensitivity to sulfonamides, anuria, hepatic coma, electrolyte imbalance
- **Caution**—severe renal disease, acute MI, diabetes mellitus, SLE, history of pancreatitis, combined with ototoxic drugs

■ **Maternal Considerations** — There are no adequate reports or well-controlled studies of **furosemide** in pregnant women. It is one of the drugs of choice for the treatment of CHF and/or pulmonary edema during pregnancy. High concentrations of **furosemide** dilate the capacitance vessels and assist the reduction in preload. The long clinical experience for the noted indications is reassuring. In one study of women with preeclampsia, **furosemide** caused a significant decrease in the intervillous blood flow. This likely reflects their already contracted intravascular volume. In rabbit studies, a high dose of **furosemide** was associated with unexplained maternal deaths.

Side effects include hypokalemia, metabolic alkalosis, orthostatic hypotension, ototoxicity, leukopenia, thrombocytopenia, pancreatitis, jaundice, SLE exacerbation, vasculitis, erythema multiforme, hemolytic anemia, dizziness, nausea, vomiting, weakness, cramps, hyperuricemia, hyperglycemia, tinnitus, paresthesias, and photosensitivity.

■ **Fetal Considerations**

There are no adequate reports or well-controlled studies in human fetuses. **Furosemide** crosses the human placenta, achieving an F:M ratio approximating unity after 8-10h. It is unclear, however, how responsive the fetal kidney is to it, and the impact of gestational age on that response. Direct administration of **furosemide** for fetal therapy, typically in association with hydrops has been frequently reported. However, no corresponding diuresis has been documented. In rodents, an effect on newborn urine concentrating ability is reported after *in utero* exposure. An increased prevalence was also noted in one mouse study. And though fetal sheep absorb it from amniotic fluid presumably via a transmembrane mechanism, direct administration fails to generate a fetal diuresis. In addition, there is no fetal diuresis after administration to the gravid ewe. In summary, the impact of furosemide on the fetus is unclear and likely small.

■ **Breastfeeding Safety**

There are no adequate reports or well-controlled studies in nursing women. **Furosemide** does enter human breast milk, but the kinetics remain to be elucidated. It is unlikely one-time or limited use would cause harm during lactation.

■ **References**

Beermann B, Groschinsky-Grind M, Fahraeus L, Lindstrom B. Clin Pharmacol Ther 1978; 24:560-2.
Suonio S, Saarikoski S, Tahvanainen K, Paakkonen A, Olkkonen H. Am J Obstet Gynecol 1986; 155:122-5.
Anandakumar C, Biswas A, Chua TM, et al. Ultrasound Obstet Gynecol 1999; 13:263-5.
Mallie JP, Boudzoumou P. Pediatr Nephrol 1996; 10:458-60.
Gilbert WM, Newman PS, Brace RA. Am J Obstet Gynecol 1995; 172:1471-6.
Ross MG, Ervin MG, Leake RD. Am J Obstet Gynecol 1985; 152:1107.
Chamberlain PF, Cumming M, Torchia MG, et al. Am J Obstet Gynecol 1985; 151:815-9.

■ **Summary** ⸻⸻⸻⸻⸻⸻⸻⸻

- **Pregnancy Category C**
- **Lactation Category S?**
- **Furosemide** should be used during pregnancy and lactation only if the benefit justifies the potential perinatal risk.
- The long clinical experience for the noted indications is reassuring.

Gabapentin (Neurontin)

- **Class** .... *Anticonvulsant*

- **Indications** .... Seizures (partial), post-herpetic neuralgia, neuropathic pain

- **Mechanism** .... Unknown

- **Dosage with Qualifiers** .... Seizures (partial)—begin 300mg PO qd ×1d, then bid ×1d, then tid; usual maintenance 1800-2400mg qd; max 3600mg/d
  Post-herpetic neuralgia—begin 300mg PO qd ×1d, then bid ×1d, then tid; max 1800mg/d
  Neuropathic pain—begin 300mg PO qd ×1d, then bid ×1d, then tid; max 3600mg/d
  NOTE—renal dosing
  - **Contraindications**—hypersensitivity to drug or class
  - **Caution**—renal dysfunction, abrupt withdrawal

- **Maternal Considerations** .... **Gabapentin** is a 2nd generation anticonvulsant used mainly as an adjunct. While there is little published experience during pregnancy and lactation, the limited study available suggests a higher safety margin relative to 1st generation agents. The dose may require adjustment during pregnancy, and should be based on both serum concentration and clinical symptoms. **Gabapentin** has been used for chronic headache during early pregnancy. While a relationship between hormones and seizure activity exists in many women, good options for catamenial epilepsy remain elusive. And while interactions between enzyme-inducing anticonvulsants and contraceptives are well documented, this is not true for **gabapentin**. Patients should be counseled to plan pregnancy, and informed of the value of **folate** supplementation, the importance of medication adherence, and the risk of teratogenicity.
  Side effects include leukopenia, dizziness, somnolence, fatigue, ataxia, tremor, blurred vision, nausea, vomiting, nervousness, dysarthria, weight gain, and dyspepsia.

- **Fetal Considerations** .... There are no adequate reports or well-controlled studies in human fetuses. It is unknown whether **gabapentin** crosses the human placenta. There was no evidence of human teratogenicity in a small post-marketing study. Rodent studies reveal fetotoxicity, and an increased prevalence of minor malformations including skeletal abnormalities (skull, spine, and limbs) and hydronephrosis.

- **Breastfeeding Safety** .... There are no adequate reports or well-controlled studies in nursing women. **Gabapentin** is excreted into human breast milk, though the content is such that the nursing neonate would be exposed to a maximum of approximately 1mg/kg/d, a dose likely to be subclinical. The infant should be monitored for possible adverse effects, the drug given at the lowest effective dose, and breastfeeding avoided at times of peak drug levels.

■ **References**

McAuley JW, Anderson GD. Clin Pharmacokinet 2002; 41:559-79.
Crawford P. CNS Drugs 2002; 16:263-72.
Marcus DA. Expert Opin Pharmacother 2002; 3:389-93.
Wilton LV, Shakir S. Epilepsia 2002; 43:983-92.
Lowe SA. Best Pract Res Clin Obstet Gynaecol 2001; 15:863-76.
Bar-Oz B, Nulman I, Koren G, Ito S. Paediatr Drugs 2000; 2:113-26.

■ **Summary**

- **Pregnancy Category C**
- **Lactation Category S?**
- Limited study suggests a higher safety margin relative to 1st generation anticonvulsants.

Gadoversetamide (Optimark)

■ **Class**

Diagnostic, nonradioactive; contrast medium

■ **Indications**

MRI

■ **Mechanism**

A component, gadolinium is paramagnetic

■ **Dosage with Qualifiers**

MRI—0.2ml/kg at 1-2ml/sec (alternatively 0.1 mmol/kg)
- **Contraindications**—hypersensitivity to drug or class
- **Caution**—hemolytic anemia, renal insufficiency

■ **Maternal Considerations**

There is no published experience with **gadoversetamide** during pregnancy.
Side effects include body discomfort, headache, abdominal pain, asthenia, back pain, flushing, nausea, vomiting, diarrhea, dyspepsia, dizziness, paresthesias, rhinitis, and taste alteration.

■ **Fetal Considerations**

There are no adequate reports or well-controlled studies in human fetuses. It is unknown whether **gadoversetamide** crosses the human placenta. It does cross the rodent placenta. Limited rodent studies are reassuring, revealing no evidence of teratogenicity or IUGR.

■ **Breastfeeding Safety**

There is no published experience in nursing women. It is unknown whether **gadoversetamide** enters human breast milk. It is excreted in rat breast milk. Breast-feeding women should consider discarding their milk after injection for 72h before resuming breastfeeding.

■ **References** .... Wible JH, Troup CM, Hynes MR, et al. Invest Radiol 2001; 36:401-12.

■ **Summary** ....
- **Pregnancy Category C**
- **Lactation Category U**
- **Gadoversetamide** should be used during pregnancy and lactation only if the benefit justifies the potential perinatal risk.

Galantamine (Reminyl)

■ **Class** .... *Alzheimer's disease*

■ **Indications** .... Alzheimer's dementia

■ **Mechanism** .... Cholinesterase inhibitor

■ **Dosage with Qualifiers** .... Alzheimer dementia—begin 4mg PO bid; increase by 4mg bid q4w to a max of 12mg bid
NOTE—renal and hepatic dosing
- **Contraindications**—hypersensitivity to drug or class
- **Caution**—peptic ulcer disease, cardiac conduction defects, seizure disorder, asthma, COPD, hepatic or renal dysfunction

■ **Maternal Considerations** .... There is no published experience in pregnancy. In light of the natural history of Alzheimer's disease, **galantamine** is unlikely to be required during pregnancy.
Side effects include AV block, bradycardia, arrhythmias, seizures, urinary obstruction, nausea, vomiting, diarrhea, anorexia, dizziness, dyspepsia, fatigue, depression, insomnia, abdominal pain, rhinitis, tremor, syncope, and hematuria.

■ **Fetal Considerations** .... There are no adequate reports or well-controlled studies in human fetuses. It is unknown whether **galantamine** crosses the human placenta. Rodent studies are reassuring, revealing no evidence of teratogenicity or IUGR despite the use of doses higher than those used clinically.

■ **Breastfeeding Safety** .... There is no published experience in nursing women. It is unknown whether **galantamine** enters human breast milk.

■ **References** .... There is no published experience in pregnancy or during lactation.

■ **Summary**
- **Pregnancy Category B**
- **Lactation Category U**
- **Galantamine** should be used during pregnancy and lactation only if the benefit justifies the potential perinatal risk.

Ganciclovir (Cytovene)

■ **Class** — Antiviral

■ **Indications** — CMV retinitis

■ **Mechanism** — Inhibits viral DNA polymerase

■ **Dosage with Qualifiers** — CMV retinitis—5mg/kg IV over 1h q12h ×14-21d; then 5mg/kg IV qd, then 1000mg PO qd
NOTE—renal dosing
- **Contraindications**—hypersensitivity to drug or class, bone marrow depression
- **Caution**—renal dysfunction

■ **Maternal Considerations** — There are no adequate reports or well-controlled studies in pregnant women. Case reports include **ganciclovir** use during the 1st trimester in one woman with a liver transplant and another with a kidney transplant, and in a third with CMV hepatitis.
Side effects include seizures, coma, thrombocytopenia, neutropenia, anemia, nephrotoxicity, fever, diarrhea, nausea, vomiting, sweating, chills, pruritus, neuropathy, paresthesias, and elevated LFTs.

■ **Fetal Considerations** — There are no adequate reports or well-controlled studies in human fetuses. **Ganciclovir** crosses the human placenta by passive diffusion. It has been administered directly to CMV-infected fetuses with sonographically detected sequelae with unclear success: the viral load declined but the fetus died. Postnatally, **ganciclovir** remains the drug of choice for the treatment of symptomatic neonatal CMV; it is not curative, but rather ameliorates sequelae. **Ganciclovir** is embryotoxic in rats and mice. In rabbits, it is associated with cleft palate, micropthalmia, renal agenesis, and hydrocephaly.

■ **Breastfeeding Safety** — There are no adequate reports or well-controlled studies in nursing women. It is unknown whether **ganciclovir** enters human breast milk. **Ganciclovir** enters rat breast milk by passive diffusion reaching near maternal serum levels. However, it is usually considered compatible with breastfeeding considering its neonatal application.

■ **References** ───────── Alcorn J, McNamara PJ. Antimicrob Agents Chemother 2002; 46:1831-6.
Bale JF, Miner L, Petheram SJ. Curr Treat Options Neurol 2002; 4:225-230.
Pescovitz MD. Transplantation 1999; 15:758-9.
Miller BW, Howard TK, Goss JA, et al. Transplantation 1995; 60:1353-4.
Miguelez M, Gonzalez A, Perez F. Scand J Infect Dis 1998; 30:304-5.
Henderson GI, Hu ZQ, Yang Y, et al. Am J Med Sci 1993; 306:151-6.

■ **Summary** ──────────
- **Pregnancy Category C**
- **Lactation Category S?**
- **Ganciclovir** should be used during pregnancy and lactation only if the benefit justifies the potential perinatal risk.

Gatifloxacin (Tequin)

■ **Class** ───────── *Antibacterial, quinolone*

■ **Indications** ───────── Bacterial infection; uncomplicated gonorrhea

■ **Mechanism** ───────── Bactericidal, inhibits DNA gyrase and topoisomerase IV

■ **Dosage with Qualifiers** ───────── Bacterial infections—200-400mg PO/IV (infuse over 60min) qd ×7-10d
Uncomplicated gonorrhea—400mg PO ×1
NOTE—renal dosing
- **Contraindications**—hypersensitivity to drug or class, prolonged QT interval
- **Caution**—cardiovascular disease, proarrhythmic condition, concurrent class IA, III antiarrhythmic agents

■ **Maternal Considerations** ───────── **Gatifloxacin** is a well-absorbed oral quinolone. There is no published experience with **gatifloxacin** during pregnancy. *Side effects* include pseudomembranous colitis, superinfection, vaginitis, increased intracranial pressure, seizures, tendonitis, toxic psychosis, nausea, vomiting, diarrhea, abdominal pain, headache, dyspepsia, dizziness, lightheadedness, insomnia, rash, anxiety, confusion, increased LFTs, agitation, and photosensitivity.

■ **Fetal Considerations** ───────── There are no adequate reports or well-controlled studies in human fetuses. It is unknown whether **gatifloxacin** crosses the human placenta. Rodent studies using multiples of the MRHD reveal an increased risk of skeletal abnormalities and neonatal death rate.

■ **Breastfeeding Safety** ···················· There is no published experience in nursing women. It is unknown whether **gatifloxacin** enters human breast milk. **Gatifloxacin** does enter rat milk and caution is recommended during lactation.

■ **References** ···················· There is no published experience in pregnancy or during lactation.

■ **Summary** ····················
- **Pregnancy Category C**
- **Lactation Category U**
- **Gatifloxacin** should be used during pregnancy and lactation only if the benefit justifies the potential perinatal risk.
- There are other agents with more experience and a higher safety profile during pregnancy and lactation.

Gemfibrozil (Lopid; Tripid)

■ **Class** ···················· *Hyperlipidemia*

■ **Indications** ···················· Hypertriglyceridemia, hypercholesterolemia (high LDL, triglycerides, low HDL)

■ **Mechanism** ···················· Decreases hepatic free fatty acid extraction, inhibits synthesis and increases the clearance of the VLDL carrier apolipoprotein B, inhibits peripheral lipolysis.

■ **Dosage with Qualifiers** ···················· Hypertriglyceridemia—600mg PO bid 30min ac
Hypercholesterolemia—600mg PO bid 30min ac
- **Contraindications**—hypersensitivity to drug or class, gallbladder disease, **cerivastatin** use, hepatic dysfunction
- **Caution**—renal dysfunction, use with other statins class agents

■ **Maternal Considerations** ···················· There are no adequate reports or well-controlled studies in pregnant women. Hyperlipidemia is a chronic illness. Discontinuation of therapy during pregnancy is unlikely to alter the long-term outcome. Case reports document uncomplicated use of **gemfibrozil** in pregnant women with either hypertriglyceridemia or familial chylomicronemia. *Side effects* include myositis, cholelithiasis, cholestatic jaundice, thrombocytopenia, anemia, rhabdomyolysis, acute appendicitis, atrial fibrillation, increased LFTs, elevated CPK, nausea, vomiting, dyspepsia, abdominal pain, diarrhea, and fatigue.

- **Fetal Considerations** .... There are no adequate and well-controlled studies in human fetuses. It is unknown whether **gemfibrozil** crosses the human placenta. Rodent studies reveal a dose-related increase in skeletal abnormalities at twice the MRHD.

- **Breastfeeding Safety** .... There are no adequate reports or well-controlled studies in nursing women. It is unknown whether **gemfibrozil** enters human breast milk. The offspring of treated rodents have reduced weight during neonatal and weaning periods.

- **References** .... Al-Shali K, Wang J, Fellows F, et al. Clin Biochem 2002; 35:125-30.
Perronne G, Critelli C. Minerva Ginecol 1996; 48:573-6.
Keilson LM, Vary CP, Sprecher DL, Renfrew R. Ann Intern Med 1987; 124:425-8.
Fitzgerald JE, Petrere JA, de la Iglesia FA. Fundam Appl Toxicol 1987; 8:454-64.

- **Summary** ....
  - **Pregnancy Category C**
  - **Lactation Category U**
  - **Gemfibrozil** should be used during pregnancy and lactation only if the benefit justifies the potential perinatal risk.

Gentamicin (G-Myticin; Garamycin; Genoptic; Gentacidin; Gentak; Ocu-Mycin)

- **Class** .... *Antibiotic, aminoglycoside; dermatologic; ophthalmologic*

- **Indications** .... Bacterial infection, endocarditis prophylaxis

- **Mechanism** .... Bactericidal, inhibits protein synthesis by binding the bacterial 30S ribosomal subunit

- **Dosage with Qualifiers** .... Bacterial infection—1-3mg/kg/d in 3 divided doses to achieve a peak 5-10mcg/ml and trough <2mcg/ml
Endocarditis prophylaxis—1.5mg/kg IV 30-60min prior to the procedure
NOTE—renal dosing; available for parenteral, topical, or ophthalmic administration
  - **Contraindications**—hypersensitivity to drug or class
  - **Caution**—renal dysfunction, nephrotoxic agents, cochlear implant, myasthenia gravis

- **Maternal Considerations** .... **Gentamicin** is commonly used in obstetric patients for the treatment of infections such as pyelonephritis. Routine monitoring of peak and trough levels are not required in otherwise healthy women with normal renal function. Coupled with **clindamycin**, it remains standard for the treatment of puerperal endomyometritis. Once a day treatment postpartum (5mg/kg) with **clindamycin** is as effective and cheaper than tid dosing. Once the endometritis has resolved on IV therapy, there is no need for further oral therapy.

Side effects include nephro- and ototoxicity, thrombocytopenia, agranulocytosis, neurotoxicity, enterocolitis, pseudotumor cerebri, nausea, vomiting, rash, pruritus, weakness, tremor, muscle cramps, anorexia, edema, headache, diarrhea, dyspepsia, tinnitus, and elevated BUN/Cr.

■ **Fetal Considerations**

There are no adequate reports or well-controlled studies in human fetuses. **Gentamicin** crosses the human placenta, reaching an F:M ratio approximating unity. In rodents, placental transfer is greater early than late gestation. It interferes with renal protein reabsorption in fetal rats, and depresses body weights, kidney weights, and median glomerular counts in newborn rats when administered systemically at multiples of the MRHD. However, the evidence for human fetal **gentamicin** toxicity is weak. There is no evidence to support the practice in some locales of using **gentamicin** for ophthalmia neonatorum prophylaxis.

■ **Breastfeeding Safety**

Gentamicin enters human breast milk, though only trace amounts can be found in the breast-feeding child.

■ **References**

Mitra AG, Whitten MK, Laurent SL, Anderson WE. Am J Obstet Gynecol 1997; 177:786-92.
Livingston JC, Llata E, Rinehart E, et al. Am J Obstet Gynecol 2003; 188:149-52.
French LM, Smaill FM. Cochrane Database Syst Rev 2002; (1):CD001067.
Briggs GG, Ambrose P, Nageotte MP. Am J Obstet Gynecol 1989; 160:309-13.
Smaoui H, Schaeverbeke M, Mallie JP, Schaeverbeke J. Pediatr Nephrol 1994; 8:447-50.
Nichoga LA, Skosyreva AM, Voropareva SD. Antibiotiki 1982; 27:46-50.
Celiloglu M, Celiker S, Guven H, et al. Obstet Gynecol 1994; 84:263-5.
Czeizel AE, Rockenbauer M, Olsen J, Sorensen HT. Scand J Infect Dis 2000; 32:309-13.

■ **Summary**

- **Pregnancy Category C**
- **Lactation Category S**
- **Gentamicin** is widely used during pregnancy and lactation without evidence of excess toxicity to mother or fetus.

Glatiramer acetate (Copaxone)

- **Class** — Immunomodulator

- **Indications** — Relapsing multiple sclerosis

- **Mechanism** — Unknown

- **Dosage with Qualifiers** — Relapsing multiple sclerosis—20mg SC qd
  - **Contraindications**—hypersensitivity to drug or class, hypersensitivity to **mannitol**
  - **Caution**—immunosuppression

- **Maternal Considerations** — There is no published experience with **glatiramer** during pregnancy.
  Side effects include injection site reactions, transient chest pain, back pain, flu-like symptoms, erythema, infection, asthenia, itching, anxiety, nausea, vomiting, insomnia, hypertonus, dyspnea, rash, sweating, and palpitations.

- **Fetal Considerations** — There are no adequate reports or well-controlled studies in human fetuses. It is unknown whether **glatiramer** crosses the human placenta. Rodent studies are reassuring, revealing no evidence of teratogenicity or IUGR despite the use of doses higher than those used clinically.

- **Breastfeeding Safety** — There is no published experience in nursing women. It is unknown whether **glatiramer** enters human breast milk.

- **References** — There is no published experience in pregnancy or during lactation.

- **Summary** —
  - **Pregnancy Category B**
  - **Lactation Category U**
  - **Glatiramer** should be used during pregnancy and lactation only if the benefit justifies the potential perinatal risk.

Glimepiride (Amaryl)

- **Class** — Hypoglycemic; sulfonylurea, 2nd generation

- **Indications** — Diabetes mellitus, type 2

- **Mechanism** — Stimulates pancreatic β cell release of insulin

- **Dosage with Qualifiers** ⸺ Diabetes mellitus, type 2—begin 1-2mg PO with first main meal of the day; max 8mg qd
  - **Contraindications**—hypersensitivity to drug or class, diabetic ketoacidosis
  - **Caution**—hypersensitivity to sulfonamides

- **Maternal Considerations** ⸺ There are no adequate reports or well-controlled studies of **glimepride** in pregnant women. The published experience is limited to a case report.
  Side effects include hypoglycemia, pancytopenia, thrombocytopenia, aplastic anemia, dizziness, asthenia, nausea, and headache.

- **Fetal Considerations** ⸺ There are no adequate reports or well-controlled studies in human fetuses. It is unknown whether **glimepiride** crosses the human placenta. There is evidence suggesting other 2nd generation sulfonylureas cross poorly. There is a single case report of a newborn with persistent hyperinsulinemic, hypoglycemia after long-term *in utero* exposure to **glimepiride**. Rodent studies are reassuring, revealing no evidence of teratogenicity or IUGR despite the use of doses higher than those used clinically. Fetal losses occurred at doses approximating 4000 times the MRHD.

- **Breastfeeding Safety** ⸺ There are no adequate reports or well-controlled studies in nursing women. It is unknown whether **glimepiride** enters human breast milk.

- **References** ⸺ Elliott BD, Schenker S, Langer O, et al. Am J Obstet Gynecol 1994; 171:653-60.
  Balaguer Santamaria JA, Feliu Rovira A, Escribano Subias J, et al. Rev Clin Esp 2000; 200:399-400.

- **Summary** ⸺
  - **Pregnancy Category C**
  - **Lactation Category U**
  - **Glimepiride** should be used during pregnancy and lactation only if the benefit justifies the potential perinatal risk.
  - A better-studied 2nd-generation agent, such as **glyburide,** is a preferable alternative if an oral hypoglycemic is necessary.

Glipizide (Glucotrol; Glucotrol XI; Minidab)

- **Class** ⸺ Hypoglycemic; *sulfonylurea, 2nd generation*

- **Indications** ⸺ Diabetes mellitus, type 2

- **Mechanism** ⸺ Stimulates pancreatic β cell release of insulin

- **Dosage with Qualifiers** ⸺ Diabetes mellitus, type 2—begin 5mg PO 30min prior to first main meal of the day; doses above 15mg/d, give in 2 divided doses 30min before meals, max 40mg qd
  NOTE—available in XL preparation (max dose 20mg/d)
  - **Contraindications**—hypersensitivity to drug or class, diabetic ketoacidosis, IDDM
  - **Caution**—hypersensitivity to sulfonamides

- **Maternal Considerations** ⸺ There is no published experience with **glipizide** during pregnancy. Some oral hypoglycemic agents are potentially attractive for the treatment of gestational or type II diabetes mellitus during pregnancy. However, their use at the present time should probably be confined to formal protocols.
  Side effects include hypoglycemia, pancytopenia, thrombocytopenia, aplastic anemia, dizziness, asthenia, nausea, and headache.

- **Fetal Considerations** ⸺ There are no adequate and well-controlled studies in human fetuses. About 6% of the maternal dose of **glipizide** crosses the isolated human placenta. Only **glyburide** transport is lower. No teratogenic effects were found in rodents, though fetal loss occurs across a range of doses.

- **Breastfeeding Safety** ⸺ There is no published experience in nursing women. It is unknown whether **glipizide** enters human breast milk.

- **References** ⸺ Elliott BD, Schenker S, Langer O, et al. Am J Obstet Gynecol 1994; 171:653-60.

- **Summary** ⸺
  - **Pregnancy Category C**
  - **Lactation Category U**
  - **Glipizide** should be used during pregnancy and lactation only if the benefit justifies the potential perinatal risk.
  - A better-studied 2nd-generation agent such as **glyburide** is a preferable alternative if an oral hypoglycemic is necessary.

Glucagon (GlucaGen [rDNA origin])

- **Class** ⸺ *Antihypoglycemic; hormone*

- **Indications** ⸺ Hypoglycemia, severe

- **Mechanism** ⸺ Converts hepatic glycogen to glucose

- **Dosage with Qualifiers** ⸺ Hypoglycemia, severe—0.5-1mg IV/IM/SC ×1; may repeat in 25min

- **Contraindications**—hypersensitivity
- **Caution**—insulinoma, pheochromocytoma

■ **Maternal Considerations** ········· There are no adequate reports or well-controlled studies in pregnant women. There is, however, a long, reassuring clinical experience of **glucagon** use during pregnancy, typically in diabetic women with insulin-induced severe hypoglycemia.
Side effects include hyperglycemia, hypotension, nausea, vomiting, urticaria, and ARDS.

■ **Fetal Considerations** ············· There are no adequate reports or well-controlled studies in human fetuses. **Glucagon** does not appear to cross the human placenta. Rodent studies are reassuring, revealing no evidence of teratogenicity or IUGR despite the use of doses higher than those used clinically.

■ **Breastfeeding Safety** ··············· There is no published experience in nursing women. It is unknown whether this drug is excreted in human breast milk. However, **glucagon** is not active when ingested, as it is destroyed in the gastrointestinal tract before absorption.

■ **References** ····················· Spellacy WN, Buhi WC. Obstet Gynecol 1976; 47:291-4.

■ **Summary** ························
- **Pregnancy Category B**
- **Lactation Category S**
- **Glucagon** is indicated for the treatment of severe hypoglycemia during pregnancy and lactation.

Glyburide (DiaBeta; Micronase)

■ **Class** ················· Hypoglycemic; *sulfonylurea, 2nd generation*

■ **Indications** ················· Diabetes mellitus, type 2

■ **Mechanism** ················· Stimulates β cell release of insulin

■ **Dosage with Qualifiers** ············· Diabetes mellitus, type 2—begin 2.5-5mg PO with first main meal of the day; usual maintenance dose 2.5-5.0 mg/d; max 20mg qd (micronized 1.5-3.0mg/d; usual maintenance dose 0.75-1.25mg/d)
NOTE—may be combined with **meformin**
- **Contraindications**—hypersensitivity to drug or class, diabetic ketoacidosis, IDDM, CrCl<50
- **Caution**—hepatic or renal dysfunction, hypersensitivity to sulfonamides, thyroid disease, adrenal insufficiency

- **Maternal Considerations** ⸺ A growing body of investigation indicates that **glyburide** is an effective alternative to insulin in women with gestational diabetes where it is more cost-effective than insulin. *Side effects* include hypoglycemia, pancytopenia, thrombocytopenia, leukopenia, aplastic or hemolytic anemia, hepatitis, nausea, epigastric pain, dizziness, blurred vision, dyspepsia, elevated LFTs, rash, photosensitivity, hyponatremia, and headache.

- **Fetal Considerations** ⸺ There are no adequate reports or well-controlled studies in human fetuses. Less than 2% of the maternal **glyburide** dose crosses the isolated perfused human placenta. Rodent studies are reassuring, revealing no evidence of teratogenicity or IUGR despite the use of doses higher than those used clinically.

- **Breastfeeding Safety** ⸺ There is no published experience in nursing women. It is unknown whether **glyburide** enters human breast milk.

- **References** ⸺ Langer O, Conway DL, Berkus MD, et al. N Engl J Med 2000; 343:1134-8.
Goetzl L, Wilkins I. J Perinatol 2002 Jul-Aug; 22(5):403-6.
Lim JM, Tayob Y O'Brien PM, Shaw RW. Med J Malaysia 1997; 52:377-81.
Elliott BD, Schenker S, Langer O, et al. Am J Obstet Gynecol 1994; 171:653-60.

- **Summary** ⸺
  - **Pregnancy Category B**
  - **Lactation Category U**
  - A potentially attractive alternative or supplement to insulin for the treatment of type 2 diabetes mellitus during pregnancy and gestational diabetes characterized by hyperglycemia.

Glycerin

- **Class** ⸺ Purgative

- **Indications** ⸺ Constipation

- **Mechanism** ⸺ Irritates mucosa, increasing peristalsis and stool water content

- **Dosage with Qualifiers** ⸺ Constipation—1 adult suppository PR prn
  - **Contraindications**—hypersensitivity to drug or class, anuria, hypovolemia, pulmonary edema
  - **Caution**—abdominal pain, hepatic or renal dysfunction

- **Maternal Considerations** ········ There are no adequate reports or well-controlled studies in pregnant women. Maternal risks are related to abuse of the product.
  Side effects include diarrhea, headache, nausea, and rectal irritation.

- **Fetal Considerations** ············· There are no adequate reports or well-controlled studies in human fetuses. However, maternal systemic absorption of **glycerin** is low.

- **Breastfeeding Safety** ············· There is no published experience in nursing women. However, maternal systemic absorption of **glycerin** is low, suggesting the risk to the breast-feeding neonate is minimal.

- **References** ························· There is no published experience in pregnancy or during lactation.

- **Summary** ·························· • **Pregnancy Category C**
  • **Lactation Category S**
  • Traditional remedy for constipation.

Glycopyrrolate (Robinul)

- **Class** ······························ Anticholinergic; *gastrointestinal, anesthetic agent*

- **Indications** ······················· Peptic ulcer disease, anesthesia adjunct, neuromuscular reversal

- **Mechanism** ······················· Antagonizes acetylcholine receptors

- **Dosage with Qualifiers** ·········· Peptic ulcer disease—1-2mg PO bid/tid; alternative 0.1-2mg IV/IM tid/qid
  Anesthesia adjunct—begin 0.004mg/kg IM 30-60min before anesthesia
  Neuromuscular reversal—0.01mg/kg, max 1mg IV for each 1mg (0.07mg/kg; max 5mg at a time) of **neostigmine**
  • **Contraindications**—hypersensitivity to drug or class, glaucoma, GI obstruction, ileus myasthenia gravis, ulcerative colitis, unstable cardiovascular system
  • **Caution**—hepatic dysfunction

- **Maternal Considerations** ········ There are no adequate reports or well-controlled studies in pregnant women. **Glycopyrrolate** reduces nausea after spinal anesthesia in pregnant women. It also reduces the prevalence of hypotension after epidural in women with normal heart rates to a similar degree as **ephedrine**. It may increase the risk of significant tachycardia when given with a betamimetic agent.

Side effects include orthostatic hypotension, constipation, dry mouth, mydriasis, blurred vision, urinary retention, nausea, insomnia, weakness, palpitations, dizziness, headache, confusion, and abdominal pain.

■ **Fetal Considerations**
There are no adequate reports or well-controlled studies in human fetuses. It is unknown whether **glycopyrrolate** crosses the human placenta. Transfer is limited in the ewe, achieving a peak F:M ratio of 0.13. Rodent studies are reassuring, revealing no evidence of teratogenicity or IUGR despite the use of doses higher than those used clinically.

■ **Breastfeeding Safety**
There is no published experience in nursing women. It is unknown whether **glycopyrrolate** enters human breast milk.

■ **References**
Ure D, James KS, McNeill M, Booth JV. Br J Anaesth 1999; 82:277-9.
Rucklidge MW, Durbridge J, Barnes PK, Yentis SM. Anaesthesia 2002; 57:4-8.
Murad SH, Conklin KA, Tabsh KM, et al. Anesth Analg 1981; 60:710-4.

■ **Summary**
• **Pregnancy Category B**
• **Lactation Category U**
• **Glycopyrrolate** is commonly used during pregnancy and lactation as an adjunct to anesthesia without apparent adverse effect.

Gold sodium thiomalate (Aurolate; Myochrysine)

■ **Class**
Arthritis

■ **Indications**
Rheumatoid arthritis

■ **Mechanism**
Unknown

■ **Dosage with Qualifiers**
Rheumatoid arthritis—begin 10mg IM qw ×1, 25mg IM qw ×1, then 25-50mg IM for an additional 10w
• **Contraindications**—hypersensitivity to drug or class, concurrent **penicillamine** use
• **Caution**—granulocytopenia or anemia secondary to drug reaction, skin rash, hepatic or renal dysfunction, moderate to severe hypertension, compromised cardiovascular or cerebral circulations

- **Maternal Considerations** ⸺ There are no adequate reports or well-controlled studies in pregnant women. It is important to perform a urinalysis before each injection because of the risk of maternal renal toxicity.

  Side effects include pruritus, exfoliative dermatitis, oral pharyngeal ulcers, metallic taste, renal toxicity, granulocytopenia, thrombocytopenia, aplastic anemia, flushing, fainting, dizziness, bradycardia, shock, and tongue swelling.

- **Fetal Considerations** ⸺ There are no adequate reports or well-controlled studies in human fetuses. Gold does cross the human placenta to a limited degree, and scant deposition occurs in the fetal liver. Rodent studies reveal an increased prevalence of multiple defects involving the CNS, abdominal wall, and limbs.

- **Breastfeeding Safety** ⸺ There are no adequate reports or well-controlled studies in nursing women. **Gold sodium thiomalate** enters human breast milk, and the slow maternal clearance of gold must be remembered. Gold was found in the serum and red blood cells of a nursing infant. In one study, the estimated weight-adjusted dose to the infant exceeded that received by the mother.

- **References** ⸺ Moller-Madsen B, Danscher G, Uldbjerg N, Allen JG. Rheumatol Int 1987; 7:47-8.
  Bennett PN, Humphries SJ, Osborne JP, et al. Br J Pharmacol 1990; 29:777-9.

- **Summary** ⸺
  - **Pregnancy Category C**
  - **Lactation Category NS?**
  - **Gold sodium thiomalate** should be used during pregnancy and lactation only if the benefit justifies the potential perinatal risk.
  - It would be reasonable to seek an alternative therapy during breastfeeding.

Granisetron hydrochloride (Kytril)

- **Class** ⸺ Antiemetic; *antivertigo; serotonin receptor antagonist*

- **Indications** ⸺ Severe nausea and vomiting secondary to chemotherapy, radiation, or spinal anesthesia

- **Mechanism** ⸺ Selective 5HT3 antagonist

■ **Dosage with Qualifiers** ⋯⋯⋯ <u>Severe nausea and vomiting of chemotherapy</u>—10mcg/kg IV over 5min, or 2mg PO qd
<u>Severe nausea and vomiting of radiation therapy</u>—2mg PO qd beginning within 30min of therapy
<u>Prophylaxis for postoperative nausea and vomiting</u>—2-4mg IV

- **Contraindications**—hypersensitivity to drug or class
- **Caution**—none

■ **Maternal Considerations** ⋯⋯ Nausea and vomiting after spinal anesthesia is common and distressing. **Granisetron** is superior to both **droperidol** and **metoclopramide** for its prevention. The addition of **dexamethasone** (8mg) further enhances its efficacy. There are several case reports of its use during pregnancy in women receiving chemotherapy.
Side effects include anemia, thrombocytopenia, leukopenia, headache, weakness, somnolence, diarrhea, constipation, fever, rash, hypertension, taste changes, alopecia, and elevated LFTs.

■ **Fetal Considerations** ⋯⋯⋯ There are no adequate reports or well-controlled studies in human fetuses. It is unknown whether **granisetron** crosses the placenta. Rodent studies are reassuring, revealing no evidence of teratogenicity or IUGR despite the use of doses higher than those used clinically.

■ **Breastfeeding Safety** ⋯⋯⋯ There is no published experience in nursing women. It is unknown whether **granisetron** enters human breast milk.

■ **References** ⋯⋯⋯⋯⋯ Fujii Y, Tanaka H, Toyooka H. Acta Anaesthesiol Scand 1998; 42:921-5.
Fujii Y, Saitoh Y, Tanaka H, Toyooka H. Anesth Analg 1999; 88:1346-50.
Merimsky O, Le Chevalier T, Missenard G, et al. Ann Oncol 1999; 10:345-50.

■ **Summary** ⋯⋯⋯⋯⋯
- **Pregnancy Category B**
- **Lactation Category S**
- An effective antiemetic during pregnancy, especially for women undergoing cancer therapy or receiving a spinal anesthetic.
- There are cheaper, often as effective, agents available for the treatment of hyperemesis.

Griseofulvin microcrystalline/ ultramicrocrystalline (Brofulin; Fulvicin U/F; Grifulin; Grifulvin V; Grisactin; Microfulvin; Microgris; Taidin/Fulvicin P/G; Fulvina; Gris-Peg; Grisactin Ultra; Griseofulvin Ultramicrosize; Sporostatin; Ultragris; Ultramicrosize Griseofulvin)

■ **Class** — *Antifungal*

■ **Indications** — Tinea corporis, tinea capitis, tinea cruris, tinea pedis, tinea unguium

■ **Mechanism** — Deposited in the keratin of precursor cells enhancing resistance to fungal invasion

■ **Dosage with Qualifiers** —
Tinea corporis—500mg PO qd
Tinea capitis—500mg PO qd
Tinea cruris—500mg PO qd
Tinea pedis—750-1000mg PO in 2 divided doses
Tinea unguium—750-1000mg PO in 2 divided doses
NOTE—micronized dose listed, 500mg = 330mg ultramicronized; avoid prolonged exposure to sunlight
- **Contraindications**—hypersensitivity to drug or class, porphyria
- **Caution**—penicillin allergy, hepatic dysfunction

■ **Maternal Considerations** — There are no adequate reports or well-controlled studies in pregnant women. Plasma concentrations of contraceptive steroids are decreased by **griseofulvin**, which stimulates their hepatic metabolism. **Griseofulvin** inhibits chromosomal distribution during cell division. Thus, men are cautioned to delay fathering children for 6mo after completing therapy, and women planning conception should wait at least 1mo.
Side effects include hepatic toxicity, granulocytopenia, nausea, headache, rash, urticaria, photosensitivity, lupus-like syndrome, oral candidasis, paresthesias, dizziness, fatigue, insomnia, proteinuria, flatulence, and diarrhea.

■ **Fetal Considerations** — There are no adequate reports or well-controlled studies in human fetuses. It is unknown whether **griseofulvin** crosses the human placenta. And while teratogenicity is suggested in horses and cats, rodent studies indicating teratogenicity were not confirmed after repetition. There are unsubstantiated reports of an association with conjoined twinning in humans.

■ **Breastfeeding Safety** — There are no adequate reports or well-controlled studies in nursing women. It is unknown whether this drug is excreted in human breast milk.

■ **References** ⸻ Scott FW, LaHunta A, Schultz RD, et al. Teratology
1975; 11:79-86.
Schutte JG, van den Ingh TS. Vet Q 1997; 19:58-60.
King CT, Rogers PD, Cleary JD, Chapman SW. Clin Infect
Dis 1998; 27:1151-60.

■ **Summary** ⸻
- **Pregnancy Category C**
- **Lactation Category U**
- There is some concern for the safety of **griseofulvin** during pregnancy, and other options exist.

Guaifenesin (Fenex La; Fenesin; Humibid L.A.; Muco-Fen LA; Mucobid-L.A.; Organidin Nr; Pneumomist; Prolex; Touro Ex; Tussin)

■ **Class** ⸻ *Antitussive, expectorant*

■ **Indications** ⸻ Cough suppression, expectorant

■ **Mechanism** ⸻ Increases the quantity and decreases the viscosity of respiratory tract secretions

■ **Dosage with Qualifiers** ⸻ Cough suppression—600-1200mg PO qd; max 2400mg/d
Expectorant—200-400mg PO q4h; max 2400mg/d
NOTE—available in tablet or syrup, and may be combined with **hydrocodone**, **phenylephrine**, or **pseudoephedrine**
- **Contraindications**—hypersensitivity to drug or class
- **Cautions**—unknown

■ **Maternal Considerations** ⸻ There are no adequate and well-controlled studies in pregnant women. Animal reproduction studies have not been conducted.
Side effects include drowsiness, nausea, vomiting, rash, and headache.

■ **Fetal Considerations** ⸻ There are no adequate reports or well-controlled studies in human fetuses. It is unknown whether **guaifenesin** crosses the human placenta. Limited epidemiological study provides no help estimating the risk of **guaifenesin**. Rodent teratogenicity studies have not been performed.

■ **Breastfeeding Safety** ⸻ There is no published experience in nursing women. It is unknown whether this drug is excreted in human breast milk.

■ **References** ⸻ Shaw GM, Todoroff K, Velie EM, Lammer EJ. Teratology
1998; 57:1-7.

■ **Summary** • **Pregnancy Category C**
• **Lactation Category U**
• **Guaifenesin** should be used during pregnancy and lactation only if the benefit justifies the potential perinatal risk.

Guanabenz acetate (Wytensin)

■ **Class** — Antihypertensive; antiadrenergic, central

■ **Indications** — Hypertension

■ **Mechanism** — Centrally acting α-2 agonist

■ **Dosage with Qualifiers** — Hypertension—begin 2-4mg PO bid; increase by 4-8mg/d q1-2w; max 32mg PO bid
• **Contraindications**—hypersensitivity to drug or class
• **Caution**—hepatic or renal dysfunction

■ **Maternal Considerations** — There is no published experience with **guanabenz** during pregnancy.
Side effects include sedation, arrhythmias, AV block, rebound hypertension, dizziness, weakness, headache, nausea, vomiting, diarrhea, constipation, chest pain, bradycardia, edema, and rash.

■ **Fetal Considerations** — There are no adequate reports or well-controlled studies in human fetuses. It is unknown whether **guanabenz** crosses the placenta. Rodent studies are generally reassuring, with only minor ossification abnormalities noted at doses many multiples of the MRHD.

■ **Breastfeeding Safety** — There is no published experience in nursing women. It is unknown whether **guanabenz** enters human breast milk.

■ **References** — No current relevant references

■ **Summary** — • **Pregnancy Category C**
• **Lactation Category U**
• **Guanabenz** should be used during pregnancy and lactation only if the benefit justifies the potential perinatal risk.
• There are many other antihypertensive agents for which is a large body of experience during pregnancy and lactation.

Guanadrel sulfate (Hylorel)

- **Class** — Antihypertensive; antiadrenergic, peripheral

- **Indications** — Hypertension

- **Mechanism** — Inhibits norepinephrine release from neuronal storage sites

- **Dosage with Qualifiers** — Hypertension—begin 5mg PO bid; adjust dose weekly until a max of 400mg/d
  NOTE—renal dosing; tolerance may develop after chronic use, requiring an increased dose
  - **Contraindications**—hypersensitivity to drug or class, suspected pheochromocytoma, recent or current use of an MAO inhibitor, CHF
  - **Caution**—asthma, anticipated major surgery, peptic ulcer disease, renal dysfunction

- **Maternal Considerations** — **Guanadrel** is an orally active antihypertensive that lowers both systolic and diastolic pressure. It is typically employed as a second-line agent following a diuretic. There is no published experience with **guanadrel** during pregnancy. *Side effects* include orthostatic hypotension, fatigue, drowsiness, headache, visual disturbances, paresthesias, constipation, nocturia, edema, and weight gain.

- **Fetal Considerations** — There are no adequate reports or well-controlled studies in human fetuses. It is unknown whether **guanadrel** crosses the placenta. Rodent studies are reassuring, revealing no evidence of teratogenicity or IUGR despite the use of doses higher than those used clinically.

- **Breastfeeding Safety** — There is no published experience in nursing women. It is unknown whether **guanadrel** enters human breast milk.

- **References** — There is no published experience in pregnancy or during lactation.

- **Summary** —
  - **Pregnancy Category B**
  - **Lactation Category U**
  - **Guanadrel** should be used during pregnancy and lactation only if the benefit justifies the potential perinatal risk.
  - There are alternative agents for which there is more experience during pregnancy and lactation.

Guanethidine monosulfate (Antipres; Declindin; Ingadine; Ismelin; Normalin; Sanotensin)

■ **Class** .... Antihypertensive; antiadrenergic, peripheral

■ **Indications** .... Hypertension, moderate to severe, including that secondary to renal disease

■ **Mechanism** .... Inhibits or interferes with catecholamine release at the neuroeffector junction, depletes norepinephrine

■ **Dosage with Qualifiers** .... Hypertension, moderate to severe:
Ambulatory—begin 10mg PO qd, increase q2-5d to achieve desired control
Hospitalized—begin 25-50mg PO qd, increasing by 25-50mg qd prn
NOTE—renal dosing; may be combined with **hydralazine** or thiazide diuretics
- **Contraindications**—hypersensitivity to drug or class, pheochromocytoma, CHF not secondary to hypertension, concurrent use of MAO inhibitors
- **Caution**—surgery, fever, chronic use (may need to reduce dose), renal dysfunction, peptic ulcer disease, recent MI, or coronary artery disease

■ **Maternal Considerations** .... This ganglionic blocker is rarely used during pregnancy, as there are other agents with fewer side effects available. Hypotension is a major concern.
Side effects include hypotension, chest pain, dyspnea, diarrhea, nausea, vomiting, dry mouth, depression, tremor, blurred vision, weakness, myalgia, dermatitis, weight gain, and increased BUN.

■ **Fetal Considerations** .... There are no adequate reports or well-controlled studies in human fetuses. It is unknown whether **guanethidine** crosses the human placenta.

■ **Breastfeeding Safety** .... There are no adequate reports or well-controlled studies in nursing women. **Guanethidine** does enter human breast milk at very low concentrations, but is probably compatible with breastfeeding.

■ **References** .... No current relevant references

■ **Summary** ....
- **Pregnancy Category C**
- **Lactation Category U**
- There are alternative agents for which there is more experience during pregnancy and lactation.

Guanfacine hydrochloride (Entulic; Tenex)

- **Class** — Antihypertensive; antiadrenergic, central

- **Indications** — Hypertension, migraine headache, heroin withdrawal

- **Mechanism** — Centrally acting α-2 agonist

- **Dosage with Qualifiers** — Hypertension—1-3mg PO qhs
  Migraine headache—1mg PO qd ×12w
  Heroin withdrawal—0.03-1.5mg PO qd
  NOTE—renal dosing
  - **Contraindications**—hypersensitivity to drug or class
  - **Caution**—hepatic dysfunction, coronary artery disease, recent MI

- **Maternal Considerations** — There are no well-controlled trials of **guanfacine** during pregnancy. It is not generally recommended for the treatment of preeclamptic hypertension, in part because of its slow onset. There is one report of 30 preeclamptic women in which only 24 responded.
  Side effects include fatigue, weakness, somnolence, dizziness, constipation, and headache.

- **Fetal Considerations** — There are no adequate reports or well-controlled studies in human fetuses.

- **Breastfeeding Safety** — There is no published experience in nursing women. It is unknown whether **guanfacine** enters human breast milk.

- **References** — Philipp E. Br J Clin Pharmacol 1980; 10:137S-140S.

- **Summary** —
  - **Pregnancy Category B**
  - **Lactation Category U**
  - There are alternative agents for which there is more experience during pregnancy and lactation.
  - Not recommended for use in women with preeclampsia.

Haemophilus influenza conjugate vaccine (ActHIB; HibTITER; OmniHIB; PedvaxHIB; ProHIBIT)

■ **Class** ································ *Vaccine*

■ **Indications** ························ Maternal susceptibility

■ **Mechanism** ······················· Immunization to capsular polysaccharides

■ **Dosage with Qualifiers** ········· <u>*Haemophilus influenza* B susceptibility</u>—0.5mg IM ×1
- **Contraindications**—hypersensitivity to drug or class, hypersensitivity to diphtheria vaccine or thimerosal, acute febrile illness
- **Caution**—immunosuppression

■ **Maternal Considerations** ······· *Haemophilus influenza* **conjugate vaccine** is a combination of capsular polysaccharides purified from HIB type B. It protects only against the B strain. There are no adequate reports or well-controlled studies in pregnant women. Maternal immunization does not interfere with subsequent neonatal immunization. *Haemophilus influenza* **conjugate vaccine** is not contraindicated in women with HIV. *Side effects* include erythema, allergic reaction, and fever.

■ **Fetal Considerations** ··········· There are no adequate and well-controlled studies in human fetuses. The H. *influenza* antibodies generated cross the placenta and provide passive immunity. In two studies, it effectively produced passive immunity in the newborn after administration to women during the 3rd trimester. While animal studies have not been conducted, there is no evidence the vaccine components either cross the placenta or pose a risk to the human fetus.

■ **Breastfeeding Safety** ··········· There is no published experience in nursing women. It is certainly possible H. *influenza* antibodies enter human breast milk. It is unknown whether they convey any protection to the nursing newborn.

■ **References** ······················· Park MK, Englund JA, Glezen WP, et al. Vaccine 1996; 14:1219-22.

■ **Summary** ·························
- **Pregnancy Category C**
- **Lactation Category U**
- A successful tool for the reduction of neonatal H. *influenza* infections in some populations.

Halcinonide topical (Dermalog; Halog; Halog-E)

■ **Class** — Corticosteroid, topical; dermatologic

■ **Indications** — Steroid-responsive dermatitis

■ **Mechanism** — Unknown

■ **Dosage with Qualifiers** — Steroid-responsive dermatitis—apply to affected area bid/tid
NOTE—available in cream, ointment, salve, 0.25% and 0.1%
- **Contraindications**—hypersensitivity to drug or class
- **Cautions**—unknown

■ **Maternal Considerations** — There is no published experience with **halcinonide** during pregnancy. **Halcinonide** reduces scar formation.
Side effects include adrenal suppression, burning, itching, contact dermatitis, folliculitis, dry skin, acne, perioral dermatitis, infection, and skin atrophy.

■ **Fetal Considerations** — While there are no adequate reports or well-controlled studies in human fetuses, the quantity of **halcinonide** absorbed systemically is unlikely to pose a risk to the fetus even if it does cross the placenta. Though some corticosteroids are teratogens in some rodents, there is no substantative evidence they act as a teratogen in humans.

■ **Breastfeeding Safety** — There is no published experience in nursing women. It is unknown whether **halcinonide** enters human breast milk. Some nonfluoridated and fluoridated corticosteroids enter human breast milk with ratios (M:P) ranging between 0.05 and 0.25.

■ **References** — There is no published experience in pregnancy or during lactation.

■ **Summary** —
- **Pregnancy Category C**
- **Lactation Category U**
- **Halcinonide** should be used during pregnancy and lactation only if the benefit justifies the potential perinatal risk.

Halobetasol topical (Ultravate)

- **Class** — Corticosteroid

- **Indications** — Steroid-responsive dermatitis, psoriasis

- **Mechanism** — Unknown

- **Dosage with Qualifiers** — Steroid-responsive dermatitis—apply qd/bid; max 50g/w
  NOTE—available in cream or ointment
  - **Contraindications**—hypersensitivity to drug or class
  - **Cautions**—unknown

- **Maternal Considerations** — There is no published experience with **halobetasol** during pregnancy. Human and animal studies indicate approximately 2% of the applied cream dose (3% ointment) enters the circulation within 96h of topical administration.
  Side effects include adrenal suppression, burning, itching, contact dermatitis, folliculitis, dry skin, acne, perioral dermatitis, infection, and skin atrophy.

- **Fetal Considerations** — While there are no adequate reports or well-controlled studies in human fetuses, the quantity of **halobetasol** absorbed systemically is unlikely to pose a risk to the fetus even if it does cross the placenta. Though some corticosteroids are teratogens in some rodents, there is no substantive evidence they act as a teratogen in humans. When given systemically to rodents at doses that are multiples of the MRHD, **halobetasol** is associated with embryotoxicity, cleft palate, and abdominal wall defects.

- **Breastfeeding Safety** — There is no published experience in nursing women. It is unknown whether **halobetasol** enters human breast milk. Considering the dose and route, it is unlikely the milk concentration will reach a clinically relevant level. Some nonfluoridated and fluoridated corticosteroids enter human breast milk with ratios (M:P) ranging between 0.05 and 0.25.

- **References** — There is no published experience in pregnancy or during lactation.

- **Summary** —
  - **Pregnancy Category C**
  - **Lactation Category S?**
  - **Halobetasol** should be used during pregnancy and lactation only if the benefit justifies the potential perinatal risk.

Haloperidol (Einalon; Haldol; Haloperidol Lactate; Pacedol; Pericate; Seranase)

■ **Class** ⸳⸳⸳⸳⸳⸳⸳⸳⸳⸳⸳⸳⸳⸳⸳⸳⸳⸳⸳⸳⸳⸳⸳⸳⸳⸳⸳⸳⸳⸳ *Antipsychotic*

■ **Indications** ⸳⸳⸳⸳⸳⸳⸳⸳⸳⸳⸳⸳⸳⸳⸳⸳⸳⸳⸳⸳⸳⸳⸳⸳ Psychosis, Tourette's syndrome

■ **Mechanism** ⸳⸳⸳⸳⸳⸳⸳⸳⸳⸳⸳⸳⸳⸳⸳⸳⸳⸳⸳⸳⸳⸳⸳⸳ Unknown

■ **Dosage with Qualifiers** ⸳⸳⸳⸳⸳⸳ Psychosis—0.5-5mg PO bid/tid; max 100mg/d; or 2.5mg IV/IM q4-8h
Tourette's syndrome—begin 0.5-1.5mg PO tid, increase 2mg/d prn; typically 9mg/d
Acute psychosis—0.5-50mg IV (slow, at 5mg/min)
NOTE—available in a depo form, **haloperidol decanoate**, 50-100mg IM qmo
- **Contraindications**—hypersensitivity to drug or class, CNS depression, coma, Parkinson's disease
- **Caution**—hepatic dysfunction, seizure disorder, thyrotoxicosis, cardiovascular disease

■ **Maternal Considerations** ⸳⸳⸳⸳ There are no adequate reports or well-controlled studies in pregnant women. There is, however, a large body of experience during pregnancy suggesting a wide margin of safety. There is one case report of an overdose at 34w treated symptomatically without detectable adverse effect. There is another case report of neuroleptic malignant syndrome during pregnancy treated successfully with **dantrolene** and **bromocriptine**. It has also been used to treat chorea gravidarum.
Side effects include arrhythmias, seizures, neuroleptic malignant syndrome, tardive dyskinesia, extrapyramidal effects, dystonia, pneumonia, fever, jaundice, insomnia, drowsiness, anxiety, menstrual irregularities, and galactorrhea.

■ **Fetal Considerations** ⸳⸳⸳⸳⸳⸳⸳ There are no adequate reports or well-controlled studies in human fetuses. **Haloperidol** crosses the human placenta and can be recovered from neonatal hair. In one case report of a maternal overdose, the fetus had an abnormal biophysical profile for 5d. **Haloperidol** is teratogenic in some rodents. In hamsters, it produces a variety of spinal abnormalities in a dose-dependent fashion. There is no substantative evidence of teratogenicity in the human.

■ **Breastfeeding Safety** ⸳⸳⸳⸳⸳⸳ There are no adequate reports or well-controlled studies in nursing women. **Haloperidol** enters human breast milk, and breast-feeding infants may reach therapeutic levels. As it is unknown whether **haloperidol** poses a risk to the neonate, breastfeeding should be permitted only with caution.

■ **References** ·············· Karageyim AY, Kars B, Dansuk R, et al. J Matern Fetal
Neonatal Med 2002; 12:353-4.
Hansen LM, Megeriaqn G, Donnenfeld AE. Obstet Gynecol
1997; 90:659-61.
Russell CS, Lang C, McCambridge M, Calhoun B. Obstet
Gynecol 2001; 98:906-8.
Uematsu T, Yamada K, Matsuno H, Nakashima M.
Ther Drug Monit 1991; 13:183-7.
Gill TS, Guram MS, Geber WF. Dev Pharmacol Ther
1982; 4:1-5.
Yoshida K, Smith B, Craggs M, Kumar R. Psychol Med
1998; 28:81-91.

■ **Summary** ·············· • **Pregnancy Category C**
• **Lactation Category S?**
• Based on clinical experience and in comparison to its
alternatives, **haloperidol** a drug of choice for the
treatment of acute or chronic psychosis during pregnancy.

Halothane (Anestane; Fluothane)

■ **Class** ·············· Anesthetic, *general*

■ **Indications** ·············· General anesthesia

■ **Mechanism** ·············· Unknown; disrupts the neuronal lipid membrane

■ **Dosage with Qualifiers** ·············· Induction of anesthesia—typically 0.5-3% (usually for
children)
Maintenance of anesthesia—typically 0.5-1.5%
NOTE—consult specialty text
• **Contraindications**—hypersensitivity to drug or class,
history of either malignant hyperthermia,
halothane-induced jaundice, or hepatitis
• **Caution**—head injury, hepatic dysfunction, arrhythmias,
prolonged QT, increased intracranial pressure,
pheochromocytoma, myasthenia gravis

■ **Maternal Considerations** ·············· **Halothane** is a halogenated inhalational agent for which
there is a long clinical experience during pregnancy. It and
related compounds relax the myometrium both *in vitro*
and *in vivo*. As a result, it should not be used for routine
vaginal delivery. Halothane is no longer routinely used by
anesthesiologists, who prefer newer agents that are not
significantly metabolized by the liver. Halothane has been
used for cesarean delivery and in instances when uterine
relaxation is important, such as acute uterine inversion,
placental entrapment, and cervical entrapment of the
after-coming head during vaginal breech delivery.

409

Currently preferred agents include nitric oxide donors. *Side effects* include malignant hyperthermia, arrhythmia, tachycardia, cardiac arrest, prolonged QT interval, asystole, cyanosis, muscle rigidity, hypotension, hypoxia, hepatic or renal toxicity, seizures, rhabdomyolysis, and carboxyhemoglobinemia.

■ **Fetal Considerations**

There are no adequate reports or well-controlled studies in human fetuses. **Halothane** rapidly crosses the human placenta reaching within minutes an F:M approaching unity. Once considered a possible anesthetic for fetal surgery, **halothane** decreases fetal cardiac output and placental blood flow, and increases total vascular resistance in sheep. Placental vascular resistance increases out of proportion to systemic vascular resistance, shunting blood away from the site of gas exchange.

■ **Breastfeeding Safety**

There is no published experience in nursing women. It is unknown whether **halothane** enters human breast milk. Considering the indication, onetime **halothane** use is unlikely to pose a clinically significant risk to the breast-feeding neonate.

■ **References**

Fahmy K. Int Surg 1977; 62:100-2.
Kangas I, Erkkola R, Kanto J, Mansikka M.
Acta Anaesthesiol Scand 1976; 20:189-94.
Sabik JF, Assad RS, Hanley FL. J Pediatr Surg 1993; 28:542-6.

■ **Summary**

- **Pregnancy Category C**
- **Lactation Category S**
- **Halothane** can be used throughout pregnancy. It is important to assure maternal oxygenation and optimal positioning for maximal uterine blood flow.

Heparin (Heparin Flush; Heparin Lok-Pak; Heparin Porcine; Hepflush; Liquaemin Sodium; Sodium Heparin)

■ **Class**

Anticoagulant

■ **Indications**

Thromboembolic disease (treatment, prophylaxis), thrombophilias (prophylaxis), antiphospholipid syndrome

■ **Mechanism**

Works synergistically with ATIII to block factor Xa activity

- **Dosage with Qualifiers** ·········· Thromboembolic disease
Treatment—80U/kg IV ×1, then 18U/kg/h IV to achieve an
aPTT 1.5-2 × baseline
Prophylaxis—5000U SC bid 1st trimester, 7500U SC bid
2nd trimester, 10,000U SC bid 3rd trimester
Thrombophilias, prophylaxis—depends on type and history
Antiphospholipid syndrome—81mg PO qd **aspirin** plus
5000U SC bid 1st trimester, 7500U SC bid 2nd trimester,
10,000U bid 3rd trimester
NOTE—may need to adjust the dose up for morbid
obesity (>120kg)
  - **Contraindications**—hypersensitivity to drug or class,
    active bleeding except DIC, vascular damage,
    conduction anesthesia
  - **Caution**—recent neuraxial anesthesia, severe
    hypertension, peptic ulcer disease, history of GI
    bleeding, renal dysfunction

- **Maternal Considerations** ········· **Heparin** consists of sulfated, long-chain acidic
mucopolysaccharides with molecular weights ranging from
4000 to 30,000 Daltons. The various low-molecular-weight
heparins are derivatives. Each is considered an
anticoagulant of choice during pregnancy, are equally
effective, and have similar risk profiles. Unfractionated
heparin has the principal advantage of low cost. Despite
the long history of clinical use, there are no adequate
reports or well-controlled studies in pregnant women.
Perhaps the greatest clinical limitation is the dose volume
that must be used considering the relatively dilute
concentrations available.
Side effects include hemorrhage, osteoporosis,
thrombocytopenia, hematoma, irritation at injection site,
ulceration, fever, chills, itching, urticaria, and rhinitis.

- **Fetal Considerations** ················· There are no adequate reports or well-controlled studies
in human fetuses. **Heparin** does not cross the placenta,
and is not associated with an adverse fetal outcome.

- **Breastfeeding Safety** ················ There is no published experience in nursing women. It is
unknown whether **heparin** enters human breast milk.

- **References** ··············· Ulander V, Stenqvist P, Kaaja R. Thromb Res 2002; 106:13.
Rai R, Cohen H, Dave M, Regan L. BMJ 1997; 314:253-7.

- **Summary** ················· • **Pregnancy Category B**
  - **Lactation Category S**
  - **Heparin**, both unfractionated and fractionated, is the
    anticoagulant of choice during pregnancy.

Hepatitis A vaccine (Havrix; Vaqta)

■ **Class** ——— *Vaccine*

■ **Indications** ——— Maternal susceptibility

■ **Mechanism** ——— Immune response to inactivated virus

■ **Dosage with Qualifiers** ——— Maternal susceptibility—1ml IM, repeat 6-8mo later
- **Contraindications**—hypersensitivity to drug or class, febrile illness
- **Caution**—immunosuppression

■ **Maternal Considerations** ——— Hepatitis A is a picornavirus, and the vaccine consists of inactivated virus. There are no adequate reports or well-controlled studies in pregnant women. There are no reported adverse effects on mother or fetus. Women either traveling to areas where hepatitis A is endemic, older than 30 years with chronic liver disease, waiting for or who have received liver transplants, or working with nonhuman primates should be vaccinated. Hepatitis A vaccination of chronic hepatitis C carrier women substantially reduces morbidity and mortality rates. The disease course is typically unaltered by pregnancy, though fulminant hepatitis is reported in the 3rd trimester. Immunoglobulin is a safe alternative for short-term protection.
Side effects include anaphylaxis, local reaction, fever, rash, pharyngitis, abdominal pain, arthralgia, elevated CPK, myalgias, lymphadenopathy, hypertonic episode, photophobia, and vertigo.

■ **Fetal Considerations** ——— There are no adequate reports or well-controlled studies in human fetuses. Hepatitis A virus is rarely transmitted to the fetus, and is not a known teratogen. The antibodies produced in response are known to cross. Rodent teratogenicity studies have not been conducted.

■ **Breastfeeding Safety** ——— There are no adequate reports or well-controlled studies in nursing women. It is unknown whether **hepatitis A vaccine** enters human breast milk. It is likely the resulting antibodies do enter breast milk, but it is unknown whether they confirm any immunity for the nursing newborn. The vaccine is generally considered compatible with breastfeeding.

■ **References** ——— Duff B, Duff P. Obstet Gynecol 1998; 91:468-71.
Jacobs RJ, Koff RS, Meyerhoff AS. Am J Gastroenterol 2002; 97:427-34.

■ **Summary**
- **Pregnancy Category C**
- **Lactation Category S**
- **Hepatitis A vaccine** should be used during pregnancy and lactation only if the benefit justifies the potential perinatal risk.

Hepatitis B immunoglobulin (BatHEP B; H-BIG; Hyperhep; Nabi-HB)

■ **Class** .... Antisera

■ **Indications** .... Post-exposure prophylaxis in susceptible women

■ **Mechanism** .... Passive immunization

■ **Dosage with Qualifiers** .... Post-exposure prophylaxis—0.06ml/kg (up to 0.5mL) IM as soon after exposure as possible (within 24h)
- **Contraindications**—hypersensitivity to drug or class
- **Caution**—history of systemic allergy to other vaccines, thrombocytopenia, or another bleeding disorder

■ **Maternal Considerations** .... **Hepatitis B immunoglobulin** is prepared from pooled plasma. Women who may benefit from inoculation include those exposed to household contacts, an infected sexual partner, and blood from infected individuals. There are no adequate reports or well-controlled studies in pregnant women. **Hepatitis B immunoglobulin** is effective in reducing perinatal transmission of hepatitis B to neonates born to infected women. **Hepatitis B immunoglobulin** should be administered concomitantly with **hepatitis B vaccine**. Women previously vaccinated but subsequently exposed should have their immune titers checked immediately, and covered with immunoglobulin if they are low.
Side effects include local reaction, swelling, erythema, headache, malaise, nausea, diarrhea, myalgia, and anaphylaxis.

■ **Fetal Considerations** .... There are no adequate reports or well-controlled studies in human fetuses. While animal studies have not been conducted, though there is no reason to expect the immunoglobulin to be harmful. Further, administration to susceptible women appears to reduce the incidence of neonatal hepatitis B. Universal vaccination is recommended postnatally.

■ **Breastfeeding Safety** .... There are no adequate reports or well-controlled studies in nursing women. Vaccinated women have higher immunoglobulin levels in their breast milk.

- **References** .... Yue Y, Yang X, Zhang S. Chin Med J (Engl) 1999; 112:37-9.
U.S. Public Health Service. MMWR Recomm Rep 2001; 50(RR-11):1-52.
Azzari C, Resti M, Rossi ME, et al. J Pediatr Gastroenterol Nutr 1990; 10:310-5.

- **Summary** ....
  - **Pregnancy Category C**
  - **Lactation Category S**
  - **Hepatitis B immunoglobulin** should be used during pregnancy and lactation only if the benefit justifies the potential perinatal risk.
  - When indicated, **hepatitis B immunoglobulin** is effective and of minimal risk to the fetus.

Hepatitis B vaccine, recombinant
(Recombivax HB; Engerix-B)

- **Class** .... *Vaccine*

- **Indications** .... Maternal susceptibility

- **Mechanism** .... Active immune response to capsular antigen

- **Dosage with Qualifiers** .... Maternal susceptibility—1ml IM; repeat at both 1mo and 6mo
  - **Contraindications**—hypersensitivity to drug or class
  - **Caution**—multiple sclerosis

- **Maternal Considerations** .... These vaccines are biotechnologically produced, consisting of nonreplicating antigens. **Hepatitis B vaccine** appears safe and immunogenic during pregnancy, and immunization may help protect the fetus. Postpartum vaccination is also effective. The number of at-risk patients is large, and many authorities recommend routine vaccination. However, vaccination can usually be delayed until after delivery for most indications. Nonimmune women in geographic locales with high endemic rates benefit from vaccination during pregnancy.
  Side effects include injection site reactions such as erythema, pruritus, swelling and nodule formation, malaise, headache, fever, nausea, vomiting, abdominal pain, rhinitis, arthralgia, myalgias, Guillain-Barré syndrome, Bell's palsy, insomnia, arthritis, and Stevens-Johnson syndrome.

- **Fetal Considerations** .... There are no adequate reports or well-controlled studies in human fetuses. Passive immunity occurs in more than half of newborns born to women vaccinated during pregnancy. Rodent teratogenicity studies have not been performed, though the native virus is not a known human teratogen.

■ **Breastfeeding Safety** ········· There are no adequate reports or well-controlled studies in nursing women. It is unknown whether **hepatitis B vaccine** enters human breast milk, but breast-fed neonates of vaccinated women have higher hepatitis B antibody levels.

■ **References** ··················· Jurema MW, Polaneczky M, Ledger WJ. Am J Obstet Gynecol 2001; 185:355-8.
Azzari C, Resti M, Rossi ME, et al. J Pediatr Gastroenterol Nutr 1990; 10:310-5.

■ **Summary** ···················· • **Pregnancy Category C**
• **Lactation Category S**
• **Hepatitis B vaccine** is noninfectious; it appears safe and effective during pregnancy and lactation.

Hexachlorophene (Phisohex)

■ **Class** ······················· Antiseptic

■ **Indications** ·················· Skin or wound preparation

■ **Mechanism** ·················· Chemical inactivation

■ **Dosage with Qualifiers** ····· Preoperative skin preparation—wash affected area 30min prior to surgery
• **Contraindications**—hypersensitivity to drug or class
• **Cautions**—unknown

■ **Maternal Considerations** ···· **Hexachlorophene** is not recommended due to narrow spectrum and the risk of percutaneous absorption. A phenol, it can be neurotoxic at high concentrations. While the wound infection rate is reduced after cleansing, and preoperative showers reduce the skin bacterial count, there are better alternatives. There are no adequate reports or well-controlled studies in pregnant women.

■ **Fetal Considerations** ········ There are no adequate reports or well-controlled studies in human fetuses. **Hexachlorophene** crosses the human placenta and in rodents accumulates in neural tube structures. Occupational exposure during pregnancy is not associated with any known adverse outcomes, though a more recent, retrospective study links exposure during pregnancy to mental retardation. **Hexachlorophene** contained in vaginal lubricants is variably absorbed across the mucosa, achieving detectable levels in both the maternal and cord sera. Because of the risk for neonatal hexachlorophene toxicity, alternative lubricants for pelvic examinations should be used during labor.

There is no published experience in nursing women. It is unknown whether **hexachlorophene** enters human breast milk.

■ **References** ┈┈┈┈┈┈┈┈┈┈┈┈┈┈┈┈┈
Baltzar B, et al. J Occup Med 1979; 21:543-8.
Roeleveld N, Zielhuis GA, Gabreels F. Br J Ind Med 1993; 50:945-54.
Zdeblick TA, Lederman MM, Jacobs MR, Marcus RE. Clin Orthop 1986; 213:211-5.
Strickland DM, Leonard RG, Stavchansky S, et al. Am J Obstet Gynecol 1983; 147:769-72.
Brandt I, Dencker L, Larsson KS, Siddall RA. Acta Pharmacol Toxicol (Copenh) 1983; 52:310-3.

■ **Summary** ┈┈┈┈┈┈┈┈┈┈┈┈┈┈┈┈┈┈┈┈
- **Pregnancy Category C**
- **Lactation Category S**
- **Hexachlorophene** should be avoided during pregnancy, but exposure requires no intervention.
- There are better alternatives such as **chlorhexidine**, **povidone-iodine** for use during pregnancy.

Hydralazine (Apresoline; Apresrex; Dralzine; Hyperex; Ipolina; Naselin; Nepresol; Solezorin; Sulesorin; Supres; Zinepress)

■ **Class** ┈┈┈┈┈┈┈┈┈┈┈┈┈┈┈┈┈┈┈┈┈┈┈
Antihypertensive; vasodilator

■ **Indications** ┈┈┈┈┈┈┈┈┈┈┈┈┈┈┈┈
Hypertension (moderate to severe), CHF

■ **Mechanism** ┈┈┈┈┈┈┈┈┈┈┈┈┈┈┈┈┈
Unknown

■ **Dosage with Qualifiers** ┈┈┈┈
Hypertension (moderate to severe)—begin 10-50mg PO qid ×2-4d, then 25mg PO qid ×1w; max 100mg PO qid; alternatively, 5-40mg IV/IM q4-6h; for chronic use, switch to PO ASAP
CHF—begin 50-75mg PO ×1, then 50-150mg PO qid; max 3000mg/d
NOTE—may be packaged with **hydrochlorothiazide**
- **Contraindications**—hypersensitivity to drug or class, coronary artery disease, mitral valve disease
- **Caution**—renal dysfunction, cardiovascular disease

■ **Maternal Considerations** ┈┈┈
Hydralazine is the most widely used drug for the treatment of acute hypertension during pregnancy. Women with severe preeclampsia whose intravascular volume is contracted are at risk for hypotension. The risk is ameliorated by the administration of appropriate intravascular volume prior to treatment. It was suggested that the incidence of hypotension is increased by continuous infusion, but that

observation may reflect a variety of other uncontrolled variables such as volume replacement and nursing protocols. More recent study suggests other commonly used agents, such as **nifedipine** or **labetolol**, are equally effective in nulliparas for the control of hypertension, and may be more effective with fewer hypotensive complications than **hydralazine** in multiparas.

Side effects include agranulocytosis, neutropenia, lupus-like syndrome, palpitations, tachycardia, headache, angina, flushing, nausea, vomiting, diarrhea, and peripheral edema.

■ Fetal Considerations

There are no adequate reports or well-controlled studies in human fetuses. **Hydralazine** crosses the human placenta, and the F:M ratio can exceed unity. The impact of the therapeutic level on the human fetus is unknown. Vascular resistance declines in the isolated perfused placenta. Limited use during the 1st trimester reveals no evidence of teratogenicity. The impact of **hydralazine** on placental blood flow is variable and greatly influenced by the occurrence of hypotension. Rodent studies reveal that **hydralazine** is teratogenic in mice at 20-30 times the MRHD and possibly in rabbits at 10-15 times the MRHD, but is not teratogenic in rats.

■ Breastfeeding Safety

There are no adequate reports or well-controlled studies in nursing women. **Hydralazine** enters human breast milk, but the amount ingested by the breast-feeding neonate would be clinically insignificant.

■ References

Aali BS, Nejad SS. Acta Obstet Gynecol Scand 2002; 81:25-30.
Magee KP, Bawdon RE. Am J Obstet Gynecol 2000; 182:167-9.
Liedholm H, Wahlin-Boll E, Hanson A, Ingemarsson I, Melander A. Eur J Clin Pharmacol 1982; 21:417-9.

■ Summary

- **Pregnancy Category C**
- **Lactation Category S**
- **Hydralazine** is a drug of choice for the treatment of acute hypertension during pregnancy.
- Other alternative agents are preferable for the treatment of chronic hypertension.

Hydrochlorothiazide (Aquazide H; Esidrix; Hydro Par; Hydrodiuril; Microzide; Oretic)

■ **Class** — Diuretic, antihypertensive

■ **Indications** — Hypertension, peripheral edema

■ **Mechanism** — Inhibits sodium and chloride reabsorption from the distal convoluted tubule

■ **Dosage with Qualifiers** — Hypertension—12.5-50mg PO qd
Peripheral edema—25-200mg PO qd
NOTE—may be packaged with **irbesartan, lisinopril, losartan, metoprolol, moexipril, propranolol, quinapril, spironolactone, telmisartan, timolol, triamterene,** or **valsartan**
- **Contraindications**—hypersensitivity to drug or class, hypersensitivity to sulfonamides, CrCl<50ml, anuria
- **Caution**—hepatic or renal dysfunction

■ **Maternal Considerations** — There are no adequate reports or well-controlled studies in pregnant women. Diuretics remain part of the regimen for the treatment of chronic hypertension. **Hydrochlorothiazide** leads to potassium loss and a transient reduction in intravascular volume when first initiated. Thereafter, intravascular volume recovers. They further reduce an already constricted maternal intravascular volume in women with preeclampsia and should be avoided. **Hydrochlorothiazide** has been used during pregnancy for the treatment of idiopathic hypoparathyroidism.
Side effects include aplastic anemia, thrombocytopenia, agranulocytosis, renal failure, hyperglycemia, hyperuricemia, hypercalcemia, hyperlipidemia, dizziness, headache, vertigo, orthostatic hypotension, nausea, vomiting, abdominal pain, paresthesias, and pancreatitis.

■ **Fetal Considerations** — **Hydrochlorothiazide** crosses the human placenta achieving an F:M ratio approximating 0.5. It is concentrated in amniotic fluid. While no evidence of teratogenicity has emerged during the long clinical experience, **hydrochlorothiazide** can cause neonatal electrolyte abnormalities, thrombocytopenia, and hyperglycemia when given around the time of delivery. Rodent studies are reassuring, revealing no evidence of teratogenicity or IUGR despite the use of doses higher than those used clinically.

■ **Breastfeeding Safety** — There are no adequate reports or well-controlled studies in nursing women. It is unknown whether **hydrochlorothiazide** enters human breast milk.

■ **References** — Kurzel RB, Hagen GA. Am J Perinatol 1990; 7:333-6.
George JD, Price CJ, Tyl RW, Marr MC, Kimmel CA.

Fundam Appl Toxicol 1995; 26:174-80.
Beermann B, Fahraeus L, Groschinsky-Grind M, Lindstrom B. Gynecol Obstet Invest 1980; 11:45-8.
IARC Monogr Eval Carcinog Risks Hum 1990; 50:293-305.

■ **Summary**

- **Pregnancy Category B**
- **Lactation Category S**
- Although diuretics are no longer first-line therapy for the treatment of hypertension during pregnancy, **hydrochlorothiazide** remains the drug of choice for the treatment of heart failure unrelated to hypertension.
- When indicated, the mother's electrolytes and hematocrit should be monitored.

Hydrocodone (Histussin-HC; Hycodan; Hycomar; Hydrocodone Compound; Hydrocone/Mycodone; Hydromet; Hydropane; Hydrotropine; Mycodone; Tussigon)

■ **Class**

Antitussive, analgesic, sedative, narcotic

■ **Indications**

Cough, acute pain

■ **Mechanism**

Binds opioid receptors in the CNS

■ **Dosage with Qualifiers**

Cough—5-10mg PO q6h prn
Acute pain—5-10mg PO q6h prn
NOTE—contains **homatropine**; may also be combined with **phenylephrine, pseudoephedrine, phenylpropanolamine, phenyltoloxamine** or **ibuprofen,** depending on the indication; available in tablet or syrup form

- **Contraindications**—hypersensitivity to drug or class, glaucoma
- **Caution**—increased intracranial pressure, hepatic or renal dysfunction, history of addiction or dependence to a drug, head injury, and abdominal pain

■ **Maternal Considerations**

Hydrocodone is a semisynthetic opioid. **Homatropine** is included at a subtherapeutic level to discourage abuse. There are no adequate reports or well-controlled studies in pregnant women. The analgesia produced by the combination is superior to that achieved with **ibuprofen** alone. Similar to **codeine**, it seems more effective for the relief of uterine cramping than episiotomy pain.
Side effects include dizziness, respiratory depression, euphoria, sedation, confusion, nausea, vomiting, constipation, dry mouth, urinary retention, itching, bradycardia, tachycardia, and increased intraocular pressure.

- ■ **Fetal Considerations** ⋯⋯⋯ There are no adequate reports or well-controlled studies in human fetuses. **Hydrocodone** presumably crosses the human placenta. Rodent studies reveal IUGR at doses below those producing maternal toxicity. In an adequate dose, it can cause neonatal depression at birth.

- ■ **Breastfeeding Safety** ⋯⋯⋯ There are no adequate reports or well-controlled studies in nursing women. It is unknown whether **hydrocodone** enters human breast milk. However, **codeine** and its metabolite **morphine** are excreted in human breast milk. Breast-feeding neonates have low plasma levels during the first few days of life, in part secondary to the low concentration in milk, and in part due to the small amount of milk produced. Thus, moderate **hydrocodone** use is probably compatible with breastfeeding.

- ■ **References** ⋯⋯⋯ Sunshine A, Olson NZ, O'Neill E, et al. J Clin Pharmacol 1997; 37:908-15.
  Beaver WT, McMillan D. Br J Clin Pharmacol 1980; 10(Suppl 2):215S-223S.

- ■ **Summary** ⋯⋯⋯
  - • **Pregnancy Category C**
  - • **Lactation Category S**
  - • **Hydrocodone** should be used during pregnancy and lactation only if the benefit justifies the potential perinatal risk.
  - • This effective analgesic combination is often used postpartum.

Hydrocortisone (Acticort; Aeroseb-Hc; Ala-Cort; Ala-Scalp; Albacort; Allercort; Alphaderm; Anusol-Hc; Balneol-Hc; Beta-Hc; Cetacort; Coracin; Coreton; Cort-Dome; Cortef; Cortenema; Cortes; Cortril; Cotacort; Dermol Hc; Eldecort; Epicort; Flexicort; Glycort; H-Cort; Hi-Cor; Hidroaltesona; Hidromar; Hidrotisona; Hycort; Hycortole; Hydro-Tex; Hydrocortemel; Hydrocortone; Hymac; Hytone; IVocort; Lacticare; Lemoderm; Lidex; Nogenic Hc; Nutracort; Otozonbase; Penecort; Procto-Hc; Proctocort; Rederm; S-T Cort; Stie-Cort; Synacort; Tega-Cort; Texacort; Topisone)

- ■ **Class** ⋯⋯⋯ *Corticosteroid; corticosteroid, topical; dermatologic*

- ■ **Indications** ⋯⋯⋯ Inflammatory disorders, ulcerative colitis, status asthmaticus, shock, steroid-responsive dermatitis, pruritus, adrenal insufficiency

- **Mechanism** ⸻ Unknown

- **Dosage with Qualifiers** ⸻ Inflammatory disorders—10-320mg PO qd in 2-4 divided doses
Ulcerative colitis—100mg qd ×2-3w, then qod
Status asthmaticus—0.5-1mg/kg IM/IV q6h
Shock—0.5-2g IM/IV q2-6h
Steroid-responsive dermatitis—apply cream bid/qid
Pruritus—apply thinly 1% or 2.5% cream to affected area tid/qid
Adrenal insufficiency—5-30mg PO bid/qid; max 80mg PO qid acutely
NOTE—available in oral, parenteral, suppository, and topical preparations; may be combined with **neomycin, oxytetracycline, pramoxine,** or **polymixin** and **neomycin**
  - **Contraindications**—hypersensitivity to drug or class, systemic fungal infection
  - **Caution**—diabetes mellitus, hypertension, seizure disorder, osteoporosis, hepatic dysfunction, tuberculosis

- **Maternal Considerations** ⸻ **Hydrocortisone** is a naturally occurring glucocorticoid. Adrenal corticosteroid secretion is increased during pregnancy. There are no adequate reports or well-controlled studies in pregnant women.
Side effects include adrenal insufficiency, steroid psychosis, immunosuppression, menstrual irregularities, CHF, peptic ulcer disease, bloating, appetite change, edema, nausea, vomiting, dyspepsia, headache, mood swings, insomnia, anxiety, acne, skin atrophy, hypokalemia, hyperglycemia, hypertension, and impaired wound healing.

- **Fetal Considerations** ⸻ There are no adequate reports or well-controlled studies in human fetuses. **Hydrocortisone** is inactivated in the placenta. Some glucocorticoids increase the risk of cleft palate in some rodents. There was no increase in registry type studies in the general frequency of malformations in offspring of women receiving a variety of corticosteroids during pregnancy. Despite placenta metabolism, 2g of **hydrocortisone** administered over 48h in divided doses improves both indices of fetal lung maturity (i.e., L:S ratio) and fetal outcomes compared to no treatment. As such, **hydrocortisone** is an alternative therapy should either **betamethasone** or **dexamethasone** be unavailable for the hastening of lung maturity. It is unknown whether repeated exposure delays myelination as has been reported in animals after either **betamethasone** or **dexamethasone**.

- **Breastfeeding Safety** ⸻ There is no published experience in nursing women. It is unknown whether **hydrocortisone** enters human breast milk. Glucocorticoids are a normal component of breast milk. It is not known whether maternal ingestion increases the concentration. The long clinical experience is reassuring.

■ **References** ⋯⋯⋯⋯⋯ Kallen B, Rydhstroem H, Aberg A. Obstet Gynecol 1999; 93:392-5.
Park-Wyllie L, Mazzotta P, Pastuszak A, et al. Teratology 2000; 62:385-92.
Moore LE, Martin JN Jr. J Perinatol 2001; 21:456-8.

■ **Summary** ⋯⋯⋯⋯⋯
- **Pregnancy Category C**
- **Lactation Category S?**
- **Hydrocortisone** should be used during pregnancy and lactation only if the benefit justifies the potential perinatal risk.
- It is a possible substitute therapy for the enhancement of fetal lung maturity should either **betamethasone** or **dexamethasone** be unavailable.

Hydromorphone (Dilaudid; Dilaudid-HP; Hydromorphone HCl; Hydrostat)

■ **Class** ⋯⋯⋯⋯⋯ Analgesic; narcotic

■ **Indications** ⋯⋯⋯⋯⋯ Pain (moderate to severe), cough

■ **Mechanism** ⋯⋯⋯⋯⋯ Binds to multiple opiate receptors

■ **Dosage with Qualifiers** ⋯⋯⋯⋯⋯ Pain (moderate to severe)—begin 1-2mg IV/IM/SC q4-6h, 2-4mg PO q4-6h
Cough—1mg PO q3-4h prn
Conduction anesthesia—see specialty texts
NOTE—available in parenteral, oral and suppository form
- **Contraindications**—hypersensitivity to drug or class, increased intracranial pressure, respiratory depression
- **Caution**—hepatic or renal dysfunction

■ **Maternal Considerations** ⋯⋯⋯⋯⋯ **Hydromorphone** plus a local anesthetic (e.g., **bupivacaine**) is popular for epidural anesthesia during labor. Similar to **morphine**, it enhances the sensory blockade, thus allowing a lower concentration of local anesthetic. The product is a decrease in motor blockade. There are no well-controlled studies of women receiving **hydromorphone** chronically.
Side effects include respiratory depression, apnea, CNS depression, sedation, drowsiness, dizziness, anorexia, nausea, vomiting, constipation, orthostatic hypotension, psychological and physical dependence, and ureteral spasm.

■ **Fetal Considerations** ⋯⋯⋯⋯⋯ There are no adequate reports or well-controlled studies in human fetuses. Systemically available **hydromorphone** rapidly crosses the placenta, achieving an F:M ratio approximating unity. Rodent studies revealed teratogenicity at doses 600 times the MRHD.

■ **Breastfeeding Safety** .... There are no adequate reports or well-controlled studies in nursing women. **Hydromorphone** enters human breast milk. After intranasal administration, the breast-fed newborn ingests approximately 0.67% of the maternal dose (adjusted for body weight). Considering the dose and pattern of clinical use, **hydromorphone** is compatible with breastfeeding.

■ **References** .... Sinatra RS, Eige S, Chung JH, et al. Anesth Analg 2002; 94:1310-1.
Halpern SH, Arellano R, Preston R, et al. Can J Anaesth 1996; 43:595-8.
Geber WF, Schramm LC. Am J Obstet Gynecol 1975; 123:705-13.
Edwards JE, Rudy AC, Wermeling DP, Desai N, McNamara PJ. Pharmacotherapy 2003; 23:153-8.

■ **Summary** ....
- **Pregnancy Category C**
- **Lactation Category S**
- **Hydromorphone** should be used during pregnancy and lactation only if the benefit justifies the potential perinatal risk.
- It is a popular agent for labor epidural analgesia in combination with a local anesthetic.

Hydroquinone topical (Aida; Banquin; Eldopaque Forte; Eldoquin Forte; Epocler; Hydroxyquinone; Melanex; Melanol; Melpaque HP; Melquin; Nuquin HP; Solaquin Forte)

■ **Class** .... Dermatologic; *depigmenting*

■ **Indications** .... Hyperpigmentation associated with pregnancy, OCPs, HRT, or trauma

■ **Mechanism** .... Suppresses melanocyte metabolism

■ **Dosage with Qualifiers** .... Hyperpigmentation—apply bid; use sunscreen
- **Contraindications**—hypersensitivity to drug or class, hypersensitivity to sulfites

■ **Maternal Considerations** .... There are no adequate reports or well-controlled studies in pregnant women. There are no indications that require use during pregnancy.
Side effects include contact dermatitis, dryness, fissures, irritation, and burning.

- **Fetal Considerations** ········· There are no adequate reports or well-controlled studies in human fetuses. **Hydroquinone** crosses the human placenta and is a teratogen in chicks and some rodents. It can cause hypoploidy in human cell culture lines. Approximately 45-50% of the topically applied dose is available for systemic absorption, or 3mcg/cm²/h.

- **Breastfeeding Safety** ········· There is no published experience in nursing women. It is unknown whether **hydroquinone** enters human breast milk. Though the systemic concentration after topical administration is likely to be low, treatment can easily be delayed until weaning.

- **References** ········· Stillman WS, Varella-Garcia M, Gruntmeir JJ, Irons RD. Leukemia 1997; 11:1540-5.
  Krasavage WJ, Blacker AM, English JC, Murphy SJ. Fundam Appl Toxicol 1992; 18:370-5.
  Burgaz S, Ozcan M, Ozkul A, Karakaya AE. Drug Chem Toxicol 1994; 17:163-74.
  Wester RC, Melendres J, Hui X, et al. J Toxicol Environ Health A 1998; 54:301-17.

- **Summary** ·········
  - **Pregnancy Category C**
  - **Lactation Category S?**
  - **Hydroquinone** should be used during pregnancy and lactation only if the benefit justifies the potential perinatal risk.
  - There are no indications that require its use during pregnancy.

Hydroxychloroquine (Plaquenil)

- **Class** ········· *Antirheumatic, antimalarial, immunomodulator*

- **Indications** ········· SLE, malaria treatment and prophylaxis, rheumatoid arthritis

- **Mechanism** ········· Unknown

- **Dosage with Qualifiers** ········· SLE—400mg PO qd/bid
  Malaria treatment—begin 800mg PO bid ×1, followed 6-8h later by 400mg PO, then 400mg PO qd ×2
  Malaria prophylaxis—begin 400mg PO qw ×2w prior to exposure, continue 4-6w after exposure
  Rheumatoid arthritis—begin 400-600mg PO qd ×4-12w, then 200-400mg PO qid
  NOTE—take with food or milk
  - **Contraindications**—hypersensitivity to drug or class, porphyria, visual field changes
  - **Caution**—unknown

- **Maternal Considerations** — There are no adequate and well-controlled studies in pregnant women. **Hydroxychloroquine** reduces serum lipids including cholesterol, triglycerides and low-density lipoproteins. Some recommend discontinuing **hydroxychloroquine** in pregnant women with connective tissue diseases, even though it has long been used for malarial prophylaxis during pregnancy in malaria-infested areas. In one randomized trial, **hydroxychloroquine** was associated with a significant reduction in the number of flare episodes in women with SLE. Thus, it may be reasonable to continue the drug considering the terminal elimination half-life may be up to 2mo and flares of SLE occur after discontinuation, and flares are detrimental to pregnancy outcome.

  Side effects include aplastic anemia, thrombocytopenia, agranulocytosis, seizures, visual changes, ototoxicity, exfoliative dermatitis, dizziness, nausea, vomiting, diarrhea, headache, ataxia, pruritus, and weight loss.

- **Fetal Considerations** — There are no adequate reports or well-controlled studies in human fetuses. While there is no substantive evidence of teratogenicity in rodents, **hydroxychloroquine** crosses the placenta and is deposited in pigmented fetal tissues. However, a large clinical experience in women with either malaria or SLE is reassuring.

- **Breastfeeding Safety** — There are no adequate reports or well-controlled studies in nursing women. The concentration of **hydroxychloroquine** entering human breast milk is apparently very low (3.2mcg in breast milk from a woman given 800mg over 48h) and should not pose a threat to the breast-fed newborn.

- **References** — Levy RA, Vilela VS, Cataldo MJ, et al. Lupus 2001; 10:401-4.
  Costedoat-Chalumeau N, Amoura Z, Aymard G, et al. Arthritis Rheum 2002; 46:1123-4.
  Borden MB, Parke AL. Drug Saf 2001; 24:1055-63.
  Levy M, Buskila D, Gladman DD, et al. Am J Perinatol 1991; 8:174-8.
  Klinger G, Morad Y, Westall CA, et al. Lancet 2001; 358:813-4.
  Ostensen M, Brown ND, Chiang PK, Aarbakke J. Eur J Clin Pharmacol 1985; 28:357.

- **Summary** —
  - **Pregnancy Category C**
  - **Lactation Category S**
  - **Hydroxychloroquine** should be used during pregnancy and lactation only if the benefit justifies the potential perinatal risk.
  - The additional risk imposed by pregnancy appears modest, and the drug should not be withheld when necessary.

Hydroxyurea (Droxea; Hydrea)

■ **Class** .... *Oncologic*

■ **Indications** .... Sickle cell disease, essential thrombocythemia, polycythemia vera, HIV, resistant CML, head and neck tumors, solid tumors

■ **Mechanism** .... Unclear, but inhibits DNA synthesis by acting as a ribonucleotide reductase inhibitor

■ **Dosage with Qualifiers** .... Sickle cell disease—15mg/kg PO qd, then increase 5mg/kd/d ×12w; max 35mg/kg/d
Essential thrombocythemia—15mg/kg PO qd; titrate to control platelet count while maintaining WBC count
Polycythemia vera—500-1500mg PO qd
HIV, adjunct therapy—500mg PO bid (use with an antiretroviral)
Resistant CML—20-30mg/kg PO qd
Solid tumors—80mg/kg PO q3d
- **Contraindications**—hypersensitivity to drug or class, bone marrow depression
- **Caution**—renal dysfunction, concurrent myelosuppressive agents

■ **Maternal Considerations** ...... There are no adequate reports or well-controlled studies in pregnant women. Published experience is limited to case reports and small series of sickle cell disease, thrombocythemia, and leukemia. The experience suggests the risk of **hydroxyurea** during human pregnancy may be greatly overestimated.
Side effects include bone marrow suppression, anemia, thrombocytopenia, leukopenia, leukemia, pulmonary fibrosis, dermatomyositis, stomatitis, anorexia, nausea, vomiting, diarrhea, constipation, erythema, dysuria, headache, dizziness, hallucinations, seizures, alopecia, and dermatitis.

■ **Fetal Considerations** .... There are no adequate reports or well-controlled studies in human fetuses. It is unknown whether **hydroxyurea** crosses the human placenta. **Hydroxyurea** is embryotoxic and a potent teratogen in a wide variety of animal models. It also causes IUGR and impaired learning in rats. However, the human experience suggests the risk of teratogenicity is somewhat overestimated.

■ **Breastfeeding Safety** .... There are no adequate reports or well-controlled studies in nursing women. **Hydroxyurea** enters human breast milk, though the kinetics require further elucidation. Considering it is a potent mutagen, **hydroxyurea** should perhaps be avoided while breastfeeding until there is additional information available.

■ References ·········· Diav-Citrin O, Hunnisett L, Sher GD, Koren G. Am J
Hematol 1999; 60:148-50.
Byrd DC, Pitts SR, Alexander CK. Pharmacotherapy
1999; 19:1459-62.
Patel M, Dukes IA, Hull JC. Am J Obstet Gynecol
1991; 165:565-6.
Koh LP, Devendra K, Tien SL. Ann Acad Med Singapore
2002; 31:353-6.
Thauvin-Robinet C, Maingueneau C, Robert E, et al.
Leukemia 2001; 15:1309-11.
Sylvester RK, Lobell M, Teresi ME, Brundage D, Dubowy R.
Cancer 1987; 60:2177-8.

■ Summary ··········
• **Pregnancy Category D**
• **Lactation Category NS?**
• **Hydroxyurea** should be used during pregnancy and
  lactation only if the benefit justifies the potential
  perinatal risk.
• The risk of **hydroxyurea** during pregnancy appears
  overestimated.

Hydroxyzine (Atarax; Atazina; Hyzine; Neucalm 50; Vistacot; Vistaril; Vistazine)

■ **Class** ·········· *Antiemetic/antivertigo; anxiolytic; sedative/hypnotic; antihistamine*

■ **Indications** ·········· Anxiety, pruritus, nausea, vomiting, sedation, insomnia

■ **Mechanism** ·········· Antagonizes central and peripheral H_1 receptors

■ **Dosage with Qualifiers** ··········
Anxiety—50-100mg PO or IM q6h prn; max 600mg/d
Pruritus—25-100mg PO q6-8h prn
Nausea, vomiting—25-100mg IM q4-6h prn; max 600mg/d
Sedation adjunct—25-100mg IM ×1
Insomnia—50-100mg PO qhs
NOTE—do not give IV
• **Contraindications**—hypersensitivity to drug or class
• **Caution**—asthma

■ **Maternal Considerations** ·········· There are no adequate reports or well-controlled studies
in pregnant women. **Hydroxyzine** remains a first-line
agent for the treatment of pruritus and nausea during
pregnancy. It is often administered with narcotic agents
to reduce the frequency of nausea. **Hydroxyzine** reduces
the pruritus associated with epidural or spinal morphine
and morphine analogs. **Hydroxyzine** is superior to
droperidol for relief of nausea associated with general
anesthesia.

> *Side effects* include seizures, wheezing, dyspnea, drowsiness, dry mouth, ataxia, headache, agitation, slurred speech, and bitter taste.

■ **Fetal Considerations** — There are no adequate reports or well-controlled studies in human fetuses. It is unknown whether **hydroxyzine** crosses the human placenta, though its administration is associated with a significant decrease in fetal heart rate variability when administered during labor. Epidemiological studies of women taking **hydroxyzine** for allergy symptoms are reassuring. In rodents, high doses of **hydroxyzine** are associated with an increased rate of malformations.

■ **Breastfeeding Safety** — There is no published experience in nursing women. It is unknown whether **hydroxyzine** enters human breast milk.

■ **References** — Juneja MM, Ackerman WE 3rd, Bellinger K. J Ky Med Assoc 1991; 89:319-21.
McKenzie R, Wadhwa RK, Uy NT, et al. Anesth Analg 1981; 60:783-8.
Einarson A, Bailey B, Jung G, et al. Ann Allergy Asthma Immunol 1997; 78:183-6.
The Drugs and Pregnancy Study Group. Ann Pharmacother 1994; 28:17-20.
Petrie RH, Yeh SY, Murata Y, et al. Am J Obstet Gynecol 1978; 130:294-9.

■ **Summary**
- **Pregnancy Category C**
- **Lactation Category U**
- **Hydroxyzine** should be used during pregnancy and lactation only if the benefit justifies the potential perinatal risk.
- The long clinical experience during pregnancy with **hydroxyzine** is reassuring.

Hyoscyamine (A-Spas S L; Anaspaz; Cystospaz-M; Donnamar; Ed-Spaz; Gastrosed; Hyco; Hyosol Sl; Hyospaz; Levbid; Levsin; Levsinex; Liqui-Sooth; Medispaz; Pasmex; Setamine; Spasdel)

■ **Class** — *Antispasmodic, anticholinergic; gastrointestinal*

■ **Indications** — GI or bladder spasm

■ **Mechanism** — Anticholinergic agent

■ **Dosage with Qualifiers** — GI tract spasm—0.125-0.25mg PO qac, qhs
Bladder spasm—0.15-0.3mg PO qid

NOTE—may be combined with **pentobarbital** or **methenamine**

- **Contraindications**—hypersensitivity to drug or class, glaucoma, ulcerative colitis, toxic megacolon, unstable cardiovascular disease, autonomic neuropathy, myasthenia gravis
- **Caution**—hepatic or renal dysfunction, hot weather, hyperthyroidism, arrhythmia, coronary artery disease, CHF, GERD, pulmonary disease

■ **Maternal Considerations**

There is no published experience with **hyoscyamine** during pregnancy.
Side effects include paralytic ileus, increased intraocular pressure, heatstroke, anticholinergic psychosis, confusion, blurred vision, urinary retention, dry mouth, constipation, tachycardia, palpitations, headache, loss of taste, and anhidrosis.

■ **Fetal Considerations**

There are no adequate reports or well-controlled studies in human fetuses. **Hyoscyamine** reportedly crosses the human placenta. Rodent teratogenicity studies have not been performed.

■ **Breastfeeding Safety**

There is no published experience in nursing women. Trace amounts of **hyoscyamine** are excreted into human breast milk, though the kinetics remain to be elucidated.

■ **References**

There are no current relevant references.

■ **Summary**

- **Pregnancy Category C**
- **Lactation Category S?**
- **Hyoscyamine** should be used during pregnancy and lactation only if the benefit justifies the potential perinatal risk.

Ibuprofen (Advil; Alaxan; Artril; Bloom; Brofen; Dolofen; Emflam; Fenspan; Ibren; Ibu-Tab; Ibugen; Ibuprohm; Ifen; Motrin; Nobafon; Paduden; Paxofen; Profen; Prontalgin; Tarein)

■ **Class** — *Analgesic*; NSAID

■ **Indications** — Mild to moderate pain, fever, dysmenorrhea, osteoarthritis, rheumatoid arthritis

■ **Mechanism** — Inhibits cyclooxygenase and lipoxygenase, leading to reduced prostaglandin synthesis

■ **Dosage with Qualifiers** —
Mild to moderate pain—400mg PO q4-6h; max 3200mg/d
Fever—200-400mg PO q4-6h; max 1200mg/d
Dysmenorrhea—400mg PO q4-6h; max 2400mg/d
Osteoarthritis or rheumatoid arthritis—300-800mg PO tid-qid; take with food, max 3200mg/d
- **Contraindications**—hypersensitivity to drug or class, ASA/NSAID-induced asthma, 3rd trimester pregnancy
- **Caution**—hypertension, CHF, history of GI bleeding, nasal polyps

■ **Maternal Considerations** — There are no adequate reports or well-controlled studies in pregnant women. In several different trials, the addition of **hydrocodone** significantly enhanced the analgesic efficacy of **ibuprofen**. In other trials, **ibuprofen** significantly reduced postabortal pain and was superior to **acetaminophen** for the treatment of postpartum pain after vaginal delivery.
Side effects include renal failure, fluid retention, dyspepsia, GI bleeding, bronchospasm, thrombocytopenia, interstitial nephritis, hepatotoxicity, Stevens-Johnson syndrome, agranulocytosis, nausea, constipation, abdominal pain, headache, dizziness, rash, increased LFTs, tinnitus, and drowsiness.

■ **Fetal Considerations** — There are no adequate reports or well-controlled studies in human fetuses. **Ibuprofen** crosses the human placenta and is found in meconium. It is linked epidemiologically to both gastroschisis and persistent pulmonary hypertension in the neonate. **Ibuprofen** is as effective as **indomethacin** in closing the ductus, but does not affect renal function to the same extent. Rodent studies are reassuring, and in cows, **ibuprofen** actually enhances the rate of implantation.

■ **Breastfeeding Safety** — There are no adequate reports or well-controlled studies in nursing women. Only small amounts of **ibuprofen** are excreted into human breast milk. Less than 1mg is excreted in the breast milk of lactating women who ingest up to 400mg q6h.

■ **References** — Windle ML, Booker LA, Rayburn WF. J Reprod Med 1989; 34:891-5.

Alano MA, Ngougmna E, Ostrea EM, Konduri GG. Pediatrics 2001; 107:519-23.
Cuzzolin L, Dal Cere M, Fanos V. Drug Saf 2001; 24:9-18.
Torfs CP, Katz EA, Bateson TF, et al. Teratology 1996; 54:84-92.
Elli M, Gaffuri B, Frigerio A, et al. Reproduction 2001; 121:151-4.
Townsend RJ, Benedetti TJ, Erickson SH, et al. Am J Obstet Gynecol 1984; 149:184-6.

■ **Summary**

- **Pregnancy Category B**
- **Lactation Category S**
- **Ibuprofen** probably poses minimal risk when taken occasionally outside the 1st trimester.
- 1st trimester exposure should be minimized until completion of future study in light of the association with gastroschisis.
- **Ibuprofen** is an excellent analgesic postpartum, though its efficacy is similar to that of other NSAIDs.

Ibutilide (Corvert)

■ **Class** — *Antiarrhythmic, class* III

■ **Indications** — Rapid conversion of recent atrial flutter/fibrillation

■ **Mechanism** — Prolongs phase 3 of the action potential

■ **Dosage with Qualifiers** — Rapid conversion of recent atrial flutter/fibrillation— 0.01mg/kg IV over 10min, may repeat after 10min if no response; max 1mg/dose
- **Contraindications**—hypersensitivity to drug or class, use of a class I or III antiarrhythmic within 4h
- **Caution**—renal or hepatic dysfunction, prolonged QT interval, hypokalemia, polymorphic ventricular tachycardia

■ **Maternal Considerations** — There is no published experience with **ibutilide** during pregnancy.
Side effects include bradycardia, sustained ventricular tachycardia, sustained polymorphic ventricular tachycardia, ventricular arrhythmias, tachycardia, prolonged QT interval, AV block, bradycardia, nausea, vomiting, headache, and hypertension.

■ **Fetal Considerations** — There are no adequate reports or well-controlled studies in human fetuses. Class III antiarrhythmic drugs, like **ibutilide** cause a spectrum of malformations in experimental teratology studies very similar to those reported for **phenytoin**. Class III antiarrhythmics decrease cardiac cell excitability by selectively blocking the rapid component of the delayed rectified potassium channel (IKr), an action shared with **phenytoin**. Malformations associated with selective and nonselective IKr-blockers may be the dose-dependent product of embryonic bradycardia/arrhythmia resulting in (1) hypoxia, explaining embryonic death and growth restriction; (2) episodes of severe hypoxia, followed by generation of reactive oxygen species within the embryo during reoxygenation, causing orofacial clefts and distal digital reductions; and (3) alterations in embryonic blood flow and blood pressure, inducing cardiovascular defects.

■ **Breastfeeding Safety** — There is no published experience in nursing women. It is unknown whether **ibutilide** enters human breast milk.

■ **References** — Danielsson BR, Skold AC, Azarbayjani F. Curr Pharm Des 2001; 7:787-802.
Marks TA, Terry RD. Teratology 1996; 54:157-64.

■ **Summary** —
- **Pregnancy Category C**
- **Lactation Category U**
- **Ibutilide** should be used during pregnancy and lactation only if the benefit justifies the potential perinatal risk.
- There are other antiarrhythmic agents available for which there is more clinical experience during pregnancy and lactation.

Idarubicin (Idamycin)

■ **Class** — Antibiotic; antineoplastic

■ **Indications** — Acute myelogenous leukemia

■ **Mechanism** — Interacts with topoisomerase II and has an inhibitory effect on DNA synthesis

■ **Dosage with Qualifiers** — AML—varies with protocols
- **Contraindications**—hypersensitivity to drug or class, prior mediastinal radiation, prior use of either **daunorubicin** or **doxorubicine**
- **Caution**—unknown

■ **Maternal Considerations** — **Idarubicin** is a analog of **daunorubicin**. There are no adequate reports or well-controlled studies in pregnant women. The published experience is limited to case reports and short series. Its efficacy is apparently uncompromised by pregnancy.

Side effects include CHF, seizures, MI, ventricular arrhythmia, extravasation necrosis, myelosuppression, bleeding, enterocolitis, abdominal pain, infection, nausea, vomiting, diarrhea, alopecia, mucositis, rash, pruritus, dyspnea, confusion, somnolence, cough, fever, and headache.

■ **Fetal Considerations**

There are no adequate reports or well-controlled studies in human fetuses. **Idarubicin** apparently crosses the human placenta, as there are multiple case reports of fetal cardiotoxicity. **Idarubicin** is embryotoxic and teratogenic in rodents at a fraction of the recommended human dose.

■ **Breastfeeding Safety**

There are no adequate reports or well-controlled studies in nursing women. It is unknown whether **idarubicin** enters human breast milk. However, considering its mechanism of action, it is perhaps best to avoid breastfeeding while **idarubicin** is administered.

■ **References**

Siu BL, Alonzo MR, Vargo TA, Fenrich AL. Int J Gynecol Cancer 2002; 12:399-402.
Achtari C, Hohlfeld P. Am J Obstet Gynecol 2000; 183:511-2.
Reynoso EE, Huerta F. Acta Oncol 1994; 33:709-10.

■ **Summary**

- **Pregnancy Category D**
- **Lactation Category U**
- **Idarubicin** should be used during pregnancy and lactation only if the benefit justifies the potential perinatal risk.
- **Idarubicin** poses a significant risk to the fetal heart.

Idoxuridine (Dendrid; Imavate; Presamine)

■ **Class**

Antiviral; *ophthalmic*

■ **Indications**

HSV keratitis

■ **Mechanism**

Inhibits DNA synthesis

■ **Dosage with Qualifiers**

HSV keratitis—begin 1 gtt q1h until improvement, then q2h during the day and q4h at night
- **Contraindications**—hypersensitivity to drug or class
- **Caution**—none

■ **Maternal Considerations**

There is no published experience with **idoxuridine** during pregnancy. The quantity of drug absorbed systemically is unknown.
Side effects include cloudy cornea, lacrimal punctual occlusions, blurred vision, and photophobia.

- **Fetal Considerations** — There are no adequate reports or well-controlled studies in human fetuses. It is unknown whether **idoxuridine** crosses the human placenta. Rodent studies reveal evidence of teratogenicity and embryotoxicity after systemic administration.

- **Breastfeeding Safety** — There is no published experience in nursing women. It is unknown whether **idoxuridine** enters human breast milk.

- **References** — There is no published experience in pregnancy or during lactation.

- **Summary**
  - **Pregnancy Category C**
  - **Lactation Category U**
  - **Idoxuridine** should be used during pregnancy and lactation only if the benefit justifies the potential perinatal risk.

Imipenem/cilastin (Primaxin)

- **Class** — Antibiotic, carbapenem

- **Indications** — Serious bacterial infection

- **Mechanism** — Bactericidal by inhibiting cell wall synthesis

- **Dosage with Qualifiers** — Serious bacterial infection—250-1000mg IM/IV q12h; max 50mg/kg/d or 4000mg/d
  NOTE—renal dosing
  - **Contraindications**—hypersensitivity to drug or class
  - **Caution**—cephalosporin allergy, renal dysfunction, seizure disorder

- **Maternal Considerations** — **Imipenem/cilastin** is broad-spectrum combination that achieves excellent pelvic tissue levels. Because of the relatively high cost, it is not considered "first-line" therapy for most obstetric and gynecologic infections. There are no adequate reports or well-controlled studies in pregnant women. The clearance of **imipenem/cilastin** is increased during pregnancy. Limited study reveals good clinical responses in women with chorioamnionitis. And while **imipenem/cilastin** provides effective prophylaxis for women undergoing nonelective cesarean delivery, it is no better than any other antibiotic agent used for this purpose. The selection of an agent for cesarean section prophylaxis typically is based on cost.
  Side effects include pseudomembranous enterocolitis, seizures, thrombocytopenia, agranulocytosis, rash, diarrhea, oliguria, phlebitis, tachycardia, candidiasis, urine discoloration, gastroenteritis, elevated LFTs, elevated BUN/Cr, nausea, and vomiting.

- **Fetal Considerations** .... There are no adequate reports or well-controlled studies in human fetuses. **Imipenem/cilastin** crosses the human placenta achieving an F:M ratio of only 0.3, while the AF:F is 0.6. Rodent studies are reassuring, revealing no evidence of teratogenicity or IUGR despite the use of doses higher than those used clinically. Adverse outcomes in animal studies share an association with adverse maternal outcomes.

- **Breastfeeding Safety** .... There are no adequate reports or well-controlled studies in nursing women. Limited concentrations of **imipenem/cilastin** are excreted into human breast milk, though the kinetics remain to be elucidated. It is generally considered compatible with breastfeeding.

- **References** .... Hcikkila A, Renkonen OV, Erkkola R. Antimicrob Agents Chemother 1992; 36:2652-5.
Chimura T. Jpn J Antibiot 1994; 47:1762-8.
Matsuda S, Suzuki M, Oh K, et al. Jpn J Antibiot 1988; 41:1731-41.

- **Summary** ....
  - **Pregnancy Category C**
  - **Lactation Category S**
  - **Imipenem/cilastin** should be used during pregnancy and lactation only if the benefit justifies the potential perinatal risk.
  - There are alternative agents for which there is more experience during pregnancy and lactation.

Imipramine (Imipramine Hcl; Imiprin; Janimine; Surplix; Tofnil; Tofranil; Tofranil-Pm)

- **Class** .... *Antidepressant; tricyclic*

- **Indications** .... Depression, chronic pain

- **Mechanism** .... Inhibits NE and serotonin reuptake

- **Dosage with Qualifiers** .... Depression—begin 25-75mg PO qhs; max 300mg/d
Chronic pain—begin 0.2-0.3mg/kg PO qhs, increase by 50% q2-3d; max 300mg/d
Panic disorder—begin 25mg PO qhs
  - **Contraindications**—hypersensitivity to drug or class, MAO inhibitor use within 14d, recovery from acute MI
  - **Caution**—history of seizure, glaucoma, coronary artery disease, thyroid disease, hepatic dysfunction, suicide risk

■ **Maternal Considerations** .... **Imipramine** is the prototype tricyclic antidepressant. There are no adequate reports or well-controlled studies in pregnant women. It has been used extensively during pregnancy for the treatment of depression. **Imipramine** has also been used during pregnancy for the treatment of panic attack.

Side effects include MI, stroke, seizures, blood dyscrasias, thrombocytopenia, agranulocytosis, dry mouth, drowsiness, confusion, disorientation, blurred vision, and increased appetite.

■ **Fetal Considerations** .... There are no adequate reports or well-controlled studies in human fetuses. **Imipramine** binds to the placental serotonin transporter, and presumably crosses the human placenta. It rapidly crosses the rodent placenta and is distributed throughout the fetus. While rodent teratogenicity studies are generally reassuring, several behavioral studies suggest prenatal exposure to **imipramine** alters postnatal adrenergic responses, serotonin uptake, and the response to stress.

■ **Breastfeeding Safety** .... There are no adequate reports or well-controlled studies in nursing women. **Imipramine** is excreted into human breast milk, though the kinetics remain to be elucidated. Only about 3% of the maternal dose (per kg) of other tricyclics is consumed by the breast-fed neonate.

■ **References** .... Ware MR, DeVane CL. J Clin Psychiatry 1990; 51:482-4.
Balkovetz DF, Tiruppathi C, Leibach FH, et al. J Biol Chem 1989; 264:2195-8.
Ali SF, Buelke-Sam J, Newport GD, Slikker W Jr. Neurotoxicology 1986; 7:365-80.
Harmon JR, Webb PJ, Kimmel GL, Delongchamp RR. Teratog Carcinog Mutagen 1986; 6:173-84.
DeVane CL, Simpkins JW. Drug Metab Dispos 1985; 13:438-42.
Sovner R, Orsulak PJ. Am J Psychiatry 1979; 136(4A):451-2.

■ **Summary** ....
- **Pregnancy Category D**
- **Lactation Category U**
- **Imipramine** should be used during pregnancy and lactation only if the benefit justifies the potential perinatal risk.
- Other, newer molecules may have better safety profiles.

Imiquimod (Aldara)

- **Class** — *Immune response modulator, antiviral, dermatologic*

- **Indications** — Genital warts

- **Mechanism** — Unknown; induces the expression of multiple cytokines

- **Dosage with Qualifiers** — <u>Genital warts</u>—apply at bedtime 3x/w, wash off after 6-10h; max 16w
  - **Contraindications**—hypersensitivity to drug or class
  - **Cautions**—unknown

- **Maternal Considerations** — There is no published experience with **imiquimod** during pregnancy. There are no studies of systemic absorption. *Side effects* include burning, hypopigmentation, pruritus, pain, fatigue, flu-like symptoms, headache, and diarrhea.

- **Fetal Considerations** — There are no adequate reports or well-controlled studies in human fetuses. It is unknown whether **imiquimod** crosses the human placenta. **Imiquimod** does not stimulate inflammatory cytokines when applied to cultured trophoblasts. Rodent studies are reassuring, revealing no evidence of teratogenicity or IUGR despite the use of doses higher than those used clinically.

- **Breastfeeding Safety** — There is no experience in nursing women. However, it is unlikely, considering the dose and route, that any significant concentration of **imiquimod** enters human breast milk.

- **References** — Manlove-Simmons JM, Zaher FM, Tomai M, et al. Infect Dis Obstet Gynecol 2000; 8:105-11.

- **Summary** —
  - **Pregnancy Category B**
  - **Lactation Category U**
  - **Imiquimod** should be used during pregnancy and lactation only if the benefit justifies the potential perinatal risk.
  - Other treatment alternatives are available.

Indapamide (Depermide; Lozol; Natralix)

- **Class** — *Diuretic, thiazide*

- **Indications** — Hypertension, CHF

- **Mechanism** — Inhibits sodium and chloride reabsorption by the distal convoluted tubule; depresses smooth muscle contractility by reducing inward calcium and sodium and outward potassium currents

- **Dosage with Qualifiers** .... Hypertension—begin 1.25mg PO qam, increase if no response after 1w; max 5mg/d
  CHF—begin 2.5mg PO qam, increase if no response after 1w; max 5mg/d
  - **Contraindications**—hypersensitivity to drug or class, hypersensitivity to sulfonamides, hepatic or renal failure, anuria

- **Maternal Considerations** .... There is no published experience with **indapamide** during pregnancy. Diuretics should not be used for the treatment of physiologic edema during pregnancy.
  Side effects include ventricular arrhythmia, hypokalemia, hyponatremia, hyperuricemia, rash, nausea, abdominal pain, orthostatic hypotension, nausea, vomiting, muscle cramps, fatigue, vertigo, and pruritus.

- **Fetal Considerations** .... There are no adequate reports or well-controlled studies in human fetuses. It is unknown whether **indapamide** crosses the human placenta. Rodent studies are reassuring, revealing no evidence of teratogenicity or IUGR despite the use of doses higher than those used clinically. However, other thiazide diuretics have neonatal sequela.

- **Breastfeeding Safety** .... There is no published experience in nursing women. It is unknown whether **indapamide** enters human breast milk.

- **References** .... There is no published experience in pregnancy or during lactation.

- **Summary** ....
  - **Pregnancy Category B**
  - **Lactation Category U**
  - **Indapamide** should be used during pregnancy and lactation only if the benefit justifies the potential perinatal risk.
  - There are alternative agents for which there is more experience during pregnancy and lactation.

Indinavir (Crixivan; MK-639)

- **Class** .... Antiviral

- **Indications** .... HIV infection

- **Mechanism** .... Protease inhibitor

- **Dosage with Qualifiers** .... HIV infection—800mg PO q8h; drink at least 1.5L water qd
  NOTE—reduce dose for hepatic dysfunction
  - **Contraindications**—hypersensitivity to drug or class, history of nephrolithiasis, concurrent use of **astemizole**, **cisapride**, **midazolam**, or **triazolam**
  - **Caution**—hepatic dysfunction, diabetes mellitus

■ **Maternal Considerations** ········ There are no adequate reports or well-controlled studies in pregnant women. **Indinavir** is effective reducing the maternal viral load to an undetectable level, especially when combined with other agents such as a nucleoside analog or a reverse transcriptase inhibitor. Pregnancy does not alter dosing.

Side effects include nephrolithiasis, diabetes mellitus, nausea, vomiting, diarrhea, abdominal pain, insomnia, headache, hyperbilirubinemia, hyperlipidemia, hyperglycemia, anorexia, dry mouth, malaise, taste changes, and the lipodystrophy syndrome.

■ **Fetal Considerations** ··········· There are no adequate reports or well-controlled studies in human fetuses. **Indinavir** does not appear to cross the human placenta. However, **indinavir** is rarely administered alone, and the fetal impact of combining it with other antiviral agents is little studied. In one series, the majority of pregnancies so treated had some adverse outcome, though the relationship of the retroviral therapies to the outcome was unclear. Certainly, the prevention of HIV transmission remains the ultimate priority. Though most premarketing rodent teratogenicity studies are reassuring, **indinavir** was associated in one study with delayed growth, and skeletal and ophthalmic abnormalities.

■ **Breastfeeding Safety** ·········· There is no published experience in nursing women. It is unknown whether **indinavir** enters human breast milk. It is excreted into rat breast milk. Regardless, breastfeeding is contraindicated in HIV-infected nursing women where formula is available to reduce the risk of neonatal transmission.

■ **References** ··········· Riecke K, Schulz TG, Shakibaei M, et al. Teratology 2000; 62:291-300.
Lorenzi P, Spicher VM, Laubereau B, et al. AIDS 1998; 12:F241-7.
Mirochnick M, Dorenbaum A, Holland D, et al. Pediatr Infect Dis J 2002; 21:835-8.

■ **Summary** ··········· • **Pregnancy Category C**
• **Lactation Category NS**
• **Indinavir** should be used during pregnancy and lactation only if the benefit justifies the potential perinatal risk.
• Reduction of the maternal viral load to undetectable levels remains the prime goal.
• Physicians are encouraged to register pregnant women under the Antiretroviral Pregnancy Registry (1-800-258-4263) for a better follow-up of the outcome while under treatment with **indinavir.**

Indomethacin (Indocin)

■ **Class** — Analgesic, non-narcotic; NSAID, antiarthritic

■ **Indications** — Dysmenorrhea, mild to moderate pain, osteoarthritis or rheumatoid arthritis

■ **Mechanism** — Inhibits cyclooxygenase and lipoxygenase leading to reduced prostaglandin synthesis

■ **Dosage with Qualifiers** — Dysmenorrhea—25mg PO tid/qid
Mild to moderate pain—25-50mg PO tid prn
Osteoarthritis or rheumatoid arthritis—begin 25mg PO bid/tid, or 50mg prn qid, increase by 25-50mg q7d; max 200mg/d
NOTE—available in liquid, tablet and suppository
- **Contraindications**—hypersensitivity to drug or class, ASA/NSAID-induced asthma, 3rd trimester pregnancy
- **Caution**—hypertension, CHF, history of GI bleeding, nasal polyps

■ **Maternal Considerations** — **Indomethacin** is used off label for the treatment of presumed preterm labor. In that scenario, it significantly prolongs gestation 48-72h, a degree similar to betamimetic agents and, in small trials, **magnesium sulfate**. The latter is relevant since in meta-analyses, **magnesium sulfate** is no better than placebo for tocolysis. The interval is adequate for the administration of corticosteroids to enhance fetal lung maturity. **Indomethacin** is no better and likely inferior to calcium-channel antagonists, such as **nifedipine**, which has a better safety profile. Continuing **indomethacin** after the successful treatment of presumed preterm labor does not further delay delivery or enhance outcome. Similarly, **indomethacin** is advocated for the treatment of the sonographically detected short cervix. Here, too, there is little quality evidence to support the practice.
Indomethacin has multiple non-prostaglandin-related actions including the inhibition of metalloprotease (MMP) 2 and 9 in amnion, chorion, and decidua. Such actions may contribute to its anti-inflammatory effect. **Indomethacin** reduces renal free water clearance and can cause abrupt maternal weight gain and edema when first initiated.
Side effects include renal failure, fluid retention, dyspepsia, GI bleeding, bronchospasm, thrombocytopenia, interstitial nephritis, hepatotoxicity, Stevens-Johnson syndrome, agranulocytosis, nausea, constipation, abdominal pain, headache, dizziness, rash, increased LFTs, tinnitus, and drowsiness.

■ **Fetal Considerations** — There are no adequate reports or well-controlled studies in human fetuses. **Indomethacin** crosses the placenta, and fetal sequelae are common. At least a third of fetuses who are exposed to **indomethacin** a week or more develop oligohydramnios. Other prostaglandin synthase inhibitors reputedly have a lower incidence of fetal sequelae when used as a tocolytic agent, though the quantity of clinical experience is much smaller than that for **indomethacin**. Because of its effect on fetal urine output, **indomethacin** is used to treat idiopathic polyhydramnios. It should not, however, be used in twin gestations complicated by the so-called "stuck twin," or the "oligo-polyhydramnios sequence." In this scenario, there is no evidence that **indomethacin** prolongs gestation, and it can lead to fetal renal shutdown. The effects of **indomethacin** on the fetal kidneys are dose- and duration-dependent. Stopping it typically results in reversal of the abnormal sonographic findings.

Indomethacin is used postnatally for the pharmacologic closure of a patent ductus arteriosus. Constriction of the fetal ductus is common when **indomethacin** is used for the treatment of preterm labor. It, too, reverses with cessation, and the long-term impact of *in utero* ductal constriction on the otherwise healthy fetus is currently unknown. In uncontrolled trials, **indomethacin** tocolysis was associated with an increased risk of IVH and NEC in the neonate. These reports remain to be confirmed. **Indomethacin** reduces the risk of IVH when given postnatally.

■ **Breastfeeding Safety** There are no adequate reports or well-controlled studies in nursing women. The quantity of **indomethacin** excreted into human breast milk is low, such that the breast-fed neonate would ingest <1% of the maternal dose per day. Neonatal plasma levels are typically below detection.

■ **References** Ulug U, Goldman S, Ben-Shlomo I, Shalev E. Mol Hum Reprod 2001; 7:1187-93.
Gyetvai K, Hannah ME, Hodnett ED, Ohlsson A. Obstet Gynecol 1999; 94:869-77.
Besinger RE, Niebyl JR, Keyes WG, Johnson TR. Am J Obstet Gynecol 1991; 164:981-6.
Newton ER, Shields L, Ridgway LE 3rd, et al. Am J Obstet Gynecol 1991; 165:1753-9.
King JF, Flenady VJ, Papatsonis DN, et al. Cochrane Database Syst Rev 2002; (2):CD002255.
Bivins HA Jr, Newman RB, Fyfe DA, et al. Am J Obstet Gynecol 1993; 169:1065-70.
Carlan SJ, O'Brien WF, O'Leary TD, Mastrogiannis D. Obstet Gynecol 1992; 79:223-8.
Restaino I, Kaplan BS, Kaplan P, et al. Am J Med Genet 1991; 39:252-7.
Robin YM, Reynaud P, Orliaguet T, et al. Pathol Res Pract 2000; 196:791-4.
Weintraub Z, Solovechick M, Reichman B, et al. Arch Dis Child Fetal Neonatal Ed 2001; 85:F13-7.
Iannucci TA, Besinger RE, Fisher SG, et al. Am J Obstet Gynecol 1996; 175:1043-6.
Suarez RD, Grobman WA, Parilla BV. Obstet Gynecol 2001; 97:921-5.
Lebedevs TH, Wojnar-Horton RE, Yapp P, et al. Br J Clin Pharmacol 1991; 32:751-4.

■ **Summary**

- **Pregnancy Category B**
- **Lactation Category S**
- **Indomethacin** is popular as a tocolytic agent allowing for the administration of corticosteroids.
- **Indomethacin** has a significant impact on the fetal and at times maternal renal and cardiovascular systems.
- Chronic therapy with **indomethacin** for short cervix or prior preterm labor does not delay delivery and is discouraged.
- **Indomethacin** should be used during pregnancy only if the benefit justifies the potential perinatal risk.

Infliximab (Remicade)

■ **Class** Anti-inflammatory, antirheumatic; Crohn's disease

■ **Indications** Crohn's disease, rheumatoid arthritis

■ **Mechanism** A chimeric monoclonal antibody that binds and inhibits TNF-α

■ **Dosage with Qualifiers** Crohn's disease, moderate to severe—5mg/kg IV ×1
Crohn's disease, fistulizing—5mg/kg IV ×1 for weeks 0, 2, 6
Rheumatoid arthritis—begin 3mg/kg IV ×1 for weeks 0, 2, 6; may increase dose to 10mg/kg or increase dose up to 10mg/kg
- **Contraindications**—hypersensitivity to drug or class, hypersensitivity to mouse proteins, active infection
- **Caution**—pregnancy, MS, chronic or recurrent infections, latent tuberculosis, demyelinating disease

■ **Maternal Considerations** There are no adequate reports or well-controlled studies; in point, there is only a single case report of **infliximab** use during pregnancy.
Side effects include sepsis, opportunistic infections, worsening of CHF, chest pain, serum sickness-like reaction, lupus-like syndrome, fever, chills, myalgias, backache, arthralgias, dizziness, nausea, vomiting, dyspepsia, pruritus, rash, URI, UTI, hypertension, hypotension, facial or hand edema, and elevated LFTs.

■ **Fetal Considerations** There are no adequate reports or well-controlled studies in human fetuses. It is unknown whether **infliximab** crosses the human placenta. Rodent teratogenicity studies have not been performed.

■ **Breastfeeding Safety** There is no published experience in nursing women. It is unknown whether **infliximab** enters human breast milk.

■ **References** ⋯⋯⋯⋯⋯⋯⋯⋯ Srinivasan R. Am J Gastroenterol 2001; 96(7):2274-5.

■ **Summary** ⋯⋯⋯⋯⋯⋯⋯⋯
- **Pregnancy Category C**
- **Lactation Category U**
- **Infliximab** should be used during pregnancy and lactation only if the benefit justifies the potential perinatal risk.

Influenza vaccine (Flu Shield; Fluimmune; Fluogen; Flushield; Fluvirin; Fluzone)

■ **Class** ⋯⋯⋯⋯⋯⋯⋯⋯⋯⋯ *Vaccine*

■ **Indications** ⋯⋯⋯⋯⋯⋯⋯⋯ Nonimmune status

■ **Mechanism** ⋯⋯⋯⋯⋯⋯⋯ Active immunity

■ **Dosage with Qualifiers** ⋯⋯⋯ Nonimmune status—0.5ml IM ×1
- **Contraindications**—hypersensitivity to drug or class, hypersensitivity to eggs, past history of Guillain-Barré syndrome, active febrile illness
- **Caution**—unknown

■ **Maternal Considerations** ⋯⋯⋯ There are no adequate reports or well-controlled studies during pregnancy. Pregnant women appear to respond to vaccination equally as well as nonpregnant women. Flu immunization is recommended during pregnancy, especially in those women with chronic pulmonary diseases.
Side effects include sepsis, opportunistic infections, worsening of CHF, chest pain, serum sickness-like reaction, lupus-like syndrome, fever, chills, myalgias, backache, arthralgias, dizziness, nausea, vomiting, dyspepsia, pruritus, rash, URI, UTI, hypertension, hypotension, facial or hand edema, and elevated LFTs.

■ **Fetal Considerations** ⋯⋯⋯ There are no adequate reports or well-controlled studies in human fetuses. It is unknown whether **influenza vaccine** crosses the human placenta. Vaccine stimulated IgG crosses the placenta, perhaps conveying some degree of passive immunity. There is no evidence heat-killed vaccine is teratogenic if given in the 1st trimester. Rodent teratogenicity studies have not been performed.

■ **Breastfeeding Safety** ⋯⋯⋯ There is no published experience in nursing women. It is unknown whether **influenza vaccine** enters human breast milk. It is likely the stimulated maternal IgG is excreted into the breast milk.

■ **References** ············· Ressel GW. Am Fam Physician 2002; 66:894-99.
Goldman RD, Koren G. Can Fam Physician 2002; 48:1768-9.
Sumaya CV, Gibbs RS. J Infect Dis 1979; 140:141-6.

■ **Summary** ············· • **Pregnancy Category C**
• **Lactation Category S?**
• Pregnant women greater than 12w gestation should be vaccinated in preparation for influenza seasons.

Insulin aspart (NovoLog)

■ **Class** ············· *Hypoglycemic, diabetes mellitus*

■ **Indications** ············· Diabetes mellitus

■ **Mechanism** ············· Stimulates peripheral glucose uptake, inhibits hepatic glucose production, inhibits adipocyte lipolysis, inhibits proteolysis, and enhances protein synthesis

■ **Dosage with Qualifiers** ············· Diabetes mellitus—individualized; should include an intermediate or long-acting insulin
NOTE—give SC <15min qac, onset <0.5h, peak 0.1-3h, max duration 3-5h
Diabetic ketoacidosis—begin 0.1U/kg IV bolus, then 0.1U/kg/h infusion; decrease infusion rate when glucose <275mg/dl
• **Contraindications**—hypersensitivity to drug or class, hypoglycemia
• **Caution**—hypokalemia, renal or hepatic dysfunction

■ **Maternal Considerations** ············· **Insulin aspart** is a rapid-acting human insulin analog whose onset is roughly twice as fast as **regular human insulin**. It is similar to **insulin lispro**, which is similar to **regular human insulin** in controlling postprandial hyperglycemia without increasing the risk of hypoglycemia. **Insulin aspart** has an added advantage over **regular human insulin** in that it can be taken immediately before the mean, rather than 30-60min. There are no adequate reports or well-controlled studies in pregnant women. Careful monitoring of glucose levels coupled with active regulation of the insulin dose is crucial for an optimal outcome.
Side effects are similar to regular recombinant human insulin and include hypoglycemia, hypokalemia, lipodystrophy, pruritus, rash, and injection site reaction.

■ **Fetal Considerations** ············· There are no adequate reports or well-controlled studies in human fetuses. Insulin does not cross the placenta. Hyperglycemia is associated with both an embryopathy and fetopathy. Women with insulin-requiring diabetes prepregnancy are at increased risk of bearing a child with a structural malformation. The magnitude of the risk correlates directly with the overall degree of hyperglycemia. Normalization of glucose prior to conception lowers the risk below control populations. Euglycemia after the embryonic stage prevents the diabetic fetopathy. While rodent teratogenicity studies reveal increased early pregnancy losses, this was likely the product of severe hypoglycemia.

■ **Breastfeeding Safety**

There is no published experience in nursing women. It is unknown whether **insulin aspart** enters human breast milk. Human insulin is a normal component of breast milk. A wide body of clinical experience with similar insulin preparations suggests it will be compatible with breastfeeding. Lactating women may require dose or meal adjustments or both.

■ **References**

Simmons D. Curr Diab Rep 2002; 2:331-6.

■ **Summary**

- **Pregnancy Category C**
- **Lactation Category S?**
- Euglycemia for the duration of pregnancy is the goal of diabetes mellitus therapy during pregnancy.
- **Insulin aspart** is a clinically attractive insulin for the control of postprandial glucose levels, though there is currently no published experience during pregnancy.
- **Insulin aspart** should be used during pregnancy and lactation only if the benefit justifies the potential perinatal risk.

Insulin glargine (Lantus)

■ **Class**

Hypoglycemic, diabetes mellitus

■ **Indications**

Diabetes mellitus

■ **Mechanism**

Stimulates peripheral glucose uptake, inhibits hepatic glucose production, inhibits adipocyte lipolysis, inhibits proteolysis, and enhances protein synthesis

■ **Dosage with Qualifiers**

Diabetes mellitus—individualized qhs (+/− rapid- or short-acting insulin) for women who require basal insulin to control hyperglycemia
NOTE—onset 1h, no true peak, max duration 24h; must not be mixed or diluted with any other insulin or solution
- **Contraindications**—hypersensitivity to drug or class, hypoglycemia, IV administration
- **Caution**—hypokalemia, renal, or hepatic dysfunction

■ **Maternal Considerations** ···· **Insulin glargine** is a long-acting recombinant insulin analog. There are no adequate reports or well-controlled studies in pregnant women. Careful monitoring of glucose levels coupled with active regulation of the insulin dose is crucial for an optimal outcome. The published experience consists of a single case report. Insulin requirements can change dramatically between 16 and 30w gestation, and the long-acting profile of **insulin glargine** renders it a poor choice for acute management.

Side effects include hypoglycemia, hypokalemia, lipodystrophy, pruritus, rash, and injection site reaction.

■ **Fetal Considerations** ·········· There are no adequate reports or well-controlled studies in human fetuses. Insulin does not cross the placenta. Hyperglycemia is associated with both an embryopathy and fetopathy. Women with insulin-requiring diabetes prepregnancy are at increased risk of bearing a child with a structural malformation. The magnitude of the risk correlates directly with the overall degree of hyperglycemia. Normalization of glucose prior to conception lowers the risk below control populations. Euglycemia after the embryonic stage prevents the diabetic fetopathy. While rodent teratogenicity studies reveal increased early pregnancy losses, this was likely the product of severe hypoglycemia.

■ **Breastfeeding Safety** ········· There is no published experience in nursing women. It is unknown whether **insulin glargine** enters human breast milk. Human insulin is a normal component of breast milk. A wide body of clinical experience with similar insulin preparations suggests it will be compatible with breastfeeding. Lactating women may require dose or meal adjustments or both.

■ **References** ···················· Devlin JT, Hothersall L, Wilkis JL. Diabetes Care 2002; 25:1095-6.
Hofmann T, Horstmann G, Stammberger I. Int J Toxicol 2002; 21:181-9.

■ **Summary** ······················ • **Pregnancy Category C**
• **Lactation Category S**
• Euglycemia for the duration of pregnancy is the goal of diabetes mellitus therapy during pregnancy.
• **Insulin glargine** is an attractive agent to provide basal insulin release for the regulation of hyperglycemia during pregnancy. Otherwise, it probably should not be used during pregnancy.

Insulin lispro (Humalog)

- **Class** — Hypoglycemic, diabetes mellitus

- **Indications** — Diabetes mellitus

- **Mechanism** — Stimulates peripheral glucose uptake, inhibits hepatic glucose production, inhibits adipocyte lipolysis, inhibits proteolysis, and enhances protein synthesis

- **Dosage with Qualifiers** — Diabetes mellitus—individualized SC administration
  NOTE—give <15min qac, onset <0.5h, peak 0.5-1.5h, max duration 4-6h
  NOTE—also available as a protamine suspension that prolongs the duration of activity, or in a mix, either 50:50 or 75:25 (75% **lispro protamine**)
  - **Contraindications**—hypersensitivity to drug or class, hypoglycemia, IV administration
  - **Caution**—hypokalemia, renal or hepatic dysfunction

- **Maternal Considerations** — **Insulin lispro** is a rapid-acting human insulin analog with the same potency as **regular human insulin**. **Insulin lispro** is superior to **regular human insulin** for the control of postprandial hyperglycemia without increasing the risk of hypoglycemia. **Insulin lispro** has an added advantage over **regular human insulin** that it can be taken immediately before the mean, rather than 30-60min. There are no adequate and well-controlled studies in pregnant women. Careful monitoring of glucose levels coupled with active regulation of the insulin dose is crucial for an optimal outcome. There is a growing body of clinical experience, which is reassuring. It suggests at least similar pregnancy outcomes are obtained with fewer hypoglycemic episodes compared to **regular human insulin**.
  Side effects include hypoglycemia, hypokalemia, lipodystrophy, pruritus, rash, and injection site reaction.

- **Fetal Considerations** — There are no adequate reports or well-controlled studies in human fetuses. Insulin does not cross the placenta. Hyperglycemia is associated with both an embryopathy and fetopathy. Women with insulin-requiring diabetes prepregnancy are at increased risk of bearing a child with a structural malformation. The magnitude of the risk correlates directly with the overall degree of hyperglycemia. Normalization of glucose prior to conception lowers the risk below control populations. Euglycemia after the embryonic stage prevents the diabetic fetopathy. While rodent teratogenicity studies reveal increased early pregnancy losses, this was likely the product of severe hypoglycemia.

- **Breastfeeding Safety** — There is no published experience in nursing women. It is unknown whether **insulin lispro** enters human breast milk. Human insulin is a normal component of breast milk.

447

A wide body of clinical experience with similar insulin preparations suggests it will be compatible with breastfeeding. Lactating women may require dose or meal adjustments or both.

■ **References**
Loukovaara S, Immonen I, Teramo KA, Kaaja R. Diabetes Care 2003; 26:1193-8.
No authors. Prescrire Int 1998; 7:67-8.
Bhattacharyya A, Brown S, Hughes S, Vice PA. QJM 2001; 94:255-60.
Buchbinder A, Miodovnik M, McElvy S, et al. Am J Obstet Gynecol 2000; 183:1162-5.
Jovanovic L, Ilic S, Pettitt DJ, et al. Diabetes Care 1999; 22:1422-7.
Jovanovic L. Endocr Pract 2000; 6:98-100.
Scherbaum WA, Lankisch MR, Pawlowski B, Somville T. Exp Clin Endocrinol Diabetes 2002; 110:6-9.

■ **Summary**
- **Pregnancy Category B**
- **Lactation Category S**
- Euglycemia for the duration of pregnancy is the goal of diabetes mellitus therapy during pregnancy.
- Growing clinical experience suggests **insulin lispro** is the rapid-acting insulin of choice during pregnancy and lactation.

Insulin, pork (Iletin I; Iletin II; Iletin II Lente Pork; Iletin II Lente(Pork); Iletin II Nph Pork; Iletin II Nph(Pork); Iletin II Protamine, Zinc(Pork); Iletin II Pzi Pork; Iletin II Reg. Pork; Iletin II Regular(Pork); Iletin II Regular(Pork)Conc; Insulatard Nph; Insulin L Purified Pork; Insulin Lente Purified Pork; Insulin N Purified Pork; Insulin Nph Purified Pork; Insulin Purified; Insulin R Purified Pork; Insulin Regular Pork; Insulin Regular Purified Pork; Mixtard; Regular Iletin II; Velosulin)

■ **Class** — *Hypoglycemic, diabetes mellitus*

■ **Indications** — Diabetes mellitus

■ **Mechanism** — Stimulates peripheral glucose uptake, inhibits hepatic glucose production, inhibits adipocyte lipolysis, inhibits proteolysis, and enhances protein synthesis

■ **Dosage with Qualifiers** — Diabetes mellitus—individualized; available in the following forms and characteristics when given SC: R(egular)—0.5-1U/kg SC qd in 3-4 divided doses: give 30-60min qac, onset 0.5h, peak 2-4h, duration 6-8h

L(ente)—give 30min before meal or qhs, onset 1-3h, peak 8-12h, duration 18-24h
N(PH)—give 30-60min before breakfast, onset 1-2h, peak 18-24h, duration 18-24h
U(ltralente) 0.5-1U/kg/d SC in 1 or 2 divided doses: give 30-60min before meal; onset 4-8h, peak 16-18h, duration >36h
Diabetic ketoacidosis—begin 0.1U/kg IV bolus of R, then 0.1U/kg/h infusion; decrease infusion rate when glucose <275mg/dl

- **Contraindications**—hypersensitivity to drug or class, hypoglycemia, IV administration (N, L)
- **Caution**—hypokalemia, renal or hepatic dysfunction, thyroid disorder

■ **Maternal Considerations**

Native insulin is isolated from the porcine pancreas and modified to produce three additional compounds with differing absorption patterns. Although it was the mainstay of diabetes therapy for decades, most diabetic patients begin therapy or switch to therapy with a human insulin analog. Careful monitoring of glucose levels coupled with active regulation of the insulin dose is crucial for an optimal outcome.
Side effects include hypoglycemia, hypokalemia, lipodystrophy, pruritus, rash, and injection site reaction.

■ **Fetal Considerations**

There are no adequate reports or well-controlled studies in human fetuses. Insulin does not cross the placenta. Hyperglycemia is associated with both an embryopathy and fetopathy. Women with insulin-requiring diabetes prepregnancy are at increased risk of bearing a child with a structural malformation. The magnitude of the risk correlates directly with the overall degree of hyperglycemia. Normalization of glucose prior to conception lowers the risk below control populations. Euglycemia after the embryonic stage prevents the diabetic fetopathy. While rodent teratogenicity studies reveal increased early pregnancy losses, this was likely the product of severe hypoglycemia.

■ **Breastfeeding Safety**

There are no adequate reports or well-controlled studies in nursing women. It is unknown whether **porcine insulin** enters human breast milk. Human insulin is a normal component of breast milk. A wide body of clinical experience with similar insulin preparations suggests it will be compatible with breastfeeding. Lactating women may require dose or meal adjustments or both.

■ **References**

No current relevant references

■ **Summary**

- **Pregnancy Category C**
- **Lactation Category U**
- Euglycemia for the duration of pregnancy is the goal of diabetes mellitus therapy during pregnancy.
- Most patients now begin therapy with a human insulin analog.

Insulin, recombinant human
(Humulin R, L, N and U)

■ **Class** ·· Hypoglycemic, diabetes mellitus

■ **Indications** ·· Diabetes mellitus

■ **Mechanism** ·· Stimulates peripheral glucose uptake, inhibits hepatic glucose production, inhibits adipocyte lipolysis, inhibits proteolysis, and enhances protein synthesis

■ **Dosage with Qualifiers** ·················· Diabetes mellitus—individualized; available in the following forms and characteristics when given SC:
R(egular)—0.5-1U/kg SC qd in 3-4 divided doses: give 30-60min qac, onset 0.5h, peak 2-4h, duration 6-8h
L(ente)—give 30min before meal or qhs, onset 1-3h, peak 8-12h, duration 18-24h
N(PH)—give 30-60min before breakfast, onset 1-2h, peak 6-12h, duration 18-24h
U(ltralente)—0.5-1U/kg/d SC in 1-2 divided doses: give 30-60min before meal; onset 4-8h, peak 16-18h, duration >36h
Diabetic ketoacidosis—begin 0.1U/kg IV bolus of R, then 0.1U/kg/h infusion; decrease infusion rate when glucose <275mg/dl
  • **Contraindications**—hypersensitivity to drug or class, hypoglycemia, IV administration (N, L, U)
  • **Caution**—hypokalemia, renal or hepatic dysfunction, thyroid disorder

■ **Maternal Considerations** ·············· **Human recombinant insulin** is synthesized from bacteria containing the human insulin gene. It is then modified to produce three additional compounds with differing absorption patterns. There is a large body of clinical experience using **human recombinant insulin** during pregnancy. Careful monitoring of glucose levels coupled with active regulation of the insulin dose is crucial for an optimal outcome.
Side effects include hypoglycemia, hypokalemia, lipodystrophy, pruritus, rash, and injection site reaction.

■ **Fetal Considerations** ···················· There are no adequate reports or well-controlled studies in human fetuses. Insulin does not cross the placenta. Hyperglycemia is associated with both an embryopathy and fetopathy. Women with insulin-requiring diabetes prepregnancy are at increased risk of bearing a child with a structural malformation. The magnitude of the risk correlates directly with the overall degree of hyperglycemia. Normalization of glucose prior to conception lowers the risk below control populations. Euglycemia after the embryonic stage prevents the diabetic fetopathy. While rodent teratogenicity studies reveal increased early pregnancy losses, this was likely the product of severe hypoglycemia.

- **Breastfeeding Safety** ⸺ There are no adequate reports or well-controlled studies in nursing women. It is unknown whether **human recombinant insulin** enters human breast milk. Human insulin is a normal component of breast milk. A wide body of clinical experience with similar insulin preparations suggests it will be compatible with breastfeeding. Lactating women may require dose or meal adjustments or both.

- **References** ⸺ No current relevant references

- **Summary** ⸺
  - **Pregnancy Category B**
  - **Lactation Category S**
  - Euglycemia for the duration of pregnancy is the goal of diabetes mellitus therapy during pregnancy.
  - **Human recombinant insulin** is a mainstay for the treatment of hyperglycemia in pregnant and lactating women with hyperglycemia.

Insulin, semisynthetic human (Velosulin BR)

- **Class** ⸺ *Hypoglycemic, diabetes mellitus*

- **Indications** ⸺ Diabetes mellitus

- **Mechanism** ⸺ Stimulates peripheral glucose uptake, inhibits hepatic glucose production, inhibits adipocyte lipolysis, inhibits proteolysis, and enhances protein synthesis

- **Dosage with Qualifiers** ⸺ Diabetes mellitus—individualized as noted; 0.5-1U/kg SC qd in 3-4 divided doses: give 30-60min qac, onset 0.5h, peak 1-3h, duration 6-8h
  - **Contraindications**—hypersensitivity to drug or class, hypoglycemia, IV administration (N, L, U)
  - **Caution**—hypokalemia, renal or hepatic dysfunction, thyroid disorder

- **Maternal Considerations** ⸺ **Human semisynthetic insulin** is synthesized from purified pork insulin, and then enzymatically modified to the human structure. It is functionally the same as **regular human insulin**. There are no published reports of its use during pregnancy or lactation. Careful monitoring of glucose levels coupled with active regulation of the insulin dose is crucial for an optimal outcome.
  Side effects include hypoglycemia, hypokalemia, lipodystrophy, pruritus, rash, and injection site reaction.

- **Fetal Considerations** — There are no adequate reports or well-controlled studies in human fetuses. Insulin does not cross the placenta. Hyperglycemia is associated with both an embryopathy and fetopathy. Women with insulin-requiring diabetes prepregnancy are at increased risk of bearing a child with a structural malformation. The magnitude of the risk correlates directly with the overall degree of hyperglycemia. Normalization of glucose prior to conception lowers the risk below control populations. Euglycemia after the embryonic stage prevents the diabetic fetopathy. While rodent teratogenicity studies reveal increased early pregnancy losses, this was likely the product of severe hypoglycemia.

- **Breastfeeding Safety** — There is no published experience in nursing women. It is unknown whether **human semisynthetic insulin** enters human breast milk. Human insulin is a normal component of breast milk. A wide body of clinical experience with similar insulin preparations suggests it will be compatible with breastfeeding. Lactating women may require dose or meal adjustments or both.

- **References** — There is no published experience in pregnancy or during lactation.

- **Summary** —
  - **Pregnancy Category B**
  - **Lactation Category S**
  - Euglycemia for the duration of pregnancy is the goal of diabetes mellitus therapy during pregnancy.
  - A reasonable alternative to regular recombinant human insulin.

Interferon alfa-2a, recombinant (Roferon A)

- **Class** — *Antineoplastic; antiviral; immunomodulator*

- **Indications** — Chronic hepatitis C, AIDS-associated Kaposi's sarcoma, hairy cell leukemia

- **Mechanism** — Unknown

- **Dosage with Qualifiers** — Chronic hepatitis C with compensated liver disease—
  3 million U/d SC/IM 3×/w for 52w
  AIDS-associated Kaposi's sarcoma—begin 36 million U/d SC/IM ×10-12w, then 3×/w
  Hairy cell leukemia—begin 3 million U/d ×16-24w, then 3×/w
  - **Contraindications**—hypersensitivity to drug or class, autoimmune hepatitis

- **Caution**—myelosuppression or myelosuppressive agents, seizure disorder, cardiac disease, severe hepatic or renal dysfunction, depression, CNS disorder, diabetes, thyroid disorders, nephrotoxic or hepatotoxic agents, autoimmune disorder

■ **Maternal Considerations** ·········· There are no adequate reports or well-controlled studies in pregnant women. Case reports document the use of **interferon alfa-2a, recombinant** during pregnancy to treat essential thrombocythemia and chronic hepatitis C. A decrease in serum estradiol and progesterone levels is reported in women receiving human leukocyte interferon. *Side effects* include leukopenia, anemia, seizures, pulmonary or hepatic toxicity, delirium, arrhythmias, cardiomyopathy, MI, GI bleeding, hypertension, flu-like symptoms, rash, anorexia, abdominal pain, diarrhea, arthralgias, dry mouth, dizziness, headache, paresthesias, emotional lability, anxiety, and injection site reaction.

■ **Fetal Considerations** ············· There are no adequate reports or well-controlled studies in human fetuses. **Interferon alfa-2a, recombinant** does not cross the isolated perfused human placenta. Rodent studies are reassuring, revealing no evidence of teratogenicity or IUGR despite the use of doses higher than those used clinically. However, it increases the risk of abortion when given at multiples of the MRHD to rhesus monkeys early in gestation. There is no detectable effect in late gestation.

■ **Breastfeeding Safety** ············· There is no published experience in nursing women. It is unknown whether **interferon alfa-2a** enters human breast milk. Breastfeeding is contraindicated in HIV-infected nursing women where formula is available to reduce the risk of neonatal transmission.

■ **References** ·························

Vantroyen B, Vanstraelen D. Acta Haematol 2002; 107:158-69.
Dumas JC, Giroux M, Teixeira MG, et al. Therapie 1993; 48:73-5.
Milano V, Gabrielli S, Rizzo N, et al. J Matern Fetal Med 1996; 5:74-8.
Waysbort A, Giroux M, Mansat V, et al. Antimicrob Agents Chemother 1993; 37:1232-7.

■ **Summary** ·························
- **Pregnancy Category C**
- **Lactation Category U**
- **Interferon alfa-2a** should be used during pregnancy and lactation only if the benefit justifies the potential perinatal risk.

Interferon alfa-2b, recombinant (Intron A)

■ **Class** ⸺ *Antineoplastic; antiviral; immunomodulator*

■ **Indications** ⸺ Condyloma acuminatum, chronic hepatitis C and B, AIDS-associated Kaposi's sarcoma, hairy cell leukemia

■ **Mechanism** ⸺ Unknown

■ **Dosage with Qualifiers** ⸺ Condyloma acuminatum—reconstitute 10 million U/1ml diluent; inject 0.1ml SC into the base of the wart 3×/w ×3w, may inject up to 5 warts per session; a 2nd course may be given 12w later
Chronic hepatitis C—3 million U SC/IM 3×/w ×16w; if a response, continue total 18-24mo
Chronic hepatitis B—10 million U SC/IM 3×/w ×16w
AIDS-associated Kaposi's sarcoma—30 million U/m² SC/IM 3×/w
Hairy cell leukemia—2 million U/m² SC/IM 3×/w
NOTE—may be combined with **ribavirin**
  ● **Contraindications**—hypersensitivity to drug or class, autoimmune hepatitis
  ● **Caution**—myelosuppression or myelosuppressive agents, seizure disorder, cardiac disease, severe hepatic or renal dysfunction, depression, CNS disorder, diabetes mellitus, thyroid disorders, nephrotoxic or hepatotoxic agents, autoimmune disorder

■ **Maternal Considerations** ⸺ There are no adequate reports or well-controlled studies in pregnant women. Case reports document the use of **interferon alfa-2b, recombinant** during pregnancy to treat essential thrombocythemia. HIV infection is not a contraindication to HCV infection therapy. Liver disease caused by chronic HCV infection is the second leading cause of death in some HIV-infected populations.
Side effects include leukopenia, thrombocytopenia, anemia, seizures, pulmonary or hepatic toxicity, delirium, suicidal ideation, arrhythmias, cardiomyopathy, MI, GI bleeding, hypertension, peripheral neuropathy, flu-like symptoms, rash, anorexia, abdominal pain, diarrhea, arthralgias, dry mouth, cough, dizziness, headache, paresthesias, emotional lability, anxiety, and injection site reaction.

■ **Fetal Considerations** ⸺ There are no adequate reports or well-controlled studies in human fetuses. It is unknown whether **interferon alfa-2b, recombinant** crosses the placenta, though other interferons do not. Rodent studies are reassuring, revealing no evidence of teratogenicity or IUGR despite the use of doses higher than those used clinically. However, it increases the risk of abortion when given at multiples of the MRHD to rhesus monkeys early in gestation.

- **Breastfeeding Safety** — There are no adequate reports or well-controlled studies in nursing women. Only a scant quantity of **interferon alfa-2b** enters human breast milk. Breastfeeding is contraindicated in HIV-infected nursing women where formula is available to reduce the risk of neonatal transmission.

- **References** — Pardini S, Dore F, Murineddu M, et al. Am J Hematol 1993; 43:78-9.
  Kumar AR, Hale TW, Mock RE. J Hum Lact 2000; 16:226-8.

- **Summary** —
  - **Pregnancy Category C**
  - **Lactation Category U**
  - **Interferon alfa-2b** should be used during pregnancy and lactation only if the benefit justifies the potential perinatal risk.

Interferon alfa-N3 (Alferon N)

- **Class** — *Immunomodulator, antiviral*

- **Indications** — Condyloma acuminatum

- **Mechanism** — Unknown

- **Dosage with Qualifiers** — Condyloma acuminatum—0.05ml (250,000U) SC at the base of each wart (max 0.5ml per session) 2×/w ×8w
  NOTE—wait at least 3mo before considering a repeat course
  - **Contraindications**—hypersensitivity to drug or class, hypersensitivity to egg proteins or **neomycin**
  - **Caution**—unstable angina, CHF, COPD, diabetes mellitus, thrombophlebitis, thrombophilia, myelosuppression, seizure disorder

- **Maternal Considerations** — **Interferon alfa-N3** is derived from human leukocytes. There is no published experience with **interferon alfa-N3** during pregnancy. It had no effect on the menstrual cycle of treated, nonpregnant women.
  Side effects include flu-like syndrome, fever, sweating, itching, dizziness, insomnia, arthralgia, myalgia, back pain, and headache.

- **Fetal Considerations** — There are no adequate reports or well-controlled studies in human fetuses. It is unknown whether **interferon alfa-N3** crosses the placenta, though other interferons do not. Rodent teratogenicity studies have not been performed.

- **Breastfeeding Safety** — There is no published experience in nursing women. It is unknown whether **interferon alfa-N3** enters human breast milk.

- **References** — There is no published experience in pregnancy or during lactation.

- **Summary** —
  - **Pregnancy Category C**
  - **Lactation Category U**
  - **Interferon alfa-N3** should be used during pregnancy and lactation only if the benefit justifies the potential perinatal risk.

Interferon alfacon-1 (Infergen)

- **Class** — *Immunomodulator, antiviral*

- **Indications** — Chronic hepatitis C infection with compensated liver disease

- **Mechanism** — Unknown

- **Dosage with Qualifiers** — Chronic hepatitis C infection—9mcg SC 2-3×w ×24w
  NOTE—a pretreatment eye exam is recommended in patients with hypertension or diabetes mellitus
  - **Contraindications**—hypersensitivity to drug or class, hypersensitivity to E. *coli*-derived products, decompensated hepatic disease, autoimmune hepatitis
  - **Caution**—preexisting cardiac disease, leukopenia, myelosuppression, autoimmune disorders

- **Maternal Considerations** — **Interferon alfacon-1** is a non-naturally occurring recombinant type-I interferon. There is no published experience during pregnancy.
  Side effects include depression, suicidal ideation, suicide, hypertension, supraventricular arrhythmias, chest pain, MI, leukopenia, granulocytopenia, thrombocytopenia, ophthalmologic disorders, and hypothyroidism.

- **Fetal Considerations** — There are no adequate reports or well-controlled studies in human fetuses. It is unknown whether **interferon alfacon-1** crosses the human placenta, though other interferons do not. While rodent studies are reassuring, revealing no evidence of teratogenicity or IUGR despite the use of doses higher than those used clinically, there is an increase in embryonic loss in both rodents and some monkeys.

- **Breastfeeding Safety** .... There is no published experience in nursing women. It is unknown whether **interferon alfacon-1** enters human breast milk.

- **References** .... There is no published experience in pregnancy or during lactation.

- **Summary** ....
  - **Pregnancy Category C**
  - **Lactation Category U**
  - **Interferon alfacon-1** should be used during pregnancy and lactation only if the benefit justifies the potential perinatal risk.

Interferon beta-1a (Avonex; Rebif)

- **Class** .... *Other neurologic, immunomodulator*

- **Indications** .... Multiple sclerosis, relapsing

- **Mechanism** .... Unknown

- **Dosage with Qualifiers** .... Multiple sclerosis, relapsing—30mcg IM qw
  - **Contraindications**—hypersensitivity to drug or class
  - **Caution**—seizure disorder, depression

- **Maternal Considerations** .... There are no adequate reports or well-controlled studies in pregnant women. Menstrual irregularities occurred in monkeys treated with 100 times the MRHD. Anovulation and decreased serum progesterone levels were also noted transiently in some animals. These effects are reversible by discontinuing the drug. Treatment with twice the recommended weekly dose had no effect on cycle duration or ovulation.
  Side effects include seizures, cardiac arrest, hemorrhage, anemia, asthenia, diarrhea, fever, chills, flu-like symptoms, increase LFTs, depression, suicidal ideation, and injection site reaction.

- **Fetal Considerations** .... There are no adequate reports or well-controlled studies in human fetuses. It is unknown whether **interferon beta-1a** crosses the placenta; other interferons do not. There was no evidence of teratogenicity in either rodent or monkey studies. However, it was embryolethal or an abortifacient in cynomolgus monkeys administered doses approximately twice the cumulative weekly human dose either during organogenesis or later in pregnancy.

■ **Breastfeeding Safety** ⋯⋯⋯ There is no published experience in nursing women. It is unknown whether **interferon beta-1a** enters human breast milk.

■ **References** ⋯⋯⋯⋯⋯ There is no published experience in pregnancy or during lactation.

■ **Summary** ⋯⋯⋯⋯⋯
- **Pregnancy Category C**
- **Lactation Category U**
- **Interferon beta-1a** should be used during pregnancy and lactation only if the benefit justifies the potential perinatal risk.

Interferon beta-1b, recombinant
(Betaferon; Betaseron)

■ **Class** ⋯⋯⋯⋯⋯⋯⋯ *Other neurologics, immunomodulator*

■ **Indications** ⋯⋯⋯⋯⋯ Multiple sclerosis, relapsing

■ **Mechanism** ⋯⋯⋯⋯⋯ Unknown

■ **Dosage with Qualifiers** ⋯⋯ Multiple sclerosis, relapsing—0.25mg (8 million U) SC qod
- **Contraindications**—hypersensitivity to drug or class
- **Caution**—seizure disorder, depression

■ **Maternal Considerations** ⋯⋯ There is no published experience with **interferon beta-1b** during pregnancy. Menstrual irregularities occur in monkeys treated with 100 times the MRHD. Anovulation and decreased serum progesterone levels were also noted transiently in some animals. These effects reversed after stopping the drug. Treatment with twice the recommended dose had no effect on cycle duration or ovulation.
Side effects include shock, seizures, cardiac arrest, arrhythmias, anemia, muscle aches, asthenia, fever, chills, flu-like symptoms, nausea, diarrhea, dyspepsia, and injection site reaction.

■ **Fetal Considerations** ⋯⋯ There are no adequate reports or well-controlled studies in human fetuses. It is unknown whether **interferon beta-1b** crosses the human placenta; other interferons do not. There is no evidence of teratogenicity in either rodent or monkey studies. However, there was a significant increase in embryolethal and abortifacient effects in cynomolgus monkeys treated with twice the weekly human dose.

■ **Breastfeeding Safety** .... There is no published experience in nursing women. It is unknown whether **interferon beta-1b** enters human breast milk.

■ **References** .... There is no published experience in pregnancy or during lactation.

■ **Summary** ....
- **Pregnancy Category C**
- **Lactation Category U**
- **Interferon beta-1b** should be used during pregnancy and lactation only if the benefit justifies the potential perinatal risk.
- It may be wise if a woman becomes pregnant or plans to become pregnant while taking **interferon beta-1b** that she consider discontinuing therapy.

Interferon gamma-1b, recombinant
(Actimmune)

■ **Class** .... *Immunomodulator*

■ **Indications** .... Chronic granulomatous disease; severe, malignant osteopetrosis

■ **Mechanism** .... Unknown

■ **Dosage with Qualifiers** .... Chronic granulomatous disease—50mcg/m^2 (1 million IU/m^2) if body surface area >0.5 m^2 and 1.5mcg/kg for those with body surface area <0.5 m^2
Severe, malignant osteopetrosis—50mcg/m^2 (1 million IU/m^2) if body surface area >0.5 m^2 and 1.5mcg/kg for those with body surface area <0.5 m^2
NOTE—expressed as 1 million IU/50mcg. *This is equivalent to what was previously expressed as units (1.5 million U/50mcg).*
- **Contraindications**—hypersensitivity to drug or class, hypersensitivity to E. *coli* products
- **Caution**—preexisting cardiac disease, myelosuppression, seizure disorder

■ **Maternal Considerations** .... There is no published experience with **interferon gamma-1b** during pregnancy.
Side effects include fever, headache, rash, chills, fatigue, diarrhea, nausea, vomiting, myalgias, arthralgias, local reactions at the injection site

■ **Fetal Considerations** .... There are no adequate reports or well-controlled studies in human fetuses. It is unknown whether **interferon gamma-1b** crosses the human placenta; other interferons do not. Studies in pregnant primates treated with intravenous doses 2-100 times the MRHD revealed no teratogenic activity. However, **interferon gamma-1b, recombinant** increased the incidence of abortion in primates given 100 times the MRHD.

■ **Breastfeeding Safety** — There is no published experience in nursing women. It is unknown whether **interferon gamma-1b, recombinant** enters human breast milk.

■ **References** — No current relevant references.

■ **Summary** —
- **Pregnancy Category C**
- **Lactation Category U**
- **Interferon gamma-1b**, recombinant should be used during pregnancy and lactation only if the benefit justifies the potential perinatal risk.
- It may be wise if a woman becomes pregnant or plans to become pregnant while taking **interferon gamma-1b** that she consider discontinuing therapy if medically feasible.

Iodoquinol (Diiodohydroxyquin; Drioquilen; Yodoxin)

■ **Class** — *Antiprotozoal, other antimicrobial*

■ **Indications** — Intestinal amebiasis

■ **Mechanism** — Amebicidal against the trophozoites and cysts of *Entamoeba histolytica*

■ **Dosage with Qualifiers** — Intestinal amebiasis—650mg PO tid after meals ×20d
- **Contraindications**—hypersensitivity to drug or class, hepatic dysfunction
- **Caution**—thyroid disease

■ **Maternal Considerations** — There is no published experience with **iodoquinol** during pregnancy.
Side effects include optic neuritis, optic atrophy, peripheral neuropathy, acne, urticaria, pruritus, nausea, vomiting, diarrhea, abdominal pain, headache, thyromegaly, and fever.

■ **Fetal Considerations** — There are no adequate reports or well-controlled studies in human fetuses. It is unknown whether **iodoquinol** crosses the human placenta. Rodent teratogenicity studies have not been performed.

- **Breastfeeding Safety** ⋯⋯ There are no adequate reports or well-controlled studies in nursing women. It is unknown whether **iodoquinol** enters human breast milk.

- **References** ⋯⋯ There is no published experience in pregnancy or during lactation.

- **Summary** ⋯⋯
  - **Pregnancy Category C**
  - **Lactation Category U**
  - **Iodoquinol** should be used during pregnancy and lactation only if the benefit justifies the potential perinatal risk.

Ipecac syrup

- **Class** ⋯⋯ *Toxicology, vitamins, minerals*

- **Indications** ⋯⋯ Emesis induction

- **Mechanism** ⋯⋯ Induces vomiting both locally and centrally

- **Dosage with Qualifiers** ⋯⋯ Emesis induction—15-30ml PO followed by 200-300ml water; repeat in 30min if no response
  - **Contraindications**—hypersensitivity to drug or class, unconscious patient
  - **Caution**—ingestion of either gasoline, kerosene, volatile oil alkali or acid, more than 1h since ingestion, <6mo of age

- **Maternal Considerations** ⋯⋯ There is no published experience with **ipecac** during pregnancy. There is, however, a long clinical experience with its use to treat patients who have ingested toxic substances. **Ipecac** is cardiotoxic if not vomited.
  Side effects include cardiotoxicity (chronic use), diarrhea, choking, drowsiness, cough, dyspepsia, CNS depression, lethargy, and myopathy.

- **Fetal Considerations** ⋯⋯ There are no adequate reports or well-controlled studies in human fetuses. It is unknown if **ipecac** crosses the human placenta. Rodent teratogenicity studies have not been performed.

- **Breastfeeding Safety** ⋯⋯ There are no adequate reports or well-controlled studies in nursing women. It is unknown whether **ipecac** enters human breast milk.

- **References** ⋯⋯ No current relevant references

■ **Summary**
- **Pregnancy Category C**
- **Lactation Category S**
- **Ipecac** is a workhorse for the treatment of acute intoxication.
- **Ipecac** should be used during pregnancy and lactation only if the benefit justifies the potential perinatal risk.

Ipratropium bromide (Atrovent; Disne-Asmol)

■ **Class** — Bronchodilator, anticholinergic

■ **Indications** — Bronchospasm, rhinitis, rhinorrhea

■ **Mechanism** — Unknown

■ **Dosage with Qualifiers** — Bronchospasm—2-3 puffs INH tid-qid; alternatively 500mcg NEB q6-8h
Rhinitis—2 sprays/nostril bid/tid (0.03%)
Rhinorrhea associated with cold—2 sprays/nostril tid/qid (0.06%)
NOTE—available in bronchial and nasal (0.03 and 0.06%) inhalers
- **Contraindications**—hypersensitivity to drug or class, hypersensitivity to soybean or peanuts
- **Caution**—narrow angle glaucoma

■ **Maternal Considerations** — There is no published experience with **ipratropium** during pregnancy. Mild asthma during pregnancy is managed with inhaled β-2 agonists; therapy for moderate asthma includes inhaled **cromolyn**, inhaled **beclomethasone** and oral **theophylline**. Severe gestational asthma should be treated with oral corticosteroids at the lowest effective dosage. The pharmacologic management of acute asthma during pregnancy includes nebulized β-2 agonists, **ipratropium**, and IV **methylprednisolone**. *Side effects* include cough, bronchospasm (nasal inhaler), headache, palpitations, nervousness, dizziness, nausea, dry mouth, pharyngitis, rash, blurred vision, and URI.

■ **Fetal Considerations** — There are no adequate reports or well-controlled studies in human fetuses. It is unknown whether **ipratropium** crosses the human placenta. Rodent studies are reassuring, revealing no evidence of teratogenicity or IUGR despite the use of doses higher than those used clinically. The highest doses (1000 times the MRHD) were associated with embryotoxicity.

- **Breastfeeding Safety** .... There is no published experience in nursing women. It is unknown whether **ipratropium** enters human breast milk. And while lipid-insoluble quaternary bases enter breast milk, it is unlikely **ipratropium** reaches the neonate to a significant degree since it is not well absorbed systematically after inhalation or oral administration.

- **References** .... Ann Allergy Asthma Immunol 2000; 84:475-80.
  Schatz M. Drug Saf 1997; 16:342-50.

- **Summary** ....
  - **Pregnancy Category B**
  - **Lactation Category S**
  - **Ipratropium** is an effective agent for the management of acute asthma.
  - There are alternative agents for which there is more experience during pregnancy and lactation.

Irbesartan (Aprovel; Avapro; Irban; Irovel)

- **Class** .... *Antihypertensive, ACE-1/A2R-antagonist*

- **Indications** .... Hypertension

- **Mechanism** .... Selectively antagonizes the AT-1 receptor

- **Dosage with Qualifiers** .... Hypertension—begin 150mg PO qd (if alone); max 300mg/d
  - **Contraindications**—hypersensitivity to drug or class, pregnancy
  - **Caution**—renal artery stenosis, history of ACE angioedema, hepatic or renal dysfunction, volume depletion, hyponatremia, CHF

- **Maternal Considerations** .... There is no published experience with **irbesartan** during pregnancy. Women taking inhibitors of renin-angiotensin should be placed on effective contraception and switched to another class of agents if they plan to or become pregnant. *Side effects* include angioedema, hypotension, hyperkalemia, dizziness, URI symptoms, back pain, diarrhea, fatigue, dyspepsia, thrombocytopenia, and neutropenia.

- **Fetal Considerations** .... There are no adequate reports or well-controlled studies in human fetuses. It is unknown whether **irbesartan** crosses the human placenta. Drugs that act directly on the renin-angiotensin system can cause perinatal morbidity and death. Adverse effects do not appear to occur if exposure is limited to the 1st trimester; 2nd and 3rd trimester morbidity includes hypotension, neonatal skull hypoplasia, anuria, and reversible or irreversible renal failure. Oligohydramnios may be associated with limb contractures, craniofacial deformation, and hypoplastic lung development. Oligohydramnios may not appear until after the fetus has sustained irreversible injury. Rarely, there is no alternative antihypertensive agent available. In these rare cases, women should be counseled on the hazards, and serial ultrasound examinations performed to assess the intraamniotic environment. If oligohydramnios is observed, **irbesartan** should be discontinued unless lifesaving for the mother. Antenatal surveillance may be appropriate depending upon gestation.

■ **Breastfeeding Safety** — There is no published experience in nursing women. While it is unknown whether **irbesartan** enters human breast milk, it is excreted at low concentration in rodent milk.

■ **References** — There is no published experience in pregnancy or during lactation.

■ **Summary** —
- **Pregnancy Category C (1st trimester), D (2nd and 3rd trimesters)**
- **Lactation Category U**
- **Irbesartan** should be used during pregnancy and lactation only if the benefit justifies the potential perinatal risk.
- Women should be counseled on the risks and switched to a different class of antihypertensives prior to conception or during the 1st trimester.

Irinotecan (Camptosar)

■ **Class** — Antineoplastic, topoisomerase inhibitor

■ **Indications** — Metastatic colon cancer

■ **Mechanism** — Topoisomerase I inhibitor

■ **Dosage with Qualifiers** — Colon cancer, metastatic—dosing protocols vary; consult specialty resources
- **Contraindications**—hypersensitivity to drug or class
- **Caution**—hyperbilirubinemia, concurrent or history of abdominal or pelvic radiation

■ **Maternal Considerations** — There is no published experience with **irinotecan** during pregnancy. Women of childbearing potential should be advised to avoid becoming pregnant while receiving **irinotecan**.
Side effects include diarrhea, nausea, vomiting, myelosuppression, anemia, thrombocytopenia, neutropenia,

leukopenia, sepsis, thromboembolism, acute renal failure, ileus, asthenia, abdominal weakness, alopecia, anorexia, fever, dyspepsia, insomnia, constipation, headache, chills, and dizziness.

■ **Fetal Considerations** — There are no adequate reports or well-controlled studies in human fetuses. It is unknown whether **irinotecan** crosses the human placenta. **Irinotecan** crosses the rat placenta. Rodent teratogen studies reveal **irinotecan** is embryotoxic and teratogenic, causing a variety of external, visceral, and skeletal abnormalities, along with decreased learning.

■ **Breastfeeding Safety** — There is no published experience in nursing women. It is unknown whether **irinotecan** enters human breast milk. **Irinotecan** is concentrated in rodent breast milk, and should probably be considered incompatible with breastfeeding until further study.

■ **References** — There is no published experience in pregnancy or during lactation.

■ **Summary** —
- **Pregnancy Category D**
- **Lactation Category NS?**
- **Irinotecan** should be used during pregnancy and lactation only if the benefit justifies the potential perinatal risk.

Isocarboxazid (Marplan)

■ **Class** — Antidepressant, MAO inhibitor

■ **Indications** — Depression

■ **Mechanism** — Nonselective hydrazine MAO inhibitor.

■ **Dosage with Qualifiers** — Depression—begin 10mg PO bid; increase by 10mg q2-3d reaching 40mg/d after 1w; thereafter, may increase by another 20mg/d for a max of 60mg/d
NOTE—reserved for patients who have not responded satisfactorily to other antidepressants
- **Contraindications**—hypersensitivity to drug or class, cerebrovascular or cardiovascular disease, pheochromocytoma, hepatic or renal disease, concurrent or recent use of MAO inhibitors, tricyclics, **bupropion**, any SSRI, **buspirone**, sympathomimetics, **meperidine**, **dextromethorphan**, foods rich in tyramine, anesthetics, antihypertensives, **caffeine,** and CNS depressant.
- **Caution**—alcohol ingestion, renal dysfunction, frequent headaches

- **Maternal Considerations** ⸺ Depression is common during and after pregnancy, but typically goes unrecognized. Pregnancy is not a reason a priori to discontinue psychotropic drugs. A major depressive episode (DSM-IV) implies a prominent and relatively persistent (almost every day for at least 2w) depressed or dysphoric mood that interferes with daily functioning. It includes at least 5 of the following 9 symptoms: depressed mood, loss of interest in usual activities, significant change in weight and/or appetite, insomnia or hypersomnia, psychomotor agitation or retardation, increased fatigue, feelings of guilt or worthlessness, slowed thinking or impaired concentration, and a suicide attempt or suicidal ideation. There are no adequate reports or well-controlled studies in pregnant women.
  Side effects include hypotension, hepatotoxicity, lower seizure threshold, dry mouth, nausea, diarrhea, dizziness and syncope.

- **Fetal Considerations** ⸺ There are no adequate reports or well-controlled studies in human fetuses. It is unknown whether **isocarboxazid** crosses the human placenta; it does cross the rat placenta. Rodent teratogenicity studies have not been performed. Prolonged treatment during rodent pregnancy is associated with behavioral changes.

- **Breastfeeding Safety** ⸺ There is no published experience in nursing women. It is unknown whether **isocarboxazid** enters human breast milk.

- **References** ⸺ Sato T, Yamamoto S, Moroi K. Jpn J Pharmacol 1972; 22:629-33.

- **Summary** ⸺
  - **Pregnancy Category C**
  - **Lactation Category U**
  - **Isocarboxazid** should be used during pregnancy and lactation only if the benefit justifies the potential perinatal risk.
  - There are alternative agents for which there is more experience during pregnancy and lactation.

Isoflurane (Forane)

- **Class** ⸺ Anesthetic

- **Indications** ⸺ Anesthesia, induction, and maintenance

- **Mechanism** ⸺ Unknown

- ■ **Dosage with Qualifiers** — Anesthesia, induction—dosing varies, typically 1.5-3% ×7-10min for surgical anesthesia. (There are few if any indications to induce anesthesia with gas in adults.) Anesthesia, maintenance—dosing varies, typically 1-2.5% with nitrous oxide, 1.5-3% with oxygen only NOTE—all commonly used muscle relaxants are markedly potentiated by isoflurane, the effect most profound with nondepolarizing agents; see specialty texts
  - **Contraindications**—hypersensitivity to drug or class, history of malignant hyperthermia
  - **Caution**—head injury, increased ICP, myasthenia gravis, cardiac risk factors

- ■ **Maternal Considerations** — There are no adequate reports or well-controlled studies in pregnant women. **Isoflurane** has been used clinically without pregnancy-related sequelae for many years. Like other halogenated anesthetic agents, **isoflurane** produces uterine relaxation.
  Side effects include malignant hyperthermia, muscle rigidity, tachycardia, cyanosis, arrhythmias, increased intracranial pressure, hepatotoxicity, laryngospasm, shivering, nausea, vomiting, delirium, and uterine relaxation.

- ■ **Fetal Considerations** — There are no adequate reports or well-controlled studies in human fetuses. **Isoflurane** rapidly crosses the human placenta achieving an F:M ratio approximating unity. It has been used for fetal surgery and to facilitate uterine maneuvers. Rodent studies are reassuring.

- ■ **Breastfeeding Safety** — There is no published experience in nursing women. It is unknown whether **isoflurane** enters human breast milk. However, considering the indications and dosing, one-time **isoflurane** use is unlikely to pose a clinically significant risk to the breast-feeding neonate.

- ■ **References** — Omae T, Uchida O, Kuro M, Chiba Y. Masui 2002; 51:49-52.

- ■ **Summary**
  - **Pregnancy Category C**
  - **Lactation Category U**
  - There is large clinical experience with **isoflurane** for general anesthesia during pregnancy. It is a reasonable selection when general anesthesia is desired.
  - **Isoflurane** should be used during pregnancy and lactation only if the benefit justifies the potential perinatal risk.

Isoniazid (Abdizide; Dipicin; Eutizon; Fetefu; INH; Isonicid; Laniazid; Niazid; Nydrazid; Nydrazyd; Rimifon)

■ **Class** .... *Antimycobacterial*

■ **Indications** .... Tuberculosis, prophylaxis and infection

■ **Mechanism** .... Inhibits lipid and nucleic acid synthesis

■ **Dosage with Qualifiers** .... Tuberculosis, prophylaxis—300mg PO qd ×6-12mo; consider the addition of 25-50mg **pyridoxine** PO qd
Tuberculosis, infection—5mg/kg PO/IM qd ×9-24mo; max 300mg/d
NOTE—may be combined with **rifampin** with or without **pyrazinamide**
  ● **Contraindications**—hypersensitivity to drug or class, acute hepatic disease
  ● **Caution**—hepatic or renal dysfunction, alcohol ingestion

■ **Maternal Considerations** .... **Isoniazid** is metabolized primarily by acetylation and dehydrazination. Approximately half of blacks and Caucasians are "slow acetylators" and the rest rapid acetylators; the majority of Eskimos and Orientals are "rapid acetylators." The rate of acetylation does not significantly alter effectiveness, but slow acetylation may lead to higher blood levels and increase toxicity. The risk of **isoniazid**-induced hepatitis is age-related and increased by alcohol ingestion. Tuberculosis is experiencing a "rebirth" in many countries and poses great risk to mother, fetus, and family. Untreated tuberculosis in pregnancy is a significant threat to mother, fetus, and family. There are no adequate reports or well-controlled studies of **isoniazid** in pregnant women. Adherence to treatment is especially difficult because of a general fear of any medication and pregnancy-related nausea. All 4 first-line drugs (**isoniazid**, **rifampin**, **ethambutol**, and **pyrazinamide**) have an excellent safety record in pregnancy.
Side effects include aplastic anemia, agranulocytosis, thrombocytopenia, leukopenia, optic neuritis, peripheral neuropathy, hepatotoxicity, seizures, nausea, vomiting, epigastric pain, diarrhea, dizziness, rash, acne, euphoria, agitation, tinnitus, and elevated LFTs.

■ **Fetal Considerations** .... There are no adequate reports or well-controlled studies in human fetuses. **Isoniazid** crosses the human placenta, but has not been associated with an increased risk of malformations. Congenital tuberculosis is rare but does occur. Rodent studies are reassuring, revealing no evidence of teratogenicity or IUGR despite the use of doses higher than those used clinically. Embryotoxicity may occur in some rodents.

■ **Breastfeeding Safety** ·················· There are no adequate reports or well-controlled studies in nursing women. Only scant amounts of **isoniazid** are excreted into human breast milk. It is generally considered compatible with breastfeeding, and is not adequate treatment for neonatal tuberculosis.

■ **References** ···················· Boggess KA, Myers ER, Hamilton CD. Obstet Gynecol 2000; 96:757-62.
Bothamley G. Drug Saf 2001; 24:553-65.
Brost BC, Newman RB. Obstet Gynecol Clin North Am 1997; 24:659-73.
Smith KC. Curr Opin Infect Dis 2002; 15:269-74.
Tran JH, Montakantikul P. J Hum Lact 1998; 14:337-40.

■ **Summary** ···················· • **Pregnancy Category C**
• **Lactation Category S**
• There is a long clinical experience with isoniazid during pregnancy. It should not be withheld when otherwise indicated.

Isoproterenol (Aerolone; Isopro Aerometer; Isuprel; Medihaler-Iso; Norisodrine; Vapo-Iso)

■ **Class** ···················· Antiarrhythmic, adrenergic agonist, bronchodilator

■ **Indications** ···················· Emergent arrhythmia, atropine-resistant bradycardia, CHB after VSD closure, bronchospasm

■ **Mechanism** ···················· Nonspecific β-adrenergic agonist

■ **Dosage with Qualifiers** ···················· Emergent arrhythmia—0.02-0.06mg IV ×1, then 2-20mcg/min IV infusion
Atropine-resistant bradycardia—2-10mcg/min IV infusion
Congenital heart block after VSD closure—0.02-0.06mg IV ×1
Bronchospasm during anesthesia—0.01-0.02mg IV ×1; may be repeated if necessary
Bronchodilator—1 deep inhalation; may repeat after 5min if necessary; max 5 inhalations/d
NOTE—available in intravenous and inhaler forms
• **Contraindications**—hypersensitivity to drug or class, hypersensitivity to sulfites, digitalis intoxication, angina
• **Caution**—renal dysfunction, CV disease, diabetes mellitus, hyperthyroidism, hypokalemia

■ **Maternal Considerations** ···················· There are no adequate reports or well-controlled studies in pregnant women. It has been suggested its addition to epidural bupivacaine and sufentanil speeds the onset of analgesia.

Side effects include hypotension, arrhythmias, cardiac arrest, bronchospasm, Stokes-Adams seizures, nervousness, insomnia, headache, tremor, angina, tachycardia, dyspepsia, nausea, vomiting, and flushing.

■ **Fetal Considerations** — There are no adequate reports or well-controlled studies in human fetuses. **Isoproterenol** crosses the human placenta, though the kinetics remain to be elucidated. It has been used (unsuccessfully) to treat fetal complete heart block. There are no reports of fetal compromise associated with **isoproterenol** despite numerous case reports and series. Rodent teratogenicity studies have not been performed.

■ **Breastfeeding Safety** — There is no published experience in nursing women. It is unknown whether **isoproterenol** enters human breast milk. Other β agonists are considered compatible with breastfeeding.

■ **References** — Marcus MA, Vertommen JD, Van Aken H, Gogarten W, Buerkle H. Anesth Analg 1998; 86:749-52.
Groves AM, Allan LD, Rosenthal E. Circulation 1995; 92:3394-6.

■ **Summary** —
- **Pregnancy Category C**
- **Lactation Category S?**
- **Isoproterenol** should be used during pregnancy and lactation only if the benefit justifies the potential perinatal risk.

Isosorbide dinitrate (Isordil; Cardio; Cedocarb; Dilatrate-Sr; Dinisor; Insucar; Isd; Iso-Bid; Isobid; Isocard; Isonate; Iso-Par; Isorbid; Isorem; Isotrate; Rigedal; Sorbitrate)

■ **Class** — Nitrates; *vasodilator*

■ **Indications** — Angina prophylaxis

■ **Mechanism** — A nitric oxide donor that stimulates cGMP production causing smooth muscle relaxation

■ **Dosage with Qualifiers** — Angina prophylaxis—begin 5mg PO qd; space doses at least 5h apart, max 80mg/d; alternatively for SR, begin 20mg PO bid
NOTE—check package insert of preparation for recommended dose, as there are variations
- **Contraindications**—hypersensitivity to drug or class, hypotension, cardiogenic shock, **sildenafil** use
- **Caution**—volume depletion

■ **Maternal Considerations** .... There are no adequate reports or well-controlled studies in pregnant women. **Isosorbide dinitrate** may be a useful alternative treatment for acute hypertension in women with severe preeclampsia (5mg SL). In one small study of preeclamptic women, sustained use was associated with a decline in the uterine artery Doppler-measured flow resistance. It was used in one instance to facilitate the manual removal of a retained placenta.

Side effects include methemoglobinemia, headache, lightheadedness, hypotension, syncope, tachycardia, flushing, peripheral edema, vomiting, fainting, and rebound hypertension.

■ **Fetal Considerations** .... There are no adequate reports or well-controlled studies in human fetuses. It is unknown whether **isosorbide dinitrate** crosses the placenta. Sublingual administration has no effect on the fetal heart rate pattern. In one small study of preeclamptic women, sustained use was associated with a decline in the umbilical artery Doppler-measured flow resistance and the maximum amniotic fluid pocket increased. Rodent studies are reassuring, revealing no evidence of teratogenicity or IUGR despite the use of doses higher than those used clinically. Embryotoxicity occurs in rodents with doses 50-100 times the MRHD.

■ **Breastfeeding Safety** .... There are no adequate reports or well-controlled studies in nursing women. It is unknown whether **isosorbide dinitrate** enters human breast milk.

■ **References** .... Martinez-Abundis E, Gonzalez-Ortiz M, Hernandez-Salazar F, Huerta-J-Lucas MT. Gynecol Obstet Invest 2000; 50:39-42.
Nakatsuka M, Takata M, Tada K, et al. J Ultrasound Med 2002; 21: 831-6.
Thaler I, Kahana H. Obstet Gynecol 2002; 100:987-91.
Thaler I, Amit A, Kamil D, Itskovitz-Eldor J. Am J Hypertens 1999; 12:341-7.

■ **Summary** ....
- **Pregnancy Category C**
- **Lactation Category U**
- **Isosorbide dinitrate** should be used during pregnancy and lactation only if the benefit justifies the potential perinatal risk.

Isosorbide mononitrate (Imdur; Imtrate; Ismo; Isopen-20; Monoket)

■ **Class** — Nitrates

■ **Indications** — Angina prophylaxis

■ **Mechanism** — Nitric oxide donor that stimulates cGMP production causing smooth muscle relaxation

■ **Dosage with Qualifiers** — Angina prophylaxis—30-60mg PO qd in one or divided doses depending on the preparation; max 240mg/d
NOTE—check package insert of preparation for recommended dose, as there are variations
- **Contraindications**—hypersensitivity to drug or class, **sildenafil** use, hypotension
- **Caution**—acute MI, hypotension, shock

■ **Maternal Considerations** — **Isosorbide mononitrate** is absorbed across the vaginal mucosa. It was investigated as a cervical ripening agent prior to 1st trimester abortion. It proved more effective than prostaglandin E_2 gel, but less effective than **misoprostol**. There are several case reports of its use in pregnant women with an acute MI.
Side effects include orthostatic hypotension, palpitations, arrhythmia, chest pain, thrombocytopenia, nausea, vomiting, headache, blurred vision, asthenia, dry mouth, constipation, abdominal pain, flatulence, bronchitis, sinusitis, and rash.

■ **Fetal Considerations** — There are no adequate reports or well-controlled studies in human fetuses. In the studies of its use either as a cervical ripening agent or treatment for preeclampsia, **isosorbide mononitrate** produced Doppler changes consistent with a maternal systemic effect. Rodent studies are reassuring, revealing no evidence of teratogenicity or IUGR despite the use of doses higher than those used clinically. Embryotoxicity occurs in rodents with doses 50-100 times the MRHD.

■ **Breastfeeding Safety** — There are no adequate reports or well-controlled studies in nursing women. It is unknown whether **isosorbide mononitrate** enters human breast milk.

■ **References** — Bates CD, Nicoll AE, Mullen AB, et al. BJOG 2003; 110:64-7.
Chanrachakul B, Herabutya Y, Punyavachira P. Int J Gynaecol Obstet 2002; 78:139-45.
Ledingham MA, Thomson AJ, Lunan CB, et al. BJOG 2001; 108:276-80.
Thaler I, Amit A, Jakobi P, Itskovitz-Eldor J. Obstet Gynecol 1996; 88:838-43.

Isotretinoin (Accutane)

■ **Class** ········· Acne

■ **Indications** ········· Acne, severe cystic and keratinization disorders

■ **Mechanism** ········· Unknown

■ **Dosage with Qualifiers** ········· Acne, severe cystic—begin 0.5-2mg/kg/d ×15-20w
Keratinization disorders—0.5-2mg/kg/d PO in divided doses bid; max 4mg/kg/d
NOTE—informed consent required
• **Contraindications**—hypersensitivity to drug or class, hypersensitivity to parabens, pregnancy
• **Caution**—psychiatric disorder, lactation, exposure to bright sunlight, seizure disorder, hyperlipidemia, history of pancreatitis, diabetes mellitus

■ **Maternal Considerations** ········· **Isotretinoin** is contraindicated during pregnancy. Patients must be capable of complying with mandatory contraceptive measures. Only manufacturer approved physicians may prescribe it. Patients should be cautioned not to self-medicate with St. Johns wort because of a possible interaction with oral contraceptives, increasing the risk of an unplanned pregnancy.
Side effects include major birth defects, depression, psychosis, suicidal ideation, hepatotoxicity, pseudotumor cerebri, allergic vasculitis, cataracts, hearing impairment, neutropenia, thrombocytopenia, agranulocytosis, hypertriglyceridemia, elevated LFTs, inflammatory bowel disease, pancreatitis, vascular thrombosis, seizures, dry skin, skin fragility, pruritus, epistaxis, conjunctivitis, photosensitivity, arthralgia, peeling of the palms, decreased night vision, tinnitus, and nail bed changes.

■ **Fetal Considerations** ········· There are no adequate reports or well-controlled studies in human fetuses. **Isotretinoin** and its active metabolites crosses the human (and subhuman primate) placenta and is a known human teratogen. Multiple organ systems are affected including CNS, cardiovascular and endocrine organs. Mental retardation without external malformation has also been reported. Similar malformations occur in rodents.

■ **References** ⋯⋯⋯⋯⋯⋯⋯⋯⋯⋯⋯

Brinker A, Trontell A, Beitz J. J Am Acad Dermatol 2002; 47:798-9.
Gorgos D. Dermatol Nurs 2002; 14:284.
Tzimas G, Nau H, Hendrickx AG, Peterson PE, Hummler H. Teratology 1996; 54:255-65.

■ **Summary** ⋯⋯⋯⋯⋯⋯⋯⋯⋯⋯⋯⋯⋯

- **Pregnancy Category X**
- **Lactation Category NS**
- **Isotretinoin** is a well documented teratogen in humans and contraindicated during pregnancy and lactation.

Isradipine (Dynacirc)

■ **Class** ⋯⋯⋯⋯⋯⋯⋯⋯⋯⋯⋯⋯⋯⋯⋯ *Antihypertensive, dihydropyridine*

■ **Indications** ⋯⋯⋯⋯⋯⋯⋯⋯⋯⋯⋯ Hypertension

■ **Mechanism** ⋯⋯⋯⋯⋯⋯⋯⋯⋯⋯⋯ Inhibits calcium influx into smooth muscle

■ **Dosage with Qualifiers** ⋯⋯⋯⋯ Hypertension—begin 2.5mg PO bid, increasing by 2.5mg PO bid q2-4w prn; max 10mg/d
NOTE—available in sustained release format
- **Contraindications**—hypersensitivity to drug or class
- **Caution**—CHF

■ **Maternal Considerations** ⋯⋯⋯ There are no adequate reports or well-controlled studies in pregnant women. Calcium-channel antagonists may be the tocolytic of choice based on their performance in meta-analyses. *In vitro*, **isradipine** is a superior tocolytic compared to **ritodrine** and **magnesium sulfate**. It has been used with success to treat preeclamptic hypertension with efficacy similar to **methyldopa** prior to delivery.
Side effects include palpitations, tachycardia, headache, hypotension, dizziness, fatigue, edema, flushing, rash, urinary frequency, nausea, and vomiting.

■ **Fetal Considerations** ⋯⋯⋯⋯⋯⋯ There are no adequate reports or well-controlled studies in human fetuses. And while **isradipine** crosses the human placenta achieving an F:M ratio of about 0.25, Doppler-measured resistances in the umbilical artery are unaltered. Rodent studies are reassuring revealing no evidence of teratogenicity despite the use of dose multiples of those used clinically. There is, however, an increased frequency of IUGR at the highest doses studied.

■ **Breastfeeding Safety** ⋯⋯⋯ There is no published experience in nursing women. It is unknown whether **isradipine** enters human breast milk.

■ **References** ⋯⋯⋯ Kantas E, Cetin A, Kaya T, Cetin M. Acta Obstet Gynecol Scand 2002; 81:825-30.
King JF, Flenady VJ, Papatsonis DN, Dekker GA, Carbonne B. Cochrane Database Syst Rev 2002; (2):CD002255.
Wide-Swensson DH, Ingemarsson I, Lunell NO, et al. Am J Obstet Gynecol 1995; 173:872-8.
Montan S, Anandakumar C, Arulkumaran S, et al. J Perinat Med 1996; 24:177-84.
Lunell NO, Bondesson U, Grunewald C, et al. Am J Hypertens 1993; 6:110S-111S.

■ **Summary** ⋯⋯⋯
- **Pregnancy Category C**
- **Lactation Category U**
- Calcium-channel antagonists are effective for the control of blood pressure, and may be the tocolytic of choice.
- **Isradipine** should be used during pregnancy and lactation only if the benefit justifies the potential perinatal risk.
- There are alternative calcium-channel antagonists for which there is more experience in pregnancy and lactation.

Itraconazole (Sporanox)

■ **Class** ⋯⋯⋯ *Antifungal*

■ **Indications** ⋯⋯⋯ Fungal infection

■ **Mechanism** ⋯⋯⋯ Inhibits cytochrome P450 dependent synthesis of ergosterol

■ **Dosage with Qualifiers** ⋯⋯⋯ Fungal infection—begin 200mg PO bid ×3d, or 200mg IV bid ×4 doses for life-threatening disease
Onchomycosis of the fingernails—200mg PO bid ×7d, off ×21d; repeat ×1
Onchomycosis of the toenails—200mg PO qd ×12w
Candidiasis, oral pharyngeal—swish first 20ml PO qd ×1-2w
Candidiasis, esophageal—swish first 10ml PO qd ×2w after symptoms resolve, total 3w
NOTE—always confirm diagnosis prior to initiating therapy; available in tablet, parenteral, and oral liquid forms; give tablets with food and solution without
- **Contraindications**—hypersensitivity to drug or class, use of either **astemizole**, **terfenadine**, **pimozide**, **quinidine**, **dofetilide,** or **cisapride**, lactation, CHF or history of CHF, LV dysfunction
- **Caution**—hepatic or renal dysfunction

- **Maternal Considerations** — There are no adequate reports or well-controlled studies in pregnant women. There several case reports of its use during pregnancy without note of diminished efficacy. There are also reports suggesting that the efficacy of oral contraceptives to block ovulation may be reduced by simultaneous use of **itraconazole**.
  Side effects include hepatic toxicity or failure, CHF, pulmonary edema, angioedema, Stevens-Johnson syndrome, nausea, vomiting, diarrhea, headache, hypertension, fatigue, fever, pruritus, hypokalemia, dizziness, anorexia, malaise, somnolence, and albuminuria.

- **Fetal Considerations** — There are no adequate reports or well-controlled studies in human fetuses. In one prospective cohort study, there was no evidence of teratogenicity or fetal sequelae. In rodents, doses of **itraconazole** 5-20 times the MRHD was associated with maternal and embryotoxicity, and teratogenicity in the survivors, consisting predominantly of skeletal defects.

- **Breastfeeding Safety** — There is no published experience in nursing women. **Itraconazole** enters human breast milk, but the pharmacokinetics is presently unclear.

- **References** — van Puijenbroek EP, Feenstra J, Meyboom RH. Ned Tijdschr Geneeskd 1998; 142:146-9.
  Aoki F, Sando Y, Tajima S, et al. Intern Med 2001; 40:1128-31.
  Bar-Oz B, Moretti ME, Bishai R, et al. Am J Obstet Gynecol 2000; 183:617-20.

- **Summary** —
  - **Pregnancy Category C**
  - **Lactation Category U**
  - **Itraconazole** should be used during pregnancy and lactation only if the benefit justifies the potential perinatal risk.

Ivermectin (Mectizan; Stromectol)

- **Class** — Antiparasitic

- **Indications** — Strongyloidiasis, onchocerciasis, scabies

- **Mechanism** — Increases cell membrane permeability in nerves and muscle

- **Dosage with Qualifiers** — Strongyloidiasis—200mcg/kg PO ×1 taken with water
  Onchocerciasis—150mcg/kg PO ×1 taken with water; re-treatment often necessary
  Scabies—200mcg/kg PO ×1

- **Contraindications**—hypersensitivity to drug or class
- **Caution**—hyperreactivity to onchderm

■ **Maternal Considerations** ⋯⋯ There are no adequate reports or well-controlled studies in pregnant women. The few published cases report no sequelae. Further, there have been several mass exposures of pregnant women during community-based treatment of onchocerciasis. There was no increase in adverse pregnancy outcomes noted.
Side effects include pruritus, fever, edema, rash, lymphadenopathy, dizziness, chest pain, abdominal distension, tachycardia, abnormal eye sensation, hypotension, and elevated LFTs.

■ **Fetal Considerations** ⋯⋯ There are no adequate reports or well-controlled studies in human fetuses. It is not known whether **ivermectin** crosses the human placenta. There have been several mass exposures of pregnant women during community-based treatment of onchocerciasis. There was no increase in pregnancy wastage or malformations observed.

■ **Breastfeeding Safety** ⋯⋯ There are no adequate reports or well-controlled studies in nursing women. Only a third of the maternal plasma **ivermectin** level is achieved in human breast milk. It is unlikely to pose a clinically significant risk to the breast-feeding infant.

■ **References** ⋯⋯ Ogbuokiri JE, Ozumba BC, Okonkwo PO. Eur J Clin Pharmacol 1993; 45:389-90.
Doumbo O, Soula G, Kodio B, Perrenoud M. Bull Soc Pathol Exot 1992; 85:247-51.
Pacque M, Munoz B, Poetschke G, et al. Lancet 1990; 336:1486-9.

■ **Summary** ⋯⋯
- **Pregnancy Category C**
- **Lactation Category S?**
- **Ivermectin** should be used during pregnancy and lactation only if the benefit justifies the potential perinatal risk.

Kanamycin (Kantrex; Klebcil)

■ **Class** — Antibiotic, aminoglycoside

■ **Indications** — Bacterial infection

■ **Mechanism** — Inhibits protein synthesis by binding the 30S ribosomal subunit leading to cell destruction

■ **Dosage with Qualifiers** — Bacterial infection—15mg/kg/d IM/IV in 2-3 divided doses
NOTE—renal dosing; peak 25-35mcg/ml, trough <10mcg/ml
- **Contraindications**—hypersensitivity to drug or class
- **Caution**—myasthenia gravis, other nephrotoxic agents, renal dysfunction, vestibular or cochlear implant

■ **Maternal Considerations** — There are no adequate reports or well-controlled studies in pregnant women. **Kanamycin** is a second-line agent for the treatment of tuberculosis, but is otherwise not used widely during pregnancy and offers no advantages over other aminoglycosides. Routine monitoring of peak and trough levels is not required in otherwise healthy women with normal renal function.
Side effects include nephrotoxicity, ototoxicity, tinnitus, enterocolitis, pseudotumor cerebri, pruritus, nausea, vomiting, diarrhea, weakness, tremor, muscle cramps, anorexia, edema, vertigo, agranulocytosis, thrombocytopenia, and elevated BUN/Cr.

■ **Fetal Considerations** — There are no adequate reports or well-controlled studies in human fetuses. **Kanamycin** crosses the placenta in rodents, and most likely in humans, as other aminoglycosides do. There is no evidence of teratogenicity for any of the aminoglycosides. In guinea pigs, doses of **kanamycin** 20 times the MRHD had no obvious side effects. However, otic nerve damage has been reported when the *in utero* treated neonate was challenged postnatally.

■ **Breastfeeding Safety** — There are no adequate reports or well-controlled studies in nursing women. **Kanamycin** enters human breast milk, but is generally considered compatible with breastfeeding.

■ **References** — Czeizel AE, Rockenbauer M, Olsen J, Sorensen HT. Scand J Infect Dis 2000; 32:309-13.
Wang Z, Liou L. Ann Otol Rhinol Laryngol 1994; 103:983-5.

■ **Summary** —
- **Pregnancy Category D**
- **Lactation Category S?**
- For most indications, there are alternative agents for which there is more experience regarding use during pregnancy and lactation.

Ketamine (Ketalar)

■ Class .... Anesthesia, *general*

■ Indications .... Induction of anesthesia

■ Mechanism .... Unknown

■ Dosage with Qualifiers .... Induction of anesthesia—1-1.5mg IV over 1min or 5-10mg/kg IM
NOTE—**atropine** may be used to decrease salivation
- **Contraindications**—hypersensitivity to drug or class, hypertension, elevated intracranial pressure, glaucoma, thyrotoxicosis, CHF, psychosis
- **Caution**—hepatic dysfunction, GERD

■ Maternal Considerations .... **Ketamine** is a rapid-acting general anesthetic agent. There are no adequate reports or well-controlled studies in pregnant women. It is popular in some locales for cesarean delivery of parturients who are either hemorrhaging, have asthma (increased catecholamine release ameliorates bronchospasm) or fetal acidemia. Compared to **thiopental**, women who receive **ketamine** during cesarean delivery have a lower need for supplemental analgesia postoperatively. The incidence of awareness to verbal commands during surgery is lower with **ketamine** compared to **thiopental**, but the frequency of recall of intraoperative events is not different. There is reportedly an increased incidence of dreaming during anesthesia, which may lead to dissatisfaction with the anesthetic experience.
Side effects include increased intracranial pressure, laryngospasm, increased intraocular pressure, hypotension, hypertension, bradycardia, myocardial depression, delirium, hypersalivation, nausea, vomiting, tremor, diplopia, nystagmus, fasciculation, depressed reflexes, and hallucinations.

■ Fetal Considerations .... There are no adequate reports or well-controlled studies in human fetuses. A number of rodent studies suggest **ketamine** may alter postnatal behavior and taste appreciation with early exposure.

■ Breastfeeding Safety .... There are no adequate reports or well-controlled studies in nursing women. It is unknown whether **ketamine** enters human breast milk. However, considering its application, it is unlikely a clinically significant amount of drug would remain in breast milk at least 48h postoperatively.

■ References .... Kee WD, Khaw KS, Ma ML, et al. Anesth Analg 1997; 85:1294-8.
Gaitini L, Vaida S, Collins G, et al. Can J Anaesth 1995; 42:377-81.

■ Summary

- **Pregnancy Category D**
- **Lactation Category U**
- **Ketamine** should be used during pregnancy and lactation only if the benefit justifies the potential perinatal risk.

Ketoconazole (Funazole; Fungazol; Fugen; Funginox; Nizoral; Zoralin)

■ **Class**	*Antifungal*
■ **Indications**	Fungal infections such as tinea versicolor, tinea capitis, tinea corporis, tinea cruris, tinea pedis, and candidiasis
■ **Mechanism**	Inhibits cell membrane ergosterol synthesis

■ **Dosage with Qualifiers**

Fungal infection—200-400mg PO qd (up to 800mg PO qd for esophageal candida or cavitary histoplasmosis)
NOTE—administer with food; soda increases absorption 50-75%; also available in topical solution and cream
- **Contraindications**—hypersensitivity to drug or class, achlorhydria, fungal meningitis, use of either **astemizole**, **cisapride**, or **terfenadine**
- **Caution**—hepatotoxic drugs, hepatic dysfunction

■ **Maternal Considerations**

There are no adequate reports or well-controlled studies in pregnant women. Although the drug is absorbed when applied topically, the systemic concentration is relatively low. **Ketoconazole** has been used to treat Cushing's syndrome during pregnancy.
Side effects include hepatic failure or toxicity, adrenal insufficiency, nausea, vomiting, diarrhea, dizziness, headache, lethargy, nervousness, somnolence, hemolytic anemia, thrombocytopenia, leukopenia, increased LFTs, and rash.

■ **Fetal Considerations**

There are no adequate reports or well-controlled studies in human fetuses. Several studies suggest **ketoconazole** interferes with ovarian synthesis of progesterone by inhibiting aromatase. As such, it could interfere with implantation and maintenance of early pregnancy. **Ketoconazole** produced maternal toxicity along with syndactyly and oligodactyly in rodents exposed to 10 times the MRHD.

■ **Breastfeeding Safety**

Only a trace amount of maternally administered **ketoconazole** enters human breast milk.

- **References** .... Amado JA, Pesquera C, Gonzalez EM, et al. Postgrad Med J 1990; 66:221-3.
  Moretti ME, Ito S, Koren G. Am J Obstet Gynecol 1995; 173:1625-6.
  Ayub M, Stitch SR. J Steroid Biochem 1986; 25:981-4.

- **Summary** ....
  - **Pregnancy Category C**
  - **Lactation Category S**
  - **Ketoconazole** should be used during pregnancy and lactation only if the benefit justifies the potential perinatal risk.

Ketoprofen (Alrhumat; Kefenid; Orudis; Oruvail)

- **Class** .... NSAID

- **Indications** .... Mild to moderate pain, fever, dysmenorrhea, osteoarthritis and rheumatoid arthritis

- **Mechanism** .... Inhibits cyclooxygenase and lipoxygenase leading to reduced prostaglandin synthesis

- **Dosage with Qualifiers** .... Mild to moderate pain—25-50mg PO q6-8h; max 75mg/d
  Fever—12.5mg PO q4-6h; max 75mg/d
  Dysmenorrhea—25-50mg PO q6-8h; max 300mg/d
  Osteoarthritis or rheumatoid arthritis—75mg PO tid, or 50mg PO qid; max 300mg/d
  NOTE—requires both renal and hepatic dosing, available in SR formulation
  - **Contraindications**—hypersensitivity to drug or class, ASA/NSAID-induced asthma
  - **Caution**—hypertension, CHF, history of GI bleeding, nasal polyps, hepatic or renal dysfunction

- **Maternal Considerations** .... There are no adequate reports or well-controlled studies in pregnant women. **Ketoprofen** provides effective analgesia after both vaginal and cesarean delivery.
  Side effects include renal failure, fluid retention, dyspepsia, GI bleeding, bronchospasm, interstitial nephritis, hepatotoxicity, Stevens-Johnson syndrome, headache, nausea, constipation, abdominal pain, dizziness, rash, agranulocytosis, increased LFTs, thrombocytopenia, tinnitus, and drowsiness.

- **Fetal Considerations** .... There are no adequate reports or well-controlled studies in human fetuses. **Ketoprofen** rapidly crosses the placenta, reaching an F:M ratio approaching unity. Most other NSAIDs can produce fetal oliguria and ductal constriction in a dose- and gestational age-dependent fashion. It is not known whether **ketoprofen** has the same actions. However, acute renal failure is reported in preterm infants whose mothers received **ketoprofen** prior to delivery. Rodent studies are reassuring, revealing no evidence of teratogenicity or IUGR.

■ **Breastfeeding Safety** ⋯⋯⋯⋯ There are no adequate reports or well-controlled studies in nursing women. Low concentrations of **ketoprofen** are found in human breast milk, but the pharmacokinetics remain to be elucidated.

■ **References** ⋯⋯⋯⋯⋯⋯ Sunshine A, Olson NZ. J Clin Pharmacol 1988; 28 (12 Suppl):S47-54.
Gouyon JB, Petion AM, Sandre D, et al. Arch Fr Pediatr 1991; 48:347-8.
De Graeve J, Frankinet C, Gielen JE. Biomed Mass Spectrom 1979; 6:249-52.

■ **Summary** ⋯⋯⋯⋯⋯⋯
- **Pregnancy Category B**
- **Lactation Category S?**
- **Ketoprofen** is an excellent agent for puerperal analgesia. There are other NSAIDs for which there is more experience regarding use during pregnancy and lactation.

Ketorolac tromethamine (Acular; Acular PF; Toradol)

■ **Class** ⋯⋯⋯⋯⋯⋯⋯⋯⋯ NSAID

■ **Indications** ⋯⋯⋯⋯⋯⋯ Moderate to severe pain

■ **Mechanism** ⋯⋯⋯⋯⋯⋯ Inhibits cyclooxygenase and lipoxygenase leading to reduced prostaglandin synthesis

■ **Dosage with Qualifiers** ⋯⋯ Moderate to severe pain—begin 60mg IM/30mg IV then repeat q6h as needed, max 120mg or 10mg PO q4-6h prn, max 40mg/d
NOTE—if transitioning from parenteral to PO, begin 20mg PO followed by 10mg PO q4-6hprn, max 40 mg/d
NOTE—do not exceed 5 days of therapy; available for ophthalmologic use
- **Contraindications**—hypersensitivity to drug or class, ASA/NSAID-induced asthma, cerebrovascular hemorrhage, preoperative use
- **Caution**—hypertension, CHF, history of GI bleeding, nasal polyps, hepatic or renal dysfunction

- **Maternal Considerations** ⸳⸳⸳⸳⸳ **Ketorolac** is indicated for the management of pain that usually would require an opioid for relief. There are no adequate reports or well-controlled studies in pregnant women.

  Side effects include renal failure, fluid retention, dyspepsia, GI bleeding, bronchospasm, interstitial nephritis, hepatotoxicity, Stevens-Johnson syndrome, nausea, constipation, abdominal pain, headache, dizziness, rash, thrombocytopenia, agranulocytosis, increased LFTs, tinnitus, and drowsiness.

- **Fetal Considerations** ⸳⸳⸳⸳⸳ There are no adequate reports or well-controlled studies in human fetuses. It is unknown whether **ketorolac** crosses the placenta. Most other NSAIDs can produce fetal oliguria and ductal constriction in a dose- and gestational age-dependent fashion. It is not known whether **ketorolac** has the same actions. Rodent studies are reassuring revealing no evidence of teratogenicity or IUGR. The perinatal mortality rate in rodents was increased in association with delayed onset of parturition.

- **Breastfeeding Safety** ⸳⸳⸳⸳⸳ Small quantities of **ketorolac** enter human breast milk. It seems relatively unlikely the breast-feeding neonate would ingest a clinically relevant amount.

- **References** ⸳⸳⸳⸳⸳ No published experience in pregnancy or during lactation

- **Summary** ⸳⸳⸳⸳⸳
  - **Pregnancy Category C**
  - **Lactation Category U?**
  - An excellent analgesic, there are other NSAIDs for which there is more experience regarding use during pregnancy and lactation.

Labetalol (Coreton; Normadate; Normodyne; Trandate)

- ■ **Class** — *Antihypertensive, adrenergic antagonist*

- ■ **Indications** — Hypertension

- ■ **Mechanism** — Selective α-1 and nonselective β-1 and -2 adrenergic receptor antagonist

- ■ **Dosage with Qualifiers** — Hypertension—begin 100mg PO bid, increase 100mg bid q2-3w; max 2.4g/d
  Acute hypertension—if diastolic BP >105mmHg, administer incremental dosing of 5-10mg IV, with a cumulative dose of 40-80mg IV over 20 min; max 300mg IV
  - **Contraindications**—hypersensitivity to drug or class, asthma, CHF, AV block, cardiogenic shock, bradycardia, hepatotoxicity, hypoglycemia
  - **Caution**—MI, angina, diabetes mellitus, hepatic or renal dysfunction, cocaine, abrupt withdrawal, major surgery

- ■ **Maternal Considerations** — Hypertensive disorders complicate 5-10% of pregnancies and are a leading cause of maternal and perinatal morbidity and death. Severe hypertension (systolic BP >170mmHg and/or diastolic BP >110mmHg) should be treated rapidly to reduce the risk of stroke, death and possibly, eclampsia in preeclamptic women. There is no consensus whether mild-to-moderate hypertension should be treated during pregnancy. The risks of transient severe hypertension, the likelihood of antenatal hospitalization, proteinuria at delivery, and neonatal RDS may be decreased by therapy. **Labetalol** reduces BP more slowly than **nifedipine**, and it does not increase the maternal cardiac index as does **nifedipine.** Thus, **labetalol** is the drug of choice for hypertensive women with tachycardia. **Labetalol** has a lower risk of hypotension than parenteral **hydralazine**. **Labetalol** is better tolerated than **methyldopa** and provides more efficient BP control. It reduces cerebral pressure without altering cerebral perfusion. **Labetalol** may also be useful for the treatment of maternal thyrotoxicosis during labor.
  Side effects include hepatic necrosis, SLE, bronchospasm, dizziness, nausea, vomiting, fatigue, dyspepsia, rhinitis, dyspnea, edema, postural hypotension, pruritus, and increased BUN/creatinine.

- ■ **Fetal Considerations** — **Labetalol** crosses the human placenta producing F:M ratios of 0.5 and AF:M ratios <0.20. Neither **labetalol** nor **hydralazine** vasodilate the perfused human cotyledon. Doppler flow studies reveal no change in umbilical, uterine, and middle cerebral resistances after treatment. Intravenous **labetalol** can cause fetal bradycardia. Hypoglycemia, bradycardia, hypotension, pericardial effusion, and myocardial hypertrophy are reported after long-term oral **labetalol**. Fetal death may also occur after a sudden drop in the maternal BP, the risk of which can be minimized by adequate hydration. Overall, neonatal outcome is similar to that achieved with **hydralazine**. **Labetalol** may be useful for the treatment of fetal thyrotoxicosis. Rodent studies are reassuring, revealing no evidence of teratogenicity or IUGR despite the use of doses higher than those used clinically. **Labetalol** reduces uteroplacental blood flow selectively in guinea pigs, perhaps explaining the increased frequency of IUGR in this model.

■ **Breastfeeding Safety**

There is no consistent relation between maternal plasma and milk concentrations either within or between individuals. The risk of hypoglycemia in breast-fed neonates is increased by **labetalol** and may be blunted with glucose-fortified formula.

■ **References**

Varon J, Marik PE. Chest 2000; 118:214-27.

Scardo JA, Vermillion ST, Newman RB, et al. Am J Obstet Gynecol 1999; 181:862-6.

Belfort MA, Tooke-Miller C, Allen JC Jr, Dizon-Townson D, Varner MA. Hypertens Pregnancy 2002; 21:185-97.

Vermillion ST, Scardo JA, Newman RB, Chauhan SP. Am J Obstet Gynecol 1999; 181:858-61.

Crooks BN, Deshpande SA, Hall C, et al. Arch Dis Child Fetal Neonatal Ed 1998; 79:F150-1.

Bowman ML, Bergmann M, Smith JF. Thyroid 1998; 8:795-6.

Gilson GJ, Kramer RL, Barada C, et al. J Matern Fetal Med 1998; 7:142-7.

el-Qarmalawi AM, Morsy AH, al-Fadly A, et al. Int J Gynaecol Obstet 1995; 49:125-30.

Petersen OB, Skajaa K, Svane D, et al. Br J Obstet Gynaecol 1994; 101:871-8.

Hjertberg R, Faxelius G, Belfrage P. Acta Obstet Gynecol Scand 1993; 72:611-5.

Hjertberg R, Faxelius G, Lagercrantz H. J Perinat Med 1993; 21:69-75.

Pickles CJ, Broughton Pipkin F, Symonds EM. Br J Obstet Gynaecol 1992; 99:964-8.

Munshi UK, Deorari AK, Paul VK, Singh M. Indian Pediatr 1992; 29:1507-12.

Olsen KS, Beier-Holgersen R. Acta Obstet Gynecol Scand 1992; 71:145-7.

Munshi UK, Deorari AK, Paul VK, Singh M. Indian Pediatr 1992; 29:1507-12.

Harper A, Murnaghan GA. Br J Obstet Gynaecol 1991; 98:453-9.

Pirhonen JP, Erkkola RU, Makinen JI, Ekblad UU. Biol Neonate 1991; 59:204-8.

Sibai BM, Mabie WC, Shamsa F, et al. Am J Obstet Gynecol 1990; 162:960-6.

Rogers RC, Sibai BM, Whybrew WD. Am J Obstet Gynecol 1990; 162:362-6.

Lunell NO, Kulas J, Rane A. Eur J Clin Pharmacol 1985; 28:597-9.

■ **Summary**

- **Pregnancy Category C**
- **Lactation Category S**
- **Labetalol** is an effective agent for the treatment of acute hypertension and thyrotoxicosis during labor.
- In many locales, **labetalol** is the preferred drug for the short-term treatment of preeclamptic hypertension.
- Hypoglycemia but not IUGR is the most common adverse neonatal effect.

Lactulose (Acilac; C-Cephulose; Cephulac; Cholac; Constilac; Constulose; Duphalac; Enulose; Evalose; Generlac; Heptalac; Laxilose)

■ **Class**

Laxative

■ **Indications**

Constipation, hepatic encephalopathy

■ **Mechanism**

Increases stool water content, traps ammonium ions

■ **Dosage with Qualifiers**

Constipation—15-30ml (10-20g/d) PO qd/bid
Hepatic encephalopathy—30-45ml PO tid/qid (20-30g tid/qid)

- **Contraindications**—hypersensitivity to drug or class, galactosemia
- **Caution**—diabetes mellitus, hypokalemia

■ **Maternal Considerations**

Constipation is common during pregnancy. **Lactulose** helps restore normal bowel habits. It is poorly absorbed, and women with **lactose** intolerance tolerate **lactulose** better in the 3rd trimester because of slow transit and bacterial adaptation.
Side effects include acidosis, abdominal distention, belching, abdominal pain, diarrhea, anorexia, nausea, vomiting, electrolyte disorders, hypernatremia, and flatulence.

■ **Fetal Considerations**

There are no adequate reports or well-controlled studies in human fetuses. Because of poor maternal absorption, it is unlikely the maternal systemic concentration will reach a clinically relevant level. Rodent studies are reassuring, revealing no evidence of teratogenicity or IUGR despite the use of doses higher than those used clinically.

■ **Breastfeeding Safety**

There is no published experience in nursing women. It is unknown whether **lactulose** enters human breast milk. Breast-feeding infants require lactase to metabolize **lactose**, the major carbohydrate in breast milk. Lactase is located on the small intestinal brush border and is extremely vulnerable to pathogenic damage.

- **References** .... Signorelli P, Croce P, Dede A. Minerva Ginecol 1996; 48:577-82.
  Szilagyi A, Salomon R, Martin M, et al. Clin Invest Med 1996; 19:416-26.
  Gattuso JM, Kamm MA. Drug Saf 1994; 10:47-65.
  Mizuno O. Endocrinol Jpn 1987; 34:449-55.
  Baglioni A, Dubini F. Boll Chim Farm 1976; 115:596-606.
  Northrop-Clewes CA, Lunn PG, Downes RM. J Pediatr Gastroenterol Nutr 1997; 24:257-63.

- **Summary** ....
  - **Pregnancy Category B**
  - **Lactation Category S**
  - Most laxatives are relatively safe during pregnancy if used intermittently as directed.

Lamivudine (Epivir; Epivir HBV; 3 TC)

- **Class** .... *Antiviral*

- **Indications** .... HIV infection, hepatitis B

- **Mechanism** .... Reverse transcriptase inhibitor

- **Dosage with Qualifiers** .... HIV infection—150mg PO bid
  Hepatitis B—100mg PO qd
  - **Contraindications**—hypersensitivity to drug or class
  - **Caution**—hepatic or renal dysfunction, pancreatitis, long-term therapy, obesity

- **Maternal Considerations** .... **Lamivudine** is rapidly absorbed after oral administration, reaching maximal serum concentrations after 30-90min. Triple therapy **(zidovudine, lamivudine, nevirapine)** is a highly effective regimen. However, there are reports of rapid development of genotypic resistance to **lamivudine**. HIV therapy that reduces the viral load significantly reduces the risk of mother-to-child transmission. There are no adequate reports or well-controlled studies of **lamivudine** in pregnant women. Hepatotoxicity, usually within 5mo of beginning therapy, is a major concern during pregnancy. It is most severe when associated with hepatitis B and C coinfection. There are presently only 2 drugs for the treatment of hepatitis B during pregnancy—**interferon alfa** and **lamivudine.** The initial response to **lamivudine** is superior to **interferon alfa**. **Lamivudine** is reportedly safe in pregnant women with chronic hepatitis B during the last weeks of pregnancy. However, resistant hepatitis B strains develop in some patients. U.S. federal government guidelines recommend **zidovudine** plus **lamivudine** for health care personnel exposed to both hepatitis B and HIV.

Side effects include acidosis, hepatic steatosis or toxicity, pancreatitis, neuropathy, neutropenia, thrombocytopenia, rhabdomyolisis, and exacerbation of hepatitis B.

■ **Fetal Considerations** .... **Lamivudine** readily crosses the human placenta, achieving F:M and Af:M ratios approaching unity. This does not necessarily prevent hepatitis B transmission to the perinate despite undetectable maternal viral DNA. Large trials are awaited. Neonatal prophylaxis with both **zidovudine** and **lamivudine** is typically initiated within 12h of birth. Mitochondrial disorders are described in children exposed *in utero* to some reverse transcriptase enzyme inhibitors (e.g., **zidovudine**). Rodent studies are reassuring, revealing no evidence of teratogenicity or IUGR despite the use of doses higher than those used clinically. Embryotoxicity occurs in rabbit. Fetal DNA damage in subhuman primates was doubled by the combination of **zidovudine** and **lamivudine** compared to **zidovudine** alone.

■ **Breastfeeding Safety** .... There are no adequate reports or well-controlled studies in nursing women. **Lamivudine** is excreted into human breast milk, though the kinetics remain to be elucidated. Its concentration in rodent milk reaches unity. Breastfeeding is contraindicated in HIV-infected nursing women where formula is available to reduce the risk of neonatal transmission.

■ **References** .... Trautwein C. Schweiz Rundsch Med Prax 2002; 91:970-6.
Kazim SN, Wakil SM, Khan LA, et al. Lancet 2002; 359:1488-9 .
Zoulim F. Drug Saf 2002; 25:497-510.
Hill JB, Sheffield JS, Zeeman GG, Wendel GD Jr. Obstet Gynecol 2001; 98:909-11.
Lee LM, Henderson DK. Drug Saf 2001; 24:587-97.
Moodley D, Pillay K, Naidoo K, et al. J Clin Pharmacol 2001; 41:732-41.
Mandelbrot L, Landreau-Mascaro A, et al. JAMA 2001; 285:2083-93.
Mandelbrot L, Peytavin G, Firtion G, Farinotti R. Am J Obstet Gynecol 2001; 184:153-8.
Olivero OA, Fernandez JJ, Antiochos BB, et al. J Acquir Immune Defic Synd 2002; 29:323-9.
Stojanov S, Wintergerst U, Belohradsky BH, Rolinski B. AIDS 2000; 14:1669.
van Nunen AB, de Man RA, Heijtink RA, et al. J Hepatol 2000; 32:1040-1.
Clarke JR, Braganza R, Mirza A, et al. J Med Virol 1999; 59:364-8.
Johnson MA, Moore KH, Yuen GJ, et al. Clin Pharmacokinet 1999; 36:41-66.
Bloom SL, Dias KM, Bawdon RE, Gilstrap LC 3rd. Am J Obstet Gynecol 1997; 176:291-3.

■ **Summary**
- Pregnancy Category C
- Lactation Category NS
- A cocktail of **zidovudine**, **lamivudine**, and **nevirapine** significantly reduces the risk of mother-to-child transmission, and remains a standard for the treatment of adult HIV infection.
- Pregnant women should be monitored closely after initiating therapy for hepatotoxicity.
- Physicians are encouraged to register pregnant women under the Antiretroviral Pregnancy Registry (1-800-258-4263) for a better follow-up of the outcome while under treatment with **lamivudine**.

Lamotrigine (Lamictal)

■ **Class** — Anticonvulsant

■ **Indications** — Seizures (partial)

■ **Mechanism** — Unknown

■ **Dosage with Qualifiers** — Seizures—begin 50mg/d, then increase up to 50-250mg PO bid; max 500mg/d
NOTE—avoid abrupt withdrawal
- **Contraindications**—hypersensitivity to drug or class, abrupt withdrawal
- **Caution**—hepatic or renal dysfunction, allergy to **valproate**

■ **Maternal Considerations** — There are no adequate reports or well-controlled studies of **lamotrigine** during pregnancy. Concerns over teratogenicity of antiepileptic drugs must be weighed against the risks to the mother and fetus of seizures. **Lamotrigine** clearance is increased during pregnancy, and many women require a higher dose to maintain therapeutic levels. Adjustments are based on clinical symptoms, not solely on serum drug levels. The impact of pregnancy on clearance reverses quickly post partum. The most frequent adverse maternal effect is skin rash, typically in the first month of treatment. Planned pregnancy and counseling before conception is crucial. Counseling should cover folate supplementation, the importance medication compliance, the risk of teratogenicity and the importance of prenatal care. **Lamotrigine** increases the metabolism of **ethinyl estradiol** and progestogens; a preparation containing at least 50mcg of **ethinylestradiol** is recommended.
Side effects include rash (0.3% and may be life-threatening), dysmenorrhea, dizziness, ataxia, somnolence, diplopia,

headache, blurred vision, nausea, vomiting, dyspepsia, rhinitis, anxiety, insomnia, pain, weight decrease, chest pain, infection, aplastic anemia, hemolytic anemia, thrombocytopenia, hepatic failure, aphasia, confusion, and nystagmus.

■ **Fetal Considerations**

There are no adequate reports or well-controlled studies in human fetuses. **Lamotrigine** crosses the human placenta achieving an F:M ratio near unity. Women taking anticonvulsant medication of any type have a 4-8% risk of delivering a child with a birth defect compared to 2-4% in the general population. **Lamotrigine** inhibits dihydrofolate reductase, an enzyme necessary for the biosynthesis of nucleic acids and proteins. Rodent studies are reassuring, revealing no evidence of teratogenicity or IUGR at doses analogous to human. The highest doses cause maternal and fetal toxicity characterized by IUGR and ventricular dilation. Registry data do not reveal a significant increase in the risk of major malformation (1.8%, 1st trimester exposure with monotherapy, 4.3% polytherapy). Use of monotherapy at the lowest effective quantity given in divided doses to minimize the peaks can minimize the risks.

■ **Breastfeeding Safety**

There are no adequate reports or well-controlled studies in nursing women. The median milk/maternal plasma concentration ratio ranges from 0.5-0.8 2-3w post partum, and nursed infants maintain plasma concentrations approximating 30% of the mother's plasma level. While no adverse effects have been reported, the infant should be monitored closely if the mother elects to breastfeed, the drug given at the lowest effective dose, and breastfeeding avoided at times of peak drug levels.

■ **References**

Williams J, Myson V, Steward S, et al. Epilepsia 2002; 43:824-31.
Tran TA, Leppik IE, Blesi K, et al. Neurology 2002; 59:251-5.
Crawford P. CNS Drugs. 2002; 16:263-72.
Tennis P, Eldridge RR. International Lamotrigine Pregnancy Registry Scientific Advisory Committee. Epilepsia 2002; 43:1161-7.
Ohman I, Vitols S, Tomson T. Epilepsia 2000; 41:709-13.
Marchi NS, Azoubel R, Tognola WA. Arq Neuropsiquiatr 2001; 59:362-4.
Bar-Oz B, Nulman I, Koren G, Ito S. Paediatr Drugs 2000; 2:113-26.
Sabers A, Gram L. Drugs 2000; 60:23-33.

■ **Summary**

- **Pregnancy Category C**
- **Lactation Category S?**
- **Lamotrigine** is well tolerated and drug interaction problems are minor with the exception of oral contraceptive failure.
- Physicians are encouraged to register patients, before fetal outcome is known (e.g., ultrasound, results of amniocentesis, birth), and can obtain information from the *Lamotrigine Pregnancy Registry* at 800-336-2176.

Lansoprazole (Lopral; Ogastro; Prevacid; Zoton)

■ **Class** — *Gastrointestinal, proton pump inhibitor*

■ **Indications** — Gastroesophageal reflex disease (GERD), esophagitis, duodenal ulcer, H. *pylori* infection, hypersecretory, stress ulcer, ulcer prophylaxis

■ **Mechanism** — Hydrogen-potassium ATPase inhibitor

■ **Dosage with Qualifiers** — GERD—15-30mg PO qd/bid ×8w
Esophagitis—30mg PO qd/bid ×8w
Gastric ulcer—30mg PO qd/ bid ×8w
Duodenal ulcer—15mg PO qd/ bid ×8w
H. *pylori* infection—30mg PO bid ×10-14d
Hypersecretory conditions—60mg PO qd; max 90mg PO bid
Stress ulcer—15-30mg PO, through feeding tube
Ulcer prophylaxis—15-30mg PO qd
- **Contraindications**—hypersensitivity to drug or class
- **Caution**—long-term use, hepatic dysfunction

■ **Maternal Considerations** — GERD and/or heartburn occur in 45-85% of women during pregnancy. The effect of estrogen and **progesterone** on lower esophageal sphincter tone is a recognized factor. The treatment of GERD consists of reducing gastric acidity following a step-up algorithm beginning with lifestyle modifications and dietary changes. Antacids or **sucralfate** are first-line medical therapy, followed by histamine receptor antagonists. **Ranitidine** is probably preferred because of its documented efficacy and safety profile in pregnancy, even in the 1st trimester. **Proton-pump** inhibitors are reserved for the woman with intractable symptoms or complicated reflux disease. There are no adequate reports or well-controlled studies of **lansoprazole** during pregnancy. However, **proton-pump** inhibitors like **lansoprazole** are generally considered effective treatment for GERD in pregnant women. Adverse effects have not been reported. Further, **proton-pump** inhibitors are first-line agents for the prevention of "aspiration syndrome" during general anesthesia.
Side effects include hepatic failure, blood dyscrasias, Stevens-Johnson syndrome, erythema multiforme, pancreatitis, toxic epidermal necrolysis, headache, diarrhea, asthenia, candidiasis, chest pain, cerebral vascual accident, hypertension/hypotension, MI, and palpitations.

■ **Fetal Considerations** — There are no adequate reports or well-controlled studies in human fetuses. It is unknown whether **lansoprazole** crosses the human placenta. Safety data are based on limited animal study and case reports. Thus, **proton-pump inhibitors** are recommended only for the treatment of severe, intractable GERD during pregnancy. Rodent studies are reassuring, revealing no evidence of teratogenicity or IUGR despite the use of doses higher than those used clinically.

■ **Breastfeeding Safety**

There is no published experience in nursing women. It is unknown whether **lansoprazole** enters human breast milk. It is excreted into rodent milk.

■ **References**

Richter JE. Gastroenterol Clin North Am 2003; 32:235-61.
Ramakrishnan A, Katz PO. Curr Treat Options Gastroenterol 2002; 5:301-310.
Broussard CN, Richter JE. Drug Saf 1998; 19:325-37.

■ **Summary**

- **Pregnancy Category B**
- **Lactation Category S?**
- **Lansoprazole** should be used during pregnancy and lactation only if the benefit justifies the potential perinatal risk.

Latanoprost (Xalatan)

■ **Class**

Ophthalmic, prostaglandin

■ **Indications**

Elevated intraocular pressure

■ **Mechanism**

Increases aqueous humor outflow

■ **Dosage with Qualifiers**

Elevated intraocular pressure—1 gtt (1.5 mcg) OS/OD qd
- **Contraindications**—hypersensitivity to drug or class
- **Caution**—asthma

■ **Maternal Considerations**

There is no published experience during pregnancy.
Side effects include epithelial keratitis, blurred vision, eyelid skin darkening, intraocular inflammation, iris pigmentation changes, macular edema, burning, hyperemia, foreign body sensation, itching, iris hyperpigmentation, dry eyes, tearing, photophobia, ocular pain, discharge, rash, lid crusting, asthma and exacerbation of asthma.

■ **Fetal Considerations**

There are no adequate reports or well-controlled studies in human fetuses. It is unknown whether **latanoprost** crosses the human placenta. Considering the dose and route, it is unlikely the maternal systemic concentration will reach a clinically relevant level. Embryotoxicity was observed in rodents treated with a dosage more than 15 times the MRHD.

■ **Breastfeeding Safety** .... There is no published experience in pregnancy. It is unknown whether **latanoprost** enters human breast milk. However, considering the dose and route, it is unlikely the breast-fed neonate would ingest clinically relevant amounts.

■ **References** .... There is no published experience in pregnancy or during lactation.

■ **Summary** ....
- **Pregnancy Category C**
- **Lactation Category S?**
- **Latanoprost** should be used during pregnancy and lactation only if the benefit justifies the potential risk.

Leflunomide (Arava)

■ **Class** .... Antirheumatic, immunomodulator

■ **Indications** .... Rheumatoid arthritis

■ **Mechanism** .... Pyrimidine synthesis inhibitor with antiproliferative activity

■ **Dosage with Qualifiers** .... Rheumatoid arthritis—begin 100mg PO qd ×3d, then 10-20mg PO qd
NOTE—check level q14d (normal above 0.02mcg/ml)
- **Contraindications**—hypersensitivity to drug or class, pregnancy
- **Caution**—immunodeficiency, blood dyscrasias, bone marrow suppression, infections, hepatitis B or C

■ **Maternal Considerations** .... There is no published experience during pregnancy. Based on animal study (see Fetal Considerations), **leflunomide** is contraindicated during pregnancy and effective contraception is a must. Women desiring pregnancy must discontinue **leflunomide** before conceiving, preferably at least 4mo before. Further, the manufacturer recommends preconception treatment with **cholestyramine** to increase drug elimination with subsequent verification that plasma levels are less than 0.02mg/L.
Side effects include hepatotoxicity, immunosuppression, leukopenia, pancytopenia, Stevens-Johnson syndrome, toxic epidermal necrolysis, erythema multiforme, diarrhea, alopecia, nausea, vomiting, headache, RDS, dyspepsia, rash, back pain, pruritus, asthenia, allergic reactions, dizziness, weight loss, and paresthesias.

- **Fetal Considerations** — There are no adequate and well-controlled studies in human fetuses. **Leflunomide** likely crosses the human placenta. No malformations are reported in infants exposed to **leflunomide**, but the number of reported pregnancy outcomes is small. The incidences of anophthalmia and micropthalmia are increased in rats treated with only 0.1 the concentration recommended in humans. In rabbits, a dose analogous to the human is associated with embryotoxicity and bony abnormalities.

- **Breastfeeding Safety** — There is no published experience in nursing women. It is unknown whether **leflunomide** enters human breast milk. In light of the animal studies, it is best to avoid breastfeeding if **leflunomide** must be prescribed.

- **References** — Kozer E, Moretti ME, Koren G. Can Fam Physician 2001; 47:721-2.
Brent RL. Teratology 2001; 63:106-12.
Prakash A, Jarvis B. Drugs 1999; 58:1137-64.

- **Summary** —
  - **Pregnancy Category X**
  - **Lactation Category U**
  - **Leflunomide** is a potent teratogen in some rodents and presently contraindicated during pregnancy.
  - Health care providers are encouraged to register patients by calling 1-877-311-8972 to improve knowledge of fetal outcomes of pregnant women exposed to **leflunomide**.
  - There are alternative agents for which there is more experience during pregnancy and lactation.

Lepirudin (Refludan)

- **Class** — Anticoagulant, thrombin inhibitor

- **Indications** — Thrombocytopenia, heparin-induced

- **Mechanism** — Direct inhibitor of thrombin independent of ATIII

- **Dosage with Qualifiers** — Heparin-induced thrombocytopenia/thrombosis—begin 0.4mg/kg, then 0.15mg/kg/h IV; max 44mg
  - **Contraindications**—hypersensitivity to drug or class
  - **Caution**—bleeding, renal dysfunction, increased risk of bleeding including AV malformations, hypertension, recent surgery

- **Maternal Considerations** — Heparin-induced thrombocytopenia is a rare but potentially life-threatening reaction to both **heparin** and low-molecular-weight heparin. It is the most common drug-induced immune-mediated thrombocytopenia. **Lepirudin** effectively treats the thrombocytopenia by inhibiting thrombin. Many patients develop antibodies (40%), and the aPTT should be monitored during long-term therapy. There is no published experience during pregnancy.

Side effects include bleeding, anemia, hematuria, intracranial hemorrhage, fever, GI bleeding, increased LFTs, and epistaxis.

■ **Fetal Considerations**
There are no adequate reports or well-controlled studies in human fetuses. It is unknown whether **lepirudin** crosses the human placenta; it does the rat. Rodent studies are reassuring, revealing no evidence of teratogenicity or IUGR despite the use of doses higher than those used clinically.

■ **Breastfeeding Safety**
There is no published experience in nursing women. It is unknown whether **lepirudin** enters human breast milk.

■ **References**
Dager WE, White RH. Ann Pharmacother 2002; 36:489-503. McCrae KR, Bussel JB, Mannucci PM, et al. Hematology (Am Soc Hematol Educ Program) 2001; 282-305.

■ **Summary**
- **Pregnancy Category B**
- **Lactation Category S?**
- Heparin-induced thrombocytopenia is the most frequently encountered drug-induced immune-mediated adverse thrombocytopenia. Therapeutic options are limited.

Letrozole (Femara)

■ **Class**
Antineoplastic, aromatase inhibitor

■ **Indications**
Breast cancer

■ **Mechanism**
Inhibits aromatase

■ **Dosage with Qualifiers**
Breast cancer—2.5mg PO qd
- **Contraindications**—hypersensitivity to drug or class
- **Caution**—renal dysfunction

■ **Maternal Considerations**
Letrozole is a nonsteroidal aromatase inhibitor that significantly lowers **estradiol** and **estrone**. It is used mostly for adjuvant therapy. **Letrozole** has also been used to treat infertility associated with poor response to FSH stimulation. There is no published experience during pregnancy.

Side effects include thromboembolism, muscular pain, nausea, vomiting, fatigue, arthralgia, vomiting, cough, chest pain, hot flashes, diarrhea, abdominal pain, viral infection, edema, hypertension, and anorexia.

- **Fetal Considerations** — There are no adequate reports or well-controlled studies in human fetuses. It is unknown whether **letrozole** crosses the human placenta. **Letrozole** is embryotoxic, fetotoxic and teratogenic in rodents even at low doses.

- **Breastfeeding Safety** — There is no published experience in nursing women. It is unknown whether **letrozole** enters human breast milk.

- **References** — Mitwally MF, Casper RF. Fertil Steril 2002; 77:776-80.

- **Summary**
  - **Pregnancy Category D**
  - **Lactation Category U**
  - **Letrozole** is an adjuvant agent for the treatment of breast cancer.
  - **Letrozole** should be used during pregnancy and lactation only if the benefit justifies the potential perinatal risk.

Leucovorin (Calcium folinate; citrovorum factor; Ledervorin-Calcium; Lerderfoline; Wellcovorin)

- **Class** — *Toxicology, antidote, vitamin*

- **Indications** — Leucovorin rescue after folate inhibition

- **Mechanism** — Counteracts folate antagonists

- **Dosage with Qualifiers** — Leucovorin rescue—15mg IV/IM/PO q6h 24h after last **methotrexate** dose
  - **Contraindications**—hypersensitivity to drug or class, vitamin B_{12} deficiency, pernicious anemia, megaloblastic anemia
  - **Caution**—seizure disorder

- **Maternal Considerations** — Gestational trophoblastic disease is a spectrum of disorders ranging from the benign complete or partial hydatidiform mole to malignant choriocarcinoma. While the preponderance of women are cured by surgery, the occasional patient requires chemotherapy. **Methotrexate**, an inhibitor of dihydrofolate reductase is the first-line agent. It can persist in human tissue for long periods. **Leucovorin** is a derivative of tetrahydrofolate and as such circumvents the block. Supplementation minimizes toxicity and can counteract inadvertent overdose. **Methotrexate** may be given as a single-dose IM, which usually does not require **leucovorin**, or in a multiple-dose regimen, which does require **leucovorin** rescue. **Methotrexate** with **leucovorin** rescue is a highly effective, well-tolerated, nonsurgical treatment for patients with ectopic pregnancy. *Side effects* include anaphylactic reaction, seizures, syncope, urticaria, nausea, and vomiting.

■ **Fetal Considerations** There are no adequate reports or well-controlled studies in human fetuses (see **folic acid**). **Folate** is quickly transferred across the placenta. Rodent teratogenicity studies have not been conducted. Periconceptional **folate** supplementation increases fertility (higher cumulative rates and of multiple births). A deficiency of **folic acid** increases the incidence of neural tube defects, and randomized studies reveal that 4mg/d of **folic acid** prior to conception prevents their recurrence. It is not known whether **leucovorin** supplementation would have the same effect.

■ **Breastfeeding Safety** There is no published experience in nursing women. It is unknown whether **leucovorin** enters human breast milk.

■ **References**

Bruno MK, Harden CL. Curr Treat Options Neurol 2002; 4:31-40.
McNeish IA, Strickland S, Holden L, et al. J Clin Oncol 2002; 20:1838-44.
Kendall A, Gillmore R, Newlands E. Curr Opin Obstet Gynecol 2002; 14:33-8.
Kwon JS, Elit L, Mazurka J, et al. Gynecol Oncol 2001; 82:367-70.
Barnhart K, Coutifaris C, Esposito M. Expert Opin Pharmacother 2001; 2:409-17.
Gillespie AM, Kumar S, Hancock BW. Br J Cancer 2000; 82:1393-5.
Newlands ES, Bower M, Holden L, et al. J Reprod Med 1998; 43:111-8.
Larson DM, Tipping SJ, Mulligan GM, et al. Wis Med J 1995; 94:664-7.
Elit L, Covens A, Osborne R, et al. Gynecol Oncol 1994; 54:282-7.
Homesley HD. J Reprod Med 1994; 39:185-92.
Czeizel AE, Dudas I, Metneki J. Arch Gynecol Obstet 1994; 255:131-9.
Wegner C, Nau H. Neurology 1992; 42:17-24.

■ **Summary**

- **Pregnancy Category C**
- **Lactation Category U**
- **Leucovorin** should be used during pregnancy and lactation only if the benefit justifies the potential perinatal risk.

Leuprolide (Lupron; Procren)

■ **Class** — Antineoplastic, hormone modifier

■ **Indications** — Endometriosis, uterine fibroids

■ **Mechanism** — Inhibits the release of the gonadotropins by suppressing ovarian steroidogenesis

■ **Dosage with Qualifiers** — Endometriosis—3.75mg IM qmo
Uterine fibroids—3.75mg IM qmo
NOTE—administer iron and check the bone mineral density if treatment extends longer than 3mo
- **Contraindications**—hypersensitivity to drug or class, undiagnosed vaginal bleeding
- **Caution**—bone metastases, osteoporosis, psychiatric disorder, depression

■ **Maternal Considerations** — Gonadotropin-releasing agonists are important for the treatment of infertility and are often used with IVF. There are no adequate reports or well-controlled studies of **leuprolide** during pregnancy, nor is there an indication for its use. *Side effects* include angina, cardiac arrhythmias, MI, pulmonary emboli, spinal cord compression, paralysis, bone density loss, erythema multiforme, libido decrease, thyroid enlargement, anxiety, blurred vision, lethargy, memory disorder, mood swings, itching, nervousness, numbness, paresthesias, cough, pleural rub, pneumonia, dry skin, ecchymosis, hair loss, local skin reactions, pigmentation, skin lesions, pulmonary fibrosis, dysuria, incontinence, leukopenia, hemoptysis, pelvic fibrosis, hair growth, and hypoproteinemia.

■ **Fetal Considerations** — There are no adequate reports or well-controlled studies in human fetuses. It is unknown whether **leuprolide** crosses the human placenta. No malformations are reported in women inadvertently exposed to **leuprolide** during pregnancy. However, early exposure of a male fetus may lead to micropenis. Rodent studies reveal a dose-dependent increase in the incidence of major malformations and IUGR.

■ **Breastfeeding Safety** — There is no published experience in nursing women. It is unknown whether **leuprolide** enters human breast milk.

■ **References** — Tay CC. Hum Fertil 2002; 5:G35-7.
McMahon DR, Kramer SA, Husmann DA. J Urol 1995; 154:825-9.

■ **Summary** —
- **Pregnancy Category X**
- **Lactation Category U**
- **Leuprolide** is currently contraindicated during pregnancy.

- Barrier contraception is recommended if therapy is initiated for indications other than infertility.
- No malformations are described in women inadvertently exposed to **leuprolide.**

Levalbuterol (Xopenex)

- **Class** — *Adrenergic agonist, bronchodilator*

- **Indications** — Bronchospasm

- **Mechanism** — Stimulates β-2 adrenergic receptors

- **Dosage with Qualifiers** — Bronchospasm—0.63-1.25mg NEB q6-8h prn
  NOTE—avoid mixing with other nebulizers
  - **Contraindications**—hypersensitivity to drug or class, MAO inhibitor <14d
  - **Caution**—arrhythmias, coronary artery disease, hypertension, hypokalemia

- **Maternal Considerations** — **Levalbuterol** is at least as effective as other β-2 adrenergic agonists for the treatment or prevention of bronchospasm. There is no published experience with **levalbuterol** during pregnancy.
  Side effects include paradoxical bronchospasm, angioedema, cardiac arrest, arrhythmia, hypokalemia, palpitation, dizziness, tremor, nervousness, headache, chest pain, and dry mouth.

- **Fetal Considerations** — There are no adequate reports or well-controlled studies in human fetuses. It is unknown whether **levalbuterol** crosses the human placenta. Maternal systemic plasma levels are low after inhalation. Rodent studies are reassuring, revealing no evidence of teratogenicity or IUGR despite the use of doses higher than those used clinically. In contrast, other β-2 adrenergic agonists (e.g., **isoproterenol** and **albuterol**) have been associated with cleft palate and NTDs.

- **Breastfeeding Safety** — There is no published experience in nursing women. It is unknown whether **levalbuterol** enters human breast milk. However, considering the indication and dosing, occasional **levalbuterol** use is unlikely to pose a clinically significant risk to the breast-feeding neonate.

- **References** — Chowdhury BA. J Allergy Clin Immunol 2002; 110:324.
  Wendel PJ, Ramin SM, Barnett-Hamm C, et al. Am J Obstet Gynecol 1996; 175:150-4.

■ **Summary**
- **Pregnancy Category C**
- **Lactation Category S?**
- **Levalbuterol** is an effective for the control and prevention of bronchospasm.
- There are alternative agents for which there is more experience during pregnancy and lactation.

Levamisole (Ascaryl; Decas; Dewormis; Ergamisol; Immunol)

■ **Class** Antineoplastic, immunomodulator

■ **Indications** Colon cancer

■ **Mechanism** Unknown

■ **Dosage with Qualifiers** Colon cancer—50mg PO q8h ×3d beginning 7-30d after surgery; repeat medication q14d ×1y
- **Contraindications**—hypersensitivity to drug or class
- **Caution**—alcohol ingestion

■ **Maternal Considerations** **Levamisole** is an immunomodulator often used as adjuvant treatment for colon cancer. It is also used as an antirheumatic and anthelmintic drug. There is no published experience during pregnancy.
Side effects include agranulocytosis, leukopenia, thrombocytopenia, dermatitis, nausea, vomiting, diarrhea, fatigue, fever, rigors, arthralgia, dizziness, headache, paresthesias, somnolence, taste change, infection, hyperpigmentation, ataxia, tearing, forgetfulness, blurred vision, conjunctivitis, and hyperbilirubinemia.

■ **Fetal Considerations** There are no adequate reports or well-controlled studies in human fetuses. It is unknown whether **levamisole** crosses the human placenta. Rodent studies are reassuring, revealing no evidence of teratogenicity or IUGR despite the use of doses higher than those used clinically. Embryotoxicity was noted in some studies.

■ **Breastfeeding Safety** There is no published experience in nursing women. It is unknown whether **levamisole** enters human breast milk. **Levamisole** is excreted into cow's milk and reportedly stimulates production.

■ **References** da Costa-Macedo LM, Rey L. Rev Inst Med Trop Sao Paulo 1990; 32:351-4.
Block E, McDonald WA, Jackson BA. J Dairy Sci 1987; 70:1080-5.
Osterdahl BG, Nordlander I, Johnsson H. Food Addit Contam 1986; 3:161-5.

Levetiracetam (Keppra)

■ **Class** ························· Anticonvulsant

■ **Indications** ················· Partial-onset seizure disorder

■ **Mechanism** ················· Unknown

■ **Dosage with Qualifiers** ········ Seizure disorder—begin 500mg PO q12h, increasing 1g/d every 2w; max 3000mg/d
• **Contraindications**—hypersensitivity to drug or class
• **Caution**—renal dysfunction, abrupt withdrawal, depression

■ **Maternal Considerations** ········ **Levetiracetam** is unrelated to other antiepileptic drugs, and is used for the treatment for partial-onset seizures. There are no adequate reports or well-controlled studies of **levetiracetam** in pregnant women. It is generally well tolerated during pregnancy. Women who become or who are planning to become pregnant while taking **levetiracetam** should supplement their **folic acid** intake. Once pregnant, dosage readjustments may be necessary and should be based on clinical symptoms, and not exclusively on serum drug concentrations.
Side effects include nausea, vomiting, suicide attempts, psychosis, leukopenia, neutropenia, pancytopenia, somnolence, asthenia, dizziness, ataxia, agitation, anxiety, behavior changes, anemia, cough, rhinitis, and diplopia.

■ **Fetal Considerations** ········ There are no adequate reports or well-controlled studies in human fetuses. It is unknown whether **levetiracetam** crosses the human placenta. Rodent studies conducted using doses in excess of the recommended maximum human dose reveal embryotoxicity and an increased prevalence of skeletal malformations.

■ **Breastfeeding Safety** ········ There is no published experience in nursing women. It is unknown whether **levetiracetam** enters human breast milk.

■ **References** ················· French J. Epilepsia 2001; 42(Suppl 4):40-3.
Harden C. Epilepsia 2001; 42(Suppl 4):36-9.
Crawford P. CNS Drugs 2002; 16:263-72.
Faught E. Epilepsia 2001; 42(Suppl 4):19-23.

■ **Summary**
- **Pregnancy Category C**
- **Lactation Category U**
- **Levetiracetam** should be used during pregnancy and lactation only if the benefit justifies the potential risk.
- There are alternative agents for which there is more experience during pregnancy and lactation.
- Physicians are encouraged to register patients, before fetal outcome is known (e.g., ultrasound, results of amniocentesis), in the Antiepileptic Drug Pregnancy Registry—telephone 888-233-2334.

Levocabastine (Livostin)

■ **Class**

Antihistamine, allergy; ophthalmic

■ **Indications**

Allergic conjunctivitis

■ **Mechanism**

Selective H_1-receptor antagonist

■ **Dosage with Qualifiers**

Allergic conjunctivitis—1 gtt OS/OD qid; max 2w
- **Contraindications**—hypersensitivity to drug or class, contact lenses
- **Caution**—unknown

■ **Maternal Considerations**

There is no published experience with **levocabastine** during pregnancy. Approximately 1/3 of childbearing-age women have allergic rhinitis. Immunotherapy, **Cromolyn** and **beclomethasone** are first-line agents because of their safety record.
Side effects include dry mouth, dyspnea, somnolence, eye burning, eyelid edema, and rash.

■ **Fetal Considerations**

There are no adequate reports or well-controlled studies in human fetuses. Considering the dose and route, it is unlikely the maternal systemic concentration reaches a clinically relevant level. In rodents, **levocabastine** caused polydactyly at doses 16,500 times the maximum recommended human ocular dose; polydactyly, hydrocephaly, brachygnathia, and embryo and maternal toxicities occur at doses 66,000 times the maximum recommended ocular human dose.

■ **Breastfeeding Safety**

There is no published experience in nursing women. The manufacturer's reports suggest a trace amount is excreted. However, considering the dose and route, it is unlikely the breast-fed neonate would ingest clinically relevant amounts.

■ **References**

Mazzotta P, Loebstein R, Koren G. Drug Saf 1999; 20:361-75.

■ **Summary**

- **Pregnancy Category C**
- **Lactation Category S?**
- **Levocabastine** is an effective agent for the treatment of allergic conjunctivitis.
- **Levocabastine** should be used during pregnancy and lactation only if the benefit justifies the potential perinatal risk.

Levodopa (Dopar; Dopastral; L-Dopa; Laradopa; Larodopa; Levotrifar; Medidopa; Prolopa)

■ **Class** — *Antiparkinsonian, dopaminergic*

■ **Indications** — Parkinson's disease

■ **Mechanism** — Dopamine precursor

■ **Dosage with Qualifiers** — Parkinson's disease—0.5-1g PO qd; max 8g/d; therapy is individualized and changed gradually
- **Contraindications**—hypersensitivity to drug or class, glaucoma, MAO inhibitor <14d, undiagnosed skin lesion
- **Caution**—severe renal and hepatic disease, cardiovascular disease, pulmonary disease

■ **Maternal Considerations** — Parkinson's disease is characterized by neuronal degeneration in the corpora nigra. Evidence suggests the symptoms are related to depletion of striatal dopamine. Parkinson's disease manifests before age 40y in about 5% of patients. Limited experience suggests symptoms often worsen during pregnancy, and may not return to baseline post partum. **Levodopa** is the first-line agent. There are no adequate reports or well-controlled studies of **levodopa** in pregnant women. Several case reports describe successful outcomes without obvious adverse effect on the pregnancy. Early reports suggested a relationship between **levodopa** during pregnancy and fulminant hepatitis.
Side effects include anorexia, nausea, vomiting, hallucinations, abdominal pain, dry mouth, dysphagia, sialorrhea, ataxia, numbness, hand tremor, headache, dizziness, weakness and faintness, bruxism, confusion, insomnia, nightmares, agitation and anxiety, malaise, fatigue, euphoria, oculogyric crises, hiccups, edema, hair loss, hoarseness, dystonic reactions, and orthostatic hypotension.

■ **Fetal Considerations** — There are no adequate reports or well-controlled studies in human fetuses. **Levodopa** crosses the human placenta. And while some studies show that **levodopa** concentrates in the fetal brain and thus has the potential to affect fetal neuronal development, the majority of studies reveal no evidence of teratogenicity. Rodent studies are generally reassuring without evidence of teratogenicity, though IUGR occurs at high doses.

■ **Breastfeeding Safety** — There are no adequate reports or well-controlled studies in nursing women. **Levodopa** is excreted into human breast milk, but the kinetics remain to be elucidated. And while it suppresses prolactin release and thus, theoretically, may interfere with lactation, the suckling stimulus seems to override any inhibitory effect on prolactin release.

■ **References** — Routiot T, Lurel S, Denis E, Barbarino-Monnier P. J Gynecol Obstet Biol Reprod 2000; 29:454-7.
Shulman LM, Minagar A, Weiner WJ. Mov Disord 2000; 15:132-5.
Nomoto M, Kaseda S, Iwata S, et al. Mov Disord 1997; 12:261.
Merchant CA, Cohen G, Mytilineou C, et al. J Neural Transm Park Dis Dement Sect 1995; 9:239-42.
Deis RP, Kann G, Martinet J. Reprod Nutr Dev 1990; 30:605-10.
Thulin PC, Woodward WR, Carter JH, Nutt JG. Neurology 1998; 50:1920-1.

■ **Summary** —
• **Pregnancy Category C**
• **Lactation Category U**
• **Levodopa** should be used during pregnancy and lactation only if the benefit justifies the potential perinatal risk.

Levorphanol (Levo-Dromoran)

■ **Class** — Analgesic, narcotic

■ **Indications** — Pain

■ **Mechanism** — Binds to opiate receptors

■ **Dosage with Qualifiers** — Pain—2mg PO q6-8h, or 1-2 mg IV q3-6h
NOTE—**naloxone** should be administered immediately in the event of overdosage
• **Contraindications**—hypersensitivity to drug or class, depressed respiratory function, MI, hypotension
• **Caution**—hepatic or renal dysfunction, drug dependency, seizure disorder

■ **Maternal Considerations** — **Levorphanol** has properties similar to **morphine**, but is 4-6 times more potent. There is no published experience during pregnancy.

Side effects include nausea vomiting, respiratory distress, bronchospasm, diplopia, mood disturbance, pruritus, flushing, rash, constipation, biliary spasm, and dry mouth.

■ **Fetal Considerations**

There are no adequate reports or well-controlled studies in human fetuses. Its chemical structure suggests **levorphanol** will rapidly cross the placenta. Adolescent rodents exposed prenatally to **morphine** are tolerant to its analgesic effect. This tolerance also occurs when the rats are exposed to **levorphanol**, a morphine congener, but not by its analgesically inactive isomer, dextromethorphan.

■ **Breastfeeding Safety**

There is no published experience in nursing women. It is unknown whether **levorphanol** enters human breast milk.

■ **References**

O'Callaghan JP, Holtzman SG. J Pharmacol Exp Ther 1977; 200:255-62.

■ **Summary**

- **Pregnancy Category C**
- **Lactation Category U**
- **Levorphanol** should be used during pregnancy and lactation only if the benefit justifies the potential risk.
- There are alternative agents for which there is more experience during pregnancy and lactation.

Levofloxacin (Cravit; Lesacin; Levaquin; Quixin)

■ **Class**

Antibiotic, quinolone

■ **Indications**

Bacterial infections (<u>aerobic gram-positive</u>: *Enterococcus faecalis, Staphylococcus aureus* [methicillin-susceptible], *Staphylococcus saprophyticus, Streptococcus pneumoniae, Streptococcus pyogenes*; <u>aerobic gram-negative</u>: *Enterobacter cloacae, Escherichia coli, Haemophilus influenzae, Haemophilus parainfluenzae, Klebsiella pneumoniae, Legionella pneumophila, Moraxella catarrhalis, Proteus mirabilis, Pseudomonas aeruginosa*; <u>other microorganisms</u>: *Chlamydia pneumoniae, Mycoplasma pneumoniae*)

■ **Mechanism**

Inhibits bacterial topoisomerase IV and DNA gyrase, required for DNA replication, transcription, repair, and recombination

■ **Dosage with Qualifiers**

<u>Bacterial infections</u>—250-500mg PO/IV qd
- **Contraindications**—hypersensitivity to drug or class, prolongation of the QT interval, concomitant usage of antiarrhythmic drugs
- **Caution**—hepatic or renal dysfunction (CrCl <50ml/min), seizure disorder, dehydration, hypokalemia, sun exposure, diabetes mellitus, bradycardia, cardiomyopathy, anemia

- ■ **Maternal Considerations** — **Levofloxacin** is indicated for the treatment of mild, moderate, and severe infections caused by a wide variety of susceptible microorganisms. Compared to other quinolones, **levofloxacin** has fewer adverse GI or CNS events and is minimally phototoxic. Recent studies report an increase sensitivity of *Chlamydia trachomatis* to **quinolone** medication. Vaginal candidiasis is more frequently associated with quinolone use than with other antibiotics. There are no adequate reports or well-controlled studies of **levofloxacin** in pregnant women. *Side effects* include nausea, vomiting, vaginitis, phototoxicity, pseudomembranous colitis, seizures, psychosis, arthropathy, restlessness, lightheadedness, anxiety, agitation, confusion, elevated LFTs, dyspepsia, and taste perversion.

- ■ **Fetal Considerations** — There are no adequate reports or well-controlled studies in human fetuses. It is unknown whether **levofloxacin** crosses the human placenta. Animal studies (mice, dogs, rabbits) reveal that several quinolones are associated with a juvenile arthropathy, and it is this toxicity that has lead to its restricted use in pregnant women. However, not all quinolones have the same potency on cartilage growth. Further, the use of quinolones during the 1st trimester of human pregnancy has not been associated with an increased risk of malformations or musculoskeletal conditions. Rodent studies with **levofloxacin** are reassuring, revealing no evidence of teratogenicity despite the use of doses higher than those used clinically. IUGR was noted.

- ■ **Breastfeeding Safety** — There is no published experience in nursing women. Based on studies of **ofloxacin**, it is likely **levofloxacin** is excreted in human milk.

- ■ **References** — Centers for Disease Control and Prevention. JAMA 2001; 286:2396-7.
Connell W, Miller A. Drug Saf 1999; 21:311-23.
Lipsky BA, Baker CA. Clin Infect Dis 1999; 28:352-64.
Loebstein R, Addis A, Ho E, et al. Antimicrob Agents Chemother 1998; 42:1336-9.
McDuffie RS Jr, Eskens JL, Gibbs RS. Obstet Gynecol 1998; 92:28-30.
Wilton LV, Pearce GL, Mann RD. Br J Clin Pharmacol 1996; 41:277-84.
Weber JT, Johnson RE. Clin Infect Dis 1995; 20(Suppl 1):S66-71.
Koul PA, Wani JI, Wahid A. Lancet 1995; 346:307-8.
Berkovitch M, Pastuszak A, Gazarian M, et al. Obstet Gynecol 1994; 84:535-8.
Siefert HM, Maruhn D, Maul W, et al. Arzneimittelforschung 1986; 36:1496-502.
Shakibaei M, Baumann-Wilschke I, Rucker M, Stahlmann R. Arch Toxicol 2002; 75:725-33.

■ **Summary**

- **Pregnancy Category C**
- **Lactation Category U**
- **Levofloxacin** should be used during pregnancy and lactation only if the benefit justifies the potential perinatal risk.
- Although quinolones appear safe during the 1st trimester, their use during the 2nd and 3rd trimesters should await further study because of the potential for juvenile arthropathy.
- There are alternative agents for which there is more experience during pregnancy and lactation.

Levothyroxine (L-Thyroxine; Levo-T; Levothroid; Levoxyl; Novothyrox; Synthroid; Synthrox; Throxinique; Thyradin; Thyroxine)

■ **Class** — *Hormone, thyroid*

■ **Indications** — Hypothyroidism, myxedema coma

■ **Mechanism** — Unknown (increases metabolism)

■ **Dosage with Qualifiers** — Hypothyroidism—50-200mcg PO qd; usual dose 75-125mcg/d
NOTE—levels should be checked q2-4w until stable, then yearly
Myxedema coma—300-500mcg IV
- **Contraindications**—hypersensitivity to drug or class, thyrotoxicosis, adrenal insufficiency
- **Caution**—hypertension, cardiovascular disease

■ **Maternal Considerations** — Hypothyroidism affects 4-10% of women. Many of the signs and symptoms of typical hypothyroidism are a normal part of pregnancy. The diagnosis of hypothyroidism (and hyperthyroidism) should be always confirmed by laboratory tests and not by symptoms. **Levothyroxine** is the standard for the treatment of hypothyroidism during pregnancy. Outside pregnancy, the adequacy of replacement is determined by TSH measurement. During pregnancy, the measurement of free T_4 may be better, since some commercial assays cross-react with placenta-derived compounds. Further, the TSH of women chronically hyper- or hypothyroid may respond much more slowly to replacement than the free T_4 level.
Side effects include weight loss, increased appetite, palpitations, nervousness, diarrhea, arrhythmias, CHF, hypertension, angina, abdominal cramps, sweating, tachycardia, tremors, insomnia, heat intolerance, fever, menstrual irregularities, and alopecia.

■ **Fetal Considerations** ⋯⋯⋯⋯ Thyroid hormones are essential for normal brain development. Both maternal and fetal thyroid hormones contribute. Though maternal thyroid hormone transport across the placenta is low, its importance is illustrated by the fact that most athyrotic newborns have no sign of hypothyroidism, and the degree of maternal hypothyroidism early and mid gestation correlates with the severity of fetal neural damage. The children of women with subclinical hypothyroidism in the first half of pregnancy have lower mean Mental Developmental Index scores during the first year of life. Fetal hypothyroidism can be diagnosed by cordocentesis. Hypothyroid fetuses are treated by weekly intra-amniotic injections of **levothyroxine**. The adequacy of therapy is determined by periodic measurement of free T_4, free T_3 and TSH compared to gestational age appropriate norms. Ultrasonographic evaluation of the fetus by biparietal diameter, cranial and abdominal circumference, and both humerus and femur length is recommended. Craniosynostosis is associated with iatrogenic hyperthyroidism in infants receiving thyroid hormone replacement therapy.

■ **Breastfeeding Safety** ⋯⋯⋯ There are no adequate reports or well-controlled studies in nursing women. **Levothyroxine** is excreted at low concentrations into human breast milk. The neonatal effect is controversial. Some reports suggest that the levels in breast milk are sufficient to treat neonatal hypothyroidism. It is unknown whether maternal supplementation increases excretion.

■ **References** ⋯⋯⋯⋯⋯⋯⋯⋯ Redmond GP. Int J Fertil Womens Med 2002; 47:123-7.
Radetti G, Zavallone A, Gentili L, et al. Minerva Pediatr 2002; 54:383-400.
Abalovich M, Gutierrez S, Alcaraz G, et al. Thyroid 2002; 12:63-8.
Glinoer D. Thyroid 2001; 11:471-81.
Gruner C, Kollert A, Wildt L, et al. Fetal Diagn Ther 2001; 16:47-51.
Smit BJ, Kok JH, Vulsma T, et al. Acta Paediatr 2000; 89:291-5.
Rotondi M, Caccavale C, Di Serio C, et al. Thyroid 1999; 9:1037-40.
van Wassenaer AG, Stulp MR, Valianpour F, et al. Clin Endocrinol (Oxf) 2002; 56:621-7.
Varma SK, Collins M, Row A, et al. J Pediatr 1978; 93:803-6.
Abbassi V, Steinour TA. J Pediatr 1980; 97:259-61.
Letarte J, Guyda H, Dussault JH, Glorieux J. Pediatrics 1980; 65:703-5.

■ **Summary** ⋯⋯⋯⋯⋯⋯⋯⋯⋯
- **Pregnancy Category A**
- **Lactation Category S**
- **Levothyroxine** is the standard treatment of hypothyroidism during pregnancy.
- Abnormalities of maternal and fetal thyroid function affect long-term neonatal neurologic development.
- Screening for thyroid deficiency during pregnancy may be warranted.

Lidocaine (Alphacaine; Leostesin; Rucaina; Xylocaina; Xylocaine)

■ **Class** — Antiarrhythmic, *class IB, anesthetics, topical/local anesthetic*

■ **Indications** — Arrhythmia (ventricular), local anesthesia, postherpetic neuralgia

■ **Mechanism** — Depress action potential phase 0, stabilizes membranes

■ **Dosage with Qualifiers** — Ventricular arrhythmia—begin 1-1.5mg/kg IV; may repeat bolus in 5min, then begin infusion 1-4mg/min IV; max 300mg ×1h
Local anesthesia—infiltrate IM/SC; max 300mg
Postherpetic neuralgia—apply topically q12h
NOTE—available in parenteral (with and without preservatives), ointment, patch, oral spray and gel formats
- **Contraindications**—hypersensitivity to drug or class, Wolff-Parkinson-White syndrome, sinoatrial or atrioventricular block, Stokes-Adams syndrome
- **Caution**—hepatic or renal dysfunction, bradycardia, CHF, hypertension

■ **Maternal Considerations** — **Lidocaine** has been used for decades for paracervical/pudendal blocks and perineal infiltration prior to episiotomy. Allergies are rare. It is often used for spinal anesthesia (saddle block) without epinephrine or epidural anesthesia with **epinephrine**. The topical application of 2% **lidocaine gel** decreases perineal pain in the immediate puerperium and in women with genital herpes. **Lidocaine** is a second option for the treatment of ventricular arrhythmias after failed electrical cardioversion.
Side effects include tinnitus, blurred vision, lightheadedness, impaired swallowing, seizures, respiratory arrest, arrhythmia, heart block, bradycardia, asthma, coma, tremor, confusion, hypotension, hallucinations, agitation, nausea, vomiting, and cardiovascular collapse.

■ **Fetal Considerations** — **Lidocaine** rapidly crosses the human placenta, and its elimination half-life after birth approximates 3h. The results of neurobehavioral exams of newborns whose mothers received continuous epidural analgesia are conflicting. Some suggest a decrease in muscle strength and tone, while others find no effect. **Lidocaine** can potentially produce neonatal CNS depression and seizures. There are no reports of associated malformations. Rodent studies are reassuring, revealing no evidence of teratogenicity or IUGR despite the use of doses higher than those used clinically.

■ **Breastfeeding Safety** ⋯⋯⋯⋯⋯ **Lidocaine** is excreted into breast milk, but the maternal systemic levels are low. Considering the dose and route, it is unlikely the breast-fed neonate would ingest clinically relevant amounts.

■ **References** ⋯⋯⋯⋯⋯⋯⋯⋯⋯⋯⋯⋯⋯ Levy BT, Bergus GR, Hartz A, et al. J Fam Pract 1999; 48:778-84.
Connelly NR, Parker RK, Lucas T, et al. Anesth Analg 2001; 93:1001-5.
Lam DT, Ngan Kee WD, Khaw KS. Anaesthesia 2001; 56:790-4.
Trappe HJ, Pfitzner P. Z Kardiol 2001; 90(Suppl 4):36-44.
Puente NW, Josephy PD. J Anal Toxicol 2001; 25:711-5.
Browne IM, Birnbach DJ. Am J Obstet Gynecol 2001; 185:1253-4.
Ng EH, Tang OS, Chui DK, Ho PC. Hum Reprod 2000; 15:2148-51.
Connelly NR, Parker RK, Vallurupalli V, et al. Anesth Analg 2000; 91:374-8.
Joglar JA, Page RL. Drug Saf 1999; 20:85-94.
Lawrie D. Aust NZ J Obstet Gynaecol 1997; 37:485-6.
Ala-Kokko TI, Pienimaki P, Herva R, et al. Pharmacol Toxicol 1995; 77:142-8.
Ortega D, Viviand X, Lorec AM, et al. Acta Anaesthesiol Scand 1999; 43:394-7.
Wiebe ER, Rawling M. Int J Gynaecol Obstet 1995; 50:41-6.
Banzai M, Sato S, Tezuka N, et al. Can J Anaesth 1995; 42:338-40.
Collins MK, Porter KB, Brook E, et al. Obstet Gynecol 1994; 84:335-7.
Guay J, Gaudreault P, Boulanger A, et al. Acta Anaesthesiol Scand 1992; 36:722-7.
Brown WU, Bell GC, Lurie AO, et al. Anesthesiology 1975; 42:698-707.
Scanlon JW, Brown WU Jr, Weiss JB, Alper MH. Anesthesiology 1974; 40:121-8.
Kuhnert BR, Philipson EH, Pimental R, et al. Anesth Analg 1986; 65:139-44.
Philipson EH, Kuhnert BR, Syracuse CD. Am J Obstet Gynecol 1984; 149:403-7.

■ **Summary** ⋯⋯⋯⋯⋯⋯⋯⋯⋯⋯⋯⋯⋯⋯⋯
- **Pregnancy Category B**
- **Lactation Category S**
- **Lidocaine** is considered safe and effective during pregnancy and lactation when used as directed.

Lincomycin (L-Mycin; Lincocin; Lincoject; Lincorex)

■ **Class** — Antibiotic, lincosamide

■ **Indications** — Bacterial infections (aerobic gram-positive cocci: *Streptococcus pyogenes*, viridans group streptococci; aerobic gram-positive bacilli: *Corynebacterium diphtheria*; anaerobic gram-positive bacteria: *Propionibacterium acnes*, *Clostridium tetani*, *Clostridium perfringens*)

■ **Mechanism** — Inhibits protein synthesis

■ **Dosage with Qualifiers** — Bacterial infection—600-1000mg q8-12h
- **Contraindications**—hypersensitivity to drug or class, pseudomembranous colitis
- **Caution**—hepatic or renal dysfunction, asthma, GI disease

■ **Maternal Considerations** — There are 2 main antibiotics in the lincosamide family— **lincomycin** and **clindamycin**. Because **lincomycin** has been associated with severe colitis that may end fatally, it should be reserved for serious infections where less toxic antimicrobial agents are ineffective. There are no adequate reports or well-controlled studies of **lincomycin** in pregnant women.
Side effects include pseudomembranous colitis, diarrhea, colitis, vaginitis, glossitis, stomatitis, nausea, vomiting, neutropenia, leukopenia, agranulocytosis, tinnitus, thrombocytopenia, aplastic anemia, angioneurotic edema, serum sickness, urticaria, rash, azotemia, oliguria, and vertigo.

■ **Fetal Considerations** — There are no adequate reports or well-controlled studies in human fetuses. It is unknown whether **lincomycin** crosses the human placenta. Rodent teratogen studies have not been performed.

■ **Breastfeeding Safety** — There are no adequate reports or well-controlled studies in nursing women. **Lincomycin** is excreted into human breast milk achieving concentrations of 0.5-2.4µg/ml. Even if a term breast-fed newborn had 100% absorption, the daily dose would be less than 2mg.

■ **References** — Czeizel AE, Rockenbauer M, Sorensen HT, Olsen J. Scand J Infect Dis 2000; 32:579-80.
Pechere JC. Pathol Biol (Paris) 1986; 34:119-28.

■ **Summary** —
- **Pregnancy Category C**
- **Lactation Category S**
- **Lincomycin** should be used during pregnancy and lactation only if the benefit justifies the potential perinatal risk.
- There are alternative agents for which there is more experience during pregnancy and lactation.

Lindane (Aphtiria; Hexicid; Kwell; Lorexane; Scabex)

■ **Class** ⋯⋯⋯⋯⋯⋯⋯⋯⋯⋯⋯⋯⋯⋯ Antiinfective, scabicides/pediculicide

■ **Indications** ⋯⋯⋯⋯⋯⋯⋯⋯⋯⋯⋯ Scabies, pediculosis

■ **Mechanism** ⋯⋯⋯⋯⋯⋯⋯⋯⋯⋯⋯ Ectoparasiticide and ovicide against *Sarcoptes scabiei* (scabies)

■ **Dosage with Qualifiers** ⋯⋯⋯⋯ Scabies—apply from neck to the feet and bathe after 8-12h; repeat treatment 1w; max 30ml per application
Pediculosis—apply 20-30ml shampoo to dry hair, wait 5min and rinse; comb hair and remove nits; may repeat in 1w
  - **Contraindications**—hypersensitivity to drug or class, inflamed skin, seizure disorder, pregnancy, breastfeeding
  - **Caution**—genitalia contact

■ **Maternal Considerations** ⋯⋯ **Lindane** is a popular over-the-counter treatment for scabies. The number of suspected adverse reactions is small considering over 10 million ounces of **1% lindane** are sold yearly. Almost all suspected adverse drug reactions involve misuse. There are no adequate reports or well-controlled studies of **lindane** in pregnant women. Rodent studies describe a reduction in uterine gap junction synthesis and, as a result, incoordination of uterine contractions.
Side effects include seizures, neurotoxicity, dizziness, eczema, dermatitis, anxiety, insomnia, and myelosuppression.

■ **Fetal Considerations** ⋯⋯⋯⋯⋯ There are no adequate reports or well-controlled studies in human fetuses. It is unknown whether **lindane** crosses the human placenta. **Lindane** is a known neurotoxin. Fortunately, the maternal systemic concentrations after topical application (cream or shampoo) are low. An increased prevalence of IUGR has been suggested. One report describes a suicide attempt with oral ingestion at 16w followed immediately by fetal death and vaginal bleeding. Transfer across the rabbit placenta occurs, but is inefficient. Rodent studies are reassuring, revealing no evidence of teratogenicity or IUGR despite the use of doses higher than those used clinically. **Lindane** transiently reduces fetal serum thyroxine in sheep.

■ **Breastfeeding Safety** ⋯⋯⋯⋯⋯ There are no adequate reports or well-controlled studies in nursing women. **Lindane** is excreted into human milk at low concentrations (0-113ppb); it is unlikely the neonate would ingest a clinically relevant amount. However, if this is a concern, the neonate may be bottle fed for 2d.

■ **References** ⋯⋯⋯⋯⋯⋯⋯⋯⋯⋯⋯ Folster-Holst R, Rufli T, Christophers E. Hautarzt 2000; 51:7-13.
Beard AP, Rawlings NC. J Toxicol Environ Health A 1999; 58:509-30.

Criswell KA, Loch-Caruso R. Reprod Toxicol 1999; 13:481-90.

Karmaus W, Wolf N. Environ Health Perspect 1995; 103:1120-5.

Konje JC, Otolorin EO, Sotunmbi PT, Ladipo OA. J Reprod Med 1992; 37:992-4.

Rasmussen JE. J Am Acad Dermatol 1981; 5:507-16.

Pompa G, Fadini L, Di Lauro F, Caloni F. Pharmacol Toxicol 1994; 74:28-34.

■ **Summary**

- **Pregnancy Category B**
- **Lactation Category S?**
- 1% **lindane** continues as the agent of choice for nearly all patients with scabies and lice during pregnancy and lactation when used as directed.

Linezolid (Zyvox)

■ **Class**

Antibiotic, oxalodinone

■ **Indications**

Bacterial infections (gram-positive bacteria: Enterococcus fecalis and E. faecium [vancomycin-resistant], Staphylococcus aureus, Streptococcus agalactiae, Streptococcus pneumoniae, Streptococcus pyogenes, viridans group streptococci; gram-negative bacteria: Pasteurella multocida and anaerobic bacteria)

■ **Mechanism**

Inhibits bacterial protein synthesis

■ **Dosage with Qualifiers**

Vancomycin-resistant enterococcal infections—600mg IV/PO q12h ×10-28d
Pneumonia—600mg IV/PO q12 ×10-28d
Skin infection—400mg PO q12 ×10-14d
NOTE—avoid tyramine-containing foods (keep tyramine content <100mg/meal); monitor the CBC count weekly

- **Contraindications**—hypersensitivity to drug or class
- **Caution**—hypertension, pheochromocytoma, carcinoid syndrome, thyroid disease, MAO inhibitors, thrombocytopenia, phenylketonuria, severe hepatic disease, myelosuppression

■ **Maternal Considerations**

Linezolid is a member of a new class of synthetic antibiotics, the oxazolidinones. It is also a nonselective MAO inhibitor. This family of drugs is useful in the treatment of aerobic gram-positive and -negative bacteria infections. There is no published experience during pregnancy with **linezolid**.

Side effects include thrombocytopenia, pseudomembranous colitis, leukopenia, pancytopenia, anemia, diarrhea, headache, nausea, vomiting, dyspepsia, localized abdominal pain, pruritus, tongue discoloration, and rash.

513

- **Fetal Considerations** ———— There are no adequate reports or well-controlled studies in human fetuses. It is unknown whether **linezolid** crosses the human placenta. Rodent studies are reassuring, revealing no evidence of teratogenicity or IUGR despite the use of doses higher than those used clinically. Embryotoxicity is noted only at doses causing maternal toxicity.

- **Breastfeeding Safety** ———— There is no published experience in nursing women. It is unknown whether **linezolid** enters human breast milk. It is excreted into rat milk achieving an M:P ratio near unity.

- **References** ———— Chin KG, Mactal-Haaf C, McPherson CE. J Hum Lact 2000; 16:351-8.

- **Summary** ————
  - **Pregnancy Category C**
  - **Lactation Category U**
  - **Linezolid** should be used during pregnancy and lactation only if the benefit justifies the potential perinatal risk.
  - There are alternative agents for which there is more experience during pregnancy and lactation.

Liothyronine (Cytomel; Triostat)

- **Class** ———— *Hormone, thyroid*

- **Indications** ———— Myxedema coma

- **Mechanism** ———— Unknown (increases metabolism)

- **Dosage with Qualifiers** ———— Myxedema coma—25-50mcg IV ×1; then 25mcg/d PO, increase 12.5-25mcg q1-2w; usual dose 25-75mcg/d
  - **Contraindications**—hypersensitivity to drug or class, MI, thyrotoxicosis, adrenal insufficiency
  - **Caution**—angina, hypertension, diabetes mellitus, renal failure

- **Maternal Considerations** ———— **Liothyronine** is synthetic T$_3$. Myxedema coma is a potentially lethal manifestation of hypothyroidism. Patients with suspected myxedema coma should be immediately admitted to an ICU for aggressive pulmonary and cardiovascular support. Most authorities recommend treatment with IV **levothyroxine** rather than IV **liothyronine**. **Hydrocortisone** is also administered until coexisting adrenal insufficiency is excluded. Advanced age, cardiac complications, and high-dose of thyroid hormone replacement (>500mcg/d) are associated with a fatal outcome within 1mo of treatment. **Amiodarone**-induced hypothyroidism may also be life threatening, and thyroid function should be tested before and during **amiodarone** therapy. There are no adequate reports or well-controlled studies of **liothyronine** in pregnant women. There are no reports of myxedema coma during pregnancy. *Side effects* include headache, irritability, nervousness, sweating, tachycardia, increased bowel motility, menstrual irregularities, shock, insomnia, tremor, arrhythmia, weight loss, heat intolerance, and diaphoresis.

■ **Fetal Considerations**
There are no adequate reports or well-controlled studies in human fetuses. Transfer of natural T_3 across the human placenta is very low.

■ **Breastfeeding Safety**
There is no published experience in nursing women. It is unknown whether **liothyronine** enters human breast milk. Several studies conclude the amount of thyroid hormone present in human milk is too low to clinically affect the neonate. It is unknown whether supplementation increases the level.

■ **References**
van Wassenaer AG, Stulp MR, Valianpour F, et al. Clin Endocrinol (Oxf) 2002; 56:621-7.
Wall CR. Am Fam Physician 2000; 62:2485-90.
Yamamoto T, Fukuyama J, Fujiyoshi A. Thyroid 1999; 9:1167-74.
Mazonson PD, Williams ML, Cantley LK, et al. Am J Med 1984; 77:751-4.
Pereira VG, Haron ES, Lima-Neto N, Medeiros-Neto GA. J Endocrinol Invest 1982; 5:331-4.

■ **Summary**
- **Pregnancy Category A**
- **Lactation Category U**
- **Liothyronine** should be used during pregnancy and lactation only if the benefit justifies the potential perinatal risk.

Liotrix (Euthroid; Thyrolar)

■ **Class**
Hormone, thyroid

■ **Indications**
Hypothyroidism

■ **Mechanism**
Unknown (increases metabolism)

■ **Dosage with Qualifiers**
Hypothyroidism—begin 50mcg PO qd, increase with 25mcg every 2-3w until replacement adequate
- **Contraindications**—hypersensitivity to drug or class, MI, thyrotoxicosis, adrenal insufficiency
- **Caution**—angina, hypertension, diabetes mellitus, renal failure

- **Maternal Considerations** .... **Liotrix** is synthetic microcrystalline **levothyroxine** (T_4) and synthetic microcrystalline liothyronine (T_3) combined in a 4:1 ratio. There are no adequate reports or well-controlled studies of **liotrix** in pregnant women. See **levothyroxine, liothyronine.**
  Side effects include headache, irritability, nervousness, sweating, tachycardia, increased bowel motility, menstrual irregularities, shock, insomnia, tremor, arrhythmia, weight loss, heat intolerance, and diaphoresis.

- **Fetal Considerations** .... There are no adequate reports or well-controlled studies in human fetuses. See **levothyroxine, liothyronine.**

- **Breastfeeding Safety** .... There are no adequate reports or well-controlled studies in nursing women. It is unknown whether **liotrix** enters human breast milk. See **levothyroxine, liothyronine.**

- **References** .... See **levothyroxine**, **liothyronine**.

- **Summary** ....
  - **Pregnancy Category A**
  - **Lactation Category S**
  - **Liotrix** should be used during pregnancy and lactation only if the benefit justifies the potential risk.

Lisinopril (Prinivil; Zestril)

- **Class** .... Antihypertensive, ACE-1, A2R-*antagonist*

- **Indications** .... Hypertension, congestive heart failure, myocardial infarct

- **Mechanism** .... Angiotensin converting enzyme inhibitor

- **Dosage with Qualifiers** .... Hypertension—10-40mg PO qd
  Congestive heart failure—5-20mg PO qd; max 40mg/d
  Myocardial infarct—5-10mg PO qd ×6w
  - **Contraindications**—hypersensitivity to drug or class, history of angioedema, pregnancy
  - **Caution**—renal artery stenosis, hepatic or renal dysfunction, hyponatremia, CHF, collagen vascular disease

- **Maternal Considerations** .... There are no adequate reports or well-controlled studies in pregnant women. In general, inhibitors of the renin angiotensin system are contraindicated during pregnancy. The lowest dose effective should be used when **lisinopril** is required during pregnancy for BP control.
  Side effects include fetal and neonatal morbidity and death, hypovolemia, asthenia, fever, paresthesias, vertigo,

dyspepsia, gastroenteritis, tachycardia, palpitation, leukopenia, hepatotoxicity, neutropenia, hyperkalemia, agranulocytosis, edema, diarrhea, chest pain, cough, elevated LFTs, pruritus, and rash.

■ **Fetal Considerations** ···············

There are no adequate reports or well-controlled studies in human fetuses. **Lisinopril** crosses the human placenta. No adverse fetal effects are reported after 1st trimester exposure. Later exposure is associated with cranial hypoplasia, anuria, reversible or irreversible renal failure, death, oligohydramnios, prematurity, IUGR, and patent ductus arteriosus. The mechanism of renal dysfunction is likely related to fetal hypotension and prolonged decreased glomerular filtration. If oligohydramnios is detected, **lisinopril** should be discontinued unless lifesaving for the mother. Antenatal surveillance should be initiated (e.g., BPP) if the fetus is potentially viable. Oligohydramnios may not appear until after the fetus has irreversible injury. Neonates exposed *in utero* to ACE inhibitors should be observed closely for hypotension, oliguria, and hyperkalemia. If oliguria occurs despite adequate pressure and renal perfusion, exchange transfusion or peritoneal dialysis may be required.

■ **Breastfeeding Safety** ···············

There is no published experience in nursing women. It is unknown whether **lisinopril** enters human breast milk. Other ACE inhibitors such as **captopril** are excreted in the milk at low concentrations.

■ **References** ···············

Tomlinson AJ, Campbell J, Walker JJ, Morgan C. Ann Pharmacother 2000; 34:180-2.
Bhatt-Mehta V, Deluga KS. Pharmacotherapy 1993; 13:515-8.
Filler G, Wong H, Condello AS, et al. Arch Dis Child Fetal Neonatal Ed 2003; 88:F154-6.
Parish RC, Miller LJ. Drug Saf 1992; 7:14-31.
Noble TA, Murray KM. Clin Pharm 1988; 7:659-69.

■ **Summary** ···············

- **Pregnancy Category C (1st trimester), D (2nd and 3rd trimesters)**
- **Lactation Category U**
- ACE inhibitors are well established in the treatment of arterial hypertension, heart failure and diabetic and/or hypertensive nephropathy with albuminuria.
- **Lisinopril** and other ACE inhibitors are to be avoided during pregnancy if possible.
- When mother's disease requires treatment with **lisinopril,** the lowest dose should be used followed by close monitoring of the fetus.

Lithium carbonate/citrate (Calith; Eskalith; Eskalith CR; Hypnorex; Hyponrex; Lilipin; Lilitin; Lithane; Litheum; Lithobid; Lithocarb; Lithonate; Lithotabs; Manialit; Phasal)

■ **Class** .... *Antipsychotic*

■ **Indications** .... Bipolar disorder, acute mania, schizoaffective disorder, neutropenia (chemotherapy)

■ **Mechanism** .... Unknown; alters Na⁺ transport at the neuronal level

■ **Dosage with Qualifiers** .... Bipolar disorder—900-1200mg/d PO; max 1800mg qd
Acute mania—600mg PO tid
Schizoaffective disorder—300mg PO tid/qid
Neutropenia (chemotherapy)—300-1000mg PO qd (slow release: 600-900mg PO bid)
NOTE—serum lithium levels should not exceed 2.0mEq/L
- **Contraindications**—hypersensitivity to drug or class, inability to monitor **lithium** level, pregnancy
- **Caution**—hepatic or renal dysfunction, hypovolemia, thyroid disorder, and coronary artery disorder

■ **Maternal Considerations** .... **Lithium** is used for the treatment of psychiatric disorders. It is typically inadequate for the rapid control of acute mania; antipsychotics, **divalproex**, or sedatives are commonly used, with or without **lithium.** The usefulness of **lithium** lies in the long-term prevention of recurrent mania and bipolar depression, and in reducing risk of suicidal behavior. Pregnancy and especially the puerperium are times high risk for recurrence of bipolar disease. Recommendations during pregnancy include discontinuing therapy for at least the 1st trimester, switching to an agent with a higher safety profile (e.g., tricyclics), using smaller doses of **lithium**, and avoiding sodium restriction or diuretics while under treatment. The dose used should be titered to maintain a serum level between 0.5-1.2mEq/L. Toxicity develops between 1.5-2.0 mEq/L. Ideally, the drug should be tapered gradually over a month. **Lithium** levels should be monitored weekly after 35w gestation, and therapy either discontinued or decreased by 1/4 2-3d before delivery.
Side effects include tremor, muscle fasciculations, twitching, clonic movements, hypertonicity, ataxia, choreo-athetotic movements, hyperactive deep tendon reflex, blackout spells, epileptiform seizures, acute distonia, cogwheel rigidity, slurred speech, dizziness, vertigo, downbeat nystagmus, incontinence of urine or feces, somnolence, psychomotor retardation, restlessness, confusion, stupor, coma, tongue movements, tics, tinnitus, hallucinations, poor memory, slowed intellectual functioning, startled response, polyuria, diarrhea, vomiting, gastritis, salivary gland swelling, abdominal pain, excessive salivation, flatulence, drowsiness, arrhythmia, hypotension,

circulatory collapse, bradycardia, glycosuria, albuminuria, oliguria, nephrogenic diabetes insipidus, alopecia, anesthesia of skin, acne, chronic folliculitis, xerosis cutis, psoriasis, goiter, myxedema, ECG changes, and hyperparathyroidism.

■ Fetal Considerations

Lithium crosses the placenta and may be a weak human teratogen. Several studies note an increased prevalence of Ebstein's anomaly, though this was not confirmed in a prospective, multicenter study. A targeted ultrasound performed by a fetal medicine expert is suggested. Other neonatal complications often attributed to **lithium** include poor respiratory effort and cyanosis, rhythm disturbances, nephrogenic diabetes insipidus, thyroid dysfunction and goiter, hypoglycemia, hypotonia and lethargy, polyhydramnios, hyperbilirubinemia, and large-for-gestational-age infant. As a result, the delivery of mother taking **lithium** should be considered a high-risk delivery. The results of long-term follow-up studies are reassuring. **Lithium** is associated with cleft palate in mice.

■ Breastfeeding Safety

Lithium is excreted into human milk and can be measured in the nursing newborn. There is no agreement whether nursing mothers should continue **lithium** while breastfeeding. There is a lack of prospective studies confounded by polypharmacy. The neonatal clearance rate is slower than in the adult; thus, the level of circulating drug might be much higher than expected. If **lithium** use must be continued during breastfeeding, it should be measured in the neonatal blood if any adverse effects are noted.

■ References

Pinelli JM, Symington AJ, Cunningham KA, Paes BA. Am J Obstet Gynecol 2002; 187:245-9.
Schou M. Bipolar Disord 1999; 1:5-10.
Grof P, Robbins W, Alda M, et al. Affect Disord 2000; 61:31-9.
Chaudron LH, Jefferson JW. J Clin Psychiatry 2000; 61:79-90.
Teixeira NA, Lopes RC, Secoli SR. Braz J Med Biol Res 1995; 28:230-9.
Maher JE, Colvin EV, Samdarshi TE, et al. Am J Perinatol 1994; 11:334-6.
Kellner CH, Beale MD, Pritchett JT. JAMA 1994; 271:1828-9.
Cohen LS, Friedman JM, Jefferson JW, et al. JAMA 1994; 271:146-50.
Troyer WA, Pereira GR, Lannon RA, et al. J Perinatol 1993; 13:123-7.
Vander Zanden JA. J Hum Lact 1991; 7:195.
Schou M. J Clin Psychiatry 1990; 51:410-3.
Ang MS, Thorp JA, Parisi VM. Obstet Gynecol 1990; 76:517-9.
Jacobson SJ, Jones K, Johnson K, et al. Lancet 1992; 339:530-3.
Stothers JK, Wilson DW, Royston N. Br Med J 1973; 3:233-4.
Silverman JA, Winters RW, Strande C. Am J Obstet Gynecol 1971; 109:934-6.

■ **Summary**

- **Pregnancy Category D**
- **Lactation Category S?**
- **Lithium** is the preferred agent for patients with typical bipolar disorder and in patients who are at high risk for suicide (severe depressions or depression combined with persistent suicidal ideas).
- **Lithium** levels should be monitored during pregnancy.
- Controversy continues regarding the potential teratogenic effect of **lithium**. Prospective studies suggest **lithium** is at worst a weak human teratogen.

Lodoxamine tromethamine (Alomide; Lomide)

■ **Class**

Mast cell stabilizer, antiallergic, ophthalmic

■ **Indications**

Vernal keratoconjunctivitis, vernal conjunctivitis, vernal keratitis

■ **Mechanism**

Inhibits the type I immediate hypersensitivity reaction of mast cells

■ **Dosage with Qualifiers**

Vernal keratoconjunctivitis—1-2 gtt OS/OD qid
Vernal conjunctivitis—1-2 gtt OS/OD qid
Vernal keratitis—1-2 gtt OS/OD qid
NOTE—treatment can last up to 3 mo

- **Contraindications**—hypersensitivity to drug or class
- **Caution**—contact lenses

■ **Maternal Considerations**

There is no published experience with **lodoxamine** during pregnancy.
Side effects include ocular itching, pruritus, blurred vision, dry eye, tearing, discharge, hyperemia, foreign body sensation, corneal ulcer, eye pain, ocular edema, ocular swelling, corneal abrasion, anterior chamber cells, keratitis, blepharitis, and allergy.

■ **Fetal Considerations**

There are no adequate reports or well-controlled studies in human fetuses. It is unknown whether **lodoxamine** crosses the human placenta. Rodent studies are reassuring, revealing no evidence of teratogenicity or IUGR despite the use of doses higher than those used clinically. Considering the dose and route, it is unlikely the maternal systemic concentration will reach a clinically relevant level.

■ **Breastfeeding Safety**

There is no published experience in nursing women. It is unknown whether **lodoxamine** enters human breast milk. However, considering the dose and route, it is unlikely the breast-fed neonate would ingest clinically relevant amounts.

- ■ **References** ⸺ There is no published experience in pregnancy or during lactation.

- ■ **Summary** ⸺
  - • **Pregnancy Category B**
  - • **Lactation Category S**
  - • **Lodoxamine** should be used during pregnancy and lactation only if the benefit justifies the potential perinatal risk.

Lomefloxacin (Maxaquin)

- ■ **Class** ⸺ Antibiotic, quinolone

- ■ **Indications** ⸺ Bacterial infections (<u>gram-positive bacteria:</u> Staphylococcus saprophyticus; <u>gram-negative bacteria:</u> Escherichia coli, Haemophilus influenzae, Klebsiella pneumoniae, Moraxella catarrhalis, Proteus mirabilis, Pseudomonas aeruginosa, Citrobacter diversus, Enterobacter cloacae)

- ■ **Mechanism** ⸺ Inhibits DNA synthesis

- ■ **Dosage with Qualifiers** ⸺ <u>Bacterial infection</u>—400mg PO qd ×10-14d
  <u>Gonorrhea</u>—400mg PO ×1
  NOTE—drink fluids liberally; renal dosing
  - • **Contraindications**—hypersensitivity to drug or class, prolongation of the QT interval, concomitant use of antiarrhythmic drugs
  - • **Caution**—hepatic or renal (CrCl <50ml/min) dysfunction, seizures, dehydration, hypokalemia, sun exposure, diabetes mellitus, bradycardia, cardiomyopathy, anemia

- ■ **Maternal Considerations** ⸺ This quinolone has poor efficacy against anaerobic infections. There are no adequate reports or well-controlled studies of **lomefloxacin** in pregnant women. *Side effects* include convulsions, coma, vaginitis, leucorrhea, intermenstrual bleeding, perineal pain, Stevens-Johnson syndrome, hyperkinesia, tremor, vertigo, paresthesias, fatigue, back pain, malaise, asthenia, chest pain, chills, allergic reaction, face edema, influenza-like symptoms, decreased heat tolerance, hypotension, hypertension, edema, syncope, tachycardia, bradycardia, arrhythmia, extrasystole, cyanosis, cardiac failure, angina pectoris, MI, PE, cerebrovascular disorder, cardiomyopathy, vomiting, flatulence, constipation, abdominal pain, dyspepsia, pseudomembranous colitis, GI inflammation, dysphagia, GI bleeding, pruritus, urticaria, eczema, dysuria, hematuria, and anuria.

- **Fetal Considerations** ⸺ There are no adequate reports or well-controlled studies in human fetuses. It is unknown whether **lomefloxacin** crosses the human placenta. Animal studies (mice, dogs, rabbits) report that several quinolones lead to arthropathy, and this toxicity resulted in the recommended restricted use in pregnant women. However, not all quinolones have the same potency on cartilage growth. Further, the use of quinolones during the 1st trimester of pregnancy is not associated with an increased risk of malformations or musculoskeletal conditions. Rodent and monkey studies are reassuring, revealing no evidence of teratogenicity or IUGR despite the use of doses higher than those used clinically. However, there was evidence of embryo and fetal toxicity at high doses.

- **Breastfeeding Safety** ⸺ There is no published experience in nursing women. Other quinolones are excreted into human breast milk.

- **References** ⸺ Tesh JM, McAnulty PA, Willoughby CR, et al. Jpn J Antibiot 1988; 41:1370-84.
Shakibaei M, Baumann-Wilschke I, Rucker M, Stahlmann R. Arch Toxicol 2002; 75:725-33.

- **Summary** ⸺
  - **Pregnancy Category C**
  - **Lactation Category U**
  - **Lomefloxacin** should be used during pregnancy and lactation only if the potential benefit justifies the perinatal risk.
  - While quinolones appear safe during the 1st trimester, their use during the 2nd and 3rd trimesters should await further study because of the potential for juvenile arthropathy.
  - There are alternative agents for which there is more experience during pregnancy and lactation.

Loperamide (Arret; Beamodium; Chisen; Hocular; Imode; Imodium; Lorico; Motilen)

- **Class** ⸺ *Gastrointestinal, antidiarrheal*

- **Indications** ⸺ Diarrhea

- **Mechanism** ⸺ Inhibits bowel peristalsis

- **Dosage with Qualifiers** ⸺ Diarrhea—begin 4mg PO ×1, then 2mg PO after each loose stool; max 16mg/d
NOTE—available in liquid or tablet forms
  - **Contraindications**—hypersensitivity to drug or class, bloody diarrhea, pseudomembranous colitis
  - **Caution**—diarrhea >48h, hepatic or renal disease

■ **Maternal Considerations** .... **Loperamide** is a popular and effective agent for the treatment of diarrhea ("traveler's diarrhea") and associated symptoms. It reduces the incidence of side effects (diarrhea, nausea) in women undergoing 2nd trimester termination.
Side effects include necrotizing enterocolitis, paralytic ileus, drowsiness, dizziness, dry mouth, abdominal pain, abdominal distention, constipation, nausea, vomiting, fatigue, and skin rash.

■ **Fetal Considerations** .... Prospective studies conducted in humans suggest that the use of **loperamide** during pregnancy is not associated with an increased risk of major malformations.

■ **Breastfeeding Safety** .... Although there are no adequate reports or well-controlled studies in nursing women, **loperamide** is generally considered safe for breast-feeding women.

■ **References** .... Jain JK, Harwood B, Meckstroth KR, Mishell DR. Contraception 2001; 63:217-21.
Einarson A, Mastroiacovo P, Arnon J, et al. Can J Gastroenterol 2000; 14:185-7.
Daugherty LM. Am Pharm 1990; 30:45-8.
Hagemann TM. J Hum Lact 1998; 14:259-62.
Nikodem VC, Hofmeyr GJ. Eur J Clin Pharmacol 1992; 42:695-6.

■ **Summary** .... • **Pregnancy Category B**
• **Lactation Category S**
• **Loperamide** is an excellent choice for the noted indications.

Loracarbef (Lorabid)

■ **Class** .... Antibiotic, 2nd-generation cephalosporin

■ **Indications** .... Bacterial infections (<u>gram-positive aerobes</u>: Staphylococcus aureus, Streptococcus pneumoniae, Streptococcus pyogenes; <u>gram-negative anaerobes</u>: Haemophilus influenzae)

■ **Mechanism** .... Bactericidal, inhibits cell wall synthesis

■ **Dosage with Qualifiers** .... <u>Bacterial infections</u>—200-400mg PO bid
NOTE—best taken on empty stomach
• **Contraindications**—hypersensitivity to drug or class, pseudomembranous colitis
• **Caution**—unknown

- **Maternal Considerations** ⸱⸱⸱⸱⸱⸱⸱ **Loracarbef** is used to treat lower respiratory tract infections, genitourinary tract infections, skin infections, septicemia, and for surgical prophylaxis. Though cephalosporins are usually considered safe during pregnancy, there is no published experience with **loracarbef** during pregnancy.
  Side effects include **penicillin** allergy, renal dysfunction, antibiotic associated colitis, and seizure.

- **Fetal Considerations** ⸱⸱⸱⸱⸱⸱⸱ There are no adequate reports or well-controlled studies in human fetuses. Other cephalosporins cross the human placenta. Rodent studies are reassuring, revealing no evidence of teratogenicity or IUGR despite the use of doses higher than those used clinically.

- **Breastfeeding Safety** ⸱⸱⸱⸱⸱⸱⸱ There is no published experience in nursing women. It is unknown whether **loracarbef** enters human breast milk. Most cephalosporins are excreted into breast milk.

- **References** ⸱⸱⸱⸱⸱⸱⸱ There is no published experience in pregnancy or during lactation.

- **Summary** ⸱⸱⸱⸱⸱⸱⸱
  - **Pregnancy Category B**
  - **Lactation Category S**
  - **Loracarbef** should be used during pregnancy and lactation only if the benefit justifies the potential perinatal risk.
  - There are alternative antibiotics for which there is more experience during pregnancy and lactation.

Loratadine (Alavert; Claritin; Claritin RediTabs)

- **Class** ⸱⸱⸱⸱⸱⸱⸱ Antihistamine

- **Indications** ⸱⸱⸱⸱⸱⸱⸱ Allergic rhinitis, urticaria

- **Mechanism** ⸱⸱⸱⸱⸱⸱⸱ Antagonizes peripheral H_1 receptors

- **Dosage with Qualifiers** ⸱⸱⸱⸱⸱⸱⸱ Allergic rhinitis—10mg PO qd
  Urticaria—10mg PO qd
  NOTE—available in orally disintegrating tablets
  - **Contraindications**—hypersensitivity to drug or class
  - **Caution**—hepatic or renal dysfunction

- **Maternal Considerations** ⸱⸱⸱⸱⸱⸱⸱ **Loratadine** is a 2nd-generation antihistamine with minimal sedating effect. It is a first-line agent for the treatment of allergic rhinorrhea. There are no adequate reports or well-controlled studies of **loratadine** in pregnant women.

Side effects include bronchospasm, hepatitis, fatigue, headache, somnolence, dry mouth, nervousness, and abdominal pain.

■ **Fetal Considerations** .... There are no adequate reports or well-controlled studies in human fetuses. It is unknown whether **loratadine** crosses the human placenta. Prospective human studies reveal no adverse outcomes. Rodent studies are reassuring, revealing no evidence of teratogenicity or IUGR despite the use of doses higher than those used clinically.

■ **Breastfeeding Safety** .... **Loratadine** and its active metabolite, descarboethoxyloratadine, pass easily into human breast milk achieving concentrations almost equivalent to maternal plasma. However, the total dose absorbed by the breast-feeding neonate is <1%.

■ **References** .... Moretti ME, Caprara D, Coutinho CJ, et al. J Allergy Clin Immunol 2003; 111:479-83.
Horak F, Stubner UP. Drug Saf 1999; 20:385-401.
Mazzotta P, Loebstein R, Koren G. Drug Saf 1999; 20:361-75.
Simons FE, Simons KJ. Clin Pharmacokinet 1991; 21:372-93.
Hilbert J, Radwanski E, Affrime MB, et al. J Clin Pharmacol 1988; 28:234-9.

■ **Summary** ....
- **Pregnancy Category B**
- **Lactation Category S**
- **Loratadine** is considered safe for the noted indications during pregnancy and lactation.

Lorazepam (Almazine; Aplacassee; Ativan; Bonton; Lorat; Lozepam; Nervistopl; Sedizepan; Wintin)

■ **Class** .... *Anxiolytic, benzodiazepine, anticonvulsant*

■ **Indications** .... Anxiety, insomnia, status epilepticus

■ **Mechanism** .... Stimulates benzodiazepine receptors

■ **Dosage with Qualifiers** .... Anxiety—0.5-2mg PO IM/IV q6-8h; max 10mg/d
Insomnia—2-4mg PO qhs
Status epilepticus—4mg IV ×1, may be repeated in 10-15min; max 8mg/12h
- **Contraindications**—hypersensitivity to drug or class, glaucoma, alcohol intoxication, depressive disorder, psychosis
- **Caution**—hepatic, pulmonary or renal dysfunction, drug abuse

■ **Maternal Considerations** ⋯⋯⋯ There is a growing appreciation that the purported risks of **lorazepam** during pregnancy are smaller than first thought. Women in need of the therapy should not be denied it solely because of the pregnancy. Although nonpharmacologic approaches to the treatment of insomnia are first-line therapy, intermediate-acting benzodiazepines such as **lorazepam** and **temazepam** may be useful in some circumstances.

Side effects include cardiovascular collapse, respiratory depression, withdrawal syndrome, blood dyscrasias, gangrene, dependency, sedation, dizziness, weakness, ataxia, depression, nausea, vomiting, antegrade amnesia, headache, sleep disturbances, diplopia, nystagmus, agitation, urinary incontinence, change in appetite, delirium, and pain at the injection site.

■ **Fetal Considerations** ⋯⋯⋯ There are no adequate reports or well-controlled studies in human fetuses. **Lorazepam** crosses the human placenta. High peak concentrations are avoided by dividing the daily dose into two or three. While there are many studies of benzodiazepine use in human pregnancy, data on teratogenicity and effects on postnatal development and behavior are limited and conflicting. Early studies suggested that 1st trimester exposure to benzodiazepines was associated with an increased risk of facial clefts and cardiac malformations. Subsequent studies contradicted that conclusion finding no clear evidence of an increase in either the overall incidence of malformations or of any particular type of defect. Benzodiazepine use in the 3rd trimester or during labor may cause the floppy infant syndrome or neonatal withdrawal. There is no increase in jaundice at term. Rodent studies are for the most reassuring, revealing no evidence of teratogenicity or IUGR despite the use of doses higher than those used clinically. In other rodent studies, prenatal exposure to some benzodiazepines is associated with behavioral and neurochemical alterations in the early postnatal period that may persist into adulthood. Studies in humans document an effect at least up to 18mo of age.

■ **Breastfeeding Safety** ⋯⋯⋯ **Lorazepam** is excreted into the human breast milk. It has been estimated the breast-fed neonate ingests <1% of the maternal dose, a dose that should be clinically insignificant. Using the lowest effective quantity in divided doses to minimize drug peaks could further minimize any theoretic risk.

■ **References** ⋯⋯⋯
Iqbal MM, Sobhan T, Ryals T. Psychiatr Serv 2002; 53:39-49.
Koff JM, Miller LG. Pharmacol Biochem Behav 1995; 51:721-4.
McElhatton PR. Reprod Toxicol 1994; 8:461-75.
Jurand A, Martin LV. Pharmacol Toxicol 1994; 74:228-35.
Laegreid L, Hagberg G, Lundberg A. Neuropediatrics 1992; 23:60-7.
Sanchis A, Rosique D, Catala J. DICP 1991; 25:1137-8.
Summerfield RJ, Nielsen MS. Br J Anaesth 1985; 57:1042-3.

Kanto JH. Drugs 1982; 23:354-80.
Humpel M, Stoppelli I, Milia S, Rainer E. Eur J Clin Pharmacol 1982; 21:421-5.
Whitelaw AG, Cummings AJ, McFadyen IR. Br Med J (Clin Res Ed) 1981; 282:1106-8.

■ **Summary**

- **Pregnancy Category D**
- **Lactation Category S?**
- Benzodiazepines historically have been prescribed in excess. They should be avoided where possible during pregnancy.
- **Lorazepam** may be an appropriate choice for women with a clear indication.
- There are alternative agents for which there is both more experience and a clearer safety profile during pregnancy and lactation.

Lovastatin (Altocor; Lofacol; Mevacor)

■ **Class**

Antihyperlipidemic, HMG CoA *reductase inhibitor*

■ **Indications**

Hypercholesterolemia, prevention of CV events

■ **Mechanism**

Inhibits HMG-CoA reductase

■ **Dosage with Qualifiers**

Hypercholesterolemia—begin 20mg PO with food, increase until desired effect; max 80mg PO qpm
Prevention of CV events—10-80mg PO qpm
NOTE—monitor hepatic transaminases at baseline, 6w after initiation, and 1mo after each increase
- **Contraindications**—hypersensitivity to drug or class, active hepatic disease, elevated transaminases, pregnancy, lactation
- **Caution**—hepatic or renal dysfunction, alcoholism

■ **Maternal Considerations**

There are no adequate reports or well-controlled studies of **lovastatin** in pregnant women. The limited information available on the effect of HMG CoA reductase inhibitors on pregnancy suggests similar outcomes as the general, nonexposed population. Hypercholesterolemia is a chronic problem. Discontinuation of **lovastatin** during pregnancy is unlikely to increase maternal morbidity.
Side effects include rhabdomyolysis, hepatotoxicity, dyspepsia, constipation, flatulence, abdominal pain, rash, asthenia, myalgias, elevated CPK, and elevated LFTs.

■ **Fetal Considerations**

Cholesterol and other products of the cholesterol biosynthesis are essential components for fetal development. There are no adequate reports or well-controlled studies in human fetuses. It is unknown whether **lovastatin** crosses the human placenta. Limited (134 pregnancies as of 1996) follow-up study of exposed fetuses is reassuring. Rodent studies, too, are generally reassuring. Skeletal abnormalities were noted when the administered dose exceeded 40 times the MRHD. Some animal studies suggest the statin drugs might be neuroprotective against hypoxic/ischemic stroke.

■ **Breastfeeding Safety** — There is no published experience in nursing women. It is unknown whether **lovastatin** enters human breast milk. Statin drugs inhibit prolactin release in the rat brain, and theoretically could interfere with the initiation of lactation.

■ **References** — Balduini W, De Angelis V, Mazzoni E, Cimino M. Stroke 2001; 32:2185-91.
Manson JM, Freyssinges C, Ducrocq MB, Stephenson WP. Reprod Toxicol 1996; 10:439-46.
Freyssinges C, Ducrocq MB. Therapie 1996; 51:537-42.

■ **Summary** —
- **Pregnancy Category X**
- **Lactation Category U**
- Pending the availability of reassuring studies, **lovastatin** is not recommended during pregnancy or lactation.

Loxapine (Loxitane)

■ **Class** — Antipsychotic

■ **Indications** — Psychosis

■ **Mechanism** — Unknown; selectively antagonizes the dopamine D_2 receptors

■ **Dosage with Qualifiers** — Psychosis—30-50mg PO bid
- **Contraindications**—hypersensitivity to drug or class, depression
- **Caution**—cardiovascular diseases, glaucoma, hepatic disease

■ **Maternal Considerations** — **Loxapine** is a tranquilizer indicated for the management of the manifestations of psychotic disorders. Galactorrhea is a common complication. There are no adequate reports or well-controlled studies of **loxapine** in pregnant women. *Side effects* include drowsiness, sedation, dizziness, faintness, staggering gait, shuffling gait, muscle twitching, weakness, insomnia, agitation, tension, seizures, akinesia, slurred speech, numbness, confusional states, parkinsonian-like symptoms, dystonic reaction, tachycardia, hypotension, hypertension, orthostatic hypotension, light-headedness, syncope, agranulocytosis, thrombocytopenia, leucopenia, dry mouth, nasal congestion, constipation, blurred vision, urinary retention, weight gain, weight loss, dyspnea, ptosis, hyperpyrexia, flushed facies, headache, paresthesia, polydipsia, nausea, and vomiting.

- ■ **Fetal Considerations** — There are no adequate reports or well-controlled studies in human fetuses. It is unknown whether **loxapine** crosses the human placenta. Rodent studies are reassuring, but are limited.

- ■ **Breastfeeding Safety** — There are no adequate reports or well-controlled studies in nursing women. **Loxapine** is excreted into human breast milk, but the kinetics have yet to be elucidated.

- ■ **References** — Gelenberg AJ. J Nerv Ment Dis 1979; 167:635-6.

- ■ **Summary** —
  - **Pregnancy Category C**
  - **Lactation Category U**
  - **Loxapine** should be used during pregnancy and lactation only if the benefit justifies the potential perinatal risk.
  - There are alternative agents for which there is more experience during pregnancy and lactation.

Lypressin (Diapid; Syntopressin)

- ■ **Class** — *Antidiuretics, hormone*

- ■ **Indications** — Diabetes insipidus

- ■ **Mechanism** — Stimulates vasopressin receptors

- ■ **Dosage with Qualifiers** — <u>Diabetes insipidus</u>—1-2 spray IN prn
  - **Contraindications**—hypersensitivity to drug or class, history of cardiovascular diseases (angina, MI)
  - **Caution**—nasal congestion, allergic rhinitis, upper respiratory infections

- ■ **Maternal Considerations** — **Lypressin** is indicated for the treatment of diabetes insipidus. It is a synthetic version of the natural porcine compound. There is no published experience during pregnancy with **lypressin**. It is a powerful vasoconstrictor when applied to isolated vessels and induces contractions in isolated myometrium from humans.
  Side effects include rhinorrhea, nasal congestion, irritation, nasal ulceration, headache, conjunctivitis, heartburn, periorbital edema, chest tightness, and dyspnea.

- **Fetal Considerations** There are no adequate reports or well-controlled studies in human fetuses. It is unknown whether **lypressin** crosses the human placenta. Rodent teratogenicity studies have not been conducted.

- **Breastfeeding Safety** There is no published experience in nursing women. It is unknown whether **lypressin** enters human breast milk. **Lypressin** stimulates mammary ejection pressure in sheep.

- **References** Landstrom G, Wallin A, Lundmark K, Noren H, Lindblom B. Hum Reprod 1999; 14:151-5.
Sala NL. Acta Physiol Lat Am 1965; 15:191-9.

- **Summary**
  - **Pregnancy Category C**
  - **Lactation Category U**
  - **Lypressin** should be used during pregnancy and lactation only if the benefit justifies the potential perinatal risk.

Magnesium chloride (Chlor-3)

■ **Class** — Electrolyte replacement

■ **Indications** — Hypomagnesemia

■ **Mechanism** — Replacement

■ **Dosage with Qualifiers** — Hypomagnesemia—4g mixed in 250ml of 5% dextrose IV no faster than 3ml/min, dose range 1-40g qd
NOTE—serum magnesium measurements should guide replacement; keep **calcium gluconate** readily available to counteract potentially serious signs of magnesium intoxication
- **Contraindications**—hypersensitivity to drug or class, renal failure, impaired myocardial function
- **Caution**—electrolyte disturbances, renal dysfunction

■ **Maternal Considerations** — There are no adequate reports or well-controlled studies of **magnesium chloride** in pregnant women.
Side effects include flushing and sweating.

■ **Fetal Considerations** — There are no adequate reports or well-controlled studies in human fetuses. Magnesium administered parenterally to the mother crosses the placenta. Rodent studies are reassuring.

■ **Breastfeeding Safety** — Magnesium is normally present in human breast milk, and its concentration is stable throughout the 1st year of lactation. It is unknown whether **magnesium chloride** increases the magnesium content of breast milk. Considering the indications, limited use is unlikely to pose a clinically significant risk to the breast-feeding neonate.

■ **References** — Oorschot DE. Magnes Res 2000; 13:265-73.
Meirowitz NB, Ananth CV, Smulian JC, Vintzileos AM. J Matern Fetal Med 1999; 8:177-83.
Nagra SA. J Trop Pediatr 1989; 35:126-8.
Martin RW, Perry KG Jr, Martin JN Jr, et al. J Miss State Med Assoc 1998; 39:180-2.
Usami M, Sakemi K, Tsuda M, Ohno Y. Eisei Shikenjo Hokoku 1996; 114:16-20.

■ **Summary** —
- **Pregnancy Category B**
- **Lactation Category S**
- **Magnesium chloride** should be used during pregnancy and lactation only for the treatment of hypomagnesemia.

Magnesium citrate

■ **Class** ⋯⋯⋯⋯⋯⋯⋯⋯⋯⋯⋯⋯⋯⋯ Laxative

■ **Indications** ⋯⋯⋯⋯⋯⋯⋯⋯⋯⋯⋯ Constipation

■ **Mechanism** ⋯⋯⋯⋯⋯⋯⋯⋯⋯⋯⋯ Unknown

■ **Dosage with Qualifiers** ⋯⋯⋯ Constipation—120-240ml PO prn
- **Contraindications**—hypersensitivity to drug or class, appendicitis, acute abdomen, GI obstruction
- **Caution**—renal dysfunction, electrolyte disturbances

■ **Maternal Considerations** ⋯⋯ **Magnesium citrate** reduces the frequency of night leg cramps in nonpregnant patients. There are no adequate reports or well-controlled studies of **magnesium citrate** in pregnant women. Its use during pregnancy increases serum magnesium.
Side effects include abdominal cramps, flatulence, diarrhea, hypotension, hypermagnesemia, and respiratory disturbances.

■ **Fetal Considerations** ⋯⋯⋯⋯ There are no adequate reports or well-controlled studies in human fetuses. Magnesium ions freely cross the placenta.

■ **Breastfeeding Safety** ⋯⋯⋯⋯ **Magnesium** is normally present in human breast milk, and its concentration is stable throughout the 1st year of lactation. It is unknown whether **magnesium citrate** increases the **magnesium** content of breast milk. Considering the indications and dosing, limited use is unlikely to pose a clinically significant risk to the breast-feeding neonate.

■ **References** ⋯⋯⋯⋯⋯⋯⋯⋯⋯⋯ Roffe C, Sills S, Crome P, Jones P. Med Sci Monit 2002; 8:CR326-30.
Ajayi GO, Fadiran EO. Clin Exp Obstet Gynecol 1998; 25:64-6.

■ **Summary** ⋯⋯⋯⋯⋯⋯⋯⋯⋯⋯⋯
- **Pregnancy Category B**
- **Lactation Category S?**
- **Magnesium citrate** should be used during pregnancy and lactation only if the benefit justifies the potential perinatal risk.

Magnesium oxide

■ **Class** .... *Electrolyte replacement*

■ **Indications** .... Hypomagnesemia

■ **Mechanism** .... Replacement

■ **Dosage with Qualifiers** .... Hypomagnesemia—1-2 tab PO bid/tid
NOTE—400mg tab = 241.3mg of elemental magnesium
- **Contraindications**—hypersensitivity to drug or class, renal failure, impaired myocardial function
- **Caution**—electrolyte disturbances, renal dysfunction

■ **Maternal Considerations** .... There are no adequate reports or well-controlled studies of **magnesium oxide** in pregnant women. Obstetricians have used oral magnesium as a tocolytic agent without demonstrable efficacy. It has also been advocated as a neuroprotectant for the acutely hypoxic fetus and to prevent preeclampsia. Neither indication can be substantiated. *Side effects* include flushing and sweating.

■ **Fetal Considerations** .... There are no adequate reports or well-controlled studies in human fetuses.

■ **Breastfeeding Safety** .... Magnesium is normally present in human breast milk, and its concentration is stable throughout the 1st year of lactation. It is unknown whether **magnesium oxide** increases the magnesium content of breast milk.

■ **References** .... Martin RW, Perry KG Jr, Martin JN Jr, et al. J Miss State Med Assoc 1998; 39:180-2.
Andreassi S, Teso A. Riv Eur Sci Med Farmacol 1992; 14:309-12.
D'Almeida A, Carter JP, Anatol A, Prost C. Womens Health 1992; 19:117-31.
Ridgway LE 3rd, Muise K, Wright JW, Patterson RM, Newton ER. Am J Obstet Gynecol 1990; 163:879-82.
Nagra SA. J Trop Pediatr 1989; 35:126-8.

■ **Summary** ....
- **Pregnancy Category B**
- **Lactation Category S**
- **Magnesium oxide** should be used during pregnancy and lactation for the treatment of hypomagnesemia. The efficacy of other applications cannot currently be substantiated.

Magnesium sulfate (Tis U Sol)

■ **Class**	*Electrolyte replacement, tocolysis, anticonvulsant*
■ **Indications**	Ventricular arrhythmia, eclampsia, hypomagnesemia
■ **Mechanism**	Inhibits Ca^{2+} release from the intracytoplasmic storage deposits, blocks Ca^{2+} influx through glutamate channels or through the N-methyl-D-aspartate receptor

■ **Dosage with Qualifiers**

Ventricular arrhythmia—3-20mg/min IV continuous IV ×6-48h

Eclampsia, prevention and treatment—begin 4g IV ×1 over 30min; then 2g/h IV maintenance rate for at least 24h postpartum, or during diuresis >200ml/h; alternatively, 10g IM loading dose followed by 5g IM q4h until at least 24h postpartum

Tocolysis—begin 6g IV ×1 over 30min, then 2-4g/h IV ×48h

Hypomagnesemia—1g IM q4-6h; alternative 5g mixed in 1L NS IV over 3h

NOTE—renal dosing; measure serum Mg every 4-6h if infusion >2g/h or oliguria or maternal symptoms of toxicity; maintain between 4-7mEq/L (4.8-8.4mg/dl)

- **Contraindications**—hypersensitivity to drug or class, renal failure, impaired myocardial function
- **Caution**—renal dysfunction, electrolyte disturbances

■ **Maternal Considerations**

Magnesium sulfate is excreted by the kidney, and a decreased GFR may lead to magnesium toxicity if not monitored closely. Begin with only 1/2 the usual load when the plasma creatinine exceeds 1.3mg/dl. Deep-tendon reflexes are decreased as the concentration exceeds 4mEq/L; they are lost as the level approaches 10mEq/L. Potentially, lethal respiratory depression may occur at 12-15mEq/L. Recent investigation suggests the measurement of total magnesium is not adequate for titration in women with either preeclampsia or preterm labor as there is poor correlation between total magnesium and the physiologically active ionized magnesium. **Calcium gluconate** should always be readily available to counteract potential serious signs of magnesium intoxication.

Preeclampsia remains a leading cause of maternal and perinatal morbidity and death. Randomized trials demonstrate **magnesium sulfate** infusion halves the risk of eclampsia and is superior to both **phenytoin** and **diazepam** for the prevention of recurrent eclamptic seizures. The anticonvulsant effect is probably exerted on the cerebral cortex. Although it is the drug of choice for the prevention and control of seizures, **magnesium sulfate** is NOT an effective antihypertensive. Approximately 10-15% of women will convulse again despite prophylaxis. An additional 2g loading dose is recommended if a woman convulses while receiving magnesium sulfate for the prevention of eclampsia.

Magnesium sulfate may also be administered IM. Prospective studies comparing magnesium levels achieved with continuous IV infusion and IM reveal that therapeutically effective levels are achieved with both.

Magnesium sulfate neither prolongs labor nor increases the oxytocin requirement in preeclamptic women.

Magnesium sulfate is often continued for at least 24h post partum, but there is little scientific support for the practice. Others suggest the duration of therapy be individualized using maternal diuresis (>200ml/h for at least 2h) as evidence the associated vasospasm has resolved. In one study, women with mild preeclampsia could receive shorter courses of **magnesium sulfate** (mean 9.5 ± 4.2h) than those with severe preeclampsia alone (mean 16 ± 5.9h), superimposed preeclampsia (mean 16 ± 5.8h), or those with atypical preeclampsia (hemolysis, elevated liver enzymes, and low platelet count) (mean 20 ± 6.7h). There was no eclampsia, and recovery room time was reduced 50%.

Preterm labor—No tocolytic agent has been proven to stop preterm labor and improve perinatal outcome. The benefit of tocolysis is based on the time gained to administer corticosteroids. **Magnesium sulfate** depresses uterine contractility both *in vitro* and *in vivo*. And although it has no effect on the labor of preeclamptic women, it is the most commonly used parenteral tocolytic in the U.S., believed effective in stopping contractions in 60-80% of patients for 48-72h. Unfortunately, the scientific support for this belief is weak, and several in-depth analyses conclude there is stronger evidence for the use of other agents with fewer side effects. There are no published placebo controlled trials with **magnesium sulfate**. Most studies compare the effectiveness of **magnesium sulfate** to betamimetics, and conclude it is at least as effective as **terbutaline** or **ritodrine** for the prevention of preterm delivery whether membranes are intact or ruptured. In other studies **magnesium sulfate** is no more effective than placebo in preventing preterm labor. **Magnesium sulfate** is not risk-free. Pulmonary edema and cardiovascular problems occur at a frequency similar to that of betamimetics (approximately 1%). Maternal infection, decreased colloid osmotic pressure and fluid overload are each predisposing risk factors. There is no evidence to support the practice of weaning the **magnesium sulfate** infusion rate when the decision is made to stop tocolysis.

Side effects include respiratory failure, cardiovascular collapse, hypothermia, depressed cardiac function, pulmonary edema, depressed reflexes, hypotension, drowsiness, nausea, vomiting, hypocalcemia, hyperkalemia, flushing, blurred vision, sweating, muscle weakness, ECG changes, sedation, and confusion.

■ **Fetal Considerations** .... Parenterally administered magnesium crosses the placenta and increases the fetal level. Though there is some controversy, there is no clear evidence of adverse effects from short-term **magnesium sulfate** therapy. Respiratory depression may occur if there is severe hypermagnesemia at delivery. Rodent studies suggest maternal seizures may be associated with fetal brain injury, an effect possibly ameliorated by **magnesium sulfate**. Some human studies also suggest a protective effect of **magnesium sulfate** against cerebral palsy in very low-birth-weight infants. However, there is as yet no confirmation based on either randomized or prospective study. Maternal administration does not protect against neonatal necrotizing enterocolitis. It remains controversial whether the intrapartum administration of **magnesium sulfate** reduces fetal heart variability and reactivity.

■ **Breastfeeding Safety** .... Some case reports describe engorgement and galactorrhea during tocolysis with intravenous **magnesium sulfate.** The mechanism remains unknown. Symptoms gradually subside after discontinuation. Magnesium is normally present in human breast milk, and its concentration stable throughout the 1st year of lactation. It is unknown whether **magnesium sulfate** increases the magnesium content of breast milk. Considering the indication and dosing, limited use is unlikely to pose a clinically significant risk to the breast-feeding neonate.

■ **References** ....

The Magpie Trial: a randomized placebo-controlled trial. Lancet 2002; 359:1877-90.

Roberts JM, Villar J, Arulkumaran S. BMJ 2002; 325:609-10.

Repke JT, Power ML, Holzman GB, Schulkin J. J Reprod Med 2002; 47:472-6.

Taber EB, Tan L, Chao CR, et al. Am J Obstet Gynecol 2002; 186:1017-21.

Chames MC, Livingston JC, Ivester TS, et al. Am J Obstet Gynecol 2002; 186:1174-7.

Lurie S, Rotmensch S, Feldman N, Glezerman M. Am J Perinatol 2002; 19:239-40.

Grether JK, Hoogstrate J, Walsh-Greene E, Nelson KB. Am J Obstet Gynecol 2000; 183:717-25.

Rasch DK, Huber PA, Richardson CJ, et al. J Pediatr 1982; 100:272-6.

Ghidini A, Espada RA, Spong CY. Acta Obstet Gynecol Scand 2001; 80:126-9.

Hennessy A, Hill I. Aust NZ J Obstet Gynaecol 1999; 39:256-7.

Hallak M, Martinez-Poyer J, Kruger ML, et al. Am J Obstet Gynecol 1999; 181:1122-7.

Szal SE, Croughan-Minihane MS, Kilpatrick SJ. Am J Obstet Gynecol 1999; 180:1475-9.

Belfort MA, Anthony J, Saade GR. Semin Perinatol 1999; 23:65-78.

Gyetvai K, Hannah ME, Hodnett ED, Ohlsson A. Obstet Gynecol 1999; 94:869-77.

Towers CV, Pircon RA, Heppard M. Am J Obstet Gynecol 1999; 180:1572-8.

Kimberlin DF, Hauth JC, Goldenberg RL, et al. Am J Perinatol 1998; 15:635-41.

Ascarelli MH, Johnson V, May WL, et al. Am J Obstet Gynecol 1998; 179:952-6.

El-Sayed YY, Riley ET, Holbrook RH Jr, et al. Obstet Gynecol 1999; 93:79-83.

Witlin AG, Sibai BM. Obstet Gynecol 1998; 92:883-9.

Mittendorf R, Dambrosia J, Pryde PG, et al. Am J Obstet Gynecol 2002; 186:1111-8.

Grether JK, Hoogstrate J, Selvin S, Nelson KB. Am J Obstet Gynecol 1998; 178:1-6.

Martin RW, Perry KG Jr, Martin JN Jr, et al. J Miss State Med Assoc 1998; 39:180-2.

Lewis DF, Bergstedt S, Edwards MS, et al. Am J Obstet Gynecol 1997; 177:742-5.

Gordon MC, Iams JD. Clin Obstet Gynecol 1995; 38:706-12.

Nelson KB, Grether JK. Pediatrics 1995; 95:263-9.

Odendaal HJ, Steyn DW, Norman K, et al. S Afr Med J 1995; 85:1071-6.

Atkinson MW, Guinn D, Owen J, Hauth JC. Am J Obstet Gynecol 1995; 173:1219-22.

Lucas MJ, Leveno KJ, Cunningham FG. N Engl J Med 1995; 333:201-5.

Hallak M, Hotra JW, Custodio D, Kruger ML. Am J Obstet Gynecol 2000; 18:793-8.

Lucas MJ, Leveno KJ, Cunningham FG. N Engl J Med 1995; 333:201-5.

Saade GR, Taskin O, Belfort MA, et al. Obstet Gynecol 1994; 84:374-8.

Atkinson MW, Belfort MA, Saade GR, Moise KJ Jr. Obstet Gynecol 1994; 83:967-70.

Belfort MA, Saade GR, Moise KJ Jr. Acta Obstet Gynecol Scand 1993; 72:526-30.

Matsuda Y, Ikenoue T, Hokanishi H. Gynecol Obstet Invest 1993; 36:102-7.

Belfort MA, Saade GR, Moise KJ Jr. Am J Obstet Gynecol 1992; 167:1548-53.

Ricci JM, Hariharan S, Helfgott A, et al. Am J Obstet Gynecol 1991; 165:603-10.

Sibai BM. Am J Obstet Gynecol 1990; 162:1141-5.

Weiner CP, Renk K, Klugman M. Am J Obstet Gynecol 1988; 159:216-22.

Martin RW, Martin JN Jr, Pryor JA, et al. Am J Obstet Gynecol 1988; 158:1440-5.

Sibai BM, Graham JM, McCubbin JH. Am J Obstet Gynecol 1984; 150:728-33.

Pritchard JA, Cunningham FG, Pritchard SA. Am J Obstet Gynecol 1984; 148:951-63.

■ **Summary**

- **Pregnancy Category A**
- **Lactation Category S**
- **Magnesium sulfate** is superior to both **phenytoin** and **diazepam** for reducing the incidence of primary and secondary eclamptic convulsions.

- Locales where eclampsia has a major impact on maternal mortality should institute policies to ensure that this inexpensive and lifesaving treatment is available, and that care providers are trained to use it safely.
- **Magnesium sulfate** is, at best, similar to betamimetics for the delay of delivery in women diagnosed with preterm labor. There are other agents such as **nifedipine** with both a superior safety profile and greater efficacy.

Mannitol (Osmitrol; Resectisol)

■ **Class** — *Diuretic, osmotic*

■ **Indications** — Oliguria from acute renal failure (prevention and treatment), cerebral edema, diuresis (forced)

■ **Mechanism** — Increases GFR

■ **Dosage with Qualifiers** —
Oliguria prevention—50-100g IV over 2h
Oliguria treatment—50-100g IV over 2h
Cerebral edema—100g IV ×2-6h
Diuresis, forced—25-100g IV over 2h
NOTE—attempt to maintain urinary output >100ml/h
- **Contraindications**—hypersensitivity to drug or class, anuria, progressive renal failure after initiation, no response to the initial bolus, pulmonary edema, severe dehydration, intracranial hemorrhage, progressive heart failure
- **Caution**—renal dysfunction

■ **Maternal Considerations** — **Mannitol** is an osmotic diuretic. It is confined to the extracellular space after IV administration and is rapidly excreted by the kidneys (80% within 3h). There are no adequate reports or well-controlled studies of **mannitol** in pregnant women. The published experience is limited to case reports of women undergoing surgery for causes unrelated to pregnancy (intracranial hemorrhage or brain tumors) or for hypermagnesemia.
Side effects include seizures, heart failure, cardiovascular collapse, pulmonary edema, acute renal failure, CNS depression, coma, fluid imbalance, tachycardia, dehydration, electrolyte disorders, acidosis, blurred vision, thrombophlebitis, urticaria, fever, infusion site infection, dryness of mouth, thirst, rhinitis, skin necrosis, angina, and water intoxication.

■ **Fetal Considerations** ⋯⋯⋯⋯ There are no adequate reports or well-controlled studies in human fetuses. **Mannitol** crosses the human placenta by diffusion. Rodent teratogenicity studies have not been performed. Studies of pregnant ewes reveal that maternal hyperosmolality influences the fetal arginine vasopressin secretion and renal function, and thus the amount of amniotic fluid.

■ **Breastfeeding Safety** ⋯⋯⋯⋯ There is no published literature in nursing women. It is unknown whether **mannitol** enters human breast milk.

■ **References** ⋯⋯⋯⋯ Chang L, Looi-Lyons L, Bartosik L, Tindal S. Can J Anaesth 1999; 46:61-5.
Bohman VR, Cotton DB. Obstet Gynecol 1990; 76:984-6.
Quraishi AN, Illsley NP. Placenta 1999; 20:167-74.
Bain MD, Copas DK, Landon MJ, Stacey TE. J Physiol 1988; 399:313-9.
Ervin MG, Ross MG, Youssef A, et al. Am J Obstet Gynecol 1986; 155:1341-7.

■ **Summary** ⋯⋯⋯⋯ • **Pregnancy Category C**
• **Lactation Category U**
• **Mannitol** should be used during pregnancy and lactation only if the benefit justifies the potential perinatal risk.

Maprotiline (Ludiomil)

■ **Class** ⋯⋯⋯⋯ *Antidepressant, tetracyclic*

■ **Indications** ⋯⋯⋯⋯ Depression

■ **Mechanism** ⋯⋯⋯⋯ Unknown; inhibits reuptake of norepinephrine

■ **Dosage with Qualifiers** ⋯⋯⋯⋯ Depression—25-50mg PO bid/tid; max 225mg PO qd ×6w
• **Contraindications**—hypersensitivity to drug or class, MI, usage of MAO inhibitor drugs within 14d
• **Caution**—seizure disorders, arrhythmias, strokes, tachycardia

■ **Maternal Considerations** ⋯⋯⋯⋯ There are no adequate reports or well-controlled studies of **maprotiline** in pregnant women.
Side effects include seizures, neuroleptic malignant syndrome, constipation, dry mouth, blurred vision, dizziness, orthostatic hypotension, drowsiness, urinary retention, tachycardia, diaphoresis, renal failure, rash, edema, dyskinesia, diarrhea, bitter taste, abdominal cramps, dysphagia, decreased libido, weakness, fatigue, insomnia, agitation, hallucinations, nightmares,

disorientation, delusions, restlessness, hypomania, mania, exacerbation of psychosis, decrease in memory, and feelings of unreality.

■ **Fetal Considerations** There are no adequate reports or well-controlled studies in human fetuses. It is unknown whether **maprotiline** crosses the human placenta. Rodent studies are reassuring, revealing no evidence of teratogenicity or IUGR despite the use of doses higher than those used clinically. Rodent and chick studies suggest **maprotiline** is less embryo and organ toxic than **imipramine** and **amitriptyline**.

■ **Breastfeeding Safety** There is no published experience in nursing women. It is unknown whether **maprotiline** enters human breast milk.

■ **References** Pinder RM, Brogden RN, Speight TM, Avery GS. Drugs 1977; 13:321-52.
Wirz-Justice A, Lichtsteiner M. J Pharm Pharmacol 1976; 28:172-5.

■ **Summary**
- **Pregnancy Category B**
- **Lactation Category U**
- **Maprotiline** should be used during pregnancy and lactation only if the benefit justifies the potential perinatal risk.

Mazindol (Mazanor; Sanorex)

■ **Class** Anorexiant, CNS stimulant

■ **Indications** Weight loss

■ **Mechanism** Appetite suppression and CNS stimulation

■ **Dosage with Qualifiers** Weight loss—1mg PO qd; dosage may be increased by max 3mg/d
NOTE—take with food or milk
- **Contraindications**—hypersensitivity to drug or class, arteriosclerosis, cardiovascular disease, hypertension, hyperthyroidism, glaucoma, anxiety
- **Caution**—drug abuse

■ **Maternal Considerations** **Mazindol** behaves like an amphetamine. Its efficacy in obese nonpregnant women is at best modest and tolerance develops. There is no published experience during pregnancy, nor are there any indications for its use. *Side effects* include palpitations, tachycardia, hypertension, psychosis, insomnia, euphoria, dyskinesia, dysphoria, tremor, headaches, Tourette's syndrome, dry mouth, diarrhea, constipation, anorexia, and decreased libido.

■ **Fetal Considerations**
There are no adequate reports or well-controlled studies in human fetuses. It is unknown whether **mazindol** crosses the human placenta. Rodent studies suggest an increase in rib abnormalities at multiples of the MRHD.

■ **Breastfeeding Safety**
There is no published experience in nursing women. It is unknown whether **mazindol** enters human breast milk.

■ **References**
There is no published experience in pregnancy or during lactation.

■ **Summary**
- **Pregnancy Category C**
- **Lactation Category U**
- There are no indications for **mazindol** during pregnancy or lactation.

Mebendazole (Vermox; Bendosan; Damaben; Drivermide; Fugacar; Ovex)

■ **Class**
Antihelmintic

■ **Indications**
Infection (pinworm, whipworm, hookworm, roundworm), capillariasis

■ **Mechanism**
Inhibition of microtubules formation; causes glucose depletion

■ **Dosage with Qualifiers**
Pinworm infection—100mg PO ×1
Whipworm infection—100mg PO bid ×3-5d
Hookworm infection—100mg PO bid ×3-5d
Roundworm infection—100mg PO bid ×3-5d
Capillariasis—200mg PO bid ×20d
- **Contraindications**—hypersensitivity to drug or class, pregnancy, children <2y
- **Caution**—pregnancy

■ **Maternal Considerations**
Treatment of reproductive-age women is strongly recommended in areas of widespread hookworm infection and its related anemia. In some endemic areas, treatment of all pregnant women after the 1st trimester is suggested as effective treatment to reduce the incidence of IUGR and perinatal death.

Side effects include angioedema, seizures, neutropenia, abdominal pain, nausea, vomiting, diarrhea, fever, dizziness, headache, rash, pruritus, alopecia, and convulsions.

■ **Fetal Considerations** .... There are no adequate reports or well-controlled studies in human fetuses. It is unknown whether **mebendazole** crosses the human placenta. Congenital helminthic infection in humans is rare. No increase in risk for congenital malformation or other adverse outcomes was noted in the largest prospective study with 140 1st trimester exposures. There are no reported sequelae from 2nd or 3rd trimester exposure. Rodent studies suggest **mebendazole** is embryotoxic and teratogenic at fairly low doses.

■ **Breastfeeding Safety** .... There is no published experience in nursing women. It is unknown whether **mebendazole** enters human breast milk.

■ **References** .... Diav-Citrin O, Shechtman S, Arnon J, Lubart I, Ornoy A. Am J Obstet Gynecol 2003; 188:282-5.
Allen H, Crompton D, de Silva N, et al. Trends Parasitol 2002; 18:381.
Dupouy-Camet J, Kociecka W, Bruschi F, et al. Expert Opin Pharmacother 2002; 3:1117-30.
Stephenson LS. Paediatr Drugs 2001; 3:495-508.
St Georgiev V. Expert Opin Pharmacother 2001; 2:223-39.
Christensen PM, Hedegaard U, Brosen K. Ugeskr Laeger 2000; 162:6552.
de Silva NR, Sirisena JL, Gunasekera DP, et al. Lancet 1999; 353:1145-9.
Fletouris D, Botsoglou N, Psomas I, Mantis A. J AOAC Int 1996; 79:1281-7.
Stoukides C. J Hum Lact 1994; 10:269.
Kurzel RB, Toot PJ, Lambert LV, Mihelcic AS. NZ Med J 1994; 107:439.

■ **Summary** .... • **Pregnancy Category C**
• **Lactation Category U**
• **Mebendazole** should be used during pregnancy and lactation only if the benefit justifies the potential perinatal risk.
• Though **mebendazole** is not associated with significant increase in the rates of congenital defects, it is best avoided during the 1st trimester.
• Treatment is beneficial for women in developing countries, where intestinal helminthiases are endemic.

Mecamylamine (Inversine)

- **Class** .... *Other antihypertensive, smoking/drug cessation*

- **Indications** .... Hypertension, malignant hypertension, smoking cessation

- **Mechanism** .... Inhibits nicotinic-cholinergic receptors (ganglion blockade)

- **Dosage with Qualifiers** .... Hypertension—begin 2.5mg PO bid and increase by 2.5mg q2d until 25mg qd
  Smoking cessation—2.5mg PO bid
  - **Contraindications**—hypersensitivity to drug or class, hypertension, history of acute MI, coronary insufficiency, uremia, pyloric stenosis, glaucoma
  - **Caution**—renal or cardiovascular dysfunction, fever, infection, anesthesia, surgery, vigorous exercise, use of alcohol or other hypertensive drugs

- **Maternal Considerations** .... There is no published experience during pregnancy.
  Side effects include dizziness, lightheadedness, fainting, hypotension, urinary retention, stroke, CHF, seizures, dizziness, ileus, constipation, nausea, vomiting, anorexia, glossitis, dry mouth, blurred vision, weakness, fatigue, tremor and choreiform movements.

- **Fetal Considerations** .... There are no adequate reports or well-controlled studies in human fetuses. Rodent teratogenicity studies have not been conducted.

- **Breastfeeding Safety** .... There is no published experience in nursing women. It is unknown whether **mecamylamine** enters human breast milk.

- **References** .... There are no current relevant references.

- **Summary** ....
  - **Pregnancy Category C**
  - **Lactation Category U**
  - **Mecamylamine** should be used during pregnancy and lactation only if the benefit justifies the potential perinatal risk.
  - There are alternative agents for which there is more experience regarding use during pregnancy and lactation.

Mechlorethamine (Mustargen)

■ **Class** ⋯⋯⋯⋯⋯⋯⋯⋯⋯⋯⋯⋯⋯ *Antineoplastic, alkylating agent*

■ **Indications** ⋯⋯⋯⋯⋯⋯⋯⋯⋯ Hodgkin's disease (stages III-IV), leukemia (chronic myelocytic and chronic lymphocytic), mycosis fungoides, polycythemia vera, lymphosarcoma

■ **Mechanism** ⋯⋯⋯⋯⋯⋯⋯⋯⋯ Alkylating agent

■ **Dosage with Qualifiers** ⋯⋯ Malignancy—0.4mg/kg/course; numerous dosing schedules exist reflecting the disease, patient response, and concomitant therapy
  • **Contraindications**—hypersensitivity to drug or class, suppurative inflammation
  • **Caution**—none

■ **Maternal Considerations** ⋯⋯ There are no adequate reports or well-controlled studies of **mechlorethamine** in pregnant women. Hodgkin's disease does not affect the normal progress of pregnancy. Termination of pregnancy is usually unnecessary. Based on limited published experience, **mechlorethamine** may be used during pregnancy with a good outcome.
Side effects include thrombosis, thrombophlebitis, anaphylaxis, nausea, vomiting, depression, hemolytic anemia, skin eruption, delayed catamenia, oligomenorrhea, and amenorrhea.

■ **Fetal Considerations** ⋯⋯⋯⋯ There are no adequate reports or well-controlled studies in human fetuses. It is unknown whether **mechlorethamine** crosses the human placenta. Children of women treated during pregnancy with a variety of cytotoxic agents including **mechlorethamine** for hematologic malignancies have normal birth weight as well as normal learning and educational performances. There is no increase in the prevalence of acute leukemia or congenital, neurologic and psychological abnormalities. Thus, chemotherapy at full doses administered during pregnancy even during the 1st trimester can end with a good outcome. **Mechlorethamine** is teratogenic in rodents.

■ **Breastfeeding Safety** ⋯⋯⋯⋯ There is no published experience in nursing women. It is unknown whether **mechlorethamine** enters human breast milk.

■ **References** ⋯⋯⋯⋯⋯⋯⋯⋯⋯ Aviles A, Neri N. Clin Lymphoma 2001; 2:173-7.
Brice P, Pautier P, Marolleau JP, et al. Nouv Rev Fr Hematol 1994; 36:387-8.
Abboud J, Nasrallah T, Chahine G, Nasnas R. J Gynecol Obstet Biol Reprod 1993; 22:783-6.

■ **Summary**
- **Pregnancy Category D**
- **Lactation Category U**
- Clinical experience reveals that **mechlorethamine** can be administered even during the 1st trimester with a good outcome.
- Long-term follow-up of children exposed *in utero* to chemotherapy is reassuring.

Meclizine (Ancolan; Antivert; Duramesan; En-Vert; Meclicot; Meclizine; Meclozine; Medivert; Yonyun)

■ **Class**
Antiemetic, antivertigo, antihistamine

■ **Indications**
Motion sickness

■ **Mechanism**
Antagonizes acetylcholine and H_1 receptors

■ **Dosage with Qualifiers**
Nausea, vomiting and dizziness due to motion sickness—25-50mg PO qd 1h before travel; repeat q24h
- **Contraindications**—hypersensitivity to drug or class
- **Caution**—GI and GU obstruction, usage of drug with CNS depressive effect

■ **Maternal Considerations**
Meclizine effectively reduces the nausea and vomiting associated with emergency hormonal contraception (Yuzpe regimen). There are no adequate reports or well-controlled studies of **meclizine** in pregnant women. *Side effects* include tachycardia, hallucinations, jaundice, ototoxicity, agitation, anxiety, hypotension, blurred vision, dry mouth, confusion, anorexia, nausea, vomiting, diarrhea, rash, and constipation.

■ **Fetal Considerations**
There are no adequate reports or well-controlled studies in human fetuses. It is unknown whether **meclizine** crosses the human placenta. Rodent studies conducted at 25-50 times the MRHD reveal cleft lip and palate. Though limited case reports suggested an increased incidence of cleft lip and cleft palate, a large clinical experience reveals little evidence that **meclizine** is a human teratogen.

■ **Breastfeeding Safety**
There are no adequate reports or well-controlled studies in nursing women. It is unknown whether **meclizine** enters human breast milk.

■ **References**
Raymond EG, Creinin MD, Barnhart KT, et al. Obstet Gynecol 2000; 95:271-7.

Shapiro S, Kaufman DW, Rosenberg L, et al. Br Med J
1978; 1:483.
Miklovich L, van den Berg BJ. Am J Obstet Gynecol 1976;
125:244-8.

■ **Summary** ──────────── • **Pregnancy Category B**
• **Lactation Category S**
• **Meclizine** should be used during pregnancy and
  lactation only if the benefit justifies the potential
  perinatal risk.

Meclofenamate (Meclomen)

■ **Class** ───────────── *Analgesic, non-narcotic*, NSAID

■ **Indications** ──────── Pain, dysmenorrhea, osteoarthritis, rheumatoid arthritis,
ankylosing spondylitis, gout

■ **Mechanism** ───────── Inhibits cyclooxygenase and lipoxygenase leading to
reduced prostaglandin synthesis

■ **Dosage with Qualifiers** ── Pain—50mg PO q4-6h; max 400mg/d
Dysmenorrhea—100mg PO tid; max 6d usage
Osteoarthritis—50-100mg PO tid/qid
Rheumatoid arthritis—50-100mg PO tid/qid
Ankylosing spondylitis—50-100mg PO tid
Gout, acute—100mg PO tid
NOTE—take with food or milk
• **Contraindications**—hypersensitivity to drug or class,
  NSAID-induced asthma
• **Caution**—nasal polyps, GI bleeding, hypertension,
  cardiac failure, asthma

■ **Maternal Considerations** ── **Meclofenamate** is a nonsteroidal agent with anti-
inflammatory, analgesic, and antipyretic activities. It has
little effect on human platelet function. There are no
adequate reports or well-controlled studies of
meclofenamate in pregnant women. In rodents,
meclofenamate induces luteolysis as indicated by the drop
in maternal **progesterone** after administration. Luteolysis
is followed by spontaneous labor. In contrast, *in vitro*
studies demonstrate **meclofenamate** inhibits myometrial
contractility. **Meclofenamate** is a popular analgesic for the
treatment of postpartum pain after vaginal delivery.
Side effects include anaphylaxis, GI bleeding,
bronchospasm, renal failure, interstitial nephritis, hepatic
failure, Stevens-Johnson syndrome, agranulocytosis,
abdominal pain, constipation, headache, dizziness, rash,
urticaria, increased LFTs, drowsiness, edema, tinnitus,
rash, lupus, and serum sickness-like symptoms.

- **Fetal Considerations** — There are no adequate reports or well-controlled studies in human fetuses. It is unknown whether **meclofenamate** crosses the human placenta. Similar class agents do cross, cause fetal ductal constriction and decreased fetal urination. Because of the potential for premature closure of the fetal ductus arteriosus after maternal use of NSAIDs, chronic **mefenamic acid** treatment during pregnancy is not recommended without fetal monitoring. Fetal exposure should be minimized until completion of future studies since **meclofenamate** may affect fetal breathing movements and pulmonary vascular resistance. Rodent studies reveal that **meclofenamate**, like **aspirin** and other nonsteroidal anti-inflammatory drugs, can cause fetotoxicity, minor skeletal malformations, e.g., supernumerary ribs and delayed ossification, but no major teratogenicity.

- **Breastfeeding Safety** — There is no published experience in nursing women. **Meclofenamate** enters human breast milk, though the kinetics remain to be elucidated.

- **References** — Facchinetti F, De Pietri R, Giunchi M, Genazzani AR. Clin J Pain 1991; 7(Suppl 1):S60-3.
Gooneratne AD, Hartmann PE, Barker I. J Reprod Fertil 1982; 65:157-62.
Cooke RG, Knifton A. Res Vet Sci 1980; 29:251-4.

- **Summary** —
  - **Pregnancy Category C (1st and 2nd trimesters), D (3rd trimester)**
  - **Lactation Category S?**
  - Similar to other NSAIDs, **meclofenamate** poses minimal risk when used occasionally.

Medroxyprogesterone (Amen; Aragest; Asconale; Clinovir; Curretab; Cycrin; Depo-Provera; Med-Pro; Provera)

- **Class** — *Hormone, contraceptive, antineoplastic*

- **Indications** — Amenorrhea, dysfunctional uterine bleeding, hormone replacement, contraception

- **Mechanism** — Inhibits gonadotropin release, stimulates transformation of proliferative into secretory endometrium

- **Dosage with Qualifiers** — Amenorrhea—5-10mg PO qd ×5 on days 16-21 of the cycle or qmo
Dysfunctional uterine bleeding—5-10mg PO qd ×5 on days 16-21 of the cycle or qmo

<u>Hormone replacement</u>—5-10mg PO qd ×12-14d
<u>Contraception</u>—150mg IM q3mo

- **Contraindications**—hypersensitivity to drug or class, thromboembolic disease, pregnancy, breast cancer, undiagnosed vaginal bleeding, thrombophlebitis, pulmonary embolism, retinal thrombosis, hepatic failure, missed abortion
- **Caution**—cerebrovascular disorders, lactation, hepatic dysfunction, cardiac failure

■ **Maternal Considerations** — A popular and effective (0.42/1000 women-years) contraceptive, irregular bleeding and amenorrhea are the most common side effects. It is estimated that 68% of women who become pregnant after discontinuing conceive within 12mo, 83% within 15mo, and 93% within 18mo. If bone density does decline, it is reversible and unlikely to adversely influence clinical events either acutely or later. Because of the noted indications, it is inevitable that numerous pregnant women are exposed to **medroxyprogesterone** since many pregnancies will not be recognized until after the 1st trimester. Progestational agents (i.e., not native **progesterone**) like **medroxyprogesterone** were long used during early pregnancy to prevent 1st trimester spontaneous abortion. The wisdom of this practice cannot be substantiated. It is speculated that progestational agents may delay spontaneous abortion in women with defective ova. While there are no adequate reports or well-controlled studies of **medroxyprogesterone** in pregnant women, epidemiologic studies are reassuring as there is not demonstrable increase in the prevalence of ectopic pregnancy.
Side effects include thromboembolism, stroke, MI, hepatic adenoma, breast cancer, gallbladder disease, cholestatic jaundice, hypertension, stroke, amenorrhea, nausea, vomiting, breast tenderness, weight gain, headache, edema, depression, rash, pruritus, libido changes, appetite changes, acne, hirsutism, galactorrhea, alopecia, and optic neuritis.

■ **Fetal Considerations** — There are no adequate reports or well-controlled studies in human fetuses. *In utero* exposure of male fetuses to progestational agents apparently doubles the risk of hypospadias. While there is insufficient data to quantify the risk for the female fetus, some progestational agents may cause mild virilization of the external genitalia. Defects outside the external genitalia are not noted in either humans or rodents. First trimester exposure is an indication for a detailed anatomic ultrasound between 18-22w.

■ **Breastfeeding Safety** — Trace amounts of **medroxyprogesterone** are excreted into human breast milk. It does not appear to either suppress lactation or affect the nursing newborn. It is typically given for contraception 3d after delivery since **progesterone** withdrawal may be one stimulus for the initiation of lactogenesis.

■ References —————— Borgatta L, Murthy A, Chuang C, et al. Contraception 2002; 66:169.

Baheiraei A, Ardsetani N, Ghazizadeh S. Int J Gynaecol Obstet 2001; 74:203-5.

FDA Med Bull 1993; 23:6-7.

Ratchanon S, Taneepanichskul S. Obstet Gynecol 2000; 96:926-8.

Carbone JP, Figurska K, Buck S, Brent RL. Teratology 1990; 42:121-30.

Prahalada S, Carroad E, Hendrickx AG. Contraception 1985; 32:497-515.

Danli S, Qingxiang S, Guowei S. Contraception 2000; 62:15-8.

Kennedy KI, Short RV, Tully MR. Contraception 1997; 55:347-50.

■ Summary ——————
- **Pregnancy Category X**
- **Lactation Category S**
- **Medroxyprogesterone** should not be administered during pregnancy.
- First trimester exposure is an indication for a detailed anatomic ultrasound between 18-22w.

Mefenamic acid (Coslan; Ponsfen; Ponstel)

■ Class —————— *Analgesic, non-narcotic, NSAID*

■ Indications —————— Pain, dysmenorrhea, osteoarthritis, rheumatoid arthritis, ankylosing spondylitis, gout

■ Mechanism —————— Inhibits cyclooxygenase and lipoxygenase reducing prostaglandin synthesis

■ Dosage with Qualifiers —————— Pain—50mg PO q4-6h; max 400mg/d
Dysmenorrhea—100mg PO tid; max 6d usage
Osteoarthritis—50-100mg PO tid/qid
Rheumatoid arthritis—50-100mg PO tid/qid
Ankylosing spondylitis—50-100mg PO tid
Gout, acute—100mg PO tid; alternatively 500mg PO, then 250mg PO q6h for not more than 7d
NOTE—take with food or milk
- **Contraindications**—hypersensitivity to drug or class, NSAID-induced asthma
- **Caution**—nasal polyps, GI bleeding, hypertension, cardiac failure, asthma

■ Maternal Considerations —————— **Mefenamic acid** is a nonsteroidal agent with anti-inflammatory, analgesic, and antipyretic action. There are no adequate reports or well-controlled studies of

mefenamic acid in pregnant women. In one small, randomized trial, the prevalence of preterm labor was significantly reduced by **mefenamic acid** compared with placebo. This observation has not subsequently been tested adequately. If the effect of **mefenamic acid** is similar to other NSAIDs, it is unlikely to be effective for the stated indication. **Mefenamic acid** rapidly decreases uterine contractility in women with dysmenorrhea.
Side effects include anaphylaxis, GI bleeding, bronchospasm, renal failure, interstitial nephritis, hepatic failure, Stevens-Johnson syndrome, agranulocytosis, abdominal pain, constipation, headache, dizziness, rash, urticaria, elevated LFTs, drowsiness, edema, tinnitus, rash, lupus and serum sickness-like symptoms.

■ **Fetal Considerations**

There are no adequate reports or well-controlled studies in human fetuses. **Mefenamic acid** crosses the human placenta achieving a F:M ratio approximating 0.32 in the 2nd trimester. There are case reports of ductal closure reported as with other NSAIDs. Rodent studies are reassuring, revealing no evidence of teratogenicity or IUGR despite the use of doses higher than those used clinically. Embryotoxicity is noted in some species. Because of the potential for premature closure of the fetal ductus arteriosus after maternal use of NSAIDs, chronic **mefenamic acid** treatment during pregnancy is not recommended without fetal monitoring.

■ **Breastfeeding Safety**

The trace amounts of **mefenamic acid** excreted into the breast milk pose no clinical risk to the nursing infant.

■ **References**

Adverse Drug Reactions Advisory Committee. Med J Aust 1998; 169:270-1.
Mital P, Garg S, Khuteta RP, et al. J R Soc Health 1992; 112:214-6.
Smith RP, Powell JR. Am J Obstet Gynecol 1982; 143:286-92.
MacKenzie IZ, Graf AK, Mitchell MD. Int J Gynaecol Obstet 1985; 23:455-8.
Buchanan RA, Eaton CJ, Koeff ST, Kinkel AW. Curr Ther Res Clin Exp 1968; 10:592-7.

■ **Summary**

- **Pregnancy Category C**
- **Lactation Category S**
- **Mefenamic acid** should be used during pregnancy and lactation only if the benefit justifies the potential perinatal risk.
- Occasional use during pregnancy appears safe, though continuous use likely has the same adverse effects as other NSAIDs.

Mefloquine (Lariam)

- **Class** ········ *Antiprotozoal*

- **Indications** ········ Malaria (prophylaxis and treatment)

- **Mechanism** ········ Unknown; acts as schizonticide

- **Dosage with Qualifiers** ········ <u>Malaria prophylaxis</u>—250mg PO qw beginning 1w before and continuing until 4w after possible exposure
  <u>Malaria treatment</u>—1250mg PO ×1 followed by treatment with **primaquine**
  NOTE—take with food and water
  - **Contraindications**—hypersensitivity to drug or class, depression, psychosis, serious life-threatening infections
  - **Caution**—seizures, psychiatric disorder, hepatic dysfunction, cardiac conduction diseases, cardiac arrhythmia

- **Maternal Considerations** ········ Malaria remains an important cause of maternal and perinatal morbidity and mortality in endemic countries. *Plasmodium falciparum* drug resistance increasingly limits the effectiveness of antimalarial therapy. **Mefloquine** is the most effective agent for the prevention of chloroquine-resistant falciparum malaria. **Mefloquine** and **quinine** are the only antimalarials generally available for the treatment of drug-resistant P. *falciparum* during pregnancy. Prospective studies show **mefloquine** (25mg/kg) in combination with **artesunate** (4mg/kg/d for 3d) is more effective than **quinine** (10mg/kg q8h) for the treatment of multidrug-resistant falciparum malaria during pregnancy. Many of the adverse effects of **mefloquine** reflect primary hepatic damage or symptomatic thyroid disturbances, which might occur either independently or as a secondary consequence of the hepatocellular injury. *Side effects* include seizures, hallucinations, ECG conduction abnormalities, erythema multiforme, Stevens-Johnson syndrome, encephalopathy, dizziness, syncope, extrasystoles, myalgia, nausea, fever, headache, vomiting, chills, diarrhea, emotional problems, pruritus, asthenia, transient emotional disturbances and hair loss.

- **Fetal Considerations** ········ Prophylactic (250mg/w) **mefloquine** during early pregnancy is not associated with an increased risk of malformations and is not an indication for pregnancy termination. Similarly, 2nd trimester exposure is not associated with adverse reactions. **Mefloquine** is associated with an increased risk of stillbirth but not abortion, IUGR, neurologic retardation, or congenital malformations. Rodent studies reveal that **mefloquine** at high doses is teratogenic and embryotoxic.

- **Breastfeeding Safety** ········· There are no adequate reports or well-controlled studies in nursing women. The detectable amounts of drug identified in the milk of mothers receiving **mefloquine** are too small to be clinically relevant.

- **References** ················· Croft AM, Herxheimer A. BMC Public Health 2002; 2:6.
  No authors. Prescrire Int 2000; 9:180-1.
  Bounyasong S. J Med Assoc Thai 2001; 84:1289-99.
  McGready R, Brockman A, Cho T, et al. Trans R Soc Trop Med Hyg 2000; 94:689-93.
  Nosten F, van Vugt M, Price R, et al. Lancet 2000; 356:297-302.
  Nosten F, Vincenti M, Simpson J, et al. Clin Infect Dis 1999; 28:808-15.
  Rosenblatt JE. Mayo Clin Proc 1999; 74:1161-75.
  Edstein MD, Veenendaal JR, Hyslop R. Chemotherapy 1988; 34:165-9.

- **Summary** ················· • **Pregnancy Category C**
  • **Lactation Category S**
  • **Mefloquine** is the most effective agent for prevention of chloroquine-resistant *falciparum malaria*.
  • Use of **mefloquine** in pregnant women has not been associated with birth defects, but the incidence of stillbirths may be increased. World Health Organization (WHO) favors **mefloquine** prophylaxis in pregnant women from 16w onward.
  • **Mefloquine** should be used during pregnancy and lactation only if the benefit justifies the potential perinatal risk.

Megestrol (Magace; Megace; Niagestine)

- **Class** ················· *Hormone, other gynecologic*

- **Indications** ············· Breast cancer, endometrial cancer (palliative), AIDS (wasting syndrome)

- **Mechanism** ············· Inhibition of pituitary gonadotropin release; stimulates transformation of proliferative endometrium to secretory; antineoplastic

- **Dosage with Qualifiers** ······· Breast cancer—40mg PO qid
  Endometrial cancer palliation—10-80mg PO qid
  AIDS wasting syndrome—800mg PO qd; alternative 400mg PO bid
  • **Contraindications**—hypersensitivity to drug or class, 1st trimester pregnancy
  • **Caution**—recurrent or metastatic cancer, thromboembolic disease

■ **Maternal Considerations**   **Megestrol** is a synthetic, progestational drug. It is used as an implantable contraceptive. There are no adequate reports or well-controlled studies of **megestrol** in pregnant women. Nor are there any indications for its use. Many case reports document successful pregnancy in women with endometrial cancer whose uterus was preserved by **megestrol**. As a treatment for weight loss in cancer patients, **megestrol** should be started only after other treatable causes are sought and addressed.
Side effects include weight increase, thrombophlebitis, pulmonary embolism, adrenal suppression, stroke, abdominal pain, amenorrhea, nausea, vomiting, breast tenderness, weight gain, headache, edema, depression, rash, pruritus, libido changes, appetite changes, acne, hirsutism, alopecia, constipation, and cardiomyopathy.

■ **Fetal Considerations**   There are no adequate reports or well-controlled studies in human fetuses. It is unknown whether **megestrol** crosses the human placenta. There are case reports of abnormalities including hypospadias.

■ **Breastfeeding Safety**   There are no adequate reports or well-controlled studies in nursing women. Small quantities of **megestrol** are excreted into human breast milk. However, **megestrol** has no clinically relevant effect on breast milk when used for contraception.

■ **References**   Lowe MP, Bender D, Sood AK, et al. Fertil Steril 2002; 77:188-9.
Kowalczyk CL, Malone J Jr, Peterson EP, et al. J Reprod Med 1999; 44:57-60.
Abdel-Aleem H, Abol-Oyoun el-S M, Shaaban MM, et al. Contraception 1996; 54:281-6.
Farrar DJ, Aromin I, Uvin SC, et al. Genitourin Med 1997; 73:226.
Lonnerdal B, Forsum E, Hambraeus L. Am J Clin Nutr 1980; 33:816-24.

■ **Summary**
- **Pregnancy Category D (tablet), X (suspension)**
- **Lactation Category S?**
- There are no indications for **megestrol** use during pregnancy.
- **Megestrol** appears compatible with breastfeeding.

Meloxicam

■ **Class** ⸺ NSAID

■ **Indications** ⸺ Osteoarthritis

■ **Mechanism** ⸺ Inhibits PGHS-II

■ **Dosage with Qualifiers** ⸺ Osteoarthritis—7.5-15mg PO qd; max 15mg/d
- **Contraindications**—hypersensitivity to drug or class, NSAID-induced asthma
- **Caution**—nasal polyps, GI bleeding, hypertension, cardiac failure, asthma

■ **Maternal Considerations** ⸺ **Meloxicam** is an NSAID with anti-inflammatory, analgesic, and antipyretic activities. There is no published clinical experience during pregnancy. *In vitro*, **meloxicam** relaxes myometrial strips from pregnant and nonpregnant women, but is less potent than **celecoxib**.
Side effects include anaphylaxis, GI bleeding, bronchospasm, renal failure, interstitial nephritis, hepatic failure, Stevens-Johnson syndrome, agranulocytosis, abdominal pain, constipation, headache, dizziness, rash, urticaria, elevated LFTs, drowsiness, edema, tinnitus, lupus, and serum sickness-like symptoms.

■ **Fetal Considerations** ⸺ There are no adequate reports or well-controlled studies in human fetuses. **Meloxicam** crosses the human placenta. The administration of high doses to rodents is associated with cardiac septal defects and embryotoxicity. RU486-stimulated labor in sheep is associated with fetal HPA activation that is attenuated by **meloxicam** treatment. Because of the potential for premature closure of the fetal ductus arteriosus after maternal use of NSAIDs, chronic **meloxicam** treatment during pregnancy is not recommended without fetal monitoring.

■ **Breastfeeding Safety** ⸺ There is no published experience in nursing women. It is unknown whether **meloxicam** enters human breast milk. It does enter rodent milk.

■ **References** ⸺ Slattery MM, Friel AM, Healy DG, Morrison JJ. Obstet Gynecol 2001; 98:563-9.
Yousif MH, Thulesius O. J Pharm Pharmacol 1998; 50:681-5.
McKeown KJ, Challis JR, Small C, et al. Biol Reprod 2000; 63:1899-904.

■ **Summary** ⸺
- **Pregnancy Category C**
- **Lactation Category U**
- **Meloxicam** should be used during pregnancy and lactation only if the benefit justifies the potential perinatal risk.
- There are alternative agents for which there is more experience regarding use during pregnancy and lactation.

Melphalan (Alkeran)

■ **Class** .... *Antineoplastic, alkylating agent*

■ **Indications** .... Multiple myeloma, ovarian cancer

■ **Mechanism** .... Alkylates and cross-links DNA

■ **Dosage with Qualifiers** ....
<u>Multiple myeloma</u>—varies depending on tumor and protocol
<u>Ovarian cancer</u>—varies depending on tumor and protocol
NOTE—the most commonly recommended dose is
10mg/d ×7-10d. Continuous maintenance therapy with
2mg/d is instituted when the WBC >4000 cells/ml and the
PLT >100,000 cells/ml.
- **Contraindications**—hypersensitivity to drug or class, hypersensitivity to **chlorambucil**, resistance to drug
- **Caution**—renal failure, leukopenia, thrombocytopenia, anemia, leukemia

■ **Maternal Considerations** ....
Melphalan is an alkylating agent. While **methotrexate** is the primary choice for uncomplicated malignant trophoblastic disease, occasional resistance to **methotrexate** requires alternative drug regimens that may include **melphalan** (e.g., **melphalan, actinomycin D,** and **methotrexate**). These regimens are more frequently associated with life-threatening hematologic toxicity compared to those regimens that include **methotrexate**. Women cured of either trophoblastic disease or ovarian cancer (usually stage 1A-C) using a drug regimen that includes **melphalan** can have successful pregnancies. **Melphalan** is also used for the treatment of primary thrombocythemia and for marrow conditioning prior to allogeneic marrow transplantation. There are no adequate and well-controlled studies of **melphalan** in pregnant women. There are only case reports of its use during an ongoing pregnancy.
Side effects include bone marrow suppression, nausea and vomiting, diarrhea, pulmonary fibrosis and interstitial pneumonitis, skin hypersensitivity, vasculitis, alopecia, hemolytic anemia, anaphylaxis, stomatitis, and sterility.

■ **Fetal Considerations** ....
There are no adequate reports or well-controlled studies in human fetuses. It is unknown whether **melphalan** crosses the human placenta. Rodent studies reveal both embryotoxicity and teratogenicity. Anomalies include CNS and skeletal defects.

■ **Breastfeeding Safety** ....
There is no published experience in nursing women. It is unknown whether **melphalan** enters human breast milk.

■ **References** ....
Curry SL, Blessing JA, DiSaia PJ, et al. Obstet Gynecol. 1989; 73:357-62.

Wiqvist N, Lundstrom V, Eneroth P. Acta Obstet Gynecol Scand 1976; 55:275-8.
Schilder JM, Thompson AM, DePriest PD, et al. Gynecol Oncol 2002; 87:1-7.

■ **Summary**
- **Pregnancy Category D**
- **Lactation Category U**
- **Melphalan** is an effective part of multiple drug regimens for the treatment of gestational trophoblastic diseases.
- It should be used during pregnancy and lactation only if the benefit justifies the potential perinatal risk.
- If possible, delay administration to the 2nd trimester.

Mepenzolate (Cantil)

■ **Class** — *Anticholinergic, gastrointestinal*

■ **Indications** — Peptic ulcer disease; adjuvant

■ **Mechanism** — Antagonizes acetylcholine receptors; decreases gastric acid and pepsin secretion

■ **Dosage with Qualifiers** — Gastric ulcer—25-50mg PO qid
- **Contraindications**—hypersensitivity to drug or class, glaucoma, pyloro-duodenal stenosis, achalasia, gastrointestinal hemorrhage, toxic megacolon, myasthenia gravis
- **Caution**—coronary heart disease, CHF, cardiac arrhythmia, tachycardia, hypertension

■ **Maternal Considerations** — There is no published experience with **mepenzolate** during pregnancy.
Side effects include vomiting, nausea, constipation, loss of taste, bloated feeling, dry mouth, tachycardia, palpitations, increased ocular tension, cycloplegia, blurred vision, dizziness, weakness, drowsiness, headache, nervousness, anaphylaxis, and urticaria.

■ **Fetal Considerations** — There are no adequate reports or well-controlled studies in human fetuses. It is unknown whether **mepenzolate** crosses the human placenta. Rodent studies are reassuring, revealing no evidence of teratogenicity or IUGR despite the use of higher doses than those used clinically.

■ **Breastfeeding Safety** — There is no published experience in nursing women. It is unknown whether **mepenzolate** enters human breast milk.

■ **References** — There is no published experience in pregnancy or during lactation.

■ **Summary** ⸺⸺⸺⸺⸺ • **Pregnancy Category B**
• **Lactation Category U**
• **Mepenzolate** should be used during pregnancy and lactation only if the benefit justifies the potential perinatal risk.
• There are alternative agents for which there is more experience regarding use during pregnancy and lactation.

Meperidine (Demerol; Doloneurin)

■ **Class** ⸺⸺⸺⸺⸺⸺⸺⸺ *Narcotic*

■ **Indications** ⸺⸺⸺⸺⸺⸺ Pain, preoperative sedation, obstetric analgesia

■ **Mechanism** ⸺⸺⸺⸺⸺⸺ Binds opioid receptors in the CNS

■ **Dosage with Qualifiers** ⸺⸺ <u>Pain</u>—50-150mg PO/SC/IM q3-4h; IM preferred over SC/IV
<u>Preoperative sedation</u>—50-100mg SC/IM ×1, 30-60min before surgery
<u>Obstetrical analgesia</u>—50-100mg SC/IM/IV q3-4h
Approximately 75mg parenteral **meperidine** = 10mg parenteral **morphine**
NOTE—available in liquid, tablet, and parenteral forms; may be combined with **promethazine**; administer slowly and adjust dose based on CrCl
• **Contraindications**—hypersensitivity to drug or class, MAO inhibitor <14d
• **Caution**—respiratory, hepatic, or renal dysfunction, seizure disorder, head injury, hypothyroidism, atrial flutter, convulsions

■ **Maternal Considerations** ⸺⸺ **Meperidine** is a synthetic narcotic qualitatively similar to **morphine**. It is metabolized to another active form, **normeperidine**. Historically, **meperidine** was perhaps the most commonly used parenteral opioid during labor for pain relief. Well-designed studies demonstrate that the incidence of cesarean delivery in nulliparous women is similar with epidural analgesia to IV **meperidine** but with superior analgesia, less maternal sedation and no need for neonatal **naloxone** as with **meperidine**. **Meperidine** does not *in vitro* have a significant effect on the spontaneous contractions of gravid human uterine muscle. Postoperatively, patient controlled epidural analgesia (PCEA) with **meperidine** offers high-quality pain relief with few side effects.
Side effects include respiratory arrest and depression, cardiac arrest, tachydysrhythmias, dependency, abuse, vomiting, sweating, shock, agitation, disorientation,

euphoria, dysphoria, weakness, dry mouth, constipation, flushing, visual disturbances, constipation, biliary tract spasm, palpitation, hypotension, syncope, pruritus, skin rashes, and pain at the site of injection.

■ **Fetal Considerations** .... **Meperidine** crosses the human placenta. It significantly decreases the number of fetal heart rate accelerations intrapartum, and is associated with insufficient fetomaternal gas exchange and fetal acidemia. **Meperidine** achieves its highest concentration in fetal tissues 2-3h after administration, correlating with the clinical observation that the maximal risk of neonatal depression occurs 2-3h after maternal injection. Respiratory depression requiring resuscitation at delivery is a risk. The interval before neonatal respiration becomes sustained increases if **meperidine** is given more than an hour before delivery. The greater the drug-to-delivery interval, the higher the fetal concentration of **normeperidine,** and the lower the newborn's performance on Brazelton Neonatal Behavioral Assessment Scale. Spontaneous behavior and cognitive performance in exposed rhesus monkeys at 3-12mo of age is altered by **meperidine**.

■ **Breastfeeding Safety** .... **Meperidine** is excreted into human breast milk, with peak levels occurring about 2h after administration. While a single dose of **meperidine** has little impact on the nursing infant, repeated administration negatively affects the newborn. Nursing infants exposed to **morphine** are more alert and oriented than those exposed repeatedly to **meperidine.** This makes **morphine** the preferred narcotic for lactating mothers.

■ **References** .... Solt I, Ganadry S, Weiner Z. Isr Med Assoc J 2002; 4:178-80.
Sharma SK, Alexander JM, Messick G, et al. Anesthesiology 2002; 96:546-51.
Head BB, Owen J, Vincent RD Jr, et al. Obstet Gynecol 2002; 99:452-7.
Yoo KY, Lee J, Kim HS, Jeong SW. Anesth Analg 2001; 92:1006-9.
Sheiner E, Shoham-Vardi I, Sheiner EK, et al. Arch Gynecol Obstet 2000; 263:95-8.
Spigset O, Hagg S. Paediatr Drugs 2000; 2:223-38.
Lurie S, Feinstein M, Heifetz C, Mamet Y. Int J Gynaecol Obstet 1999; 65:125-7.
Gambling DR, Sharma SK, Ramin SM, et al. Anesthesiology 1998; 89:1336-44.
Clark A, Carr D, Loyd G, et al. Am J Obstet Gynecol 1998; 179:1527-33.
Sharma SK, Sidawi JE, Ramin SM, et al. Anesthesiology 1997; 87:487-94.
Ngan Kee WD, Lam KK, Chen PP, Gin T. Anesth Analg 1997; 85:380-4.
Ngan Kee WD, Lam KK, Chen PP, Gin T. Anesthesiology 1996; 85:289-94.

Ramin SM, Gambling DR, Lucas MJ, et al. Obstet Gynecol 1995; 86:783-9.

Paech MJ, Moore JS, Evans SF. Anesthesiology 1994; 80:1268-76.

Vincent RD Jr, Chestnut DH. Am Fam Physician 1998; 58:1785-92.

Chestnut DH. Reg Anesth 1997; 22:495-9.

Wittels B, Glosten B, Faure EA, et al. Anesth Analg 1997; 85:600-6.

Golub MS, Donald JM. Biol Neonate 1995; 67:140-8.

Nguyen Thi TV, Orliaguet G, et al. Reg Anest. 1994; 19:386-9.

Paech MJ, Moore JS, Evans SF. Anesthesiology 1994; 80:1268-76.

Herbst A, Wolner-Hanssen P, Ingemarsson I. Obstet Gynecol 1997; 90:125-30.

Thorp JA, Hu DH, Albin RM, et al. Am J Obstet Gynecol 1993; 169:851-8.

Kariniemi V, Rosti J. J Perinat Med 1986; 14:131-5.

Kuhnert BR, Linn PL, Kennard MJ, Kuhnert PM. Anesth Analg 1985; 64:335-42.

Kuhnert BR, Kuhnert PM, Philipson EH, Syracuse CD. Am J Obstet Gynecol 1985; 151:410-5.

Belfrage P, Boreus LO, Hartvig P, et al. Acta Obstet Gynecol Scand 1981; 60:43-9.

Peiker G, Muller B, Ihn W, Noschel H. Zentralbl Gynakol 1980; 102:537-41.

■ **Summary**

- **Pregnancy Category B**
- **Lactation Category S?**
- There is a long clinical experience with **meperidine** during pregnancy and lactation that is reassuring overall.
- Repeated use during labor leads to the accumulation of **meperidine** and normeperidine in fetal tissues, reaching a maximum about 3h after administration.
- Neonatal depression may occur 2-3h after maternal administration.
- **Morphine** is preferred when postpartum analgesia is required in breastfeeding women.

Mephentermine (Wyamine)

■ **Class** — *Pressor, adrenergic agonist*

■ **Indications** — Hypotension

■ **Mechanism** — Stimulates the release of norepinephrine/epinephrine

■ **Dosage with Qualifiers** — Hypotension shock—1mg/ml IV solution in D_5W; may also be given as a stock solution of 30mg/ml IV ×1

Hypotension spinal anesthesia—15mg IVP ×1; may be repeated in 30min; maintenance of BP accomplished by a continuous infusion of a 0.1% solution of **mephentermine** in D₅W (1mg/ml solution)

NOTE—not distributed in the U.S.

- **Contraindications**—hypersensitivity to drug or class, hypotension induced by **chlorpromazine**, MAO inhibitor <14d
- **Caution**—general anesthesia, CV diseases, hypertension, hyperthyroidism

■ Maternal Considerations

Mephentermine is a synthetic sympathomimetic used for treatment of hypotension. **Mephentermine** increases stroke volume and thus increases both systolic and diastolic blood pressures. There is also a variable degree of peripheral vasoconstriction. **Mephentermine** increases HR by the release of epinephrine. There are no adequate reports or well-controlled studies of **mephentermine** in pregnant women. It was previously used during pregnancy to restore or support uteroplacental blood flow after spinal or epidural analgesia, but has largely been abandoned in favor of **ephedrine**.

Side effects include nervousness, anxiety, arrhythmias, transient extrasystoles, AV block, and hypertension.

■ Fetal Considerations

There are no adequate reports or well-controlled studies in human fetuses. It is unknown whether **mephentermine** crosses the human placenta. Rodent teratogenicity studies have not been performed. Studies in animals and humans reveal fetal hypoxia after **mephentermine** presumably secondary to uterine artery constriction and decreased uterine blood flow. Transient fetal hypertension (mean arterial blood pressure >20% of control) is also reported.

■ Breastfeeding Safety

There is no published experience in nursing women. It is unknown whether **mephentermine sulfate** enters human breast milk.

■ References

Chestnut DH, Ostman LG, Weiner CP, et al. Anesthesiology 1988; 68:363-6.
Lauckner W, Schwarz R, Retzke U. Zentralbl Gynakol 1978; 100:217-21.
Ralston DH, Shnider SM, DeLorimier AA. Anesthesiology 1974; 40:354-70.
Senties L, Arellano G, Casellas A, et al. Am J Obstet Gynecol 1970; 107:892-7.
James FM 3rd, Greiss FC Jr, Kemp RA. Anesthesiology 1970; 33:25-34.

■ Summary

- **Pregnancy Category C**
- **Lactation Category U**
- **Mephentermine** was previously used to prevent hypotensive episodes following spinal and epidural analgesia. It has largely been replaced by **ephedrine**.

Mephenytoin (Mesantoin)

■ **Class**	Anticonvulsant
■ **Indications**	Seizure disorder
■ **Mechanism**	Modulates neuronal voltage-dependent sodium and calcium channels
■ **Dosage with Qualifiers**	Seizure disorder—begin with 50-100mg qd and increase 50-100mg qw until desired effect; max 800mg/d in divided doses • **Contraindications**—hypersensitivity to drug or class • **Caution**—unknown
■ **Maternal Considerations**	Seizure control should be sought prior to pregnancy. **Mephenytoin** should be used only after safer anticonvulsants are given an adequate trial and failed. There are no adequate reports or well-controlled studies of **mephenytoin** in pregnant women. Drug clearance increases between preconception and the 2nd and 3rd trimesters. Thus, many pregnant women require higher doses to maintain therapeutic levels. *Side effects* include leukopenia, thrombocytopenia, agranulocytosis, pancytopenia, neutropenia, neuroleptic malignant syndrome, exfoliative dermatitis, Stevens-Johnson syndrome, pulmonary fibrosis, drowsiness, nausea, vomiting, insomnia, dizziness, alopecia, weight gain, edema, photophobia, conjunctivitis, ataxia, diplopia, nystagmus, dysarthria, fatigue, irritability, choreiform movements, depression, tremor, nervousness, gum hyperplasia, and SLE.
■ **Fetal Considerations**	There are no adequate reports or well-controlled studies in human fetuses. It is unknown whether **mephenytoin** crosses the human placenta. The great majority of mothers on anticonvulsant medication deliver normal infants. Rodent studies suggest that the other hydantoins may not have the same behavioral and teratogenic effects as **phenytoin.**
■ **Breastfeeding Safety**	There is no published experience in nursing women. It is unknown whether **mephenytoin** enters human breast milk.
■ **References**	Minck DR, Acuff-Smith KD, Vorhees CV. Teratology 1991; 43:279-93. Wells PG, Kupfer A, Lawson JA, Harbison RD. J Pharmacol Exp Ther 1982; 221:228-34.
■ **Summary**	• **Pregnancy Category C** • **Lactation Category U** • **Mephenytoin** should be used during pregnancy and lactation only if the benefit justifies the potential perinatal risk.

- **Mephenytoin** should be used only after safer anticonvulsants are given an adequate trial and fail.

Mephobarbital (Mebaral)

- **Class** — Anticonvulsant, barbiturate, sedative/hypnotic

- **Indications** — Seizure disorder (grand mal and petit mal epilepsy), anxiety

- **Mechanism** — Alters sensory cortex, cerebellar and motor activities; induces sedation, hypnosis, and anesthesia

- **Dosage with Qualifiers** — Seizure disorder—400-600mg PO qd
  Anxiety—50mg PO tid/qid
  - **Contraindications**—hypersensitivity to drug or class, porphyria, psychological dependence on barbiturates
  - **Caution**—rickets, osteomalacia, vitamin K or C deficiencies, hepatic dysfunction

- **Maternal Considerations** — Seizure control should be sought prior to pregnancy. There are no adequate reports or well-controlled studies of **mephobarbital** in pregnant women. Clearance is altered by pregnancy and may require frequent adjustment through the puerperium. **Mephobarbital** must be increased in 85% of pregnancies to maintain therapeutic levels. Barbiturates are hepatic enzyme inducers and alter the clearance of many other drugs. *Side effects* include drowsiness, sedation, hypnosis, marked excitement, depression, confusion, respiratory depression, erythema multiforme, Stevens-Johnson syndrome, angioedema, megaloblastic anemia, TTP, urticaria, blood dyscrasias, thrombophlebitis, necrosis, dependence, hepatitis, and swelling.

- **Fetal Considerations** — There are no adequate reports or well-controlled studies in human fetuses. Barbiturates rapidly cross the human placenta reaching F:M ratios approaching unity. Retrospective, case-controlled studies suggested a connection between the maternal consumption of barbiturates and a higher than expected incidence of fetal abnormalities. The great majority of women on anticonvulsant medication deliver normal infants. Rodent teratogenicity studies have not apparently been conducted with **mephobarbital.**

- **Breastfeeding Safety** — There is no published experience in nursing women. It is unknown whether **mephobarbital** enters human breast milk. Small amounts of other barbiturates are excreted.

■ References .... Lander CM, Eadie MJ. Epilepsia 1991; 32:257-66.

■ Summary ....
- **Pregnancy Category D**
- **Lactation Category U**
- **Mephobarbital** should be used during pregnancy and lactation only if the benefit justifies the potential perinatal risk.
- There are alternative agents for which there is more experience during pregnancy and lactation.

Meprobamate (Amosene; Atacin; Disatral; Equanil; Mepriam; Meproban-400; Meprospan; Miltown; Neuramate; Oasil-Simes; Probate; Procalmadiol; Sinanin; Trancot; Tranmep)

■ **Class** .... Anxiolytic

■ **Indications** .... Anxiety

■ **Mechanism** .... Unknown; has effects on multiple CNS sites including thalamus and limbic system

■ **Dosage with Qualifiers** .... Anxiety—400mg PO bid; max 2400mg/d
- **Contraindications**—hypersensitivity to drug or class, alcohol consumption
- **Caution**—job requiring driving or operating machinery

■ **Maternal Considerations** .... There are no adequate reports or well-controlled studies of **meprobamate** in pregnant women. **Meprobamate** decreases clearance of alcohol in rodents during pregnancy.
Side effects include dependence, ataxia, slurred speech, vertigo, anxiety, anorexia, insomnia, vomiting, ataxia, tremors, muscle twitching, confusional states, hallucinosis, convulsive seizures, paresthesias, impairment of visual accommodation, euphoria, overstimulation, paradoxic excitement, palpitation, tachycardia, arrhythmia, transient ECG changes, syncope, hypotension, maculopapular rash, leukopenia, acute nonthrombocytopenic purpura, petechiae, ecchymoses, eosinophilia, peripheral edema, adenopathy, fever, anaphylaxis, exfoliative dermatitis, stomatitis, Stevens-Johnson syndrome, agranulocytosis, aplastic anemia, thrombocytopenic purpura, coma, shock, vasomotor and respiratory collapse.

■ **Fetal Considerations** .... There are no adequate reports or well-controlled studies in human fetuses. **Meprobamate** crosses the human placenta. Several studies suggest an increased prevalence of malformations associated with the 1st trimester use of minor tranquilizers such as **meprobamate**, **chlordiazepoxide**, and **diazepam**. Monotherapy and the lowest effective quantity given in divided doses to minimize the peaks might minimize the risks. While rodent studies reveal that **meprobamate** reduces the learning ability of mature rodent offspring, this effect is not seen in humans.

■ **Breastfeeding Safety** ⋯⋯⋯⋯ The small amount of **meprobamate** entering breast milk and ingested by the nursing newborn (approximately 4% of the weight-adjusted maternal dose) does not pose a clinically significant risk.

■ **References** ⋯⋯⋯⋯⋯⋯⋯⋯ Leonard BE. Arch Toxicol Suppl 1982; 5:48-58.
Rawat AK. Adv Exp Med Biol 1980; 132:561-8.
Belafsky HA, Breslow S, Hirsch LM, et al. Obstet Gynecol 1969; 34:378-86.
Rosenberg JM. NY State J Med 1975; 75:1334-5.
Hartz SC, Heinonen OP, Shapiro S, Siskind V, Slone D. N Engl J Med 1975; 292:726-8.
Nordeng H, Zahlsen K, Spigset O. Ther Drug Monit 2001; 23:298-300.

■ **Summary** ⋯⋯⋯⋯⋯⋯⋯⋯⋯⋯ • **Pregnancy Category D**
• **Lactation Category S**
• **Meprobamate** should be used during pregnancy and lactation only if the benefit justifies the potential perinatal risk.
• It is rarely required during pregnancy and should be avoided at least during the 1st trimester.

Mercaptopurine (Purinethol)

■ **Class** ⋯⋯⋯⋯⋯⋯⋯⋯⋯⋯⋯ *Antineoplastic, antimetabolite; immunomodulatory*

■ **Indications** ⋯⋯⋯⋯⋯⋯⋯⋯ Leukemia (acute lymphocytic and acute myelogenous), Crohn's disease, ulcerative colitis

■ **Mechanism** ⋯⋯⋯⋯⋯⋯⋯⋯ Unknown; multiple biochemical effects leading to cell death

■ **Dosage with Qualifiers** ⋯⋯ Acute lymphocytic leukemia—numerous dosing schedules depending on disease, response and concomitant therapy
Acute myelogenous leukemia—numerous dosing schedules depending on disease, response and concomitant therapy
Crohn's disease—75-125mg PO qd; max 1.5mg/kg/d
Ulcerative colitis—begin with 50mg PO qd; typical dose 75-125mg PO qd; max 1.5mg/kg/d

NOTE—monitor CBC qw ×4 then qmo and LFTs q3mo after induction or during maintenance of remission; discontinue temporarily with evidence of an abnormally large decrease in WBC or platelet count, or Hb concentration
- **Contraindications**—hypersensitivity to drug or class, renal dysfunction
- **Caution**—bone marrow suppression

■ **Maternal Considerations** ⋯⋯⋯ Mercaptopurine and **azathioprine** are the most commonly used immunomodulatory agents. Their clinical effect is probably identical, and both drugs require caution. In addition to the listed indications, **mercaptopurine** is used as an adjunct to prevent organ rejection after transplant. There are no adequate reports or well-controlled studies of **mercaptopurine** in pregnant women. Inflammatory bowel disease can be challenging. Women with quiescent disease are likely to have an uncomplicated pregnancy, whereas those with active disease are more likely to suffer spontaneous abortion, stillbirth, and exacerbation of disease. This is truer for patients with Crohn's disease than those with ulcerative colitis. In women considering pregnancy, an active episode should be treated aggressively and remission accomplished before pregnancy attempted. A woman who unexpectedly conceives while her disease is active should be treated aggressively, as remission provides the greatest hope for a favorable outcome. The treatment of acute myelogenous leukemia typically involves a complex drug regimen that includes **mercaptopurine**. Multiple case reports suggest the use of **mercaptopurine** can produce a complete and sustained remission culminating in the delivery of a normally developed infant.
Side effects include leukopenia, thrombocytopenia, anemia, hepatotoxicity, urate nephropathy, nephrolithiasis, diarrhea, fever, nausea, vomiting, anorexia, jaundice, abdominal pain, anemia, edema, and bleeding.

■ **Fetal Considerations** ⋯⋯⋯⋯ There are no adequate reports or well-controlled studies in human fetuses. It likely crosses the human placenta as transient, but severe neonatal bone marrow hypoplasia is reported. The impact of **mercaptopurine** use during the 1st trimester on development is controversial. Retrospective studies conclude there is no increased prevalence of anomalies. However, a more recent population-based cohort study concluded the risk of malformation is increased more than 6-fold. In a second recent report, the incidence of fetal loss was higher in women with inflammatory bowel disease previously treated with 6-MP compared to those who had not been so treated. Whether this was related to their older age at conception, longer duration of disease, initially more severe disease, or use of 6-MP could not be determined. Although it was suggested **mercaptopurine** increases the risk of spontaneous abortion, it proved a poor abortifacient in one prospective trial. Exposure during the

2nd and 3rd trimesters does affect the fetal immune system, and birthweight may be reduced. Toxic effects on the neonatal pancreas, liver, and lymphocytes are reported. Rodent studies reveal teratogenicity perhaps mediated by DNA modification or drug-induced changes in mineral metabolism (zinc). Malformations include cleft palate, micrognathia and agnathia, microglossia, short limbs, and gut herniation. Zinc supplementation reduces the risk of an adverse effect.

■ **Breastfeeding Safety** There is no published experience in nursing women. It is unknown whether **mercaptopurine** enters human breast milk. Until such data become available, it is perhaps best to avoid immunosuppressive medications while breastfeeding.

■ **References**

Zlatanic J, Korelitz BI, Rajapakse R, et al. J Clin Gastroenterol 2003; 36:303-9.
Norgard B, Pedersen L, Fonager K, Rasmussen SN, Sorensen HT. Aliment Pharmacol Ther 2003; 17:827-34.
Francella A, Dyan A, Bodian C, et al. Gastroenterology 2003; 124:9-17.
Nielsen OH, Vainer B, Rask-Madsen J. Aliment Pharmacol Ther 2001; 15:1699-708.
Rajapakse R, Korelitz BI. Curr Treat Options Gastroenterol 2001; 4:245-51.
Modigliani R. Eur J Gastroenterol Hepatol 1997; 9:854-7.
Ramsey-Goldman R, Schilling E. Rheum Dis Clin North Am 1997; 23:149-67.
Little BB. Semin Perinatol 1997; 21:143-8.
Platzek T, Schwabe R, Rahm U, Bochert G. Chem Biol Interact 1994; 93:59-71.
Davis AR, Miller L, Tamimi H, Gown A. Obstet Gynecol 1999; 93:904-9.
Amemiya K, Keen CL, Hurley LS. Teratology 1986; 34:321-34.
Shah RM, Burdett DN. Can J Physiol Pharmacol 1979; 57:53-8.

■ **Summary**

- **Pregnancy Category D**
- **Lactation Category U**
- **Mercaptopurine** is one of the most commonly used drugs for the treatment of inflammatory bowel disease.
- Women with ulcerative colitis should be advised to conceive when their disease is quiescent.
- **Mercaptopurine** should be used during pregnancy only if the benefit justifies the potential perinatal risk. It is contraindicated during lactation.
- Zinc supplementation may reduce the risk of an adverse perinatal effect.

Meropenem (Merrem IV)

■ **Class** — Antibiotic, *carbapenem*

■ **Indications** — Bacterial infections (<u>gram-positive aerobes</u>: *Streptococcus pneumoniae, Streptococcus viridians* ; <u>gram-negative aerobes</u>: *Escherichia coli, Haemophilus influenzae* [β-lactamase and non-β-lactamase-producing], *Klebsiella pneumoniae, Neisseria meningitidis, Pseudomonas aeruginosa*; <u>anaerobes</u>: *Bacteroides fragilis, Bacteroides thetaiotaomicron, Peptostreptococcus* species), appendicitis, peritonitis, bacterial meningitis

■ **Mechanism** — Bactericidal; inhibits bactericidal cell wall synthesis

■ **Dosage with Qualifiers** — <u>Bacterial infections</u>—appendicitis: 1g IV q8h; peritonitis: 1g IV q8h; bacterial meningitis: 2g IV q8h
NOTE—renal dosing
  • **Contraindications**—hypersensitivity to drug or class, penicillin allergy
  • **Caution**—seizure disorder, renal dysfunction

■ **Maternal Considerations** — There are no adequate reports or well-controlled studies of **meropenem** in pregnant women. One multicenter study concluded **meropenem** is an effective and safe alternative to **clindamycin/gentamicin** for the treatment of women with acute obstetric infections. There is a case report of its successful use to treat pyogenic sacroilitis in pregnancy. *Side effects* include seizures, C. *difficile* colitis, pain, abdominal pain, chest pain, sepsis, shock, fever, abdominal enlargement, back pain, hepatic failure, CHF, tachycardia, hypertension, MI, pulmonary embolus, bradycardia, hypotension, syncope, anemia, peripheral edema, hypoxia, insomnia, agitation, delirium, confusion, dizziness, seizure, renal failure, dysuria, dyspnea, injection site reaction, rash, pruritus, and constipation.

■ **Fetal Considerations** — There are no adequate reports or well-controlled studies in human fetuses. It is unknown whether **meropenem** crosses the human placenta. Rodent and monkey studies are reassuring, revealing no evidence of teratogenicity or IUGR despite the use of doses higher than those used clinically.

■ **Breastfeeding Safety** — There is no published experience in nursing women. It is unknown whether **meropenem** enters human breast milk.

■ **References** — Chimura T, Banzai M, Yamakawa M, et al. Jpn J Antibiot 2001; 54:491-6.
Chimura T, Murayama K, Oda T, et al. Jpn J Antibiot 2001; 54:1-7.
Hemsell DL, Martens MG, Faro S, et al. Clin Infect Dis 1997; 24(Suppl 2):S222-30.

■ **Summary**
- **Pregnancy Category B**
- **Lactation Category U**
- **Meropenem** should be used during pregnancy and lactation only if the benefit justifies the potential perinatal risk.
- There are alternative agents for which there is more experience with during pregnancy and lactation.

Mesalamine (Asacol; Pentasa; Rowasa)

■ **Class** — Gastrointestinal, salicylate

■ **Indications** — Ulcerative colitis, Crohn's disease

■ **Mechanism** — Unknown

■ **Dosage with Qualifiers** — Ulcerative colitis—1000mg PO qid ×8w; alternatively, rectal dosing 4g qh ×3-6w
Crohn's disease—1000mg PO qid ×8w
- **Contraindications**—hypersensitivity to drug or class, hypersensitivity to salicylates
- **Caution**—renal or hepatic dysfunction, pyloric stenosis, bowel movement suppressants

■ **Maternal Considerations** — Inflammatory bowel disease can be challenging. Women with quiescent disease are likely to have an uncomplicated pregnancy, whereas those with active disease are more likely to suffer spontaneous abortion, stillbirth, and exacerbation of disease. This is truer for patients with Crohn's disease than those with ulcerative colitis. In women considering pregnancy, an active episode should be treated aggressively and remission accomplished before pregnancy attempted. A woman who unexpectedly conceives while her disease is active should be treated aggressively, as remission provides the greatest hope for a favorable outcome. **Mesalamine** is a byproduct of **5-aminosalicylic acid** bound to **sulfapyridine.** Most patients with adverse effects from **sulfasalazine** will tolerate **mesalamine. Mesalamine** is at least equivalent or superior to **sulfasalazine**, and superior to placebo, with a dose-response benefit, in inducing remission of acute inflammatory bowel disease. It is also comparable to **sulfasalazine** and superior to placebo for long-term maintenance of remission.
Side effects include bloody diarrhea, fever, headache, rash, anaphylaxis, thrombocytopenia, leukopenia, anemia, agranulocytosis, interstitial nephritis, peptic ulcer, nephropathy, myocarditis, hepatitis, peripheral neuropathy, Stevens-Johnson syndrome, headache,

abdominal pain, dyspepsia, nausea, vomiting, flatulence, constipation, asthenia, diarrhea, back pain, arthralgia, rhinitis, dry mouth, elevated LFTs, elevated BUN, elevated creatinine, dysmenorrhea, hair loss, and flu-like symptoms.

■ **Fetal Considerations** ············· There are no adequate reports or well-controlled studies in human fetuses. While it is unknown whether **mesalamine** crosses the human placenta, only trace amounts of the active metabolite, **5-aminosalicylic acid** can be found in the fetus. Rodent studies are reassuring, revealing no evidence of teratogenicity or IUGR despite the use of doses higher than those used clinically. Perhaps the greatest threat to a normal conception is active disease. Ulcerative colitis is associated with decreased birthweight (−330g, adjusted 95% CI: −509 to −150g, p <0.001); the birthweight is even lower if **mesalamine** or steroids are required.

■ **Breastfeeding Safety** ············· There are no adequate reports or well-controlled studies in nursing women. While it is unknown whether **mesalamine** enters human breast milk, only trace amounts of its active metabolite, **5-aminosalicylic acid** are excreted.

■ **References** ············· Schroeder KW. Scand J Gastroenterol Suppl 2002; 236:42-7.
Stein RB, Hanauer SB. Drug Saf 2000; 23:429-48.
Saubermann LJ, Wolf JL. Inflamm Bowel Dis 1999; 5:148-9.
Marteau P, Tennenbaum R, Elefant E, et al. Aliment Pharmacol Ther 1998; 12:1101-8.
Diav-Citrin O, Park YH, Veerasuntharam G, et al. Gastroenterology 1998; 114:23-8.
Ludvigsson JF, Ludvigsson J. Acta Paediatr 2002; 91:145-51.
Bell CM, Habal FM. Am J Gastroenterol 1997; 92:2201-2.
Ambrosius Christensen L, Rasmussen SN, Hansen SH, et al. Acta Obstet Gynecol Scand 1987; 66:433-5.
Christensen LA, Rasmussen SN, Hansen SH. Acta Obstet Gynecol Scand 1994; 73:399-402.
Jenss H, Weber P, Hartmann F. Am J Gastroenterol 1990; 85:331.
Mulder CJ, Tytgat GN, Weterman IT, et al. Gastroenterology 1988; 95:1449-53.

■ **Summary** ·············
● **Pregnancy Category B**
● **Lactation Category S**
● **Mesalamine** is a first-line agent for the treatment of inflammatory bowel disease during pregnancy.
● **Mesalamine** does not appear to pose a teratogenic risk when used at recommended doses.

Mesoridazine (Serentil)

■ **Class** — Antipsychotic, phenothiazine

■ **Indications** — Anxiety, alcoholism

■ **Mechanism** — Unknown; dopamine D_2 antagonist

■ **Dosage with Qualifiers** — Anxiety—30-150mg PO qd; max 150mg/d
Alcoholism—begin 25mg PO bid; max 200mg/d
- **Contraindications**—hypersensitivity to drug or class, cardiac arrhythmia, CNS depression, coma, prolonged QT interval, arrhythmia, hypotension, glaucoma, paralytic ileus, GI obstruction, bone marrow depression
- **Caution**—renal or hepatic dysfunction, CV disease, Parkinson's disease, seizure disorder, CNS depression

■ **Maternal Considerations** — Because of its proarrhythmic effect, **mesoridazine** is indicated for the management of schizophrenic patients who first fail to respond adequately to other antipsychotic drugs. There are no adequate reports or well-controlled studies of **mesoridazine** in pregnant women.
Side effects include thrombocytopenia, leukopenia, aplastic anemia, agranulocytosis, neuroleptic malignant syndrome, dystonia, fever, laryngeal edema, angioneurotic edema, asthma, ECG QT interval prolongation, torsades de pointes, arrhythmia, nausea, vomiting, jaundice, biliary stasis, blurred vision, rash, tachycardia, tardive dyskinesia, phototoxicity, miosis, anorexia, and sudden death.

■ **Fetal Considerations** — There are no adequate reports or well-controlled studies in human fetuses. It is unknown whether **mesoridazine** crosses the human placenta. Rodent teratogenicity studies have not been performed.

■ **Breastfeeding Safety** — There is no published experience in nursing women. It is unknown whether **mesoridazine** enters human breast milk.

■ **References** — No published experience in pregnancy or during lactation.

■ **Summary** —
- **Pregnancy Category C**
- **Lactation Category U**
- **Mesoridazine** should be used during pregnancy and lactation only if the benefit justifies the potential perinatal risk.
- There are alternative agents for which there is more experience regarding use during pregnancy and lactation.

Mestranol (Genora; Micronor; Nelova; Norethin; Norinyl; Ortho-Novum)

■ **Class**	Hormone
■ **Indications**	Contraception, dysmenorrhea, dysfunctional uterine bleeding, endometriosis, polycystic ovary syndrome
■ **Mechanism**	Inhibits gonadotropin release leading to anovulation and changes in the proprieties of cervical mucus and endometrium
■ **Dosage with Qualifiers**	Contraception—1 tab PO qd Dysmenorrhea—1 tab PO qd Dysfunctional uterine bleeding—1 tab PO qd Endometriosis—1 tab PO qd Polycystic ovary syndrome—1 tab PO qd NOTE—combined with **norethindrone** • **Contraindications**—hypersensitivity to drug or class, pregnancy, hepatic carcinoma, smoker >35 years of age, undiagnosed vaginal bleeding, breast cancer, endometrial cancer, CAD, stroke, history of hepatic dysfunction, or a history of cholestatic jaundice with other OCPs or pregnancy • **Caution**—hepatic dysfunction, diabetes, hyperlipidemia, depression, breastfeeding, migraine
■ **Maternal Considerations**	**Mestranol** is the estrogen component of several popular oral contraceptives. The use of OCs containing **mestranol** is causally related to an increased incidence of benign liver adenomas and a decreased incidence of benign breast disease. These adenomas are not necessarily worsened by pregnancy. There is sufficient evidence in experimental animals to conclude **mestranol** is a potential carcinogen. Other estrogens are implicated as human carcinogens. It is now well recognized that there are differences in the physiologic responses to native and synthetic estrogens. There is no indication for **mestranol** during pregnancy and lactation. *Side effects* include thromboembolism, MI, stroke, hypertension, cholestatic jaundice, hepatic adenoma, nausea, vomiting, abdominal pain, bloating, changes in menstrual flow, amenorrhea, breast tenderness, edema, migraine, weight changes, cervical secretions changes, emotional lability, headache, breakthrough bleeding, vaginal candidiasis, acne, rash, and glucose intolerance.
■ **Fetal Considerations**	There are no adequate reports or well-controlled studies in human fetuses. The observation that maternal administration of **mestranol** inhibits **testosterone** synthesis in the rodent fetal testes suggests it crosses the rodent placenta. Limited rodent studies are otherwise reassuring, revealing no evidence of teratogenicity after early pregnancy exposure.

There are no adequate reports or well-controlled studies in nursing women. **Mestranol** enters human breast milk, though the kinetics remains to be detailed. Lactation and infant weight gain is reduced when **mestranol** is given during the immediate postpartum period. As a result, it is generally considered incompatible with breastfeeding until the milk reflex is well established.

■ **References** Vido I, Cepicky P. Cesk Gynekol 1989; 54:654-61.
Varma SK, Bloch E. Acta Endocrinol 1987; 116:193-9.
Christensen SE, Andersen VR, Vilstrup H. Acta Obstet Gynecol Scand 1981; 60:519.
Wallace ME, Badr FM, Badr RS. J Med Genet 1979; 16:206-9.

■ **Summary**
- **Pregnancy Category X**
- **Lactation Category NS**
- **Mestranol** is an effective contraceptive when combined with a progestational agent.
- There are no indications during pregnancy for its use.

Metaproterenol (Alupent; Arm-A-Med; Dey-Dose; Metaprel; Prometa)

■ **Class** *Adrenergic agonist, bronchodilator*

■ **Indications** Asthma

■ **Mechanism** β-2 adrenergic agonist

■ **Dosage with Qualifiers** Asthma—2-3 puffs INH q3-4h; max 12 puffs/d; or 0.2-0.3ml 5% sol NEB q4h; or 20mg PO tid/qid
NOTE—available for inhalation, and for PO as a tablet or syrup
- **Contraindications**—hypersensitivity to drug or class, arrhythmia, tachycardia, hyperthyroidism, seizure disorder
- **Caution**—hypertension, hypokalemia, heart disease, diabetes, cirrhosis, concomitant use of cardiac glycosides

■ **Maternal Considerations** **Metaproterenol** is a bronchodilator popular during pregnancy for the treatment of asthma. Similar to other betamimetic agents, **metaproterenol** increases pulse, lowers blood pressure, and alters the ECG pattern. There are no adequate reports or well-controlled studies of **metaproterenol** in pregnant women. It has been used as a tocolytic agent (a.k.a. **fenoterol, partusisten**), but there is no evidence its provides any unique advantage. *In vitro*, β-2 adrenergic agonists are equally potent inhibiting myometrial contractility as **nitroglycerin**. There are only case reports of its use during pregnancy in asthmatic women requiring ICU admission. **Metaproterenol**-saline solution irrigation is used for bronchoalveolar lavage to facilitate restoration of the bronchial function.

Side effects include tachycardia, nervousness, cardiac arrest, tremor, headache, palpitation, nausea, vomiting, dizziness, asthma exacerbation, insomnia, and diarrhea.

■ Fetal Considerations

There are no adequate reports or well-controlled studies in human fetuses. While it is unknown whether **metaproterenol** crosses the human placenta, other betamimetic agents do. In rabbits, **metaproterenol** is a teratogen given at doses more than 50 times the MRHD; there is no adverse effect on other rodents. Studies in animals and humans reveal no evidence that β-2 adrenergic agonists pose a cardiovascular risk for the fetus and neonate. It may be that β-2 adrenoreceptor ontogenesis is completed near term.

■ Breastfeeding Safety

There is no published experience in nursing women. It is unknown whether **metaproterenol** enters human breast milk.

■ References

David M, Hamann C, Chen FC, et al. J Perinat Med 2000; 28:232-42.
Ivanov S. Akush Ginekol 1997; 36:9-10.
Kast A, Hermer M. J Perinat Med 1993; 2:97-106.
Schreier L, Cutler RM, Saigal V. Am J Obstet Gynecol 1989; 160:80-1.

■ Summary

- **Pregnancy Category C**
- **Lactation Category U**
- **Metaproterenol** is an effective bronchodilator for women with bronchial asthma and reversible bronchospasm.
- **Metaproterenol** should be used during pregnancy and lactation only if the benefit justifies the potential perinatal risk.

Metaraminol (Aramine)

- **Class** — *Adrenergic agonist*

- **Indications** — Shock

- **Mechanism** — Mixed α- and β-1 adrenergic agonist

- **Dosage with Qualifiers** — Shock—0.5-5mg IV
  - **Contraindications**—hypersensitivity to drug or class, general anesthesia with **halothane** or **cyclopropane**
  - **Caution**—CV disease, thyroid disease, diabetes, history of malaria

- **Maternal Considerations** — **Metaraminol** is a potent sympathomimetic that increases both systolic and diastolic pressures. There are no adequate reports or well-controlled studies of **metaraminol** in pregnant women. **Metaraminol** has been used to maintain arterial pressure during spinal anesthesia before cesarean delivery, and for cardiovascular support in women with septic shock. *In vitro*, **metaraminol** is a more potent constrictor of the uterine arteries than **ephedrine**. The effect is more pronounced in uterine compared to femoral arteries. For that reason, many prefer **ephedrine** prior to spinal anesthesia. However, a recent randomized controlled trial suggests **metaraminol** given as a continuous infusion provides a superior clinical result compared to a continuous infusion of **ephedrine.** Confirmation of this study would be helpful.
  Side effects include cardiac arrest, pulmonary edema, hypertension, seizures, arrhythmia, cerebral hemorrhage, anxiety, restlessness, dizziness, headache, nausea, vomiting, flushing, pallor, and sweating.

- **Fetal Considerations** — There are no adequate reports or well-controlled studies in human fetuses. It is unknown whether **metaraminol** crosses the human placenta. Rodent teratogenicity studies have not been performed. Fetal bradycardia or late decelerations are well-recognized complications of untreated spinal/epidural analgesia induced hypotension. They are a product of hypotension secondary to peripheral sympathetic blockade. In studies of spinal anesthesia, **metaraminol** treated pregnancies may have a lower incidence of neonatal acidosis compared to **ephedrine.**

- **Breastfeeding Safety** — There is no published experience in nursing women. It is unknown whether **metaraminol** enters human breast milk. However, considering the dose and route, it is unlikely the breast-fed neonate would ingest clinically relevant amounts.

- **References** — Ngan Kee WD, Khaw KS, Lee BB, et al. Br J Anaesth 2001; 87:772-4.

Ngan Kee WD, Khaw KS, Lee BB, et al. Anesth Analg 2001; 93:703-8.
Ngan Kee WD, Lau TK, Khaw KS, Lee BB. Anesthesiology 2001; 95:307-13.
Tong C, Eisenach JC. Anesthesiology 1992; 76:792-8.
James FM 3rd, Greiss FC Jr, Kemp RA. Anesthesiology 1970; 33:25-34.
Cavanagh D, McLeod AG. Am J Obstet Gynecol 1966; 96:913-8.
Speroff L. Am J Obstet Gynecol 1966; 95:139-51.

■ Summary
- **Pregnancy Category C**
- **Lactation Category S?**
- **Metaraminol** effectively maintains arterial pressure during spinal/epidural analgesia.

Metaxalone (Skelaxin)

■ **Class** — Muscle relaxant

■ **Indications** — Muscle spasm

■ **Mechanism** — Unknown

■ **Dosage with Qualifiers** — Muscle spasm—800mg PO tid/qid on an empty stomach
- **Contraindications**—hypersensitivity to drug or class, hemolytic anemia
- **Caution**—renal or hepatic dysfunction

■ **Maternal Considerations** — There is no published experience during pregnancy. **Side effects** include hemolytic anemia, leukopenia, hepatotoxicity, dizziness, drowsiness, lightheadedness, paradoxical stimulation, abdominal pain, nausea, vomiting, headache, and nervousness.

■ **Fetal Considerations** — There are no adequate reports or well-controlled studies in human fetuses. It is unknown whether **metaxalone** crosses the human placenta. Rodent teratogenicity studies have not been performed. Post-marketing surveys do not suggest any increase in adverse fetal outcomes.

■ **Breastfeeding Safety** — There is no published experience in nursing women. It is unknown whether **metaxalone** enters human breast milk.

■ **References** — There is no published experience in pregnancy or during lactation.

■ **Summary** ──────────────── • **Pregnancy Category C**
• **Lactation Category U**
• **Metaxalone** should be used during pregnancy and lactation only if the benefit justifies the potential perinatal risk.
• There are alternative agents for which there is more experience during pregnancy and lactation.

Metformin (Glucophage; Glucophage XR)

■ **Class** ──────────────── Hypoglycemic, biguanide

■ **Indications** ──────────────── Diabetes mellitus type 2, polycystic ovary syndrome

■ **Mechanism** ──────────────── Increases insulin sensitivity, decreases hepatic glucose production and intestinal glucose absorption; decrease serum insulin and androgen levels

■ **Dosage with Qualifiers** ──────────────── Diabetes mellitus—begin 850mg PO qd or 500mg PO bid; usual dose 850mg PO bid; max 2550mg/d. Alternatively, XR format; 500mg PO qd with evening meal, increase 500mg qw up to 2000mg qd.
Polycystic ovary syndrome—500mg PO tid
NOTE—renal dosing; hold for iodinated contrast study
• **Contraindications**—hypersensitivity to drug or class, renal or hepatic dysfunction, metabolic acidosis, CHF, acute MI, concurrent use of iodinated contrast
• **Caution**—pulmonary disease, hepatic dysfunction

■ **Maternal Considerations** ──────────────── **Metformin** is an insulin-sensitizing agent effective in women with PCOS who have significant insulin resistance. PCOS is one of the most common endocrinopathies with approximately 5% of women being affected. Seventy percent of those women taking only **metformin** and who ovulate conceive in less than 6mo. **Metformin** also improves the outcome of *in vitro* fertilization in women with **clomiphene**-resistant PCOS. There are no adequate reports or well-controlled studies of **metformin** in pregnant women. **Metformin** therapy in women with PCOS is associated with a decreased rate of spontaneous abortions and an approximately 10-fold reduction in the incidence of gestational diabetes. **Metformin** and **glibenclamide** are proposed as alternatives to **insulin** in controlling gestational diabetes. Their use remains exciting but investigational.
Side effects include flatulence, diarrhea, nausea, vomiting, asthenia, indigestion, abdominal discomfort, headache, megaloblastic anemia, anorexia, altered taste, and rash.

■ Fetal Considerations

There are no adequate reports or well-controlled studies in human fetuses. It is unknown whether **metformin** crosses the human placenta. It does not limit placental glucose uptake and transport in the isolated cotyledon perfusion model. In limited clinical study, **metformin** was not teratogenic, and did not adversely affect birthweight, height, weight, motor and social development at 3 and 6mo of life. Newborns of women who had their serum glucose levels controlled by **metformin** do not develop hypoglycemic episodes more frequently than newborns delivered of women treated by **insulin** alone. Rodent studies are reassuring, revealing no evidence of teratogenicity or IUGR despite the use of doses higher than those used clinically. There is evidence of poor placental transport in the rat.

■ Breastfeeding Safety

Only 0.28% of the weight-normalized maternal dose of **metformin** enters human breast milk. In rodents, the **metformin** concentration in milk approaches that of the maternal plasma. This is well below the 10% level usually expected for the concentration to have a clinical impact.

■ References

Stadtmauer LA, Toma SK, Riehl RM, Talbert LM. Reprod Biomed Online 2002; 5:112-6.
Glueck CJ, Wang P, Goldenberg N, Sieve-Smith L. Hum Reprod 2002; 17:2858-64.
Legro RS. Minerva Ginecol 2002; 54:97-114.
Seli E, Duleba AJ. Curr Opin Obstet Gynecol 2002; 14:245-54.
Heard MJ, Pierce A, Carson SA, Buster JE. Fertil Steril 2002; 77:669-73.
Glueck CJ, Wang P, Kobayashi S, et al. Fertil Steril 2002; 77:520-5.
Phipps WR. Obstet Gynecol Clin North Am 2001; 28:165-82.
Elliott BD, Langer O, Schuessling F. Am J Obstet Gynecol 1997; 176:527-30.
Glueck CJ, Phillips H, Cameron D, et al. Fertil Steril 2001; 75:46-52.
Coetzee EJ, Jackson WP. Diabetes Res Clin Pract 1986; 1:281-7.
Coetzee EJ, Jackson WP. S Afr Med J 1984; 65:635-7.
Hale TW, Kristensen JH, Hackett LP, et al. Diabetologia 2002; 45:1509-14.

■ Summary

- **Pregnancy Category B**
- **Lactation Category S**
- **Metformin** therapy throughout pregnancy in women with PCOS reduces the high rate of 1st trimester spontaneous abortion and gestational diabetes.
- Further studies are necessary to determine whether metformin and other hypoglycemic agents will be safe and effective in women with gestational diabetes.

Methacholine (Provocholine)

- **Class** — _Cholinergic, diagnostic, nonradioactive_

- **Indications** — Diagnosis of bronchial airway hyperreactivity

- **Mechanism** — Stimulates cholinergic receptors

- **Dosage with Qualifiers** — <u>Diagnosis of bronchial airway hyperreactivity</u>—5 breaths (neb); measure FEV_1 at baseline and after 5 breaths
  NOTE—diagnostic purpose only. **Methacholine** inhalation challenge should be performed only under the supervision of a physician trained in and throughly familiar with all aspects of the technique.
  - **Contraindications**—hypersensitivity to drug or class, asthma, concurrent usage of β-blocker, FEV<70 %
  - **Caution**—cardiovascular disease, epilepsy, thyroid disease

- **Maternal Considerations** — **Methacholine** is the β-methyl homolog of acetylcholine and differs primarily in its greater duration and selectivity. It is more slowly hydrolyzed by acetylcholinesterase and is almost totally resistant to nonspecific cholinesterase or pseudocholinesterase inactivation. There are no adequate reports or well-controlled studies of **methacholine** in pregnant women. Pregnancy is associated with an improvement in airway responsiveness in asthmatic women.
  Side effects include respiratory distress, headache, lightheadedness, chest tightness, dyspnea, cough, throat irritation, wheezing, and pruritus.

- **Fetal Considerations** — There are no adequate reports or well-controlled studies in human fetuses. Rodent teratogenicity studies have not been conducted. Based on its physiologic actions, it is unlikely limited exposure to **methacholine** during a diagniostic procedure would pose a significant risk to the fetus.

- **Breastfeeding Safety** — There is no published experience in nursing women. It is unknown whether **methacholine** enters human breast milk. However, considering the dose and route, it is unlikely the breast-fed neonate would ingest clinically relevant amounts.

- **References** — Juniper EF, Daniel EE, Roberts RS, et al. Am Rev Respir Dis 1989; 140:924-31.

- **Summary** —
  - **Pregnancy Category C**
  - **Lactation Category S?**
  - **Methacholine** should be used during pregnancy and lactation only if the benefit justifies the potential perinatal risk.

Methadone (Dolophine; Dolophine HCL; Methadone HCl; Methadose; Tussol; Westadone)

■ **Class** ⋯⋯⋯⋯⋯⋯⋯⋯⋯ *Analgesic, narcotic*

■ **Indications** ⋯⋯⋯⋯⋯⋯⋯ Pain, opiate addiction

■ **Mechanism** ⋯⋯⋯⋯⋯⋯⋯ Partial opiate-receptor agonist

■ **Dosage with Qualifiers** ⋯⋯ Pain—2.5-10mg PO q3-4h
Opiate addiction—15-20mg PO qd; max 120mg qd
Opiate addiction maintenance—20-120mg PO qd
NOTE—equianalgesic: PO = 2 × IV dose
- **Contraindications**—hypersensitivity to drug or class
- **Caution**—renal or hepatic dysfunction, hypothyroidism, Addison's disease, acute abdominal pain, concomitant use of **rifampin**, **pentazocin**, **desipramine**, or **MAO inhibitors**, acute abdominal pain

■ **Maternal Considerations** ⋯⋯ **Methadone** is a synthetic narcotic analgesic with many actions quantitatively similar to **morphine** except its intense euphoria. **Methadone** is a first-line agent for the treatment of heroin addiction. The goal of maintenance is to relieve the narcotic craving, suppress withdrawal, and block the euphoric effects associated with **heroin**. The majority of patients require 80-120mg/d or more. Treatment continues for an indefinite period of time. Illicit drug use during pregnancy is a major perinatal health issue worldwide. Some 200,000 addicted infants are born each year in the U.S. Because most drug-addicted women use a variety of illicit agents, the impact of **methadone** alone is difficult to ascertain. The practice of placing all **heroin** users on **methadone** during pregnancy perhaps needs to be revisited. While suitable for those women who stabilize their illicit **heroin** use at or shortly after conception, its advisability for women who show little desire or likelihood of moving away from regular **heroin** use and its associated lifestyle is questionable. **Methadone** is nonsedating and safe during pregnancy. A major problem with opiate-addicted women is postoperative pain management. It is generally recommended that **methadone** treatment be continued while short-acting narcotics are given as necessary (preferably on a fixed schedule) to relieve the pain. Opiate antagonists must be avoided. The elimination rate constant of **methadone** is higher and the half-life lower during pregnancy, perhaps because of a decrease in the fraction absorbed. **Methadone** is not recommended for obstetric analgesia because its long duration of action increases the probability of neonatal respiratory depression.
Side effects include euphoria, dysphoria, weakness, insomnia, agitation, visual disturbances, headache,

disorientation, seizures, shock, cardiac arrest, respiratory depression or arrest, dizziness, sedation, nausea, vomiting, sweating, dry mouth, flushing, urinary retention, rash, and thrombocytopenia.

■ **Fetal Considerations** — Women (and rodents) who continue **heroin** use throughout pregnancy have a greater likelihood of preterm birth and IUGR. Infants whose mothers are on **methadone** maintenance have higher mean birth weights and head circumferences than those of untreated addicted women. It is not associated with respiratory depression. However, the withdrawal is more intense in the **methadone**-treated group compared to **heroin**-exposed babies without **methadone** treatment (convulsions 47.1% vs. 27.1%). Maternal **methadone** dosage is related to the duration of neonatal hospitalization, neonatal abstinence score, and treatment for withdrawal. Heroin supplementation does not alter this dose-response relationship. In selected pregnancies, lowering the maternal **methadone** dose is associated with both decreased incidence and severity of neonatal withdrawal. **Methadone** does not appear detrimental for fetal brain development. Some reports suggest an increased incidence of SIDS in neonates delivered of mothers who use **methadone** during pregnancy. This association may be more circumstantial.

■ **Breastfeeding Safety** — Only small quantities of **methadone** are excreted into human breast milk. It is estimated the average newborn would ingest only 0.05mg **methadone** per day, an amount too small to reliably prevent neonatal withdrawal. The risk of an adverse event with either breastfeeding or weaning is low. Pregnant women on methadone maintenance therapy are to be encouraged to nurse if they are HIV-negative.

■ **References** —
Langlois NE, Ellis PS, Little D, Hulewicz B. Am J Forensic Med Pathol 2002; 23:162-6.
Hulse GK, O'Neill G. Aust NZ J Obstet Gynaecol 2001; 41:329-32.
Sinha C, Ohadike P, Carrick P, et al. Int J Gynaecol Obstet 2001; 74:241-6.
Gressens P, Mesples B, Sahir N, et al. Semin Neonatol 2001; 6:185-94.
Scimeca MM, Savage SR, Portenoy R, Lowinson J. Mt Sinai J Med 2000; 67:412-22.
Joseph H, Stancliff S, Langrod J. Mt Sinai J Med 2000; 67:347-64.
Dashe JS, Sheffield JS, Olscher DA, et al. Obstet Gynecol 2002; 100:1244-9.
McCarthy JJ, Posey BL. J Hum Lact 2000; 16:115-20.
Ziegler M, Poustka F, von Loewenich V, Englert E. Nervenarzt 2000; 71:730-6.
Sarman I. Lakartidningen 2000; 97:2182-4, 2187-8, 2190.
Jarvis MA, Wu-Pong S, Kniseley JS, Schnoll SH. J Addict Dis 1999; 18:51-61.
Begg EJ, Malpas TJ, Hackett LP, Ilett KF. Br J Clin Pharmacol 2001; 52:681-5.

Geraghty B, Graham EA, Logan B, Weiss EL. J Hum Lact 1997; 13:227-30.
Kunko PM, Smith JA, Wallace MJ, et al. J Pharmacol Exp Ther 1996; 277:1344-51.
Pierson PS, Howard P, Kleber HD. JAMA 1972; 220:1733-4.

■ **Summary**

- **Pregnancy Category B**
- **Lactation Category S**
- **Methadone** maintenance is not a curative treatment for heroin addiction and should be undertaken only in specialized centers.
- **Methadone** maintenance reduces and/or eliminates the use of heroin, reduces the death rates and criminality associated with heroin use, and allows patients to improve their health and social productivity.
- Enrollment in a **methadone** maintenance program has the potential to reduce the transmission of infectious diseases associated with heroin injection.

Methamphetamine (Desoxyn; Methampex)

■ **Class**

Anorexiant, CNS *stimulant, amphetamine*

■ **Indications**

Attention-deficit disorder, weight loss, narcolepsy

■ **Mechanism**

Appetite suppression and CNS stimulation

■ **Dosage with Qualifiers**

Attention-deficit disorder—20-25mg PO qd
Weight loss—5-10mg PO tid; treatment should not exceed few weeks
Narcolepsy—5-60mg/d in divided doses
- **Contraindications**—hypersensitivity to drug or class, glaucoma, arteriosclerosis, cardiovascular disease, severe hypertension, hyperthyroidism, agitation, drug abuse
- **Caution**—hypertension

■ **Maternal Considerations**

Methamphetamine is a CNS stimulant that has no medical indications during pregnancy. The illicit use of **methamphetamine**, also called *crystal, meth,* or *speed* is a major health care problem in some locales. It may be injected, smoked, snorted, or ingested orally. Prolonged use leads to dependence. The use of a variant of methamphetamine, Ecstasy (3,4-methylenedioxymethamphetamine) is also becoming more common during pregnancy. Maternal death is associated with usage. Ecstasy users during pregnancy tend to be young, single, report psychological morbidity, have a higher rate of unplanned pregnancies, and a higher likelihood of using other potentially harmful substances (smoking, heavy alcohol intake, and polydrug usage).

Side effects include tachycardia, palpitation, dizziness, dysphoria, overstimulation, euphoria, insomnia, tremor, restlessness, headache, diarrhea, constipation, dry mouth, unpleasant taste, urticaria, decreased libido, stroke, cardiac arrhythmia, stomach cramps, shaking, anxiety, insomnia, paranoia, hallucinations, structural changes to the brain, and suppression of growth.

■ **Fetal Considerations**

There are no adequate reports or well-controlled studies in human fetuses. **Methamphetamine** crosses the human placenta and produces significant and long-lasting maternal and fetal cardiovascular effects, including a decrease in fetal PaO_2 after maternal administration. The latter reflects decreased uteroplacental perfusion, whereas the observed changes in fetal blood pressure and fetal pH are a direct result of **methamphetamine**. Children of abusers are at risk for IUGR and preterm birth. Antenatal **methamphetamine** exposure is associated with postnatal developmental disorders associated with neuronal damage, enduring cognitive deficits and greater risks of neglect and abuse postnatally. These changes are also associated with abnormalities of brain energy metabolism. The neuronal damage may be mediated by free-radical formation, affect the serotoninergic and monoamine oxidase systems, and differ by fetal gender. Rodent studies reveal embryotoxicity and an increased incidence of microcephaly, neural tube defects, incomplete rotation of the body axis, and a tortuous spinal cord. Increased frequencies of clefting, cardiac anomalies, and IUGR are reported in humans. Reliable and sensitive screening procedures are available using meconium to identify prenatal exposure to illicit drugs.

■ **Breastfeeding Safety**

There is no published experience in nursing women. It is unknown whether **methamphetamine** enters human breast milk.

■ **References**

Ho E, Karimi-Tabesh L, Koren G. Neurotoxicol Teratol 2001; 23:561-7.
Anglin MD, Burke C, Perrochet B, et al. J Psychoactive Drugs 2000; 32:137-41.
Perez JA Jr, Arsura EL, Strategos S. J Emerg Med 1999; 17:469-71.
Plessinger MA. Obstet Gynecol Clin North Am 1998; 25:119-38.
Yamamoto Y, Yamamoto K, Hayase T, et al. Reprod Toxicol. 1998; 12:133-7.
Stewart JL, Meeker JE. J Anal Toxicol 1997; 21:515-7.
Stek AM, Baker RS, Fisher BK, et al. Am J Obstet Gynecol 1995; 173:1592-8.
Catanzarite VA, Stein DA. West J Med 1995; 162:454-7.
Smith LM, Chang L, Yonekura ML, et al. Neurology 2001; 57:255-60.
Moriya F, Chan KM, Noguchi TT, Wu PY. J Anal Toxicol 1994; 18:41-5.

Stek AM, Fisher BK, Baker RS, et al. Am J Obstet Gynecol 1993; 169:888-97.
De Vito MJ, Wagner GC. Psychopharmacology (Berl) 1989; 97:432-5.

■ **Summary**
- **Pregnancy Category C**
- **Lactation Category U**
- **Methamphetamine** is the most common illicitly abused amphetamine; it can be inhaled, injected intravenously, or smoked. More and more pregnant women report use of 3,4-methylenedioxymethamphetamine (Ecstasy) during pregnancy.
- **Methamphetamine** increases the risk of adverse outcome and congenital malformations.

Methantheline (Banthine)

■ **Class**
Gastrointestinal, anticholinergic

■ **Indications**
Peptic ulcer, adjunctive treatment

■ **Mechanism**
Cholinergic antagonist; reduces GI motility and gastric acid secretion

■ **Dosage with Qualifiers**
Peptic ulcer—50-100mg PO qid; may decrease dose to 25-50mg for maintenance therapy
- **Contraindications**—hypersensitivity to drug or class, glaucoma, achalasia, paralytic ileus, bowel obstruction, pyloric stenosis, ulcerative colitis, toxic megacolon, myasthenia gravis
- **Caution**—autonomic neuropathy, hepatic or renal disease, coronary heart disease, CHF, tachyarrhythmias, hypertension, hiatal hernia, hyperthyroidism

■ **Maternal Considerations**
There is no published experience during pregnancy. *Side effects* include drowsiness, blurred vision, dry mouth, decreased sweating, mydriasis, cycloplegia, increased ocular tension, tachycardia, palpitations, loss of the sense of taste, headache, nervousness, mental confusion, weakness, dizziness, insomnia, nausea, vomiting, constipation, bloated feeling, suppression of lactation, and urticaria.

■ **Fetal Considerations**
There are no published studies in human fetuses. It is unknown whether **methantheline** crosses the human placenta. Rodent teratogenicity studies have not been performed.

■ **Breastfeeding Safety**
There is no published experience in nursing women. It is unknown whether **methantheline** enters human breast milk.

Methazolamide (MZM; Neptazane)

■ **Class** ———————————————— *Carbonic anhydrase inhibitor*

■ **Indications** ————————— Glaucoma

■ **Mechanism** ———————— Carbonic anhydrase inhibitor

■ **Dosage with Qualifiers** ————— <u>Glaucoma</u>—50-100mg bid/tid; may be used concomitantly with miotic and osmotic agents
- **Contraindications**—hypersensitivity to drug or class, hyponatremia, hypokalemia, depressed respiratory function, cirrhosis, hyperchloride acidosis, adrenocortical insufficiency
- **Caution**—cirrhosis, hepatic dysfunction, pulmonary obstruction, emphysema

■ **Maternal Considerations** ——— There is no published experience during pregnancy. It is well absorbed orally.
Side effects include aplastic anemia, Stevens-Johnson syndrome, toxic epidermal necrolysis, fulminant hepatitis, paresthesias, loss of appetite, taste changes, hearing dysfunction, tinnitus, fatigue, malaise, loss of appetite, taste alteration, nausea, vomiting, diarrhea, drowsiness, confusion, metabolic acidosis, electrolyte imbalance, dyspepsia, and polyuria.

■ **Fetal Considerations** ————— There are no adequate reports or well-controlled studies in human fetuses. It is unknown whether **methazolamide** crosses the human placenta. **Methazolamide** causes skeletal abnormalities in rodents when given at high multiples of the MRHD.

■ **Breastfeeding Safety** ———— There is no published experience in nursing women. It is unknown whether **methazolamide** enters human breast milk.

■ **References** ———————— No published experience in pregnancy or during lactation.

■ Summary
- **Pregnancy Category C**
- **Lactation Category U**
- **Methazolamide** should be used during pregnancy and lactation only if the benefit justifies the potential perinatal risk.

Methenamine (Hexydal; Lemandine; Mandameth; Mandelamine; Metanamin; Methenamine)

■ **Class** — Antibiotic, other

■ **Indications** — Bacterial infections (<u>gram-positive aerobes</u>: *Streptococcus pneumoniae, Streptococcus viridans*; <u>gram-negative aerobes</u>: *Escherichia coli, Klebsiella, Enterobacter, Proteus mirabilis, Morganella morganii*); urinary tract infection

■ **Mechanism** — Bactericidal; hydrolyzed to ammonia and bactericidal formaldehyde

■ **Dosage with Qualifiers** — <u>Bacterial infections, urinary</u>—1g PO qid
NOTE—ineffective for some infections with *Proteus vulgaris* and urea-splitting strains of *Pseudomonas aeruginosa* and A. *aerogenes*
- **Contraindications**—hypersensitivity to drug or class, renal insufficiency, hypovolemia, sulfonamide usage
- **Caution**—unknown

■ **Maternal Considerations** — There are no adequate reports or well-controlled studies of **methenamine** in pregnant women. **Methenamine** is used for chronic suppressive treatment of bacteriuria during pregnancy. Approximately 80% of the oral dose is excreted into the urine within 24h. Pathogens resistant to other antibacterial agents may respond to **methenamine** because of the nonspecific effect of formaldehyde formed in the acid urine.
Side effects include edema, lipoid pneumonitis, nausea, vomiting, cramps, bladder irritation, proteinuria, dysuria, urinary urgency, headache, hematuria, stomatitis, and anorexia.

■ **Fetal Considerations** — There are no adequate reports or well-controlled studies in human fetuses. **Methenamine** crosses the human placenta. The concentration of **methenamine** in umbilical cord plasma is low, approximating that in maternal plasma after 4h. Low concentrations of **methenamine** are also found in amniotic fluid. Rodent teratogenicity studies have not been conducted.

- **Breastfeeding Safety** .... **Methenamine** enters human breast milk at a concentration similar to maternal plasma. It is generally considered compatible with breastfeeding.

- **References** .... Allgen LG, Holmberg G, Persson B, Sorbo B. Acta Obstet Gynecol Scand 1979; 58:287-93.

- **Summary** .... • **Pregnancy Category C**
  • **Lactation Category S**
  • **Methenamine** should be used during pregnancy and lactation only if the benefit justifies the potential perinatal risk.

Methicillin (Staphcillin)

- **Class** .... *Antibiotic, penicillin*

- **Indications** .... Bacterial infections (penicillinase-resistant staphylococci)

- **Mechanism** .... Bactericidal; inhibits cell wall synthesis

- **Dosage with Qualifiers** ...... Bacterial infections—1-2g IM/IV q4-6h
  • **Contraindications**—hypersensitivity to drug or class
  • **Caution**—renal or hepatic dysfunction

- **Maternal Considerations** ...... Pregnant women often have mixed vaginal flora of both **methicillin**-sensitive S. *aureus* (MSSA) and **methicillin**-resistant S. *aureus* (MRSA). Strains of MRSA are a major cause of nosocomial infection. Chorioamnionitis with MRSA is a rare complication of pregnancy. There are no adequate reports or well-controlled studies in pregnant women.
  Side effects include anaphylactic reaction (angioneurotic edema, laryngospasm, bronchospasm, hypotension, vascular collapse, death), serum sickness-like symptoms (fever, malaise, urticaria, myalgia, arthralgia, abdominal pain), nausea, vomiting, diarrhea, stomatitis, hairy tongue, interstitial nephritis, agranulocytosis, neutropenia, and bone marrow depression.

- **Fetal Considerations** ...... There are no adequate reports or well-controlled studies in human fetuses. **Methicillin** crosses the human placenta achieving an M:F ratio approximating unity. Rodent studies are reassuring, revealing no evidence of teratogenicity or IUGR despite the use of doses higher than those used clinically. Routine surveillance reveals a rising incidence of MRSA infections in neonatal intensive care units. Maternal-neonatal transmission of MRSA is documented.

■ **Breastfeeding Safety** ⋯⋯⋯ There are no adequate reports or well-controlled studies in nursing women. **Methicillin** enters human breast milk, though the kinetics remain to be elucidated. There is only limited published experience in women with mastitis. Most are secondary to **methicillin**-sensitive staphylococci. Mastitis secondary to MRSA is reported, as is toxic shock syndrome. **Methicillin** is generally considered compatible for breastfeeding based on this clinical experience.

■ **References** ⋯⋯⋯⋯⋯⋯

Morel AS, Wu F, Della-Latta P, et al. Am J Infect Control 2002; 30:170-3.
Fujiwara Y, Endo S. Kansenshogaku Zasshi 2001; 75:898-903.
Novak FR, Almeida JA, Warnken MB, et al. Mem Inst Oswaldo Cruz 2000; 95:29-33.
Andre P, Thebaud B, Guibert M, et al. Am J Perinatol 2000; 17:423-7.
Geisler JP, Horlander KM, Hiett AK. Clin Exp Obstet Gynecol 1998; 25:119-20.
Mitsuda T, Arai K, Fujita S, Yokota S. Eur J Pediatr 1996; 155:194-9.
Pacifici GM, Nottoli R. Clin Pharmacokinet 1995; 28:235-69.
Zueva VS, Dmitrenko OA, Gladkova KK, Zueva EA. Zh Mikrobiol Epidemiol Immunobiol 1994; 2:20-3.
Gaufberg VV, Moroz AZ, Gurtovoi BL. Antibiotiki 1975; 20:445-51.
Nau H. Dev Pharmacol Ther 1987; 10:174-98.
Ziv G, Storper M. J Vet Pharmacol Ther 1985; 8:276-83.
Ziv G, Soback S, Bor A. J Vet Pharmacol Ther 1983; 6:41-7.
Kulakov VI, Zak IR, Kulikova NN, Smekuna FA. Antibiotiki 1981; 26:110-3.

■ **Summary** ⋯⋯⋯⋯⋯⋯
- **Pregnancy Category B**
- **Lactation Category S**
- **Methicillin** should be used during pregnancy and lactation only if the benefit justifies the potential perinatal risk.
- MRSA must be considered when chorioamnionitis or refractory endometritis is encountered.

Methimazole (Antitroide-GW; Favistan; Mercaptizol; Mercazole; Tapazole)

■ **Class** ⋯⋯⋯ *Antithyroid agent, hormone*

■ **Indications** ⋯⋯⋯ Hyperthyroidism secondary to thyroid-stimulating immunoglobulin

■ **Mechanism** ⋯⋯⋯ Inhibits thyroid hormone synthesis

■ **Dosage with Qualifiers** ⋯⋯⋯ <u>Hyperthyroidism</u>—begin 5-20mg PO q8h, then 5-15mg
PO qd
NOTE—take with food
- **Contraindications**—hypersensitivity to drug or class,
  lactation
- **Caution**—pregnancy, agranulocytosis, bone marrow
  suppression

■ **Maternal Considerations** ⋯⋯ Several clinical aspects of hyperthyroidism have received
special attention in the recent past. Hyperthyroidism
associated with *hyperemesis gravidarium* was originally
believed secondary to inappropriate secretion of β-hCG.
More recently, a mutation in the thyrotropin-releasing
hormone receptor was discovered. It does not require
treatment. The most common cause of maternal
hyperthyroidism during pregnancy is Graves' disease. The
mainstay of treatment is an antithyroid drug, either
propylthiouracil (PTU) or **methimazole**. Thyroid function
tests should be obtained during gestation in women
suffering from hyperthyroidism and the dose of
methimazole adjusted accordingly to keep T_3 and T_4
within the upper normal range for these women. The
lowest effective dose is recommended. Women previously
treated with either a radioactive cocktail or thyroidectomy
may still be producing thyroid-stimulating
immunoglobulin even though they are themselves
euthyroid. If the level is elevated, the fetus
is at risk and should be referred to a fetal center for
evaluation (see **PTU**).
Side effects include agranulocytosis, leukopenia,
thrombocytopenia, nephritis, hypoprothrombinemia,
anemia, and periarteritis.

■ **Fetal Considerations** ⋯⋯⋯⋯ There are no adequate reports or well-controlled studies in
human fetuses. **Methimazole** crosses the human placenta
and is an alternative to **propylthiouracil (PTU)** for the
treatment of fetal hyperthyroidism secondary to thyroid-
stimulating immunoglobulin. The fetal response is often
different than the maternal and some recommend it be
tested directly. **Methimazole** can induce fetal goiter and
even cretinism in a dose-dependent fashion. Recent studies
of exposed children followed until 3-11 years reveal no
deleterious effects on either thyroid function or physical
and intellectual development with doses up to 20mg daily.
However, rare instances of aplasia cutis (manifest as scalp
defects), esophageal atresia with tracheoesophageal fistula,
and choanal atresia with absent/hypoplastic nipples
(**methimazole** syndrome) are reported suggesting
methimazole may be a weak human teratogen. This
reinforces the designation of **PTU** as the drug of choice.

■ **Breastfeeding Safety** ⋯⋯⋯ **Methimazole** is excreted in human breast milk, but the
kinetics remain to be clarified. Several recent studies
observe no deleterious effects on neonatal thyroid function
or on physical and intellectual development of breast-fed
infants whose mothers were treated with up to 20mg daily.

■ References

Azizi F, Khamseh ME, Bahreynian M, Hedayati M.
J Endocrinol Invest 2002; 25:586-9.
Shepard TH, Brent RL, Friedman JM, et al. Teratology
2002; 65:153-61.
Di Gianantonio E, Schaefer C, Mastroiacovo PP, et al.
Teratology 2001; 64:262-6.
De Santis M, Carducci B, Cavaliere AF, et al. Drug Saf
2001; 24:889-901.
Azizi F, Khoshniat M, Bahrainian M, Hedayati M. J Clin
Endocrinol Metab 2000; 85:3233-8.
Mortimer RH, Cannell GR, Addison RS, et al. J Clin
Endocrinol Metab 1997; 82:3099-102.
Mestman JH. Curr Opin Obstet Gynecol 1999; 11:167-75.
Becks GP, Burrow GN. Med Clin North Am 1991; 75:121-50.
Cooper DS. Am J Obstet Gynecol 1987; 157:234-5.
Johansen K, Andersen AN, Kampmann JP, et al. Eur J Clin
Pharmacol 1982; 23:339-41.

■ Summary

- **Pregnancy Category D**
- **Lactation Category S?**
- **Methimazole** may be a weak human teratogen and should be avoided during embryogenesis.
- **Methimazole** is an effective alternative to **propylthiouracil** for the management of maternal Graves' disease or fetal hyperthyroidism secondary to maternal thyroid-stimulating immunoglobulin if PTU is contraindicated.

Methocarbamol (Bolaxin; Carbacot; Forbaxin; Methocarb; Miolaxin; Robaxin; Skedesin; Traumacut; Tresortil)

■ **Class** — Muscle relaxant

■ **Indications** — Muscle spasm

■ **Mechanism** — Unknown (centrally acting muscle relaxant)

■ **Dosage with Qualifiers** — Muscle spasm—1-1.5g PO qid
- **Contraindications**—hypersensitivity to drug or class, renal dysfunction, seizures
- **Caution**—unknown

■ **Maternal Considerations** — There is no published experience during pregnancy. **Methocarbamol** has no direct effect on the contractile mechanism of striated muscle, the motor end plate or the nerve fiber.
Side effects include seizures, anaphylaxis, lightheadedness, dizziness, urticaria, nausea, vomiting, rash, conjunctivitis, blurred vision, headache, fever, bradycardia, hypotension, and thrombophlebitis.

■ **Fetal Considerations** ⋯⋯⋯ There are no adequate reports or well-controlled studies in human fetuses. It is unknown whether **methocarbamol** crosses the human placenta. Rodent teratogen studies have not been performed.

■ **Breastfeeding Safety** ⋯⋯⋯ There is no published experience in nursing women. It is unknown whether **methocarbamol** enters human breast milk.

■ **References** ⋯⋯⋯ No published experience in pregnancy or during lactation.

■ **Summary** ⋯⋯⋯
- **Pregnancy Category C**
- **Lactation Category U**
- **Methocarbamol** should be used during pregnancy and lactation only if the benefit justifies the potential perinatal risk.
- There are alternative agents for which there is more experience during pregnancy and lactation.

Methotrexate (Abitrexate; Emtexate; Folex; Mexate; Rheumatrex; Tremetex)

■ **Class** ⋯⋯⋯ *Antimetabolite, antineoplastic, antirheumatic*

■ **Indications** ⋯⋯⋯ Ectopic pregnancy, trophoblastic disease, rheumatoid arthritis, psoriasis, mycosis fungoides, chemotherapy

■ **Mechanism** ⋯⋯⋯ Inhibits dihydrofolate reductase and lymphocyte proliferation; immunosuppressant

■ **Dosage with Qualifiers** ⋯⋯⋯ Ectopic pregnancy—50mg/m^2 IM ×1; may be repeated in 1w if HCG rising
Trophoblastic disease—15-30mg PO/IM qd ×5d; repeat ×3-5 at >1w intervals; administer with **folic acid** 1mg PO qd or **leukovorin** 5mg qw
Rheumatoid arthritis—7.5-25mg PO/IM/SC qw; alternatively 2.5-7.5mg PO q12h 3×/w; max 30mg/w
Psoriasis—10-25mg PO/IM/SC qw; alternatively 2.5-7.5mg PO q12h 3×/w; max 30mg/w
Mycosis fungoides—5-50mg PO/IV qw; alternatively 15-37.5mg PO 2×/w
Chemotherapy—numerous dosing schedules depending on disease, response, and concomitant therapy
NOTE—renal dosing
- **Contraindications**—hypersensitivity to drug or class, alcohol consumption, hepatic failure, infection, pleural effusion, immunodeficiency syndrome
- **Caution**—renal or hepatic dysfunction, bone marrow depression, ulcerative colitis, peptic ulcer

■ Maternal Considerations

Methotrexate is an antimetabolite with multiple uses in reproductive-age women including the treatment of ectopic pregnancy, neoplastic disease, autoimmune disorders, and inflammatory conditions.

Ectopic pregnancy—Ectopic pregnancy is a major cause of maternal morbidity and mortality. Its treatment remains primarily surgical, but medical treatment is routine in some locales. Criteria include: serum β-hCG titer <5000IU/L, at most moderate free fluid (i.e., confined to the pelvis), and pregnancy diameter <3.5cm. Surgery is preferred after tubal rupture, or with a high potential for rupture, hypotension, and anemia, or a pregnancy >3.5cm diameter. Some report that **methotrexate** is safe and effective for the treatment of a hemodynamically stable ectopic characterized by an adnexal mass up to 5cm, or a β-hCG titer >5000IU/L. Larger trials are needed for confirmation. Treatment often leads to an increase in mass size and should not be considered a sign of failure. Severe abdominal/pelvic pain may follow, and the surgeon must determine whether the pain is secondary to medical treatment or failure of the **methotrexate** and rupture of the ectopic. Persistent ectopic pregnancy is usually diagnosed when there is abdominal pain, intra-abdominal hemorrhage or plateau β-hCG titers. In those situations, **methotrexate** can be administered a 2nd time. Ten to 20% of treated women ultimately require surgery. Though the greatest experience is with a tubal ectopic, there are case reports supporting its use in cervical, corneal, interstitial and uterine incision scar ectopic pregnancies. Oral **methotrexate** ($60mg/m^2$) may also be successful, though the body of clinical experience is small. Local injection of **methotrexate** reduces the frequency of persistent ectopic pregnancy after linear salpingostomy.

Gestational trophoblastic disease (GTD)—**Methotrexate** is a first-line agent for uncomplicated malignant trophoblastic disease. Occasionally, resistance to **methotrexate** is encountered requiring the use of alternative drug regimens (see **melphalan**). Prognostic factors useful for treatment decisions divide women into low-, medium-, and high-risk groups. Low-risk patients are treated by a single agent, preferably **methotrexate**. Medium- to high-risk populations require multidrug regimens that frequently include **methotrexate**. Women should avoid pregnancy until their β-hCG titer is normal for 1y.

Medical abortion—**Methotrexate** has been used to induce a medical abortion of an intrauterine pregnancy. It is more effective combined with **misoprostol** than alone. As it is not 100% effective, women must be followed clinically until there is complete normalization of β-hCG titers from their serum.

Side effects include thrombocytopenia, leukopenia, anemia (severe or aplastic), hepatic and renal dysfunction, immunosuppression, opportunistic infection, leukoencephalopathy, seizures, neurotoxicity, arachnoiditis, myelopathy, Stevens-Johnson syndrome, pulmonary fibrosis, erythema multiforme, elevated LFTs, nausea, vomiting, exfoliative dermatitis, fever, dizziness, diarrhea, pruritus, alopecia, and photosensitivity.

■ **Fetal Considerations** ⋯⋯⋯⋯⋯ There are no adequate reports or well-controlled studies in human fetuses. It is unknown whether **methotrexate** crosses the human placenta. **Methotrexate** is rapidly taken up by the trophoblast in a fashion that does not interfere with folate uptake, and then extruded. It seems reasonable to conclude that 1st trimester exposure results in an increased risk of internal and external malformations (craniofacial, axial skeletal, cardiopulmonary, and GI abnormalities) and developmental delay, though most pregnancies exposed to low doses are successful. Others report no association between later pregnancy exposure and congenital abnormalities.

■ **Breastfeeding Safety** ⋯⋯⋯⋯⋯ There are no adequate reports or well-controlled studies in nursing women. It is unknown whether **methotrexate** enters human breast milk. Despite the lack of information, **methotrexate** is generally considered contraindicated in nursing mothers.

■ **References** ⋯⋯⋯⋯⋯⋯⋯⋯⋯⋯⋯ Kaya H, Babar Y, Ozmen S, et al. J Am Assoc Gynecol Laparosc 2002; 9:464-7.
Gamzu R, Almog B, Levin Y, et al. Hum Reprod 2002; 17:2585-7.
Gerulath AH, Ehlen TG, Bessette P, et al. J Obstet Gynaecol Can 2002; 24:434-46.
Lipscomb GH, Meyer NL, Flynn DE, et al. Am J Obstet Gynecol 2002; 186:1192-5.
el-Lamie IK, Shehata NA, Kamel HA. J Reprod Med 2002; 47:144-50.
Nijman RG, Mantingh A, Aarnoudse JG. BJOG 2002; 109:587-8.
Nguyen C, Duhl AJ, Escallon CS, Blakemore KJ. Obstet Gynecol 2002; 99:599-602.
Chew S, Anandakumar C. Singapore Med J 2001; 42:537-9.
Gracia CR, Brown HA, Barnhart KT. Fertil Steril 2001; 76:1191-5.
Shufaro Y, Nadjari M. Fertil Steril 2001; 75:1217.
Barnhart K, Coutifaris C, Esposito M. Expert Opin Pharmacother 2001; 2:409-17.
Margolis K. Aust NZ J Obstet Gynaecol 2000; 40:347-9.
Ostensen M, Hartmann H, Salvesen K. J Rheumatol 2000; 27:1872-5.
Mussalli GM, Shah J, Berck DJ, et al. J Perinatol 2000; 20:331-4.
Sweiry JH, Yudilevich DL. Biochim Biophys Acta 1985; 821:497-501.
Riggs JC, Jahshan A, Schiavello HJ. J Reprod Med 2000; 45:595-8.
Sheiner E, Yanai I, Yohai D, Katz M. Harefuah 1999; 137:537-40.
Del Campo M, Kosaki K, Bennett FC, Jones KL. Teratology 1999; 60:10-2.
Lipscomb GH, McCord ML, Stovall TG, et al. N Engl J Med 1999; 341:1974-8.
Newlands ES, Bower M, Holden L, et al. Int J Gynaecol Obstet 1998; 60:S65-70.

Ostensen M, Ramsey-Goldman R. Drug Saf 1998; 19:389-410.
Flam F, Karlstrom PO, Carlsson B, Garoff L. Eur J Obstet Gynecol Reprod Biol 1999; 83:127-9.
Creinin MD, Darney PD. Contraception 1993; 48:339-48.
Newlands ES, Bagshawe KD, Begent RH, et al. Br J Obstet Gynaecol 1991; 98:550-7.
Kozlowski RD, Steinbrunner JV, MacKenzie AH, et al. Am J Med 1990; 88:589-9.
Johns DG, Rutherford LD, Leighton PC, Vogel CL. Am J Obstet Gynecol 1972; 112:978-80.

■ **Summary**

- **Pregnancy Category X**
- **Lactation Category NS?**
- **Methotrexate** is contraindicated during ongoing pregnancy and lactation because of its teratogenic potential.
- **Methotrexate** is effective for the medical treatment of ectopic pregnancy in selected women. A high serum β-hCG is the single most important factor predictive of single-dose **methotrexate** treatment failure.
- **Methotrexate** is the drug of choice for low-risk malignant trophoblastic disease.

Methotrimeprazine (Levoprome)

■ **Class**
Analgesics, non-narcotic

■ **Indications**
Preanesthetic medication, acute pain, obstetric pain or postoperative analgesia

■ **Mechanism**
Suppresses sensory impulses, reduces motor activity, sedates and tranquilizes, raises the pain threshold and produces amnesia

■ **Dosage with Qualifiers**
Preanesthetic medication—2-20mg IM q45min-3h
Pain, acute—10-20mg IM q4-6h
Obstetric analgesia—15-20mg IM q4-6h prn
Postoperative analgesia—2.5-7.5mg IM q4-6h
- **Contraindications**—hypersensitivity to drug or class, antihypertensive medication, MAO inhibitors <14d, CNS depression, severe cardiac, renal or hepatic dysfunction, MI, hypotension
- **Caution**—infertility

■ **Maternal Considerations**
Methotrimeprazine is a phenothiazine derivative that produces sedation and tranquilization. There are no adequate reports or well-controlled studies of **methotrimeprazine** in pregnant women.

Side effects include orthostatic hypotension, disorientation, dizziness, weakness, jaundice, biliary stasis, abdominal discomfort, nausea, vomiting, nasal congestion, chills, uterine atony, dry mouth, amenorrhea, agranulocytosis, pancytopenia, leukopenia, eosinophilia, thrombocytopenia, constipation, cardiac arrest, tachycardia, dyskinesia, dystonia, parkinsonism, opisthotonos, hyperreflexia, photosensitivity, itching, erythema, urticaria, pigmentation, rash, exfoliative dermatitis, lenticular and corneal deposits, pigmentary retinopathy, edema, and asthma.

■ **Fetal Considerations**
There are no adequate reports or well-controlled studies in human fetuses. It is unknown whether **methotrimeprazine** crosses the human placenta. Rodent teratogenicity studies have not been performed.

■ **Breastfeeding Safety**
There is no published experience in nursing women. It is unknown whether **methotrimeprazine** enters human breast milk.

■ **References**
There are no current relevant references.

■ **Summary**
- **Pregnancy Category C**
- **Lactation Category U**
- **Methotrimeprazine** should be used during pregnancy and lactation only if the benefit justifies the potential perinatal risk.
- There are alternative agents for which there is more experience regarding use during pregnancy and lactation.

Methoxamine (Vasoxyl)

■ **Class**
Antihypotensive, adrenergic agonist

■ **Indications**
Hypotension

■ **Mechanism**
α-adrenergic agonist

■ **Dosage with Qualifiers**
Hypotension—3-5mg IV; alternative 10-15mg IM before or at the time of spinal anesthesia
- **Contraindications**—hypersensitivity to drug or class, hypertension
- **Caution**—concomitant use of tricyclic antidepressants or oxytocic agents or MAO inhibitor <14d, heart block, hyperthyroidism, bradycardia, myocardial disease, arteriosclerosis

■ **Maternal Considerations** ········ Neuraxial analgesia is frequently accompanied by hypotension. If untreated, there are many well-described maternal and fetal effects. Perioperative hypotension may be controlled by **methoxamine** should **ephedrine** fail. There are no adequate reports or well-controlled studies of **methoxamine** in pregnant women. It decreases uterine blood flow in pregnant ewes and monkeys at doses similar to human. In rats, **methoxamine** increases uterine contractility in a dose-dependent fashion. It is unclear whether the same occurs in humans. **Methoxamine** was used in one study to alter afterload as part of an evaluation of women thought recovered from peripartal cardiomyopathy. If used to correct hypotension during labor and delivery, oxytocic drugs like **vasopressin**, **ergotamine**, **ergonovine**, and **methylergonovine** may cause severe hypertension.

Side effects include uterine hypertonus, fetal bradycardia, hypertension, nausea, vomiting, headache, anxiety, sweating, piloerection, and urinary urgency.

■ **Fetal Considerations** ············· There are no adequate reports or well-controlled studies in human fetuses. It is unknown whether **methoxamine** crosses the human placenta. It decreases uterine blood flow and, consequently, causes fetal bradycardia and acidemia when given to pregnant ewes and monkeys at doses similar to human doses. Doppler studies reveal a brief increase in uterine artery pulsatility index after **methoxamine** for epidural-related hypotension, whereas **ephedrine** has no effect. This short-lived effect is small compared to the effect of the hypotension.

■ **Breastfeeding Safety** ············ There is no published experience in nursing women. It is unknown whether **methoxamine** enters human breast milk.

■ **References** ························· Tamura T, Kobashigawa T, Morishige Y, et al. Masui 1998; 47:1212-6.
Morgan P. Can J Anaesth 1994; 41:404-13.
Lampert MB, Weinert L, Hibbard J, et al. Am J Obstet Gynecol 1997; 176:189-95.
Wright PM, Iftikhar M, Fitzpatrick KT, et al. Anesth Analg 1992; 75:56-63.
Palop V, Tarazona E, Martinez-Mir I, et al. Gynecol Obstet Invest 1992; 34:1-5.
Estan L, Morales-Olivas FJ, Rubio E, Esplugues J. Gynecol Obstet Invest 1985; 19:53-6.

■ **Summary** ····························
- **Pregnancy Category C**
- **Lactation Category U**
- **Methoxamine** should be used during pregnancy and lactation only if the benefit justifies the potential perinatal risk.
- **Ephedrine** remains the first drug of choice for hypotension associated with neuraxial anesthesia.

Methoxsalen (8-MOP; Deltasoralen; Houva-Caps; Oxsoralen)

■ **Class** — *Photosensitizer, psoralen*

■ **Indications** — Psoriasis, severe

■ **Mechanism** — Unknown; photosensitizes to UV radiation probably by DNA damage decreasing cell proliferation

■ **Dosage with Qualifiers** — Psoriasis, severe—20mg PO with food 4h before UVA light exposure; treat only on alternate days
NOTE—each patient should be first evaluated to determine the minimum phototoxic dose and phototoxic peak time after drug administration; available in cream.
- **Contraindications**—hypersensitivity to drug or class, invasive squamous cell carcinomas, melanoma
- **Caution**—SLE, *porphyria cutanea tarda*, erythropoietic protoporphyria, variegate porphyria, xeroderma pigmentosum, albinism

■ **Maternal Considerations** — There are no adequate reports or well-controlled studies of **methoxsalen** in pregnant women.
Side effects include ocular damage, skin aging, skin cancer, skin burn, nervousness, insomnia, depression, nausea, vomiting, pruritus, erythema, edema, dizziness, headache, malaise, hypopigmentation, vesiculation, rash, herpes simplex, miliaria, urticaria, folliculitis, GI disturbances, cutaneous tenderness, leg cramps, hypotension, and extension of psoriasis.

■ **Fetal Considerations** — There are no adequate reports or well-controlled studies in human fetuses. It is unknown whether **methoxsalen** crosses the human placenta. Rodent teratogenicity studies have not been performed. In one limited study, there was no increase in the risk of specific defects after exposure to **methoxsalen**.

■ **Breastfeeding Safety** — There is no published experience in nursing women. It is unknown whether **methoxsalen** enters human breast milk.

■ **References** — Stern RS, Lange R. Arch Dermatol 1991; 127:347-50.
Nietsche UB. Int J Dermatol 1978; 17:149-57.

■ **Summary** —
- **Pregnancy Category C**
- **Lactation Category U**
- **Methoxsalen** should be used during pregnancy and lactation only if the benefit justifies the potential perinatal risk.

Methscopolamine (Pamine)

- **Class** — Anticholinergic, gastrointestinal

- **Indications** — Peptic ulcer, adjunctive treatment

- **Mechanism** — Acetylcholine antagonist; inhibits GI propulsive motility and decreases gastric acid secretion

- **Dosage with Qualifiers** — Peptic ulcer—2.5mg PO qac, qhs
  - **Contraindications**—hypersensitivity to drug or class, ulcerative colitis, glaucoma, GI obstruction, paralytic ileus, acute hemorrhage, toxic megacolon, myasthenia gravis
  - **Caution**—high temperature, hyperthyroidism, coronary heart disease, CHF, tachyarrhythmias, tachycardia, hypertension

- **Maternal Considerations** — There are no adequate reports or well-controlled studies of **methscopolamine** in pregnant women. See **scopolamine**. *Side effects* include tachycardia, palpitation, nausea, vomiting, constipation, decreased sweating, urticaria, blurred vision, headaches, nervousness, mental confusion, drowsiness, and dizziness.

- **Fetal Considerations** — There are no adequate reports or well-controlled studies in human fetuses. It is unknown whether **methscopolamine** crosses the human placenta. Rodent teratogenicity studies have not been performed. See **scopolamine**.

- **Breastfeeding Safety** — There is no published experience in nursing women. It is unknown whether **methscopolamine** enters human breast milk. See **scopolamine**.

- **References** — See **scopolamine**.

- **Summary**
  - **Pregnancy Category C**
  - **Lactation Category U**
  - **Methscopolamine** should be used during pregnancy and lactation only if the benefit justifies the potential perinatal risk.
  - There are superior agents for which there is more experience regarding use during pregnancy and lactation.

Methsuximide (Celontin)

- **Class** — Anticonvulsant, *succinimide*

- **Indications** — Seizures (petit mal)

- **Mechanism** — Depresses the motor cortex and elevates the CNS threshold to convulsive stimuli

- **Dosage with Qualifiers** — Seizures (petit mal)—300mg PO qd; increase 300mg qw until desired effect; max 1.2g qd
  - **Contraindications**—hypersensitivity to drug or class
  - **Caution**—blood dyscrasias, hepatic dysfunction

- **Maternal Considerations** — **Methsuximide** is indicated for the control of absence (petit mal) seizures refractory to other drugs. There is no published experience during pregnancy.
  Side effects include nausea, vomiting, anorexia, diarrhea, weight loss, abdominal pain, constipation, eosinophilia, leukopenia, monocytosis, pancytopenia, irritability, nervousness, headache, blurred vision, photophobia, hiccups, insomnia, drowsiness, ataxia, dizziness, urticaria, Stevens-Johnson syndrome, hyperemia, proteinuria, and periorbital edema.

- **Fetal Considerations** — There are no adequate reports or well-controlled studies in human fetuses. It is unknown whether **methsuximide** crosses the human placenta. Rodent teratogenicity studies have not been conducted. Many anticonvulsants are associated with an increased risk of malformation. The limited experience with **methsuximide** precludes comment. As for most anticonvulsant drugs, using monotherapy and the lowest effective quantity given in divided doses to minimize the peaks can minimize the risks.

- **Breastfeeding Safety** — There is no published experience in nursing women. It is unknown whether **methsuximide** enters human breast milk.

- **References** — There is no published experience in pregnancy or during lactation.

- **Summary** —
  - **Pregnancy Category C**
  - **Lactation Category U**
  - **Methsuximide** should be used during pregnancy and lactation only if the benefit justifies the potential perinatal risk.
  - There are alternative agents for which there is more experience regarding use during pregnancy and lactation.

Methyclothiazide (Aquatensen; Enduron; Thiazidil; Urimor)

■ **Class** — Diuretic, thiazide

■ **Indications** — Hypertension (chronic), edema

■ **Mechanism** — Inhibits resorption of sodium and chloride

■ **Dosage with Qualifiers** — Chronic hypertension—2.5-5mg PO qd; if no control 8-12w, add a 2nd agent
Edema (peripheral)—2.5-10mg PO qd; max 10mg PO qd
NOTE—may be combined with **reserpine**
- **Contraindications**—hypersensitivity, electrolyte imbalances, anuria
- **Caution**—hypersensitivity to sulfonamides

■ **Maternal Considerations** — There are no adequate reports or well-controlled studies of **methyclothiazide** in pregnant women. Thiazides and other diuretics are inappropriate treatment for physiologic edema of pregnancy. They are not indicated for the treatment of preeclampsia. See **chlorothiazide**.
Side effects include renal failure, hyponatremia, hypochloremia, hypomagnesemia, glucose intolerance, hyperlipidemia, and photosensitivity.

■ **Fetal Considerations** — There are no adequate reports or well-controlled studies in human fetuses. It is unknown whether **methyclothiazide** crosses the human placenta. Other thiazide diuretics do cross. Rodent studies are reassuring, revealing no evidence of teratogenicity or IUGR despite the use of doses higher than those used clinically. See **chlorothiazide**.

■ **Breastfeeding Safety** — There are no adequate reports or well-controlled studies in nursing women. It is unknown whether **methyclothiazide** enters human breast milk. Other thiazide diuretics are excreted into milk. See **chlorothiazide**.

■ **References** — No current relevant references. See **chlorothiazide**.

■ **Summary** —
- **Pregnancy Category B**
- **Lactation Category S?**
- **Thiazide** diuretics are contraindicated during pregnancy except for women with CHF (see chlorothiazide).

Methylcellulose

■ **Class** — *Laxative*

■ **Indications** — Constipation

■ **Mechanism** — Increases stool bulk

■ **Dosage with Qualifiers** — Constipation—1 tbsp PO qd-tid
- **Contraindications**—hypersensitivity to drug or class, appendicitis, fecal impaction, acute abdomen
- **Caution**—unknown

■ **Maternal Considerations** — There are no adequate reports or well-controlled studies of **methylcellulose** in pregnant women. **Methylcellulose** is frequently used in the gel preparations for local application of prostaglandin or relaxin. Systemic absorption is likely low.
Side effects include nausea, diarrhea, and abdominal cramps.

■ **Fetal Considerations** — There are no adequate reports or well-controlled studies in human fetuses. Based on molecular size, it is unlikely **methylcellulose** crosses the human placenta. Rodent studies are reassuring, revealing no evidence of teratogenicity or IUGR despite the use of doses higher than those used clinically. **Methylcellulose** did not influence behavior, appearance, or growth postnatally.

■ **Breastfeeding Safety** — There are no adequate reports or well-controlled studies in nursing women. It is unknown whether **methylcellulose** enters human breast milk. Animal studies reveal no evidence that **methylcellulose** adversely affects lactation.

■ **References** — Elliott JP, Clewell WH, Radin TG. J Reprod Med 1992; 37:713-6.
Buttino LT Jr, Garite TJ. J Reprod Med 1990; 35:155-8.
Hoshi N, Ueno K, Igarashi T, et al. J Toxicol Sci 1985; 10(Suppl 2):203-34.

■ **Summary** —
- **Pregnancy Category B**
- **Lactation Category S**
- **Methylcellulose** is a suitable vehicle for suspending pharmacologic materials during pregnancy.

Methyldopa (Aldomet; Alfametildopa; Dimal; Elanpres; Highprepin; Hypermet; Medomet; Methyldopum; Modepres; Prodop; Scandopa)

- **Class** ⋯⋯⋯⋯⋯⋯⋯⋯⋯⋯⋯⋯⋯⋯ *Antihypertensive, central antiadrenergic*

- **Indications** ⋯⋯⋯⋯⋯⋯⋯⋯⋯⋯⋯⋯ Hypertension

- **Mechanism** ⋯⋯⋯⋯⋯⋯⋯⋯⋯⋯⋯⋯ Central α-2 adrenergic agonist

- **Dosage with Qualifiers** ⋯⋯⋯⋯ <u>Hypertension</u>—250-500mg PO bid; begin 250mg PO bid and adjust q2d; max 3g/d; alternative 250-500mg IV q6h×4, then PO
  NOTE—obtain a CBC, Coombs' test, and LFTs before beginning
  - **Contraindications**—hypersensitivity to drug or class, acute hepatitis, cirrhosis
  - **Caution**—usage of other antihypertensives or levodopa, renal dysfunction, MAO inhibitor <14d, positive Coombs' test, hemolytic anemia

- **Maternal Considerations** ⋯⋯ One to 6% of young women have chronic hypertension. **Methyldopa** is perhaps the best-studied antihypertensive agent during pregnancy. It remains a first-line agent for the treatment of moderate to mild hypertension. **Methyldopa** requires 48-72h to exert its effect. The delay can be reduced to less than 12h if the patient is loaded either parenterally or orally. Hypertension predating pregnancy should be differentiated from preeclampsia. While treatment is indicated for women with a systolic blood pressure >170mmHg and/or a diastolic blood pressure >109mmHg, there is no consensus whether lesser degrees of hypertension require treatment during pregnancy. In women with mild to moderate chronic hypertension, antihypertensive therapy improves the maternal but apparently not the fetal outcome. In such patients, **methyldopa** prolongs pregnancy by some 10d compared to placebo, but does not decrease the prevalence of superimposed preeclampsia. **Methyldopa** is less effective than **metoprolol,** but as effective as **nifedipine, labetalol** and **ketanserin,** in decreasing both systolic and diastolic blood pressure in women with chronic hypertension. On average, **methyldopa** decreases the maternal MAP 10.0mmHg and the mean heart rate by 6.0 beats/min. The uterine artery pulsatility index is generally unchanged. Neither short- nor long-term use of **methyldopa** is associated with adverse maternal effects. Rare, sporadic cases of reactive hepatitis are reported in women treated with **methyldopa** during pregnancy. In chronically hypertensive women, **methyldopa** increases prolactin, thyrotropin, and triiodothyronine in a dose-dependent fashion indicating decreased dopaminergic inhibition of pituitary hormone release.

In contrast, **methyldopa** decreases plasma **thyroxine** levels.

Side effects include hemolytic anemia, myocarditis, thrombocytopenia, leukopenia, bradycardia, pancreatitis, headache, sedation, angina, weakness, CHF, nausea, vomiting, pancreatitis, reactive hepatitis, diarrhea, bone marrow suppression, black tongue, pericarditis, myocarditis, arthralgia, myalgia, jaundice, amenorrhea, breast enlargement, decreased libido, and hepatic dysfunction.

■ **Fetal Considerations**

Most antihypertensive agents cross the placental barrier. **Methyldopa** is the only drug accepted for use during the 1st trimester of pregnancy. Neither short- nor long-term effects on the fetus or the neonate are reported after long-term **methyldopa** use. **Methyldopa** does not significantly alter fetal cardiac activity or produce any fetal hemodynamic changes as measured by Doppler flow studies. In contrast, **methyldopa** decreases placental vascular resistance in mild preeclampsia and in chronic hypertension. Longitudinal studies revealed no developmental disturbances at 3y in children exposed *in utero*. Rodent studies are reassuring, revealing no evidence of teratogenicity or IUGR despite the use of doses higher than those used clinically.

■ **Breastfeeding Safety**

Methyldopa enters human breast milk, but the M/P ratio is low. Breast-fed neonates delivered by women who are using **methyldopa** are normotensive.

■ **References**

Borghi C, Esposti DD, Cassani A, et al. J Hypertens 2002; 20(Suppl 2):S52-6.
Magee LA. Best Pract Res Clin Obstet Gynaecol 2001; 15:827-45.
Khedun SM, Maharaj B, Moodley J. Paediatr Drugs 2000; 2:419-36.
Hung JH, Yen MY, Pan YP, Hsu LP. Ultrasound Obstet Gynecol 2000; 15:513-9.
Kirsten R, Nelson K, Kirsten D, Heintz B. Clin Pharmacokinet 1998; 35:9-36.
Rath W. Z Geburtshilfe Neonatol 1997; 201:240-6.
Smith GN, Piercy WN. Am J Obstet Gynecol 1995; 172:222-4.
Jayawardana J, Lekamge N. Ceylon Med J 1994; 39:87-90.
Wide-Swensson D, Montan S, Arulkumaran S, et al. Am J Obstet Gynecol 1993; 169:1581-5.
Montan S, Anandakumar C, Arulkumaran S, et al. Am J Obstet Gynecol 1993; 168:152-6.
Rey E. Obstet Gynecol 1992; 80:783-7.
Sibai BM. Obstet Gynecol 1991; 78:451-61.
Sibai BM, Mabie WC, Shamsa F, et al. Am J Obstet Gynecol 1990; 162:960-6; discussion 966-7.
Oumachigui A, Verghese M, Balachander J. Indian Heart J 1992; 44:39-41.
Sulyok E, Bodis J, Hartman G, Ertl T. Acta Paediatr Hung 1991; 31:53-65.
De Andrade J. Arq Bras Cardiol 1990; 55:137-9.

Voto LS, Zin C, Neira J, et al. J Cardiovasc Pharmacol 1987; 10(Suppl 3):S101-3.

Plouin PF, Breart G, Maillard F, et al. Br J Obstet Gynaecol 1988; 95:868-76.

Weitz C, Khouzami V, Maxwell K, Johnson JW. Int J Gynaecol Obstet 1987; 25:35-40.

Hauser GJ, Almog S, Tirosh M, Spirer Z. Helv Paediatr Acta 1985; 40:83-6.

White WB, Andreoli JW, Cohn RD. Clin Pharmacol Ther 1985; 37:387-90.

Henderson-Smart DJ, Horvath JS, Phippard A, et al. Clin Exp Pharmacol Physiol 1984; 11:351-4.

Beardmore KS, Morris JM, Gallery ED. Hypertens Preg 2002; 21:85-95.

■ Summary

- **Pregnancy Category B**
- **Lactation Category S**
- **Methyldopa** is an agent of choice for the treatment of hypertension during pregnancy.
- There is no evidence of adverse effects on the progeny when observed long-term after exposure to **methyldopa**.

Methylene blue (Methylthioninium Chloride; Urolene Blue)

■ Class — Antidote

■ Indications — Methemoglobinemia

■ Mechanism — Converts ferrous iron to ferric iron, producing methemoglobin

■ Dosage with Qualifiers — Methemoglobinemia—1-2mg/kg IV over 5min
NOTE—usually not recommended for cyanide poisoning
- **Contraindications**—hypersensitivity to drug or class, renal insufficiency, intraspinal or intrathecal injection, SC injection
- **Caution**—G6PD deficiency, prolonged use

■ Maternal Considerations — **Methylene blue** causes smooth muscle contraction of many vessels including the uterine arteries by inhibiting guanylate cyclase. In the past, **methylene blue** was injected intra-amniotically to facilitate the diagnosis of PPROM and to demonstrate independent sacs were sampled during amniocentesis of a multiple gestation. Based on concerns of vasoconstriction and case reports of methemoglobinemia in susceptible women, **methylene blue** has been largely replaced by **indigo carmine** for amniocentesis.

Side effects include nausea, abdominal or precordial pain, dizziness, headache, profuse sweating, mental confusion, methemoglobin, necrotic abscess, fecal discoloration, urine discoloration, hypertension, chest pain, dizziness, nausea, vomiting, abdominal pain, fever, skin coloration, bladder irritation, diaphoresis, and mental confusion.

■ **Fetal Considerations**

There are no adequate reports or well-controlled studies in human fetuses. **Methylene blue** crosses the human placenta after intra-amniotic injection and is excreted in the maternal urine. Preterm neonates with G6PD deficiency exposed *in utero* may experience severe hemolysis and hyperbilirubinemia requiring exchange transfusion. A specific syndrome is described that includes hemolytic anemia, hyperbilirubinemia, and methemoglobinemia. Photosensitization is reported in very low-birth-weight neonates exposed prenatally. **Methylene blue** use for 2nd trimester amniocentesis in twin gestation is associated with a dose-dependent increased risk of fetal intestinal atresia and/or death. In rodents, **methylene blue** given late gestation induces preterm delivery and IUGR.

■ **Breastfeeding Safety**

There are no adequate reports or well-controlled studies in nursing women. It is unknown whether **methylene blue** enters human breast milk. It is excreted into the milk of cows and goats.

■ **References**

Mhaskar R, Mhaskar AM. Int J Gynaecol Obstet 2002; 77:41-2.
Gauthier TW. J Matern Fetal Med 2000; 9:252-4.
Sirisena J, Lanerolle SD. Ceylon Med J 2000; 45:44-5.
Cragan JD. Teratology 1999; 60:42-8.
Porat R, Gilbert S, Magilner D. Pediatrics 1996; 97:717-21.
Kidd SA, Lancaster PA, Anderson JC, et al. Prenat Diagn 1996; 16:39-47.
Izumi H, Makino Y, Shirakawa K, Garfield RE. Am J Obstet Gynecol 1995; 172:1477-84.
Thompson LP, Weiner CP. Am J Physiol 1993; 264:H1139-45.
van der Pol JG, Wolf H, Boer K, et al. Br J Obstet Gynaecol 1992; 99:141-3.
Lopes P, Aubron F, Le Neel JC, et al. Presse Med 1991; 20:1568-9.
Weiner C, Liu KZ, Thompson L, et al. Am J Physiol 1991; 261:H1275-83.
Nicolini U, Monni G. Lancet 1990; 336:1258-9.
Crooks J. Arch Dis Child 1982; 57:872-3.

■ **Summary**

- **Pregnancy Category C**
- **Lactation Category U**
- **Methylene blue** is contraindicated for obstetric procedures because of its fetal risks.

Methylergonovine (Methergine)

- **Class** — Ergot alkaloid derivative, oxytocic, uterine stimulant

- **Indications** — Postpartum bleeding

- **Mechanism** — 5-HT agonist; acts directly on myometrium to increase tone, rate, and amplitude of contractions

- **Dosage with Qualifiers** — Postpartum bleeding—emergent: 0.2mg IM q2-4h; max 5 doses; nonemergent: 0.2-0.4mg PO q6-12h; max duration 7d
  - **Contraindications**—hypersensitivity to drug or class, hypertension, toxemia, pregnancy
  - **Caution**—sepsis

- **Maternal Considerations** — Postpartum hemorrhage remains a leading cause of maternal death and morbidity. **Oxytocin, methylergonovine**, and several prostaglandin agents are the pharmacologic agents most frequently used to prevent or treat postpartum hemorrhage. There is a long clinical experience with **methylergonovine**. It is effective and inexpensive. Unfortunately, its shelf life is compromised in tropical climates where **misoprostol** may be preferable. **Methylergonovine** is typically administered in the immediate postpartum period when **oxytocin** alone fails to control myometrial atony. However, it is not effective prophylaxis for atony after delivery, and its administration with delivery of the anterior shoulder may actually increase the risk of a retained placenta. The half-life of **methylergonovine** is 1-3min, its onset of action 2-5min after IM and 5-10min after oral administration. IM is more effective than PO for the treatment of atony; the IV route is usually avoided unless the dose is diluted and infused slowly due to potential hypertension (perhaps causing stroke or MI) or vascular/tissue damage due to extravasation. There are potential interactions of **methylergonovine** and vasoactive agents, which perhaps have been administered to treat hemorrhagic hypotension. Therefore there must be communication between the obstetrician and anesthesiologist at an operative delivery with unexpected blood loss before the **methylergonovine** is given. The combination of **oxytocin** and **methylergonovine** is more effective than **oxytocin** and **misoprostol** with fewer side effects. Given late postpartum, **methylergonovine** accelerates involution but enhances maternal cramping. A combination of **misoprostol** and **methylergonovine** is an extremely efficient abortifacient in the 2nd trimester.
Side effects include MI, nausea, vomiting, diarrhea, headache, hallucinations, hypertension, chest pain, tinnitus, nasal congestion, hematuria, dyspnea, thrombophlebitis and dizziness.

- **Fetal Considerations** ⸱⸱⸱⸱⸱⸱⸱⸱⸱⸱⸱⸱⸱⸱⸱⸱⸱ There are no adequate reports or well-controlled studies in human fetuses. It is unknown whether **methylergonovine** crosses the human placenta. Rodent teratogenicity studies have not been performed. Inadvertent administration during pregnancy is followed by tetanic contractions and fetal bradycardia.

- **Breastfeeding Safety** ⸱⸱⸱⸱⸱⸱⸱⸱⸱⸱⸱⸱⸱⸱ There are no adequate reports or well-controlled studies in nursing women. The concentrations of **methylergonovine** in human breast milk are clinically insignificant. While some reports suggest **methylergonovine** may decrease milk production, it has been used for decades PO tid/qid up to a week to prevent postpartum hemorrhage without adverse effects on either lactation or the newborn.

- **References** ⸱⸱⸱⸱⸱⸱⸱⸱⸱⸱⸱⸱⸱⸱⸱⸱⸱⸱⸱⸱⸱⸱⸱⸱⸱

Caliskan E, Meydanli MM, Dilbaz B, et al. Am J Obstet Gynecol 2002; 187:1038-45.

Amant F, Spitz B, Timmerman D, et al. Br J Obstet Gynaecol 1999; 106:1066-70.

Andersen B, Andersen LL, Sorensen T. Acta Obstet Gynecol Scand 1998; 77:54-7.

de Groot AN, van Dongen PW, Vree TB, et al. Drugs 1998; 56:523-35.

Hogerzeil HV, Walker GJ. Eur J Obstet Gynecol Reprod Biol 1996; 69:25-9.

Ko WJ, Ho HN, Chu SH. Int J Cardiol 1998; 63:81-4.

Yaegashi N, Miura M, Okamura K. Int J Gynaecol Obstet 1999; 64:67-8.

de Groot AN. Eur J Obstet Gynecol Reprod Biol 1996; 69:31-6.

Hammer M, Bostrom K, Borgvall B. Gynecol Obstet Invest 1990; 30:91-3.

Bugalho A, Bique C, Pereira C, et al. Acta Obstet Gynecol Scand 1996; 75:270-3.

Fujiwara Y, Yamanaka O, Nakamura T, et al. Jpn Heart J 1993; 34:803-8.

Moise KJ Jr, Carpenter RJ Jr. J Reprod Med 1988; 33:771-3.

Arabin B, Ruttgers H, Kubli F. Geburtshilfe Frauenheilkd 1986; 46:215-20.

Scapin F, Calistri D, Tronconi G, et al. Gynecol Obstet Invest 1983; 15:185-90.

Mantyla R, Kanto J. Int J Clin Pharmacol Ther Toxicol 1981; 19:386-91.

- **Summary** ⸱⸱⸱⸱⸱⸱⸱⸱⸱⸱⸱⸱⸱⸱⸱⸱⸱⸱⸱⸱⸱⸱⸱⸱⸱⸱
  - **Pregnancy Category C**
  - **Lactation Category S**
  - There are no indications for **methylergonovine** during a continuing pregnancy.
  - While **oxytocin** remains the drug of choice to prevent and treat postpartum uterine atony, **methylergonovine** rapidly treats most women should **oxytocin** fail.

Methylphenidate (Concerta; Metadate CD; Metadate ER; Ritalin; Ritalin-SR; Ritalin LA)

- **Class** — CNS *stimulant, amphetamine*

- **Indications** — Attention-deficit/hyperactivity disorder (ADHD), narcolepsy

- **Mechanism** — Unknown (CNS stimulation)

- **Dosage with Qualifiers** — ADHD—begin 20mg PO qd before the am meal; increase 20mg PO qw; max 60mg qd
  Narcolepsy—begin 5-10mg PO bid; increase 10mg/d q7d
  NOTE—do not crush/chew
  - **Contraindications**—hypersensitivity to drug or class, glaucoma, Tourette's syndrome, anxiety, MAO inhibitor <14d
  - **Caution**—hypertension, seizure disorder, psychosis, CV disease, alcohol/drug abuse

- **Maternal Considerations** — There are no adequate reports or well-controlled studies of **methylphenidate** in pregnant women. The clinical experience consists of limited case reports of narcolepsy and substance abuse.
  Side effects include seizures, growth suppression, psychosis, leukopenia, thrombocytopenic purpura, Tourette's syndrome, exfoliative dermatitis, drug dependency, arrhythmia, erythema multiforme, neuroleptic malignant syndrome, cerebral arteritis, hepatic dysfunction, nervousness, insomnia, abdominal pain, nausea, vomiting, blurred vision, tachycardia, motor tics, weight loss, angina, rash, fever, urticaria, drowsiness, and dyskinesia.

- **Fetal Considerations** — There are no adequate reports or well-controlled studies in human fetuses. It is unknown whether **methylphenidate** crosses the human placenta. However, maternal abuse of **pentazocine** and **methylphenidate** is associated with preterm birth, IUGR and evidence of neonatal withdrawal, but no malformations or developmental delay. Rodent teratogen studies reveal skeletal abnormalities in rabbits treated with 40 times the MRHD. IUGR was seen in lower doses.

- **Breastfeeding Safety** — There is no published experience in nursing women. It is unknown whether **methylphenidate** enters human breast milk.

- **References** — Hoover-Stevens S, Kovacevic-Ristanovic R. Clin Neuropharmacol 2000; 23:175-81.
  Debooy VD, Seshia MM, Tenenbein M, Casiro OG. Am J Dis Child 1993; 147:1062-5.

■ **Summary** ──────── • **Pregnancy Category C**
• **Lactation Category U**
• **Methylphenidate** should be used during pregnancy and lactation only if the benefit justifies the potential perinatal risk.

Methylprednisolone (Medlone; Medrol; Metrocort Summicort)

■ **Class** ──────────────── Corticosteroid

■ **Indications** ──────────── Inflammatory disorders, collagen vascular diseases, congenital adrenal hyperplasia, rheumatic disorders, allergy, respiratory diseases, hematologic disorders

■ **Mechanism** ──────────── Unknown

■ **Dosage with Qualifiers** ──── Inflammatory disorders—2-60mg PO qd
Congenital adrenal hyperplasia—2-60mg PO qd
Rheumatic disorders, adjunctive treatment—2-60mg PO qd
Collagen vascular diseases—2-60mg PO qd
Allergy—2-60mg PO qd
Respiratory diseases—2-60mg PO qd
Hematologic disorders—2-60mg PO qd
Multiple sclerosis—acute exacerbations 200mg PO qd ×7d, then 80mg PO qod ×1m
NOTE—4mg **methylprednisolone** = 5mg **prednisolone**
• **Contraindications**—hypersensitivity to drug or class, systemic fungal infection
• **Caution**—CHF, seizure disorder, diabetes, hypertension, osteoporosis, tuberculin, hepatic dysfunction

■ **Maternal Considerations** ──── **Methylprednisolone** is effective treatment for a wide range of disorders that occur during pregnancy. The large number prevents a detailed list here. **Methylprednisolone** is effective and believed safe during pregnancy for the treatment of acute asthma, lupus, nephrotic syndrome with mixed connective tissue disease, immune glomerulonephritis, alloimmune thrombocytopenia, immune thrombocytopenia, inflammatory bowel disease, Bell's palsy, gestational herpes, and for a "stress" dose in labor and delivery to chronically suppressed patients, among many. Other inflammatory disorders such as Quervain's disease of pregnancy can be treated successfully. First trimester hyperemesis gravidarium refractory to conventional treatments may respond well to **methylprednisolone**. Steroids may also be useful reducing the severity and speeding the recovery of women who develop atypical preeclampsia, or HELLP syndrome. **Methylprednisolone** reduces the risk of ovarian hyperstimulation during ovulation induction for *in vitro* fertilization.

Side effects include immunosuppression, menstrual irregularities, hypertension, peptic ulcer, CHF, adrenal insufficiency, steroid psychosis, pancreatitis, pseudotumor cerebri, nausea, vomiting, headache, dizziness, dyspepsia, mood swings, insomnia, anxiety, hypokalemia, edema, appetite change, skin changes, acne, cushingoid features, hyperglycemia, and ecchymosis.

■ **Fetal Considerations**

There are no adequate reports or well-controlled studies in human fetuses. **Methylprednisolone** does not cross the placenta. Rodent teratogenicity studies have not been performed, but there is no clinical evidence it is teratogenic. The effect of bolus doses of **methylprednisolone** on the fetus is unknown.

■ **Breastfeeding Safety**

There are no adequate reports or well-controlled studies in nursing women. It is unknown whether **methylprednisolone** enters human breast milk. What little evidence exists suggests the quantity of corticosteroid excreted into breast milk is not clinically relevant for the newborn.

■ **References**

Lainas T, Petsas G, Stavropoulou G, et al. Fertil Steril 2002; 78:529-33.

Avci S, Yilmaz C, Sayli U. J Hand Surg 2002; 27:322-4.

Moore LE, Martin JN Jr. J Perinatol 2001; 21:456-8.

Mallmann F, Fernandes AK, Avila EM, et al. Braz J Med Biol Res 2002; 35:39-47.

Schlembach D, Munz W, Fischer T. J Perinat Med 2000; 28:502-5.

Horita Y, Tsunoda S, Inenaga T, et al. Nephron 2001; 89:354-6.

Radoncic E, Delmis J, Pfeifer D, Mayer D. Acta Med Croatica 2000; 54:125-7.

Mari I, Pouchot J, Grasland A, Vinceneux P. Presse Med 2000; 29:2213-5.

Ponnighaus JM, Ziegler H, Kowalzick L. Zentralbl Gynakol 1998; 120:548-50.

Safari HR, Fassett MJ, Souter IC, et al. Am J Obstet Gynecol 1998; 179:921-4.

Lockshin MD, Sammaritano LR. Scand J Rheumatol Suppl 1998; 107:136-8.

Ozsoylu S. Am J Obstet Gynecol 1998; 178:1368.

Fischer T, Wallukat G, Schneider MP, et al. Eur J Obstet Gynecol Reprod Biol 2001; 97:255-7.

Futami H, Kodaira M, Furuta T, et al. J Gastroenterol 1998; 33:408-11.

Safari HR, Alsulyman OM, Gherman RB, Goodwin TM. Am J Obstet Gynecol 1998; 178:1054-8.

Faedda R, Palomba D, Satta A, et al. Clin Nephrol 1995; 44:367-75.

Isler CM, Barrilleaux PS, Magann EF, et al. Am J Obstet Gynecol 2001; 184:1332-7.

Martin JN Jr, Perry KG Jr, Blake PG, et al. Am J Obstet Gynecol 1997; 177:1011-7.

Magann EF, Perry KG Jr, Meydrech EF, et al. Am J Obstet Gynecol 1994; 171:1154-8.

■ **Summary**
- **Pregnancy Category C**
- **Lactation Category S?**
- **Methylprednisolone** is generally considered safe during pregnancy and lactation for recognized medical indications.

Methyltestosterone (Android; Androral; Fopou; Forton; Madiol; Metandren; Metestone; Oreton Methyl; Primotest; Testo-B; Testred; Vigorex; Virilon; Virormone)

■ **Class** Hormone

■ **Indications** Breast cancer

■ **Mechanism** Unknown

■ **Dosage with Qualifiers** Breast cancer—50-200mg PO qd; alternatively 25-100mg buccal qd
- **Contraindications**—hypersensitivity to drug or class, pregnancy
- **Caution**—renal, cardiac and hepatic dysfunction

■ **Maternal Considerations** **Methyltestosterone** is used with modest results for the treatment of endometriosis in infertile women. It is used for palliation with advancing inoperable breast cancer known or believed to be estrogen-sensitive. **Methyltestosterone** is also used in combination with estrogen to enhance libido in women. There are no adequate reports or well-controlled studies of **methyltestosterone** in pregnant women, nor are there indications for its use.
Side effects include amenorrhea, breast tenderness, edema, virilism, hypertension, hepatic dysfunction, nausea, vomiting, hirsutism, cholestatic jaundice, decreased libido, increased libido, hypercholesterolemia, clitoral enlargement, acne, leukopenia, hypercalcemia, and polycythemia.

■ **Fetal Considerations** There are no adequate reports or well-controlled studies in human fetuses. It is unknown whether **methyltestosterone** crosses the human placenta. It does increase placental estradiol synthesis *in vitro*. Animal studies (rodents, dog) reveal pseudohermaphroditism in female fetuses exposed to **methyltestosterone**.

■ **Breastfeeding Safety**

There is no published experience in nursing women. It is unknown whether **methyltestosterone** enters human breast milk. It is ineffective for suppressing lactation.

■ **References**

Hammond MG, Hammond CB, Parker RT. Fertil Steril 1978; 29:651-4.
Kawashima K, Nakaura S, Nagao S, et al. Endocrinol Jpn 1977; 24:77-81.
Biggs JS, Hacker N, Andrews E, Munro C. Med J Aust 1978; 2:23-5.
Shane BS, Dunn HO, Kenney RM, et al. Biol Reprod 1969; 1:41-8.

■ **Summary**

- **Pregnancy Category X**
- **Lactation Category U**
- **Methyltestosterone** is contraindicated during pregnancy.

Methysergide (Deseril; Sansert)

■ **Class**

Ergot alkaloid

■ **Indications**

Migraine headache, diarrhea secondary to carcinoid

■ **Mechanism**

Nonspecific 5HT antagonist

■ **Dosage with Qualifiers**

Migraine headache—begin 2mg PO qd; typical dose 4-8mg PO qd; drug-free interval of 3-4w q6mo
Diarrhea (carcinoid)—begin 2mg PO tid; typical dose 4-16mg PO tid
- **Contraindications**—hypersensitivity to drug or class, arteriosclerosis, renal or hepatic dysfunction, hypertension, CAD, collagen disease, valvular heart disease
- **Caution**—retroperitoneal fibrosis, pulmonary insufficiency

■ **Maternal Considerations**

Methysergide is a semisynthetic, ergot ergometrine alkaloid derivative that constricts cranial and peripheral blood vessels. It is used prophylactically to treat migraine headache. There are no adequate reports or well-controlled studies of **methysergide** in pregnant women. Despite the limited clinical data to provide guidance, **methysergide** is generally considered contraindicated during pregnancy because of its vasoconstrictive effects.
Side effects include retroperitoneal, pleural, pulmonary or cardiac fibrosis, thickening of the aortic root, aortic and

mitral valve fibrosis, nausea, vomiting, diarrhea, heartburn, abdominal pain, insomnia, drowsiness, mild euphoria, dizziness, ataxia, lightheadedness, hyperesthesia, facial flush, telangiectasia, increased hair loss, peripheral edema, neutropenia, eosinophilia, arthralgia, and myalgia.

■ **Fetal Considerations** .... There are no adequate reports or well-controlled studies in human fetuses. It is unknown whether **methysergide** crosses the human placenta. Rodent studies reveal evidence of embryotoxicity and bradycardia when administered at high doses. It is suspected that the toxic effects are vascularly mediated, and not a direct myocardial effect.

■ **Breastfeeding Safety** .... There is no published experience in nursing women. It is unknown whether **methysergide** enters human breast milk.

■ **References** .... Silberstein SD. Cephalalgia 1998; 18:421-35.
Noguchi H. Nippon Sanka Fujinka Gakkai Zasshi 1986; 38:1026-32.
Roberts GT, Rand MJ. Mutat Res 1978; 50:317-25.

■ **Summary** ....
  • **Pregnancy Category X**
  • **Lactation Category U**
  • **Methysergide** is generally considered contraindicated during pregnancy and lactation.
  • There are alternative agents for which there is more experience during pregnancy and lactation.

Metoclopramide (Reglan)

■ **Class** .... *Antiemetic, antivertigo, gastrointestinal*

■ **Indications** .... Nausea (vomiting), nausea (vomiting) associated with chemotherapy, GERD, gastroparesis (diabetes)

■ **Mechanism** .... Stimulates GI motility

■ **Dosage with Qualifiers** .... <u>Nausea, vomiting</u>—5-10mg PO/IM/IV q6-8h
<u>Nausea, vomiting (chemo)</u>—1-2mg/kg IV/PO q2-4h
<u>GERD</u>—5-15mg PO/IV/IM qac, qhs
<u>Gastroparesis (diabetes)</u>—10mg IV/PO qac, qhs
NOTE—may be given 30min before meals; adjust dose based on CrCl
  • **Contraindications**—hypersensitivity to drug or class, pheochromocytoma, seizure disorder, GI bleeding, GI obstruction, concomitant usage of drugs likely to cause extrapyramidal reactions

- **Caution**—cirrhosis, CHF, renal or hepatic dysfunction, Parkinson's disease, hypertension, psychosis, depression, breast CA

■ **Maternal Considerations** ⋯⋯ Nausea and vomiting are common during the 1st trimester. **Metoclopramide** effectively reduces the incidence and severity, but may be associated with an increased risk of preterm delivery. It is unclear whether this relationship is related to **metoclopramide** or to the underlying disease. The insufficient data on the safety of **metoclopramide** makes it a second-line agent for the treatment of hyperemesis or gastroesophageal reflux. **Metoclopramide** is highly effective controlling nausea and vomiting during surgery in women undergoing cesarean section. It reduces gastric secretions but does not decrease the quantity of narcotics used to control pain postoperatively. In contrast, **metoclopramide** significantly reduces the duration of labor and the total PCA **morphine** requirements of women undergoing prostaglandin-induced abortion. To reduce the risk of dystonia, patients may be premedicated with **dyphenhydramine**. **Metoclopramide** is also helpful for the treatment of migraine, and enhances erythropoiesis in women with Diamond-Blackfan anemia.
Side effects include suicidal ideation, seizures, neutropenia, agranulocytosis, bronchospasm, dystonic reactions, galactorrhea, amenorrhea, hypotension, changes in libido, tardive dyskinesia, CHF, hypotension, hypertension, arrhythmia, porphyria, methemoglobinemia, diarrhea, irritability, urinary frequency, anxiety, rash, dizziness, hyperprolactinemia, urticaria, insomnia, headache, confusion, and neuroleptic malignant syndrome.

■ **Fetal Considerations** ⋯⋯ There are no adequate reports or well-controlled studies in human fetuses. **Metoclopramide** crosses the human placenta, though the kinetics remain to be elucidated. Its use in the 1st trimester does not appear to be associated with an increased risk of malformations, spontaneous abortions, or decreased fetal birth weight. Rodent studies are reassuring, revealing no evidence of teratogenicity or IUGR despite the use of doses higher than those used clinically.

■ **Breastfeeding Safety** ⋯⋯ There are no adequate reports or well-controlled studies in nursing women. It is unknown whether **metoclopramide** enters human breast milk. **Metoclopramide** augments milk production without having any effect on the prolactin or sodium concentrations.

■ **References** ⋯⋯
Berkovitch M, Mazzota P, Greenberg R, et al. Am J Perinatol 2002;19:311-6.
Magee LA, Mazzotta P, Koren G. Am J Obstet Gynecol 2002; 185:S256-61.
Gabay MP. J Hum Lact 2002; 18:274-9.
Hagen EM, Farbu E, Bindoff L. Tidsskr Nor Laegeforen 2001; 121:2162-3.
Poortinga E, Rosenthal D, Bagri S. Psychosomatics 2001; 42:153-6.

Biervliet FP, Maguiness SD, Hay DM, et al. Hum Reprod 2001; 16:581-3.

Stefos T, Sotiriadis A, Tsirkas P, et al. Acta Obstet Gynecol Scand 2001; 80:34-8.

Berkovitch M, Elbirt D, Addis A, et al. N Engl J Med 2000; 343:445-6.

Sorensen HT, Nielsen GL, Christensen K, et al. Br J Clin Pharmacol 2000; 49:264-8.

Aube M. Neurology 1999; 53:S26-8.

Pfaffenrath V, Rehm M. Drug Saf 1998; 19:383-8.

Broussard CN, Richter JE. Drug Saf 1998; 19:325-37.

Danzer BI, Birnbach DJ, Stein DJ, et al. Reg Anesth 1997; 22:424-7.

Stuart JC, Kan AF, Rowbottom SJ, et al. Anaesthesia 1996; 51:415-21.

Rosenblatt WH, Cioffi AM, Sinatra R, Silverman DG. Anesth Analg 1992; 75:760-3.

Riggs KW, Rurak DW, Taylor SM, et al. J Pharm Sci 1990; 79:1056-61.

■ **Summary**

- **Pregnancy Category B**
- **Lactation Category S**
- **Metoclopramide** complements other antiemetic drugs for the management of nausea and vomiting during pregnancy. It is a second-line agent.
- **Metoclopramide** increases prolactin secretion during both labor and postpartum. These properties make it a useful galactagogue.

Metolazone (Diulo; Metenix; Mykrox; Zaroxolyn)

■ **Class**

Diuretic, antihypertensive, thiazide

■ **Indications**

CHF, peripheral edema, hypertension

■ **Mechanism**

Inhibits resorption sodium and chloride in the proximal convoluted tubule

■ **Dosage with Qualifiers**

Zaroxolyn (see NOTE)
CHF—5-20mg PO qd
Peripheral edema—5-20mg PO qd
Hypertension—2.5-5mg PO qd
Mykrox (more rapid bioavailability; see NOTE)
Hypertension—begin 0.5mg PO qd; max 1mg PO qd
NOTE—Mykrox and other brands of **metolazone** are not therapeutically equivalent. Consult the package insert.
- **Contraindications**—hypersensitivity to drug, class, or sulfonamides; hyponatremia, hypokalemia, anuria, hepatic coma
- **Caution**—hypersensitivity to thiazide, renal or hepatic dysfunction, gout

- ■ **Maternal Considerations** — The use of diuretics in an otherwise healthy woman is inappropriate and exposes mother and fetus to unnecessary hazard. Diuretics do not prevent the development of preeclampsia, and there is no evidence that they are useful in the treatment of those with the disease. See **chlorothiazide**.
  Side effects include hyponatremia, hypokalemia, hypomagnesemia, hypercalcemia, agranulocytosis, aplastic anemia, neuropathy, pancreatitis, hypotension, dizziness, headache, palpitations, fatigue, dyspepsia, nausea, vomiting, constipation, anorexia, muscle cramps, rash, photosensitivity, hyperuricemia, and urticaria.

- ■ **Fetal Considerations** — There are no adequate reports or well-controlled studies in human fetuses. It is unknown whether **metolazone** crosses the human placenta. Rodent studies are reassuring, revealing no evidence of teratogenicity or IUGR despite the use of doses higher than those used clinically. See **chlorothiazide**.

- ■ **Breastfeeding Safety** — There are no adequate reports or well-controlled studies in nursing women. **Metolazone** enters human breast milk, but the kinetics remain to be elucidated. See **chlorothiazide**.

- ■ **References** — There are no current relevant references.
  See **chlorothiazide**.

- ■ **Summary**
  - **Pregnancy Category B**
  - **Lactation Category U**
  - **Thiazide** diuretics are contraindicated during pregnancy except in women with CHF.
  - There are alternative agents for which there is more experience regarding use during pregnancy and lactation.

Metoprolol (Betalor; Bloxan; Cardoxone; Lopressor; Metolar; Seloxen; Toprol XL)

- ■ **Class** — Antiadrenergic, β-blocker

- ■ **Indications** — Hypertension, acute MI, angina

- ■ **Mechanism** — Selective β-1 adrenergic antagonist

- ■ **Dosage with Qualifiers** — Hypertension—50-200mg PO bid
  Acute MI—begin 5mg IV q2min ×3; after the 3rd dose, begin 50mg PO q6h × 48h; then 100mg PO bid or 25-50mg PO q6h
  Angina—50-200mg PO bid; max 400mg qd

- **Contraindications**—hypersensitivity to drug or class, bronchospastic disease, sinus bradycardia, cardiogenic shock, AV block 1st degree or severe, CHF, hypotension, depressed respiratory function
- **Caution**—asthma, diabetes, major surgery, hyperthyroidism

■ **Maternal Considerations** ┄┄┄┄ **Metoprolol** is effective for the treatment of mild to moderate chronic hypertension, stable angina, arrhythmia and post-MI patients. **Metoprolol** was extensively tested during pregnancy and proved safe. Its clearance is increased during pregnancy, and the dose may require upward revision each trimester. **Metoprolol** is more effective than **methyldopa** in decreasing both systolic and diastolic blood pressures in women with chronic hypertension, but less effective than **nicardipine**. There are many case reports of its use during pregnancy without apparent adverse effects. In principle, the management of an arrhythmia is similar whether the patient is pregnant or not. **Metoprolol** has been used successfully to correct supraventricular arrhythmias. It may also reduce the frequency of migraine headache during pregnancy when given prophylactically. **Metoprolol** is as effective as **propranolol** in controlling symptoms of hyperthyroidism. *Side effects* include bradycardia, CHF, bronchospasm, depression, dyspnea, fatigue, dizziness, abdominal pain, dry mouth, agranulocytosis, nonthrombocytopenic purpura, thrombocytopenic purpura, nausea, vomiting, dyspepsia, flatulence, constipation, diarrhea, pruritus, headache, somnolence, nightmares, insomnia, musculoskeletal pain, blurred vision, decreased libido, and tinnitus.

■ **Fetal Considerations** ┄┄┄┄ There are no adequate reports or well-controlled studies in human fetuses. **Metoprolol** crosses the human placenta, but does not adversely affect the fetal heart rate. Some studies of β-blockers in pregnancy reveal an increased risk of IUGR. While true with **atenolol** and **propranolol,** it is not noted with **metoprolol**. Current study suggests the cause of the IUGR is excessive β blockade, producing a decrease in maternal cardiac output. Rodent studies are reassuring, revealing no evidence of teratogenicity or IUGR despite the use of doses higher than those used clinically. High doses are associated with embryotoxicity.

■ **Breastfeeding Safety** ┄┄┄┄ Small quantities of **metoprolol** are excreted into human breast milk. The neonatal plasma level is either very low or undetectable between breast-feeding periods. Feeding 3-4h after the maternal dose further reduces the neonatal risk.

■ **References** ┄┄┄┄ Benfield P, Clissold SP, Brogden RN. Drugs 1986; 31:376-429.
Pfaffenrath V, Rehm M. Drug Saf 1998; 19:383-8.

Kaaja R, Hiilesmaa V, Holma K, Jarvenpaa AL. Int J Gynaecol Obstet 1992; 38:195-9.
Lindeberg S, Lundborg P, Regardh CG, Sandstrom B. Eur J Clin Pharmacol 1987; 33:363-8.
Hogstedt S, Lindberg B, Peng DR, et al. Clin Pharmacol Ther 1985; 37:688-92.
Feely J, Peden N. Drugs 1984; 27:425-46.
Kulas J, Lunell NO, Rosing U, et al. Acta Obstet Gynecol Scand Suppl 1984; 118:65-9.
Lindeberg S, Sandstrom B, Lundborg P, Regardh CG. Acta Obstet Gynecol Scand Suppl 1984; 118:61-4.

■ **Summary**
- **Pregnancy Category C**
- **Lactation Category S**
- **Metoprolol** is generally considered safe during pregnancy and lactation for the noted indications and doses.

Metronidazole (Flagyl)

■ **Class** — Antibiotic, antiprotozoal

■ **Indications** — Bacterial infections (<u>anaerobic gram-negative bacilli</u>: *Bacteroides fragilis* species [B. *distasonis*, B. *ovatus*, B. *thetaiotaomicron*, B. *vulgatus*]; <u>anaerobic gram-positive bacilli</u>: *Clostridium* species and *Eubacterium* species; <u>anaerobic gram-positive cocci</u>: *Peptococcus* species, *Peptostreptococcus* species; <u>other microorganisms</u>: *Trichomonas vaginalis*, amebae)

■ **Mechanism** — Unknown; inhibits DNA synthesis

■ **Dosage with Qualifiers** — <u>Bacterial infections</u>—500mg PO q6-8h ×7-14d; alternative 15mg/kg/IV ×1 followed by 7.5mg/kg IV q5h; max 1g/dose
<u>Amebic abscess</u>—500-750mg PO tid ×5-10d
<u>Bacterial vaginosis</u>—2g PO ×1, alternative 500mg PO bid ×7d
<u>Giardiasis</u>—250mg PO tid ×5-7d; alternative 2g PO qd ×3d
<u>C. *difficile* colitis</u>—500mg PO tid ×7-14d; alternative 250mg PO qid ×7-14d
<u>Rosacea</u>—topical gel application bid ×9w
<u>Vaginal trichomoniasis</u>—2g PO ×1; alternative 500mg PO bid ×7d, 1g PO bid ×1d (partner treatment is critical)
NOTE—available also in gel (0.75%) or cream (0.75%)
- **Contraindications**—hypersensitivity to drug or class, alcohol consumption
- **Caution**—hepatic dysfunction, blood dyscrasia, seizures, neuropathies

■ Maternal Considerations ········· **Metronidazole** is used widely during pregnancy and has multiple therapeutic benefits.

Bacterial vaginosis—Bacterial vaginosis (BV) is associated with preterm rupture of membrane, preterm labor and delivery, and postpartum endometritis. Systemic and local therapy with **metronidazole** effectively treats BV. Several large randomized trials seeking to determine whether successful treatment of BV reduced the prevalence of adverse outcomes ended in controversy. Women who deliver preterm with symptomatic BV have a lower risk of preterm birth in a subsequent pregnancy if treated with **metronidazole**. Unfortunately, the treatment of women with asymptomatic BV and no prior preterm birth apparently does not alter their preterm delivery rate. High-risk conditions that require treatment of BV with **metronidazole** include: women with prior preterm birth, body mass index below 19.8kg/m^2 and women with evidence of endometritis before pregnancy. A "test of cure" should be obtained 1mo later. Small trials suggest that the combination of **ampicillin** and **metronidazole** successfully prolongs pregnancy in women with threatened idiopathic preterm labor. Similar results are reported when **metronidazole** is combined with **erythromycin**. Large clinical trials with **metronidazole**, threatened preterm labor and intact membranes have yet to be accomplished. And as already noted, the randomized trials clearly show **metronidazole** does not reduce the incidence of preterm labor. In fact, women with asymptomatic BV who took **metronidazole** before 26w gestation had a higher incidence of preterm labor than controls. BV treatment may offer other benefits. Prophylactic IV **metronidazole** reduces infectious morbidity postoperatively after a clinically indicated cesarean section. Similar results are obtained when the **metronidazole** is applied per vagina. **Metronidazole** also decreases the risk of upper genital tract infection after 1st trimester suction curettage.

Trichomoniasis is associated with an increased incidence of adverse outcomes of pregnancy. A single dose of **metronidazole** cures 90%. The cure rate is higher if both partners are treated. Unfortunately, the treatment of pregnant women with asymptomatic *trichomoniasis* does not prevent preterm delivery. It is not known whether the result is different for symptomatic disease.

Other diseases such as inflammatory bowel disease, *Clostridium difficile* colitis, anaerobic and protozoal infections are successfully treated during pregnancy with short-term courses of **metronidazole**.

Side effects include seizures, peripheral neuropathy, metallic taste, glossitis, stomatitis, neutropenia, overgrowth of *Candida*, ECG changes, dizziness, vertigo, incoordination, ataxia, confusion, irritability, depression, weakness, insomnia, erythematous rash, flushing, nasal congestion, mucous membrane dryness, fever, dysuria, cystitis, polyuria, incontinence, dyspareunia, decrease of libido, distress, nausea, vomiting, and headache.

■ **Fetal Considerations** **Metronidazole** crosses the human placenta. Though achieving an F:M ratio near unity, it does not pose a major teratogenic risk when used in the recommended doses. The safety of drug therapy for inflammatory bowel disease during pregnancy is an important clinical concern. **Metronidazole** appears safe if used for short durations. The possible fetal adverse effects related with long-term exposure as required by this condition remain unknown. Rodent studies are reassuring, revealing no evidence of teratogenicity or IUGR despite the use of doses higher than those used clinically. Embryotoxicity occurs.

■ **Breastfeeding Safety** **Metronidazole** is excreted into human breast milk reaching an M:P ratio greater than unity, but is not associated with adverse effects in breast-fed neonates.

■ **References**

Saling E, Schreiber M, al-Taie T. J Perinat Med 2001; 29:199-211.
Koumans EH, Markowitz LE, Hogan V. Clin Infect Dis 2002; 35:S152-72.
Gerstner G, Kofler E, Huber J. Z Geburtshilfe Perinatol 1980; 184:418-23.
Gulmezoglu AM. Cochrane Database Syst Rev 2002; CD000220.
Carey JC, Klebanoff MA. Curr Womens Health Rep 2001; 1:14-9.
Odendaal HJ, Popov I, Schoeman J, et al. S Afr Med J 2002; 92:231-4.
Pitt C, Sanchez-Ramos L, Kaunitz AM. Obstet Gynecol 2001; 98:745-50.
Klebanoff MA, Carey JC, Hauth JC, et al. N Engl J Med 2001; 345:487-93.
Goldenberg RL, Klebanoff M, Carey JC, Macpherson C. Am J Obstet Gynecol 2001; 185:485-6.
Diav-Citrin O, Shechtman S, Gotteiner T, et al. Teratology 2001; 63:186-92.
Crowley T, Low N, Turner A, et al. BJOG 2001; 108:396-402.
Einarson A, Ho E, Koren G. Can Fam Physician 2000; 46:1053-4.
McGregor JA, French JI. Obstet Gynecol Surv 2000; 55:S1-19.
Gulmezoglu AM. Cochrane Database Syst Rev 2000; CD000220.
Carey JC, Klebanoff MA, Hauth JC, et al. N Engl J Med 2000; 342:534-40.
National guideline for the management of Trichomonas vaginalis. Sex Transm Infect 1999; 75(Suppl 1):S21-3.
National guideline for the management of bacterial vaginosis. Sex Transm Infect 1999; 75(Suppl 1):S16-8.
Connell W, Miller A. Drug Saf 1999; 21:311-23.
Woodrow N, Lamont RF. Hosp Med 1998; 59:447-50.
Zhang Y, Zhang Q, Xu Z. Zhonghua Fu Chan Ke Za Zhi 1997; 32:288-92.
Czeizel AE, Rockenbauer M. Br J Obstet Gynaecol 1998; 105:322-7.
McDonald HM, O'Loughlin JA, Vigneswaran R, et al. Br J Obstet Gynaecol 1997; 104:1391-7.

Freeman CD, Klutman NE, Lamp KC. Drugs 1997;
54:679-708.
James AH, Katz VL, Dotters DJ, Rogers RG. South Med J
1997; 90:889-92.
Svare J, Langhoff-Roos J, Andersen LF, et al. Br J Obstet
Gynaecol 1997; 104:892-7.
Hauth JC, Goldenberg RL, Andrews WW, et al. N Engl
J Med 1995; 333:1732-6.
Ferris DG, Litaker MS, Woodward L, et al. J Fam Pract
1995; 41:443-9.

■ **Summary**

- **Pregnancy Category B**
- **Lactation Category S**
- **Metronidazole** is a first-line treatment for bacterial vaginosis.
- Although there is a strong association between BV, *Trichomonas vaginalis*, and preterm birth, the largest randomized trials with **metronidazole** failed to show benefit in treating asymptomatic women.
- The treatment of women with a prior preterm birth and symptomatic bacterial vaginosis or T. *vaginalis* reduces the risk of recurrence in a subsequent pregnancy.

Mexiletine (Mexitil)

■ **Class** — *Antiarrhythmic, class* IB

■ **Indications** — Arrhythmia, diabetic neuropathy

■ **Mechanism** — Stabilizes membranes and depresses phase 0 action potential

■ **Dosage with Qualifiers** — Arrhythmia (ventricular)—200mg PO q8h; alternative 400mg PO, then 200mg PO q8-12h
Diabetic neuropathy—begin 150mg qd ×3d, 300mg qd ×3d followed by 10mg/kg
NOTE—plasma levels >0.5 mcg/ml are generally considered therapeutic.
- **Contraindications**—hypersensitivity to drug or class, cardiogenic shock
- **Caution**—1st degree AV block, seizure disorder

■ **Maternal Considerations** — **Mexiletine** is a local anesthetic structurally similar to **lidocaine**, but active orally. There are no adequate reports or well-controlled studies of **mexiletine** in pregnant women. The published experience during pregnancy is limited to a few case reports where the drug was used throughout gestation to treat symptomatic PVCs. The dose requires monitoring to ensure that therapeutic levels are maintained. **Mexiletine** has also been used for the treatment of chronic neuropathic pain.

Side effects include arrhythmia, dyspepsia, dizziness, tremor, insomnia, diarrhea, dyspnea, rash, tinnitus, nervousness, headache, depression, palpitations, dry mouth, arthralgia, fever, anorexia, angina, and fatigue.

■ **Fetal Considerations** — There are no adequate reports or well-controlled studies in human fetuses. It is unknown whether **mexiletine** crosses the human placenta. Rodent studies are reassuring, revealing no evidence of teratogenicity or IUGR despite the use of doses higher than those used clinically. Some embryotoxicity was noted at doses that were multiples of the recommended human doses.

■ **Breastfeeding Safety** — **Mexiletine** is excreted into human breast milk achieving an M:P ratio greater than unity. However, the neonate does not reach a clinically relevant level because of the volume of distribution.

■ **References** — Gregg AR, Tomich PG. J Perinatol 1988; 8:33-5.
Lownes HE, Ives TJ. Am J Obstet Gynecol 1987; 157:446-7.
Lewis AM, Patel L, Johnston A, Turner P. Postgrad Med J 1981; 57:546-7.
Timmis AD, Jackson G, Holt DW. Lancet 1980; 2:647-8.

■ **Summary** —
- **Pregnancy Category C**
- **Lactation Category S**
- **Mexiletine** should be used during pregnancy and lactation only if the benefit justifies the potential perinatal risk.

Mezlocillin (Mezlin)

■ **Class** — Antibiotic, penicillin

■ **Indications** — Bacterial infections (gram-negative aerobes: *Escherichia coli, Klebsiella* species, *Proteus mirabilis, Enterobacter, Proteus vulgaris, Shigella, Morganella morganii, Pseudomonas aeruginosa, Providencia rettgeri, Haemophilus influenzae, Providencia stuartii, H. parainfluenzae, Citrobacter, Neisseria* species; gram-positive aerobes: *Staphylococcus aureus*, beta-hemolytic streptococci, *Streptococcus pneumoniae, S. faecalis*; anaerobic bacteria: *Peptococcus* species, *Peptostreptococcus* species, *Clostridium* species, *Bacteroides* species, *Fusobacterium* species, *Veillonella* species, *Eubacterium* species)

■ **Mechanism** — Bactericidal; inhibits bacterial wall mucopeptide synthesis

■ **Dosage with Qualifiers** — Bacterial infections—3-4gIV/IM q4-6h; alternative 200-350mg/kg/d IV in divided doses; max 24g/d

- **Contraindications**—hypersensitivity to drug or class
- **Caution**—bleeding, uremia, hypokalemia

■ **Maternal Considerations**

Mezlocillin, alone or in combination with other antibiotics, is effective as treatment or prophylaxis for a variety of diseases during pregnancy, including pyelonephritis, puerperal endomyometritis, PPROM, or cesarean section prophylaxis. In several small trials, **mezlocillin** prolonged the latency interval after PPROM. **Mezlocillin** is as safe and effective as **cefoxitin** and **clindamycin/gentamicin** for treatment of postpartum endometritis. A single perioperative dose of **mezlocillin** is as effective as a 3-dose regimen of either **mezlocillin** or **cefoxitin** in preventing postoperative endometritis after a cesarean section. Because there is no antibiotic that provides superior post-cesarean prophylaxis, the decision is usually based on cost.
Side effects include rash, pruritus, urticaria, drug fever, unpleasant taste, seizures, neutropenia, thrombocytopenia, hemolytic anemia, leukopenia, pseudomembranous colitis, pain, phlebitis, nausea, vomiting, eosinophilia, fever, elevated LFTs, and thrombophlebitis.

■ **Fetal Considerations**

There are no adequate reports or well-controlled studies in human fetuses. **Mezlocillin** crosses the placenta and is found in low concentrations in fetal blood and amniotic fluid. Rodent studies are reassuring, revealing no evidence of teratogenicity or IUGR despite the use of doses higher than those used clinically.

■ **Breastfeeding Safety**

There are no adequate reports or well-controlled studies in nursing women. Low concentrations of **mezlocillin** are found in human breast milk, too low to achieve clinically relevant level in the fetus. Other penicillins are generally considered compatible with breastfeeding.

■ **References**

Meyrier A, Guibert J. Drugs 1992; 44:356-67.
Pastorek JG 2nd, Sanders CV Jr. Rev Infect Dis 1991; 13(Suppl 9):S752-7.
Johnston MM, Sanchez-Ramos L, Vaughn AJ, et al. Am J Obstet Gynecol 1990; 163:743-7.
Boemi P, Reitano S, Cilano L, et al. Minerva Ginecol 1989; 41:359-63.
Faro S. Obstet Gynecol Clin North Am 1988; 15:685-95.
Conturso R, Valsecchi A, De Lalla F. Chemioterapia 1987; 6:611-3.
Faro S, Phillips LE, Baker JL, et al. Obstet Gynecol 1987; 69:760-6.
Singlas E. Nouv Presse Med 1982; 11:373-6.
Crombleholme WR, Green JR, Ohm-Smith M, et al. Am J Reprod Immunol Microbiol 1987; 13:71-5.
Saltzman DH, Eron LJ, Tuomala RE, et al. J Reprod Med 1986; 31:709-12.
Jaffe R, Altaras M, Loebel R, Ben-Aderet N. Chemotherapy 1986; 32:173-7.

■ Summary
- **Pregnancy Category B**
- **Lactation Category S**
- **Mezlocillin** is effective treatment and prophylaxis for a variety of bacterial infections during pregnancy.

Miconazole (Fungoid; Monistat; Ony-Clear; Tara)

■ **Class**	*Antifungal, dermatologic*
■ **Indications**	Yeast and mold infections (<u>Candida species</u>: C. *albicans*; <u>dermatophytes species</u>: T*richophyton*, *Microsporum*, E*pidermophyton*; <u>fungal infections, systemic</u>: coccidioidomycosis, candidiasis, cryptococcosis, petriellidiosis, paracoccidioidomycosis, mucocutaneous candidiasis)
■ **Mechanism**	Inhibits ergosterol biosynthesis, essential for the fungal cell wall
■ **Dosage with Qualifiers**	<u>Vulvovaginal candidiasis</u>—numerous dosing schedules reflecting disease, response, concomitant therapy, and commercial brand <u>Trichophyton rubrum (tinea pedis, tinea cruris, tinea corporis)</u>—numerous dosing schedules reflecting disease, response, concomitant therapy, and commercial brand <u>Epidermophyton floccosum, cutaneous candidiasis (moniliasis), tinea versicolor</u>—numerous dosing schedules reflecting disease, response, concomitant therapy and commercial brand NOTE—available in intravaginal suppository/cream/soft gel or dermatologic cream forms <u>Severe systemic fungal infections</u>—400-1200mg IV q8h • **Contraindications**—hypersensitivity to drug or class • **Caution**—unknown
■ **Maternal Considerations**	*Candida* vaginitis is perhaps the most common female genital tract infection. The vaginal milieu during pregnancy predisposes to C. *albicans* overgrowth. There are no adequate reports or well-controlled studies of **miconazole** in pregnant women. There is controversy whether the various imidazole compounds differ in efficacy for mycotic vaginitis. Studies conducted immediately after **miconazole** was released suggested it was significantly better than **nystatin**, **clotrimazole**, and **butoconazole** for the treatment of vaginal candidiasis during gestation. However, no randomized trial substantiates that conclusion. There is no significant difference in cure rates achieved after 7-14d of therapy. Significantly more patients relapsed after cure in the **nystatin** and

clotrimazole groups than in the **miconazole** groups. **Miconazole** is as effective as oral therapy with **fluconazole** for vulvovaginal candidiasis. Though women frequently prefer oral medication, **fluconazole** is not recommended during pregnancy.

Side effects include anaphylaxis, thrombocytopenia, cardiac arrest, vulvovaginal burning, itching, hives, rash, irritation, burning, maceration, phlebitis, pruritus, nausea, vomiting, fever, drowsiness, diarrhea, anorexia, and flushing.

■ **Fetal Considerations**

There are no adequate reports or well-controlled studies in human fetuses. It is unknown whether **miconazole** crosses the human placenta, but it has been used successfully in newborns. *In vitro*, **miconazole** effectively inhibits placental and fetal adrenal steroid aromatase. **Miconazole** is absorbed systemically after vaginal application, reaching peak levels approximating 10ng/mL. In contrast, parenteral levels of **miconazole** exceed 1mcg/ml. Post-marketing studies are reassuring, revealing no excess rates of adverse outcomes. Rodent studies are reassuring, revealing no evidence of teratogenicity or IUGR despite the use of doses higher than those used clinically. Embryotoxicity is associated with doses that also produce maternal toxicity.

■ **Breastfeeding Safety**

There is no published experience in nursing women. It is unknown whether **miconazole** enters human breast milk. However, considering the dose and route, it is unlikely the breast-fed neonate of a woman being treated for vaginitis would ingest clinically relevant amounts.

■ **References**

Timonen H. Mycoses 1992; 35:317-20.
Ainsworth RE. West J Med 1987; 147:599-600.
Mason JI, Carr BR, Murry BA. Steroids 1987; 50:179-89.
Eliot BW, Howat RC, Mack AE. Br J Obstet Gynaecol 1979; 86:572-7.
McNellis D, McLeod M, Lawson J, Pasquale SA. Obstet Gynecol 1977; 50:674-8.
Hilton AL, Warnock DW, Milne JD, Scott AJ. Curr Med Res Opin 1977-78; 5:295-8.
Qualey JR, Cooper C. J Reprod Med 1975; 15:123-5.

■ **Summary**

- **Pregnancy Category C**
- **Lactation Category U**
- **Miconazole** cream is effective for the treatment of pregnant women with confirmed candidiasis.
- **Miconazole** should be used during pregnancy and lactation only if the benefit justifies the potential perinatal risk.

Midazolam (Midolam; Versed)

■ **Class** ⋯⋯⋯⋯⋯⋯⋯⋯⋯ *Sedative, hypnotic, anxiolytic, benzodiazepine (short-acting)*

■ **Indications** ⋯⋯⋯⋯⋯⋯ Sedation

■ **Mechanism** ⋯⋯⋯⋯⋯⋯ Binds benzodiazepine receptors and enhances GABA effects

■ **Dosage with Qualifiers** ⋯⋯⋯ Sedation, preoperative—5mg IM 1h preoperatively; alternatively, 0.07-0.08mg/kg IM ×1
Surgical sedation—0.5-1mg IV q2-3min prn; max 5mg
General anesthesia induction—0.3mg/kg IV over 20-30sec
Mechanical ventilation, sedation—0.02-0.1mg/kg/h IV prn
  • **Contraindications**—hypersensitivity to drug or class, glaucoma, shock, CNS depression
  • **Caution**—history of substance abuse, COPD, CHF, renal or hepatic dysfunction

■ **Maternal Considerations** ⋯⋯⋯ Outpatient surgery demands rapid recovery with minimal delay. The short-acting sedation of **midazolam** makes it one of the most frequently used benzodiazepines for short, surgical procedures. It is most appropriate for those who are particularly anxious. Conscious sedation with **midazolam** and **fentanyl** significantly improves patient satisfaction with 1st trimester termination performed under local anesthesia. Similar results are obtained in women undergoing outpatient procedures such as oocyte retrieval procedure or GIFT. In rodents, **midazolam** suppresses uterine contractility *in vitro*.
Side effects include respiratory and or cardiac arrest, withdrawal, habituation, nausea, vomiting, confusion, euphoria, involuntary movements, hypotension, sedation, agitation, retrograde amnesia, hallucinations, marked aggressiveness, ataxia, urticaria, rash, dizziness, metallic taste, dry mouth, and constipation.

■ **Fetal Considerations** ⋯⋯⋯ There are no adequate reports or well-controlled studies in human fetuses. **Midazolam** crosses the human placenta somewhat more slowly than **diazepam**, achieving an F:M concentration ratio approaching unity 30-60min after maternal injection. Postnatally, its elimination half-life is 6-7h. The reported effects of benzodiazepines on development are inconsistent. Studies in the 1970s suggested 1st trimester exposure to benzodiazepines increased the risk of facial clefts, cardiac malformations, and other multiple malformations. Yet, no syndrome could be described. **Diazepam** and **chlordiazepoxide** were most frequently implicated. However, an increased risk was not confirmed in recent studies. **Midazolam** use during the 3rd trimester or labor may be associated with floppy infant syndrome, or symptoms of neonatal withdrawal. These symptoms vary from mild sedation, hypotonia, apneic spells, cyanosis, impaired metabolic responses to cold stress, and reluctance to suck, and may persist for hours to months after birth.

Midazolam is excreted at low concentrations into human breast milk with an M:P ratio approximating 0.15. Considering the dose and route, it is unlikely the breast-fed neonate would ingest clinically relevant amounts.

■ **References**

Wong CY, Ng EH, Ngai SW, Ho PC. Hum Reprod 2002; 17:1222-5.

Sen A, Rudra A, Sarkar SK, Biswas B. J Indian Med Assoc 2001; 99:683-4.

Karsli B, Kaya T, Cetin A. Pol J Pharmacol 1999; 51:505-10.

Hammadeh ME, Wilhelm W, Huppert A, et al. Arch Gynecol Obstet 1999; 263:56-59.

Milki AA, Tazuke SI. Fertil Steril 1997; 68:128-32.

Valentine JM, Lyons G, Bellamy MC. Eur J Anaesthesiol 1996; 13:589-93.

Bach V, Carl P, Crawford ME, et al. Anesth Analg 1989; 68:238-42.

Soussis I, Boyd O, Paraschos T, et al. Fertil Steril 1995; 64:1003-7.

Rossi AE, Lo Sapio D, Oliva O, et al. Minerva Anesthesiol 1995; 61:265-9.

McElhatton PR. Reprod Toxicol 1994; 8:461-75.

Martinez-Telleria A, Cano ME, Carlos R. Rev Esp Anestesiol Reanim 1992; 39:379-80.

Chambrier C, Zayneh E, Pouyau A, et al. Ann Fr Anesth Reanim 1991; 10:81-3.

Hamar O, Garamvolgyi G. Acta Chir Hung 1990; 31:63-8.

Camann W, Cohen MB, Ostheimer GW. Anesthesiology 1986; 65:441.

Matheson I, Lunde PK, Bredesen JE. Br J Clin Pharmacol 1990; 30:787-93.

■ **Summary**

- **Pregnancy Category D**
- **Lactation Category S**
- **Midazolam** is a useful agent during pregnancy and lactation for the indications cited.

Midodrine (ProAmatine)

■ **Class** — *Adrenergic agonist*

■ **Indications** — Hypotension, urinary incontinence

■ **Mechanism** — α-1 adrenergic agonist

■ **Dosage with Qualifiers** — Hypotension (orthostatic)—10mg PO tid
Urinary incontinence—2.5mg PO bid/tid
- **Contraindications**—hypersensitivity to drug or class, renal dysfunction, thyrotoxicosis, pheochromocytoma
- **Caution**—hepatic dysfunction, diabetes

- **Maternal Considerations** .... **Midodrine** increases vascular tone and elevates blood pressure. There is no published experience during pregnancy. Rodent studies reveal no effect on uterine contractility *in vitro*.
  Side effects include bradycardia, erythema multiforme, pruritus, dysuria, paresthesias, piloerection, anxiety, dry mouth, nervousness, vasodilatation, chills, confusion, headache, nausea, vomiting, hypertension; paresthesias, visual field defect, dry skin, impaired urination, asthenia, backache, flatulence, and leg cramps.

- **Fetal Considerations** .... There are no adequate reports or well-controlled studies in human fetuses. It is unknown whether **midodrine** crosses the human placenta. Though no evidence of teratogenicity was found in rodent studies, there was an increased prevalence of embryo resorption and IUGR.

- **Breastfeeding Safety** .... There is no published experience in nursing women. It is unknown whether **midodrine** enters human breast milk.

- **Reference** .... Pittner H. Arzneimittelforschung 1987; 37:794-6.

- **Summary** ....
  - **Pregnancy Category C**
  - **Lactation Category U**
  - **Midodrine** should be used during pregnancy and lactation only if the benefit justifies the potential perinatal risk.
  - None of the indicated uses is urgent. Thus, its use can likely be delayed until delivery.

Mifepristone (Mifeprex; RU-486)

- **Class** .... *Abortifacient, stimulant, uterine contractility*

- **Indications** .... Abortion

- **Mechanism** .... Progesterone receptor antagonist

- **Dosage with Qualifiers** .... Abortion—200-600mg PO ×1
  NOTE—pregnancy <49d from LMP; often combined with **misoprostol**
  - **Contraindications**—hypersensitivity to drug, class, or prostaglandins; ectopic pregnancy, IUD in place, anticoagulation, corticosteroid use, chronic adrenal failure, bleeding disorder, porphyria, no access to emergent health care, noncompliance with the treatment
  - **Caution**—unknown

■ Maternal Considerations

Sheep studies demonstrate that **progesterone** suppresses uterine/placental secretion of **PGF-2α,** and that critical progesterone:estradiol-17β and PGE:PGF-2α ratios are necessary for continuation of the pregnancy. **Mifepristone** causes **progesterone** withdrawal. In 1996 the FDA Advisory Committee for Reproductive Health Drugs concluded **mifepristone** was safe and effective for early pregnancy termination. In 2000, the FDA approved **mifepristone** to induce abortion in pregnancies <49 days from the LMP. The most popular treatment schedule is **mifepristone** 200-600mg followed 36-48h later by oral **misoprostol** (0.4-0.6mg) in pregnancies up to 49d, and vaginal **gemeprost** (1.0mg) or **misoprostol** (0.8mg) if the pregnancy dates from 49-63d since the LMP. The addition of 2 doses of **misoprostol** beginning 48h after **mifepristone** significantly reduces the ongoing pregnancy rate compared to **mifepristone** alone. β-hCG and **progesterone** concentrations continue to increase for 48h after **mifepristone**. After **misoprostol,** the β-hCG and **progesterone** levels decline in 24h by 70 and 60%, respectively. Treated women should expect some bleeding for 9-16d. All women experience some form of adverse reaction. Eight percent of treated women bleed 30d or more. The duration of bleeding increases with gestational age at termination. There are only a few randomized studies comparing medical and surgical termination, and the definitions of successful outcome (complete abortion), adverse effects, and complications vary. The three most common reasons a woman chooses a medical abortion are "avoidance of surgery," "avoidance of general anesthesia," and "the method being more natural." The duration of bleeding, degree of blood loss, frequency of uterine pain, vomiting, and diarrhea are all greater with **mifepristone** abortion. On the other hand, the incidence of major complications such as blood transfusion and pelvic infection does not seemingly differ between the two. Surgical complications, such as uterine perforation and cervical tears, are less common in women who choose medical abortion. **Mifepristone** helps preserve fertility and avoid major maternal complications (death, hysterectomy) in women with either cervical or uterine scar ectopic pregnancy. At term, **mifepristone** has a modest impact on cervical ripening if given 24h before labor induction. **Mifepristone** appears to reduce the need for **misoprostol** and **oxytocin** compared with placebo. More recent studies address the potential role of **mifepristone** as emergency contraception. Low-dose **mifepristone** (either 25mg PO ×1, or 10mg PO ×1 followed by levonorgestrel 1.5mg PO 12h later) is 80% effective.

Side effects include vaginal bleeding, abdominal cramps, incomplete abortion, fetal malformation, hemorrhage, nausea, vomiting, anxiety, fever, rigors, dyspepsia, fainting, vaginitis, asthenia, leucorrhoea, and insomnia.

■ Fetal Considerations

There are no adequate reports or well-controlled studies in human fetuses. **Mifepristone** does cross the primate placenta. The human experience with continued pregnancy after failed medical termination is limited. Normal outcomes are reported. And while Mobius syndrome is increased after failed **misoprostol** termination, the same cannot be said for **mifepristone**.

■ **Breastfeeding Safety** ⋯⋯⋯⋯ There are no adequate reports or well-controlled studies in nursing women. It is unknown whether **mifepristone** enters human breast milk. Rodent studies suggest that **mifepristone** enhances lactation.

■ **References** ⋯⋯⋯⋯ Schaff EA, Fielding SL, Eisinger S, Stadalius L. Contraception 2001; 63:251-4.
Bartley J, Baird DT. BJOG 2002; 109:1290-4.
Ashok PW, Templeton A, Wagaarachchi PT, Flett GM. BJOG 2002; 109:1281-9.
Bygdeman M, Danielsson KG. Drugs 2002; 62:2459-70.
Weems YS, Bridges PJ, Sasser RG, et al. Prostaglandins Other Lipid Mediat 2002; 70:195-208.
Schaff EA, Fielding SL, Westhoff C. Contraception 2002; 66:247-50.
VonHertzen H, Piaggio G, Ding J, et al. Lancet 2002; 360:1803-10.
Omokanye S. J Fam Plann Reprod Health Care 2001; 27:102.
Fox MC, Creinin MD, Harwood B. Contraception 2002; 66:225-9.
Li FF, Chen YX, Tang JH. Di Yi Jun Yi Da Xue Xue Bao 2002; 22:466-6.
Changhai H, Youlun G, Jie Y, et al. Contraception 2002; 66:221-4.
No author. Reprod Freedom News 1996; 5:7-8.
Honkanen H, Ranta S, Ylikorkala O, Heikinheimo O. Hum Reprod 2002; 17:2315-9.
Turner AN, Ellertson C. Drug Saf 2002; 25:695-706.
Honkanen H, von Hertzen H. Contraception 2002; 65:419-23.
Ashok PW, Stalder C, Wagaarachchi PT, et al. BJOG 2002; 109:553-60.
Ellertson C, Waldman SN. Curr Womens Health Rep 2001; 1:184-90.
Weimin W, Wenqing L. Int J Gynaecol Obstet 2002; 77:201-7.
Jain JK, Dutton C, Harwood B, et al. Hum Reprod. 2002; 17:1477-82.
Sexton C, Sharp N. Aust NZ J Obstet Gynaecol 2002; 42:211-3.
Wing DA, Fassett MJ, Mishell DR. Obstet Gynecol 2000; 96:543-8.
Elliott CL, Brennand JE, Calder AA. Obstet Gynecol 1998; 92:804-9.
Frydman R, Lelaidier C, Baton-Saint-Mleux C, et al. Obstet Gynecol 1992; 80:972-5.
Cabrol D, Carbonne B, Bienkiewicz A, et al. Prostaglandins 1991; 42:71-9.
Wolf JP, Sinosich M, Anderson TL, et al. Am J Obstet Gynecol 1989; 160:45-7.

Wolf JP, Chillik CF, Itskovitz J, et al. Am J Obstet Gynecol 1988; 159:238-42.
Soaje M, de Di Nasso EG, Deis RP. J Endocrinol 2002; 172:255-61.

■ **Summary**

- **Pregnancy Category X**
- **Lactation Category S**
- **Mifepristone** is an effective abortifacient either alone or in combination with a prostaglandin analog.
- **Mifepristone** is contraindicated in women planning to continue pregnancy.
- The fetal impact of continuing the pregnancy after a failed medical termination remains unclear.

Miglitol (Glyset)

■ **Class** Antidiabetic agent, α-glucosidase inhibitor

■ **Indications** Diabetes mellitus type 2

■ **Mechanism** Reversibly inhibits intestinal α-glucoside hydrolase decreasing glucose absorption

■ **Dosage with Qualifiers** Diabetes—begin 25mg PO prior to each meal; max 100mg PO tid
- **Contraindications**—hypersensitivity to drug or class, DKA, inflammatory bowel disease, colonic ulceration, intestinal obstruction
- **Caution**—hypoglycemia, loss of diabetic control, renal dysfunction

■ **Maternal Considerations** Because it inhibits glucose absorption, **miglitol** is additive to the hypoglycemic effect of other agents such as sulfonylureas. There is no evidence that systemic absorption contributes to its effect. There are no adequate reports or well-controlled studies of **miglitol** in pregnant women. **Insulin** is the currently recommended hypoglycemic agent of choice during pregnancy, though a growing body of work suggests a promising future for some oral hypoglycemic agents.
Side effects include abdominal pain, diarrhea, flatulence, and hypoglycemia.

■ **Fetal Considerations** There are no adequate reports or well-controlled studies in human fetuses. It is unknown whether **miglitol** crosses the human placenta. Considering poor absorbtion, it is unlikely the maternal systemic concentration will reach clinically relevant level. Rodent studies are reassuring, revealing no evidence of teratogenicity, though there was a small increase in IUGR at doses in multiples of those used clinically. Placental transport studies in the rat indicate limited transport even after parenteral administration.

■ **Breastfeeding Safety** — There is no published experience in nursing women. The breast-feeding newborn is exposed to less than 0.5% of the maternal dose of **miglitol**, a dose that should not have a clinically relevant effect on the neonate.

■ **References** — Ahr HJ, Boberg M, Brendel E, et al. Arzneimittelforschung 1997; 47:734-45.

■ **Summary** —
- **Pregnancy Category B**
- **Lactation Category S**
- **Miglitol** is a potentially attractive agent for use during pregnancy and breastfeeding.
- It should be used during pregnancy and lactation only if the benefit justifies the potential perinatal risk.
- There are alternative agents for which there is more experience during pregnancy.

Milrinone (Primacor)

■ **Class** — *Inotrope, vasodilator*

■ **Indications** — CHF

■ **Mechanism** — Selective inhibitor of the cAMP phosphodiesterase in cardiac and vascular muscle

■ **Dosage with Qualifiers** — CHF—load 50mcg/kg IV over 10min, then 0.375mcg/kg/min and titrate to desired response; max 0.75mcg/kg/min
NOTE—renal dosing
- **Contraindications**—hypersensitivity to drug or class, aortic valve disease, pulmonary valve disease, MI
- **Caution**—atrial fibrillation, atrial flutter, renal dysfunction

■ **Maternal Considerations** — **Milrinone** is an ionotropic agent for the short-term management of CHF. There is no published experience during pregnancy.
Side effects include ventricular arrhythmia, ventricular ectopy, headache, chest pain, hypotension, angina, hypokalemia, and thrombocytopenia.

■ **Fetal Considerations** — There are no adequate reports or well-controlled studies in human fetuses. It is unknown whether **milrinone** crosses the human placenta. While **milrinone** does cross the baboon placenta, placental transfer in the ewe is low. In the latter, **milrinone** increases uterine blood flow. Rodent studies are reassuring, revealing no evidence of teratogenicity or IUGR despite the use of doses higher than those used clinically. There was some evidence of embryotoxicity at high doses in rabbits.

■ **Breastfeeding Safety** ⸺ There is no published experience in nursing women. It is unknown whether **milrinone** enters human breast milk.

■ **References** ⸺ Kitazawa T, Takaoka K, Taneike T. J Auton Pharmacol 1999; 19:65-75.
Atkinson BD, Fishburne JI Jr, Hales Ka, et al. Am J Obstet Gynecol 1996; 174:895-6.
Santos AC, Baumann AL, Wlody D, et al. Am J Obstet Gynecol 1992; 166:257-62.

■ **Summary** ⸺
- **Pregnancy Category C**
- **Lactation Category S**
- **Milrinone** should be used during pregnancy and lactation only if the benefit justifies the potential perinatal risk.
- There are alternative agents for which there is more experience regarding use during pregnancy and lactation.

Minocycline (Arestin; Dynacin; Lederderm; Minocin, Vectrin)

■ **Class** ⸺ *Antibiotic, tetracycline*

■ **Indications** ⸺ Bacterial infections (gram-negative microorganisms: *Haemophilus ducreyi* [chancroid], *Yersinia pestis, Francisella tularensis, Pasteurella pestis, P. tularensis, Bartonella, Bacteroides* species, *Vibrio comma, V. fetus, Brucella, Escherichia coli, Enterobacter aerogenes, Shigella, H. influenzae, Klebsiella*; gram-positive microorganisms: *Streptococcus pyogenes, S. faecalis, S. pneumoniae, Staphylococcus aureus, Neisseria gonorrhoeae, Listeria monocytogenes, Clostridium* species, *bacillus anthracis, Fusobacterium fusiforme* [Vincent's infection]; rickettsiae, *Treponema pallidum, Actinomyces,* amebiasis)

■ **Mechanism** ⸺ Bacteriostatic; inhibits protein synthesis

■ **Dosage with Qualifiers** ⸺ Bacterial infections, acne vulgaris—50mg PO qd/tid
Gonorrhea—100mg PO bid ×5d; alternative 100-200mg ×1 followed by 50mg PO qid
Syphilis—100mg PO bid ×15d
Mycobacterium marinum infection—100mg PO bid ×6-8w

- **Contraindications**—hypersensitivity to drug or class
- **Caution**—renal or hepatic dysfunction

■ **Maternal Considerations** ········· There are no adequate reports or well-controlled studies of **minocycline** in pregnant women. Case reports note its use for the treatment of recurrent pemphigoid gestationis. Similar to other tetracyclines, concern has been raised that it might lower the effectiveness of low-dose oral contraceptive agents. See **tetracycline**.
Side effects include thrombocytopenia, hepatotoxicity, neutropenia, Jarisch-Herxheimer reaction, enterocolitis, fatty liver disease, pseudomembranous colitis, skeletal abnormalities, hemolytic anemia, hepatic or renal dysfunction, increased BUN, glossitis, ataxia, vertigo, tinnitus, pseudotumor cerebri, and vaginal candidiasis.

■ **Fetal Considerations** ················· There are no adequate reports or well-controlled studies in human fetuses. It is unknown whether **minocycline** crosses the human placenta. It is unlikely the maternal systemic concentration will reach clinically relevant level if applied topically for acne. Other tetracyclines cross the human placenta and are associated with tooth discoloration and in rodents, increased embryo resorption. See **tetracycline**.

■ **Breastfeeding Safety** ················· There are no adequate reports or well-controlled studies in nursing women. It is unknown whether **minocycline** enters human breast milk. Milk discoloration is reported. See **tetracycline**.

■ **References** ················· Loo WJ, Dean D, Wojnarowska F. Clin Exp Dermatol 2001; 26:726-7.
Hunt MJ, Salisbury EL, Grace J, Armati R. Br J Dermatol 1996; 134:943-5.
See **tetracycline**.

■ **Summary** ················· • **Pregnancy Category D**
- **Lactation Category U**
- The tetracyclines are generally contraindicated during pregnancy because of fetal tooth discoloration.
- There are alternative agents during pregnancy for almost all indications.

Minoxidil (Alopexil; Alostil; Loniten; Lonolax; Mintop; Modil; Rogaine)

■ **Class** — Antihypertensive, vasodilator

■ **Indications** — Hypertension, baldness

■ **Mechanism** — Unknown; peripheral vessel vasodilator

■ **Dosage with Qualifiers** — Hypertension—40 mg/d in divided doses; max 100mg PO qd
Baldness (alopecia androgetica)—apply 1ml to scalp bid (2.5% solution)
- **Contraindications**—hypersensitivity to drug or class, pheochromocytoma, pericardial effusion
- **Caution**—renal or hepatic dysfunction, MI

■ **Maternal Considerations** — There are no adequate reports or well-controlled studies of **minoxidil** in pregnant women. **Minoxidil** is no longer often used for the treatment of hypertension, but rather is used for balding. Balding can be a normal physiologic occurrence in women taking oral contraceptives or after parturition. It can be treated with either **progesterone** or **minoxidil**.
Side effects include CHF, Stevens-Johnson syndrome, pericardial effusion, angina, edema, tachycardia, hypertrichosis, headache, breast tenderness, paresthesias, weight gain, thrombocytopenia, EEG changes, contact dermatitis, itching, skin irritation, and leukopenia.

■ **Fetal Considerations** — There are no adequate reports or well-controlled studies in human fetuses. It is unknown whether **minoxidil** crosses the human placenta. Caudal regression syndrome was reported in a mother taking **minoxidil** long before and during gestation. Fetal hypertrichosis is also reported in fetuses whose mothers used **minoxidil** topically throughout pregnancy. Rodent studies are reassuring, revealing no evidence of teratogenicity or IUGR despite the use of doses higher than those used clinically. Embryotoxicity was seen with high doses.

■ **Breastfeeding Safety** — There are no adequate reports or well-controlled studies in nursing women. **Minoxidil** enters human breast milk, but the kinetics remain to be elucidated.

■ **References** — Burke KE. Postgrad Med 1989; 85:52-8, 67-73, 77.
Kaler SG, Patrinos ME, Lambert GH, et al. Pediatrics 1987; 79:434-6.
Veyrac G, Chiffoleau A, Bailly C, et al. Therapie 1995; 50:474-6.
Valdivieso A, Valdes G, Spiro TE, Westerman RL. Ann Intern Med 1985; 102:135.

Mirtazapine (Remeron)

■ **Class** ⎯⎯⎯⎯⎯⎯⎯⎯⎯⎯⎯⎯⎯⎯⎯⎯ *Antidepressant, tricyclic*

■ **Indications** ⎯⎯⎯⎯⎯⎯⎯⎯⎯⎯⎯ Depression

■ **Mechanism** ⎯⎯⎯⎯⎯⎯⎯⎯⎯⎯ Unknown; antagonizes α-2 adrenergic and serotonin receptors

■ **Dosage with Qualifiers** ⎯⎯⎯ Depression—15-45mg PO qhs; begin 15mg PO qhs
● **Contraindications**—hypersensitivity to drug or class, MAO inhibitors <14d
● **Caution**—advanced age, renal or hepatic dysfunction, mania, hypomania, seizures, cardiovascular disease, CV disease, consumption of alcohol

■ **Maternal Considerations** ⎯⎯ Depression is common during and after pregnancy, but typically goes unrecognized. Pregnancy is not a reason a priori to discontinue psychotropic drugs. **Mirtazapine** is one option for patients unresponsive to, or intolerant of SSRIs. There is no published experience with **mirtazapine** during pregnancy.
Side effects include agranulocytosis, orthostatic hypotension, torsades de pointes, increased appetite, weight gain, hypercholesterolemia, dry mouth, somnolence, dyspnea, confusion, tremor, abnormal thinking, abnormal dreams, dizziness, asthenia, constipation, flu-like symptoms, elevated LFTs, urinary frequency, myalgia, and back pain.

■ **Fetal Considerations** ⎯⎯⎯⎯ There are no adequate reports or well-controlled studies in human fetuses. It is unknown whether **mirtazapine** crosses the human placenta.

■ **Breastfeeding Safety** ⎯⎯⎯⎯ There is no published experience in nursing women. It is unknown whether **mirtazapine** enters human breast milk.

■ **Reference** ⎯⎯⎯⎯⎯⎯⎯⎯⎯⎯⎯ Brown CS. Obstet Gynecol Clin North Am 2001; 28:241-68.

- **Pregnancy Category C**
- **Lactation Category U**
- **Mirtazapine** should be used during pregnancy and lactation only if the benefit justifies the potential perinatal risk.
- There are alternative agents for which there is more experience regarding use during pregnancy and lactation.

Misoprostol (Cytotec)

■ **Class** ································· *Gastrointestinal, abortifacient, stimulant uterine contractility*

■ **Indications** ······························ NSAID-induced gastric ulcer, constipation, cervical ripening, abortion

■ **Mechanism** ······························ Inhibits gastric acid secretions; protects gastric mucosa; stimulates uterine contractility

■ **Dosage with Qualifiers** ············ NSAID-induced gastric ulcers—100-200mcg PO qid
Constipation—600-2400mcg/d PO bid-qid
Cervical ripening—25mcg vaginally q3-6h; wait at least 4h before initiating **oxytocin**; max 50mcg/dose
Abortion—400mcg PO ×1; may repeat q4-6h
NOTE—take with meals; **misoprostol** is often used with **mifepristone** for 1st trimester termination
- **Contraindications**—hypersensitivity to drug or class, pregnancy (for GI indications)
- **Caution**—childbearing potential (GI indications), prior cesarean section, myomectomy or other uterine surgery, fetal macrosomia, grand multiparity

■ **Maternal Considerations** ········ **Misoprostol** is a **prostaglandin E** analog. The only FDA-approved indication is the treatment and prevention of intestinal ulcer disease resulting from **NSAID** drug use. Although still not approved by the FDA for other indications, **misoprostol** is well studied and widely used for both cervical ripening and the induction of labor during either the 2nd or 3rd trimesters.
Early to mid-pregnancy termination—Combined with **mifepristone**, **misoprostol** is safe and effective for medical termination of early pregnancy. Typically, **misoprostol** is given per vaginam 48h after **mifepristone**. The administration of 2 doses of **misoprostol** after **mifepristone** significantly reduces the risk of failed abortion compared to **mifepristone** alone. Vaginal **misoprostol** shortens the time from induction to delivery compared to PO. A wide range of dosing regimens has been suggested for 2nd trimester termination. 400mcg PO or 200mcg per vaginam q4h are common. **Misoprostol**

does not reduce the blood loss and the time for placental expulsion after 2nd trimester termination.

Term pregnancy— **Misoprostol** is commonly used to induce cervical ripening and labor. The manufacturer of **misoprostol** issued in August 2000 a warning letter to American health care providers, cautioning against the use of **misoprostol** in pregnant women secondary to the lack of safety data for its use in obstetric practice. The ACOG took issue with that position, as there was a multitude of studies supporting its use. **Misoprostol** is effective in ripening the cervix and inducing labor at term when given either per vaginam or PO. It is inexpensive and stable at room temperature. Debate continues on the optimal dose, regimen, route of administration, and concurrent use of ancillary ripening methods (laminaria, Foley balloon, **dinoprostone gel**). Low-dose **misoprostol** (25mcg) is effective for cervical ripening and labor induction. Uterine tachysystole is more common after 50mcg or more given vaginally or orally. Clinical trials report increased frequencies of meconium passage, neonatal acidemia and cesarean delivery due to fetal distress if high doses are used. Some trials report no decrease in the overall rate of cesarean delivery, though the frequency of failed induction as an indication is reduced. **Misoprostol** is effective for the induction of labor in women with preterm premature rupture of the membranes (PPROM), intrauterine fetal demise, or preeclampsia. Parity, initial cervical dilatation, and gestational age are the most useful predictors of successful cervical ripening and labor induction if administered per vaginam. The most common side effects during labor induction are shivering and uterine tachysystole. Because of the tachysystole, low-dose **oxytocin** may be preferred in the high-risk parturient whose fetus is at increased risk for fetal intolerance to labor. In 2002, the ACOG Committee Opinion on Obstetric Practice concluded the risk of uterine rupture during VBAC is substantially increased by the use of various prostaglandin cervical ripening agents. They are specifically discouraged in favor of mechanical methods. Rectal **misoprostol** (400mcg) may be similar to **oxytocin** (10IU with the anterior shoulder), while either rectal or oral **misoprostol** are significantly less effective than **oxytocin** plus **methylergometrine** for the prevention and treatment of postpartum hemorrhage.

Side effects include abortion, uterine rupture, uterine hyperstimulation, diarrhea, constipation, abdominal pain, nausea, vomiting, flatulence, dyspepsia, hypermenorrhea, dysmenorrhea, and headache.

■ **Fetal Considerations** ············· There are no adequate reports or well-controlled studies in human fetuses. **Misoprostol** is associated with a higher rate of uterine hyperstimulation, more variable decelerations, and likely as a result, a higher prevalence of meconium. However, compared to **oxytocin**, there is no increase in the incidence of cesarean section for fetal distress or umbilical acidemia. A recent meta-analysis concluded there was no difference in the frequencies of uterine hyperstimulation with fetal heart rate changes whether **misoprostol** was given PO or intravaginally. **Misoprostol** is not embryotoxic or teratogenic in rodents at doses 625 and 63 times the MRHD, respectively. Congenital defects after unsuccessful medical abortions are reported, but a mechanism has yet to be demonstrated. Several reports in the literature associate the use of **misoprostol** during the 1st trimester with skull defects, cranial nerve palsies, facial malformations, and limb defects. In rodents, prostaglandins but not **oxytocin** stimulate intestinal smooth muscle.

■ **Breastfeeding Safety**   There is no published experience in nursing women. It is unknown whether **misoprostol** enters human breast milk.

■ **References**

Zikopoulos KA, Papanikolaou EG, Kalantaridou SN, et al. Hum Reprod 2002; 17:3079-83.
Bartley J, Baird DT. BJOG 2002; 109:1290-4.
Ashok PW, Templeton A, Wagaarachchi PT, Flett GM. BJOG 2002; 109:1281-9.
Schaff EA, Fielding SL, Westhoff C. Contraception 2002; 66:247-50.
Ferguson JE 2nd, Head BH, Frank FH, et al. Am J Obstet Gynecol 2002; 187:273-9.
Bebbington MW, Kent N, Lim K, et al. Am J Obstet Gynecol 2002; 187:853-7.
Matonhodze BB, Katsoulis LC, Hofmeyr GJ. J Perinat Med 2002; 30:405-10.
Gulmezoglu AM, Forna F, Villar J, Hofmeyr GJ. Cochrane Database Syst Rev 2002; CD000494.
Wing DA. Drug Saf 2002; 25:665-76.
Shetty A, Mackie L, Danielian P, et al. BJOG 2002; 109:645-50.
Wing DA, Tran S, Paul RH. Am J Obstet Gynecol 2002; 186:1237-40.
Barrilleaux PS, Bofill JA, Terrone DA, et al. Am J Obstet Gynecol 2002; 186:1124-9.
Hall R, Duarte-Gardea M, Harlass F. Obstet Gynecol 2002; 99:1044-8.
Jain JK, Dutton C, Harwood B, et al. Hum Reprod 2002; 17:1477-82.
ACOG Committee Opinion. Obstet Gynecol 2002; 99:679-80.
Ozden S, Delikara MN, Avci A, Ficicioglu C. Int J Gynaecol Obstet 2002; 77:109-15.
Wagaarachchi PT, Ashok PW, Smith NC, Templeton A. BJOG 2002; 109:462-5.
Sahin HG, Sahin HA, Kocer M. Acta Obstet Gynecol Scand 2002; 81:252-7.
Carlan SJ, Blust D, O'Brien WF. Am J Obstet Gynecol 2002; 186:229-33.
Karkanis SG, Caloia D, Salenieks ME, et al. J Obstet Gynaecol Can 2002; 24:149-154.
Shetty A, Danielian P, Templeton A. Am J Obstet Gynecol 2002; 186:72-6.

Pandis GK, Papageorghiou AT, Otigbah CM, et al.
Ultrasound Obstet Gynecol 2001; 18:629-35.
Alfirevic Z. Cochrane Database Syst Rev 2001;
(2):CD001338.
Rozenberg P, Chevret S, Goffinet F, et al. BJOG 2001;
(1) 08:1255-62.
Has R, Batukan C, Ermis H, et al. Gynecol Obstet Invest
2002; 53:16-21.
Elsheikh A, Antsaklis A, Mesogitis S, et al. Arch Gynecol
Obstet 2001; 265:204-6.

■ **Summary**

- **Pregnancy Category X**
- **Lactation Category U**
- **Misoprostol** is an effective adjunct to **mifepristone** for medical abortion during early pregnancy. Two doses of **misoprostol** compared to one significantly reduce the failed abortion rate.
- **Misoprostol** induction of cervical ripening or labor at term is a common practice.
- Oral **misoprostol** is more convenient than vaginal, but may increase the risk of tachysystole.
- **Misoprostol** should not be used for either ripening or labor induction in women undergoing VBAC.

Mitomycin (Mutamycin)

■ **Class** — Antineoplastic, antibiotic

■ **Indications** — Stomach and pancreatic CA

■ **Mechanism** — Inhibits DNA synthesis

■ **Dosage with Qualifiers** — Stomach CA—numerous dosing schedules exist and depend on disease, response, and concomitant therapy
Pancreatic CA—numerous dosing schedules exist and depend on disease, response, and concomitant therapy

- **Contraindications**—hypersensitivity to drug or class, thrombocytopenia, coagulopathy, herpes zoster, renal dysfunction
- **Caution**—unknown

■ **Maternal Considerations** — **Mitomycin** is an alkylating agent used as adjunct therapy and is not recommended as single-agent, primary therapy. There are no adequate reports or well-controlled studies of **mitomycin** in pregnant women.
Side effects include thrombocytopenia, leukopenia, hemolytic-uremic syndrome, renal dysfunction, interstitial pneumonitis, sepsis, nausea, vomiting, alopecia, anorexia, diarrhea, and cardiac or renal toxicity.

- **Fetal Considerations** .... There are no adequate reports or well-controlled studies in human fetuses. It is unknown whether **mitomycin** crosses the human placenta. It crosses the rodent placenta in a limited fashion reaching F:M ratios less than 10%. In rodents, **mitomycin** is a potent teratogen damaging the preimplantation blastocyst leading to embryo loss. Later exposure produces a myriad of bony malformations. Its effect is enhanced by **caffeine**. There are no reports in humans.

- **Breastfeeding Safety** .... There is no published experience in nursing women. It is unknown whether **mitomycin** enters human breast milk.

- **References** .... Nagao T, Saitoh Y, Yoshimura S. Teratology 2000; 61:248-61.
  Rahman ME, Ishikawa H, Watanabe Y, Endo A. Reprod Toxicol 1996; 10:485-9.
  Boike GM, Deppe G, Young JD, et al. Gynecol Oncol 1989; 34:187-90.
  Sivak A. Regul Toxicol Pharmacol 1994; 19:1-13.

- **Summary** ....
  - **Pregnancy Category C**
  - **Lactation Category U**
  - **Mitomycin** should be used during pregnancy and lactation only if the benefit justifies the potential perinatal risk.
  - This drug should be assumed a human teratogen until proved otherwise.

Mitoxantrone (Novantrone)

- **Class** .... *Antineoplastic, miscellaneous*

- **Indications** .... Acute myelogenous leukemia, multiple sclerosis

- **Mechanism** .... Multiple actions that disturb DNA synthesis

- **Dosage with Qualifiers** .... Acute myelogenous leukemia—numerous dose schedules depending on disease, response, and concomitant therapy
  Multiple sclerosis—12mg/m² IV over 5-15min q3mo
  NOTE—an evaluation of left ventricular function and a CBC should precede each dose.
  - **Contraindications**—hypersensitivity to drug or class, prior **doxorubicine** exposure, CHF, myelosuppression
  - **Caution**—unknown

- **Maternal Considerations** .... There are no adequate reports or well-controlled studies of **mitoxantrone** in pregnant women. The published experience is limited to a case report. More recently,

mitoxantrone has been advocated as a treatment for multiple sclerosis, a disease common in reproductive-age women.

Side effects include seizures, arrhythmia, myocardial toxicity, CHF, myelosuppression, renal failure, nausea, vomiting, fever, abdominal pain, GI bleeding, alopecia, diarrhea, sepsis, stomatitis, conjunctivitis, pneumonia, UTI, headache, cough, and fungal infection.

■ **Fetal Considerations**

There are no adequate reports or well-controlled studies in human fetuses. It is unknown whether **mitoxantrone** crosses the human placenta. Rodent studies are reassuring, revealing no evidence of teratogenicity, but the doses studied were too low.

■ **Breastfeeding Safety**

There is no published experience in nursing women. **Mitoxantrone** enters human breast milk reaching a significant concentration, though the kinetics remain unclear. It should probably be considered incompatible with breastfeeding pending additional study.

■ **References**

Jain KK. Expert Opin Investig Drugs 2000; 9:1139-49.
Requena A, Velasco JG, Pinilla J, Gonzalez-Gonzalez A. Eur J Obstet Gynecol Reprod Biol 1995; 63:139-41.

■ **Summary**

- **Pregnancy Category D**
- **Lactation Category NS?**
- **Mitoxantrone** should be used during pregnancy and lactation only if the benefit justifies the potential perinatal risk.

Modafinil (Provigil)

■ **Class**

CNS *stimulant, analeptic*

■ **Indications**

Narcolepsy, multiple sclerosis

■ **Mechanism**

Unknown

■ **Dosage with Qualifiers**

Narcolepsy—200mg PO qam; max 400mg qd
Multiple sclerosis—200mg PO qam; max 400mg qd
NOTE—hepatic dosing
- **Contraindications**—hypersensitivity to drug or class, left ventricular hypertrophy
- **Caution**—coronary artery disease, hypertension, renal or hepatic dysfunction, history of psychosis, alcohol use

- **Maternal Considerations** ········ **Modafinil** is an inducer of cytochrome P450 enzymes. Thus, the effectiveness of oral contraceptives may be reduced during therapy and for 1mo after discontinuation. Multiple sclerosis is fairly common in reproductive-age women. There is no published experience with **modafinil** during pregnancy.

  Side effects include arrhythmia, MI, headache, nausea, vomiting, palpitations, insomnia, anxiety, euphoria, tachycardia, chest pain, rhinitis, pharyngitis, and epistaxis.

- **Fetal Considerations** ········ There are no adequate reports or well-controlled studies in human fetuses. It is unknown whether **modafinil** crosses the human placenta. Adequate rodent teratogenicity studies have not been performed. Those that have been done suggest an increased rate of embryotoxicity. The manufacturer reports seven exposures during pregnancy without apparent adverse effects.

- **Breastfeeding Safety** ········ There is no published experience in nursing women. It is unknown whether **modafinil** enters human breast milk.

- **References** ········ There is no published experience in pregnancy or during lactation.

- **Summary** ········
  - **Pregnancy Category C**
  - **Lactation Category U**
  - **Modafinil** should be used during pregnancy and lactation only if the benefit justifies the potential perinatal risk.

Moexipril (Univasc; Fampress)

- **Class** ········ Antihypertensive, ACE inhibitor

- **Indications** ········ Hypertension

- **Mechanism in action** ········ Inhibits angiotensin-converting enzyme

- **Dosage with Qualifiers** ········ Hypertension—7.5-30mg PO qd
  - **Contraindications**—hypersensitivity to drug or class, history of ACE-inhibitor angioedema, hereditary angioedema, idiopathic angioedema, pregnancy
  - **Caution**—renal artery stenosis, severe cardiac failure, collagen vascular disease, renal dysfunction, hypotension

- **Maternal Considerations** ········ There is no published experience with **moexipril** during pregnancy.

Side effects include hypotension, postural hypotension, syncope, abdominal pain, constipation, vomiting, appetite change, dry mouth, pancreatitis, hepatic dysfunction, bronchospasm, dyspnea, renal insufficiency, oliguria, drowsiness, sleep disturbances, nervousness, mood changes, anxiety, tinnitus, sweating, malaise, arthralgia, and hemolytic anemia.

■ **Fetal Considerations** — There are no adequate reports or well-controlled studies in human fetuses. It is unknown whether **moexipril** crosses the human placenta. Other inhibitors of the rennin angiotensin system cross and can cause fetal renal failure. They are generally considered contraindicated during pregnancy unless there is no other therapeutic option.

■ **Breastfeeding Safety** — There is no published experience in nursing women. It is unknown whether **moexipril** enters human breast milk.

■ **References** — There is no published experience in pregnancy or during lactation.

■ **Summary**
- **Pregnancy Category C (1st trimester), D (2nd and 3rd trimesters)**
- **Lactation Category U**
- **Moexipril** should be used during pregnancy and lactation only if the benefit justifies the potential perinatal risk, and after other antihypertensive agents have failed.
- There are alternative agents for which there is more experience regarding use during pregnancy and lactation.

Molindone (Moban)

■ **Class** — Antipsychotic

■ **Indications** — Schizophrenia

■ **Mechanism** — Unknown (selectively antagonizes dopamine D_2 receptors)

■ **Dosage with Qualifiers** — Schizophrenia—begin 50-75mg qd divided tid/qid; increase to 100mg qd every 3-5d; max 225mg/d
- **Contraindications**—hypersensitivity to drug or class, CNS depression
- **Caution**—seizures

■ **Maternal Considerations** — Acute schizophrenia presents several difficult management decisions during pregnancy and a careful risk-benefit analysis is required. There are no adequate reports or well-controlled studies of **molindone** in pregnant women. The published experience consists of isolated case reports.

Side effects include constipation, extrapyramidal effects, blurred vision, tardive dyskinesia, neuroleptic malignant syndrome, leukopenia, decreased sweating, dry mouth, akinesia, tachycardia, depression, hyperactivity and euphoria.

■ **Fetal Considerations** ⋯⋯⋯ There are no adequate reports or well-controlled studies in human fetuses. It is unknown whether **molindone** crosses the human placenta. Rodent studies are reassuring, revealing no evidence of teratogenicity or IUGR despite the use of doses higher than those used clinically.

■ **Breastfeeding Safety** ⋯⋯⋯ There is no published experience in nursing women. It is unknown whether **molindone** enters human breast milk.

■ **References** ⋯⋯⋯ Pinkofsky HB. Ann Clin Psychiatry 1997; 9:175-9.
Kahn JL. Am J Psychiatry 1979; 136:1617-8.
Wesp CE Jr, Annitto W, Feinsod R. Am J Psychiatry 1979; 136:975.

■ **Summary** ⋯⋯⋯
- **Pregnancy Category C**
- **Lactation Category U**
- **Molindone** should be used during pregnancy and lactation only if the benefit justifies the potential perinatal risk.

Mometasone (Elocon)

■ **Class** ⋯⋯⋯ Corticosteroid

■ **Indications** ⋯⋯⋯ Allergic rhinitis, dermatitis

■ **Mechanism** ⋯⋯⋯ Unknown (anti-inflammatory)

■ **Dosage with Qualifiers** ⋯⋯⋯ Allergic rhinitis—2 sprays/nostril qd; begin 2w before the allergy season
Dermatitis—apply qd
NOTE—available as spray and cream
- **Contraindications**—hypersensitivity to drug or class
- **Caution**—unknown

■ **Maternal Considerations** ⋯⋯⋯ Allergic rhinitis affects 1/3 of women of childbearing age. There are no adequate reports or well-controlled studies of **mometasone** in pregnant women.
Side effects include adrenal suppression, skin atrophy, dryness, folliculitis, pruritus, irritation, and burning.

- **Fetal Considerations** ⋯⋯⋯ There are no adequate reports or well-controlled studies in human fetuses. It is unknown whether **mometasone** crosses the human placenta. There are no documented epidemiologic studies with intranasal corticosteroids (e.g., **budesonide, fluticasone, mometasone**) during pregnancy. However, inhaled corticosteroids (e.g., **beclomethasone**) are not incriminated as teratogens. Considering the dose and route, it is unlikely the maternal systemic concentration will reach clinically relevant level.

- **Breastfeeding Safety** ⋯⋯⋯ There is no published experience in nursing women. It is unknown whether **mometasone** enters human breast milk. However, considering the indications, dose, and route, it is unlikely the breast-fed neonate would ingest clinically relevant amounts.

- **References** ⋯⋯⋯ Mazzotta P, Loebstein R, Koren G. Drug Saf 1999; 20:361-75.

- **Summary** ⋯⋯⋯
  - **Pregnancy Category C**
  - **Lactation Category S?**
  - **Mometasone** should be used during pregnancy and lactation only if the benefit justifies the potential perinatal risk.

Moricizine (Ethmozine)

- **Class** ⋯⋯⋯ Antiarrhythmic, class IB

- **Indications** ⋯⋯⋯ Ventricular arrhythmia

- **Mechanism** ⋯⋯⋯ Stabilizes membranes and depresses phase 0 action potential

- **Dosage with Qualifiers** ⋯⋯⋯ Ventricular arrhythmia—200-300mg PO q8h
  - **Contraindications**—hypersensitivity to drug or class, cardiogenic shock, 2nd and 3rd degree AV block
  - **Caution**—unknown

- **Maternal Considerations** ⋯⋯⋯ There is no published experience with **moricizine** during pregnancy.
  Side effects include arrhythmia, ECG changes, CHF, cardiac arrest, nausea, vomiting, dizziness, dry mouth, headache, fatigue, palpitations, chest pain, dyspnea, blurred vision, nervousness, insomnia, dysuria, urinary incontinence, kidney pain, decreased libido, leg pain, hyperventilation, apnea, asthma, pharyngitis, cough, sinusitis, anorexia, bitter taste, dysphagia, flatulence, ileus, hypothermia, thrombocytopenia, drug fever, eye pain, rash, pruritus, dry skin, urticaria, swelling of lips and tongue, and periorbital edema.

- **Fetal Considerations** — There are no adequate reports or well-controlled studies in human fetuses. It is unknown whether **moricizine** crosses the human placenta. Rodent studies are reassuring, revealing no evidence of teratogenicity or IUGR despite the use of doses higher than those used clinically.

- **Breastfeeding Safety** — There are no adequate reports or well-controlled studies in nursing women. **Moricizine** enters human and rodent breast milk, but the kinetics remain to be elucidated.

- **References** — No published experience in pregnancy or during lactation.

- **Summary**
  - **Pregnancy Category B**
  - **Lactation Category U**
  - **Moricizine** should be used during pregnancy and lactation only if the benefit justifies the potential perinatal risk.
  - There are alternative agents for which there is more experience regarding use during pregnancy and lactation.

Morphine (Avinza; Kadian; MS Contin; MSIR; Oramorph; Roxanol)

- **Class** — *Analgesic, narcotic*

- **Indications** — Severe pain

- **Mechanism** — Binds to opiate receptors

- **Dosage with Qualifiers** — Pain—2.5-10mg IV slowly over 5-15min; alternative 5-20mg IM/SC or 10-30mg PO q4h
  Post-cesarean section analgesia—intrathecal 100-250mcg, epidural 2-5 mg
  NOTE—do not use solution if dark, discolored, or contains precipitate
  - **Contraindications**—hypersensitivity to drug or class, respiratory depression, asthma, ileus
  - **Caution**—COPD, head injury, CNS depression, seizure disorder, acute pancreatitis, pseudomembranous colitis, hypotension, hepatic or renal dysfunction, biliary disease, alcoholism

- **Maternal Considerations** — **Morphine** is one of the most frequently used opioids for pain control during human parturition. The elimination half-life of **morphine** is shorter and the plasma clearance quicker in the parturients than in nonpregnant women. **Morphine** as part of an epidural or PCA regimen is common. It is also administered intrathecally after cesarean section for relief of postoperative pain for the first 48h. There is a long clinical experience supporting the relative safety of **morphine** for the listed indications. The combination of small doses of opioids and **bupivacaine** for spinal anesthesia eliminates intraoperative discomfort and reduces postoperative analgesic requirements in women undergoing either vaginal or cesarean delivery. The two most frequently used agents are **fentanyl** and **morphine.** Patient-controlled analgesia (PCA), which provides pain relief through self-administration of intravenous doses of opioids, is widely available and advocated as an effective analgesic modality. **Morphine** PCA offers a good quality of analgesia with minimal side effects during both the ante- and postnatal periods. **Morphine** does not affect the spontaneous contractility *in vitro* of human myometrium. It is one of the most frequently used opioids to achieve pain relief during an ambulatory surgical procedure. Patients receiving **morphine** and **diazepam** are to be cautioned against operating machinery or driving. *Side effects* include addiction, seizures, respiratory depression, hypotension, shock, apnea, cardiac arrest, bradycardia, toxic megacolon, ileus, abdominal pain, miosis, itching, dry mouth, decreased libido, biliary spasm, paresthesias, pruritus, itching, flushing, urinary retention, and asthenia.

■ **Fetal Considerations**

Morphine readily crosses the term human placenta. Rapid maternal clearance shortens the fetal exposure. Alterations in fetal biophysical profile parameters such as fetal breathing movements and fetal heart rhythm should be expected as **morphine** decreases fetal heart variability and breathing frequency. It is not clear whether **morphine** decreases gross or fine fetal movements. Placental retention of **morphine** may prolong fetal exposure explaining at least in part its prolonged effect on fetal behavior relative to the maternal concentration.

Morphine has been combined with benzodiazepines (e.g., **diazepam**) for the relief of pain and anxiety during fetal surgical procedures. While there is no evidence **morphine** is a human teratogen, uncontrolled retrospective studies of neonates chronically exposed to other opioids note reduced brain volume at birth that normalizes during the 1st month of life. Infants born to opioid-abusing mothers are more often SGA, have decreased ventilatory responses to CO_2 and increased risk of sudden infant death syndrome. Neonatal abstinence syndrome due to opiate withdrawal produces sleep-wake abnormalities, feeding difficulties, weight loss, and seizures. Rodent teratogen studies have not been performed. Other rodent studies suggest *in utero* exposure causes long-term alterations in adult brain and behavior. These changes affect both the norepinephrine and opioid systems of several brain areas including those involved in memory, stress responses, and the maintenance of homeostatic balance with the external environment.

■ **Breastfeeding Safety** ⸻ **Morphine** is excreted in human breast milk, and the M:P area under the curve ratio after parenteral administration approximates 2.5:1. The amount taken by the neonate depends on the maternal plasma concentration, quantity of milk ingested, and the extent of first-pass metabolism. In general, **morphine** is preferred to **meperidine** in breast-feeding women. Intrathecal **morphine** is not associated with clinically relevant maternal plasma and milk **morphine** concentrations. The colostrum concentration of **morphine** and its active metabolites in women using patient-controlled analgesia (PCA) after cesarean delivery is small, supporting the safety of breastfeeding in mothers using a **morphine** PCA.

■ **References** ⸻ Cowan CM, Kendall JB, Barclay PM, Wilkes RG. Br J Anapest 2002; 89:452-8.
Iberia I, Nuns F, Ghana M. Act Med Port 2001; 14:395-8.
Bake NE, Bayou F, Boutros MJ, Laxenaire MC. Anesth Analg 2002; 94:184-7.
Vathy I. Psychoneuroendocrinology 2002; 27:273-83.
Slamberova R, Schindler CJ, Pometlova M, et al. Physiol Behav 2001; 73:93-103.
Yoo KY, Lee J, Kim HS, Jeong SW. Anesth Analg 2001; 92:1006-9.
Kopecky EA, Simone C, Knie B, Koren G. Life Sci 1999; 65:2359-71.
Kopecky EA, Ryan ML, Barrett JF, et al. Am J Obstet Gynecol 2000; 183:424-30.
Farrell T, Owen P, Harrold A. Clin Exp Obstet Gynecol 1996; 23:144-6.
McIntosh DG, Rayburn WF. Obstet Gynecol 1991; 78:1129-35.
Gerdin E, Salmonson T, Lindberg B, Rane A. J Perinat Med 1990; 18:479-87.
Oberlander TF, Robeson P, Ward V, et al. J Hum Lact 2000; 16:137-42.
Wittels B, Glosten B, Faure EA, et al. Anesth Analg 1997; 85:600-6.
Robieux I, Koren G, Vandenbergh H, Schneiderman J. J Toxicol Clin Toxicol 1990; 28:365-70.

■ **Summary** ⸻ • **Pregnancy Category C**
  • **Lactation Category S**
  • **Morphine** provides safe and effective analgesia for pregnant and breast-feeding women when used as indicated.

Moxifloxacin (Avelox)

■ **Class** — Antibiotic, quinolone

■ **Indications** — Bacterial infections (<u>aerobic gram-positive</u>: *Enterococcus faecalis, Staphylococcus aureus* [methicillin-susceptible], *S. saprophyticus, Streptococcus pneumoniae, S. pyogenes*; <u>aerobic gram-negative</u>: *Enterobacter cloacae, Escherichia coli, Haemophilus influenzae, H. parainfluenzae, Klebsiella pneumoniae, Legionella pneumophila, Moraxella caterrhalis, Proteus mirabilis, Pseudomonas aeruginosa*; <u>other microorganisms</u>: *Chlamydia pneumoniae, Mycoplasma pneumoniae*)

■ **Mechanism** — Bactericidal; inhibits DNA synthesis

■ **Dosage with Qualifiers** — <u>Bacterial infections</u>—400mg PO/IV qd
- **Contraindications**—hypersensitivity to drug or class, ECG modification, concomitant usage of antiarrhythmic medication (class IA, III), age <18yr
- **Caution**—advanced age, seizure disorder, CNS disorder, dehydration

■ **Maternal Considerations** — There is no published experience with **moxifloxacin** during pregnancy.
Side effects include vaginitis, photosensitivity, pseudomembranous colitis, seizures, increased intracranial pressure, headache, psychosis, nausea, vomiting, diarrhea, abdominal pain, dyspepsia, dizziness, insomnia, agitation, tendonitis, arthralgias, and increased LFTs.

■ **Fetal Considerations** — There are no adequate reports or well-controlled studies in human fetuses. It is unknown whether **moxifloxacin** crosses the human placenta. Animal studies in rodents and dogs reveal that fetal exposure to quinolone antibiotics is associated with an acute arthropathy of the weight-bearing joints. Although arthropathy has only rarely been observed in humans, the toxicity observed in immature animals has lead to the restricted use of quinolones in pregnant women. There was no evidence of teratogenicity in monkeys fed 2.5 times the MRHD, though there was an increase in IUGR. Recent studies conclude that the use of fluoroquinolones during embryogenesis is not associated with an increased risk of major malformations.

■ **Breastfeeding Safety** — There is no published experience in nursing women. It is unknown whether **moxifloxacin** enters human breast milk. It is excreted into rodent milk.

■ **References** — There is no published experience in pregnancy or during lactation.

■ **Summary** ———————————— • **Pregnancy Category C**
- **Lactation Category U**
- **Moxifloxacin** should be used during pregnancy and lactation only if the benefit justifies the potential perinatal risk.
- There are alternative agents for which there is more experience regarding use during pregnancy and lactation.

Nabumetone (Nabuco; Relafen)

- **Class** — *Analgesic*, NSAID

- **Indications** — Osteoarthritis or rheumatoid arthritis, anti-inflammatory

- **Mechanism** — Inhibits cyclooxygenase- and lipoxygenase-reducing prostaglandin synthesis

- **Dosage with Qualifiers** — Osteoarthritis—1g PO qd-bid
  Rheumatoid arthritis—1g PO qd-bid
  Anti-inflammatory—1g bid ×7-14d; begin 2g/d ×1d;
  max 2g/d
  - **Contraindications**—hypersensitivity to drug or class, NSAID asthma
  - **Caution**—nasal polyps, GI bleeding, hypertension, CHF

- **Maternal Considerations** — There is no published experience with **nabumetone** during pregnancy.
  Side effects include thrombocytopenia, GI bleeding, renal failure, Stevens-Johnson syndrome, interstitial nephritis, hepatotoxicity, agranulocytosis, abdominal pain, diarrhea, constipation, increased sweating, nervousness, insomnia, somnolence, tinnitus, cholestatic jaundice, duodenal ulcer, dysphagia, gastric ulcer, gastroenteritis, increased appetite, increased LFTs, melena, edema, urticaria, rash, dizziness, and headache.

- **Fetal Considerations** — There are no adequate reports or well-controlled studies in human fetuses. It is unknown whether **nabumetone** crosses the human placenta. Rodent studies are reassuring, revealing no evidence of teratogenicity or IUGR despite the use of doses higher than those used clinically. There is evidence, however, of increased embryo resorption.

- **Breastfeeding Safety** — There is no published experience in nursing women. It is unknown whether **nabumetone** enters human breast milk.

- **References** — There is no published experience in pregnancy or during lactation.

- **Summary** —
  - **Pregnancy Category C**
  - **Lactation Category U**
  - **Nabumetone** should be used during pregnancy and lactation only if the benefit justifies the potential perinatal risk.
  - There are alternative agents for which there is more experience regarding use during pregnancy and lactation.

Nadolol (Corgard)

- **Class** — Antiadrenergic, β-blocker

- **Indications** — Hypertension, angina, arrhythmia, headache prophylaxis (vascular)

- **Mechanism** — Nonselective β-adrenergic receptor antagonist

- **Dosage with Qualifiers** — Hypertension—begin 20-40mg/d; increase 40-80mg qd 2-14d; max 240-320mg/d
  Angina—begin 20-40mg/d; increase 40-80mg qd 3-7d; max 160-240mg/d
  Arrhythmia—60-640mg PO qd
  Headache prophylaxis (vascular)—20-80mg PO qd; max 120mg/d
  - **Contraindications**—hypersensitivity to drug or class, sinus bradycardia, asthma, AV block 2nd-3rd degree
  - **Caution**—diabetes mellitus, hepatic failure, CHF

- **Maternal Considerations** — **Nadolol** is a nonselective β-blocker offering the advantage of once a day dosing. There are no adequate reports or well-controlled studies of **nadolol** in pregnant women. In one instance, it was used to treat hypertension associated with primary hyperaldosteronism.
  Side effects include fatigue, dizziness, slurred speech, bradycardia, rash, CHF, bronchospasm, constipation, dry mouth, nausea, diarrhea, weight gain, cough, nasal stuffiness, sweating, tinnitus, facial swelling, and blurred vision.

- **Fetal Considerations** — There are no adequate reports or well-controlled studies in human fetuses. It is unknown whether **nadolol** crosses the human placenta. Other drugs in this class do cross. Scattered case reports suggest fetal exposure may increase the risk of cardiorespiratory depression, mild hypoglycemia, and IUGR. The long duration of action of **nadolol** and the fact that it is only 30% protein bound make it less desirable during pregnancy than other β-blockers such as **propranolol**. **Nadolol** crosses the rodent placenta. Rodent studies are generally reassuring, revealing no evidence of teratogenicity despite the use of doses higher than those used clinically. There is evidence of embryotoxicity and IUGR.

- **Breastfeeding Safety** — There is no published experience in nursing women. **Nadolol** is excreted into human breast milk. It is estimated the nursing newborn would ingest 2-7% of the daily maternal dose. Thus, there is a small but real potential for a clinical effect depending upon neonatal clearance. If a woman elects to continue nursing while taking **nadolol**, the child should be observed for evidence of β blockade.

■ References .... Solomon CG, Thiet M, Moore F Jr, Seely EW. J Reprod Med 1996; 41:255-8.
Fox RE, Marx C, Stark AR. Am J Obstet Gynecol 1985; 152:1045-6.
Wilson AL, Matzke GR. Drug Intell Clin Pharm 1981; 15:21-6.
Devlin RG, Duchin KL, Fleiss PM. Br J Clin Pharmacol 1981; 12:393-6.

■ Summary ....
- **Pregnancy Category C**
- **Lactation Category S?**
- **Nadolol** should be used during pregnancy and lactation only if the benefit justifies the potential perinatal risk.
- There are alternative agents for which there is more experience regarding use during pregnancy and lactation.

Nafcillin (Nafcil; Nallpen; Unipen)

■ **Class** .... *Antibiotic, penicillin*

■ **Indications** .... Bacterial infections, especially penicillinase-producing *Staphylococcus*

■ **Mechanism** .... Bactericidal; inhibits cell wall synthesis

■ **Dosage with Qualifiers** .... Bacterial infections—500mg-2g IV/IM q4-6h; max 12g/d IM or 20g/d IV
NOTE—hepatic and renal dosing; concurrent administration of **nafcillin** and **probenecid** increases and prolongs serum levels
- **Contraindications**—hypersensitivity to drug or class
- **Caution**—cephalosporin allergy, renal or hepatic dysfunction, neonate

■ **Maternal Considerations** .... **Nafcillin** is a penicillinase-resistant penicillin eliminated primarily by nonrenal routes, namely hepatic inactivation and excretion in the bile. There are no adequate reports or well-controlled studies of **nafcillin** in pregnant women. The published literature consists of scattered case reports. Other penicillins have proved safe during pregnancy.
Side effects include pain, swelling, inflammation, interstitial nephritis, pseudomembranous colitis, hepatotoxicity, seizures, tissue necrosis, nausea, vomiting, diarrhea, candidiasis, urticaria, thrombophlebitis, neutropenia, leukopenia, thrombocytopenia, hypokalemia, and rash.

■ **Fetal Considerations** .... There are no adequate reports or well-controlled studies in human fetuses. It is unknown whether **nafcillin** crosses the human placenta. Rodent studies are reassuring, revealing no evidence of teratogenicity or IUGR despite the use of doses higher than those used clinically.

- **Breastfeeding Safety** — There is no published experience in nursing women. It is unknown whether **nafcillin** enters human breast milk. It is generally considered compatible with breastfeeding. **Nafcillin** is frequently used for the treatment of mastitis of cows.

- **References** — Takeba K, Fujinuma K, Miyazaki T, et al. 1998; 812:205-11.

- **Summary** —
  - **Pregnancy Category B**
  - **Lactation Category S?**
  - **Nafcillin** is an alternative for the treatment of puerperal mastitis.
  - There are alternative agents if necessary during pregnancy for almost all indications.

Naftifine (Naftin)

- **Class** — *Antifungal topical, dermatologic*

- **Indications** — Fungal and candidal infections (underline: fungal infections: *Trichophyton rubrum*, T. *mentagrophytes*, T. *tonsurans*, *Epidermophyton floccosum*, Microsporum canis, M. *audouini*, M. *gypseum*; candida species: *Candida albicans*), skin infections

- **Mechanism** — Inhibits biosynthesis of **ergosterol**, and thus the fungal cell wall

- **Dosage with Qualifiers** — Skin infections—apply affected area qd
  NOTE—available as 1% cream or gel
  - **Contraindications**—hypersensitivity to drug or class
  - **Caution**—unknown

- **Maternal Considerations** — There is no published experience with **naftifine** during pregnancy.
  Side effects include burning, dryness, erythema, and itching.

- **Fetal Considerations** — There are no adequate reports or well-controlled studies in human fetuses. It is unknown whether **naftifine** crosses the human placenta. Considering the dose and route, it is unlikely the maternal systemic concentration will reach a clinically relevant level. Rodent studies are reassuring, revealing no evidence of teratogenicity or IUGR despite the use of doses higher than those used clinically.

- **Breastfeeding Safety** — There is no published experience in nursing women. It is unknown whether **naftifine** enters human breast milk. However, considering the dose and route, it is unlikely to pose a clinically significant risk to the breast-feeding neonate.

■ **References** .... There is no published experience in pregnancy or during lactation.

■ **Summary** ....
- **Pregnancy Category B**
- **Lactation Category U**
- **Naftifine** should be used during pregnancy and lactation only if the benefit justifies the potential perinatal risk.

Nalbuphine (Nubain)

■ **Class** .... *Analgesic, narcotic agonist-antagonist*

■ **Indications** .... Pain, anesthesia (adjunct)

■ **Mechanism** .... Binds to opiate receptors

■ **Dosage with Qualifiers** .... Pain—10mg IV/IM/SC q3-6h prn; max 20mg/dose or 160mg/d
Anesthesia (adjunct)—0.25-0.5mg/kg prn; begin 0.3-3mg/kg IV
- **Contraindications**—hypersensitivity to drug or class
- **Caution**—opiate dependency, renal, hepatic or pulmonary dysfunction, biliary surgery, sulfite allergy

■ **Maternal Considerations** .... **Nalbuphine** is a analgesic whose potency is essentially equivalent to **morphine** on a milligram basis. It acts within minutes after IV administration, and <15min after SC or IM injection; the duration of analgesia ranges from 3-6h. There are no adequate reports or well-controlled studies of **nalbuphine** in pregnant women. It is a popular agent for analgesia during labor comparable to **meperidine**. Due to its ability to bind the same opiate receptor as **morphine**, IV **nalbuphine** is sometimes used for the treatment of intrathecal **morphine**-induced pruritus after cesarean delivery.
Side effects include headache, nervousness, depression, restlessness, crying, floating, hostility, unusual dreams, confusion, euphoria, faintness, hallucinations, dysphoria, feeling of heaviness, numbness, tingling, dizziness, bradycardia, hypotension, respiratory depression, dyspepsia, nausea, vomiting, sweating, dry mouth, urticaria, cramps, dyspnea, asthma, bitter taste, speech difficulty, urinary urgency, blurred vision, pruritus, and substance abuse.

■ **Fetal Considerations** .... There are no adequate reports or well-controlled studies in human fetuses. **Nalbuphine** crosses the human placenta achieving an F:M ratio approximating 0.75. **Nalbuphine** decreases the number of fetal heart rate accelerations and variability, but does not affect the fetal response to vibroacoustic stimulation. The neonatal half-life is

655

estimated at 4h. **Nalbuphine** can cause respiratory depression, and should be used with caution in women delivering preterm. Rodent studies are reassuring, revealing no evidence of teratogenicity or IUGR despite the use of doses higher than those used clinically.

■ **Breastfeeding Safety** — Though **nalbuphine** is excreted into human milk, the nursing newborn would receive less than 0.05% of the administered dose.

■ **References** — Frank M, McAteer EJ, Cattermole R, et al. Anaesthesia 1987; 42:697-703.
Charuluxananan S, Kyokong O, Somboonviboon W, et al. Anesth Analg 2001; 93:162-5.
Culebras X, Gaggero G, Zatloukal J, et al. Anesth Analg 2000; 91:601-5.
Somrat C, Oranuch K, Ketchada U, et al. J Obstet Gynaecol Res 1999; 25:209-13.
Giannina G, Guzman ER, Lai YL, et al. Obstet Gynecol 1995; 86:441-5.
Nicolle E, Devillier P, Delanoy B, et al. Eur J Clin Pharmacol 1996; 49:485-9.
Poehlmann S, Pinette M, Stubblefield P. J Reprod Med 1995; 40:707-10.
Sherer DM, Cooper EM, Spoor C, et al. Am J Perinatol 1994; 11:367-8.
Wischnik A, Wetzelsberger N, Lucker PW. Arzneimittelforschung 1988; 38:1496-8.

■ **Summary** —
- **Pregnancy Category B**
- **Lactation Category S**
- **Nalbuphine** is a popular labor analgesic and an efficacious treatment of side effects secondary to epidural **morphine**.

Nalidixic acid (Enexina; Faril; Nalidixio; Nalydixine; NegGram; Nevigramon; Notricel; Urodic; Winlomylon)

■ **Class** — *Antibiotic, quinolone*

■ **Indications** — Bacterial infections (<u>aerobic gram-positive</u>: *Enterococcus faecalis, Staphylococcus aureus (methicillin-susceptible), Staphylococcus saprophyticus, Streptococcus pneumoniae, Streptococcus pyogenes;* <u>aerobic gram-negative</u>: *Enterobacter cloacae, Escherichia coli, Haemophilus influenzae, Haemophilus parainfluenzae, Klebsiella pneumoniae, Legionella pneumophila, Moraxella catarrhalis, Proteus mirabilis, Pseudomonas aeruginosa;* <u>other microorganisms</u>: *Chlamydia pneumoniae, Mycoplasma pneumoniae*)

■ **Mechanism** .... Bactericidal; inhibits DNA synthesis

■ **Dosage with Qualifiers** .... Bacterial infections—1g PO qid; alternatively, 2g PO qd for chronic suppression
- **Contraindications**—hypersensitivity to drug or class, seizures
- **Caution**—renal or hepatic dysfunction, impaired pulmonary function, cardiovascular disease, excessive sunlight exposure

■ **Maternal Considerations** .... Asymptomatic bacteriuria is a common during pregnancy. Perhaps a third of affected pregnant women will develop symptomatic disease (hemorrhagic cystitis or pyelonephritis). **Nalidixic acid** is one treatment alternative for asymptomatic bacteriuria of pregnancy. *Side effects* include vaginitis, photosensitivity, pseudomembranous colitis, seizures, increased intracranial pressure, headache, psychosis, nausea, vomiting, diarrhea, abdominal pain, dyspepsia, dizziness, insomnia, agitation, tendonitis, arthralgia, and elevated LFTs.

■ **Fetal Considerations** .... There are no adequate reports or well-controlled studies in human fetuses. **Nalidixic acid** crosses the human placenta, though the kinetics remain to be elucidated. Rodent and canine teratogenicity studies reveal the older quinolones such as **nalidixic acid**, **flumequine**, and **pipemidic acid** are associated with acute arthropathy of the weight-bearing joints. Although arthropathy is rare in adult humans, toxicity was observed in immature animals, leading to the restricted use of these agents during pregnancy. More recent studies conclude that **nalidixic acid** is not associated with any increased risks of spontaneous abortion, prematurity, IUGR or postnatal disorders. A small increase in the risk of pyloric stenosis cannot be excluded.

■ **Breastfeeding Safety** .... **Nalidixic acid** is excreted into human breast milk. However, the nursing newborn would ingest <0.05% of the maternal dose.

■ **References** .... Czeizel AE, Sorensen HT, Rockenbauer M, Olsen J. Int J Gynaecol Obstet 2001; 73:221-8.
No authors. Prescrire Int 1999; 8:29-31.
Pedler SJ, Bint AJ. Drugs 1987; 33:413-21.
Peiker G, Traeger A. Pharmazie 1983; 38:613-5 .
Traeger A, Peiker G. Arch Toxicol Suppl 1980; 4:388-90.

■ **Summary** ....
- **Pregnancy Category C**
- **Lactation Category S**
- **Nalidixic acid** should be used during pregnancy only if the benefit justifies the potential perinatal risk.
- It is a reasonable first-line drug for the treatment of asymptomatic bacteriuria during the 2nd and 3rd trimesters.

Nalmefene (Cervene; Revex)

■ **Class** — *Antagonist, narcotic; antidote*

■ **Indications** — Opiate overdose, postoperative opiate reversal

■ **Mechanism** — Opiate receptor antagonist

■ **Dosage with Qualifiers** — Opiate overdose—0.5mg IV; over 70kg, dose individually; max 1.5mg
Postoperative opiate reversal—0.25mcg/kg IV; increase 0.25mcg/kg increments q2-5min; max 1mcg/kg IV
● **Contraindications**—hypersensitivity to drug or class
● **Caution**—renal or hepatic dysfunction, opiate addiction, concomitant usage of cardiotoxic drugs

■ **Maternal Considerations** — **Nalmefene** is a long-acting opioid antagonist used for the treatment of overdose. It was also used to provide long-term relief from side effects of intrathecal **morphine sulfate.** However, **nalmefene** failed in one prospective trial to reduce the incidence of pruritus, nausea, vomiting, and the level of sedation, but increased the need for supplemental analgesics.
Side effects include arrhythmia, tachycardia, bradycardia, fever, postoperative pain, nausea, vomiting, headache, vasodilatation, dizziness, somnolence, confusion, and chills.

■ **Fetal Considerations** — There are no adequate reports or well-controlled studies in human fetuses. It is unknown whether **nalmefene** crosses the human placenta. Rodent studies are reassuring, revealing no evidence of teratogenicity or IUGR despite the use of doses higher than those used clinically.

■ **Breastfeeding Safety** — There is no published experience in nursing women. **Nalmefene** is excreted into human breast milk, though the kinetics remain to be elucidated. However, considering the indication and dosing, one-time **nalmefene** use is unlikely to pose a clinically significant risk to the breast-feeding neonate.

■ **References** — Pellegrini JE, Bailey SL, Graves J, et al. AANA J 2001; 69:199-205.

■ **Summary** — ● **Pregnancy Category B**
● **Lactation Category S?**
● **Nalmefene** should be used during pregnancy and lactation only if the benefit justifies the potential perinatal risk.
● There are superior agents to treat the side effects of intrathecal morphine.

Naloxone (Narcan)

- ■ **Class** — Antagonist, narcotic, antidote

- ■ **Indications** — Opiate overdose, postoperative opiate reversal

- ■ **Mechanism** — Antagonizes various opiate receptors (opiate antagonist)

- ■ **Dosage with Qualifiers** — Opiate overdose—0.4-2mg SC/IV/IM q2-3min; if no response by 10min, the diagnosis should be questioned
Postoperative opiate reversal—0.1-0.2mg IV q2-3min prn
  - **Contraindications**—hypersensitivity to drug or class
  - **Caution**—opiate addiction, renal or hepatic dysfunction, cardiotoxic drugs

- ■ **Maternal Considerations** — There are no adequate reports or well-controlled studies of **naloxone** in pregnant women. Pregnant **heroin** users have poor maternal and neonatal outcome. Medically supervised **heroin** withdrawal is generally discouraged during pregnancy because of the fetal risk and a high likelihood of failure with return to regular illicit **heroin** use. More recently, a number of withdrawal procedures were developed using **naloxone** or **naltrexone** that have met with some success in users who continue the antagonist throughout pregnancy. Maternal respiratory arrest is a rare but potentially life-threatening complication associated with intrathecal opioids for labor analgesia. Resuscitation should include IV **naloxone**. Very low-dose intravenous **naloxone** is often used to treat neuraxially-injected **morphine**-associated pruritus.
Side effects include cardiac arrest, ventricular fibrillation, tachycardia, hypertension, hypotension, seizures, nausea, vomiting, tremor, diaphoresis, pulmonary edema, withdrawal symptoms, and sweating.

- ■ **Fetal Considerations** — There are no adequate reports or well-controlled studies in human fetuses. It is unknown whether **naloxone** crosses the human placenta. **Naloxone** does not alter the placental transfer or clearance of **morphine** in humans. Neonates of women given parenteral opioids in labor that require **naloxone** have lower 1min Apgar scores than neonates whose mothers have epidural analgesia. Physicians practicing in community vs. university hospitals use **naloxone** more often to resuscitate the neonate. It is unclear whether this increased use reflects adherence to the American Academy of Pediatrics' guidelines for resuscitation, or whether the neonates delivered in community hospital require resuscitation more frequently. Porcine studies suggest that increased opioid "tonus" lowers the fetal heart rate and decreases fetal movement. **Naloxone** antagonizes the inhibitory effect of **morphine** on fetal heart rhythm and stimulates fetal hypermotility. Rodent studies are reassuring, revealing no evidence of teratogenicity or IUGR despite the use of doses higher than those used clinically.

■ **Breastfeeding Safety** ⋯⋯⋯⋯ There are no adequate reports or well-controlled studies in nursing women. It is unknown whether **naloxone** enters human breast milk. However, considering the indication and dosing, one-time **naloxone** use is unlikely to pose a clinically significant risk to the breastfeeding neonate. Endogenous opioids inhibit oxytocin neurons until parturition, and **naloxone** increases oxytocin secretion in pregnant rats. In humans, oxytocin secretion is inhibited in breastfeeding women by exogenous **morphine** compared to control. **Naloxone** does not reverse the process.

■ **References** ⋯⋯⋯⋯⋯⋯⋯⋯⋯ Leighton BL, Halpern SH. Am J Obstet Gynecol 2002; 186(Suppl):S69-77.
Leighton BL, Halpern SH. Semin Perinatol 2002; 26:122-35.
Douglas AJ, Leng G, Russell JA. Reproduction 2002; 123:543-52.
Head BB, Owen J, Vincent RD Jr, et al. Obstet Gynecol 2002; 99:452-7.
Hulse GK, O'Neill G, Pereira C, Brewer C. Aust NZ J Obstet Gynaecol 2001; 41:424-8.
Herschel M, Khoshnood B, Lass NA. Pediatrics 2000; 106:831-4.
Kopecky EA, Simone C, Knie B, Koren G. Life Sci 1999; 65:2359-71.
Douglas AJ, Neumann I, Meeren HK, et al. J Neurosci 1995; 15:5049-57.
Douglas AJ, Bicknell RJ, Russell JA. Adv Exp Med Biol 1995; 395:381-94.
Katsiris S, Williams S, Leighton BL, Halpern S. Can J Anaesth 1998; 45:880-3.
Lindow SW, Hendricks MS, Nugent FA, et al. Gynecol Obstet Invest 1999; 48:33-7.

■ **Summary** ⋯⋯⋯⋯⋯⋯⋯⋯⋯ ● **Pregnancy Category B**
● **Lactation Category S**
● **Naloxone** reverses the effect of narcotics on the fetus and newborn. It should be given within minutes of delivery.

Naltrexone (ReVia; Trexan)

■ **Class** ⋯⋯⋯⋯⋯⋯⋯⋯⋯⋯⋯ *Antagonist, narcotic, antidote*

■ **Indications** ⋯⋯⋯⋯⋯⋯⋯⋯ Opiate addiction, alcohol dependence

■ **Mechanism** ⋯⋯⋯⋯⋯⋯⋯⋯ Opioid receptor antagonist

- **Dosage with Qualifiers** ···········
Opiate addiction—begin 25mg PO ×1, repeat in 1h if no withdrawal; alternative 100mg PO qd, then 150mg PO q3d
NOTE—patient must be opiate free ×7-10d and pass **naloxone** challenge test
Alcohol dependence—50mg PO qd
  - **Contraindications**—hypersensitivity to drug or class, opiate use, failed **naloxone** challenge, failed **naltrexone** challenge, acute hepatitis, hepatic failure, opiate dependence, acute opiate withdrawal
  - **Caution**—unknown

- **Maternal Considerations** ··········
Naltrexone is a synthetic congener of **oxymorphone** with no opioid agonist properties. There are no adequate reports or well-controlled studies of **naltrexone** in pregnant women. Pregnant heroin users have poor maternal and neonatal outcome. Medically supervised heroin withdrawal is generally discouraged during pregnancy because of the fetal risk and a high likelihood of failure with return to regular illicit heroin use. Recently, a number of withdrawal procedures were developed using **naloxone** or **naltrexone** that have met with some success in users who continue the antagonist throughout pregnancy. More recently, implants have been studied as a vehicle for sustained release. Ovarian failure of hypothalamic origin is a consequence of an inappropriate increase in opioid tone of the neurons that release GnRH in a pulsatile manner. **Naltrexone** administration to these women can lead to pregnancy. After cesarean section **naltrexone** is effective against the pruritus and vomiting associated with intrathecal **morphine** for analgesia, but shortens the duration of analgesia.
Side effects include suicidal ideation, opiate withdrawal symptoms, insomnia, nausea, vomiting, headache, anxiety, chills, anorexia, somnolence, constipation, abdominal pain, muscle aches, rash, dizziness, fatigue, restlessness, bone or joint pain, myalgia, and nasal symptoms.

- **Fetal Considerations** ··········
There are no adequate reports or well-controlled studies in human fetuses. **Naltrexone** crosses the human and rodent placenta. Rodent studies are generally reassuring, revealing no evidence of teratogenicity or IUGR despite the use of doses higher than those used clinically. There is evidence of embryo and early fetal toxicity. Rodents exposed to **naltrexone** during prenatal life are larger in weight and length, confirming that native opioids are important growth-inhibiting regulators. **Naltrexone** has no behavioral affect on exposed rabbit pups.

- **Breastfeeding Safety** ··········
There is no published experience in nursing women. It is unknown whether **naltrexone** enters human breast milk. It does enter rodent milk. However, considering the indication and dosing, one-time **naltrexone** use is unlikely to pose a clinically significant risk to the breast-feeding neonate.

■ **References** ·················· Hulse G, O'Neil G. Aust NZ J Obstet Gynaecol 2002; 42:569-73.

Hulse GK, O'Neill G, Pereira C, Brewer C. Aust NZ J Obstet Gynaecol 2001; 41:424-8.

Zagon IS, Hurst WJ, McLaughlin PJ. Life Sci 1998; 62:221-8.

Zagon IS, Hurst WJ, McLaughlin PJ. Life Sci 1997; 61:1261-7.

McLaughlin PJ, Tobias SW, Lang CM, Zagon IS. Physiol Behav 1997; 62:501-8.

Wildt L, Leyendecker G, Sir-Petermann T, Waibel-Treber S. Hum Reprod 1993; 8:350-8.

Abboud TK, Lee K, Zhu J, et al. Anesth Analg 1990; 71:367-70.

Christian MS. J Clin Psychiatry 1984; 45:7-10.

■ **Summary** ··················
- **Pregnancy Category C**
- **Lactation Category U**
- **Naltrexone** reduces the adverse symptoms associated with morphine analgesia, but shortens the duration.
- **Naltrexone** should be used during pregnancy and lactation only if the benefit justifies the potential perinatal risk.

Naphazoline (Ak-Con; Albalon; Allersol; I-Naphline; Murine; Muro's Opcon; Nafazair; Naphacel; Naphazole; Naphcon Forte; Nazil; Ocu-Zoline; Opcon; Spectro-Con; Vasocon)

■ **Class** ·················· *Decongestant, nasal, ophthalmic, sympathomimetic*

■ **Indications** ·················· Ocular congestion

■ **Mechanism** ·················· Stimulates α-adrenergic receptors (sympathomimetic)

■ **Dosage with Qualifiers** ·················· Ocular congestion—1-2 gtt OS/OD q3-4h; max 4 doses/d
- **Contraindications**—hypersensitivity to drug or class, glaucoma
- **Caution**—cardiovascular disease, diabetes mellitus, hyperthyroidism, hypertension

■ **Maternal Considerations** ·················· There are no adequate reports or well-controlled studies of **naphazoline** in pregnant women. Considering the dose and route, it is unlikely that when used as directed the maternal systemic concentration associated will reach a clinically relevant level.

Side effects include hyperemia, headache, dizziness, blurred vision, large pupils, increased sweating, weakness, and nervousness.

- **Fetal Considerations** — There are no adequate reports or well-controlled studies in human fetuses. It is unknown whether **naphazoline** crosses the human placenta. Considering the dose and route, it is unlikely the maternal systemic concentration associated with systemic use will reach clinically relevant level.

- **Breastfeeding Safety** — There is no published experience in nursing women. It is unknown whether **naphazoline** enters human breast milk. However, considering the indication and dosing, occasional **naphazoline** use is unlikely to pose a clinically significant risk to the breast-feeding neonate.

- **References** — There are no current relevant references.

- **Summary**
  - **Pregnancy Category C**
  - **Lactation Category S?**
  - **Naphazoline** should be used during pregnancy and lactation only if the benefit justifies the potential perinatal risk.

Naproxen (EC-Naprosyn; Ec-Naprosyn; Flexipen; Napoton; Napren; Naprosyn; Sutony)

- **Class** — *Analgesic*, NSAID

- **Indications** — Osteoarthritis or rheumatoid arthritis, dysmenorrhea, pain, ankylosing spondilitis, anti-inflammatory effect

- **Mechanism** — Inhibits cyclooxygenase and lipoxygenase leading to reduced prostaglandin synthesis

- **Dosage with Qualifiers** — Osteoarthritis—250-500mg PO bid; max 1500mg/d ×3-5d
  Rheumatoid arthritis—250-500mg PO bid; max 1500mg/d ×3-5d
  Dysmenorrhea—250mg PO q6-8h prn; begin 500mg ×1; max 1250mg/d
  Pain—250-500mg PO bid; max 1500mg/d ×3-5d
  Ankylosing spondilitis—250-500mg PO bid; max 1500mg/d ×3-5d
  Anti-inflammatory effect—250-500mg PO bid; max 1500mg/d ×3-5d
  - **Contraindications**—hypersensitivity to drug or class, NSAID-induced asthma, renal or hepatic dysfunction
  - **Caution**—GI bleeding, hypertension, CHF, nasal polyps, chronic alcoholic liver disease, anemia

- **Maternal Considerations** — NSAIDs are widely distributed in over-the-counter preparations, and their use during pregnancy is underestimated. There are no adequate reports or well-controlled studies of **naproxen** in pregnant women. **Naproxen** offers no distinct clinical advantage over other NSAIDs on the market. It provides analgesic relief similar to **acetaminophen** after vaginal delivery. One randomized trial suggests the addition of plus regular doses of **naproxen** to prn requests for **acetaminophen codeine** provides small reductions in pain on day two after cesarean delivery, with the greatest effects at 36h, when pain typically peaks.

Side effects include headache, dyspnea, dizziness, drowsiness, lightheadedness, vertigo, skin eruption, ecchymosis, sweating, purpura, edema, palpitations, tinnitus, hearing disturbances, visual disturbances, renal failure, bronchospasm, Stevens-Johnson syndrome, interstitial nephritis, hepatotoxicity, thrombocytopenia, agranulocytosis, constipation, rash, increased hepatic transaminases, urticaria, and fluid retention.

■ **Fetal Considerations**

There are no adequate reports or well-controlled studies in human fetuses. **Naproxen** crosses the human placenta, achieving an F:M ratio of 0.92 during the 2nd trimester. Other NSAIDs can cause premature closure of the fetal ductus arteriosus. While the ductal response to **naproxen** remains to be studied, there are several case reports of neonatal pulmonary hypertension after its use in the 3rd trimester. Rodent studies are reassuring, revealing no evidence of teratogenicity or IUGR despite the use of doses higher than those used clinically.

■ **Breastfeeding Safety**

Although **naproxen** is excreted into human breast milk, the amount of drug transferred is only a small fraction of the maternal dose and should not pose a risk to the nursing newborn.

■ **References**

Angle PJ, Halpern SH, Leighton BL, et al. Anesth Analg 2002; 95:741-5.
Skovlund E, Fyllingen G, Landre H, Nesheim BI. Eur J Clin Pharmacol 1991; 40:539-42.
Siu SS, Yeung JH, Lau TK. Hum Reprod 2002; 17:1056-9.
Talati AJ, Salim MA, Korones SB. Am J Perinatol 2000; 17:69-71.
Davies NM, Anderson KE. Clin Pharmacokinet 1997; 32:268-93.

■ **Summary**

- **Pregnancy Category B**
- **Lactation Category S**
- **Naproxen** should be used during pregnancy and lactation only if the benefit justifies the potential perinatal risk.
- There are alternative agents for which there is more experience during pregnancy and lactation.

Naratriptan (Amerge)

- **Class** — *Serotonin receptor agonist*

- **Indications** — Migraine headache

- **Mechanism** — Selective 5HT-1D and -1B agonist

- **Dosage with Qualifiers** — Migraine headache—1-2.5mg PO ×1; may repeat in 4h after 1st dose; max 5mg/d
  - **Contraindications**—hypersensitivity to drug or class, hypertension, CAD, hepatic failure, significant renal or hepatic dysfunction, MAO inhibitors <14d, ergot derivatives <24h
  - **Caution**—CVD, mild hepatic dysfunction

- **Maternal Considerations** — Migraine headaches are a frequent complaint during pregnancy, and ergot compounds are generally considered contraindicated. From 55-90% of pregnant women experience an improvement in headache symptoms during the 2nd and 3rd trimesters. A higher percentage of women with menstrual migraine find they improve during pregnancy. There are no adequate reports or well-controlled studies of **naratriptan** in pregnant women. The clearance of **naratriptan** is modestly reduced (22%) in women on oral contraceptives; clearance during pregnancy is unstudied. Smoking increases clearance by a third. The manufacturer, Glaxo-Wellcome, maintains a registry for postmarketing information on pregnancy outcomes. *Side effects* include malaise, fatigue, abnormal ECG, acute MI, stroke, coronary vasospasm, cardiac arrest, palpitations, tachyarrhythmia, hypertensive crisis, colonic ischemia, hyposalivation, vomiting, tracheitis, asthma, pleuritis, tremors, cognitive function disorders, sleep disorders, disorders of equilibrium, anxiety, depression, hallucinations, panic, inflammation of the breast, vagina, or bladder, polyuria, and diuresis.

- **Fetal Considerations** — There are no adequate reports or well-controlled studies in human fetuses. It is unknown whether **naratriptan** crosses the human placenta. Rodent studies reveal embryotoxicity and skeletal abnormalities at doses producing maternal plasma levels only a few multiples of the MRHD. However, the frequencies of these adverse outcomes are not dose-dependent.

- **Breastfeeding Safety** — There is no published experience in nursing women. It is unknown whether **naratriptan** enters human breast milk. It does enter rodent milk. However, considering the indication and dosing, one-time **naratriptan** use is unlikely to pose a clinically significant risk to the breast-feeding neonate. The patient may choose to pump her breasts for 24h for added safety.

■ **References** ———————— Pfaffenrath V, Rehm M. Drug Saf 1998; 19:383-8.

■ **Summary** ————————
- **Pregnancy Category C**
- **Lactation Category U**
- **Naratriptan** should be used during pregnancy and lactation only if the benefit justifies the potential perinatal risk.
- Physicians are encouraged to register pregnant women under the **Naratriptan** Pregnancy Registry (1-800-336-2176) for a better follow-up of outcome while under treatment with **naratriptan**.
- There are alternative agents for which there is more experience during pregnancy and lactation.

Nateglinide (Starlex)

■ **Class** ———————— Antidiabetic agent, biguanide

■ **Indications** ———————— Diabetes mellitus type 2

■ **Mechanism** ———————— Stimulates pancreatic β-cell insulin release

■ **Dosage with Qualifiers** ———— Diabetes mellitus—begin 30-60mg PO qac if HbA1c close to normal; use as monotherapy or in combination with **metformin**
NOTE—do not use with insulin secretagogues; take 30min before meal and skip dose if no meal taken
- **Contraindications**—hypersensitivity to drug or class, diabetes mellitus type 1, diabetic ketoacidosis
- **Caution**—hepatic dysfunction

■ **Maternal Considerations** ——— **Insulin** remains the hypoglycemic agent of choice during pregnancy, though some oral agents are emerging as viable alternatives in women with type 2 diabetes mellitus. **Nateglinide** is a D-phenylalanine derivative that helps reduce postprandial hyperglycemia. There is no published experience during pregnancy.
Side effects include upper respiratory infection, arthropathy, bronchitis, hypoglycemia, diarrhea, and dizziness.

■ **Fetal Considerations** ———— There are no adequate reports or well-controlled studies in human fetuses. It is unknown whether **nateglinide** crosses the human placenta. Rodent studies are generally reassuring, though some note an increase in gallbladder agenesis at doses 40 times the MRHD.

■ **Breastfeeding Safety** ———— There is no published experience in nursing women. It is unknown whether **nateglinide** enters human breast milk. It is excreted into rodent milk, and the maternal administration of high doses slows pup weight gain. It is unknown whether the reduced growth reflects only maternal hypoglycemia.

■ **References** — There is no published experience in pregnancy or during lactation.

■ **Summary** —
- **Pregnancy Category C**
- **Lactation Category U**
- Insulin remains the hypoglycemic agent of choice during pregnancy.
- **Nateglinide** should be used during pregnancy and lactation only if the benefit justifies the potential perinatal risk.

Nedocromil (Alocril; Tilade)

■ **Class** — *Mast cell stabilizer*

■ **Indications** — Asthma, chronic; allergic conjunctivitis

■ **Mechanism** — Inhibits release of various inflammatory cell mediators

■ **Dosage with Qualifiers** —
Asthma, chronic—2 puffs INH qid
Allergic conjunctivitis—1-2 gtt OS/OD bid
NOTE—2% solution; may reduce dose 50% if clinical improvement
- **Contraindications**—hypersensitivity to drug or class, acute asthma attack
- **Caution**—unknown

■ **Maternal Considerations** — There is no published experience with **nedocromil** during pregnancy. **Nedocromil** is effective long-term maintenance therapy for bronchial asthma.
Side effects include bronchospasm, headache, bitter taste, cough, pharyngitis, rhinitis, bronchitis, dyspnea, nausea, vomiting, dry mouth, dyspepsia, and fatigue.

■ **Fetal Considerations** — There are no adequate reports or well-controlled studies in human fetuses. It is unknown whether **nedocromil** crosses the human placenta. Considering the dose and route, it is unlikely the maternal systemic concentration will reach clinically relevant level. Rodent studies are reassuring, revealing no evidence of teratogenicity or IUGR despite the use of doses higher than those used clinically.

- **Breastfeeding Safety** There is no published experience in nursing women. It is unknown whether **nedocromil** enters human breast milk. However, considering the indication and dosing, occasional **nedocromil** use is unlikely to pose a clinically significant risk to the breast-feeding neonate.

- **References** There is no published experience in pregnancy or during lactation.

- **Summary**
  - **Pregnancy Category B**
  - **Lactation Category U**
  - **Nedocromil** should be used during pregnancy and lactation only if the benefit justifies the potential perinatal risk.
  - There are alternative agents for which there is more experience during pregnancy and lactation.

Nefazodone (Serzone)

- **Class** *Antidepressants*

- **Indications** Depression

- **Mechanism** Inhibits norepinephrine and 5HT reuptake; antagonizes 5HT receptor

- **Dosage with Qualifiers** Depression—begin 100mg PO bid, 150-300mg PO bid; max 600mg/d
  - **Contraindications**—hypersensitivity to drug or class, active hepatic disease, MAO inhibitor <14d, **cisapride** use
  - **Caution**—unknown

- **Maternal Considerations** Depression is common during and after pregnancy, but typically goes unrecognized. Pregnancy is not a reason *a priori* to discontinue psychotropic drugs. The serotonin reuptake inhibitors are first-line treatment for most depressive and anxiety disorders. **Nefazodone** is unrelated to SSRIs, tricyclics, or MAO inhibitors. There is no published experience with **nefazodone** during pregnancy.
  Side effects include hepatotoxicity, seizures, hypomania, hepatic failure, insomnia, asthenia, dizziness, lightheadedness, headache, dry mouth, dyspepsia, constipation, diarrhea, pharyngitis, abnormal vision, blurred vision, confusion, orthostatic hypotension, increased appetite, and paresthesias.

- **Fetal Considerations** — There are no adequate reports or well-controlled studies in human fetuses. It is unknown whether **nefazodone** crosses the human placenta. A prospective case control study was reassuring, revealing no evidence of an adverse fetal effect. Rodent studies are generally reassuring, revealing no signs of teratogenicity or IUGR despite the use of doses higher than those used clinically. There is an unexplained increase in early pup death.

- **Breastfeeding Safety** — There are no adequate reports or well-controlled studies in nursing women. **Nefazodone** enters human breast milk, and neonatal drowsiness, lethargy and poor feeding that resolves when breastfeeding stops are reported. If the mother elects to breastfeed, the infant should be monitored for possible adverse effects, the drug given at the lowest effective dose, and breastfeeding avoided at times of peak drug levels.

- **References** — Einarson A, Bonari L, Voyer-Lavigne S, et al. Can J Psychiatry 2003; 48:106-10.
  Yapp P, Ilett KF, Kristensen JH, et al. Ann Pharmacother 2000; 34:1269-72.
  Dodd S, Buist A, Burrows GD, et al. J Chromatogr B Biomed Sci Appl 1999; 730:249-55.

- **Summary**
  - **Pregnancy Category C**
  - **Lactation Category NS?**
  - **Nefazodone** should be used during pregnancy and lactation only if the benefit justifies the potential perinatal risk.
  - There are alternative agents for which there is more experience during pregnancy and lactation.

Nelfinavir (Viracept)

- **Class** — Antiviral, *protease inhibitor*

- **Indications** — HIV infection

- **Mechanism** — Protease inhibitor

- **Dosage with Qualifiers** — HIV infection—1250mg PO with food bid in combination with other antiretroviral agents; alternatively, 750mg PO tid
  NOTE—do not mix with juice or acidic food
  - **Contraindications**—hypersensitivity to drug or class, **astemizole** use, **midazolam** use, **rifampin** use, phenylketonuria
  - **Caution**—hepatic dysfunction

■ **Maternal Considerations** .... The incidence of both the AIDS syndrome and opportunistic infections has declined over the last few years due to advances in drug regimens. Triple therapy **(zidovudine, lamivudine, nevirapine)** remains the standard of care for the management of HIV infection in adults because of its high efficacy. Some study protocols use **nelfinavir** as the protease inhibitor. The treatment of HIV during pregnancy dramatically reduces the risk of mother-to-child transmission in proportion to the maternal viral load. There are no adequate reports or well-controlled studies of **nelfinavir** in pregnant women. Careful monitoring for hepatotoxicity during therapy with **nelfinavir** is recommended. The association between combination antiviral therapy with protease inhibitors and an increased risk of very low birth weight requires confirmation.

Side effects include nausea, vomiting, flatulence, diarrhea, hepatitis, seizures, rash, asthenia, abdominal pain, arthralgia, myalgias, myopathy, dyslipidemia, hyperglycemia, leukopenia, thrombocytopenia, and pruritus.

■ **Fetal Considerations** .... There are no adequate reports or well-controlled studies in human fetuses. Like most protease inhibitors, **nelfinavir** crosses the human placenta but only achieves subtherapeutic levels. The transfer is probably limited by a high degree of plasma protein binding and backward transport by placental P-glycoprotein. While low protease inhibitor concentrations in the fetus decreases the likelihood of teratogenic and toxic effects, they may fail to provide protection from transplacental or intrapartum transmission of HIV-1 virus. Rodent studies are reassuring, revealing no evidence of teratogenicity or IUGR despite the use of doses higher than those used clinically.

■ **Breastfeeding Safety** .... There is no published experience in nursing women. It is unknown whether **nelfinavir** enters human breast milk. It is excreted into rodent milk. Breastfeeding is contraindicated in HIV-infected nursing women where formula is available to reduce the risk of neonatal transmission.

■ **References** .... Mirochnick M, Dorenbaum A, Holland D, et al. Pediatr Infect Dis J 2002; 21:835-8.
Marzolini C, Rudin C, Decosterd LA, et al. AIDS 2002; 16:889-93.
Hill JB, Sheffield JS, Zeeman GG, Wendel GD Jr. Obstet Gynecol 2001; 98:909-11.
Rachel Jordan, Lisa Gold, Carole Cummins, Chris Hyde. BMJ 2002; 324:757.
Tuomala RE, Shapiro DE, Mofenson LM, et al. N Engl J Med 2002 Jun 13; 346:1863-70.

■ Summary ··· • **Pregnancy Category B**
• **Lactation Category NS**
• Triple therapy consisting of **nevirapine**, **lamivudine**, and **zidovudine** significantly reduces the risk of mother-to-child transmission and remains the standard of care for management of HIV infection in adults.
• Pregnant women require careful monitoring for hepatotoxicity during antiretroviral therapy.
• Physicians are encouraged to register pregnant women under the Antiretroviral Pregnancy Registry (1-800-258-4263) for a better follow-up of the outcome while under treatment with **nelfinavir**.

Neomycin (Mycifradin; Myciguent; Neo-Rx; Qrp)

■ **Class** ·· *Antibiotic, aminoglycoside*

■ **Indications** ·································· Hepatic coma, bacterial infections (<u>aerobic gram-negative</u>: *Enterobacter cloacae, Escherichia coli, Klebsiella, Enterobacter*)

■ **Mechanism** ·································· Bactericidal; inhibits protein synthesis reducing ammonia forming bacteria in the gut

■ **Dosage with Qualifiers** ··········· <u>Hepatic coma</u>—4-12g/d PO; minimize protein in diet
<u>Bacterial infections</u>—apply topically qd/tid; max 1w
NOTE—available in combination with **bacitracin** and **polymyxin B** as Neosporin
• **Contraindications**—hypersensitivity to drug or class, GI obstruction, inflammatory and ulcerative GI disease, severe dermatologic diseases
• **Caution**—hepatic dysfunction

■ **Maternal Considerations** ········· There are no adequate reports or well-controlled studies of **neomycin** in pregnant women. **Neomycin** is poorly absorbed in the bowel, though repeated dosing can lead to accumulation especially in the inner ear. Clearance can take weeks. The U.S. CDC recommends the use of a selective broth culture to improve detection of genital tract or anorectal carriage of group B streptococci (GBS) in pregnant women. The addition of **neomycin** to **nalidixic acid** in a selective broth medium improves the sensitivity of screening cultures for the detection of GBS carriage in women.
Side effects include nausea, vomiting, diarrhea, malabsorbtion syndrome, nephrotoxicity, ototoxicity, and neuromuscular blockage.

- **Fetal Considerations** ⸻ There are no adequate reports or well-controlled studies in human fetuses. It is unknown whether **neomycin** crosses the human placenta. While there is no evidence that it is a human teratogen, some aminoglycosides (e.g., **streptomycin**) have been associated with irreversible deafness after *in utero* exposure. Considering the dose and route, it is unlikely the maternal systemic concentration will reach clinically relevant level after topical administration. Rodent teratogenicity studies have not been performed. **Neomycin** is used for prophylaxis of ophthalmia neonatorum, though efficacy has not been tested through clinical trials.

- **Breastfeeding Safety** ⸻ There are no adequate reports or well-controlled studies in nursing women. It is unknown whether **neomycin** enters human breast milk. **Neomycin** is excreted into both ovine and rat breast milk. However, considering the indication and dosing, occasional topical use is unlikely to pose a clinically significant risk to the breast-feeding neonate.

- **References** ⸻ Assadian O, Assadian A, Aspock C et al. Wien Klin Wochenschr 2002; 114:194-9.
  Czeizel AE, Rockenbauer M, Olsen J, Sorensen HT. Scand J Infect Dis 2000; 32:309-13.
  Dunne WM Jr. J Clin Microbiol 1999; 37:3705-6.
  Dunne WM Jr, Holland-Staley CA. J Clin Microbiol 1998; 36:2298-300.
  Scheer M. Arzneimittelforschung 1976; 26:778-81.

- **Summary** ⸻
  - **Pregnancy Category D**
  - **Lactation Category S?**
  - **Neomycin** should be used during pregnancy and lactation only if the benefit justifies the potential perinatal risk.

Neostigmine (Prostigmin)

- **Class** ⸻ *Cholinesterase inhibitor, muscle stimulant*

- **Indications** ⸻ Myasthenia gravis, neuromuscular reversal, urinary retention

- **Mechanism** ⸻ Inhibits cholinesterase activity

- **Dosage with Qualifiers** ⸻ <u>Myasthenia gravis treatment</u>—15-375mg PO qd; 10mg SC/IV/IM qd; 0.5-2.5mg SC/IV/IM q2-3h prn; max 375mg PO qd
  <u>Myasthenia gravis diagnostic</u>—0.02mg/kg IM ×1 with **atropine**

Neuromuscular reversal—0.07mg/kg IV, max 5mg; give slow IV push with **atropine** and **glycopyrrolate**
Urinary retention treatment—0.5-1mg SC/IM ×1; if no output after 1h, catheterize bladder and give 0.5mg SC/IM q3h ×5 doses
Urinary retention prophylaxis—0.25mg SC/IM q4-6h ×2-3d; begin immediately postoperatively to prevent bladder distention/atony
NOTE—renal dosing
- **Contraindications**—hypersensitivity to drug or class, GI obstruction, urinary tract obstruction, peritonitis
- **Caution**—epilepsy, asthma, bradycardia, recent MI, hyperthyroidism, peptic ulcer disease

■ **Maternal Considerations**

There are case reports of its use throughout pregnancy for the treatment of maternal myasthenia gravis.
Side effects include cholinergic crisis, cardiac arrest, arrhythmia, respiratory paralysis, bronchospasm, respiratory secretions, salivation, drowsiness, fasciculation, nausea, vomiting, abdominal pain, flatulence, diarrhea, dizziness, seizures, syncope, hypotension, rash, weakness, flushing, and urinary frequency.

■ **Fetal Considerations**

There are no adequate reports or well-controlled studies in human fetuses. It is unknown whether **neostigmine** crosses the human placenta. Twenty to 30% offspring of women suffering from myasthenia gravis have transient neonatal motor symptoms, suggesting maternal antibodies cross the placenta. Newborns with myasthenia gravis require **neostigmine** until complete recovery of the motor handicap. Rodent teratogenicity studies have not been performed.

■ **Breastfeeding Safety**

There are no adequate reports or well-controlled studies in nursing women. It is unknown whether **neostigmine** enters human breast milk. However, considering the indication and dosing, occasional use is unlikely to pose a clinically significant risk to the breast-feeding neonate. It is generally considered compatible with breastfeeding.

■ **References**

Licht C, Model P, Kribs A, et al. Nervenarzt 2002; 73:774-8.
Owen MD, Ozsarac O, Sahin S, et al. Anesthesiology 2000; 92:361-6.
Nelson KE, D'Angelo R, Foss ML, et al. Anesthesiology 1999; 91:1293-8.
Klamt JG, Garcia LV, Prado WA. Anaesthesia 1999; 54:27-31.
Mitchell PJ, Bebbington M. Obstet Gynecol 1992; 80:178-81.
Mercier FJ, Benhamou D. Baillieres Clin Obstet Gynaecol 1998; 12:397-407.
Chung CJ, Kim JS, Park HS, Chin YJ. Anesth Analg 1998; 87:341-6.
Clark RB, Brown MA, Lattin DL. Anesthesiology 1996; 84:450-2.
Rolbin WH, Levinson G, Shnider SM, Wright RG. Anesth Analg 1978; 57:441-7.

■ **Summary** • **Pregnancy Category C**
• **Lactation Category S**
• **Neostigmine** should be used during pregnancy only if the benefit justifies the potential perinatal risk.

Nesiritide (Natrecor)

■ **Class** — *Cardiovascular, natriuretic peptide, type-B human*

■ **Indications** — Acute CHF

■ **Mechanism** — Stimulates *c*GMP production and thus vascular smooth muscle relaxation

■ **Dosage with Qualifiers** — Acute CHF— begin 2mcg/kg IV bolus, then 0.01mcg/kg/min IV; decrease or discontinue if hypotension; max 0.03mcg/kg/min
- **Contraindications**—hypersensitivity to drug or class, cardiogenic shock, systolic blood pressure below 90mmHg, cardiac tamponade, restrictive cardiomyopathy, obstructive cardiomyopathy, constrictive pericarditis
- **Caution**—renal dysfunction, hypotension, volume depletion, concomitant use of other hypotensive agents

■ **Maternal Considerations** — **Nesiritide** is human recombinant BNP. There is no published experience with **nesiritide** during pregnancy. *Side effects* include hypotension, tachycardia, ventricular extrasystoles, dizziness, elevated creatinine, headache, hypotension, back pain, nausea, vomiting, insomnia, anxiety, and angina.

■ **Fetal Considerations** — There are no adequate reports or well-controlled studies in human fetuses. It is unknown whether **nesiritide** crosses the human placenta. Rodent teratogen studies have not been performed.

■ **Breastfeeding Safety** — There is no published experience in nursing women. It is unknown whether **nesiritide** enters human breast milk.

■ **References** — There are no current relevant references.

■ **Summary** — • **Pregnancy Category C**
• **Lactation Category U**
• **Nesiritide** should be used during pregnancy and lactation only if the benefit justifies the potential perinatal risk.
• There are alternative agents for which there is more experience during pregnancy and lactation.

Netilmicin (Netromycin)

■ **Class** — Antibiotic, aminoglycoside

■ **Indications** — Bacterial infections of the skin, sepsis, intra-abdominal, and respiratory tract (aerobic gram-negative: *Enterobacter cloacae, Escherichia coli, Haemophilus influenzae,* H. *parainfluenzae, Klebsiella* species, *Legionella pneumophila, Moraxella caterrhalis, Proteus mirabilis;* aerobic gram-positive: *Enterococcus faecalis, Staphylococcus aureus* [methicillin-susceptible], S. *saprophyticus, Streptococcus pneumoniae,* S. *pyogenes*)

■ **Mechanism** — Bactericidal; inhibits protein synthesis

■ **Dosage with Qualifiers** — Bacterial infections—4-6.5mg/kg/IV qd divided q8-12h
  • **Contraindications**—hypersensitivity to drug or class
  • **Caution**—unknown

■ **Maternal Considerations** — There are no adequate reports or well-controlled studies of **netilmicin** in pregnant women. It is the 1st alternative to **gentamicin** for the treatment of brucellosis. There are case reports of its use for listeriosis.
Side effects include nephrotoxicity, ototoxicity, rash, neuromuscular blockade, elevation of the liver enzyme, elevation of the bilirubin, elevation of the alkaline phosphatase, hypomagnesemia, thrombocytosis, pain at injection site, tinnitus, nystagmus, and hearing loss.

■ **Fetal Considerations** — There are no adequate reports or well-controlled studies in human fetuses. It is unknown whether **netilmicin** crosses the human placenta. While there is no evidence that **netilmicin** is a human teratogen, some aminoglycosides (e.g., **streptomycin**) have been associated with irreversible deafness after *in utero* exposure. Rodent teratogenicity studies have not been performed. Transfer across the term rat placenta appears low. In the guinea pig, **netilmicin** had significantly less effect on the cochlea compared to **gentamicin**. In the rat, the impact of **netilmicin** on renal function after *in utero* exposure is similar to **gentamicin** and greater than **amikacin**.

■ **Breastfeeding Safety** — There is no published experience in nursing women. A small amount of **netilmicin** enters human breast milk, but the kinetics remain to be elucidated.

■ **References** — Bonacorsi S, Doit C, Aujard Y, et al. Clin Infect Dis 1993; 17:139-40.
Kawasaki H, Yamada Y, Takei T, Akiyoshi M. Jpn J Antibiot 1982; 35:1553-61.
Mallie JP, Coulon G, Billerey C, et al. Kidney Int 1988; 33:36-44.
Fujino A, Uda F, Nomura A, Tokiwa T. Jpn J Antibiot 1982; 35:979-86.

■ Summary
- • **Pregnancy Category D**
- • **Lactation Category U**
- • **Netilmicin** should be used during pregnancy and lactation only if the benefit justifies the potential perinatal risk.
- • There are alternative agents for which there is more experience during pregnancy and lactation.

Nevirapine (Viramune)

■ **Class** — *Antiviral, non-nucleoside reverse transcriptase inhibitor*

■ **Indications** — HIV

■ **Mechanism** — Inhibits reverse transcriptase

■ **Dosage with Qualifiers** — <u>HIV infection</u>—200mg PO qd ×14d; continue treatment with 200mg PO bid in combination with nucleoside antiretrovirals
- • **Contraindications**—hypersensitivity to drug or class
- • **Caution**—renal or hepatic dysfunction

■ **Maternal Considerations** — **Nevirapine** should not typically be used alone, except in unusual circumstances, such as to prevent infection after accidental HIV exposure because of the potential for side effects. The incidence of both the AIDS syndrome and opportunistic infection has decreased dramatically over the last years because of advances in drug regimens. Triple therapy **(zidovudine, lamivudine, nevirapine)** remains the standard of care for the management of HIV infection in adults because of its high efficacy. A single dose of **nevirapine** (200mg PO) given at the onset of labor dramatically reduces perinatal HIV transmission in women receiving no other antenatal, antiretroviral therapy. It is more effective (in the absence of regular antiretroviral therapy) than an intrapartum and postpartum regimen of **zidovudine** if given to both women at the onset of labor and their newborns within 72h of birth. **Nevirapine** resistance does occur from this approach. Maternal risk factors include a low CD$_4$ cell count and a high viral load at delivery. The addition of **nevirapine** during the labor of women receiving antiretroviral therapy during pregnancy does not further reduce perinatal HIV transmission if cesarean section is available. Cost and identification of women with HIV infection during pregnancy represents a significant problem in many developing countries. As a result, it is proposed that in high HIV prevalence areas, "triple therapy" be offered routinely to all pregnant women and their infants without prior HIV testing. The association between combination therapy that includes a protease inhibitor, and an increased risk of very low birth weight requires confirmation. Hepatotoxicity usually does not manifest before 5mo of therapy.

Side effects include Stevens-Johnson syndrome, fever, hepatotoxicity, hepatitis, neutropenia, peripheral neuropathy, nausea, vomiting, abdominal pain, diarrhea, rash, myalgias, headache, arthralgia, and stomatitis.

■ **Fetal Considerations**

There are no adequate reports or well-controlled studies in human fetuses. The safety of many approved antiretroviral agents during pregnancy is not established. In contrast to other protease inhibitors, **nevirapine** rapidly crosses the human placenta. A single 2mg/kg dose administered to the newborn at 48-72h after birth achieves serum **nevirapine** concentrations 10 times the *in vitro* 50% inhibitory concentration against wild-type HIV-1 throughout the 1st week of life. This limited regimen is well tolerated and reduces the risk of mother-to-child transmission by nearly 50% in women and infants receiving no other antiretrovirals. However, neonatal plasma concentrations decrease more rapidly after maternal **nevirapine** therapy during pregnancy suggesting *in utero* liver enzyme induction.

■ **Breastfeeding Safety**

There are no adequate reports or well-controlled studies in nursing women. **Nevirapine** is excreted into human breast milk with an M:P ratio approximating 0.6. However, breastfeeding is contraindicated in HIV-infected nursing women when formula is available to reduce the risk of neonatal transmission.

■ **References**

Cunningham CK, Chaix ML, Rekacewicz C, et al. J Infect Dis 2002; 186:181-8.
Dorenbaum A, Cunningham CK, Gelber RD, et al. JAMA 2002; 288:189-98.
Brocklehurst P, Volmink J. Cochrane Database Syst Rev 2002;CD003510.
Eshleman SH, Jackson JB. AIDS Rev 2002; 4:59-63.
AIDS Treat News 2001;6-8.
Morris L, Pillay C, Gray G, McIntyre J. SADJ 2001; 56:614-6.
Podzamczer D, Fumero E. Expert Opin Pharmacother 2001; 2:2065-78.
Edwards SG, Larbalestier N, Hay P, et al. HIV Med 2001; 2:89-91.
Mirochnick M, Siminski S, Fenton T, et al. Pediatr Infect Dis J. 2001; 20:803-5.
Hankins C. Reprod Health Matters 2000; 8:87-92.
Mirochnick M. Ann NY Acad Sci 2000; 918:287-97.
McGowan JP, Shah SS. Curr Opin Obstet Gynecol 2000; 12:357-67.
Mirochnick M, Clarke DF, Dorenbaum A. Clin Pharmacokinet 2000; 39:281-93.

■ **Summary** ················· • **Pregnancy Category C**
• **Lactation Category NS**
• **Nevirapine** given at the onset of labor and to newborns within 72h of birth is more effective than intrapartum and postpartum **zidovudine** for women who have not received the regular antiretroviral therapy during prenatal period.
• Physicians are encouraged to register pregnant women under the Antiretroviral Pregnancy Registry (1-800-258-4263) for a better follow-up of the outcome while under treatment with **nevirapine**.

Niacin (Acido Nicotinico; Akotin; Niaspan; Nicolar; Niconacid; Nicotinic Acid; Nikacid; Nikotime; Novo-Niacin; Slo Niacin; Span Niacin; Vitaplex; Wampocap)

■ **Class** ·································· *Antihyperlipidemic, vitamin/mineral*

■ **Indications** ························· Hypercholesterolemia, mixed dyslipidemia, hypertriglyceridemia, pellagra

■ **Mechanism** ························ Decreases hepatic LDL/VLDL production and triglyceride esterification, inhibits lipolysis, increases lipoprotein lipase activity

■ **Dosage with Qualifiers** ·········· Hypercholesterolemia—begin 250mg PO qd, increase 250mg q4-7d based on effect/tolerance; max 6g/d
Mixed dyslipidemia—begin 500mg/d PO qhs ×4w and then 1g/d q4w; max 2g/d
Hypertriglyceridemia—begin 500mg/d PO qhs ×4w and then 1g/d q4w; max 2g/d
Pellagra—300-500mg PO qd; available SC
NOTE—**aspirin** may reduce the flushing; LFTs at baseline, q6-12w ×1y, then q3-6mo; do not cut/crush/chew
• **Contraindications**—hypersensitivity to drug or class, bleeding, hypotension, active ulcer disease, severe hepatic dysfunction
• **Caution**—gout, mild hepatic dysfunction, diabetes mellitus, coronary artery disease, hypotension

■ **Maternal Considerations** ········ **Niacin** is a water-soluble B complex vitamin with essential roles in lipid metabolism, tissue respiration and glycogenolysis. The higher death rate from pellagra in women compared to men is attributed to an estrogen-mediated decrease in the formation of **niacin** from tryptophan. Pregnancy imposes a metabolic stress, which grows with advancing gestation. The recommended dose of **niacinamide** (a by-product of **niacin**) varies between

15-17mg/d and it is usually found in prenatal vitamins. There are no adequate reports or well-controlled studies of **niacin** in pregnant women. Despite routine vitamin supplementation, a high percent of **vitamin A**, **B$_6$**, **niacin**, **thiamin** and **B$_{12}$** hypovitaminemia occurs during pregnancy. **Niacin** deficiency is particularly common during the 1st trimester and its prevalence increases subsequently. Combination deficits of **niacin**, **thiamin**, **vitamins A**, **B$_6$**, **B$_{12}$** occur in each trimester. There is no evidence that supplementation changes pregnancy outcome. **Niacin** deficiencies were once thought associated with preeclampsia and hyperemesis gravidarium, but these associations were not confirmed by well-designed studies.

Side effects include rhabdomyolysis, atrial fibrillation, cardiac arrhythmias, orthostatic hypotension, dyspepsia; vomiting, peptic ulceration, elevated LFTs, jaundice, diarrhea, flushing, dry skin, decrease glucose tolerance, gout, hyperuricemia, macular edema, amblyopia, and headache.

■ **Fetal Considerations**
There are no adequate reports or well-controlled studies in human fetuses. **Niacin** crosses the human placenta, though the kinetics remain to be elucidated. Rodent teratogen studies have not been conducted.

■ **Breastfeeding Safety**
There are no adequate reports or well-controlled studies in nursing women. **Niacin** is excreted into human breast milk. It is not known whether supplementation increases both the milk and neonatal concentration. It is generally considered compatible with breastfeeding.

■ **References**
Baker H, DeAngelis B, Holland B, et al. J Am Coll Nutr 2002; 21:33-7.
Hobson W. J Hyg 1948; 46:198-216.
Hart BF, McConnell WT. Am J Obstet Gynecol 1943; 46:283-7.
Deodhar AD, Rajalakshmi R, Ramakrishnan CV. Acta Paediatr Scand 1964; 53:42-8.

■ **Summary**
- **Pregnancy Category C**
- **Lactation Category S**
- **Niacin** is a component of most prenatal vitamins.
- Many pregnant women are deficient despite supplementation.

Nicardipine (Cardene)

- **Class** — Antihypertensive, antiarrhythmic, calcium-channel blocker

- **Indications** — Hypertension, angina

- **Mechanism** — Inhibits calcium influx into vascular smooth muscle and myocardium

- **Dosage with Qualifiers** — Hypertension—20-40mg PO tid; max 40mg PO tid
  Angina—begin 20mg PO tid; max 40mg PO tid
  Acute hypertension—5mg/hr, increase 2.5mg/hr q5-15min prn, titrate down to effect
  NOTE—hepatic dosing
  - **Contraindications**—hypersensitivity to drug or class, aortic stenosis
  - **Caution**—renal or hepatic dysfunction, CHF, cardiac conduction disease

- **Maternal Considerations** — *Hypertension during pregnancy*—Hypertension remains a significant cause of maternal and fetal morbidity and death. Severe hypertension during pregnancy (BP >170/110mmHg) should be treated immediately to improve both the maternal and fetal outcome. An uncontrolled reduction in BP may lead to coma, stroke, MI, acute renal failure, and death. Pregnancy further complicates the treatment of an acute hypertensive episode because an acute decrease in BP might adversely affect the fetus. Thus, the goal is not just to decrease BP, but to do so with minimal adverse effects while preserving organ function. Randomized trials reveal that **nicardipine** is safe and effective for the treatment of severe hypertension during pregnancy. It is more efficient than **metoprolol** and similar to **labetalol**. Although the definitive treatment for severe preeclampsia remains delivery, some practitioners attempt to temporize in hopes of reducing the complications of prematurity. Preliminary study indicates the long-term treatment with **nicardipine** for severe preeclampsia is effective and safe. **Nicardipine** has also been used during pregnancy to treat hypertension due to pheochromocytoma and autonomic hyperreflexia. *Preterm labor*—**Nicardipine** abolishes *in vitro* contractility of the smooth muscle strips. It causes a modest decline in systolic (9mmHg) and diastolic (7mmHg) pressures in normotensive patients as peripheral resistance falls. The reflex increase in heart rate is usually small, but may occasionally be pronounced. One prospective clinical trial concluded that **nicardipine** is an effective, safe, and well-tolerated tocolytic agent. It arrests preterm labor more rapidly than **magnesium sulfate**, and women treated with **nicardipine** have fewer adverse medication effects and episodes of recurrent preterm labor compared to those treated with **magnesium sulfate**. Any treatment related maternal hypotension is not associated with fetal distress. In another clinical trial, **nicardipine** lead to a greater percentage of women delivering more than 7d after diagnosis compared to **salbutamol**, and there were fewer maternal side effects. **Nicardipine** seems especially attractive in women with hypertension, diabetes mellitus or maternal cardiomyopathy. See **nifedipine**.

Side effects include edema, flushing, asthenia, malaise, nausea, vomiting, dyspnea, palpitations, tachycardia, dizziness, dry mouth, constipation, nervousness, nocturia, ECG abnormalities, and orthostatic hypotension.

■ **Fetal Considerations** ········· There are no adequate reports or well-controlled studies in human fetuses. It is unknown whether **nicardipine** crosses the human placenta. Transfer across the nonhuman primate placenta is poor, and there is no effect on fetal cardiovascular parameters after maternal administration. **Nicardipine** may have some beneficial effect on fetoplacental blood flow resistances in animals and humans. Rodent studies are reassuring, revealing no evidence of teratogenicity or IUGR despite the use of doses higher than those used clinically. Embryotoxicity occurred at doses 50 times the MRHD.

■ **Breastfeeding Safety** ········· There is no published experience in nursing women. It is unknown whether **nicardipine** enters human breast milk. It is excreted into rodent milk.

■ **References** ·········

Elatrous S, Nouira S, Ouanes Besbes L, et al. Intensive Care Med 2002; 28:1281-6.
Seki H, Takeda S, Kinoshita K. Int J Gynaecol Obstet 2002; 76:135-41.
Economy KE, Abuhamad AZ. Semin Perinatol 2001; 25:264-71.
Larmon JE, Ross BS, May WL, et al. Am J Obstet Gynecol 1999; 181:1432-7.
Jannet D, Abankwa A, Guyard B, et al. Eur J Obstet Gynecol Reprod Biol 1997; 73:11-6.
Kasai Y, Tsutsumi O, Taketani Y, et al. J Physiol 1995; 486:373-84.
Jannet D, Carbonne B, Sebban E, Milliez J. Obstet Gynecol 1994; 84:354-9.
Ducsay CA, Thompson JS, Wu AT, Novy MJ. Am J Obstet Gynecol 1987; 157:1482-6.
Carbonne B, Jannet D, Touboul C, et al. Obstet Gynecol 1993; 81:908-14.
Ichihara J, Izumi H, Koyama Y, et al. Nippon Sanka Fujinka Gakkai Zasshi 1991; 43:1249-54.
Marin J, Reviriego J. Arch Int Pharmacodyn Ther 1989; 302:209-19.
Csapo AI, Puri CP, Tarro S, et al. Am J Obstet Gynecol 1982; 142:483-91.

■ Summary ———————— • **Pregnancy Category C**
- **Lactation Category U**
- Calcium-channel blockers have excellent safety profiles and a high degree of efficacy for the treatment of acute and chronic hypertension.
- Calcium-channel blockers are considered the agents of choice for tocolysis.
- There is more experience with **nifedipine** than **nicardipine** for tocolysis.

Nicotine (Habitrol; NicoDerm; Nicotrol; ProStep; Quit Spray; Stubit)

■ **Class** ———————— CNS *stimulant*

■ **Indications** ———————— Smoking cessation

■ **Mechanism** ———————— Stimulates nicotinic-cholinergic receptors localized in various CNS and peripheral sites

■ **Dosage with Qualifiers** ———— Smoking cessation—begin 21mg/d transdermal patches ×6w, 14mg/d ×2w, then 7mg/d ×2w; alternatively, 14mg/d ×6w if <100 lb, <$^{1}/_{2}$ ppd, or signs of cardiac disease
NOTE—available in patches that release 7, 14, 21mg/d
- **Contraindications**—hypersensitivity to drug or class, nonsmokers, recent history acute MI, arrhythmia, angina, allergy to menthol, Buerger's disease, Prinzmetal's variant angina, Raynaud's phenomenon, hyperthyroidism, pheochromocytoma, insulin-dependent diabetes mellitus
- **Caution**—CAD, peptic ulcer disease

■ **Maternal Considerations** ———— Cigarette smoking is directly linked to an array of health care problems whose costs to society are staggering. It increases the rate of subfertility and failed IVF. Cigarette smoking is the single largest modifiable risk for pregnancy-related morbidity and death in the U.S. Addiction to **nicotine** is a primary contributor to tobacco use. **Nicotine** replacement facilitates cessation by relieving the physiologic symptoms of withdrawal. **Nicotine** delivery systems include gum, patch, nasal spray, and vapor inhaler. Because **nicotine** medications do not deliver the toxins and carcinogens delivered by cigarettes, they are safer than smoking if used as directed. Women should be advised to stop smoking completely during pregnancy, and that a simple reduction in the number of cigarettes smoked, or switching to so-called low tar or **nicotine** concentration cigarettes does not significantly reduce the perinatal risks. **Nicotine** patch therapy may help some pregnant smokers, but the success rate during pregnancy is low. Yet, despite the failure of large numbers of treated women to quit, the average birthweight is increased by therapy. The success rate may be enhanced by the addition of an SSRI and formal counseling. Preliminary study suggests women who cannot quit smoking after the 1st trimester metabolize **nicotine** more rapidly than those who can. Thus, the optimal response may be to raise the support level during pregnancy, not lower it. Social support systems can enhance the likelihood of long-term success in women who do quit smoking during pregnancy. The initial dose of **nicotine** during replacement therapy should approximate the dose of **nicotine** being consumed. Intermittent-use formulations of NRT (gum, spray, inhaler) are preferred as the total dose of **nicotine** delivered to the fetus is less than with continuous-use formulations (transdermal patch). *Side effects* include ventricular arrhythmia, atrial fibrillation, MI, vasculitis, dependence, local erythema, local pruritus, nausea, vomiting, diarrhea, insomnia, headache, nervousness, abnormal dreams, dizziness, and rash.

■ Fetal Considerations

Cigarette smoke contains thousands of chemicals, many of which are well-documented reproductive toxins (e.g., **nicotine**, carbon monoxide, and lead). **Nicotine** rapidly crosses the placenta and the fetuses of mothers who smoke are exposed to higher concentrations than their mothers. Smoking during pregnancy is a major risk factor for spontaneous abortion, preterm placental abruption, IUGR, late fetal death, neonatal polycythemia, and SIDS. The increased miscarriage rate among mothers who smoke may be related to direct adverse effects of **nicotine**, cadmium, or the polyaromatic hydrocarbons on trophoblast invasion and proliferation. The mean reduction in birthweight in smokers is 200g. Longitudinal studies in humans suggest that prenatal exposure to **nicotine** increases the risks for cognitive deficits, attention deficit/hyperactivity disorder, conduct disorder, criminality in adulthood, and a predisposition of the offspring to abuse tobacco and alcohol. Sheep and human studies reveal that prenatal **nicotine** blunts elements of the fetal cardiorespiratory defense for hypoxia (heart rate, ventilatory and arousal responses), and has long-term effects on the postnatal breathing pattern. The newborn unable to maximize cardiac output during times of stress is at increased risk for morbidity and possible death. Acute exposure to **nicotine** significantly decreases fetal heart reactivity. Median epinephrine and norepinephrine concentrations in the umbilical cord are significantly lower in smokers compared with nonsmokers. The significance of this finding is unclear, but could reflect depletion. Rodent studies show that **nicotine** exposure compromises neuronal maturation, leading to long-lasting structural alterations in key brain regions involved with cognition, learning, and memory.

■ **Breastfeeding Safety** .... **Nicotine** is excreted in human milk at low concentrations. Milk cotinine (a by-product of **nicotine**) levels do not correlate with the number of cigarettes smoked. Newborns breastfed by smoking women are exposed not only to environmental ("passive") smoke, but also by ingesting **nicotine** metabolites and toxin byproducts present in the milk. Nicotine replacement therapy is considered compatible with breastfeeding.

■ **References** .... Oncken CA, Henry KM, Campbell WA, et al. Pediatr Res 2003; 53:119-124.

Hafstrom O, Milerad J, Sundell HW. Am J Respir Crit Care Med 2002; 166:1544-9.

Nattie E, Kinney H. Am J Respir Crit Care Med 2002; 166:1530-1.

Schroeder DR, Ogburn PL Jr, Hurt RD, et al. J Matern Fetal Neonatal Med 2002; 11:100-7.

Hellstrom-Lindahl E, Nordberg A. Respiration 2002; 69:289-93.

Hafstrom O, Milerad J, Sundell HW. Am J Respir Crit Care Med 2002; 166:92-7.

Mitchell EA, Thompson JM, Robinson E, et al. Acta Paediatr 2002; 91:323-8.

Dempsey D, Jacob P 3rd, Benowitz NL. J Pharmacol Exp Ther 2002; 301:594-8.

Oncken C, Kranzler H, O'Malley P, et al. Obstet Gynecol 2002; 99:751-5.

Roy TS, Seidler FJ, Slotkin TA. J Pharmacol Exp Ther 2002; 300:124-33.

Koren G. Can Fam Physician 2001; 47:1971-2.

Weitzman M, Byrd RS, Aligne CA, Moss M. Neurotoxicol Teratol 2002; 24:397-406.

Narayanan U, Birru S, Vaglenova J, Breese CR. Neuroreport 2002; 13:961-3.

Klesges LM, Johnson KC, Ward KD, Barnard M. Obstet Gynecol Clin North Am 2001; 28:269-82.

Paszkowski T, Wojewoda K. Ginekol Pol 2001; 72:945-9.

Haustein KO. Int J Clin Pharmacol Ther 1999; 37:417-27.

Dempsey DA, Benowitz NL. Drug Saf 2001; 24:277-322.

al-Alawi E, Jenkins D. Ir Med J 2000; 93:175-6.

Wisborg K, Henriksen TB, Jespersen LB, et al. Obstet Gynecol 2000; 96:967-71.

Oncken CA, Pbert L, Ockene JK, et al. Obstet Gynecol 2000; 96:261-5.

Fant RV, Owen LL, Henningfield JE. Prim Care 1999; 26:633-52.

Anderson HA, Wolff MS. J Expo Anal Environ Epidemiol 2000; 10:755-60.

■ **Summary** ....
- **Pregnancy Category D**
- **Lactation Category S**
- All pregnant women should be advised to stop smoking completely during pregnancy.
- Pregnant smokers unable to stop smoking without medical treatment can be offered **nicotine** replacement therapy.

- The exposed pregnant woman subjects herself and her pregnancy to risks including IUGR and increased perinatal mortality.
- Prenatal **nicotine** exposure is associated with higher rates of behavior problems (increased activity, decreased attention) diminished intellectual abilities, and school failure.

Nifedipine (Adalat; Adalat CC; Alonix; Corinfar; Ecodipin-E; Procardia; Procardia XL)

■ **Class** *Antihypertensive, antiarrhythmic, calcium-channel blocker*

■ **Indications** Angina

■ **Mechanism** Inhibits Ca^{2+} influx into vascular smooth muscle and myocardium

■ **Dosage with Qualifiers** Hypertension—begin 10mg PO tid, titer to effect; max 180mg/d
Angina, Prinzmetal's—begin 10mg PO tid, titer to effect; max 180mg/d
Angina variant—begin 10mg PO tid, titer to effect; max 180mg/d
- **Contraindications**—hypersensitivity to drug or class
- **Caution**—CHF

■ **Maternal Considerations** *Hypertension during pregnancy*—Hypertension remains a significant cause of maternal and fetal morbidity and death. Severe hypertension during pregnancy (BP >170/110mmHg) should be treated immediately to improve both the maternal and fetal outcome. An uncontrolled reduction in BP may lead to coma, stroke, MI, acute renal failure, and death. Treatment of an acute hypertensive episode during pregnancy further complicates the process because an acute decrease in BP might adversely affect the fetus. Thus, the goal is not just to decrease BP, but to do so with minimal adverse effects while preserving organ function. **Nifedipine** is proven safe and effective. The antihypertensive effect of **nifedipine** does not correlate with the serum concentration. Given PO or SL, **nifedipine** (8-10mg ×1) has a longer duration of action and is more effective than either IV **hydralazine** (5-10mg ×1) or IV **labetolol** (20mg ×1). In randomized trials, **nifedipine** *retard* was as effective as the *rapidly acting* format, though women given the *retard* form required a 2nd dose more frequently. One approach is to observe the patient 24h to learn the proper timing of **nifedipine**. This is based on the observation hypertension is more pronounced at night in women with preeclampsia compared to chronic hypertension. Maternal cerebral blood flow is influenced by antihypertensive treatment.

A reduction in middle cerebral artery flow velocities after **nifedipine** and **methyldopa** confirms that cerebral vasospasm occurs in preeclamptic women. In contrast to the middle cerebral artery, there is no change in uteroplacental Doppler determined resistances in severe preeclamptic women treated with **nifedipine.**

Preterm labor—No tocolytic agent actually stops preterm labor or alone improves perinatal outcome. Tocolysis changes perinatal outcome by allowing time for corticosteroid administration. When compared to placebo and any other tocolytic agent, calcium-channel blockers and specifically **nifedipine** reduce the number of women giving birth within 48h or 7d of diagnosis. The doses used ranged widely from 30-240mg/d until contractions stop; 40-80mg PO q6h seem the typical starting dose. The frequency of drug discontinuation for adverse effects is also dramatically reduced for **nifedipine** compared to all other tocolytic agents. The use of **nifedipine** with **magnesium sulfate** is potentially dangerous; the combination is more frequently associated with severe hypotension, neuromuscular blockade, and cardiac depression. Similar to all other agents, maintenance therapy with oral **nifedipine** after the successful treatment of presumed preterm labor does not alter the timing of delivery. Several case reports note the occurrence of acute MI during the use of **nifedipine** for tocolysis. A short interval between cessation of betamimetic therapy and the start of **nifedipine** may have had a role.

Pulmonary hypertension—The treatment of pulmonary hypertension during pregnancy remains controversial in part because of its rarity and complexity. Some authors consider PO **nifedipine** and IV **prostacyclin**, guided by right pulmonary artery catheterization and Doppler measurements of cardiac output, effective.

Side effects include flushing, CHF, pulmonary edema, dyspnea, MI, headache, nausea, vomiting, dizziness, peripheral edema, nervousness, weakness, wheezing, nasal congestion, pruritus, and muscle cramps.

■ **Fetal Considerations**

There are no adequate reports or well-controlled studies in human fetuses. **Nifedipine** crosses the human placenta achieving an F:M ratio approximating 0.75. Newborns exposed to **nifedipine** have lower NICU admission rates, lower incidences of RDS, intracranial bleeding, and neonatal jaundice. Part of the benefit, but not all, appears to be prolongation of pregnancy. A beneficial effect of **nifedipine** on placental blood flow cannot be excluded. **Nifedipine** is teratogenic and embryotoxic in rodents, increasing the prevalence of skeletal abnormalities, cleft palate, and IUGR. Its use in subhuman primates is associated with small placentas. In the ewe, **nifedipine** is associated with a fetal acidemia despite little change in uteroplacental blood flows.

■ **Breastfeeding Safety** ⋯⋯⋯⋯ **Nifedipine** is excreted into human breast milk achieving an M:P ratio approximating 0.3. It is unlikely the nursing newborn would ingest a clinically relevant amount.

■ **References** ⋯⋯⋯⋯⋯⋯⋯⋯⋯

Brown MA, Buddle ML, Farrell T, et al. Am J Obstet Gynecol 2002; 187:1046-50.

Borghi C, Esposti DD, Cassani A, et al. J Hypertens 2002; 20 (Suppl 2):S52-6.

King JF, Flenady VJ, Papatsonis DN, et al. Cochrane Database Syst Rev 2002;CD002255.

Aali BS, Nejad SS. Acta Obstet Gynecol Scand 2002; 81:25-30.

Tsatsaris V, Carbonne B. J Gynecol Obstet Biol Reprod 2001; 30:246-51.

Tsatsaris V, Papatsonis D, Goffinet F, et al. Obstet Gynecol 2001; 97:840-7.

Khedun SM, Maharaj B, Moodley J. Paediatr Drugs 2000; 2:419-36.

Papatsonis DN, Kok JH, van Geijn HP, et al. Obstet Gynecol 2000; 95:477-81.

Haghighi L. Int J Gynaecol Obstet 1999; 66:297-8.

Oei SG, Mol BW, de Kleine MJ, Brolmann HA. Acta Obstet Gynecol Scand 1999; 78:783-8.

Scardo JA, Vermillion ST, Newman RB, et al. Am J Obstet Gynecol 1999; 181:862-6.

Easterling TR, Ralph DD, Schmucker BC. Obstet Gynecol 1999; 93:494-8.

Carr DB, Clark AL, Kernek K, Spinnato JA. Am J Obstet Gynecol 1999; 181:822-7.

Oei SG, Oei SK, Brolmann HA. N Engl J Med 1999; 340:154.

Kwawukume EY, Ghosh TS. Int J Gynaecol Obstet 1995; 49:265-9.

Magann EF, Bass JD, Chauhan SP, Perry et al. J Soc Gynecol Investig 1994; 1:210-4.

Norman JE, Ward LM, Martin W, et al. J Reprod Fertil 1997; 110:249-54.

Benedetto C, Zonca M, Giarola M, et al. Br J Obstet Gynaecol 1997; 104:682-8.

Serra-Serra V, Kyle PM, Chandran R, et al. Br J Obstet Gynaecol 1997; 104:532-7.

Kook H, Yoon YD, Baik YH. J Korean Med Sci 1996; 11:250-7.

Visser W, Wallenburg HC. J Hypertens 1995; 13:791-5.

Sullivan CA, Morrison JC. Obstet Gynecol Clin North Am 1995; 22:197-214.

Belfort MA, Saade GR, Suresh M, et al. Am J Obstet Gynecol 1995; 172:1395-403.

Kiss H, Egarter C, Asseryanis E, et al. Am J Obstet Gynecol 1995; 172:1052-4.

Blea CW, Barnard JM, Magness RR, et al. Am J Obstet Gynecol 1997; 176:922-30.

Saade GR, Taskin O, Belfort MA, et al. Obstet Gynecol 1994; 84:374-8.

Fried G, Liu YA. Acta Physiol Scand 1994; 151:477-84.

Manninen AK, Juhakoski A. Int J Clin Pharmacol Res 1991; 11:231-6.

Danielsson BR, Danielson M, Reiland S, Teratology 1990; 41:185-93 .
Yoshida T, Kanamori S, Hasegawa Y. Toxicol Lett 1988; 40:127-32.

■ **Summary**

- **Pregnancy Category C**
- **Lactation Category S?**
- **Nifedipine** is safe and effective in controlling BP in women with severe preeclampsia.
- Current evidence supports the conclusion that calcium-channel blockers, and **nifedipine** specifically, are the most effective tocolytic agents with the highest maternal/fetal safety profile.
- **Nifedipine** should be considered a first-line tocolytic agent.

Nimodipine (Nimotop)

■ **Class** — *Calcium-channel blocker*

■ **Indications** — Subarachnoid hemorrhage with vasospasm

■ **Mechanism** — Inhibits Ca^{2+} influx into vascular smooth muscle and myocardium

■ **Dosage with Qualifiers** — Subarachnoid hemorrhage—begin 60mg PO q4h within 96h of hemorrhage ×21d
NOTE—hepatic dosing
- **Contraindications**—hypersensitivity to drug or class
- **Caution**—hepatic dysfunction

■ **Maternal Considerations** — **Nimodipine** is a calcium-channel blocker with selective cerebrovascular effect.
Hypertension during pregnancy—Hypertension remains a significant cause of maternal and fetal morbidity and death. Severe hypertension during pregnancy (BP >170/110mmHg) should be treated immediately to improve both the maternal and fetal outcome. An uncontrolled reduction in BP may lead to coma, stroke, MI, acute renal failure, and death. Pregnancy further complicates the treatment of an acute hypertensive episode since an acute decrease in BP might adversely affect the fetus. Thus, the goal is not just to decrease BP, but to do so with minimal adverse effects while preserving organ function. Cerebral perfusion pressure may be either high or low in women with preeclampsia and eclampsia. **Nimodipine** is under investigation in women with severe preeclampsia. It appears an effective, easily administered antihypertensive agent with significant maternal and fetal cerebral vasodilator activity. It significantly reduces

Doppler measured resistances of the retinal vessels. Compared to **magnesium sulfate, nimodipine** increases cerebral perfusion pressure in women with severe preeclampsia. While once suggested as an agent to prevent eclampsia, it is inferior to **magnesium sulfate** as prophylaxis.

Preterm labor—No tocolytic agent actually stops preterm labor and improves perinatal outcome. Tocolysis changes perinatal outcome by allowing time for corticosteroid administration. When compared with any other tocolytic agent, calcium-channel blockers reduce the number of women giving birth within 48h or 7d of diagnosis. The frequency of drug discontinuation for adverse effects is also dramatically reduced. There are no adequate reports or well-controlled studies of **nimodipine** for tocolysis in pregnant women. It is an effective inhibitor of uterine contractions *in vitro*. Either **nifedipine** or **nicardipine** would be preferable.

Psychiatric disorders—**Nimodipine** may be an alternative to **lithium** in pregnant women with bipolar disease.

Side effects include hypotension, tachycardia, bradycardia, arrhythmia, ECG abnormalities, AV conduction abnormalities, GI bleeding, thrombocytopenia, thromboembolism, elevated LFTs, diarrhea, edema, dyspnea, headache, rash, dyspepsia, anemia, acne, muscle aches, and flushing.

■ **Fetal Considerations**

There are no adequate reports or well-controlled studies in human fetuses. **Nimodipine** crosses the human placenta reaching an F:M ratio approaching unity within several hours. Maternal administration reduces both maternal and fetal cerebral resistances. Rodent studies are somewhat conflicting. Placental transfer is inefficient. Embryotoxicity, teratogenicity, and IUGR are reported in some models, but it occurs in a non-dose-dependent fashion.

■ **Breastfeeding Safety**

There are no adequate reports or well-controlled studies in nursing women. **Nimodipine** enters human breast milk. In one case report, the M:P ratio approximated 0.1. It was estimated the breast-fed newborn would ingest a clinically insignificant amount ranging between 0.008% and 0.092% of the weight-adjusted maternal dose.

■ **References**

Belfort MA, Anthony J, Saade GR, et al. N Engl J Med 2003; 348:304-11

Yingling DR, Utter G, Vengalil S, et al. Am J Obstet Gynecol 2002; 187:1711-2.

Kaya T, Cetin A, Cetin M, Sarioglu Y. J Reprod Med 1999; 44:115-21.

Belfort MA, Saade GR, Yared M, et al. Am J Obstet Gynecol 1999; 181:402-7.

Belfort MA, Anthony J, Saade GR. Semin Perinatol 1999; 23:65-78.

Anthony J, Mantel G, Johanson R, Dommisse J. Br J Obstet Gynaecol 1996; 103:518-22.
Kaya T, Cetin A, Cetin M, Sarioglu Y. Eur J Pharmacol 1998; 346:65-9.
Tonks AM. Aust NZ J Surg 1995; 65:693-4.
Belfort MA, Saade GR, Moise KJ Jr, et al. Am J Obstet Gynecol 1994; 171:417-24.
Belfort MA, Carpenter RJ Jr, Kirshon B, et al. Am J Obstet Gynecol 1993; 169:204-6.
Suwelack D, Weber H, Maruhn D. Arzneimittelforschung 1985; 35:1787-94.
Carcas AJ, Abad-Santos F, de Rosendo JM, Frias J. Ann Pharmacother 1996; 30:148-50.

■ **Summary**

- **Pregnancy Category C**
- **Lactation Category S?**
- **Nimodipine** should be used during pregnancy and lactation only if the benefit justifies the potential perinatal risk.
- There are alternative agents for which there is more experience during pregnancy and lactation.

Nisoldipine (Sular)

■ **Class** — *Antihypertensive, calcium-channel blocker*

■ **Indications** — Hypertension

■ **Mechanism** — Inhibits Ca^{2+} influx into vascular smooth muscle and myocardium

■ **Dosage with Qualifiers** — Hypertension—20-40mg PO qd; max 60mg/d
- **Contraindications**—hypersensitivity to drug or class
- **Caution**—unknown

■ **Maternal Considerations** — Hypertension remains a significant cause of maternal and fetal morbidity and death. Severe hypertension during pregnancy (BP >170/110mmHg) should be treated immediately to improve both the maternal and fetal outcome. An uncontrolled reduction in BP may lead to coma, stroke, MI, acute renal failure, and death. Treatment of an acute hypertensive episode during pregnancy further complicates the process, because an acute decrease in BP might adversely affect the fetus. Thus, the goal is not just to decrease BP, but to do so with minimal adverse effects while preserving organ function. In one study, **nisoldipine** was used to treat preeclamptic women with severe postpartum hypertension. A rapid and significant fall in BP was seen within 30min, and maintained successfully

by repeating **nisoldipine** for the duration of the study period. There were no adverse reactions.
Side effects include vasodilatation, headache, palpitation, chest pain, CHF, 1st degree AV block, dizziness, pharyngitis, edema, rash, nausea, vomiting, increased LFTs, sinusitis, and malaise.

■ **Fetal Considerations**
There are no adequate reports or well-controlled studies in human fetuses. It is unknown whether **nisoldipine** crosses the human placenta. **Nisoldipine** was unassociated with changes in the fetal heart rate despite maternal bradycardia. Rodent studies conducted at doses that cause maternal toxicity were associated with embryotoxicity.

■ **Breastfeeding Safety**
There is no published experience in nursing women. It is unknown whether **nisoldipine** enters human breast milk.

■ **References**
Belfort MA, Kirshon B. S Afr Med J 1992; 81:267-70.

■ **Summary**
- **Pregnancy Category C**
- **Lactation Category U**
- **Nisoldipine** should be used during pregnancy and lactation only if the benefit justifies the potential perinatal risk.
- There are alternative agents for which there is more experience during pregnancy and lactation.

Nitrofurantoin (Furadantin; Furalan; Furan; Furanite; Furantoina; Furatoin; Nitrofan; Nitrofuracot)

■ **Class**
Antibiotic, nitrofuran

■ **Indications**
Urinary tract infection

■ **Mechanism**
Bactericidal at high concentrations; inhibits protein and cell wall synthesis

■ **Dosage with Qualifiers**
Urinary tract infection—100mg PO bid; alternative 50-100mg PO qid
Urinary tract infection suppression—50-100mg PO qhs
NOTE—renal dosing
- **Contraindications**—hypersensitivity to drug or class, CrCl <50ml/h
- **Caution**—asthma, anemia, G6PD deficiency

■ Maternal Considerations ········ Urinary tract infection (UTI) is common during pregnancy and all pregnant women should be screened. Treatment of asymptomatic bacteriuria and recurrent cystitis during pregnancy reduces the risk of pyelonephritis. **Ampicillin** should not be used because of the high prevalence of resistant *E. coli*. **Nitrofurantoin** is highly soluble in urine. It is safe and effective for the treatment of asymptomatic bacteriuria as well as acute and recurrent UTIs. Resistance rates are <10%. Women with recurrent UTI are candidates for long-term antibiotic prophylaxis. Neither gravidity nor pyelonephritis alters the renal excretion or blood concentration of **nitrofurantoin**. However, labor reduces renal excretion and increases the blood level. Thus, **nitrofurantoin** is a poor selection for therapy during labor. Acute pulmonary reactions to **nitrofurantoin,** presumably immune mediated, are uncommon but may be life-threatening. Symptoms include fever, chills, cough, pleuritic chest pain, dyspnea, pleural effusion, and pulmonary hemorrhage. The drug should be discontinued and corticosteroids initiated for severe reactions. Irreversible pulmonary fibrosis is also reported. Patients with G6PD *deficiency* may experience hemolytic reactions. It remains unclear how long a woman with asymptomatic bacteriuria should be treated, and there are no randomized studies. Some suggest that short-term administration combined with continued surveillance for recurrent bacteriuria is sufficient. Pyelonephritis occurs in approximately 7% of women despite adequate treatment.

Side effects include acute pulmonary hypersensitivity, hepatitis, pancreatitis, cholestatic jaundice, nausea, vomiting, flatulence, peripheral neuropathy, exfoliative dermatitis, erythema multiforme, Stevens-Johnson syndrome, lupus-like syndrome, angioedema, urticaria, rash, agranulocytosis, leukopenia, granulocytopenia, hemolytic anemia, thrombocytopenia, interstitial pneumonitis, and arthralgia.

■ Fetal Considerations ················ There are no adequate reports or well-controlled studies in human fetuses. It is unknown whether **nitrofurantoin** crosses the human placenta. There is no evidence **nitrofurantoin** is a human teratogen. Although contraindicated in labor and in infants <1mo, there are no well-documented cases of hemolytic reactions in neonates. Rodent studies are reassuring, revealing no evidence of teratogenicity or IUGR despite the use of doses higher than those used clinically.

■ Breastfeeding Safety ················ The long clinical experience is reassuring, though the literature is conflicting. One study whose subjects received 100mg concluded **nitrofurantoin** is actively transported into human milk, and that a nursing newborn could ingest 6% of the maternal dose. Another study whose subjects received 50mg found a much lower M:P ratio and concluded the likelihood of a nursing newborn ingesting a clinically relevant amount of **nitrofurantoin**

was low. Thus, concern remains for breastfeeding women treated therapeutically with **nitrofurantoin** if they have a family history of G6PD deficiency or sensitivity to **nitrofurantoin**.

■ **References**

Dwyer PL, O'Reilly M. Curr Opin Obstet Gynecol 2002; 14:537-43.

Akerele P, Abhulimen F, Okonofua J. J Obstet Gynaecol 2001; 21:141-4.

Christensen B. J Antimicrob Chemother 2000; 46(Suppl 1):29-34.

Delzell JE Jr, Lefevre ML. Am Fam Physician 2000; 61:713-21.

Boggess KA, Benedetti TJ, Raghu G. Obstet Gynecol Surv 1996; 51:367-70.

Ben David S, Einarson T, Ben David Y, et al. Fundam Clin Pharmacol 1995; 9:503-7.

Philpot J, Muntoni F, Skellett S, Dubowitz V. Neuromuscul Disord 1995; 5:67-9.

Bint AJ, Hill D. J Antimicrob Chemother 1994; 33(Suppl A):93-7.

Pons G, Rey E, Richard MO, et al. Dev Pharmacol Ther 1990; 14:148-52.

Nicolle LE. Am J Med 2002; 113(Suppl 1A):35S-44S.

Gait JE. DICP 1990; 24:1210-3.

Cunha BA. Obstet Gynecol Surv 1989; 44:399-406.

Van Dorsten JP, Lenke RR, Schifrin BS. J Reprod Med 1987; 32:895-900.

Gilstrap LG 3rd, Hankins GD, Snyder RR, Greenberg RT. Compr Ther 1986; 12:38-42.

Stamm WE. Am J Med 1984; 76:148-54.

Czeizel AE, Rockenbauer M, Sorensen HT, Olsen J. Eur J Obstet Gynecol Reprod Biol 2001; 95:119-26.

Prytherch JP, Sutton ML, Denine EP. J Toxicol Environ Health 1984; 13:811-23.

Lenke RR, VanDorsten JP, Schifrin BS. Am J Obstet Gynecol 1983; 146:953-7.

Hailey FJ, Fort H, Williams JC, Hammers B. J Int Med Res. 1983; 11:364-9.

Noschel H, Schroder S, Eichhorn KH, Peiker G. Pharmazie 1982; 37:204-5.

Whalley PJ, Cunningham FG. Obstet Gynecol 1977; 49:262-5.

Gerk PM, Kuhn RJ, Desai NS, McNamara PJ. Pharmacotherapy 2001; 21:669-75.

Pons G, Rey E, Richard MO, et al. Dev Pharmacol Ther 1990; 14:148-52.

■ **Summary**

- **Pregnancy Category B**
- **Lactation Category S?**
- **Nitrofurantoin** a first-line agent for both the treatment of urinary tract infection and outpatient prophylaxis.

Nitroglycerin (Deponit; Glyceryl; Mi-Trates; Minitran; Natirose; Nitrek; Nitro; Nitro-Bid; Nitrocap T.D.; Nitrocine; Nitrocot; Nitro-Dur; Nitro-Par; Nitro-Time; Nitrodisc; Nitrogard; Nitroglyn; Nitrol; Nitrolin; Nitrolingual; Nitronal; Nitrong; Nitrorex; Nitrospan; Nitrostat; NTS; NTG; Transderm-Nitro; Transiderm; Tridil)

■ **Class** ⋯⋯⋯⋯⋯⋯⋯⋯⋯⋯⋯⋯⋯⋯⋯ *Vasodilator*

■ **Indications** ⋯⋯⋯⋯⋯⋯⋯⋯⋯⋯⋯⋯ Angina

■ **Mechanism** ⋯⋯⋯⋯⋯⋯⋯⋯⋯⋯⋯⋯ NO donor relaxing vascular smooth muscle via cGMP

■ **Dosage with Qualifiers** ⋯⋯⋯⋯ Angina, acute—0.3-0.6mg SL q5min; max 3 doses within 15min
Angina, prophylaxis—0.3-0.6mg SL ×1; take 5-10min before strenuous activity
NOTE—available in 2% cream, tablets, aerosol spray, parenteral or patch formats; store tablets in original glass container
- **Contraindications**—hypersensitivity to drug or class, anemia, methemoglobinemia, increase intracranial pressure, head trauma, cerebral hemorrhage, recent **sildenafil**
- **Caution**—hypotension, hypovolemia, chronic heart failure, acute MI

■ **Maternal Considerations** ⋯⋯⋯ *Hypertension during pregnancy*—Hypertension remains a significant cause of maternal and fetal morbidity and death. Severe hypertension during pregnancy (BP >170/110mmHg) should be treated immediately to improve both the maternal and fetal outcome. An uncontrolled reduction in BP may lead to coma, stroke, MI, acute renal failure, and death. Treatment of a hypertensive episode during pregnancy further complicates the process because an acute decrease in BP might adversely affect the fetus. Thus, the goal is not just to decrease BP, but to do so with minimal adverse effects while preserving organ function. It is suggested nitric oxide donors may have a therapeutic role in preeclampsia. Doppler studies are conflicting. Some investigators report vascular smooth muscle sensitivity to **nitroglycerin** is unaltered by preeclampsia, while others observe that **nitroglycerin** produces a more profound decrease in the BP of preeclamptic women compared to normal subjects. **Nitroglycerin** also causes a fall in the resistance indices of the uterine arteries whether administered acutely or chronically. It is unknown whether the decline in resistance is associated with an increase in perfusion. Low-dose prophylactic **nitroglycerin** beginning in the 2nd trimester does not reduce the incidence of preeclampsia or IUGR.
Cervical ripening and tocolysis—The nitric oxide-cGMP relaxation pathway is present in the human cervix and uterus.

High doses of sublingual or IV **nitroglycerin** have been used acutely as a uterine relaxant to assist fetal surgery, fetal extraction at cesarean section, external version, internal intrapartum podalic version of the 2nd twin, manual exploration of the uterus to remove a retained placenta, and replacement of an inverted uterus. Yet placebo controlled trials demonstrate **nitroglycerin** is no better than placebo for the facilitation of fetal extraction at cesarean section, or for external version. IV **nitroglycerin** currently continues to be used intra- and postoperatively to facilitate uterine relaxation during or after open uterine fetal surgery. Pulmonary edema is the most common complication. The short half-life (2.5min) of **nitroglycerin** makes long-term therapy difficult, and tolerance is associated with longer-acting donors. It has also been postulated that nitric oxide may have a physiologic role in uterine quiescence and cervical ripening. While **nitroglycerin** reduces the force necessary to dilate the cervix for a 1st trimester termination, it is less effective than prostaglandins for cervical ripening. **Nitroglycerin** has also proved a poor tocolytic. It does not inhibit uterine contractility in sheep. And in laboring women, 800mcg/dose reduces BP but has no effect on either uterine tone or contractility. Controversy continues regarding the ability of **nitroglycerin** to prevent preterm labor. **Nitroglycerin** is more effective than placebo but similar to a β-**agonist** or **magnesium sulfate** as a tocolytic agent. Its purported ability to delay labor was gestational age dependent.

Side effects include hypotension, methemoglobinemia, anaphylactic reactions, bradycardia, headache, tolerance/dependence, lightheadedness, burning oral sensation, tingling oral sensation, reflex tachycardia, postural hypotension, dizziness, flushing, and edema.

■ **Fetal Considerations**

There are no adequate reports or well-controlled studies in human fetuses. When given to women with mild preeclampsia, **nitroglycerin** is associated with a decrease in the resistance in fetoplacental circulation approximately 20-30min after administration. Low levels of **nitroglycerin** are found in the fetus after its use to facilitate an acute obstetric procedure. Sheep studies reveal no adverse fetal effects after maternal administration. There is no effect on fetal carotid blood flow. Rodent teratogenicity studies are reassuring, but limited by dose and format.

■ **Breastfeeding Safety**

There is no published experience in nursing women. It is unknown whether **nitroglycerin** enters human breast milk. However, considering the indication, dosing, and clearance rate, limited **nitroglycerin** use is unlikely to pose a clinically significant risk to the breast-feeding neonate.

■ References

Rosen MA, Andreae MH, Cameron AG. Anesth Analg 2003; 96:698-700.

Leszczynska-Gorzelak B, Laskowska M, et al. Ginekol Pol 2002; 73:666-71.

Buhimschi CS, Buhimschi IA, Malinow AM, Weiner CP. Am J Obstet Gynecol 2002; 187:235-8.

Choi JW, Im MW, Pai SH. Ann Clin Lab Sci 2002; 32:257-63.

Caponas G. Anaesth Intensive Care 2001; 29:163-77.

Schleussner E, Richter S, Gross W, et al. Z Geburtshilfe Neonatol 2001; 205:189-94.

David M, Nierhaus M, Schauss B, Vetter K. Z Geburtshilfe Neonatol 2001; 205:137-42.

Buhimschi I, Yallampalli C, Dong YL, Garfield RE. Am J Obstet Gynecol 1995; 172:1577-84.

Wetzka B, Schafer WR, Stehmans A, et al. Gynecol Endocrinol 2001; 15:34-42.

Lau LC, Adaikan PG, Arulkumaran S, Ng SC. BJOG 2001; 108:164-8.

Yanny H, Johanson R, Balwin KJ, et al. BJOG 2000; 107:562-4.

O'Grady JP, Parker RK, Patel SS. J Perinatol 2000; 20:27-33.

David M, Walka MM, Schmid B, et al. Am J Obstet Gynecol 2000; 182:955-61.

Mirabile CP Jr, Massmann GA, Figueroa JP. Am J Obstet Gynecol 2000; 183:191-8.

Ekerhovd E, Brannstrom M, Weijdegard B, Norstrom A. Am J Obstet Gynecol 2000; 183:610-6.

Chanrachakul B, Herabutya Y, Punyavachira P. Obstet Gynecol 2000; 96:549-53.

Luzi G, Caserta G, Iammarino G, Ultrasound Obstet Gynecol 1999; 14:101-9.

Smith GN, Walker MC, McGrath MJ. Br J Obstet Gynaecol 1999; 106:736-9.

Skarsgard ED, VanderWall KJ, Morris JA, et al. Am J Obstet Gynecol 1999; 181:440-5.

Lees CC, Lojacono A, Thompson C, et al. Obstet Gynecol 1999; 94:403-8.

Black RS, Lees C, Thompson C, et al. Obstet Gynecol 1999; 94:572-6.

El-Sayed YY, Riley ET, Holbrook RH Jr, et al. Obstet Gynecol 1999; 93:79-83.

Anumba DO, Ford GA, Boys RJ, Robson SC. Am J Obstet Gynecol 1999; 181:1479-84.

Smith GN, Brien JF. Obstet Gynecol Surv 1998; 53:559-65.

DiFederico EM, Burlingame JM, Kilpatrick SJ, et al. Am J Obstet Gynecol 1998; 179:925-33.

Kirsten R, Nelson K, Kirsten D, Heintz B. Clin Pharmacokinet 1998; 35:9-36.

Cacciatore B, Halmesmaki E, Kaaja R, et al. Am J Obstet Gynecol 1998; 179:140-5.

Lees C, Valensise H, Black R, et al. Ultrasound Obstet Gynecol 1998; 12:334-8.

Dufour P, Vinatier D, Puech F. Arch Gynecol Obstet 1997; 261:1-7.

Weiner CP, Thompson LP. Semin Perinatol 1997; 21:367-80.

Rowlands S, Trudinger B, Visva-Lingam S. Aust NZ J Obstet Gynaecol 1996; 36:377-81.

Vinatier D, Dufour P, Berard J. Int J Gynaecol Obstet 1996; 55:129-34.

Houlihan C, Knuppel RA. Clin Perinatol 1996; 23:91-116.

DiFederico EM, Harrison M, Matthay MA. Chest 1996; 109:1114-7.

Buhimschi I, Ali M, Jain V, Hum Reprod 1996; 11:1755-66.

Dufour P, Vinatier D, Bennani S, et al. J Gynecol Obstet Biol Reprod 1996; 25:617-22.

Wessen A, Elowsson P, Axemo P, Acta Anaesthesiol Scand 1995; 39:847-9.

Lees C, Campbell S, Jauniaux E, et al. Lancet 1994; 343:1325-6.

Ramsay B, De Belder A, Campbell S, et al. Eur J Clin Invest 1994; 24:76-8.

Weiner CP, Knowles RG, Nelson SE, Stegink LD. Endocrinology 1994; 135:2473-8.

Belfort MA. S Afr Med J 1993; 83:656.

Yallampalli C, Garfield RE. Am J Obstet Gynecol 1993; 169:1316-20.

■ **Summary**

- **Pregnancy Category C**
- **Lactation Category U**
- **Nitroglycerin** should be used during pregnancy and lactation only if the benefit justifies the potential perinatal risk.
- In emergent situations, IV **nitroglycerin** may provide short-term uterine relaxation.
- There are superior options for cervical ripening.
- **Nitroglycerin** is a poor agent for tocolysis and does not provide effective prophylaxis for either preterm labor or preeclampsia.

Nitroprusside (Nipride; Nitropress)

■ **Class** — *Vasodilator*

■ **Indications** — Hypertension, heart failure

■ **Mechanism** — NO donor relaxing vascular smooth muscle via cGMP

■ **Dosage with Qualifiers** — Hypertension—begin 0.25-0.3mcg/kg/min IV; max 10 mcg/kg/min
Heart failure—0.3-10mcg/kg/min IV; max 10mcg/kg/min
NOTE—check serum thiocyanate levels with prolonged usage
- **Contraindications**—hypersensitivity to drug or class, poor cerebral or coronary perfusion, optic atrophy, tobacco-induced amblyopia
- **Caution**—increased ICP

■ **Maternal Considerations** .... The metabolism of **nitroprusside** is important to remember. One molecule of **nitroprusside** combines with hemoglobin to produce one molecule of cyanmethemoglobin and four CN⁻ ions. Thiosulfate reacts with cyanide to produce thiocyanate. Thiocyanate is eliminated in the urine. Cyanide not otherwise removed binds to cytochromes. Cyanide is much more toxic than methemoglobin or thiocyanate.

Hypertension during pregnancy—Hypertension remains a significant cause of maternal and fetal morbidity and death. Severe hypertension during pregnancy (BP >170/110mmHg) should be treated immediately to improve both the maternal and fetal outcome. An uncontrolled reduction in BP may lead to coma, stroke, MI, acute renal failure, and death. Treatment of an acute hypertensive episode during pregnancy further complicates the process because an acute decrease in BP might adversely affect the fetus. Thus, the goal is not just to decrease BP, but to do so with minimal adverse effects while preserving organ function. It has been suggested nitric oxide donors could have a therapeutic role in preeclampsia. IV **nitroprusside** is an excellent hypotensive agent with the added advantage of a titratable effect. **Nitroprusside** exerts its relaxant effect by an endothelium-independent mechanism. Pharmacologic studies reveal that *in vitro* vasorelaxation to **nitroprusside** is attenuated in vessels obtained from preeclamptic women. On the other hand, many severe preeclampsia patients are relatively or absolutely hypovolemic. In these patients, systemic BP may be extremely sensitive to small doses. Therefore, some clinicians begin therapy at lower rates of infusion (e.g., 0.5-0.1mcg/m).

Cervical ripening—The nitric oxide-cGMP relaxation pathway is present in the human and cervix uterus. **Nitroprusside** decreases collagen cross-links in the guinea pig cervix. It reduces the force necessary to dilate the cervix for a 1st trimester termination.

Side effects include increased ICP, dizziness, nausea, vomiting, cyanide or thiocyanate toxicity, bradycardia, reflex tachycardia, ileus, diaphoresis, abdominal pain, headache, muscle twitching, acidosis, and flushing.

■ **Fetal Considerations** .... There are no adequate reports or well-controlled studies in human fetuses. It is unknown whether **nitroprusside** crosses the human placenta. **Nitroprusside** dilates the fetal vascular bed of the isolated perfused placenta, and that its efficacy is unaffected by preeclampsia or IUGR. Fetal cyanide toxicity occurs in sheep after maternal administration. It is reversed by maternal administration of **sodium thiosulfate**, which unfortunately does not cross the human placenta. Rodent teratogenicity studies have not been performed.

■ **Breastfeeding Safety** ⸱⸱⸱⸱⸱⸱⸱⸱⸱⸱⸱ There is no published experience in nursing women. It is unknown whether **nitroprusside** enters human breast milk. However, considering the indication, dosing, and clearance rate, limited **nitroprusside** use is unlikely to pose a clinically significant risk to the breast-feeding neonate.

■ **References** ⸱⸱⸱⸱⸱⸱⸱⸱⸱⸱⸱⸱⸱⸱⸱⸱

Ong SS, Crocker IP, Warren AY, Baker PN. Hypertens Pregnancy 2002; 21:175-83.
Keeble JE, Poyser NL. Reproduction 2002; 124:317-22.
Boujedaini N, Liu J, Thuillez C, et al. Eur J Pharmacol 2001; 427:143-9.
Xiao D, Pearce WJ, Zhang L. Am J Physiol Heart Circ Physiol 2001; 281:H183-90.
Longo M, Jain V, Vedernikov YP, et al. Am J Obstet Gynecol 2001; 184:971-8.
Wetzka B, Schafer WR, Stehmans A, et al. Gynecol Endocrinol 2001; 15:34-42.
Zhang XQ, Kwek K, Read MA. Placenta 2001; 22:337-46.
Fittkow CT, Shi SQ, Bytautiene E, et al. J Perinat Med 2001; 29:535-43.
Facchinetti F, Piccinini F, Volpe A. Hum Reprod 2000; 15:2224-7.
Shi L, Shi SQ, Saade GR, et al. Mol Hum Reprod 2000; 6:382-9.
Thompson LP, Aguan K, Pinkas G, Weiner CP. Am J Physiol Regul Integr Comp Physiol 2000; 279:R1813-20.
Thompson LP, Weiner CP. Am J Obstet Gynecol 1999; 181:105-11.
Graeme KA, Curry SC, Bikin DS, et al. Anesth Analg 1999; 89:1448-52.
Ekerhovd E, Weidegard B, Brannstrom M, Norstrom A. Obstet Gynecol 1999; 93:987-94.
Chwalisz K, Shao-Qing S, Garfield RE, Beier HM. Hum Reprod 1997; 12:2093-101.
Curry SC, Carlton MW, Raschke RA. Anesth Analg 1997; 84:1121-6.
Gregg AR, Thompson LP, Herrig JE, Weiner CP. J Vasc Res 1995; 32:106-11.
Thompson LP, Weiner CP. Pediatr Res 1996; 40:192-7.
Prisant LM, Carr AA, Hawkins DW. Postgrad Med 1993; 93:92-6, 101-4, 108-10.
Silver HM. Med Clin North Am 1989; 73:623-38.
Shoemaker CT, Meyers M. Am J Obstet Gynecol 1984; 149:171-3.
Read MA, Giles WB, Leitch IM, et al. Reprod Fertil Dev 1995; 7:1557-61.

■ **Summary** ⸱⸱⸱⸱⸱⸱⸱⸱⸱⸱⸱⸱⸱⸱⸱⸱⸱⸱⸱

- **Pregnancy Category C**
- **Lactation Category U**
- **Nitroprusside** should be used during pregnancy and lactation only if the benefit justifies the potential perinatal risk.
- The prudent use of **nitroprusside** is excellent for the rapid treatment of a hypertensive crisis during pregnancy.
- There are superior options for cervical ripening.

Nizatidine (Axid)

■ Class — *Gastrointestinal, antihistamine*

■ Indications — GERD, duodenal ulcer

■ Mechanism — Competitive, reversible peripheral H_2 receptor antagonist

■ Dosage with Qualifiers — GERD—150mg PO bid
Duodenal ulcer, maintenance—150mg PO qhs
Duodenal ulcer, active—300mg PO qhs
NOTE—renal dosing
- **Contraindications**—hypersensitivity to drug or class
- **Caution**—renal dysfunction

■ Maternal Considerations — Gastroesophageal reflux and heartburn are reported by 45-85% of women during pregnancy. There are no adequate reports or well-controlled studies of **nizatidine** in pregnant women. **Nizatidine** should be reserved for patients with severe symptoms.
Side effects include hepatitis, thrombocytopenic purpura, exfoliative dermatitis, rhinitis, headache, nausea, vomiting, anorexia, dyspepsia, abdominal pain, constipation, agitation, increased LFTs, pharyngitis, agitation, confusion, somnolence, insomnia, sinusitis, dry mouth, leukopenia, and anemia.

■ Fetal Considerations — There are no adequate reports or well-controlled studies in human fetuses. It is unknown whether **nizatidine** crosses the human placenta *in vivo*. It freely crosses the isolated perfused cotyledon. Rodent studies are reassuring, revealing no evidence of teratogenicity or IUGR despite the use of doses higher than those used clinically.

■ Breastfeeding Safety — There are no adequate reports or well-controlled studies in nursing women. **Nizatidine** is excreted into human breast milk. On average, less than 0.1% of the maternal dose is secreted during a 12h interval after either single or multiple doses. This is less than either **cimetidine** or **ranitidine**. Thus, it is unlikely the breast-feeding newborn would ingest a clinically relevant quantity. The relevance of the observation that pups reared by **nizatidine** treated lactating rats had poor growth is unclear.

■ References — Broussard CN, Richter JE. Drug Saf 1998; 19:325-37.
Hagemann TM. J Hum Lact 1998; 14:259-62.
Obermeyer BD, Bergstrom RF, Callaghan JT, et al. Clin Pharmacol Ther 1990; 47:724-30.
Dicke JM, Johnson RF, Henderson GI, et al. Am J Med Sci 1988; 295:198-206.

- **Pregnancy Category B**
- **Lactation Category S?**
- **Nizatidine** should be used during pregnancy and lactation only if the benefit justifies the potential perinatal risk.

Norethindrone (Dianor; Micronor; Nor-QD; Norethisterone; Norlutin; Primulut)

■ **Class** — *Hormone, contraceptive*

■ **Indications** — Contraception, dysmenorrhea, dysfunctional uterine bleeding, endometriosis, polycystic ovarian syndrome

■ **Mechanism** — Inhibits pituitary gonadotropin release, transforms proliferative to secretory endometrium, thickens cervical mucus

■ **Dosage with Qualifiers** — Contraception—1 tab PO qd; take at same time every day
Dysmenorrhea—1 tab PO qd
Dysfunctional uterine bleeding—1 tab PO qd
Endometriosis—1 tab PO qd
Polycystic ovarian syndrome—1 tab PO qd
NOTE—available in combination with **ethinyl estradiol** (35mcg/1mg or 50mcg/1mg)
- **Contraindications**—hypersensitivity to drug or class, pregnancy, breast or hepatic cancer, CAD, abnormal vaginal bleeding, acute hepatic disease
- **Caution**—smoking

■ **Maternal Considerations** — **Norethindrone** is the progestogen in several popular oral contraceptives. The use of oral contraceptives containing **norethindrone** is causally related to an increased incidence of breakthrough bleeding. A slight increase in the incidence of ectopic pregnancy may occur with progesterone-only contraceptives. There is no indication for **norethindrone** during pregnancy and lactation.
Side effects include irregular vaginal bleeding, altered menstrual bleeding, amenorrhea, acne, hirsuitism, weight gain, headache, breast tenderness, nausea, thromboembolism, MI, hypertension, vomiting, hepatic adenoma, nausea, edema, melasma, rash, and dizziness.

■ **Fetal Considerations** — There are no adequate reports or well-controlled studies in human fetuses. **Norethindrone** likely crosses the human placenta since there are scattered cases of masculinized female fetuses reported. Most consist of clitoral hypertrophy not requiring surgical treatment. First trimester exposure is an indication for a detailed anatomic ultrasound between 18-22w. **Norethindrone** is not teratogenic in rodents.

■ **Breastfeeding Safety** ················· Small amounts of **norethindrone** pass into the breast milk, resulting in steroid levels of 1-6% that of maternal plasma in the infant. Long-term follow-up studies reveal that progestogen-only contraceptives popular during lactation do not adversely affect breastfeeding and infant development.

■ **References** ·············· van Vliet HA, Grimes DA, Helmerhorst FM, et al. Contraception 2002; 65:321-4.
Van Vliet H, Grimes D, Helmerhorst F. Cochrane Database Syst Rev 2001:CD003283.
WHO, Task Force for Epidemiological Research on Reproductive Health; Special Programme of Research, Development, and Research Training in Human Reproduction. Contraception 1994; 50:55-68.
Beischer NA, Cookson T, Sheedy M, et al. Aust NZ J Obstet Gynaecol 1992; 32:233-8.
Shaaban MM. J Steroid Biochem Mol Biol 1991; 40:705-10.
Cooke ID, Back DJ, Shroff NE. Contraception 1985; 31:611-21.
Maier WE, Herman JR. Regul Toxicol Pharmacol 2001; 34:53-61.

■ **Summary** ····························· • **Pregnancy Category X**
• **Lactation Category S**
• **Norethindrone** is an effective contraceptive when used as directed.
• There are no indications for its use during pregnancy.

Norfloxacin (Chibroxin; Floxenor; Norofin; Noroxin; Norxacin; Oroflox)

■ **Class** ················· *Antibiotic, quinolone*

■ **Indications** ··················· Bacterial infections (aerobic gram-positive: *Enterococcus faecalis, Staphylococcus aureus* [methicillin-susceptible], *S. saprophyticus, Streptococcus pneumoniae, S. pyogenes*; aerobic gram-negative: *Enterobacter cloacae, Escherichia coli, Haemophilus influenzae, H. parainfluenzae, Klebsiella pneumoniae, Legionella pneumophila, Moraxella catarrhalis, Proteus mirabilis, Pseudomonas aeruginosa*; other microorganisms: *Chlamydia pneumoniae, Mycoplasma pneumoniae*), gonorrhea, gastroenteritis, traveler's diarrhea)

■ **Mechanism** ··················· Bactericidal; inhibits DNA synthesis

- **Dosage with Qualifiers** ········ Bacterial infections—400mg PO bid
Gonorrhea—800mg PO ×1; consult most recent CDC STD guidelines
Gastroenteritis—400mg PO bid ×5d
Traveler's diarrhea—400mg PO bid ×3d
NOTE—renal dosing
  - **Contraindications**—hypersensitivity to drug or class
  - **Caution**—renal, hepatic or pulmonary dysfunction, cardiovascular disease, CNS disorder, seizure disorder, diabetes mellitus, G6PD deficiency, myasthenia gravis

- **Maternal Considerations** ······· There are no adequate reports or well-controlled studies of **norfloxacin** in pregnant women. See **ciprofloxacin**. *Side effects* include photosensitivity, pseudomembranous colitis, vaginitis, seizures, increased, ICP, headache, psychosis, nausea, vomiting, diarrhea, abdominal pain, dyspepsia, dizziness, insomnia, agitation, tendonitis, arthralgia, tendon rupture, restlessness, and elevated LFTs.

- **Fetal Considerations** ·············· There are no adequate reports or well-controlled studies in human fetuses. It is unknown whether **norfloxacin** crosses the human placenta. The limited human experience is reassuring, as 1st trimester use does not appear to be associated with an increased risk of malformations or musculoskeletal problems. Animal studies (rodent, monkey) are reassuring, revealing no evidence of teratogenicity or IUGR despite the use of doses 6-50 times higher than those used clinically.

- **Breastfeeding Safety** ············ There is no published experience in nursing women. It is unknown whether **norfloxacin** enters human breast milk.

- **References** ·············· Loebstein R, Addis A, Ho E, et al. Antimicrob Agents Chemother 1998; 42:1336-9.
Berkovitch M, Pastuszak A, Gazarian M, et al. Obstet Gynecol 1994; 84:535-8.
Mani VR, Vidya KC. J Indian Med Assoc 1997; 95:416-7, 421.
Gips M, Soback S. J Vet Pharmacol Ther 1999; 22:202-8.

- **Summary** ··············
  - **Pregnancy Category C**
  - **Lactation Category U**
  - **Norfloxacin** should be used during pregnancy and lactation only if the benefit justifies the potential perinatal risk.
  - There are alternative agents for which there is more experience during pregnancy and lactation.

Norgestrel (Ovrette; Norplant)

■ **Class** .... *Hormone, contraceptive*

■ **Indications** .... Contraception, dysmenorrhea, dysfunctional uterine bleeding, endometriosis, polycystic ovarian syndrome

■ **Mechanism** .... Inhibition of the pituitary gonadotropin release, stimulates transformation of the proliferative endometrium into secretory, alters cervical mucus

■ **Dosage with Qualifiers** .... Contraception—1 tab PO qd; take at same time every day
Dysmenorrhea—1 tab PO qd
Dysfunctional uterine bleeding—1 tab PO qd
Endometriosis—1 tab PO qd
Polycystic ovarian syndrome—1 tab PO qd
NOTE—each tab contains 0.75mg; also combined with a variety of estrogens for combination oral contraceptives
● **Contraindications**—hypersensitivity to drug or class, pregnancy, breast CA, hepatic CA, CAD, abnormal vaginal bleeding, acute hepatic disease
● **Caution**—smoking

■ **Maternal Considerations** .... **Norgestrel** is a synthetic progestogen that alone or in combination with estrogen is used in several popular oral, slow release, and local (IUD) forms of contraception. It is pharmacologically similar to **levonorgestrel**. Progestin-only emergency contraception (1 tab PO q12h ×2) is available as a prepackaged product. The **levonorgestrel**-only regimen prevents 85% of unintended pregnancies compared with 57% for the Yuzpe regimen (2 tablets each with 50mcg **ethinyl estradiol** and 0.25mg **levonorgestrel**, repeated 12h later). **Levonorgestrel** implants are contraindicated in women with a history of seizures. There is no indication for **norgestrel** during pregnancy. *Side effects* include irregular vaginal bleeding, acne, hirsuitism, weight gain, headache, breast tenderness, nausea, thromboembolism, MI, hypertension, hepatic adenoma, vomiting, edema, breakthrough bleeding, altered menstrual bleeding, amenorrhea, melasma, rash, and dizziness.

■ **Fetal Considerations** .... There are no adequate reports or well-controlled studies in human fetuses. *In utero* exposure of male fetuses to progestational agents may double the risk of hypospadias. While there are insufficient data to quantify the risk for the female fetus, some progestational agents may cause mild virilization of the external genitalia. Defects outside the external genitalia are not reported in either humans or rodents. First trimester exposure is an indication for a detailed anatomic ultrasound between 18-22w.

■ **Breastfeeding Safety** .... **Norgestrel** is excreted into maternal milk. Maintaining a time interval between mini-pill intake and breastfeeding results in higher levels in breast milk, thus exposing the newborn to a bolus of drug in a "single-delayed" feed. Long-term follow-up studies reveal that progestogen-only contraceptives popular during lactation do not adversely affect breastfeeding and infant development.

■ **References** .... Dolan LM, Mulholland M, Price J. J Fam Plann Reprod Health Care 2001; 27:19-21.
Schwartz JL. Curr Womens Health Rep 2001; 1:191-5.
Toddywalla VS, Patel SB, Betrabet SS, et al. Contraception 1995; 51:193-5.

■ **Summary** ....
- **Pregnancy Category X**
- **Lactation Category S**
- **Norgestrel** is an effective contraceptive when used as directed.
- There are no indications for its use during pregnancy.

Nortriptyline (Allergron; Lisunim; Pamelor)

■ **Class** .... *Antidepressant, tricyclic*

■ **Indications** .... Depression

■ **Mechanism** .... Unknown (inhibits norepinephrine and serotonin reuptake)

■ **Dosage with Qualifiers** .... Depression—begin 25-50mg PO qhs or tid/qid, increase q2-3w until desired effect; max 150mg/d
- **Contraindications**—hypersensitivity to drug or class, recovery from acute MI, MAO inhibitors <14d
- **Caution**—hepatic dysfunction, CAD, suicide risk, thyroid disease, glaucoma, seizure history

■ **Maternal Considerations** .... Depression is common during and after pregnancy, but typically goes unrecognized. Pregnancy is not a reason *a priori* to discontinue psychotropic drugs. There are no adequate and well-controlled studies of **nortriptyline** in pregnant women. Women who experienced one episode of postpartum-onset major depression are at high risk for subsequent recurrence. Unfortunately, **nortriptyline** is no different than placebo as prophylaxis for the prevention of recurrent postpartum depression in a high-risk population. Cigarette smoking during pregnancy is the single largest modifiable risk for pregnancy-related morbidity and death in the U.S. Although **nicotine** replacement therapy (gum, patch, nasal spray, and inhaler) combined with **bupropion** has the highest rate of success, **nortriptyline** also has a positive impact on smoking cessation rates. **Nortriptyline** is used for the treatment of neuropathic pain, chronic pain, and panic disorder. Its use for these indications may be avoidable during pregnancy.

Side effects include seizures, MI, stroke, thrombocytopenia, agranulocytosis, confusion, disorientation, constipation, tachycardia, dizziness, increased appetite, blurred vision, drowsiness, and dry mouth.

■ **Fetal Considerations**

There are no adequate reports or well-controlled studies in human fetuses. Only about 6% of the **nortriptyline** dose crosses the isolated perfused human placenta. Fetal exposure may be limited because of its lipophilicity.

A case report suggested an association between **nortriptyline** and limb anomalies. There is no other support for this possibility. Rodent teratogenicity studies have yielded conflicting results.

■ **Breastfeeding Safety**

Nortriptyline is excreted at low concentration into human breast milk, and it is estimated the newborn would ingest only 2.5% of the corresponding maternal weight corrected dose. Further, **nortriptyline** levels are typically at or below the level of detection in the nursing newborn.

Nortriptyline is generally considered a drug of choice for breast-feeding women suffering from depression.

■ **References**

Kotlyar M, Hatsukami DK. J Dent Educ 2002; 66:1061-73.
Wisner KL, Perel JM, Peindl KS, et al. J Clin Psychiatry 2001; 62:82-6.
Heikkinen T, Ekblad U, Laine K. Psychopharmacology 2001; 153:450-4.
Wisner KL, Perel JM, Findling RL, et al. Psychopharmacol Bull 1997; 33:249-51.
Wisner KL, Perel JM. Am J Psychiatry 1996; 153:1132-7.
Matheson I, Skjaeraasen J. Eur J Clin Pharmacol 1988; 35:217-20.
Bourke GM. Lancet 1974; 1:98.
McBride WG. Med J Aust 1972; 1:492.

■ **Summary**

- **Pregnancy Category D**
- **Lactation Category S**
- Serotonin reuptake inhibitors are first-line agents for the treatment of most depressive and anxiety disorders.
- **Nortriptyline** should be used during pregnancy and lactation only if the benefit justifies the potential perinatal risk.
- **Nortriptyline** is generally considered a drug of choice for breast-feeding women suffering from depression.

Novobiocin (Albamycin)

■ **Class** — Anti-infective, urinary

■ **Indications** — Bacterial infections (<u>aerobic gram-positive</u>: *Staphylococcus aureus*; <u>aerobic gram-negative</u>: *Proteus mirabilis*)

■ **Mechanism** — Unknown

■ **Dosage with Qualifiers** — <u>Bacterial infections</u>—250mg PO tid; max1g q12h
NOTE—**novobiocin** should be used only after other antibiotics with lower toxicity have failed
  • **Contraindications**—hypersensitivity to drug or class
  • **Caution**—unknown

■ **Maternal Considerations** — There are no adequate reports or well-controlled studies of **novobiocin** in pregnant women. **Novobiocin** should be used only after other antibiotics with lower toxicity have failed.
Side effects include urticaria, erythematous maculopapular rash, scarlatiniform rash, Stevens-Johnson syndrome, leukopenia, eosinophilia, hemolytic anemia, pancytopenia, agranulocytosis, thrombocytopenia, jaundice, increased LFTs, nausea, vomiting and diarrhea.

■ **Fetal Considerations** — There are no adequate reports or well-controlled studies in human fetuses. It is unknown whether **novobiocin** crosses the human placenta. Rodent teratogenicity studies have not been performed.

■ **Breastfeeding Safety** — There is no published experience in nursing women. It is unknown whether **novobiocin** enters human breast milk. Studies in animals (cows, mice) report **novobiocin** is excreted into breast milk and can be used to treat bovine mastitis.

■ **References** — There are no current relevant references.

■ **Summary** —
  • **Pregnancy Category C**
  • **Lactation Category U**
  • **Novobiocin** should be used during pregnancy and lactation only if the benefit justifies the potential perinatal risk.

Nystatin (Barstatin; Bio-Statin; Candex; Candio-Hermal; Korostatin; Mycostatin; Mykinac; Nilstat; Nysert; Nystex; Nystop; O-V Statin; Pedi-Dry; Statin; Vagistat)

■ **Class** — Antifungal, *dermatologic*

■ **Indications** — Yeast infections (Candida species: Candida *albicans*)

■ **Mechanism** — Inhibits biosynthesis of **ergosterol**, and thus the fungal cell wall

■ **Dosage with Qualifiers** — Candidiasis oral—0.5-1 million U PO tid; continue treatment at least 48h after resolution of the symptoms
Candidiasis cutaneous—apply bid/tid
• **Contraindications**—hypersensitivity to drug or class

■ **Maternal Considerations** — Candida vaginitis is perhaps the most common female genital tract infection. **Nystatin** is an antifungal, antibiotic that is both fungistatic and fungicidal *in vitro* against a wide variety of yeasts and yeast-like fungi. It is a polyene antibiotic obtained from *Streptomyces noursei*. The vaginal milieu during pregnancy predisposes to C. *albicans* overgrowth. In *vitro*, **nystatin** is highly effective against 83% of sensitive strains of tested C. *albicans*. There are no adequate reports or well-controlled studies of **nystatin** in pregnant women. It is not clear whether the various imidazole compounds differ in efficacy for mycotic vaginitis. **Nystatin** is thought less effective than **miconazole** for the treatment of vaginal candidiasis during pregnancy, though there are no randomized trials to substantiate this conclusion. There is no significant difference in the cure rates achieved after 7d or 14d of therapy. More patients relapsed after a cure with **nystatin** than with **miconazole**. *Side effects* include Stevens-Johnson syndrome, local irritation, nausea, vomiting, and diarrhea.

■ **Fetal Considerations** — There are no adequate reports or well-controlled studies in human fetuses. It is unknown whether **nystatin** crosses the human placenta. 1st trimester use of **nystatin** (and imidazole agents) is unassociated with an increased prevalence of spontaneous abortion or fetal malformation. Congenital candidiasis of the neonate's skin rarely occurs, and **nystatin** is used to treat this infection and avoid septicemia. Rodent teratogenicity studies are limited to a single report where fetal losses were associated with maternal toxicity.

■ **Breastfeeding Safety** — There are no adequate reports or well-controlled studies in nursing women. It is unknown whether **nystatin** enters human breast milk. However, considering the indication and dosing, limited **nystatin** use is unlikely to pose a clinically significant risk to the breast-feeding neonate. **Nystatin** is not effective treatment of nipple candidiasis.

■ **References**

Young GL, Jewell D. Cochrane Database Syst Rev 2001; CD000225.

Lisiak M, Klyszejko C, Marcinkowski Z, et al. Ginekol Pol 2000; 71:959-63.

Laskus A, Mendling W, Runge K, Schmidt A. Mycoses 1998; 41 Suppl 2:37-40.

Bodley V, Powers D. J Hum Lact 1997; 13:307-11.

Lee CR, McKenzie CA, Nobles A. Am Pharm 1991; NS31:44-6.

Broberg A, Thiringer K. Int J Dermatol 1989; 28:464-5.

Rosa FW, Baum C, Shaw M. Obstet Gynecol 1987; 69:751-5.

Weisberg M. Clin Ther 1986; 8:563-7.

Renault F, Roy C, Costil J, Girouin D. Nouv Presse Med 1982; 11:1863-5.

Eliot BW, Howat RC, Mack AE. Br J Obstet Gynaecol 1979; 86:572-7.

Rudolph N, Tariq AA, Reale MR, et al. Arch Dermatol 1977; 113:1101-3.

Slonitskaia NN, Mikhailets GA. Antibiotiki 1975; 20:45-7.

■ **Summary**

- **Pregnancy Category B**
- **Lactation Category S**
- **Nystatin** is effective for the treatment of candidiasis.
- Topical imidazole agents may be more effective than **nystatin** for treating symptomatic vaginal candidiasis in pregnancy.
- A 7d treatment regimen may be necessary during pregnancy rather than the shorter courses more commonly used in nonpregnant women.

Oatmeal (Aveeno)

- **Class** — Other dermatologic

- **Indications** — Contact dermatitis, e.g., poison ivy/oak

- **Mechanism** — Forms a moisturizing, colloidal suspension

- **Dosage with Qualifiers** — Contact dermatitis—apply tid/qid prn; may also mix in bath water and soak
  - **Contraindications**—hypersensitivity to drug or class
  - **Caution**—unknown

- **Maternal Considerations** — There is no published experience with topical **oatmeal** during pregnancy.
  Side effects have not been reported.

- **Fetal Considerations** — There are no adequate reports or well-controlled studies in human fetuses. Absorption is likely insignificant.

- **Breastfeeding Safety** — There are no adequate reports or well-controlled studies in nursing women. As a traditional food substance, oatmeal is unlikely to pose a clinically significant risk to the nursing infant.

- **References** — No current relevant references

- **Summary** —
  - **Pregnancy Category A**
  - **Lactation Category S**

Octreotide acetate (Sandostatin)

- **Class** — Other endocrine, antidiarrheal, gastrointestinal

- **Indications** — Secretory diarrhea, carcinoid tumor, acromegaly, esophageal varices

- **Mechanism** — Somatostatin-like activities include inhibition of GH, LH, insulin, glucagon, and VIP

- **Dosage with Qualifiers** — Secretory diarrhea—50-100mcg SC or IV qd/tid; max 1500mcg/d
  Carcinoid tumor symptoms—50-100mcg SC or IV qd/tid; max 1500mcg/d
  Carcinoid tumor crisis—50mcg/h IV ×8-24h acutely; 250mcg-500mcg IV ×1, 1-2h preoperatively for prevention

Acromegaly—50mcg SC or IV tid; max 1500mcg/d
Esophageal varices—begin 25-50mcg IV ×1 for bleeding, then 25-50mcg/h
- **Contraindications**—hypersensitivity to drug or class
- **Caution**—biliary disease, renal dysfunction, diabetes mellitus

■ **Maternal Considerations**

There are no adequate reports or well-controlled studies in pregnant women. **Octreotide** has pharmacologic actions that mimic the natural hormone somatostatin, but is more potent. There are multiple case reports of **octreotide** use during pregnancy without obvious adverse effect, typically for the treatment of acromegaly. Depressed vitamin B_{12} levels and abnormal Schilling's tests are observed in some patients, and monitoring of vitamin B_{12} is recommended. **Octreotide** reportedly improves implantation in supraovulated mice.
Side effects include arrhythmias, edema, cholecystitis, cholelithiasis, ascending cholangitis, nausea, vomiting, diarrhea, steatorrhea, flushing, hyperglycemia, myalgias, arthralgias, and headache.

■ **Fetal Considerations**

There are no adequate reports or well-controlled studies in human fetuses. It is not known whether **octreotide** crosses the human placenta. It does not affect placental GH production. Rodent studies are reassuring, revealing no evidence of teratogenicity or IUGR despite the use of doses higher than those used clinically.

■ **Breastfeeding Safety**

There are no adequate reports or well-controlled studies in nursing women. **Octreotide** enters human breast milk, but the reported concentrations are unlikely to have a clinically significant effect on the nursing infant.

■ **References**

Blackhurst G, Strachan MW, Collie D, et al. Clin Endocrinol 2002; 57:401-4.
Mikhail N. Mayo Clin Proc 2002; 77:297-8.
Katagiri S, Moon YS, Yuen BH. Hum Reprod 1997; 12:671-6.
Caron P, Buscail L, Beckers A, et al. J Clin Endocrinol Metab 1997; 82:3771-6.
Castronovo FP Jr, Stone H, Ulanski J. Nucl Med Commun 2000; 21:695-9.

■ **Summary**

- **Pregnancy Category B**
- **Lactation Category S?**
- **Octreotide** is considered safe during pregnancy and lactation if the benefit justifies the potential perinatal risk.

Ofloxacin (Floxin)

- **Class** — *Antibiotic, quinolone*

- **Indications** — Bacterial infection with gram-positive and -negative aerobes, uncomplicated gonorrhea (urethritis, cervicitis, rectal), chlamydial infections, bacterial conjunctivitis, corneal ulcer, otitis externa

- **Mechanism** — Bactericidal; inhibits topoisomerase IV and DNA gyrase.

- **Dosage with Qualifiers** — Bacterial infections—200-400mg PO/IV q12h
  Uncomplicated gonorrhea—400mg PO ×1
  Bacterial conjunctivitis—1-2 gtt q2-4h each eye ×2d, then qid ×5d
  Corneal ulcer—1-2 gtt q30min each eye ×2d, then 1h ×5d, then qid ×2d
  Otitis externa—10 gtt bid ×10d
  NOTE—renal dosing; available in otic, ophthalmic, and parenteral preparations
  - **Contraindications**—hypersensitivity to drug or class
  - **Caution**—hepatic or renal dysfunction, seizure disorder, CNS abnormalities, diabetes mellitus, dehydration, sun exposure

- **Maternal Considerations** — There are no adequate reports or well-controlled studies in pregnant women. **Ofloxacin** achieves high tissue penetration. It is not effective prophylaxis for infection after therapeutic abortion; **doxycycline** is preferred.
  Side effects include vaginitis, photosensitivity, pseudomembranous colitis, seizures, increased ICP, headache, psychosis, nausea, vomiting, diarrhea, abdominal pain, dyspepsia, dizziness, insomnia, agitation, tendonitis, arthralgias, and elevated LFTs.

- **Fetal Considerations** — There are no adequate reports or well-controlled studies in human fetuses. **Ofloxacin** crosses the human placenta reaching potentially therapeutic levels in amniotic fluid and sera, making it a candidate for fetal therapy if otherwise safe. In humans, fluoroquinolones are not associated with an increased risk of malformation. Neither ophthalmic nor otic application results in significant systemic drug levels. In general, rodent studies are reassuring, though some rodent models using otic application revealed minor skeletal abnormalities and IUGR. The administration of very high multiples of the MRHD is associated with fetal toxicity.

- **Breastfeeding Safety** — There are no adequate reports or well-controlled studies in nursing women. **Ofloxacin** reaches concentrations in human breast milk similar to or above plasma and is generally considered incompatible with breastfeeding.

■ **References** ⋯⋯⋯⋯⋯ Nielsen IK, Engdahl, Larsen T. Acta Obstet Gynecol Scand 1993; 72:556-9.
Loebstein R, Addis A, Ho E, et al. Antimicrob Agents Chemother 1998; 42:1336-9.
Giamarellou H, Kolokythas E, Petrikkos G, et al. Am J Med 1989; 87:49S-51S.

■ **Summary** ⋯⋯⋯⋯⋯
- **Pregnancy Category C**
- **Lactation Category NS**
- **Ofloxacin** should be used during pregnancy if the benefit justifies the potential perinatal risk.
- Though the fetal risk may not be as great as once thought, there are alternative agents during pregnancy for almost all indications.

Olanzapine (Zyprexa)

■ **Class** ⋯⋯⋯⋯⋯ *Antipsychotic, class* 4

■ **Indications** ⋯⋯⋯⋯⋯ Bipolar disorder, psychosis

■ **Mechanism** ⋯⋯⋯⋯⋯ Unknown; high affinity for 5HT 2a/c and dopamine receptors

■ **Dosage with Qualifiers** ⋯⋯⋯ <u>Bipolar disorder</u>—begin 5-10mg qd, increasing 5mg/d prn; max 20mg/d
<u>Psychosis</u>—begin 5-10mg qd, increasing 5mg/d prn; max 20mg/d
NOTE—available in an orally disintegrating tablet form
- **Contraindications**—hypersensitivity to drug or class
- **Caution**—seizure disorder, narrow angle glaucoma, paralytic ileus, hypotension, hypovolemia, hepatic dysfunction, cardiovascular or cerebrovascular disease

■ **Maternal Considerations** ⋯⋯ **Olanzapine** clearance is 30% lower in women, but there are no apparent differences in effectiveness or side effects. While there are no adequate reports or well-controlled studies in pregnant women, the growing body of clinical experience with **olanzapine** during pregnancy is reassuring. *Side effects* include hypotension, tachycardia, menstrual irregularities, hyperprolactinemia, tardive dyskinesia, extrapyramidal symptoms, diabetes mellitus, hyperglycemia, somnolence, weight gain, constipation, dry mouth, dyspepsia, rhinitis, fever, and elevated LFTs.

■ **Fetal Considerations** ⋯⋯⋯ There are no adequate reports or well-controlled studies in human fetuses. Less than 20% of the maternal dose crosses the human placenta, though there is no information on accumulation in the fetal compartment.

As for most psychotropic drugs, monotherapy and the lowest effective quantity given in divided doses to minimize the peaks can minimize the risks. Rodent studies are reassuring, revealing no evidence of teratogenicity despite the use of doses higher than those used clinically. Embryo and fetal toxicities were seen with high doses. There was no effect of intrauterine exposure on postnatal learning.

■ **Breastfeeding Safety**   There are no adequate reports or well-controlled studies in nursing women. **Olanzapine** enters human breast milk.

■ **References**   Ernst CL, Goldberg JF. J Clin Psychiatry 2002; 63(Suppl 4):42-55.
Rosengarten H, Quartermain D. Pharmacol Biochem Behav 2002; 72:575-9.
Goldstein DJ, Corbin LA, Fung MC. J Clin Psychpharacol 2000; 20:399-400.
Schenker S, Yang Y, Mattiuz E, et al. Clin Exp Pharmacol Physiol 1999; 26:691-7.
Kasper SC, Mattiuz EL, Swanson SP, et al. J Chromatogr B Biomed Sci Appl 1999; 726:203-9.

■ **Summary**   • **Pregnancy Category C**
• **Lactation Category U**
• **Olanzapine** should be used during pregnancy and lactation only if the benefit justifies the potential perinatal risk

Olmesartan medoxomil (Benicar)

■ **Class**   Antihypertensive, ACE-1, A2R-antagonist

■ **Indications**   Hypertension

■ **Mechanism**   Selectively AT-1 receptor antagonist

■ **Dosage with Qualifiers**   Hypertension—begin 20-40mg PO qd if monotherapy, lower if on diuretic; max 40mg/d
• **Contraindications**—hypersensitivity to drug or class, pregnancy
• **Caution**—hepatic or renal dysfunction, CHF, renal artery stenosis, ACE angioedema, hyponatremia, volume depletion

■ **Maternal Considerations**   There is no published experience with **olmesartan** during pregnancy. The lowest effective dose should be used when **olmesartan** is required during pregnancy for blood pressure control.

Side effects include severe hypotension, angioedema, hyperkalemia, dizziness, fatigue, URI symptoms, back pain, diarrhea, and dyspepsia.

■ **Fetal Considerations** ⋯⋯⋯⋯ There are no adequate reports or well-controlled studies in human fetuses. It is unknown whether **olmesartan** crosses the human placenta. Inhibitors of the renin angiotensin system as a group cross the human placenta. While no adverse fetal effects are reported after 1st trimester exposure, later exposure is associated with cranial hypoplasia, anuria, reversible or irreversible renal failure, death, oligohydramnios, prematurity, IUGR, and patent ductus arteriosus. In those rare instances when these inhibitors are necessary, women should be apprised of the potential hazards and serial ultrasound examinations conducted. If oligohydramnios is detected, **olmesartan** should be discontinued unless lifesaving for the mother and antenatal surveillance initiated. Oligohydramnios may not appear until after irreversible injury. Neonates with *in utero* exposure should be closely observed for hypotension, oliguria and hyperkalemia.

■ **Breastfeeding Safety** ⋯⋯⋯ There is no published experience in nursing women. It is unknown whether **olmesartan** enters human breast milk, though it is secreted at low concentration in rat milk.

■ **References** ⋯⋯⋯⋯⋯⋯⋯ No current relevant references are available.

■ **Summary** ⋯⋯⋯⋯⋯⋯⋯⋯
- **Pregnancy Category C (1st trimester), D (2nd and 3rd trimesters)**
- **Lactation Category U**
- **Olmesartan** and other inhibitors of the renin angiotensin system should be avoided during pregnancy if possible.
- When mother's disease requires treatment with **olmesartan**, the lowest doses should be used followed by close monitoring of the fetus.

Olopatadine hydrochloride (Patanol)

■ **Class** ⋯⋯⋯⋯⋯⋯⋯⋯⋯⋯ *Antihistamine, allergy*

■ **Indications** ⋯⋯⋯⋯⋯⋯⋯ Allergic conjunctivitis

■ **Mechanism** ⋯⋯⋯⋯⋯⋯ Selective H₁ receptor antagonist and inhibits mast cell release of histamine

■ **Dosage with Qualifiers** ⋯⋯ Allergic conjunctivitis—1-2 gtt each eye bid 6-8h apart
- **Contraindications**—hypersensitivity to drug or class
- **Caution**—unknown

- **Maternal Considerations** — There is no published experience with **olopatadine** during pregnancy.
  Side effects include dry eyes, headache, burning, eyelid edema, keratitis, hyperemia, rhinitis, and sinusitis.

- **Fetal Considerations** — There are no adequate reports or well-controlled studies in human fetuses. It is unknown whether **olopatadine** crosses the human placenta. Rodent studies are reassuring, revealing no evidence of teratogenicity or IUGR despite the use of doses higher than those used clinically. Very high multiples of the MRHD are associated with fetal toxicity.

- **Breastfeeding Safety** — There is no published experience in nursing women. It is unknown whether **olopatadine** enters human breast milk, though it has been found in rodent milk. However, considering the dose and route, it is unlikely nursing could result in a clinically significant level in the neonate.

- **References** — No current relevant references are available.

- **Summary**
  - **Pregnancy Category C**
  - **Lactation Category S?**
  - **Olopatadine** should be used during pregnancy and lactation only if the benefit justifies the potential perinatal risk

Olsalazine (Dipentum)

- **Class** — *Gastrointestinal, inflammatory bowel, salicylate*

- **Indications** — Ulcerative colitis

- **Mechanism** — Unknown; appears to work directly on the gut

- **Dosage with Qualifiers** — Ulcerative colitis—500mg PO bid
  - **Contraindications**—hypersensitivity to drug or class, hypersensitivity to salicylates
  - **Caution**—renal dysfunction

- **Maternal Considerations** — There are no adequate reports or well-controlled studies in pregnant women. Limited published experience consists predominantly of case reports and small series. It suggests that **olsalazine** retains efficacy during pregnancy.
  Side effects include hepatotoxicity, interstitial nephritis, pancreatitis, bone marrow suppression, nausea, vomiting, dyspepsia, diarrhea, abdominal pain, arthralgias, bloating, anorexia, itching, fatigue, depression, and dizziness.

- ■ **Fetal Considerations** ⋯⋯⋯⋯⋯ There are no adequate reports or well-controlled studies in human fetuses. Limited quantities of **olsalazine** and its metabolites cross the human placenta. Rodent studies conducted at multiples of the MRHD revealed IUGR, delayed skeletal and organ maturation.

- ■ **Breastfeeding Safety** ⋯⋯⋯⋯ There are no adequate reports or well-controlled studies in nursing women. In a single study, neither **olsalazine** nor its main active metabolite was detected in breast milk up to 48h after ingestion. However, oral administration to lactating rats in doses 5-20 times the MRHD reduced growth in the pups.

- ■ **References** ⋯⋯⋯⋯⋯⋯⋯⋯ Tennenbaum R, Marteau P, Elefant, et al. Gastroenterol Clin Biol 1999; 23:464-9.
Miller LG, Hopkinson JM, Motil KJ, et al. J Clin Pharmacol 1993; 33:703-6.
Christensen LA. Dan Med Bull 2000; 47:20-41.

- ■ **Summary** ⋯⋯⋯⋯⋯⋯⋯⋯⋯
  - **Pregnancy Category C**
  - **Lactation Category U**
  - **Olsalazine** should be used during pregnancy and lactation only if the benefit justifies the potential perinatal risk.

Omeprazole (Losec; Omid; Prilosec; Roweprazol)

- ■ **Class** ⋯⋯⋯⋯⋯⋯⋯⋯⋯⋯⋯ *Gastrointestinal, antiulcer, proton pump inhibitor*

- ■ **Indications** ⋯⋯⋯⋯⋯⋯⋯⋯ GERD, GI ulcer, erosive esophagitis, H. *pylori* treatment

- ■ **Mechanism** ⋯⋯⋯⋯⋯⋯⋯⋯ Inhibits hydrogen-potassium ATPase in the gastric parietal cells

- ■ **Dosage with Qualifiers** ⋯⋯ GERD—20-40mg PO before eating qd ×4-8w, then 10mg PO qd; max 80mg/d
  GI ulcer (gastric or duodenal)—40mg PO before eating qd ×4-8w
  Erosive esophagitis—20-40mg PO before eating qd ×4-8w, max 80mg/d
  H. *pylori* treatment—20mg PO bid ×10d if combined with **amoxicillin** and **clarithromycin**
  NOTE—hepatic dosing
  - **Contraindications**—hypersensitivity to drug or class
  - **Caution**—hepatic dysfunction, long-term use

- ■ **Maternal Considerations** ⋯⋯ **Omeprazole** is effective treatment for a number of hypersecretory disorders, and effective preoperative prophylaxis (20-40mg PO qd) against aspiration pneumonitis. While there are no adequate reports or well-controlled studies in pregnant women, **omeprazole** appears to retain its efficacy during pregnancy. And though it increases human myometrial contractility in isolated muscle strips, there are no reports of an increased prevalence of preterm delivery. **Omeprazole** is advocated to lower gastric pH prior to cesarean section, but the results of the randomized trials are inconsistent, perhaps reflecting dose and route of delivery. Further, it and similar agents require 20-30min to take effect. Thus, **Bicitra** (citric acid/sodium citrate solution), perhaps with **metoclopramide** to enhance lower esophageal sphincter tone remain agents of choice for emergent procedures. *Side effects* include headache, diarrhea, hepatic dysfunction, Stevens-Johnson syndrome, and blood dyscrasias.

■ **Fetal Considerations**

There are no adequate reports or well-controlled studies in human fetuses. It is unknown whether **omeprazole** crosses the human placenta. Proton pump inhibitors in general, and **omeprazole** specifically are not associated with an increased risk of malformations. In the ewe, the F:M ratio approximates 0.5, and is strongly related to the rate of maternal clearance. Rodent studies are generally reassuring, revealing no evidence of teratogenicity despite the use of doses higher than those used clinically. However, embryo and fetal toxicity are noted in some models when multiples of the MRHD are used.

■ **Breastfeeding Safety**

There are no adequate reports or well-controlled studies in nursing women. **Omeprazole** enters human breast milk, but milk concentrations are less than 10% of the maternal serum level. Thus, the nursing infant is unlikely to ingest a clinically significant amount.

■ **References**

Yildirim K, Sarioglu Y, Kaya T, et al. Life Sci 2001; 69:435-42.
Lin CJ, Huang CL, Hsu HW, Chen TL. Acta Anaesthesiol Sin 1996; 34:179-84.
Tripathi A, Somwanshi M, Singh B, Bajaj P. Can J Anaesth 1995; 42:797-800.
Ruigomez A, Garcia Rodriguez LA, Cattaruzzi C, et al. Am J Epidemiol 1999; 150:476-81.
Nikfar S, Abdollahi M, Moretti ME, et al. Dig Dis Sci 2002; 47:1526-9.
Kallen BA. Eur J Obstet Gynecol Reprod Biol 2001; 96:63-8.
Ching MS, Morgan DJ, Mihaly GW, et al. Dev Pharmacol Ther 1986; 9:323-31.
Marshall JK, Thompson AB, Armstrong D. Can J Gastroenterol 1998; 12:225-7.

■ **Summary**

- **Pregnancy Category C**
- **Lactation Category S?**
- **Omeprazole** should be used during pregnancy only if the benefit justifies the unknown potential perinatal risk.

Ondansetron (Zofran)

- **Class** — *Antiemetic, nausea and vomiting, serotonin receptor antagonist*

- **Indications** — Severe nausea and vomiting

- **Mechanism** — Selectively inhibits the 5HT-3 receptors

- **Dosage with Qualifiers** — <u>Severe nausea and vomiting</u>—postoperative: 4mg IM/IV ×1; pre-chemotherapy: 24mg PO or 32mg IV 30min before initiating chemotherapy; radiation therapy: begin 8mg PO 1-2h before radiation, continue q8h ×2d
  NOTE—renal dosing; also available in orally disintegrating tablets
  - **Contraindications**—hypersensitivity to drug or class
  - **Caution**—hepatic dysfunction

- **Maternal Considerations** — There are no adequate reports or well-controlled studies in pregnant women. **Ondansetron** is effective for nausea and vomiting of pregnancy, but the published experience is inadequate to yet consider it first-line therapy. A single IV dose (4mg) given prophylactically significantly reduces the nausea and vomiting after cesarean delivery, though the same may be accomplished with other less expensive antiemetic agents. Since **ondansetron** (0.1mg/kg IV ×1) significantly reduces the pruritus associated with intrathecal **morphine**, some clinicians choose this agent as their antiemetic of choice no matter what the cost; others use less expensive alternative agents. It is no better than **metoclopramide** as prophylaxis for nausea and vomiting after minor gynecologic surgery, but superior to it for patients undergoing chemotherapy.
  Side effects include bronchospasm, extrapyramidal symptoms, oculogyric crisis, headache, fatigue, constipation, diarrhea, agitation, pruritus, and dizziness.

- **Fetal Considerations** — There are no adequate reports or well-controlled studies in human fetuses. It is not known whether **ondansetron** crosses the human placenta. Rodent studies are reassuring, revealing no evidence of teratogenicity or IUGR despite the use of doses higher than those used clinically.

- **Breastfeeding Safety** — There is no published experience in nursing women. It is unknown whether **ondansetron** enters human breast milk. It is detectable in rat milk.

- **References** — Abouleish EI, Rashid S, Haque S, et al. Anaesthesia 1999; 54:479-82.
  Yeh HM, Chen LK, Lin CJ, et al. Anesth Analg 2000; 91:172-5.
  Monagle J, Barnes R, Goodchild C, Hewitt M. Eur J Anaesthesiol 1997; 14:604-9.
  Magee LA, Mazzotta P, Koren G. Am J Obstet Gynecol 2002; 185:S256-61.

- **Summary** .... • **Pregnancy Category B**
  - **Lactation Category U**
  - **Ondansetron** is a reasonable (though relatively expensive) prophylactic agent for the prevention of postoperative nausea and vomiting. It is indicated for the "rescue" treatment of postoperative nausea and vomiting that fails to respond to first-line agents.
  - It is superior to most first-line agents for the treatment of nausea and vomiting associated with chemotherapy.

Oprelvekin (Neumega)

- **Class** .... *Hematopoietic agents*

- **Indications** .... Myelosuppressive chemotherapy for nonmyeloid malignancies at high risk of severe thrombocytopenia

- **Mechanism** .... Directly stimulating hematopoietic stem cells and megakaryocyte progenitor cells

- **Dosage with Qualifiers** .... Myelosuppressive chemotherapy—50mcg/kg qd SC beginning 6-24h after completing chemotherapy; monitor platelet counts at time of expected nadir; continue until post-nadir platelet count >50,000 cells/ccl
  NOTE—should be used within 3h of reconstitution
  - **Contraindications**—hypersensitivity to drug or class
  - **Caution**—CHF, arrhythmia, chronic diuretic therapy, chemotherapy greater than 5d duration, chemotherapy associated with delayed myelosuppression

- **Maternal Considerations** .... **Oprelvekin** is genetically engineered IL-11. There is no published experience with it during pregnancy.
  Side effects include fluid retention, weight gain, tachycardia, palpitations, atrial fibrillation, blurred vision, papilledema, transient rash, oral monilia, dyspnea, and pleural effusion.

- **Fetal Considerations** .... There are no adequate reports or well-controlled studies in human fetuses. IL-11 is an endogenous cytokine with many actions and interactions. **Oprelvekin** is embryocidal in some rodents at doses analogous to those used in humans. IUGR and reduced ossification is also reported.

- **Breastfeeding Safety** .... There is no published experience in nursing women. It is unknown whether **oprelvekin** enters human breast milk.

- **References** .... No current relevant references

■ Summary
• **Pregnancy Category C**
• **Lactation Category U**
• **Oprelvekin** should be used during pregnancy and lactation only if the benefit justifies the potential perinatal risk.

Orlistat (Xenical)

■ **Class** — *Gastrointestinal, lipase inhibitor, metabolism*

■ **Indications** — Obesity

■ **Mechanism** — Inhibits gastric and pancreatic lipases

■ **Dosage with Qualifiers** — Obesity—120mg PO tid; take during meals with fat
NOTE—separate **orlistat** from fat-soluble vitamin supplements by at least 2h
• **Contraindications**—hypersensitivity to drug or class, cholestasis, chronic malabsorbtion syndromes
• **Caution**—history of renal stones

■ **Maternal Considerations** — **Orlistat** is a reversible lipase inhibitor for obesity management that acts by inhibiting the absorption of dietary fats. There is no published experience with it during pregnancy. It has been suggested but unproven **orlistat** might interfere with the absorption of oral contraceptives and thus diminish their efficacy.
Side effects include diarrhea, flatulence, steatorrhea, fecal incontinence, nausea, and vomiting.

■ **Fetal Considerations** — There are no adequate reports or well-controlled studies in human fetuses. It is unknown whether **orlistat** crosses the human placenta. However, the mother absorbs little systemically (peak plasma levels at the limit of detection). Rodent studies are reassuring, revealing no evidence of teratogenicity or IUGR despite the use of doses higher than those used clinically. Some dilation of the cerebral ventricles was noted.

■ **Breastfeeding Safety** — There is no published experience in nursing women. Considering the maternal systemic level, it is unlikely a clinically relevant concentration of **orlistat** enters human breast milk. It is not known whether the milk components are altered.

■ **References** — Peleg R. Isr Med Assoc J 2000; 2:712.

■ **Summary** • • Pregnancy Category B
                 • Lactation Category S?
                 • Though there are no clear contraindications for
                   orlistat during pregnancy, there are also no indications
                   for a weight loss regimen that would necessitate it.

Orphenadrine citrate (Banflex; Flexoject; Flexon; Flexor; Marflex; Mio-Rel; Myolin; Myophen; Myotrol; Neocyten; Noradex; Norflex; O'Flex; Orflagen; Orfro; Orphenate; Qualaflex; Tega-Flex)

■ **Class** .... *Muscle relaxant*

■ **Indications** .... Muscle spasm

■ **Mechanism** .... Unknown

■ **Dosage with Qualifiers** ...... Muscle spasm—60-100mg PO bid; also available for
injection
  • **Contraindications**—hypersensitivity to drug or class,
    glaucoma, pyloric or duodenal obstruction, myasthenia
    gravis
  • **Caution**—cardiovascular disease, sulfite allergy,
    arrhythmia

■ **Maternal Considerations** ...... There is no published experience with **orphenadrine**
during pregnancy.
Side effects include drowsiness, nausea, vomiting, dry
mouth, aplastic anemia, lightheadedness, and headache.

■ **Fetal Considerations** .... There are no adequate reports or well-controlled studies
in human fetuses. It is unknown whether **orphenadrine**
crosses the human placenta. There is some passage
across the ovine placenta. Rodent teratogen studies have
not been conducted.

■ **Breastfeeding Safety** .... There is no published experience in nursing women. It is
unknown whether **orphenadrine** enters human breast milk.

■ **References** .... Yoo SD, Axelson JE, Rurak DW. J Chromatogr 1986;
378:385-93.

■ **Summary** .... • Pregnancy Category C
                 • Lactation Category U
                 • **Orphenadrine** should be used during pregnancy and
                   lactation only if the benefit justifies the potential
                   perinatal risk.

Oseltamivir phosphate (Tamiflu)

▪ Class .... *Antiviral*

▪ Indications .... Influenza A and B virus prophylaxis and treatment

▪ Mechanism .... Blocks influenza neuraminidase altering virus aggregation and release

▪ Dosage with Qualifiers .... Influenza A/B prophylaxis—75mg PO qd; initiate at outbreak
Influenza A/B treatment—75mg PO bid ×5d beginning within 48h symptoms
NOTE—renal dosing
- **Contraindications**—hypersensitivity to drug or class
- **Caution**—hepatic dysfunction

▪ Maternal Considerations .... There is no published experience with **oseltamivir** during pregnancy. Evidence of evolving viral resistance is emerging. Prophylaxis is not a substitute for vaccination (CDC Immunization Practices Advisory Committee). *Side effects* include nausea, vomiting, bronchitis, insomnia, and vertigo.

▪ Fetal Considerations .... There are no adequate reports or well-controlled studies in human fetuses. It is unknown whether **oseltamivir** crosses the human placenta. Rodent studies are reassuring, revealing no evidence of teratogenicity despite the use of doses higher than those used clinically. Maternal toxicity is noted along with a non-significant increase in skeletal abnormalities.

▪ Breastfeeding Safety .... There is no published experience in nursing women. It is unknown whether **oseltamivir** enters human breast milk.

▪ References .... No current relevant references are available.

▪ Summary ....
- **Pregnancy Category C**
- **Lactation Category U**
- **Oseltamivir** should be used during pregnancy and lactation only if the benefit justifies the potential perinatal risk.

Oxacillin (Bactocill; Dicloxal OX; Prostaphlin; Staphaloxin; Wydox)

■ **Class** — Antibiotic, penicillin

■ **Indications** — Bacterial infection, especially with penicillinase-producing *Staphylococcus*

■ **Mechanism** — Bactericidal; inhibits cell wall synthesis

■ **Dosage with Qualifiers** — Bacterial infection—1-2g IV/IM q4-6h, or 500-1000mg PO q4-6h
NOTE—renal dosing
- **Contraindications**—hypersensitivity to drug or class
- **Caution**—unknown

■ **Maternal Considerations** — **Oxacillin** is penicillinase-resistant, acid-resistant, semisynthetic penicillin suitable for oral administration. There is a long clinical experience with **oxacillin** during pregnancy.
Side effects include neutropenia, granulocytopenia, eosinophilia, hemolytic anemia, thrombocytopenia, nausea, vomiting, diarrhea, pseudomembranous colitis, oral lesions, fever, chills, rash, lethargy, urticaria, interstitial nephritis, and elevated LFTs.

■ **Fetal Considerations** — There are no adequate reports or well-controlled studies in human fetuses. Most penicillin compounds cross the human placenta. There is no evidence **oxacillin** is teratogenic in humans after a long clinical experience. Rodent studies are reassuring, revealing no evidence of teratogenicity or IUGR despite the use of doses higher than those used clinically. There are a number of interesting studies in rodents suggesting *in utero* exposure alters *in utero* and postnatal immune responses. The implications are unclear.

■ **Breastfeeding Safety** — There are no adequate reports or well-controlled studies in nursing women. **Oxacillin** is concentrated in human breast milk exceeding the typical MIC making it suitable for the treatment of puerperal mastitis. It is generally considered compatible with breastfeeding.

■ **References** — Czeizel AE, Rockenbauer M, Sorensen HT, Olsen J. Scand J Infect Dis 1999; 31:311-2.
Dostal M, Horka I, Tuma O, Soukupova D. Funct Dev Morphol 1994; 4:67-75.
Peiker G, Schroder S. Pharmazie 1986; 41:793-5.

■ **Summary** —
- **Pregnancy Category B**
- **Lactation Category S**
- **Oxacillin** is an alternative for the treatment of puerperal mastitis.
- There are alternative agents for almost all indications.

Oxaprozin (Daypro)

- **Class** — *Analgesic*, NSAID

- **Indications** — Osteoarthritis and rheumatoid arthritis, mild to moderate pain

- **Mechanism** — Inhibits cyclooxygenase and lipoxygenase leading to reduced prostaglandin synthesis

- **Dosage with Qualifiers** — Osteoarthritis or rheumatoid arthritis—1200mg PO qd with food; max 1800mg/d
  Mild to moderate pain—1200mg PO qd
  - **Contraindications**—hypersensitivity to drug or class, hypersensitivity to aspirin, aspirin/NSAID-induced asthma
  - **Caution**—hypertension, CHF, history of GI bleeding, nasal polyps

- **Maternal Considerations** — **Oxaprozin** is a NSAID with anti-inflammatory, analgesic, and antipyretic properties. There is no published experience with **oxaprozin** during pregnancy.
  Side effects include fluid retention, thrombocytopenia, agranulocytosis, acute renal failure, interstitial nephritis, hepatotoxicity, bronchospasm, nausea, vomiting, dyspepsia, abdominal pain, headache, dizziness, rash, drowsiness, elevated LFTs and tinnitus.

- **Fetal Considerations** — There are no adequate reports or well-controlled studies in human fetuses. It is unknown whether **oxaprozin** crosses the human placenta. Other NSAIDs cross the human placenta and are associated with decreased fetal urination and ductal constriction. Malformed fetuses were observed in rabbits but not mice treated with doses analogous to the human. Pup survival was also reduced.

- **Breastfeeding Safety** — There is no published experience in nursing women. It is unknown whether **oxaprozin** enters human breast milk. It does enter rodent milk.

- **References** — No current relevant references exist.

- **Summary** —
  - **Pregnancy Category C**
  - **Lactation Category U**
  - **Oxaprozin** should be used during pregnancy and lactation only if the benefit justifies the potential perinatal risk.
  - There are alternative agents for which there is more experience regarding use during pregnancy and lactation.

Oxazepam (Murelax; Serax; Wakezepam)

- **Class** — *Benzodiazepine, short-acting*

- **Indications** — Anxiety, alcohol withdrawal

- **Mechanism** — Binds to benzodiazepine receptors augmenting GABA responses

- **Dosage with Qualifiers** — Anxiety, short-term relief—10-30mg PO tid or qid
  Alcohol withdrawal—15-30mg PO tid or qid
  - **Contraindications**—hypersensitivity to drug or class, psychosis
  - **Caution**—none

- **Maternal Considerations** — Alcoholism is an often-unrecognized problem during pregnancy that poses a clear hazard to mother and child. **Oxazepam** has a wide safety range compared to other benzodiazepines. There are no adequate reports or well-controlled studies in pregnant women. Some also considers **oxazepam** a second-line agent for the treatment of pruritus during pregnancy, despite the lack of study for this indication. It is highly effective for the short-term relief of anxiety. Physical and psychological dependency is a risk with chronic usage.
  Side effects include nausea, hepatic dysfunction, jaundice, leukopenia, dizziness, syncope, vertigo, headache, edema, tremor, rash, and lethargy.

- **Fetal Considerations** — Benzodiazepines are lipophilic molecules that easily penetrate membranes. There are no adequate reports or well-controlled studies in human fetuses. **Oxazepam** crosses the human placenta at a slower rate than **diazepam,** reaching an F:M ratio during the 1st trimester of 0.5 after 4h. The impact of benzodiazepines in human pregnancy appears in general to have been overestimated. Long-term follow-up studies are for the most part reassuring. Fetal exposure can be minimized by qid dosing to reduce peak levels. Subtle behavioral affects of *in utero* **oxazepam** exposure are reported in rodents.

- **Breastfeeding Safety** — There are no adequate reports or well-controlled studies in nursing women. **Oxazepam** enters human breast milk in low concentrations unlikely to be clinically significant for the breast-feeding infant.

- **References** — Drugs and Pregnancy Study Group. Ann Pharmacother 1994; 28:17-20.
  Jorgensen NP, Thurmann-Nielsen E, Walstad RA. Acta Obstet Gynecol Scand 1988; 67:493-7.
  Fiore M, Dell'Omo G, Alleva E, Lipp HP. Psychopharmacology 1995; 122:72-7
  McElhatton PR. Reprod Toxicol 1994; 8:461-75.
  Wretlind M. Eur J Clin Pharmacol 1987; 33:209-10.

■ **Summary**
- **Pregnancy Category D**
- **Lactation Category S?**
- **Oxazepam** should be used during pregnancy and lactation only if the benefit justifies the potential perinatal risk.
- Though unnecessary treatment should be avoided, appropriate candidates should not be denied therapy solely because they are pregnant.

Oxcarbazepine (Trileptal)

■ **Class** — *Anticonvulsant, 2nd generation*

■ **Indications** — Seizure disorder

■ **Mechanism** — Unknown; block voltage sensitive sodium channels

■ **Dosage with Qualifiers** — Seizure disorder—begin at 300mg PO bid, increasing by 300mg/d q3d; max 2400mg/d
NOTE—renal dosing
- **Contraindications**—hypersensitivity to drug or class
- **Caution**—renal dysfunction

■ **Maternal Considerations** — **Oxcarbazepine** is an enzyme-inducing agent. Thus, either a higher dose oral contraceptive or a second method of contraception is recommended. Planned pregnancy and counseling on the importance of folate supplementation and medication adherence are important. There are no adequate reports or well-controlled studies in pregnant women. Vitamin K (10mg qd) is recommended for the last 4w of gestation in women taking enzyme-inducing agents such as **oxcarbazepine**, **phenytoin**, **phenobarbital**, **carbamazepine**, and **topiramate**.
Side effects include hyponatremia, thrombocytopenia, leukopenia, Stevens-Johnson syndrome, toxic epidermal necrolysis, nausea, vomiting, dyspepsia, abdominal pain, somnolence, dizziness, diplopia, fatigue, nystagmus, acne, alopecia, and elevated LFTs.

■ **Fetal Considerations** — There are no adequate reports or well-controlled studies in human fetuses. **Oxcarbazepine** crosses the human placenta reaching an F:M ratio approximating unity with the placenta taking an active role in its metabolism. The frequency of neonatal bleeding complications is not increased, calling into question the necessity of vitamin K supplementation. **Oxcarbazepine** is closely related structurally to **carbamazepine**, which is considered teratogenic in humans. Polytherapy increases the risk. If feasible, the number of agents used during pregnancy should be reduced. Rodent studies performed at doses analogous to the human demonstrate embryo lethality, IUGR and a variety of malformations (craniofacial, cardiovascular, and skeletal).

■ **Breastfeeding Safety** — There are no adequate reports or well-controlled studies in nursing women. Though the concentrations of **oxcarbazepine** and its major metabolites in human breast milk are low, and neonatal concentrations decline despite breastfeeding, periodic monitoring of the infant concentration is suggested by some.

■ **References** — Bruno MK, Harden CL. Curr Treat Options Neurol 2002; 4:31-40.
Myllynen P, Pienimaki P, Jouppila P, Vahakangas K. Epilepsia 2001; 42:1482-5.
Pienimaki P, Lampela E, Hakkola J, et al. Epilepsia 1997; 38:309-16.
Kaaja E, Kaaja R, Matila R, Hiilesmaa V. Neurology 2002; 58:549-53.
Bulau P, Paar WD, von Unruh GE. Eur J Clin Pharmacol 1988; 34:311-3.

■ **Summary** —
- **Pregnancy Category C**
- **Lactation Category S?**
- **Oxcarbazepine** should be used during pregnancy and lactation only if the benefit justifies the potential perinatal risk.
- As for most psychotropic drugs, monotherapy and the lowest effective quantity, given in divided doses to minimize the peaks, can minimize the risks.

Oxiconazole nitrate (Oxistat; Oxizole)

■ **Class** — Antifungal, *dermatologic*

■ **Indications** — Skin fungal infection due to *Epidermophyton floccosum, Trichophyton mentagrophytes, Trichophyton rubrum, Malassezia furfur*

■ **Mechanism** — Inhibits ergosterol biosynthesis, which is critical for cellular membrane integrity

■ **Dosage with Qualifiers** — Skin fungal infection—apply to affected and surrounding area bid
NOTE—available in cream or lotion; for dermatologic use only
- **Contraindications**—hypersensitivity to drug or class, vaginal or ophthalmologic infections
- **Caution**—unknown

- ■ **Maternal Considerations** ········· There is no published experience with **oxiconazole** during pregnancy. However, less than 1% of the applied dose is absorbed systemically.
  Side effects include skin irritation and itching.

- ■ **Fetal Considerations** ················· There are no adequate reports or well-controlled studies in human fetuses. It is unknown whether **oxiconazole** crosses the human placenta. However, the maternal systemic concentration is not likely to reach a clinically relevant level. Rodent studies are reassuring, revealing no evidence of teratogenicity or IUGR despite the use of doses higher than those used clinically.

- ■ **Breastfeeding Safety** ·················· There is no published experience in nursing women. It is unknown whether **oxiconazole** enters human breast milk. Because less than 1% of the applied dose is absorbed systemically, it is unlikely the breast-feeding newborn would absorb a clinically relevant amount.

- ■ **References** ········· There are no current relevant references.

- ■ **Summary** ·········
  - Pregnancy Category B
  - Lactation Category S
  - **Oxiconazole** should be used during pregnancy and lactation if the benefit justifies the potential perinatal risk.

Oxtriphylline (Brondecon; Choledyl; Cholegyl)

- ■ **Class** ·········· Bronchodilator, xanthine

- ■ **Indications** ·········· Bronchospasm, asthma, bronchitis, emphysema

- ■ **Mechanism** ·········· Direct smooth muscle relaxant possibly by phosphodiesterase inhibition

- ■ **Dosage with Qualifiers** ·········· Bronchospasm in otherwise healthy nonsmoking adults—7.8mg/kg PO load, then 4.7mg/kg PO q8h; 10-20mcg/ml the target range
  NOTE—check standard reference as dose varies by age and whether or not the patient is already taking **theophylline**; laboratory monitoring is essential to assure appropriate dosing is essential
  NOTE—0.8mg **oxtriphylline** = 0.5mg **theophylline.**
  - **Contraindications**—hypersensitivity to drug or class, active peptic ulcer disease, untreated seizure disorder
  - **Caution**—arrhythmias

- **Maternal Considerations** ⋯ **Oxtriphylline** is the choline salt of **theophylline**. Its clearance is increased in cigarette smokers, in patients with CHF, hepatic dysfunction and those taking a variety of other drugs such as **erythromycin, phenytoin, cimetidine, lithium,** and oral contraceptives. There is no published experience with **oxtriphylline** during pregnancy. See **theophylline**.
Side effects include arrhythmias, palpitations, hypotension, convulsions, nausea, vomiting, epigastric pain, headaches, restlessness, insomnia, frequent urination, tachypnea, and hyperglycemia.

- **Fetal Considerations** ⋯ There are no adequate reports or well-controlled studies in human fetuses. It is unknown whether **oxtriphylline** crosses the human placenta. Rodent studies have not been conducted. See **theophylline**.

- **Breastfeeding Safety** ⋯ There is no published experience in nursing women. While it is unknown whether **oxtriphylline** enters human breast milk, **theophylline** is distributed into breast milk and may cause irritability or other signs of toxicity in nursing infants. See **theophylline**.

- **References** ⋯ There are no current relevant references. See **theophylline**.

- **Summary** ⋯
  - **Pregnancy Category C**
  - **Lactation Category U**
  - **Oxtriphylline** should be used during pregnancy and lactation only if the benefit justifies the potential perinatal risk

Oxybutynin chloride (Ditropan)

- **Class** ⋯ *Anticholinergic, antispasmodic*

- **Indications** ⋯ Bladder spasm

- **Mechanism** ⋯ Direct antispasmodic effect; inhibits muscarinic effects of acetylcholine

- **Dosage with Qualifiers** ⋯ Bladder spasm—5mg PO bid/tid; max 5mg PO qid
  - **Contraindications**—hypersensitivity to drug or class, glaucoma, ulcerative colitis, GI obstruction or ileus, myasthenia gravis
  - **Caution**—hepatic or renal dysfunction

- **Maternal Considerations** ⋯⋯ There is no published experience with **oxybutynin** during pregnancy.
  Side effects include tachycardia, vasodilation, rash, constipation, decreased sweating, dry mouth, drowsiness, hallucinations, restlessness, cycloplegia, and insomnia.

- **Fetal Considerations** ⋯⋯ There are no adequate reports or well-controlled studies in human fetuses. It is not known whether **oxybutynin** crosses the human placenta. Rodent studies are reassuring, revealing no evidence of teratogenicity or IUGR despite the use of doses higher than those used clinically.

- **Breastfeeding Safety** ⋯⋯ There is no published experience in nursing women. It is unknown whether **oxybutynin** enters human breast milk.

- **References** ⋯⋯ There are no current relevant references.

- **Summary** ⋯⋯
  - **Pregnancy Category B**
  - **Lactation Category U**
  - **Oxybutynin** should be used during pregnancy and lactation only if the benefit justifies the potential perinatal risk.

Oxycodone (OxyContin—slow release; Roxicodone—immediate release)

- **Class** ⋯⋯ Analgesic, narcotic (schedule II)

- **Indications** ⋯⋯ Moderate to severe pain

- **Mechanism** ⋯⋯ Binds to opiate receptors

- **Dosage with Qualifiers** ⋯⋯ Moderate to severe pain—immediate release 5-30mg PO q4h prn; slow release 10mg bid, increase as needed
  NOTE—hepatic and renal dosing
  NOTE—Tablets are to be swallowed whole, not broken, chewed, or crushed to release the drug rapidly. A fatal overdose may result.
  - **Contraindications**—hypersensitivity to drug or class
  - **Caution**—history opiate abuse, hepatic dysfunction, acute abdomen, GI obstruction or ileus

- **Maternal Considerations** ⋯⋯ Thirty milligrams (30mg) of **oxycodone** is approximately equal to 10mg **morphine**. **Oxycodone** is not intended for use as a prn analgesic. Women have, on average, plasma **oxycodone** concentrations up to 25% higher than men on a body-weight-adjusted basis. There are no adequate reports or well-controlled studies in pregnant women. Its effects should be similar to **morphine**.

Side effects include dependency, hepatotoxicity, seizures, respiratory depression, dizziness, sedation, nausea, vomiting, pruritus, rash, dysphoria, and constipation.

- **Fetal Considerations** .... There are no adequate reports or well-controlled studies in human fetuses. Other drugs in its class readily cross the human placenta. **Oxycodone** abuse during pregnancy may be associated with neonatal withdrawal.

- **Breastfeeding Safety** .... There are no adequate reports or well-controlled studies in nursing women. **Oxycodone** can be detected in human breast milk, though the kinetics remain to be elucidated.

- **References** .... Rao R, Desai NS. J Perinatol 2002; 22:324-5.
  Dickson PH, Lind A, Studts P, et al. J Forensic Sci 1994; 39:207-14.

- **Summary** ....
  - **Pregnancy Category C**
  - **Lactation Category U**
  - **Oxycodone** should be used during pregnancy and lactation only if the benefit justifies the potential perinatal risk.
  - There are alternative agents for which there is more experience during pregnancy and lactation.

Oxymetazoline, nasal (Afrin)

- **Class** .... Nasal spray

- **Indications** .... Nasal congestion

- **Mechanism** .... α-2 adrenergic agonist

- **Dosage with Qualifiers** .... Nasal congestion—2-3 sprays each nostril bid; max 6 sprays per nostril/d
  - **Contraindications**—hypersensitivity to drug or class, glaucoma
  - **Caution**—preeclampsia, hypertension, hyperthyroidism, diabetes mellitus, eye injury

- **Maternal Considerations** .... Allergic rhinitis affects about 1/3 of reproductive-age women. **Oxymetazoline** is available over the counter and the prevalence of its use during pregnancy and lactation are unknown. Chronic abuse may lead to rebound rhinitis. Because there are no adequate reports or well-controlled studies in pregnant women, it should be considered a second-line agent behind 1st generation antihistamines such as **chlorpheniramine**. **Oxymetazoline** binds to human myometrium, and can *in vitro* cause contraction of both the myometrium and the umbilical artery. Preeclamptic women may experience an acute rise in blood pressure after administration.

Side effects include hypertension, cardiovascular collapse, rebound rhinitis, nasal irritation, burning, and sneezing.

- **Fetal Considerations** — There are no adequate reports or well-controlled studies in human fetuses. It is suggested that some vasoactive decongestants may be involved in the etiology of gastroschisis, including **oxymetazoline**. It can also constrict the umbilical artery, and is suggested as a cause of a nonreactive NST. However, another study of healthy pregnancies could detect no effect of **oxymetazoline** on fetal Doppler flows in a variety of vessels.

- **Breastfeeding Safety** — There are no adequate reports or well-controlled studies in nursing women. It is unknown whether **oxymetazoline** enters human breast milk. However, considering the dose, route, and frequency, it is unlikely the breast-feeding neonate would absorb clinically relevant quantities.

- **References** — Mazzotta P, Loebstein R, Koren G. Drug Saf 1999; 20:361-75.
  Adolfsson PI, Dahle LO, Berg G, Svensson SP. Gynecol Obstet Invest 1998; 45:145-50.
  Torfs CP, Katz EA, Bateson TF, et al. Teratology 1996; 54:84-92.
  Baxi LV, Gindoff PR, Pregenzer GJ, Parras MK. Am J Obstet Gynecol 1985; 153:799-800.
  Rayburn WF, Anderson JC, Smith CV, et al. Obstet Gynecol 1990; 76:180-2.

- **Summary** —
  - **Pregnancy Category C**
  - **Lactation Category S?**
  - **Oxymetazoline** should be used during pregnancy and lactation only if the benefit justifies the potential perinatal risk.
  - There are alternative agents for which there is more experience during pregnancy and lactation.

Oxymorphone (Numorphan)

- **Class** — *Analgesic, narcotic, schedule* II

- **Indications** — Moderate to severe pain, labor analgesia

- **Mechanism** — Binds opiate receptors

- **Dosage with Qualifiers** — Moderate to severe pain—0.5-1.5mg SC/IM q4-6h; 0.5mg IV q4-6h

<u>Labor analgesia</u>—0.5-1mg SC/IM
- **Contraindications**—hypersensitivity to drug or class
- **Caution**—pulmonary, hepatic, or renal dysfunction, head trauma, seizure disorder, history substance abuse

■ **Maternal Considerations** ⋯⋯ **Oxymorphone** was at one time popular for labor analgesia. It provides similar pain relief with less pruritus compared to **morphine** when used with epidural analgesia. **Oxymorphone** is an alternative to **morphine** administered by PCA after cesarean section, but may be associated with an increase in nausea. The level of sedation is similar.
Side effects include abuse or addiction, constipation, hypotension, respiratory depression, sedation, confusion, nausea, vomiting, dizziness, sweating, nervousness, and hallucinations.

■ **Fetal Considerations** ⋯⋯ There are no adequate reports or well-controlled studies in human fetuses. See **morphine**.

■ **Breastfeeding Safety** ⋯⋯ There is no published experience in nursing women. It is unknown whether **oxymorphone** enters human breast milk. Only limited quantities of morphine enter breast milk.

■ **References** ⋯⋯ Celleno D, Capogna G, Sebastiani M, et al. Reg Anesth 1991; 16:79-83.
Sinatra R, Chung KS, Silverman DG, et al. Anesthesiology 1989; 71:502-7.

■ **Summary** ⋯⋯
- **Pregnancy Category C**
- **Lactation Category U**
- **Oxymorphone** should be used during pregnancy and lactation only if the benefit justifies the potential perinatal risk.

Oxytetracycline (E.P. Mycin; Clinmycin; Oxy-Kesso-Tetra; Terramycin; Tija; Uri-Tet)

■ **Class** ⋯⋯ *Antibiotic, tetracycline*

■ **Indications** ⋯⋯ Bacterial infections with gram-negative and -positive bacteria including *Rickettsia, Mycoplasma pneumoniae, Borrelia recurrentis, Haemophilus ducreyi* (chancroid), *Pasteurella pestis* and *Pasteurella tularensis, Bartonella bacilliformis, Bacteroides* species, *Vibrio comma* and *Vibrio fetus, Escherichia coli, Enterobacter aerogenes* (formerly *Aerobacter aerogenes*), *Shigella* species, *Mima* species and *Herellea* species, *Haemophilus influenzae* (respiratory infections), *Klebsiella* species (respiratory and urinary infections), and the agents of psittacosis, ornithosis, lymphogranuloma venereum, and granuloma inguinale.

- **Mechanism** .... Bacteriostatic

- **Dosage with Qualifiers** .... <u>Bacterial infections</u>—250-500mg PO bid depending on severity, or 250mg IM qd
  <u>Gonorrhea when penicillin is contraindicated</u>—1.5g PO ×1, then 500mg PO qid for a total of 9g
  <u>Syphilis when penicillin is contraindicated</u>—500mg PO qid ×10-15d
  NOTE—renal dosing; IM formulation contains 2% **lidocaine**
  - **Contraindications**—hypersensitivity to drug or class
  - **Caution**—concomitant anticoagulant or penicillin therapy

- **Maternal Considerations** .... When penicillin is contraindicated, tetracyclines are alternative drugs for the treatment of N. *gonorrhoeae*, T. *pallidum* and T. *pertenue* (syphilis and yaws), *Listeria monocytogenes*. *Clostridium* species, *Bacillus anthracis*. *Fusobacterium fusiforme* (Vincent's infection), and *Actinomyces* species. There are no adequate reports or well-controlled studies in pregnant women. Tetracyclines are generally considered contraindicated during pregnancy because of their effect on the fetal teeth.
  Side effects include nausea, vomiting, diarrhea, glossitis, rash, photosensitivity, renal toxicity, urticaria, angioneurotic edema, hemolytic anemia, eosinophilia, thrombocytopenia, and neutropenia.

- **Fetal Considerations** .... There are no adequate reports or well-controlled studies in human fetuses. **Oxytetracycline** rapidly crosses the placenta and blood-brain barrier. Epidemiologic study links 1st trimester use of oxytetracycline with NTDs, cleft palate, and cardiovascular malformations. Tetracyclines in general are known to cause tooth discoloration when given in the second half of pregnancy and during the neonatal period. They are incorporated into fetal bones in a reversible fashion. Rodent studies are reassuring, revealing no evidence of teratogenicity despite the use of doses higher than those used clinically. However, **oxytetracycline** produced dose-dependent maternal and embryo toxicity.

- **Breastfeeding Safety** .... There is no published experience in nursing women. It is unknown whether **oxytetracycline** enters human breast milk. Other tetracyclines are excreted in breast milk.

- **References** .... Czeizel AE, Rockenbauer M. Eur J Obstet Gynecol Reprod Biol 2000; 88:27-33.
  Morrissey RE, Tyl RW, Price CJ, et al. Fundam Appl Toxicol 1986; 7:434-43.

■ **Summary**

- **Pregnancy Category D**
- **Lactation Category U**
- **Oxytetracycline** should be used during pregnancy and lactation only if the benefit justifies the potential perinatal risk.
- There is reason to suspect **oxytetracycline** is a weak teratogen in humans.
- There are alternative agents for which there is more experience regarding use during pregnancy and lactation.

Oxytocin (Pitocin; Syntocinon; Xitocin)

■ **Class**
Hormone, uterotonic

■ **Indications**
Labor induction, postpartum bleeding, lactation aid

■ **Mechanism**
Binds oxytocin receptors

■ **Dosage with Qualifiers**
Labor induction—1-2mIU/min IV; double q20-30min until 8mIU/min, then increase by 1-2mIU/min; max 200mIU/min
Postpartum bleeding—10-40IU/L at a rate titrated to control bleeding
Lactation aid—1-2 sprays per nostril 2-3min before feeding or pumping during the 1st week after delivery
NOTE—available for either parenteral use or as a nasal spray

- **Contraindications**—hypersensitivity to drug or class, nonpolar lie, CPD, fetal distress, placenta previa, vasa previa, umbilical cord prolapse, fetal bradycardia, other contraindications to vaginal delivery
- **Caution**—prior uterine scar, breech presentation

■ **Maternal Considerations**
The physiologic role of **oxytocin** in the stimulation and maintenance of human labor remains unclear. Though the search continues for new oxytocin receptor antagonists, large trials conducted with one antagonist revealed it was at best no better than many of the tocolytic agents already available. **Oxytocin** is usually effective stimulating rhythmic uterine contractions and is the drug of choice for either the induction and augmentation of labor. In some geographic locales, an oxytocin challenge test (OCT) is still used to assess placental reserve in the at-risk pregnancy. It is unclear whether routine amniotomy enhances the efficacy of **oxytocin**. High-dose **oxytocin** (4.5mIU/min initially, increased by 4.5mIU/min q30min) is associated with significantly shorter labors without demonstrable adverse fetal or neonatal effect compared to a low-dose **oxytocin** (1.5mIU/min initially, increased by 1.5mIU/min q30min)

protocol. Low-dose **oxytocin** (1-4mIU/min) is equivalent to **misoprostol** for cervical ripening. **Oxytocin** is also important for the management of postpartum bleeding. **Oxytocin** infused at 2667mU/min (80mIU/500ml over 30min) for the first 30min post partum reduces the need for additional uterotonic agents after cesarean delivery compared to an infusion of 333mU/min (10mIU/500ml over 30min) at cord clamping. And while it is often given (10mIU IV) with the delivery of the anterior shoulder, there is no clinical advantage to its administration then compared to after placental delivery for the reduction of 3rd stage hemorrhage. Injection into the umbilical vein after delivery has little impact on the 3rd stage of labor. Electronic fetal heart rate monitoring is indicated for all antepartal infusions.

Side effects include uterine tetany, arrhythmia, uterine rupture, placental abruption, fetal distress, SIADH, nausea, and vomiting.

■ **Fetal Considerations** — **Oxytocin** is used only to end pregnancy, and as such poses only labor-associated risks to the fetus. There are no indications for its use in the 1st trimester, and animal teratogen studies have not been conducted.

■ **Breastfeeding Safety** — There are no adequate reports or well-controlled studies in nursing women. Endogenous **oxytocin** is essential for the initiation of lactation, and synthetic oxytocin can aid the establishment of a milk reflex.

■ **References** — Choy CM, Lau WC, Tam WH, Yuen PM. BJOG 2002; 109:173-7.
Merrill DC, Zlatnik FJ. Obstet Gynecol 1999; 94:455-63.
Jackson KW Jr, Allbert JR, Schemmer G, et al. Am J Obstet Gynecol 2001; 185:873-7.
Carroli G, Bergel E. Cochrane Database Syst Rev 2001; (4):CD001337.
Howarth GR, Botha DJ. Cochrane Database Syst Rev 2001; (3):CD003250.
Munn MB, Owen J, Vincent R, et al. Obstet Gynecol 2001; 98:386-90.
Ferguson JE 2d, Head BH, Frank FH, et al. Am J Obstet Gynecol 2002; 187:273-9; discussion 279-80.

■ **Summary** —
- **Pregnancy Category X**
- **Lactation Category S**
- **Oxytocin** is the drug of choice for labor augmentation.
- It remains a first-line agent for induction and the treatment of puerperal hemorrhage.

Paclitaxel (Onxol; Taxol)

■ **Class**	*Antineoplastic, other oncologic*
■ **Indications**	Malignancy, metastatic ovarian or breast, lung (non-small cell), and HIV-related Kaposi's sarcoma
■ **Mechanism**	Inhibits mitosis by promoting assembly and stabilization of microtubules
■ **Dosage with Qualifiers**	<u>Metastatic ovarian or breast, lung (non-small cell), and HIV-related Kaposi's sarcoma</u>—dosing regimens vary • **Contraindications**—hypersensitivity to drug or class, hypersensitivity to **castor oil**, neutropenia • **Caution**—radiation therapy, pregnancy
■ **Maternal Considerations**	**Paclitaxel** is a natural product. It is usually combined with **cisplatin** as first-line therapy. There are no adequate reports or well-controlled studies in pregnant women. The published experience is limited to a single case report where therapy was initiated at 27w and ended with a good neonatal outcome. *Side effects* include alopecia, neutropenia, leukopenia, thrombocytopenia, nausea, vomiting, diarrhea, anemia, arthralgia, myalgia, peripheral neuropathy, infection, elevated LFTs, and injection site reactions.
■ **Fetal Considerations**	There are no adequate reports or well-controlled studies in human fetuses. It is unknown whether **paclitaxel** crosses the human placenta. Rodent studies reveal embryotoxicity, and IUGR, but no teratogenicity.
■ **Breastfeeding Safety**	There is no published experience in nursing women. It is unknown whether **paclitaxel** enters human breast milk. **Paclitaxel** is concentrated in rat milk.
■ **References**	Sood AK, Shahin MS, Sorosky JI. Gynecol Oncol 2001; 83:599-600. Kai S, Kohmura H, Hiraiwa E, et al. J Toxicol Sci 1994; 19(Suppl 1):69-111.
■ **Summary**	• **Pregnancy Category D** • **Lactation Category U** • **Paclitaxel** should be used during pregnancy and lactation only if the benefit justifies the potential perinatal risk. • Initiate therapy after organogenesis if possible.

Pamidronate (Aredia)

- **Class** — Biphosphonate

- **Indications** — Paget's disease, malignant hypercalcemia, osteolytic lesions

- **Mechanism** — Inhibits osteoclast bone resorption

- **Dosage with Qualifiers** — Paget's disease—30mg IV infused over 4h qd ×3d
  Hypercalcemia secondary to malignancy—60-90mg IV infused over 24h ×1; wait 7d between treatments
  Osteolytic lesions—90mg IV infused over 4h qmo
  - **Contraindications**—hypersensitivity to drug or class
  - **Caution**—renal dysfunction

- **Maternal Considerations** — There are no adequate reports or well-controlled studies in pregnant women. The published experience consists of a single case report during the 3rd trimester to treat hypercalcemia secondary to metastatic breast carcinoma. There was no apparent adverse effect. In animal studies, **pamidronate** inhibits bone resorption at the recommended dose for hypercalcemia apparently without inhibiting bone formation and mineralization.
  Side effects include nausea, vomiting, dyspepsia, seizures, hypertension, thrombocytopenia, leukopenia, hypokalemia, hypocalcemia, hypomagnesemia, hypophosphatemia, tachycardia, anorexia, fever, confusion, psychosis, pain, and fatigue.

- **Fetal Considerations** — There are no adequate reports or well-controlled studies in human fetuses. It is unknown whether **pamidronate** crosses the human placenta. Rodent studies revealed maternal toxicity presumably associated with hypocalcemia, fetal skeletal retardation, but no evidence of teratogenicity. The delayed skeletal formation suggests **pamidronate** crosses the rodent placenta.

- **Breastfeeding Safety** — There are no reports or well-controlled studies in nursing women. **Pamidronate** is not excreted into human breast milk. Women with hereditary hyperphosphatasia, a rare bone disorder characterized by increased bone turnover, may develop symptomatic hypercalcemia during lactation.

- **References** — Illidge TM, Hussey M, Godden CW. Clin Oncol (R Coll Radiol) 1996; 8:257-8.
  Graepel P, Bentley P, Fritz H, et al. Arzneimittelforschung 1992; 42:654-67.
  Siminoski K, Fitzgerald AA, Flesch G, Gross MS. J Bone Miner Res 2000; 15:2052-5.

■ **Summary**
- **Pregnancy Category C**
- **Lactation Category S**
- **Pamidronate** should be used during pregnancy and lactation only if the benefit justifies the potential perinatal risk.

Pancrelipase (Amylase; Amylase Lipase Protease; Cotazym-S; Creon; Creon 5; Donnazyme; Encron 10; Entolase; Enzymase 16; Festalan; Ilozyme; Ku-Zyme HP; Lipase; Panase; Pancote; Pancrease; Pancreatic Enzyme; Pancreatin 10; Pancrelipase 10000; Pancrelipase Mt 16; Pancrelipase Mt-16; Pancron 10; Panokase; Promylin; Protease; Protilase; Protilase Mt 16; Ultrase; Ultrase Mt; Vio-Moore; Zymase)

■ **Class** — *Digestive enzymes*

■ **Indications** — Pancreatic insufficiency

■ **Mechanism** — Disintegrates into trypsin, amylase, and lipase

■ **Dosage with Qualifiers** — Pancreatic insufficiency—1-3 tabs PO swallowed quickly with meals depending on preparation
NOTE—do not cut, crush, or chew
- **Contraindications**—hypersensitivity to drug or class, allergy to pork, acute pancreatitis
- **Caution**—unknown

■ **Maternal Considerations** — The enzymes in **pancrelipase** act locally in the GI, where they may be either digested, or constituents partially absorbed and subsequently excreted in the urine. Undigested enzymes are excreted in the feces. There is no published experience in pregnancy.
Side effects include nausea, vomiting, diarrhea, stomatitis, oral ulceration, rash, urticaria, hyperuricemia, and perianal irritation.

■ **Fetal Considerations** — There are no adequate reports or well-controlled studies in human fetuses. The enzymes are not absorbed in a functional format and pose no risk to the fetus. Rodent studies are reassuring, revealing no evidence of teratogenicity or IUGR despite the use of doses higher than those used clinically.

■ **Breastfeeding Safety** — There is no published experience in nursing women. However, the enzymes are not absorbed systemically and are unlikely to enter human breast milk.

■ **References** — There are no current relevant references.

Pancuronium (Pavulon)

■ **Class** ⋯⋯⋯⋯⋯⋯⋯⋯⋯⋯⋯⋯⋯⋯⋯ *Neuromuscular blocker, nondepolarizing*

■ **Indications** ⋯⋯⋯⋯⋯⋯⋯⋯⋯⋯⋯ Anesthesia, paralysis

■ **Mechanism** ⋯⋯⋯⋯⋯⋯⋯⋯⋯⋯⋯ Blocks acetylcholine motor endplate receptors

■ **Dosage with Qualifiers** ⋯⋯⋯⋯ Paralysis—0.04-0.1mg/kg IV
Paralysis, fetal—0.03mg/kg fetal IM or IV into the umbilical vein
- **Contraindications**—hypersensitivity to drug or class
- **Caution**—hypovolemia, hepatic dysfunction

■ **Maternal Considerations** ⋯⋯⋯ There are no adequate reports or well-controlled studies in pregnant women. **Pancuronium** is approximately 1/3 less potent than **vecuronium**, though its duration is longer at equipotent doses. As compared to **vecuronium, pancuronium** is also vagolytic with accompanying tachycardia; unwanted in some adults but perhaps desired during fetal transfusion. **Magnesium sulfate** enhances the neuromuscular blockade, and reversal may be incomplete. Neuromuscular blockade is reversed by anticholinesterase agents like **pyridostigmine**, **neostigmine**, and **edrophonium**.
Side effects include arrhythmia, hypertension, tachycardia, rash, increased salivation, and pruritus.

■ **Fetal Considerations** ⋯⋯⋯⋯⋯ There are no adequate reports or well-controlled studies in human fetuses. There is minimal transport across the human placenta. **Pancuronium** is often used for fetal paralysis to facilitate intrauterine procedures (0.3-0.6mg IV or IM). Because it increases heart rate, **pancuronium** blunts the normal decline in cardiac output after fetal intravascular transfusion. Fetal paralysis modestly reduces oxygen consumption.

■ **Breastfeeding Safety** ⋯⋯⋯⋯ There is no published experience in nursing women. It is unknown whether **pancuronium** enters human breast milk. However, it is unlikely a significant amount would enter the breast milk given once for the described indications.

■ **References** ⋯⋯⋯⋯⋯⋯⋯⋯⋯⋯⋯ Dailey PA, Fisher DM, Shnider SM, et al. Anesthesiology 1984; 60:569-74.
Higashi T, Kamo N, Naitou H, Tada K. Masui 1996; 45:96-8.

Wilkening RB, Boyle DW, Meschia G. Am J Physiol 1989;
257:H734-8.

■ **Summary** — • **Pregnancy Category C**
• **Lactation Category U**
• **Pancuronium** should be used during pregnancy and lactation only if the benefit justifies the potential perinatal risk.

Pantoprazole (Protonix; Somac)

■ **Class** — *Gastrointestinal, antiulcer, proton pump inhibitor*

■ **Indications** — Erosive esophagitis, hypersecretory conditions

■ **Mechanism** — Inhibits gastric parietal cell hydrogen-potassium ATPase

■ **Dosage with Qualifiers** — Erosive esophagitis—40mg PO qd/bid ×8w; may repeat course followed by maintenance of 40mg/d
Hypersecretory conditions—begin 40mg PO bid; max 240mg qd
NOTE—do not crush, cut, or chew tablet
• **Contraindications**—hypersensitivity to drug or class
• **Caution**—long-term use

■ **Maternal Considerations** — There is no published experience in pregnancy.
Side effects include headache, diarrhea, pancreatitis, blood dyscrasias, hepatic dysfunction, toxic epidermal necrolysis, and erythema multiforme.

■ **Fetal Considerations** — There are no adequate report or well-controlled studies in human fetuses. It is unknown whether **pantoprazole** crosses the human placenta. Rodent studies are reassuring, revealing no evidence of teratogenicity or IUGR despite the use of doses higher than those used clinically.

■ **Breastfeeding Safety** — There is no published experience during lactation. It is unknown whether **pantoprazole** enters human breast milk; it is excreted into rodent milk.

■ **References** — There are no current relevant references.

■ **Summary** — • **Pregnancy Category B**
• **Lactation Category U**
• **Pantoprazole** should be used during pregnancy and lactation only if the benefit justifies the potential perinatal risk.
• There are alternative agents for which there is more experience during pregnancy and lactation.

Pantothenic acid

- ■ **Class** — *Vitamin*

- ■ **Indications** — Supplementation

- ■ **Mechanism** — Unknown

- ■ **Dosage with Qualifiers** — Supplementation—RDA not established
  - **Contraindications**—hypersensitivity to drug or class
  - **Caution**—unknown

- ■ **Maternal Considerations** — **Pantothenic acid** is a water-soluble B vitamin. There are no adequate reports or well-controlled studies of **pantothenic acid** in pregnant women. Its level may decline modestly during pregnancy.
  Side effects are not reported.

- ■ **Fetal Considerations** — There are no adequate reports or well-controlled studies in human fetuses. **Pantothenic acid** is actively transported across the placenta. It is not known whether maternal supplementation increases the fetal concentration. Supplementation reduces the incidence of neural tube defects in mice treated with **valproate**.

- ■ **Breastfeeding Safety** — There are no adequate reports or well-controlled studies in nursing women. **Pantothenic acid** enters human breast milk and the concentration in term milk correlates with maternal serum, dietary intake, and urinary excretion. Maternal serum levels may decline modestly during lactation without supplementation.

- ■ **References** — Sato M, Shirota M, Nagao T. Teratology 1995; 52:143-8.
  Song WO, Wyse BW, Hansen RG. J Am Diet Assoc 1985; 85:192-8.
  Song WO, Chan GM, Wyse BW, Hansen RG. Am J Clin Nutr 1984; 40:317-24.

- ■ **Summary** —
  - **Pregnancy Category A**
  - **Lactation Category S**
  - **Pantothenic** acid is a common component of prenatal vitamins.

Paregoric

■ **Class** .... Antidiarrheal, narcotic

■ **Indications** .... Diarrhea

■ **Mechanism** .... Binds opioid receptors

■ **Dosage with Qualifiers** .... Diarrhea—5-10ml qd/qid prn loose stools
  - **Contraindications**—hypersensitivity to drug or class, hypersensitivity to **morphine**, diarrhea secondary to toxic metal poisoning
  - **Caution**—head injury, abdominal pain of unknown origin

■ **Maternal Considerations** .... **Paregoric** is a mixture of opium powder (anhydrous **morphine**) and **alcohol**. There are no adequate reports or well-controlled studies in pregnant women. It does not delay or inhibit preterm labor. See **morphine**.
Side effects include hypotension, convulsions and supraventricular tachycardia.

■ **Fetal Considerations** .... There are no adequate reports or well-controlled studies in human fetuses. Rodent teratogenicity studies have not been conducted, though the large clinical experience is reassuring. **Paregoric** is used postnatally for the treatment of neonatal withdrawal. See **morphine**.

■ **Breastfeeding Safety** .... There are no adequate reports or well-controlled studies in nursing women. See **morphine**.

■ **References** .... Levy M, Spino M. Pharmacotherapy 1993; 13:202-11.

■ **Summary** ....
  - **Pregnancy Category B**
  - **Lactation Category S**
  - **Paregoric** should be used during pregnancy and lactation only if the benefit justifies the potential perinatal risk.
  - There are alternative agents for which there is more experience during pregnancy and lactation.

Paricalcitol (Zemplar)

- **Class** — Nutritional, calcium metabolism

- **Indications** — Hyperparathyroidism typically secondary to dialysis

- **Mechanism** — Stimulates intestinal calcium and phosphorus absorption, bone mineralization, reduces PTH

- **Dosage with Qualifiers** — Secondary hyperparathyroidism—0.04-0.1mcg/kg IV 3×/w; max 0.24mcg/kg
  - **Contraindications**—hypersensitivity to drug or class, vitamin D toxicity, hypercalcemia
  - **Caution**—none reported

- **Maternal Considerations** — **Paricalcitol** is a synthetic vitamin D analog. There is no published experience in pregnancy.
  Side effects include hypercalcemia, nausea, vomiting, fever, chills, edema, sepsis, light-headedness, pneumonia, GI bleeding, palpitations, and dry mouth.

- **Fetal Considerations** — There are no adequate reports or well-controlled studies in human fetuses. It is unknown whether **paricalcitol** crosses the human placenta. The results of rodent studies are mixed. Sequelae may reflect hypocalcemia rather than the drug.

- **Breastfeeding Safety** — There is no published experience during lactation. It is unknown whether **paricalcitol** enters human breast milk.

- **References** — There are no current relevant references.

- **Summary** —
  - **Pregnancy Category C**
  - **Lactation Category U**
  - **Paricalcitol** should be used during pregnancy and lactation only if the benefit justifies the potential perinatal risk.

Paromomycin (Humatin)

- **Class** — Antibiotic, aminoglycoside, antiprotozoal

- **Indications** — Intestinal amebiasis, management of hepatic coma

- **Mechanism** — Bactericidal—inhibits protein synthesis by binding the bacterial 30S ribosomal subunit

- **Dosage with Qualifiers** .... <u>Intestinal amebiasis</u>—25-35mg/kg/d PO with meals ×5-10d
  <u>Management (adjunctive) of hepatic coma</u>—4g PO tid ×5-6d
  - **Contraindications**—hypersensitivity to drug or class, intestinal obstruction
  - **Caution**—bowel ulcerations

- **Maternal Considerations** .... **Paromomycin** closely parallels **neomycin** and is poorly absorbed orally—nearly 100% is recoverable from the stool. There are no adequate reports or well-controlled studies in pregnant women. A single case report documents the successful treatment of giardiasis.
  Side effects include nausea, vomiting, abdominal cramps, and diarrhea.

- **Fetal Considerations** .... There are no adequate reports or well-controlled studies in human fetuses. It is unknown whether **paromomycin** crosses the human placenta. However, it is unlikely the maternal systemic concentration will reach clinically relevant level.

- **Breastfeeding Safety** .... There are no adequate reports or well-controlled studies in nursing women. It is unknown whether **paromomycin** enters human breast milk. However, it is generally considered compatible with breastfeeding because of the poor oral absorption.

- **References** .... Kreutner AK, Del Bene VE, Amstey MS. Am J Obstet Gynecol 1981; 140:895-901.

- **Summary** ....
  - **Pregnancy Category C**
  - **Lactation Category S**
  - **Paromomycin** should be used during pregnancy and lactation only if the benefit justifies the potential perinatal risk.

Paroxetine (Paxil)

- **Class** .... *Depression*, SSRI

- **Indications** .... Depression, OCD, panic disorder, anxietal disorders, post-traumatic stress, chronic headache, diabetic neuropathy

- **Mechanism** .... Selectively inhibits serotonin reuptake

- **Dosage with Qualifiers** .... <u>Depression</u>—begin 20mg PO qam increasing by 10mg/d qw; max 60mg/d

<u>OCD</u>—begin 20mg PO qam increasing by 10mg/d qw; max 60mg/d

<u>Panic disorder</u>—begin 10mg PO qam increasing by 10mg/d qw; max 60mg/d

<u>Anxietal disorders</u>—begin 20mg PO qam increasing by 10mg/d qw; max 60mg/d

<u>Post-traumatic stress</u>—begin 20mg PO qam increasing by 10mg/d qw; max 60mg/d

<u>Chronic headache</u>—begin 10mg PO qam increasing by 10mg/d qw; max 60mg/d

<u>Diabetic neuropathy</u>—begin 10mg PO qam increasing by 10mg/d qw; max 60mg/d

NOTE—taper gradually

- **Contraindications**—hypersensitivity to drug or class, MAO inhibitor use within 14d, **thioridazine** use
- **Caution**—abrupt withdrawal, mania, history of seizures, hepatic or renal dysfunction, narrow angle glaucoma, suicide risk

■ **Maternal Considerations** .... Depression is common during and after pregnancy, but typically goes unrecognized. Pregnancy is not a reason *apriori* to discontinue psychotropic drugs. There are no adequate reports or well-controlled studies of **paroxetine** in pregnant women. About 2/3 of women taking SSRIs during pregnancy for major depression must increase their dose to maintain efficacy. Women should not feel or be compelled to stop **paroxetine** when they become pregnant. If, after receiving appropriate evidence-based information, she decides to stop, it should be tapered gradually to avoid the abrupt discontinuation syndrome. *Side effects* include serotonin or withdrawal syndromes, extrapyramidal symptoms, mania, seizures, nausea, diarrhea, headache somnolence, dizziness, diarrhea, weakness, constipation, tremor, flatulence, anxiety, sweating, decreased libido, blurred vision, appetite changes, and flushing.

■ **Fetal Considerations** .... There are no adequate reports or well-controlled studies in human fetuses. **Paroxetine** apparently crosses the human placenta since neonatal withdrawal symptoms are documented. Recent epidemiologic studies indicate relative safety. Rodent studies are reassuring, revealing no evidence of teratogenicity or IUGR despite the use of doses higher than those used clinically.

■ **Breastfeeding Safety** .... There are no adequate reports or well-controlled studies in nursing women. **Paroxetine** is excreted into human breast milk with the highest concentrations in the hind milk. However, the levels are variable, and no breast-fed child studied to date has had clinically relevant levels detected.

■ **References** .... Kulin NA, Pastuszak A, Sage SR, et al. JAMA 1998; 279:609-10.

Hostetter A, Stowe ZN, Strader JR Jr, et al. Depress Anxiety 2000; 11:51-7.

747

Nijhuis IJ, Kok-Van Rooij GW, Bosschaart AN. Arch Dis Child Fetal Neonatal Ed 2001; 84:F77.
Rayburn WF, Gonzalez CL, Christensen HD, et al. J Matern Fetal Med 2000; 9:136-41.
Stowe ZN, Cohen LS, Hostetter A, et al. Am J Psychiatry 2000; 157:185-9.

■ **Summary**
- **Pregnancy Category C**
- **Lactation Category S?**
- **Paroxetine** should be used during pregnancy only if the benefit justifies the potential perinatal risk.

Pegfilgrastim (Neulasta)

■ **Class** — *Hematopoeitic agent*

■ **Indications** — Post-chemotherapy neutropenia

■ **Mechanism** — Stimulates granulocyte and macrophage proliferation and differentiation

■ **Dosage with Qualifiers** — Post-chemotherapy neutropena—6mg SC ×1 >24h after chemotherapy completed
NOTE—do not give within 14d of next chemotherapy course
- **Contraindications**—hypersensitivity to drug or class, hypersensitivity to E. *coli* proteins
- **Caution**—myelodysplasia, sickle cell disease, myeloid malignancy

■ **Maternal Considerations** — There is no published experience in pregnancy.
Side effects include thrombocytopenia, splenic rupture, splenomegaly, ARDS, muscular and skeletal pain, headache, abdominal pain, flank pain, elevated LDH or uric acid or alkaline phosphatase, and injection site reaction.

■ **Fetal Considerations** — There are no adequate reports or well-controlled studies in human fetuses. It is unknown whether **pegfilgrastim** crosses the human placenta. Rodent studies reveal increased post implantation resorption and abortion rates and IUGR often at doses in excess of that recommended and in association with maternal toxicity.

■ **Breastfeeding Safety** — There is no published experience during lactation. It is unknown whether **pegfilgrastim** enters human breast milk.

■ **References** — There is no published experience in pregnancy or during lactation.

■ **Summary**

- **Pregnancy Category C**
- **Lactation Category U**
- **Pegfilgrastim** should be used during pregnancy and lactation only if the benefit justifies the potential perinatal risk.

Peginterferon alfa-2b (PEG-Intron)

■ **Class** — *Immunomodulator, antiviral*

■ **Indications** — Hepatitis C

■ **Mechanism** — Inhibits viral replication via multiple antiviral, antiproliferative and immunomodulatory effects

■ **Dosage with Qualifiers** — Chronic hepatitis C—1mg/kg/wk SC ×1y
NOTE—anemia and neutropena dosing; restricted access in U.S.
- **Contraindications**—hypersensitivity to drug or class, autoimmune hepatitis, decompensated hepatic disease
- **Caution**—myelosuppression, diabetes mellitus, psychiatric disorders, thyroid disease, colitis, cardiac or pulmonary disease, ophthalmologic disorders

■ **Maternal Considerations** — Interferons bind to specific cell surface membrane receptors to initiate a complex sequence of intracellular events. Alpha interferons, including **peginterferon alfa-2b**, may cause or aggravate fatal or life-threatening neuropsychiatric, autoimmune, ischemic, and infectious disorders. Patients should be monitored closely with periodic clinical and laboratory evaluations. Therapy should be discontinued in women with persistently severe or worsening signs or symptoms. In many, but not all, instances, these disorders resolve after discontinuation. There is no published experience in pregnancy. Irregular menstrual cycles occurred in cynomolgus monkeys treated SC with doses in multiples of the MRHD.
Side effects include psychosis, suicidal ideation, anemia, neutropenia, thrombocytopenia, thyroid dysfunction, cardiomyopathy, arrhythmias, MI, pancreatitis, retinal thrombosis, retinal hemorrhage, headache, nausea, vomiting, fatigue, rigors, fever, depression, abdominal pain, diarrhea, and injection site reactions.

■ **Fetal Considerations** — There are no adequate reports or well-controlled studies in human fetuses. It is unknown whether **peginterferon alfa-2b** crosses the human placenta. High doses of native interferon alfa-2b were associated with abortion in cynomolgus monkeys.

- **Breastfeeding Safety** — There is no published experience during lactation. It is unknown whether **peginterferon alfa-2b** enters human breast milk. Unlike HIV, breastfeeding is not considered a risk for the newborns of hepatitis C-infected women.

- **References** — There is no published experience in pregnancy or during lactation.

- **Summary** —
  - **Pregnancy Category C**
  - **Lactation Category U**
  - **Peginterferon alfa-2b** should be used during pregnancy and lactation only if the benefit justifies the potential perinatal risk.

Pemirolast ophthalmic (Alamast)

- **Class** — *Allergy; mast cell stabilizer*

- **Indications** — Allergic conjunctivitis

- **Mechanism** — Inhibits mast cell degranulation

- **Dosage with Qualifiers** — Allergic conjunctivitis—1-2 gtt each eye qid for max 4w
  - **Contraindications**—hypersensitivity to drug or class
  - **Caution**—unknown

- **Maternal Considerations** — There is no published experience in pregnancy. **Side effects** include headache, dry eyes, burning or other ocular discomfort, and respiratory symptoms.

- **Fetal Considerations** — There are no adequate reports or well-controlled studies in human fetuses. It is unknown whether **pemirolast** crosses the human placenta. However, considering the dose and route, it is unlikely the maternal systemic concentration would achieve a clinically relevant level. Rodent teratogenicity studies revealed skeletal abnormalities following the systemic administration of doses 20,000 times or more above the MRHD.

- **Breastfeeding Safety** — There is no published experience during lactation. It is unknown whether **pemirolast** enters human breast milk. However, considering the dose and route, it is unlikely the breast-fed neonate will ingest clinically relevant amounts. It is concentrated in rodent milk.

- **References** — There are no current relevant references.

■ **Summary**

- **Pregnancy Category C**
- **Lactation Category S?**
- **Pemirolast** should be used during pregnancy and lactation only if the benefit justifies the potential perinatal risk.

Pemoline (Cylert)

■ **Class** — Anorexiant, stimulant

■ **Indications** — ADHD, narcolepsy

■ **Mechanism** — Stimulates CNS by unknown mechanisms

■ **Dosage with Qualifiers** — ADHD—begin 37.5mg PO qam, increasing by 18.75mg qw; max 112.5mg/d
Narcolepsy—25-100mg PO bid
NOTE—check ALT at baseline and q2w
- **Contraindications**—hypersensitivity to drug or class, hepatic dysfunction, Tourette's syndrome, dependency
- **Caution**—seizure disorder, renal dysfunction

■ **Maternal Considerations** — **Pemoline** has a pharmacological activity similar to other known CNS stimulants; however, it has minimal sympathomimetic effects. There are no adequate reports or well-controlled studies in pregnant women. It has been used to treat narcolepsy during pregnancy.
Side effects include seizures, aplastic anemia, ototoxicity, nausea, vomiting, abdominal pain, headache, rash, insomnia, drowsiness, irritability, Tourette's syndrome, dyskinesia, and elevated LFTs.

■ **Fetal Considerations** — There are no adequate reports or well-controlled studies in human fetuses. It is unknown whether **pemoline** crosses the human placenta. Rodent studies are reassuring, revealing no evidence of teratogenicity or IUGR despite the use of doses higher than those used clinically.

■ **Breastfeeding Safety** — There is no published experience in nursing women. It is unknown whether **pemoline** enters human breast milk.

■ **References** — Hoover-Stevens S, Kovacevic-Ristanovic R. Clin Neuropharmacol 2000; 23:175-81.

■ **Summary**

- **Pregnancy Category B**
- **Lactation Category U**
- **Pemoline** should be used during pregnancy and lactation only if the benefit justifies the potential perinatal risk.

Penbutolol (Levatol)

- **Class** — Antiadrenergic; antihypertensive, β-blocker

- **Indications** — Hypertension

- **Mechanism** — Nonspecific β-adrenergic receptor antagonist

- **Dosage with Qualifiers** — Hypertension—begin 20mg PO qd; max 80mg PO qd
  NOTE—avoid abrupt discontinuation
  - **Contraindications**—hypersensitivity to drug or class, AV block, sinus bradycardia, cardiac insufficiency
  - **Caution**—COPD, diabetes mellitus

- **Maternal Considerations** — Hypertensive disorders complicate 5-10% of pregnancies and are a leading cause of maternal and perinatal morbidity and death. There are no adequate reports or well-controlled studies of **penbutolol** in pregnant women. The free fraction of **penbutolol** increases during pregnancy because of altered protein binding.
  Side effects include nausea, vomiting, diarrhea, abdominal pain, dyspepsia, headache, dizziness, fatigue, URI, CHF, asthenia, insomnia, and sweating.

- **Fetal Considerations** — There are no adequate reports or well-controlled studies in human fetuses. It is unknown whether **penbutolol** crosses the human placenta. Other β-blockers are associated with IUGR and fetal/neonatal bradycardia. The former is dose-dependent and appears to reflect an excessive drop in maternal cardiac output. Other neonatal sequelae associated with β-blockade include hypoglycemia and hyperbilirubinemia. Rodent studies are reassuring, revealing no evidence of teratogenicity or IUGR despite the use of doses higher than those used clinically. Fetal toxicity was noted.

- **Breastfeeding Safety** — There is no published experience in nursing women. It is unknown whether **penbutolol** enters human breast milk.

- **References** — Aquirre C, Rodriguez-Sasiain JM, Navajas P, Calvo R. Eur J Drug Metab Pharmacokinet 1988; 13:23-6.

- **Summary** —
  - **Pregnancy Category C**
  - **Lactation Category U**
  - **Penbutolol** should be used during pregnancy and lactation only if the benefit justifies the potential perinatal risk.
  - There are alternative agents for which there is more experience during pregnancy and lactation.

Penciclovir topical (Denavir)

- **Class** — Antiviral, *dermatologic*

- **Indications** — Herpes labialis

- **Mechanism** — Inhibits DNA polymerase

- **Dosage with Qualifiers** — Herpes labialis—apply q2h ×4d
  - **Contraindications**—hypersensitivity to drug or class
  - **Caution**—immune deficiency

- **Maternal Considerations** — There is no published experience in pregnancy. There is little systemic absorption after topical application. *Side effects* include headache, pruritus, taste changes, and erythema.

- **Fetal Considerations** — There are no adequate reports or well-controlled studies in human fetuses. It is unknown whether **penciclovir** crosses the placenta. However, considering the dose and route, it is unlikely the maternal systemic concentration will reach clinically relevant levels. Rodent studies are reassuring, revealing no evidence of teratogenicity or IUGR despite the use of doses higher than those used clinically.

- **Breastfeeding Safety** — There is no published experience in nursing women. It is unknown whether **penciclovir** enters human breast milk. However, considering the dose and route, it is unlikely the breast-fed neonate would ingest clinically relevant amounts.

- **References** — There is no published experience in pregnancy or during lactation.

- **Summary** —
  - **Pregnancy Category B**
  - **Lactation Category S?**
  - **Penciclovir** should be used during pregnancy only if the benefit justifies the potential perinatal risk.

Penicillamine (Cuprimine; Depen; Mercaptyl)

- **Class** — Antirheumatoid, *Wilson's disease, cystinuria*

- **Indications** — Wilson's disease, cystinuria, rheumatoid arthritis, heavy-metal poisoning

- **Mechanism** — Unknown for arthritis; chelates copper

- **Dosage with Qualifiers** ········ Wilson's disease—250-500mg PO tid/qid 30min before meals
  Cystinuria—250-1000mg PO qid 30min before meals
  Rheumatoid arthritis (unresponsive to conventional agents)—250mg PO bid/tid 30min before meals; requires 3-6mo for max effect
  Heavy-metal poisoning—125-600mg PO tid 30min before meals
    - **Contraindications**—hypersensitivity to drug or class, gold salt, antimalarial or immunosuppressant use, history of **penicillamine**-related anemia
    - **Caution**—renal dysfunction, penicillin allergy

- **Maternal Considerations** ······· There are no adequate reports or well-controlled studies in pregnant women. **Penicillamine** is contraindicated during pregnancy except for the treatment of Wilson's disease and some cases of cystinuria. Zinc induces intestinal cell metallothionein that binds copper and prevents its transfer into blood, may be a suitable adjunct or alternative therapy.
  Side effects include thrombocytopenia, aplastic anemia, agranulocytosis, pancreatitis, exfoliative dermatitis, myasthenia gravis, SLE-like syndrome, rash, pruritus, nausea, vomiting, dyspepsia, proteinuria, glossitis, taste changes, stomatitis, and hirsutism.

- **Fetal Considerations** ············ There are no adequate reports or well-controlled studies in human fetuses. **Penicillamine** apparently crosses the human placenta, since congenital cutis laxa and associated defects are reported in neonates of treated women. **Penicillamine** is teratogenic in rodents at doses 6 times the MRHD. Adverse effects include skeletal deformities, cleft palate, and embryotoxicity.

- **Breastfeeding Safety** ············ There is no published experience in nursing women. It is unknown whether **penicillamine** enters human breast milk.

- **References** ································ Furman B, Bashiri A, Wiznitzer A, et al. Eur J Obstet Gynecol Reprod Biol 2001; 96:232-4.
  Brewer GJ, Johnson VD, Dick RD, et al. Hepatology 2000; 31:364-70.
  Martinez-Frias ML, Rodriguez-Pinilla E, Bermejo E, Blanco M. Am J Med Genet 1998; 76:274-5.

- **Summary** ···································
    - **Pregnancy Category D**
    - **Lactation Category U**
    - **Penicillamine** should be used during pregnancy only if the benefit justifies the potential perinatal risk.
    - It is probably best to avoid breastfeeding.

Penicillin G, aqueous

■ **Class** ⋯⋯⋯⋯⋯⋯⋯⋯⋯⋯⋯⋯⋯⋯ *Antibiotic, penicillin*

■ **Indications** ⋯⋯⋯⋯⋯⋯⋯⋯⋯⋯⋯ Systemic infection (moderate to severe), anthrax

■ **Mechanism** ⋯⋯⋯⋯⋯⋯⋯⋯⋯⋯⋯ Bactericidal—inhibits cell wall mucopeptide synthesis

■ **Dosage with Qualifiers** ⋯⋯⋯ <u>Systemic infection (moderate to severe)</u>—4 million units IM/IV q4h
<u>Anthrax</u>—4million units IV q4h as part of a multidrug regimen ×60d for oral, GI or inhalational; 4 million units IV q4h ×7-10d for cutaneous, then switch to PO for 60d
NOTE—renal dosing
- **Contraindications**—hypersensitivity to drug or class
- **Caution**—renal dysfunction, cephalosporin allergy, seizure disorder

■ **Maternal Considerations** ⋯⋯ Though there is a long clinical experience that is reassuring, there are no adequate reports or well-controlled studies in pregnant women.
Side effects include thrombocytopenia, seizures, Stevens-Johnson syndrome, hemolytic anemia, neutropenia, interstitial nephritis, nausea, vomiting, abdominal pain, diarrhea, rash, fever, and thrombophlebitis.

■ **Fetal Considerations** ⋯⋯⋯⋯ There are no adequate reports or well-controlled studies in human fetuses. Most penicillins cross the human placenta to some extent. Rodent studies are reassuring, revealing no evidence of teratogenicity or IUGR despite the use of doses higher than those used clinically.

■ **Breastfeeding Safety** ⋯⋯⋯⋯ There are no adequate reports or well-controlled studies in nursing women. Only trace amounts of **penicillin G** enter human breast milk. It is generally considered compatible with breastfeeding.

■ **References** ⋯⋯⋯⋯⋯⋯⋯⋯⋯⋯ Matsuda S. Biol Res Pregnancy Perinatol 1984; 5:57-60.

■ **Summary** ⋯⋯⋯⋯⋯⋯⋯⋯⋯⋯⋯
- **Pregnancy Category B**
- **Lactation Category S**
- **Penicillin G** has been used for decades during pregnancy and lactation.
- Though there is little objective study, it is generally considered safe for listed indications.
- **Penicillin** resistance is a growing disadvantage.

Penicillin G, benzathine (Bicillin LA; Pen-Di-Ben; Permapen)

■ **Class** — *Antibiotic, penicillin*

■ **Indications** — Syphilis, group A streptococcus

■ **Mechanism** — Bactericidal—inhibits cell wall mucopeptide synthesis

■ **Dosage with Qualifiers** — Syphilis—2.4 million units IM ×1 if <1y duration, qw ×3 if >1y duration
Group A streptococcus—1.2 million units IM ×1
- **Contraindications**—hypersensitivity to drug or class
- **Caution**—renal dysfunction, cephalosporin allergy, seizure disorder

■ **Maternal Considerations** — There are no adequate reports or well-controlled studies in pregnant women. **Benzathine penicillin** remains the drug of choice for syphilis during pregnancy. There is some concern it may not prevent neurosyphilis, but the overall risk appears low. Partner notification is mandatory to prevent the spread of the disease. About 40% of patients experience a Jarisch-Herxheimer reaction; treated women should be warned of the possibility and monitored closely for the first 48h.
Side effects include thrombocytopenia, seizures, rash, Stevens-Johnson syndrome, fever, hemolytic anemia, neutropenia, interstitial nephritis, nausea, vomiting, abdominal pain, diarrhea, and thrombophlebitis.

■ **Fetal Considerations** — There are no adequate reports or well-controlled studies in human fetuses. Most penicillins cross the human placenta to some extent. The currently recommended dose of **benzathine penicillin** is effective preventing congenital syphilis in most settings, although some additional study regarding dose modification is needed. **Azithromycin** and **ceftriaxone** are potential alternatives for penicillin-allergic women, but there is insufficient data on efficacy, which limits their use in pregnancy. Rodent studies are reassuring, revealing no evidence of teratogenicity or IUGR despite the use of doses higher than those used clinically.

■ **Breastfeeding Safety** — There are no adequate reports or well-controlled studies in nursing women. Only trace amounts of **benzathine penicillin** enter human breast milk. It is generally considered compatible with breastfeeding.

■ **References** — Wendel Jr GD, Sheffield JS, Hollier LM, et al. Clin Infect Dis 2002; 35(Suppl 2):S200-9.
Sheffield JS, Sanchez PJ, Morris G, et al. Am J Obstet Gynecol 2002; 186:569-73.

Myles TD, Elam G, Park-Hwang E, Nguyen T. Obstet Gynecol 1998; 92:859-64.
Watson-Jones D, Gumodoka B, Weiss H, et al. J Infect Dis 2002; 186:948-57.
Matsuda S. Biol Res Pregnancy Perinatol 1984; 5:57-60.

■ **Summary**

- **Pregnancy Category B**
- **Lactation Category S**
- **Benzathine penicillin G** has been used for decades during pregnancy and lactation.
- Though there is little objective study, it is generally considered safe for listed indications.
- It remains the drug of choice for the treatment of syphilis.

Penicillin G, procaine (Wycillin; Crysticillin AS; Duracillin AS; Pfizerpen AS; Provaine Pencillin)

■ **Class** — Antibiotic, penicillin

■ **Indications** — Systemic infection (moderate to severe), pneumococcal pneumonia, gonorrhea

■ **Mechanism** — Bactericidal—inhibits cell wall mucopeptide synthesis

■ **Dosage with Qualifiers** — Systemic infection (moderate to severe)—0.6-1.2million units IM qd
Uncomplicated gonorrhea—4.8million units IM ×1 30min after 1g **probenecid** PO
Pneumococcal pneumonia—0.6-1.2million units IM qd
- **Contraindications**—hypersensitivity to drug or class, IV injection
- **Caution**—renal dysfunction, cephalosporin allergy, seizure disorder

■ **Maternal Considerations** — There are no adequate reports or well-controlled studies in pregnant women. **Penicillin G** may be used in place of **benzathine penicillin** for the treatment of syphilis, but has no advantage.
Side effects include thrombocytopenia, seizures, rash, Stevens-Johnson syndrome, Jarisch-Herxheimer reaction, myocardial depression, hemolytic anemia, neutropenia, interstitial nephritis, nausea, vomiting, abdominal pain, diarrhea, fever, sterile abscess, vasodilation, and thrombophlebitis.

■ **Fetal Considerations** — There are no adequate reports or well-controlled studies in human fetuses. Most penicillins cross the human placenta to some extent. The large clinical experience is reassuring, as are the rodent studies, which reveal no evidence of teratogenicity or IUGR despite the use of doses higher than those used clinically.

■ **Breastfeeding Safety** .... There are no adequate reports or well-controlled studies in nursing women. Only trace amounts of **procaine penicillin G** enter human breast milk. It is generally considered compatible with breastfeeding.

■ **References** .... Paryani SG, Vaughn AJ, Crosby M, Lawrence S. J Pediatr 1994; 125:471-5.
Matsuda S. Biol Res Pregnancy Perinatol 1984; 5:57-60.

■ **Summary** ....
- **Pregnancy Category B**
- **Lactation Category S**
- **Procaine penicillin G** has been used for decades during pregnancy and lactation.
- Though there is little objective study, it is generally considered safe for listed indications.
- Penicillin resistance is a growing disadvantage.

Penicillin VK (Pen-Vee K; Veetids)

■ **Class** .... *Antibiotic, penicillin*

■ **Indications** .... Group A streptococcus, pneumococcal pneumonia or rheumatic fever prophylaxis

■ **Mechanism** .... Bactericidal—inhibits cell wall mucopeptide synthesis

■ **Dosage with Qualifiers** .... Group A streptococcus—250-500mg PO q6-8h ×10d
Pneumococcal pneumonia prophylaxis—250mg PO bid
Rheumatic fever prophylaxis—250mg PO bid
NOTE—to be taken 1h before or 2h after meals
- **Contraindications**—hypersensitivity to drug or class
- **Caution**—renal dysfunction, cephalosporin allergy, seizure disorder, PKU

■ **Maternal Considerations** .... There are no adequate reports or well-controlled studies in pregnant women. However, there is a long clinical experience that is reassuring.
Side effects include thrombocytopenia, seizures, rash, Stevens-Johnson syndrome, hemolytic anemia, neutropenia, interstitial nephritis, nausea, vomiting, abdominal pain, diarrhea, pseudomembranous colitis, and fever.

■ **Fetal Considerations** .... There are no adequate reports or well-controlled studies in human fetuses. Most penicillins cross the human placenta to some extent. The large clinical experience is reassuring, as are the rodent studies, which reveal no evidence of teratogenicity or IUGR despite the use of doses higher than those used clinically.

■ **Breastfeeding Safety** — There are no adequate reports or well-controlled studies in nursing women. Only trace amounts of **penicillin VK** enter human breast milk. It is generally considered compatible with breastfeeding.

■ **References** — Dencker BB, Larsen H, Jensen ES, et al. Clin Microbiol Infect 2002; 8:196-201.
Matsuda S. Biol Res Pregnancy Perinatol 1984; 5:57-60.

■ **Summary** —
- **Pregnancy Category B**
- **Lactation Category S**
- **Penicillin VK** has been used for decades during pregnancy and lactation.
- Though there is little objective study, it is generally considered safe for listed indications.
- Penicillin resistance is a growing disadvantage.

Pentamidine (Nebupent; Pentam 300)

■ **Class** — *Antiprotozoal*

■ **Indications** — PCP prophylaxis and treatment

■ **Mechanism** — Unknown

■ **Dosage with Qualifiers** — PCP prophylaxis—300mg NEB q4wk
PCP treatment—4mg/kg IV/IM qd ×14-21d
- **Contraindications**—hypersensitivity to drug or class
- **Caution**—hepatic or renal dysfunction, hypertension, hypotension, leukopenia, hypoglycemia

■ **Maternal Considerations** — There are no adequate reports or well-controlled studies in pregnant women. Withholding appropriate PCP prophylaxis can adversely affect maternal and fetal outcomes. PCP during pregnancy may have a more aggressive course with increased morbidity and death. Maternal and fetal outcomes are poor. Treatment with **sulfamethoxazole-trimethoprim** may improve outcome compared to other therapies. Aerosolized **pentamidine** does not appear to pose a significant risk to pregnant health care workers.
Side effects include renal failure, leukopenia, thrombocytopenia, hypoglycemia, Stevens-Johnson syndrome, bronchospasm, fatigue, nausea, dyspepsia, decreased appetite, fever, rash, cough, and dizziness.

- **Fetal Considerations** ⸻ There are no adequate reports or well-controlled studies in human fetuses. There are no published human reports of concern, and human placental transport of **pentamidine** across the isolated cotyledon is limited. **Pentamidine** crosses the rodent placenta and penetrates all fetal compartments. Rodent studies are in general reassuring, revealing embryotoxicity but no teratogenicity or IUGR.

- **Breastfeeding Safety** ⸻ There is no published experience in nursing women. It is unknown whether **pentamidine** enters human breast milk. Breastfeeding is contraindicated in HIV-infected nursing women where formula is available to reduce the risk of neonatal transmission.

- **References** ⸻ Ahmad H, Mehta NJ, Manikal VM, et al. Chest 2001; 120:666-71.
Ito S, Koren G. Chest 1994; 106:1460-2.
Fortunato SJ, Bawdon RE. Am J Obstet Gynecol 1989; 160:759-61.
Little BB, Harstad TH, Bawdon RE, et al. Am J Obstet Gynecol 1991; 164:927-30.
Harstad TW, Little BB, Bawdon RE, et al. Am J Obstet Gynecol 1990; 163:912-6.

- **Summary** ⸻
  - **Pregnancy Category C**
  - **Lactation Category NS**
  - **Pentamidine** should be used during pregnancy and lactation only if the benefit justifies the potential perinatal risk.
  - Withholding appropriate PCP prophylaxis can adversely affect maternal and fetal outcomes.

Pentazocine (Talwin)

- **Class** ⸻ Analgesic; *narcotic agonist-antagonist*

- **Indications** ⸻ Moderate to severe pain, obstetric analgesia, anesthesia adjunct

- **Mechanism** ⸻ Binds opiate receptors producing both agonist and antagonist effects

- **Dosage with Qualifiers** ⸻ Moderate to severe pain—30mg IM/IV/SC q3-4h prn; max 60mg/dose
Obstetric analgesia—20mg IV (or 30mg IM) q2-4h prn
Anesthesia adjunct—20mg IV (or 30mg IM) q2-4h prn
NOTE—SC injections may cause severe tissue damage and are best avoided.

- **Contraindications**—hypersensitivity to drug or class
- **Caution**—opiate dependence, head injury, hepatic or renal or pulmonary dysfunction, post MI

■ **Maternal Considerations** ········ **Pentazocine** is a potent analgesic; 30-45mg is equianalgesic to **morphine** 10mg and **meperidine** 75-100mg. There are no adequate reports or well-controlled studies in pregnant women. **Pentazocine** is a poor choice for labor analgesia because of greater maternal respiratory depression than the alternatives. Some patients receiving narcotics, including **methadone** experience withdrawal symptoms since **pentazocine** is a weak narcotic antagonist. *Side effects* include addiction, respiratory depression, hypotension, seizures, granulocytopenia, nausea, vomiting, dizziness, euphoria, hallucinations, sedation, headache, constipation, blurred vision, miosis, tremor, irritability, facial edema, flushing, and pruritus.

■ **Fetal Considerations** ············· There are no adequate reports or well-controlled studies in human fetuses. **Pentazocine** crosses the human placenta. The addictive combination of **pentazocine** and **tripelennamine** (T's and blues) remains popular in some locales. Infants of women who use T's and blues throughout pregnancy have similar interactive deficits and withdrawal as **methadone**-addicted newborns. In general, rodent studies are reassuring, revealing no evidence of teratogenicity or IUGR despite the use of doses higher than those used clinically. A single study in hamsters suggested an increased risk of CNS malformations.

■ **Breastfeeding Safety** ············· There is no published experience in nursing women. While it is unknown whether **pentazocine** enters human breast milk, the clinical experience is reassuring.

■ **References** ························· Wahab SA, Askalani AH, Amar RA, et al. Int J Gynaecol Obstet 1988; 26:75-80.
Chasnoff IJ, Hatcher R, Burns WJ, Schnoll SH. Dev Pharmacol Ther 1983; 6:162-9.
Geber WF, Schramm LC. Am J Obstet Gynecol 1975; 123:705-13.

■ **Summary** ·························
- **Pregnancy Category C**
- **Lactation Category U**
- **Pentazocine** should be used during pregnancy and lactation only if the benefit justifies the potential perinatal risk.
- There are less addictive but equally effective analgesics available for most indications.

Pentobarbital (Carbrital; Nembutal)

■ **Class** ---- *Barbiturate, anticonvulsant, sedative, anxiolytic*

■ **Indications** ---- Sedation, insomnia, barbiturate coma

■ **Mechanism** ---- Depresses the sensory and motor cortex and alters cerebellar function

■ **Dosage with Qualifiers** ---- Sedation—20-40mg PO bid/qid
Insomnia—100mg PO qhs prn for short-term therapy
Barbiturate coma—load with 5mg/kg over 30min then 1-3mg/kg/h IV; systemic arterial BP must be supported (e.g., inotropic support)
- **Contraindications**—hypersensitivity to drug or class, decreased respiratory function, porphyria
- **Caution**—hepatic dysfunction, history of substance abuse, suicidal ideation

■ **Maternal Considerations** ---- Barbiturates produce CNS mood alteration ranging from excitation to sedation, to hypnosis, and deep coma. As a sleep aid, barbiturates are of limited value beyond the short-term as they lose effectiveness after 1-2w. There are superior agents that have less effect on the sleep cycle. There are no adequate reports or well-controlled studies in pregnant women. Hypnotic doses do not impair uterine activity during labor.
Side effects include addiction, respiratory depression, Stevens-Johnson syndrome, SLE, angioedema, confusion, agitation, hyperkinesias, ataxia, CNS depression, hallucinations, dizziness, apnea, bradycardia, hypotension, syncope, nausea, vomiting, constipation, and headache.

■ **Fetal Considerations** ---- There are no adequate reports or well-controlled studies in human fetuses. **Pentobarbital** rapidly crosses the human placenta. The highest concentrations are found in placenta, liver, and brain. Its administration during labor can cause neonatal respiratory depression. Preterm infants are particularly susceptible, and resuscitation equipment should be available. Chronic use during the 3rd trimester can yield addicted neonates who have an extended withdrawal syndrome. Retrospective, case-controlled studies suggest a connection between barbiturates and an increased risk of fetal abnormalities. However, there are no such reports specifically for **pentobarbital**, and the rodent studies are reassuring. There is a single study suggesting a reduction in fertility.

■ **Breastfeeding Safety** ---- There are no adequate reports or well-controlled studies in nursing women. Only small amounts of **pentobarbital** enter human breast milk, and it is generally considered compatible with breastfeeding.

- **References** .... Ito T, Ingalls TH. Arch Environ Health 1981; 36:316-20.

- **Summary** ....
  - **Pregnancy Category D**
  - **Lactation Category S**
  - **Pentobarbital** should be used during pregnancy and lactation only if the benefit justifies the potential perinatal risk.
  - For all but coma, there are other agents with superior safety profiles during pregnancy.

Pentosan polysulfate sodium (Elmiron)

- **Class** .... *Other, genitourinary*

- **Indications** .... Interstitial cystitis

- **Mechanism** .... Unknown

- **Dosage with Qualifiers** .... Interstitial cystitis—100mg PO tid 1h before or 2h after meals
  - **Contraindications**—hypersensitivity to drug or class
  - **Caution**—hepatic or splenic disorders

- **Maternal Considerations** .... There is no published experience in pregnancy. *Side effects* include hepatotoxicity, diarrhea, nausea, vomiting, headache, dyspepsia, abdominal pain, dizziness, depression, alopecia, and elevated LFTs.

- **Fetal Considerations** .... There are no adequate reports or well-controlled studies in human fetuses. **Pentosan** does not appear to cross the human placenta and should pose little risk during pregnancy.

- **Breastfeeding Safety** .... There are no published studies in nursing women. It is unknown whether **pentosan polysulfate** enters human breast milk.

- **References** .... Forestier F, Fischer AM, Daffos F, et al. Thromb Haemost 1986; 56:247-9.

- **Summary** ....
  - **Pregnancy Category B**
  - **Lactation Category U**
  - **Pentosan polysulfate** should be used during pregnancy and lactation only if the benefit justifies the potential perinatal risk.

Pentostatin (Nipent)

■ **Class** Antineoplastic, antimetabolite

■ **Indications** Hairy cell leukemia

■ **Mechanism** Inhibits adenosine deaminase

■ **Dosage with Qualifiers** Hairy cell leukemia—4mg/m² IV qw
- **Contraindications**—hypersensitivity to drug or class, concomitant **fludarabine** use
- **Caution**—active infection, renal dysfunction

■ **Maternal Considerations** There is no published experience in pregnancy. *Side effects* include nausea, vomiting, arrhythmia, hemorrhage, leukopenia, thrombocytopenia, fatigue, anorexia, diarrhea, headache, rash, bronchitis, fever, chills, hematuria, and somnolence.

■ **Fetal Considerations** There are no adequate reports or well-controlled studies in human fetuses. It is unknown whether **pentostatin** crosses the human placenta. The developing mouse allantois is quite sensitive to **pentostatin**, and interference with allantois development leads to embryo lethality. Late exposure in rodent pregnancy is associated with neural tube, craniofacial, and limb defects.

■ **Breastfeeding Safety** There is no published experience during lactation. It is unknown whether **pentostatin** enters human breast milk.

■ **References** Airhart MJ, Robbins CM, Knudsen TB, et al. Teratology 1996; 53:361-73.
Airhart MJ, Robbins CM, Knudsen TB, et al. Teratology 1993; 47:17-27.

■ **Summary**
- **Pregnancy Category D**
- **Lactation Category U**
- **Pentostatin** should be used during pregnancy and lactation only if the benefit justifies the potential perinatal risk.

Pentoxifylline (Ebisanin; Sipental; Techlon; Trental)

- **Class** — *Other hematologic*

- **Indications** — Claudication

- **Mechanism** — Decreases blood viscosity, improves RBC membrane flexibility

- **Dosage with Qualifiers** — Claudication—400mg PO tid with meals
  - **Contraindications**—hypersensitivity to drug or class, methylxanthine intolerance
  - **Caution**—recent retinal or cerebral hemorrhage

- **Maternal Considerations** — **Pentoxifylline** and its metabolites improve the flow properties of blood by decreasing viscosity. It is used with **tocopherol** to treat IVF patients with a thin endometrium. It also enhances sperm motility prior to IVF or IUI. In rodents, long-term use is associated with the development of mammary fibroadenomas. There are no adequate reports or well-controlled studies during pregnancy. Clearance is unaltered by pregnancy.
  Side effects include arrhythmia, angina, nausea, vomiting, diarrhea, dyspepsia, dizziness, headache, insomnia, blurred vision, drowsiness, and agitation.

- **Fetal Considerations** — There are no adequate reports or well-controlled studies in human fetuses. It is unknown whether **pentoxifylline** crosses the human placenta. Rodent studies are reassuring, revealing no evidence of teratogenicity or IUGR despite the use of doses higher than those used clinically. Embryo toxicity was noted.

- **Breastfeeding Safety** — There are no adequate reports or well-controlled studies in nursing women. **Pentoxifylline** enters human breast milk achieving near unity with maternal plasma. It is perhaps wise to avoid **pentoxifylline** while breastfeeding because of its association with mammary fibroadenomas in rodents.

- **References** — Boiko SS, Zherdev VP, Vikhliaeva EM, Supriaga OM. Eksp Klin Farmakol 1992; 55:52-5.
  Ledee-Bataille N, Olivennes F, Lefaix JL, et al. Hum Reprod 2002; 17:1249-53.
  Terriou P, Hans E, Giorgetti C, et al. J Assist Reprod Genet 2000; 17:194-9.
  Witter FR, Smith RV. Am J Obstet Gynecol 1985; 151:1094-7.

- **Summary**
  - **Pregnancy Category C**
  - **Lactation Category NS?**
  - **Pentoxifylline** should be used during pregnancy only if the benefit justifies the potential perinatal risk.
  - There is no published experience during pregnancy except in infertility patients.

Pergolide mesylate (Permax)

■ **Class** .... Antiparkinsonism; dermatologics; ergot alkaloids and derivatives

■ **Indications** .... Parkinsonism

■ **Mechanism** .... Dopamine receptor (1 and 2) agonist

■ **Dosage with Qualifiers** .... Parkinsonism—0.05mg qd ×2d when used as an adjunct with **levodopa** or **carbidopa**, increase by 0.1mg/d q3d ×12; then 0.25mg q3d ×12d then adjust; max dose 3.5mg/d) max 5mg/d
   • **Contraindications**—hypersensitivity to drug or class
   • **Caution**—unknown

■ **Maternal Considerations** .... **Pergolide** is effective primary treatment for pituitary macroprolactinomas. It is 10-1000 times more potent a dopamine agonist than **bromocriptine**. There are no adequate reports or well-controlled studies in pregnant women.
Side effects include ventricular arrhythmia, MI, hypotension, nausea, vomiting, dyskinesia, rhinitis, confusion, dizziness, somnolence, hallucinations, diarrhea, dyspepsia, tremor, syncope, and anemia.

■ **Fetal Considerations** .... There are no adequate reports or well-controlled studies in human fetuses. It is unknown whether **pergolide** crosses the human placenta. Rodent studies are reassuring, revealing no evidence of teratogenicity or IUGR despite the use of doses higher than those used clinically.

■ **Breastfeeding Safety** .... There is no published experience in nursing women. It is unknown whether **pergolide** enters human breast milk. The pharmacologic action of **pergolide** suggests it may interfere with lactation, and thus should be avoided at least until the milk reflex is well established.

■ **References** .... Orrego JJ, Chandler WF, Barkan AL. Pituitary 2000; 3:251-6.

■ **Summary** ....
   • **Pregnancy Category B**
   • **Lactation Category U**
   • **Pergolide** should be used during pregnancy and lactation only if the benefit justifies the potential perinatal risk.

Perindopril erbumine (Aceon)

■ **Class**	Antihypertensive, ACE-1/A2R-antagonist
■ **Indications**	Hypertension, CHF
■ **Mechanism**	ACE inhibitor
■ **Dosage with Qualifiers**	Hypertension—begin 4mg PO qd; max 16mg/d CHF—begin 2mg PO qd NOTE—renal dosing; lower dose if on a diuretic • **Contraindications**—hypersensitivity to drug or class, history of ACEI angioedema or idiopathic angioedema • **Caution**—renal dysfunction, renal artery stenosis, severe CHF, collagen vascular disease, volume depletion, hyponatremia, pregnancy
■ **Maternal Considerations**	There is no published experience with **perindopril** during pregnancy. The lowest dose effective should be used when it is required during pregnancy for pressure control. *Side effects* include fetal or neonatal death, angioedema, hypotension, renal failure, hyperkalemia, neutropena, agranulocytosis, pancreatitis, cough, nausea, vomiting, musculoskeletal pains, dizziness, fatigue, and elevated BUN/Cr.
■ **Fetal Considerations**	There are no adequate reports or well-controlled studies in human fetuses. It is unknown whether **perindopril** crosses the human placenta. Inhibitors of the renin angiotensin system cross the human placenta. No adverse fetal effects are reported after 1st trimester exposure. Subsequent exposure to other inhibitors is associated with cranial hypoplasia, anuria, reversible or irreversible renal failure, death, oligohydramnios, prematurity, IUGR, and patent ductus arteriosus. There is no reason to expect **perindopril** is different.
■ **Breastfeeding Safety**	There is no published experience in nursing women. It is unknown whether **perindopril** enters human breast milk.
■ **References**	Moulin B, Morin JP, Seurin-Toutain P, et al. Int J Tissue React 1990; 12:309-17.
■ **Summary**	• **Pregnancy Category C (1st trimester), D (2nd and 3rd trimesters)** • **Lactation Category U** • **Perindopril** and other inhibitors of the renin angiotensin system should be avoided during pregnancy if possible. • There are alternative agents for which there is more experience during pregnancy and lactation. • When the mother's disease requires treatment with **perindopril**, the lowest dose should be used and coupled with close monitoring of the fetus.

Permethrin topical (Elimite; Nix)

■ **Class**	*Dermatologic, antiparasitic*
■ **Indications**	Scabies
■ **Mechanism**	Disrupts nerve cell sodium channel currents in parasite
■ **Dosage with Qualifiers**	Scabies—massage into skin from head to toe, allow to remain 8-14h before bathing • **Contraindications**—hypersensitivity to drug or class • **Caution**—unknown
■ **Maternal Considerations**	**Permethrin** is rapidly metabolized by to inactive metabolites that are excreted primarily in the urine. Although the amount of **permethrin** absorbed after a single application has not been precisely determined, preliminary study suggests it is less than 2% of the amount applied. There are no adequate reports or well-controlled studies in pregnant women. Published experience is limited to case reports and reviews. *Side effects* include burning, numbness, tingling, pruritus, and erythema.
■ **Fetal Considerations**	There are no adequate reports or well-controlled studies in human fetuses. It is unknown whether **permethrin** crosses the human placenta. It is unlikely the maternal systemic concentration reaches a clinically relevant level. Rodent studies are reassuring, revealing no evidence of teratogenicity or IUGR despite the use of doses higher than those used clinically.
■ **Breastfeeding Safety**	There are no adequate reports or well-controlled studies in nursing women. It is unknown whether **permethrin** enters human breast milk. Considering the route and frequency of use, it is unlikely the maternal clinically relevant systemic concentration will be reached and sustained.
■ **References**	Judge MR, Kobza-Black A. Br J Dermatol 1995; 132:116-9. Imamura L, Hasegawa H, Kurashina K, et al. Arch Toxicol 2002; 76:392-7.
■ **Summary**	• **Pregnancy Category B** • **Lactation Category S?** • **Permethrin topical** should be used during pregnancy and lactation only if the benefit justifies the potential perinatal risk. • A long clinical experience is reassuring.

Perphenazine (Trilifan; Trilafon)

■ **Class** .... Antipsychotic; antiemetic/antivertigo; phenothiazine

■ **Indications** .... Psychosis, severe nausea and vomiting

■ **Mechanism** .... Unknown; antagonizes D_2 receptors

■ **Dosage with Qualifiers** .... Psychosis—8-16mg PO bid/qid; max 64mg/d
Severe nausea and vomiting—begin 5mg IM or PO
(avoid IV); max 24mg/d
- **Contraindications**—hypersensitivity to drug or class,
  CNS depression, blood dyscrasias, bone marrow
  depression, hepatic disease, coma, subcortical damage
- **Caution**—unknown

■ **Maternal Considerations** .... **Perphenazine** increases circulating prolactin levels in
both humans and rodents. There are no adequate reports
or well-controlled studies in pregnant women.
Side effects include cardiac arrest, tachycardia, seizures,
hepatotoxicity, hemolytic anemia, agranulocytosis,
thrombocytopenia, neuroleptic malignant syndrome,
extrapyramidal effects, tardive dyskinesia, sedation,
drowsiness, dry mouth, blurred vision, nausea, vomiting,
rash, and anorexia.

■ **Fetal Considerations** .... There are no adequate reports or well-controlled studies
in human fetuses. It is unknown whether **perphenazine**
crosses the human placenta. However, peroxidative
bioactivation of **perphenazine** by human placental
peroxidase occurs and may be one mechanism of the
reported toxicity of other phenothiazines. Postnatal
behavioral abnormalities are suggested. Rodent
teratogenicity studies have apparently not been
conducted.

■ **Breastfeeding Safety** .... There is no published experience in nursing women. It is
unknown whether **perphenazine** enters human breast milk.

■ **References** .... Yang X, Kulkarni AP. Teratog Carcinog Mutagen 1997;
17:139-51.
Handal M, Matheson I, Bechensteen AG, Lindemann R.
Tidsskr Nor Laegeforen 1995; 115:2539-40.

■ **Summary** ....
- **Pregnancy Category C**
- **Lactation Category U**
- **Perphenazine** should be used during pregnancy and
  lactation only if the benefit justifies the potential
  perinatal risk.
- There are alternative agents for which there is more
  experience regarding use during pregnancy and lactation.

Phenacemide (Phenurone)

- **Class** .... Anticonvulsant

- **Indications** .... Seizures

- **Mechanism** .... Unknown; elevates seizure threshold

- **Dosage with Qualifiers** .... Seizures (complex partial resistant to other drugs)—begin 500mg PO tid ×7d before adjusting; usual dose 2-3g/d
  NOTE—Measure hepatic transaminases and a CBC before and periodically during therapy; *the total number of each cell type per mm³ is a better index of a possible blood dyscrasia than the % of cells.* Marked depression of the blood count is an indication for withdrawal.
  - **Contraindications**—hypersensitivity to drug or class, blood dyscrasias
  - **Caution**—personality disorder, suicidal ideation, hepatic dysfunction, allergy

- **Maternal Considerations** .... There are no adequate reports or well-controlled studies in pregnant women. Mouse studies reveal synergy when **phenacemide** is administered with either **mephenytoin**, **phenobarbital**, or **trimethadione**.
  Side effects include personality changes, hepatotoxicity, nephritis, aplastic anemia, death, neutropenia, loss of interest, depression, aggressiveness, sore throat, fever, malaise, blood dyscrasia, anorexia, weight loss, rash, Stevens-Johnson syndrome, fatigue, fever, muscle pain, elevated creatinine, and palpitations.

- **Fetal Considerations** .... There are no adequate reports or well-controlled studies in human fetuses. It is unknown whether **phenacemide** crosses the human placenta. While it is difficult to separate the possible teratogenic effects from the anticonvulsant agents used concurrently, limited rodent study suggests **phenacemide** is a teratogen.

- **Breastfeeding Safety** .... There is no published experience in nursing women. It is unknown whether **phenacemide** enters human breast milk.

- **References** .... Fabro S, Shull G, Brown NA. Teratog Carcinog Mutagen 1982; 2:61-76.

- **Summary** ....
  - **Pregnancy Category D**
  - **Lactation Category U**
  - **Phenacemide** should be used during pregnancy and lactation only if the benefit justifies the potential perinatal risk.
  - There are alternative agents with a superior safety profile for which there is more experience during pregnancy and lactation.

Phenazopyridine (Azo-Standard; Eridium; Geridium; Phenazodine; Pyridiate; Pyridium; Ro-Pyridine; Urodine; Urodol; Uropyridine; Viridium)

- **Class** — *Analgesic, non-narcotic; other genitourinary*

- **Indications** — Dysuria

- **Mechanism** — Unknown

- **Dosage with Qualifiers** — Dysuria—100-200mg PO tid pc ×2d
  NOTE—turns urine red/orange; may be combined with **sulfamethoxazole** (Azo-Gantanol) or **sulfisoxazole** (Azo-Gantrisin; Azo-Sulfisoxazole; Azo-Truxazole; Sul-Azo)
  - **Contraindications**—hypersensitivity to drug or class, renal insufficiency, uremia, hepatitis, glomerulonephritis, pyelonephritis during pregnancy
  - **Caution**—unknown

- **Maternal Considerations** — **Phenazopyridine** has a topical analgesic effect on urinary tract mucosa, helping to relieve pain, burning, urgency and frequency. There are no adequate reports or well-controlled studies in pregnant women.
  Side effects include anemia, headache, nausea, vomiting, dyspepsia, pruritus, and stained contact lenses.

- **Fetal Considerations** — There are no adequate reports or well-controlled studies in human fetuses. **Phenazopyridine** crosses the human placenta. Rodent studies are reassuring, revealing no evidence of teratogenicity or IUGR despite the use of doses higher than those used clinically.

- **Breastfeeding Safety** — There are no adequate reports or well-controlled studies in nursing women. It is unknown whether **phenazopyridine** enters human breast milk. However, it is generally considered compatible with breastfeeding based on long clinical experience.

- **References** — Meyer BA, Gonik B, Creasy RK. Am J Perinatol 1991; 8:297-9.

- **Summary** —
  - **Pregnancy Category B**
  - **Lactation Category S**
  - **Phenazopyridine** has been used for decades during pregnancy and lactation.
  - Though there is little objective study, it is generally considered safe for listed indications.

Phendimetrazine (Adipost; Anorex; Appecon; Bontril; Cam-Metrazine; Dital; Melfiat; Metra; Obalan; Obezine; P.D.M.; Phenazine; Phendiet; Phendimetrazine Bitartrate; Plegine; Prelu-2; PT 105; Statobex; X-Trozine)

■ **Class** — *Anorexiant, stimulant*

■ **Indications** — Obesity

■ **Mechanism** — CNS stimulant

■ **Dosage with Qualifiers** — Obesity—35mg PO bid-tid; individualize to the lowest effective dose
NOTE—for short-term use only coupled to calorie restriction; tolerance occurs within weeks
- **Contraindications**—hypersensitivity to drug or class, substance abuse, advanced arteriosclerosis, symptomatic cardiovascular disease, moderate or severe hypertension, hyperthyroidism, glaucoma, ingestion of other CNS stimulants, agitation
- **Caution**—mild hypertension, diabetes mellitus

■ **Maternal Considerations** — **Phendimetrazine** is a phenylalkylamine sympathomimetic with pharmacologic activity similar to **amphetamine**. Obese adult patients given dietary instruction and treated with "anorectic" drugs lose a fraction of a pound a week more during short-term trials compared to those treated with placebo and diet. There is no published experience in pregnancy, and no indications for its use.
Side effects include restlessness, insomnia, agitation, flushing, tremor, sweating, dizziness, headache, psychosis, blurred vision, tachycardia, hypertension, dry mouth, nausea, diarrhea, constipation, stomach pain, urinary frequency, dysuria, and libido change.

■ **Fetal Considerations** — There are no adequate reports or well-controlled studies in human fetuses. It is unknown whether **phendimetrazine** crosses the human placenta. Similar compounds do. Rodent teratogenicity studies have apparently not been performed.

■ **Breastfeeding Safety** — There are no published studies in nursing women. It is unknown whether **phendimetrazine** enters human breast milk.

■ **References** — There is no published experience in pregnancy or during lactation.

■ **Summary** —————————————
- **Pregnancy Category C**
- **Lactation Category U**
- There are no indications for the use of **phendimetrazine** during pregnancy and lactation.
- **Phendimetrazine** is of limited value for the treatment of obesity in nonpregnant women.

Phenelzine (Nardil)

■ **Class** —————————————— *Antidepressant, MAO inhibitor*

■ **Indications** ———————————— Depression, bulimia

■ **Mechanism** ————————————— Inhibits monoamine oxidase

■ **Dosage with Qualifiers** ————— Depression—15mg PO tid; response may take at least 4w
Bulimia—begin 15mg PO tid; max 30mg PO tid
NOTE—wait >4w after stopping an SSRI before initiating
- **Contraindications**—hypersensitivity to drug or class, CHF, hypertension, pheochromocytoma, hepatic disease, general anesthesia or **cocaine** use within 10d, **bupropion** use
- **Caution**—unknown

■ **Maternal Considerations** ———— Depression is common during and after pregnancy, but typically goes unrecognized. Pregnancy is not a reason *apriori* to discontinue psychotropic drugs. **Phenelzine** is often effective in treating depression characterized as atypical, nonendogenous, or neurotic. These patients frequently have anxiety and depression mixed with phobic or hypochondriacal features. There are no adequate reports or well-controlled studies of **phenelzine** in pregnant women. Most publications consist of case reports or small series. Many drugs interact with MAO inhibitors. Well-documented and potentially fatal interactions between MAO inhibitors and opioids, notably **meperidine**, require that labor analgesia be well planned in advance. Pressor agents should be avoided as even indirect-acting drugs can produce severe hypertension. *Side effects* include hypertensive crisis, intracranial hemorrhage, seizures, hypermetabolic syndrome, hypomania, respiratory or CNS depression, coma, leukopenia, SLE-like syndrome, headache, dizziness, weakness, tremor, constipation, dry mouth, dyspepsia, elevated LFTs, weight gain, orthostatic hypotension, hyperreflexia, nystagmus, and edema.

■ **Fetal Considerations** ————— There are no adequate reports or well-controlled studies in human fetuses. It is unknown whether **phenelzine** crosses the human placenta. As for most psychotropic drugs, monotherapy and the smallest effective quantity given in divided doses to may reduce risk by minimizing the systemic peaks. Rodent teratogenicity studies have apparently not been performed.

- **Breastfeeding Safety** — There is no published experience in nursing women. It is unknown whether **phenelzine** enters human breast milk.

- **References** — Gracious BL, Wisner KL. Depress Anxiety 1997; 6:124-8. Pavy TJ, Kliffer AP, Douglas MJ. Can J Anaesth 1995; 42:618-20.

- **Summary**
  - **Pregnancy Category C**
  - **Lactation Category U**
  - **Phenelzine** should be used during pregnancy and lactation only if the benefit justifies the potential perinatal risk.

Phenobarbital (Barbita; Dormiral; Luminal Sodium; Luminaletten; Phenobarbital Sodium; Phenobarbitone; Sedofen; Solfoton)

- **Class** — *Anticonvulsant, barbiturate*

- **Indications** — Seizure disorder, status epilepticus, sedation

- **Mechanism** — Nonselective CNS depressant of the sensory cortex, motor activity, and alters cerebellar function

- **Dosage with Qualifiers** — Seizure disorder—load with 15-20mg/kg IV, then 60mg PO bid/tid
  Status epilepticus—10-20mg/kg IV ×1; may repeat if necessary
  Sedation—10-40mg PO/IM/IV tid
  NOTE—avoid abrupt withdrawal; may be combined with **phenytoin** or **belladona** or **ergotrate**
  - **Contraindications**—hypersensitivity to drug or class, history of porphyria, hepatic or respiratory dysfunction
  - **Caution**—uremia, depression or suicidal ideation

- **Maternal Considerations** — Less time is spent in REM during barbiturate-induced sleep compared to normal sleep. Abrupt cessation may trigger increased dreaming, nightmares, and/or insomnia. Barbiturates provide little analgesia at subanesthetic doses; in fact, they may increase the reaction to painful stimuli. There are no adequate reports or well-controlled studies in pregnant women. Several investigations indicate clearance is increased and that periodic dose adjustment may be necessary. All adjustments should be guided by clinical symptoms. **Phenobarbital** is not effective for the treatment of cholestasis of pregnancy. Planned pregnancy and counseling before conception are crucial. It is important to discuss folic acid supplementation, medication adherence, the risk of teratogenicity, and the importance of prenatal care.

Side effects include respiratory depression, habituation, erythema multiforme, Stevens-Johnson syndrome, hepatitis, angioedema, megaloblastic anemia, blood dyscrasias, TTP, drowsiness, lethargy, nausea, vomiting, rash, urticaria, pain, necrosis, thrombophlebitis, swelling, and necrosis.

■ **Fetal Considerations**

There are no adequate reports or well-controlled studies in human fetuses. Barbiturates readily cross the human placental barrier and are distributed throughout fetal tissues, with highest concentration found in the placenta, fetal liver, and brain. The F:M ratio approximates unity. Withdrawal symptoms can occur in neonates exposed to barbiturates throughout the 3rd trimester. Case-controlled studies suggest a relationship between barbiturate use and a higher than expected incidence of birth defects (oral clefting and cardiac malformations). Antenatal **phenobarbital** exposure does not affect the neurodevelopmental outcome of preterm infants at 18-22mo of age. It also does not reduce the risk of neonatal IVH.

■ **Breastfeeding Safety**

Phenobarbital enters human breast milk, and the magnitude is altered by polypharmacy especially early in breastfeeding. Breastfeeding is controversial because of the potential for slow elimination by some neonates. Infant sedation is possible, and the infant should be observed closely. Serum monitoring may be advisable if **phenobarbital** is continued during breastfeeding.

■ **References**

Gomita Y, Furuno K, Araki Y, et al. Am J Ther 1995; 2:968-971.

Jenkins JK, Boothby LA. Ann Pharmacother 2002; 36:1462-5.

Dessens AB, Cohen-Kettenis PT, Mellenbergh GJ, et al. Teratology 2001; 64:181-8.

Arpino C, Brescianini S, Robert E, et al. Epilepsia 2000; 41:1436-43.

Shankaran S, Papile LA, Wright LL, et al. Am J Obstet Gynecol 2002; 187:171-7.

Crowther CA, Henderson-Smart DJ. Cochrane Database Syst Rev 2001; (2):CD000164.

Bar-Oz B, Nulman I, Koren G, Ito S. Paediatr Drugs 2000; 2:113-26.

Kuhnz W, Koch S, Helge H, Nau H. Dev Pharmacol Ther 1988; 11:147-54.

■ **Summary**

- **Pregnancy Category D**
- **Lactation Category S?**
- **Phenobarbital** should be used during pregnancy and lactation only if the benefit justifies the potential perinatal risk.

Phenoxybenzamine (Dibenzyline)

■ **Class** ————————————————— *Other antihypertensive, α-adrenergic antagonist*

■ **Indications** ————————————— Pheochromocytoma

■ **Mechanism** ————————————— Nonspecific α antagonist

■ **Dosage with Qualifiers** ————— Pheochromocytoma—begin 10mg PO bid, increasing by
10mg qod until target BP achieved
- **Contraindications**—hypersensitivity to drug or class
- **Caution**—renal dysfunction, CAD

■ **Maternal Considerations** ——— **Phenoxybenzamine** is a long-acting, α-receptor
antagonist that creates a "chemical sympathectomy." It
increases blood flow to the skin, mucosa, and abdominal
organs, and lowers both supine and erect blood pressures. It
has no effect on the parasympathetic system. There are no
adequate reports or well-controlled studies in pregnant
women. Though there are numerous case reports confirming
its efficacy for pheochromocytoma during pregnancy, it does
not reverse the acute decrease in maternal cardiac output
associated with a hypertensive episode.
Side effects include hypotension, CHF, reflex tachycardia,
nasal congestion, miosis, dyspepsia, and fatigue.

■ **Fetal Considerations** ————— There are no adequate reports or well-controlled studies
in human fetuses. **Phenoxybenzamine** crosses the human
placenta and is concentrated in the fetal plasma, achieving
an F:M ratio of 3:1. Appropriate rodent studies have
apparently not been conducted.

■ **Breastfeeding Safety** ————— There is no published experience in nursing women. It is
unknown whether **phenoxybenzamine** enters human
breast milk.

■ **References** ————————————— Martinez Brocca MA, Acosta Delgado D, Quijada D, et al.
Gynecol Endocrinol 2001; 15:439-42.
Lyons CW, Colmorgen GH. Obstet Gynecol 1988; 72:450-1.
Combs CA, Easterling TR, Schmucker BC, Benedetti TJ.
Obstet Gynecol 1989; 74:439-41.
Santeiro ML, Stromquist C, Wyble L. Ann Pharmacother
1996; 30:1249-51.

■ **Summary** ————————————— • **Pregnancy Category C**
- **Lactation Category U**
- **Phenoxybenzamine** should be used during pregnancy
and lactation only if the benefit justifies the potential
perinatal risk.

Phensuximide (Milontin)

- **Class** — Anticonvulsant; anorexiant

- **Indications** — Absence (petit mal) seizures

- **Mechanism** — Unknown

- **Dosage with Qualifiers** — Absence (petit mal) seizures—0.5-1g PO bid/tid
NOTE—avoid abrupt withdrawal
  - **Contraindications**—hypersensitivity to drug or class
  - **Caution**—hepatic or renal dysfunction, SLE

- **Maternal Considerations** — **Phensuximide** suppresses the paroxysmal, 3 cycles/sec spike and wave activity associated with the lapse of consciousness common in absence (petit mal) seizures. There is no published experience with **phensuximide** during pregnancy. Consideration may be given to stopping **phensuximide** if the severity and frequency are such they do not pose a serious threat to the patient. However, even minor seizures pose some hazard to the embryo and fetus. *Side effects* include pruritus, severe blood dyscrasias, granulocytopenia, transient leukopenia, pancytopenia with or without bone marrow suppression, sore throat, fever, evaluated LFTs, muscle weakness, nausea, vomiting, anorexia, drowsiness, dizziness, ataxia, headache, dreamlike state, lethargy, skin eruptions, erythema multiforme, Stevens-Johnson syndrome, erythematous rashes, and alopecia.

- **Fetal Considerations** — There are no adequate reports or well-controlled studies in human fetuses. It is unknown whether **phensuximide** crosses the human placenta. It is difficult to separate the impact of **phensuximide** from other agents used concurrently and the potential impact of the seizures. The sole published estimate is that the risk is similar to **ethosuximide**. Limited rodent studies are reassuring.

- **Breastfeeding Safety** — There is no published experience in nursing women. It is unknown whether **phensuximide** enters human breast milk.

- **References** — Fabro S, Shull G, Brown NA. Teratog Carcinog Mutagen 1982; 2:61-76.

- **Summary**
  - **Pregnancy Category D**
  - **Lactation Category U**
  - **Phensuximide** should be used during pregnancy and lactation only if the benefit justifies the potential perinatal risk.
  - **Ethosuximide** is probably the drug of first choice in absence seizures.

Phentermine (Adipex-P; Dapex-37.5; Fastin; Obe-Nix; Oby-Cap; Oby-Trim; Ona-Mast; Panbesyl; Phentercot; Phentride; T-Diet; Teramine; Tora; Umi-Pex 30; Zantryl)

■ **Class** — Anorexiant; CNS *stimulant*

■ **Indications** — Obesity

■ **Mechanism** — Sympathomimetic

■ **Dosage with Qualifiers** — Obesity—8mg PO tid
- **Contraindications**—hypersensitivity to drug or class, severe hypertension, symptomatic cardiovascular disease, MAO use <14d, glaucoma, agitated states, history of substance abuse
- **Caution**—unknown

■ **Maternal Considerations** — **Phentermine** is a sympathomimetic similar to **amphetamine**. It is indicated only for short-term monotherapy, and the associated weight loss is typically modest. Tachyphylaxis and tolerance occur with **phentermine** and all related drugs. Serious regurgitant disease of the aortic, mitral, and tricuspid valves occur in patients taking a combination of **phentermine** and **fenfluramine**. The latter was withdrawn from the U.S. market, but it is not definitive which drug was at fault. There are no adequate reports or well-controlled studies in pregnant women, and there is probably no indication for its use during either pregnancy or lactation. In one case control study, the rate of gestational diabetes was significantly greater in the women who took **phentermine** and **fenfluramine** during the 1st trimester. In the guinea pig, **mephentermine** reduces uterine blood flow.
Side effects include hypertension, insomnia, palpitations, dry mouth, headache, dizziness, excitation, constipation, diarrhea, and urticaria.

■ **Fetal Considerations** — There are no adequate reports or well-controlled studies in human fetuses. It is unknown whether **phentermine** crosses the human placenta. Similar agents do cross. There was no significant increase in pregnancy wastage or major malformations in almost 100 women who took **phentermine** and **fenfluramine** during pregnancy. Rodent teratogenicity studies have not been performed. A decrease in serotonergic axons in the hippocampus and mitral valve thickening was observed postnatally in the pups of rats exposed to the combination antenatally.

■ **Breastfeeding Safety** — There is no published experience in nursing women. It is unknown whether **phentermine** enters human breast milk.

■ **References** —————————— Jones KL, Johnson KA, Dick LM, et al. Teratology 2002; 65:125-30.
Chestnut DH, Ostman LG, Weiner CP, et al. Anesthesiology 1988; 68:363-6.
Bratter J, Gessner IH, Rowland NE. Eur J Pharmacol 1999; 369:R1-3.

■ **Summary** —————————————
- **Pregnancy Category C**
- **Lactation Category U**
- There are no indications for phentermine during pregnancy and lactation.

Phentolamine (Regitine)

■ **Class**———————————————— *Other antihypertensive, adrenergic antagonist*

■ **Indications** ———————————— Pheochromocytoma (preoperation), hypertensive crisis, extravasation necrosis

■ **Mechanism**————————————— α-adrenergic antagonist

■ **Dosage with Qualifiers** ————— Pheochromocytoma (preoperation)—5mg IM/IV 1-2h preoperatively; may repeat as necessary
Hypertensive crisis—5mg IV/IM
Extravasation necrosis—5-10mg/10ml NaCl injected into affected area
- **Contraindications**—hypersensitivity to drug or class, MI, coronary artery disease
- **Caution**—peptic ulcer disease

■ **Maternal Considerations** ——— **Phentolamine** is a short-acting α antagonist with direct iono- and chronotropic actions. There are no adequate reports or well-controlled studies in pregnant women. There are a number of case reports documenting efficacy for the noted indications. Rodent studies suggest **phentolamine** reduces uterine contractility postpartum, but there is no clinical evidence of such activity in women. *Side effects* include MI, stroke, hypotension, arrhythmia, tachycardia, peptic ulceration, weakness, dizziness, flushing, nausea, vomiting, diarrhea, abdominal pain, and nasal congestion.

■ **Fetal Considerations** —————— There are no adequate reports or well-controlled studies in human fetuses. It is unknown whether **phentolamine** crosses the human placenta. Rodent studies are reassuring for the most part. Only in the mouse was there evidence of IUGR and skeletal delay after the maternal dose exceeded 25 times the MRHD.

■ **Breastfeeding Safety** ————— There is no published experience in nursing women. It is unknown whether **phentolamine** enters human breast milk.

■ **References** ································· O'Halloran T, McGreal G, McDwermott E, O'Higgins N. Ir Med J 2001; 94:200-3.
Takahashi K, Sai Y, Nosaka S. Eur J Anaesthesiol 1998; 15:364-6.
Zupko I, Gaspar R, Kovacs L, Falkay G. Life Sci 1997; 61:PL159-63.

■ **Summary** ····························· • **Pregnancy Category C**
• **Lactation Category U**
• **Phentolamine** should be used during pregnancy and lactation only if the benefit justifies the potential perinatal risk.

Phenylephrine (Ah-Chew D; Ak-Dilate; Dilatair; Efrin; Fenilefrina; I-Phrine; Minims; Mydfrin; Neo-Synephrine; Neofrin; Ocu-Phrin; Phenylephrine HCl; Pupiletto-Forte; Ricobid-D; Spectro-Dilate; Spectro-Nephrine; Storz-Fen)

■ **Class** ································· *Pressor, ionotrope, sympathomimetic*

■ **Indications** ························· Shock, nasal congestion, hypotension after neuraxial anesthesia

■ **Mechanism** ······················· α-adrenergic agonist

■ **Dosage with Qualifiers** ········· Shock—40-180mcg/min infusion, or 50mcg IV bolus
Nasal congestion—2-3 gtt per nostril q4h; do not exceed 0.25% for more than 3d
Hypotension, spinal or epidural—50-100mcg IV bolus for aggressive support of arterial blood pressure at cesarean delivery
NOTE—frequently combined with a large range of preparations symptom relief and with topical anesthetics to prolong their duration of action; available in ophthalmic solutions
• **Contraindications**—hypersensitivity to drug or class, hypertension, ventricular tachycardia
• **Caution**—diabetes mellitus, thyroid disease

■ **Maternal Considerations** ········· Allergic rhinitis affects about a third of reproductive-age women. More than 170 over-the-counter preparations contain a sympathomimetic agent as their active ingredient. **Phenylephrine** should be considered a second-line agent behind 1st and 2nd generation antihistamines. It is popular for the prevention of hypotension following neuraxial anesthesia during cesarean delivery especially when ephedrine might be contraindicated (e.g., maternal cardiac disease).

Side effects include arrhythmia, MI, asthma exacerbation, hypertension, palpitations, headache, PVCs, tissue necrosis, and excitability.

■ **Fetal Considerations**
There are no adequate reports or well-controlled studies in human fetuses. It is unknown whether **phenylephrine** crosses the human placenta. **Pseudoephedrine** is associated with intestinal atresias, but the same has yet to be reported for **phenylephrine**. The combination of **pseudoephedrine**, **phenylephrine** and **phenylpropanolamine** (Triaminic) may be associated with distal limb reduction.

■ **Breastfeeding Safety**
There is no published experience in breastfeeding women. It is unknown whether **phenylephrine** enters human breast milk. However, considering the frequency of use, the dose and route, it seems unlikely the breast-fed neonate would ingest a clinically relevant amount.

■ **References**
Mazzotta P, Loebstein R, Koren G. Drug Saf 1999; 20:361-75.
Lee A, Ngan Kee WD, Gin T. Anesth Analg 2002; 94:920-6.
Ayorinde BT, Buczkowski P, Brown J, et al. Br J Anaesth 2001; 86:372-6.
Thomas DG, Robson SC, Redfern N, et al. Br J Anaesth 1996; 76:61-5.
Werler MM, Sheehan JE, Mitchell AA. Am J Epidemiol 2002; 155:26-31.
Gilbert-Barness E, Drut RM. Vet Hum Toxicol 2000; 42: 168-71.

■ **Summary**
- **Pregnancy Category C**
- **Lactation Category S?**
- **Phenylephrine** should be used during pregnancy and lactation only if the benefit justifies the potential perinatal risk.
- A 1st or 2nd generation antihistamine is preferred for the symptomatic relief of nasal congestion.

Phenylpropanolamine (Kleer; Propan; Rhindecon)

■ **Class**
Decongestant

■ **Indications**
Nasal decongestant

■ **Mechanism**
Sympathomimetic amine

■ **Dosage with Qualifiers**
Nasal congestion—75mg PO q12h prn (extended release tabs); alternatively, 25mg PO q4h (immediate release)
NOTE—previously included in a range of over-the-counter preparations, the U.S. FDA is requiring the removal of

phenylpropanolamine from the market because of the associated risk of stroke.

- **Contraindications**—hypersensitivity to drug or class, severe hypertension, severe CAD, concurrent MAO inhibitor use
- **Caution**—hypertension, diabetes mellitus, ischemic heart disease, increased intraocular pressure, hyperthyroidism, hyperreactivity to **ephedrine**

■ **Maternal Considerations**

More than 170 over-the-counter preparations contain a sympathomimetic agent as their active ingredient. An estimated 5 billion doses of **phenylpropanolamine** are taken each year. There are no adequate reports or well-controlled studies in pregnant women. Ventricular arrhythmia during pregnancy and intracranial hemorrhage postpartum are reported in association with **phenylpropanolamine**.

Side effects include tachycardia, palpitations, headache, dizziness, nausea, vomiting, fear, anxiety, weakness, pallor, insomnia, hallucinations, CNS depression, stroke, arrhythmia, and cardiovascular collapse.

■ **Fetal Considerations**

There are no adequate reports or well-controlled studies in human fetuses. It is unknown whether **phenylpropanolamine** crosses the human placenta. Rodent reproduction and teratogenicity studies have not been conducted. **Pseudoephedrine** is associated with intestinal atresias, but similar data for **phenylpropanolamine** is not available. The combination of **pseudoephedrine**, **phenylephrine** and **phenylpropanolamine** (Triaminic) is associated with distal limb reduction.

■ **Breastfeeding Safety**

There are no adequate reports or well-controlled studies in nursing women. It is unknown whether **phenylpropanolamine** enters human breast milk.

■ **References**

Onuigbo M, Alikhan M. South Med J 1998; 91:1153-5.
Maher LM, Peterson PL, Dela-Cruz C. Neurology 1987; 37:1686.
Werler MM, Sheehan JE, Mitchell AA. Am J Epidemiol 2002; 155:26-31.
Gilbert-Barness E, Drut RM. Vet Hum Toxicol 2000; 42:168-71.

■ **Summary**

- **Pregnancy Category C**
- **Lactation Category U**
- **Phenylpropanolamine** is being withdrawn from the U.S. market, though the magnitude of risk is unclear.
- **Phenylpropanolamine** may increase the risk of fetal intestinal atresias. A 1st or 2nd generation antihistamine is preferred for the symptomatic relief of nasal congestion.

Phenytoin (Aladdin; Aleviatin; Dantoin; Decatona; Dilantin; Ditoin; Ditomed; Epilantin-E; Eptoin; Hidantoina; Hydantol; Neosidantoina; Phenilep; Zentropil)

■ **Class** — Anticonvulsant, *hydantoin*

■ **Indications** — Seizure disorder, status epilepticus

■ **Mechanism** — Regulates motor cortex neuronal voltage-dependent sodium and calcium channels

■ **Dosage with Qualifiers** — Seizure disorder—load with 400mg, 300mg, and 300mg PO 2-4h apart, then 300-400mg PO qd (or divided bid), alternatively, 10-20mg/kg; IV ×1, then 4-6mg/kg IV qd
Status epilepticus—15-20mg/kg IV q30min prn; max 1500mg/d
NOTE—therapeutic level 10-20mcg/ml; recommend continuous ECG during load and not to exceed 50mg/min IV; avoid abrupt withdrawal; available in oral and parenteral forms
- **Contraindications**—hypersensitivity to drug or class, SA or AV block (IV), sinus bradycardia (IV), Adams-Stokes syndrome (IV)
- **Caution**—hepatic or renal dysfunction, hypotension, cardiovascular disease, diabetes mellitus, porphyria, thyroid disease, alcohol use

■ **Maternal Considerations** — **Phenytoin** is a 1st generation, enzyme-inducing anticonvulsant. Stable **phenytoin** serum levels are achieved in most, though there is wide variability with equivalent doses. Patients with unusually low levels may be either noncompliant or hypermetabolizers. Unusually high levels can result from hepatic disease, congenital enzyme deficiency or other drugs that interfere with metabolism. Clearance is increased during pregnancy, with concentrations declining to half of prepregnancy if the dose is not adjusted. Dose adjustments should be based on clinical symptoms, and not solely serum drug concentrations. **Phenytoin** may impair the effect of **corticosteroids**, **coumadin**, **digitoxin**, **doxycycline**, **estrogens**, **furosemide**, oral contraceptives, **quinidine**, **rifampin**, **theophylline**, and **vitamin D**. Drug interactions between enzyme-inducing anticonvulsants such as **phenytoin** and contraceptives are well documented. Either a higher dose oral contraceptive or a second contraceptive method is recommended. Planned pregnancy and counseling before conception is crucial, and should include information on the risk of teratogenicity, need for folate supplementation, and the importance of prenatal care.
Side effects include fibrillation (IV), hypotension (IV), cardiovascular collapse (IV), hepatotoxicity, hepatitis, gingival hyperplasia, thrombocytopenia, leukopenia,

agranulocytosis, pancytopenia, megaloblastic anemia, exfoliative dermatitis, periarteritis nodosa, gingival hyperplasia, Stevens-Johnson syndrome, toxic epidermal necrolysis, tissue necrosis (IV), hypersensitivity syndrome, lymphoma, SLE, osteomalacia, nausea, vomiting, rash, nystagmus, ataxia, slurred speech, dizziness, confusion, somnolence, constipation, headache, insomnia, tremor, osteomalcia, hyperglycemia, and coarse facies.

■ **Fetal Considerations**

There are no adequate reports or well-controlled studies in human fetuses. **Phenytoin** crosses the human placenta. The risk of major malformations in the offspring of women receiving antiepileptic drugs is double the general population. Risk factors include dose and polytherapy. **Phenytoin** is specifically associated with congenital heart defects and cleft palate. There is evidence that a **phenytoin**-induced embryonic arrhythmia is one mechanism of teratogenicity. The arrhythmia reflects the ability of **phenytoin** to inhibit a specific potassium channel (Ikr), and may cause embryonic ischemia/reperfusion injury with the generation of reactive oxygen species. Exposure to **phenytoin** *in utero* may lead to subtle psychomotor delay. Prior reports of an increased risk of neonatal intracranial hemorrhage after *in utero* phenytoin exposure due to **vitamin K** deficiency have not been substantiated. As with most psychotropic drugs, the risks may be minimized by monotherapy and the smallest effective quantity given in divided doses to minimize the serum peaks.

■ **Breastfeeding Safety**

There are no adequate reports or well-controlled studies in nursing women. The transfer of **phenytoin** into human breast milk appears relatively low and it is generally considered safe for breastfeeding.

■ **References**

McAuley JW, Anderson GD. Clin Pharmacokinet 2002; 41:559-79.
Leppik IE, Rask CA. Semin Neurol 1988; 8:240-6.
Crawford P. CNS Drugs 2002; 16:263-72.
Wide K, Henning E, Tomson T, Winbladh B. Acta Paediatr 2002; 91:409-14.
Azarbayjani F, Danielsson BR. Epilepsia 2002; 43:457-68.
Beghi E, Annegers JF; The Collaborative Group for the Pregnancy Registries in Epilepsy. Epilepsia 2001; 42:1422-5.
Nau H, Kuhn W, Egger HJ, et al. Clin Pharacokinet 1982; 7:508-43.
Kaaja E, Kaaja R, Matila R, Hiilesmaa V. Neurology 2002; 58:549-53.
Shimoyama R, Ohkubo T, Sugawara K, et al. J Pharm Biomed Anal 1998; 17:863-9.
Steen B, Rane A, Lonnerholm G, et al. Ther Drug Monit 1982; 4:331-4.

- **Summary**
  - Pregnancy Category D
  - Lactation Category S
  - **Phenytoin** should be used during pregnancy and lactation only if the benefit justifies the potential perinatal risk.
  - As with most psychotropic drugs, the risks may be minimized by monotherapy and the smallest effective quantity given in divided doses to minimize the serum peaks.

Physostigmine (Antilirium; Eserine Salicylate; Isopto Eserine)

- **Class** — *Cholinesterase inhibitor*

- **Indications** — Glaucoma, open-angle

- **Mechanism** — Reversible cholinesterase inhibitor prolonging the effect of acetylcholine

- **Dosage with Qualifiers** — Glaucoma, open-angle—1-2 gtt per eye tid/qid
  Reversal of anticholinergic syndrome—2mg IM or slow IV
  Post-anesthesia care—0.5-1.0mg IM or slow IV; repeat at intervals of 10-30min as needed for response
  NOTE—0.25% and 0.5% ophthalmic solutions
  - **Contraindications**—hypersensitivity to drug or class, acute uveitis, corneal abrasion, glaucoma (closed angle), asthma, gangrene, diabetes mellitus, cardiovascular disease
  - **Caution**—unknown

- **Maternal Considerations** — There are no adequate reports or well-controlled studies in pregnant women. The published experience is confined to the scattered case report.
  Side effects include irritation, blurred vision, ocular pain, tearing, redness, and headache.

- **Fetal Considerations** — There are no adequate reports or well-controlled studies in human fetuses. Considering the indications, dose, and route, it is unlikely the maternal systemic concentration will reach clinically relevant level unless the woman is being treated for the anticholinergic syndrome.

- **Breastfeeding Safety** — There is no published experience in nursing women. It is unknown whether **physostigmine** enters human breast milk. However, considering the indication and dosing, **physostigmine** use is unlikely to pose a clinically significant risk to the breast-feeding neonate.

- **References** —————— There are no current relevant references.

- **Summary** —————
  - **Pregnancy Category C**
  - **Lactation Category S?**
  - **Physostigmine** should be used during pregnancy and lactation only if the benefit justifies the potential perinatal risk.

Phytonadione (Aqua-Mephyton; Konakion; Vitamin K$_1$; Mephyton)

- **Class** ———— Bleeding disorders, vitamin/mineral

- **Indications** ———— Hypoprothrombinemia, vitamin K deficiency

- **Mechanism** ———— Co-factor for hepatic synthesis of factors II, VII, IX, X

- **Dosage with Qualifiers** ———— Hypoprothrombinemia—10mg SC/IM/IV ×1; may repeat in 6-8h based on INR; or 2.5-25mg PO qd-qwk, max 25mg/dose
  NOTE—severe reactions, including fatalities, are reported after IV use
  - **Contraindications**—hypersensitivity to drug or class, hereditary hypoprothrombinemia
  - **Caution**—heparin anticoagulation

- **Maternal Considerations** ———— Hypoprothrombinemia may result from anticoagulation, antibiotic therapy, or GI disease, or may be drug-induced. The drugs listed are each vitamin K products with some pharmacologic differences. There are no adequate reports or well-controlled studies in pregnant women.
  Side effects include anticoagulant resistance, hypotension, taste changes, flushing, diaphoresis, dyspnea, edema, and injection site hematoma or pain.

- **Fetal Considerations** ———— There are no adequate reports or well-controlled studies in human fetuses. While **phytonadione** crosses the human placenta, it varies with the compound, and is limited seeming to preclude a significant fetal effect. Placental transport is more efficient in the rat. Animal teratogenicity studies have apparently not been conducted.

- **Breastfeeding Safety** ———— **Phytonadione** is concentrated in human breast milk, and may be useful as a supplement for the preterm, breastfeeding neonate. It is generally considered compatible with breastfeeding.

■ **References** ································· Anai T, Hirota Y, Yoshimatsu J, et al. Obstet Gynecol 1993; 81:251-4.
Kazzi NJ, Ilagan NB, Liang KC, et al. Obstet Gynecol 1990; 75:334-7.
Saga K, Terao T. Nippon Sanka Fujinka Gakkai Zasshi 1989; 41:1713-9.
Gullaumont MJ, Durr FM, Combet JM, et al. Dev Pharmacol Ther 1988; 11:57-64.

■ **Summary** ································· • **Pregnancy Category C**
• **Lactation Category S**
• **Phytonadione** should be used during pregnancy and lactation only if the benefit justifies the potential perinatal risk.

Pilocarpine (Adsorbocarpine; Akarpine; I-Pilopine; Isopto Carpine; Ocu-Carpine; Pilokair; Pilopine HS; Pilosol; Pilostat; Salagen; Spectro-Pilo; Storzine)

■ **Class** ································· Miotic; *ophthalmic*

■ **Indications** ································· Xerostomia secondary to Sjögren syndrome or head/neck cancer

■ **Mechanism** ································· Cholinergic agonist

■ **Dosage with Qualifiers** ················· Xerostomia secondary to Sjögren syndrome—5mg PO qid; response may take 6w
Xerostomia secondary to head/neck cancer—begin 5mg PO tid; max 30mg/d
NOTE—hepatic dosing
• **Contraindications**—hypersensitivity to drug or class, acute asthma, narrow-angle glaucoma, acute iritis, severe hepatic dysfunction
• **Caution**—moderate hepatic dysfunction, asthma, COPD, chronic bronchitis, biliary disease, nephrolithiasis, psychiatric illness

■ **Maternal Considerations** ············· There is no published experience in pregnancy.
Side effects include pulmonary edema, visual impairment, impaired fertility, bradycardia, tachycardia, hypotension, hypertension, cholecystitis, biliary spasm, shock, sweating, chills, nausea, vomiting, flushing, rhinitis, dizziness, weakness, diarrhea, headache, dyspepsia, edema, tremor, dysphagia, and voice changes.

- **Fetal Considerations** — There are no adequate reports or well-controlled studies in human fetuses. It is unknown whether **pilocarpine** crosses the human placenta. In rabbits, pilocarpine accelerates fetal lung maturation.

- **Breastfeeding Safety** — There is no published experience during lactation. It is unknown whether **pilocarpine** enters human breast milk.

- **References** — Smith DM, Shelley SA, Balis JU. Anat Rec 1982; 202:23-31.

- **Summary** —
  - **Pregnancy Category C**
  - **Lactation Category S**
  - **Pilocarpine** should be used during pregnancy and lactation only if the benefit justifies the potential perinatal risk.

Pimecrolimus, topical (Elidel)

- **Class** — Other dermatologic, immunosuppressant

- **Indications** — Atopic dermatitis

- **Mechanism** — Inhibits T-lymphocyte activation

- **Dosage with Qualifiers** — Atopic dermatitis (mild-moderate)—for resistant cases, apply topically bid for up to 6w
  - **Contraindications**—hypersensitivity to drug or class, local infection, Netherton syndrome
  - **Caution**—HIV, VZV, or HSV infections, sun exposure

- **Maternal Considerations** — There is no published experience in pregnancy. *Side effects* include viral reactivation, lymphadenopathy, skin burning, headache, cough, pharyngitis, skin papilloma, erythema, and pruritus.

- **Fetal Considerations** — There are no adequate reports or well-controlled studies in human fetuses. It is unknown whether **pimecrolimus** crosses the human placenta. Considering the dose and route, it is unlikely the maternal systemic concentration will reach clinically relevant level. Rodent studies utilizing a topical application are reassuring, revealing no evidence of toxicity, teratogenicity, or IUGR despite the use of doses higher than those used clinically. **Pimecrolimus** does cross the rodent placenta after oral administration.

- **Breastfeeding Safety** — There are no published reports of **pimecrolimus** use during breastfeeding. It is unknown whether it enters human breast milk.

- **References** ⬛ There is no published experience in pregnancy or during lactation.

- **Summary**
  - **Pregnancy Category C**
  - **Lactation Category U**
  - **Pimecrolimus** should be used during pregnancy and lactation only if the benefit justifies the potential perinatal risk.
  - There are alternative agents for which there is more experience regarding use during pregnancy and lactation.

Pimozide (Orap; Pimodac)

- **Class** — *Antipsychotic*

- **Indications** — Tourette's syndrome

- **Mechanism** — Dopamine D_2 antagonist plus multiple other actions

- **Dosage with Qualifiers** — Tourette's syndrome—begin 1-2mg PO qd; max 10mg/d; alternatively 0.2mg/kg/d; max 10mg/d
  NOTE—may cause sedation
  - **Contraindications**—hypersensitivity to drug or class, CNS depression, arrhythmia, prolonged QT interval syndrome, coma
  - **Caution**—unknown

- **Maternal Considerations** — There is no published experience in pregnant women. **Pimozide** produces a dose-dependent increase in pituitary tumors in rats.
  Side effects include amenorrhea, neuroleptic malignant syndrome, seizure, arrhythmia, tachycardia, palpitations, hypotension, tremor, rigidity, akinesia, nausea, vomiting, dyspepsia, rash, urticaria, increased salivation, diarrhea, constipation, sedation, lethargy, and dystonic reactions.

- **Fetal Considerations** — There are no adequate reports or well-controlled studies in human fetuses. It is unknown whether **pimozide** crosses the human placenta. Rodent studies are reassuring, revealing no evidence of teratogenicity, though IUGR and increased embryo resorption were noted at doses 8 times the MRHD.

- **Breastfeeding Safety** — There are no published reports of **pimozide** use in nursing women. It is unknown whether **pimozide** enters human breast milk. **Pimozide** stimulates prolactin secretion.

- **References** — There are no current relevant references.

■ **Summary** ···································
- **Pregnancy Category C**
- **Lactation Category U**
- **Pimozide** should be used during pregnancy and lactation only if the benefit justifies the potential perinatal risk.

Pindolol (Bedrrenal; Betadren; Visken)

■ **Class** ······················· *β-blocker*

■ **Indications** ·················· Hypertension, chronic stable angina

■ **Mechanism** ················· Nonselective β-blocker with intrinsic sympathomimetic activity

■ **Dosage with Qualifiers** ······ Hypertension—begin 5mg PO bid, increase by 10mg/d q3-4w; max 60mg/d
Chronic stable angina—15-40mg PO qd; hepatic dosing
- **Contraindications**—hypersensitivity to drug or class, asthma, severe bradycardia, 2nd or 3rd degree AV block, CHF, severe COPD, cardiogenic shock
- **Caution**—past history of CHF, abrupt withdrawal, major surgery, diabetes mellitus, thyrotoxicosis, hepatic dysfunction

■ **Maternal Considerations** ······ There are no adequate reports or well-controlled studies in pregnant women. **Pindolol** is considered a second-line drug (**alpha methyldopa, labetolol,** or calcium-channel blockers are first-line) for the treatment of nonsevere, chronic hypertension during pregnancy. It does not increase uterine contractility. **Pindolol** is superior to **propranolol** for the control of preeclamptic hypertension when **hydralazine** alone is inadequate. Women with preeclampsia treated with **pindolol** reportedly have a greater decline in Doppler-determined uterine artery flow resistance compared to women treated with **propranolol**. *Side effects* include CHF, severe bradycardia, bronchospasm, peripheral vascular disease, insomnia, dizziness, fatigue, muscle aches, joint pain, peripheral edema, nervousness, dyspnea, and elevated LFTs.

■ **Fetal Considerations** ·········· There are no adequate reports or well-controlled studies in human fetuses. **Pindolol** crosses the human placenta achieving an F:M ratio approximating 0.5 measured 6h. Doppler flow studies are reassuring with no detectable impact on fetal hemodynamics when given to women with mild preeclampsia. Rodent studies are reassuring, revealing no evidence of teratogenicity or IUGR despite the use of doses higher than those used clinically.

- **Breastfeeding Safety** ⋯⋯⋯ There are no adequate reports or well-controlled studies in nursing women. **Pindolol** enters human breast milk achieving a M:P ratio approximating 0.5.

- **References** ⋯⋯⋯ Rey E, LeLorier J, Burgess E, et al. CMAJ 1997; 157:1245-54.
Paran E, Holzberg G, Mazor M, et al. Int J Pharmacol Ther 1995; 33:119-23.
Meizner I, Paran E, Katz M, et al. J Clin Ultrasound 1992; 20:115-9.
Rasanen J, Jouppila P. Eur J Obstet Reprod Biol 1995; 62:195-201.
Montan S, Ingemarsson I, Marsal K, Sjoberg NO. BMJ 1992; 304:946-9.
Goncalves PV, Matthes AC, Da Cunha SP, Lanchote VL. Chirality 2002; 14:683-7.
Krause W, Stoppelli I, Milia S, Rainer E. Eur J Pharmacol 1982; 22:53-5.

- **Summary** ⋯⋯⋯
  - **Pregnancy Category B**
  - **Lactation Category U**
  - **Pindolol** should be used during pregnancy and lactation only if the benefit justifies the potential perinatal risk.
  - It is a reasonable choice for the treatment of women with chronic hypertension, and maybe of use in some preeclamptic women.

Pioglitazone (Actos)

- **Class** ⋯⋯⋯ *Antidiabetic, thiazolidinediones*

- **Indications** ⋯⋯⋯ Diabetes mellitus, type 2

- **Mechanism** ⋯⋯⋯ Increases insulin sensitivity and inhibits hepatic gluconeogenesis by activating peroxisome proliferator-activated receptor-gamma

- **Dosage with Qualifiers** ⋯⋯⋯ Diabetes mellitus, type 2—15-30mg PO qd, increase dose after 12w if no response; max 45mg/d
NOTE—check ALT periodically; may be combined with other oral agents; caution with insulin
  - **Contraindications**—hypersensitivity to drug or class, diabetes mellitus type 1, ketoacidosis, CHF class III or IV NYHA
  - **Caution**—CHF class I or II NYHA, hepatic dysfunction, hypertension, edema

- **Maternal Considerations** ⋯⋯⋯ **Pioglitazone** improves glycemic control while decreasing circulating insulin and free fatty acid levels and increasing HDL and LDL. When used alone, it is slightly less potent than the sulfonylureas and **metformin**. Clearance is increased by 20-60% in nonpregnant women compared to men. There is no published experience in pregnancy. **Insulin** remains the hypoglycemic agent of choice during pregnancy.

Side effects include hepatotoxicity, CHF, anemia, fluid retention, edema, weight gain, URI, headache, sinusitis, myalgia, pharyngitis, dyspepsia, and hypoglycemia.

■ **Fetal Considerations**

There are no adequate reports or well-controlled studies in human fetuses. It is unknown whether **pioglitazone** crosses the human placenta. Rodent studies are for the most part reassuring, revealing no evidence of teratogenicity, or functional or behavioral abnormalities despite the use of doses higher than those used clinically. There is evidence of embryotoxicity.

■ **Breastfeeding Safety**

There is no published experience with **pioglitazone** during lactation. It is unknown whether it enters human breast milk. **Pioglitazone** is excreted into rat breast milk.

■ **References**

There is no published experience in pregnancy or during lactation.

■ **Summary**

- **Pregnancy Category C**
- **Lactation Category U**
- There are alternative agents for which there is more experience during pregnancy and lactation.

Piperacillin (Pipracil)

■ **Class**

Antibiotic, penicillin

■ **Indications**

Susceptible bacterial infections including intra-abdominal, gonococcus, lower respiratory and urinary tracts, skin and bone

■ **Mechanism**

Bactericidal; inhibits cell wall and septum mucopeptide synthesis

■ **Dosage with Qualifiers**

Bacterial infections (pseudomonas, intra-abdominal or sepsis)—3-4g IV/IM q4-6h ×3-10d
Post-gynecologic or cesarean prophylaxis—2g IV 30min preoperatively or at umbilical cord clamping, then q4-6h ×2
Gonorrhea, uncomplicated—1g **probenecid** PO 30min before 2g IM ×1
NOTE—renal dosing; may be combined with the β-lactamase inhibitor **tazobactam** (Tazosyn; Zosyn)

- **Contraindications**—hypersensitivity to drug or class
- **Caution**—cephalosporin allergy, uremia, hypokalemia, seizure disorder, nephrotoxic agents, renal dysfunction, sodium restriction

■ **Maternal Considerations**

Piperacillin is widely distributed including therapeutic levels in bone, heart, bile, and the CSF during inflammation. It is best studied during pregnancy for the treatment of gonorrhea, PPROM, and cesarean section prophylaxis. **Piperacillin** pharmacokinetics reveals a larger volume of distribution and higher clearance rate during pregnancy. This suggests higher doses are necessary for effective treatment of serious infections in pregnant women near term and in the puerperium. In reference to prophylaxis, no single antibiotic proved effective for prophylaxis (**ampicillin**, **cefazolin**, **piperacillin**, and **cefotetan**) is superior to the other; cost and convenience are the deciding variables. **Piperacillin** may be given as a single 4g dose at cord clamping with little loss of efficacy. Several reports support the use of **piperacillin** (3-4g IV q6h x 72h) to prolong the latency interval between PPROM and the onset of labor.
Side effects include thrombocytopenia, seizures, fever, pseudomembranous enterocolitis, interstitial nephritis, neutropena, hemolytic anemia, prolonged bleeding time, rash, bleeding, hypokalemia, headache, dizziness, fatigue, phlebitis, hyperbilirubinemia, and elevated LFTs.

■ **Fetal Considerations**

There are no adequate reports or well-controlled studies in human fetuses. Placental transfer is rapid, achieving an F:M ratio between 0.25 and 0.3. The concentration in amniotic fluid is similar to fetal serum. Rodent studies are reassuring, revealing no evidence of teratogenicity or IUGR despite the use of doses higher than those used clinically.

■ **Breastfeeding Safety**

There are no adequate reports or well-controlled studies in nursing women. Only small amounts of **piperacillin** enter human breast milk, and it is usually considered compatible with breastfeeding.

■ **References**

Heikkila A, Erkkola R. J Antimicrob Chemother 1991; 28:419-23.
Ford LC, Hammil HA, Lebherz TB. Am J Obstet Gynecol 1987; 157:506-10.
Shah S, Mazher Y, John IS. Int J Gynaecol Obstet 1998; 62:23-9.
Charles D, Larsen B. Gynecol Obstet Invest 1985; 20:194-8.
Gall SA, Hill GB. Am J Obstet Gynecol 1987; 157:502-6.
Lockwood CJ, Costigan K, Ghidini A, et al. Am J Obstet Gynecol 1993; 169:970-6.
Brown CE, Christmas JT, Bawdon RE. Am J Obstet Gynecol 1990; 163:938-43.

■ **Summary**
- **Pregnancy Category B**
- **Lactation Category S**
- **Piperacillin** should be used during pregnancy and lactation only if the benefit justifies the potential perinatal risk.
- It is an excellent agent for cesarean prophylaxis and the treatment of gonorrhea.
- Routine administration of **piperacillin** to women with PPROM may prolong latency, though erythromycin is better-studied and preferred.

Piperacillin/tazobactam (Tazosyn; Zosyn)

■ **Class**

Antibiotic, penicillin

■ **Indications**

Susceptible bacterial infections including intra-abdominal, gonococcus, lower respiratory and urinary tracts, skin and bone

■ **Mechanism**

Bactericidal; inhibits cell wall and septum mucopeptide synthesis

■ **Dosage with Qualifiers**

Bacterial infections (pseudomonas, intra-abdominal, or sepsis)—3.375g IV q6h ×3-10d
Postpartum endomyometritis or pelvic inflammatory disease—3.375g IV q6h ×3-10d
Community-acquired pneumonia—3.375g IV q6h × 3-10d
NOTE—renal dosing
- **Contraindications**—hypersensitivity to drug or class
- **Caution**—cephalosporin allergy, uremia, hypokalemia, seizure disorder, nephrotoxic agents, renal dysfunction, sodium restriction

■ **Maternal Considerations**

Tazobactam is a β-lactamase inhibitor with no significant antibacterial activity; its addition expands the antibacterial spectrum of **piperacillin**.
Piperacillin/tazobactam is active against most strains of the following **piperacillin**-resistant β-lactamase-producing microorganisms: *Staphylococcus aureus* (not methicillin-resistant), *Escherichia coli*, *Haemophilus influenzae* (not ampicillin-resistant β-lactamase), and *Bacteroides fragilis* group (B. *fragilis*, B. *ovatus*, B. *thetaiotaomicron*, or B. *vulgatus*). Clearance of the combination appears enhanced during pregnancy. It is similar to **ampicillin/gentamicin** in efficacy for the treatment of postpartum endometritis.
Side effects include thrombocytopenia, seizures, fever, cholestatic jaundice, erytheme multiforme, pseudomembranous enterocolitis, interstitial nephritis,

neutropena, hemolytic anemia, prolonged bleeding time, prolonged INR, rash, bleeding, hypokalemia, headache, dizziness, fatigue, phlebitis, hyperbilirubinemia, and elevated LFTs.

■ **Fetal Considerations** ⋯⋯ There are no adequate reports or well-controlled studies in human fetuses. Placental transfer is rapid reaching an F:M ratio between 0.25 and 0.3. The concentration in amniotic fluid is similar to fetal serum. Rodent studies at doses up to 4 times the MRHD are reassuring showing no evidence of impaired fertility or teratogenicity.

■ **Breastfeeding Safety** ⋯⋯ There are no adequate reports or well-controlled studies in nursing women. Only small amounts of **piperacillin** enter human breast milk, and it is usually considered compatible with breastfeeding. It is not known whether **tazobactam** enters human breast milk.

■ **References** ⋯⋯ Bourget P, Sertin A, Lesne-Hulin A, et al. Eur J Obstet Gynecol Reprod Biol 1998; 76:21-7.
Figueroa-Damian R, Villagrana-Zesati R, San Martin Herrasti JM, Arredondo-Garcia JL. Ginecol Obstet Mex 1996; 64:214-8.

■ **Summary** ⋯⋯
- **Pregnancy Category B**
- **Lactation Category S?**
- **Piperacillin/tazobactam** should be used during pregnancy and lactation only if the benefit justifies the potential perinatal risk.

Piperazine (Aloxin; Antcucs; Antepar; Ascalix; Expellin; Multifuge; Rotape; Vermidol; Vermizine; Worm)

■ **Class** ⋯⋯ Anthelmintic, Sympathomimetic

■ **Indications** ⋯⋯ Treatment of intestinal ascariasis (2nd to *Ascaris lumbricoides*, "roundworms"); Enterobiasis due to *Enterobius vermicularis* ("pinworms")

■ **Mechanism** ⋯⋯ Produces worm paralysis allowing expulsion

■ **Dosage with Qualifiers** ⋯⋯ Ascariasis—3.5g PO before breakfast qd ×2
Enterobiasis—65mg/kg before breakfast qd ×7d; max 2.5g/d
- **Contraindications**—hypersensitivity to drug or class, renal dysfunction, convulsive disorders
- **Caution**—hepatic dysfunction, malnutrition, anemia

- **Maternal Considerations** ---- There are no adequate reports or well-controlled studies in pregnant women. The long clinical experience is reassuring.
  Side effects include nausea, vomiting, abdominal cramps, diarrhea, urticaria, erythema multiforme, purpura, fever, arthralgia headache, vertigo, ataxia, tremors, choreiform movement, muscular weakness, hyporeflexia, paresthesia, blurred vision, convulsions, EEG abnormalities, and memory deficit.

- **Fetal Considerations** ---- There are no adequate reports or well-controlled studies in human fetuses. It is unknown whether **piperazine** crosses the human placenta.

- **Breastfeeding Safety** ---- There is no published experience in nursing women. It is unknown whether **piperazine** enters human breast milk.

- **References** ---- Villar MA, Sibai BM. Am J Obstet Gynecol 1992; 166:549-50.

- **Summary** ----
  - **Pregnancy Category B**
  - **Lactation Category U**
  - **Piperazine** should be used during pregnancy and lactation only if the benefit justifies the potential perinatal risk.

Pirbuterol acetate (Maxair)

- **Class** ---- Bronchodilator, sympathomimetic

- **Indications** ---- Bronchospasm

- **Mechanism** ---- β-2 adrenergic agonist

- **Dosage with Qualifiers** ---- Bronchospasm—1-2 puffs (200mcg/puff) INH q4-6h; max 12 puffs/d
  NOTE—currently unavailable in the U.S.
  - **Contraindications**—hypersensitivity to drug or class
  - **Caution**—diabetes mellitus, hyperthyroidism, seizures, cardiovascular disease, hypokalemia

- **Maternal Considerations** ---- There is no published experience in pregnancy.
  Side effects include arrhythmia, angina, anorexia, severe hypertension, tremor, nervousness, nausea, vomiting, diarrhea, headache, vertigo, and taste changes.

- **Fetal Considerations** ---- There are no adequate reports or well-controlled studies in human fetuses. Rodent studies, both inhalational and oral are reassuring, revealing no evidence of teratogenicity or

IUGR despite the use of doses higher than those used clinically. Fetal toxicity was noted at the higher doses tested.

■ **Breastfeeding Safety**
There is no published experience or during lactation. It is unknown whether **pirbuterol** enters human breast milk.

■ **References**
There are no current relevant references.

■ **Summary**
- **Pregnancy Category C**
- **Lactation Category U**
- **Pirbuterol** should be used during pregnancy and lactation only if the benefit justifies the potential perinatal risk.
- There are alternative agents for which there is more experience during pregnancy and lactation.

Piroxicam (Brexicam; Feldene; Feline)

■ **Class**
NSAID, oxicam

■ **Indications**
Osteoarthritis and rheumatoid arthritis, mild to moderate pain, dysmenorrhea

■ **Mechanism**
Inhibits prostaglandin biosynthesis

■ **Dosage with Qualifiers**
Osteoarthritis and rheumatoid arthritis—20-40mg PO qd with food
Dysmenorrhea—begin 40mg qd ×2d, then 20mg PO qd ×3d
Mild to moderate pain—20mg PO qd
- **Contraindications**—hypersensitivity to drug or class, aspirin- or NSAID-induced asthma
- **Caution**—GI bleeding, nasal polyps, hypertension, CHF

■ **Maternal Considerations**
Piroxicam is an orally absorbed oxicam with anti-inflammatory, analgesic, and antipyretic properties. There are no adequate reports or well-controlled studies in pregnant women.
Side effects include GI bleeding, acute renal failure, bronchospasm, thrombocytopenia, Stevens-Johnson syndrome, interstitial nephritis, hepatotoxicity, agranulocytosis, dyspepsia, nausea, abdominal pain, constipation, headache, dizziness, rash, drowsiness, tinnitus, fluid retention, and elevated LFTs.

■ **Fetal Considerations**
There are no adequate reports or well-controlled studies in human fetuses. **Piroxicam** presumably crosses the human

placenta, as similar to other NSAIDs, it is associated with severe fetal oligohydramnios in case reports. **Piroxicam** increases the incidence of dystocia and delayed parturition in animals if administered continuously late into pregnancy.

■ **Breastfeeding Safety** There are no adequate reports or well-controlled studies in nursing women. Only trace quantities of **piroxicam** is excreted into human breast milk, and does not pose a threat to the breast-feeding neonate.

■ **References** Powell JG Jr, Cochrane RL. Prostaglandins 1982; 23:469-88.
Voyer LE, Drut R, Mendez JH. Pediatr Nephrol 1994; 8:592-4.
Ostensen M, Matheson I, Laufen H. Eur J Clin Pharmacol 1988; 35:567-9.

■ **Summary**
- **Pregnancy Category B (first 20w; D thereafter)**
- **Lactation Category S**
- **Piroxicam** should be used during pregnancy and lactation only if the benefit justifies the potential perinatal risk.
- There are alternative agents for which there is more experience during pregnancy.

Plicamycin (Mithracin; Mithramycin)

■ **Class** *Antibiotic, antineoplastic*

■ **Indications** Hypercalcemia

■ **Mechanism** Unknown; complexes with DNA, inhibits cellular and enzymatic RNA synthesis

■ **Dosage with Qualifiers** Hypercalcemia—25mcg/kg IV qd given over 4-6h for 3-4d
- **Contraindications**—hypersensitivity to drug or class, thrombocytopenia, bleeding disorder, herpes zoster, recent varicella, pregnancy
- **Caution**—unknown

■ **Maternal Considerations** There is no published experience in pregnancy.
Side effects include hypocalcemia, hypophosphatemia, leukopenia, thrombocytopenia, bleeding, renal or hepatic dysfunction, nausea, vomiting, anorexia, diarrhea, stomatitis, somnolence, phlebitis, rash, and flushing.

■ **Fetal Considerations** There are no adequate reports or well-controlled studies in human fetuses. It is unknown whether **plicamycin** crosses the human placenta. Rodent teratogenicity studies have apparently not been performed.

Pneumococcal vaccine (Pneumovax 23; Pnu-Imune 23)

■ **Class** ⋯⋯⋯⋯⋯⋯⋯⋯ Vaccine

■ **Indications** ⋯⋯⋯⋯⋯⋯ Enhanced susceptibility to pneumococcus

■ **Mechanism** ⋯⋯⋯⋯⋯⋯ Active immunization

■ **Dosage with Qualifiers** ⋯⋯ Immunocompetent patients with increased pneumococcal susceptibility—0.5ml IM ×1
NOTE—avoid IV or intradermal administration
- **Contraindications**—hypersensitivity to any component of the vaccine, Hodgkin's disease treated with either immunosuppressive or radiotherapy
- **Caution**—unknown

■ **Maternal Considerations** ⋯⋯ Pneumococcal infection is a leading cause of death and a major cause of pneumonia, meningitis, and otitis media. **Pneumococcal vaccine** is a mixture of highly purified capsular polysaccharides from the 23 clinically relevant pneumococcal types accounting for at least 90% of pneumococcal blood isolates. The antibody induced by the vaccine may persist for as long as 5 years. Susceptible patients at increased risk include HIV-infected women. *Side effects* include local injection site soreness, erythema and swelling, rash, urticaria, arthritis, arthralgia, serum sickness, adenitis, and fever.

■ **Fetal Considerations** ⋯⋯ There are no adequate reports or well-controlled studies in human fetuses. Stimulated antibodies are transferred across the placenta. And while gestational age affects the efficiency of antibody transfer, vaccination is efficient and newborns of treated women have higher titers during the first year of life. Maternal immunization does not alter the neonatal response to vaccination.

Rodent teratogenicity studies have not been performed, though there is no reason to expect an adverse fetal effect. Vaccinated rodents transfer enough antibody to their offspring to protect against otitis media.

■ **Breastfeeding Safety**   There are no adequate reports or well-controlled studies in nursing women. It is unknown whether **pneumococcal vaccine** enters human breast milk. However, the IgA antibody level for many of the serotypes included are enhanced and provide enhanced neonatal protection.

■ **References**   Lehmann D, Pomat WS, Combs B, et al. Vaccine 2002; 20:1837-45.
Munoz FM, Englund JA, Cheesman CC, et al. Vaccine 2001; 20:826-37.
Okoko BJ, Wesumperuma LH, Hart AC. Vaccine 2001; 20:647-50.
Yoon JK, Lee HH, Choi BM, et al. J Korean Med Sci 2001; 16:9-14.
Shahid NS, Steinhoff MC, Hoque SS, et al. Lancet 1995; 346:1252-7.
Hajek DM, Quartey M, Giebink GS. Acta Otolaryngol 2002; 122:262-9

■ **Summary**
- **Pregnancy Category C**
- **Lactation Category S**
- **Pneumococcal vaccine** may be beneficial for mother and newborn in some patient populations.

Podofilox (Condylox)

■ **Class**   Antiviral, *dermatologic*

■ **Indications**   Genital or perianal warts

■ **Mechanism**   Unknown; antimitotic

■ **Dosage with Qualifiers**   Genital or perianal warts—apply topically bid ×3d; repeat weekly for up to 4w
- **Contraindications**—hypersensitivity to drug or class
- **Caution**—unknown

■ **Maternal Considerations**   **Podofilox** is related to **podophyllum**. There are no adequate reports or well-controlled studies in pregnant women. Toxicity with overuse is reported, but systemic absorption of doses up to 1.5ml is low. **Podofilox** should not be used to treat large lesions during pregnancy. Though an effective agent, there are other therapies such as laser and cryotherapy, which pose fewer risks.
Side effects include burning and inflammation.

- **Fetal Considerations** .... There are no adequate reports or well-controlled studies in human fetuses. And while many antimitotic drugs are embryotoxic, topical applications of 0.1-1.5ml produce peak serum levels <17ng/ml 1-2h after the application. The elimination half-life is <4.5h and it does not accumulate after multiple treatments. Considering the dose and route, it is unlikely the maternal systemic concentration will reach a clinically relevant level after the treatment of small warts. Limited rodent studies are reassuring, revealing no evidence of teratogenicity or IUGR despite the use of doses higher than those used clinically.

- **Breastfeeding Safety** .... There are no adequate reports or well-controlled studies in nursing women. It is unknown whether **podofilox** enters human breast milk. However, considering the indication and dosing, **podofilox** use is unlikely to pose a clinically significant risk to the breast-feeding neonate.

- **References** .... There are no current relevant references.

- **Summary** ....
  - **Pregnancy Category C**
  - **Lactation Category S?**
  - **Podofilox** should be used during pregnancy and lactation only if the benefit justifies the potential perinatal risk.
  - The risk when used during pregnancy for small lesions is low.
  - There are other therapies such as laser and cryotherapy, which pose even fewer risks.

Podophyllum resin (Podoben; Podocon-25; Pododerm; Podofin)

- **Class** .... Antiviral, *dermatologic*

- **Indications** .... Genital or perianal warts

- **Mechanism** .... Unknown; antimitotic

- **Dosage with Qualifiers** .... Condylomata acuminata—apply qw for up to 3w
  - **Contraindications**—hypersensitivity to drug or class, diabetes mellitus, patients chronically receiving corticosteroids
  - **Caution**—unknown

- **Maternal Considerations** .... **Podophyllum resin** is a mixture of resins from the mandrake (*Podophyllum peltatum Linné*), a perennial plant of northern and middle U.S. It is made exclusively from American podophyllin, which has a lower level of

podophyllotoxin than the Indian resin. There are no adequate reports or well-controlled studies in pregnant women. Though systemic absorption of doses up to 1.5ml is low, toxicity is reported with overuse. Thus, **podophyllum** should not be used during pregnancy for large lesions. Though an effective agent, there are other therapies, such as laser and cryotherapy, which pose fewer risks.
Side effects include paresthesia, polyneuritis, paralytic ileus, pyrexia, leukopenia, thrombocytopenia, coma and death.

■ **Fetal Considerations**

There are no adequate reports or well-controlled studies in human fetuses. It is unknown whether **podophyllum** crosses the human placenta. Considering the dose and route, it is unlikely the maternal systemic concentration will reach a clinically relevant level after the treatment of small warts. There are reports of complications associated with the topical use of podophyllin on condylomata of pregnant patients including birth defects, fetal death, and stillbirth. The relationship of outcome to the use of **podophyllum** is unclear.

■ **Breastfeeding Safety**

There are no adequate reports or well-controlled studies in nursing women. It is unknown whether **podophyllum** enters human breast milk. However, considering the indications and dosing, **podophyllum** use is unlikely to pose a clinically significant risk to the breast-feeding neonate.

■ **References**

Moher LM, Maurer SA. J Fam Pract 1979; 9:237-40.
Karol MD, Conner CS, Watanabe AS, Murphrey KJ. Clin Toxicol 1980; 16:283-6.

■ **Summary**

- **Pregnancy Category X**
- **Lactation Category S?**
- **Podophyllum** should be used during pregnancy and lactation only if the benefit justifies the potential perinatal risk.
- The risk when used during pregnancy for small lesions is low.
- There are other therapies such as laser and cryotherapy, which pose even fewer risks.

Poliovirus vaccine, inactivated (Ipol; Poliovax)

■ **Class** — Vaccine

■ **Indications** — Poliovirus susceptibility

■ **Mechanism** — Active immunization

■ **Dosage with Qualifiers** ⋯⋯⋯ Poliovirus susceptibility, adult—1 vial IM in the deltoid; repeat 1-2mo later and again in 6-12mo
  - **Contraindications**—hypersensitivity to drug or class, hypersensitivity to **neomycin**, **streptomycin** and **polymyxin B**, acute febrile illness
  - **Caution**—unknown

■ **Maternal Considerations** ⋯⋯⋯ **Inactivated poliovirus vaccine** is a sterile suspension of three types [type 1 (Mahoney), type 2 (MEF-1), and type 3 (Saukett)] grown in culture and inactivated with formaldehyde. **Neomycin**, **streptomycin**, and **polymyxin B** are each used in vaccine production. Paralytic poliomyelitis has not been reported after vaccination. Routine primary poliovirus vaccination of adults (>18y) living in the U.S. is not recommended. Adults at increased risk of exposure but not previously immunized should be vaccinated. This group includes travelers to regions where poliomyelitis is endemic or epidemic, health care workers in close contact with patients who may be excreting polioviruses, laboratory workers handling specimens that may contain polioviruses, members of groups with disease caused by wild polioviruses, and incompletely vaccinated or unvaccinated adults in contact with children given **oral poliovirus vaccine**. Vaccination during pregnancy is effective and the antibodies are detectable in the fetus.
Side effects include erythema at the injection site, fever, and decreased appetite.

■ **Fetal Considerations** ⋯⋯⋯ There are no adequate reports or well-controlled studies in human fetuses. Poliovirus antibodies cross the human placenta and may offer some perinatal protection. Rodent teratogenicity studies have not been conducted, though an inactivated virus should not pose a significant fetal risk.

■ **Breastfeeding Safety** ⋯⋯⋯ There are no adequate reports or well-controlled studies in nursing women. While it is unknown whether **inactivated poliovirus vaccine** enters human breast milk, the resulting antibodies might. However, it appears the oral vaccine is superior for the stimulation of IgA.

■ **References** ⋯⋯⋯ Munoz FM, Englund JA. Pediatr Clin North Am 2000; 47:449-63.
Hanson LA, Carlsson B, Jalil F, et al. Rev Infect Dis 1984; 6(Suppl 2):S356-60.

■ **Summary** ⋯⋯⋯
  - **Pregnancy Category C**
  - **Lactation Category S**
  - **Inactivated poliovirus vaccine** should be used during pregnancy and lactation only if the benefit justifies the potential perinatal risk.

Poliovirus vaccine, oral live (Orimune)

■ **Class** .... *Vaccine*

■ **Indications** .... Poliovirus susceptibility

■ **Mechanism** .... Active immunization

■ **Dosage with Qualifiers** .... Poliovirus 1-3 susceptibility—0.5ml PO repeated 8w later, with a 3rd dose 6-12mo after the 2nd
- **Contraindications**—hypersensitivity to drug or class, hypersensitivity to **neomycin**, **streptomycin,** and **polymyxin B**, immune deficiency states or altered immunity due to disease or therapy, acute febrile illness
- **Caution**—none

■ **Maternal Considerations** .... **Oral poliovirus vaccine** is a live, trivalent mixture of three types of attenuated polioviruses grown in monkey kidney cell culture. **Oral poliovirus vaccine** simulates natural infection, inducing active mucosal and systemic immunity without producing symptoms of disease. Routine primary poliovirus vaccination of adults (>18y) living in the U.S. is not recommended. Adults who are at increased risk of exposure and who have not been adequately immunized should receive poliovirus vaccination. This group includes travelers to regions where poliomyelitis is endemic or epidemic, health care workers in close contact with patients who may be excreting polioviruses, laboratory workers handling specimens that may contain polioviruses, and members of groups with disease caused by wild polioviruses. **Oral poliovirus vaccine** is used for epidemic control. Vaccination during pregnancy is effective and does not increase the risk of a pregnancy complication.
Side effects include paralytic disease (1/1.2 million 1st doses, 1/25 million 2nd or 3rd doses), and Guillain-Barré syndrome.

■ **Fetal Considerations** .... There are no adequate reports or well-controlled studies in human fetuses. Maternal vaccination results in a level of passive immunity for the newborn. There is no evidence of teratogenicity or fetal toxicity. Rodent teratogenicity studies have not been performed.

■ **Breastfeeding Safety** .... There are no adequate reports or well-controlled studies in nursing women. Antibodies are found in breast milk. While it is unknown whether **oral poliovirus vaccine** enters human breast milk, the resulting IgA antibodies do and may offer a level of neonatal protection. It is generally considered compatible with breastfeeding.

■ **References** .... Harjulehto-Mervaala T, Hovi T, Aro T, et al. Acta Obstet Gynecol Scand 1995; 74:262-5.

Bavdekar SB, Naik S, Nadkarni SS, et al. Indian J Pediatr 1999; 66:45-8.

Harjulehto-Mervaala T, Aro T, Hiilesmaa VK, et al. Clin Infect Dis 1994; 18:414-20.

Hanson LA, Carlsson B, Jalil F, et al. Rev Infect Dis 1984; 6(Suppl 2):S356-60.

■ **Summary**
- **Pregnancy Category C**
- **Lactation Category S**
- Although one might intuit that a live vaccine should be avoided during pregnancy in favor of an inactivated preparation, the largest studies are reassuring.

Polyethylene glycol (MiraLax)

■ **Class** — Laxative

■ **Indications** — Constipation

■ **Mechanism** — Unknown; osmotic agent which causes water retention in stool

■ **Dosage with Qualifiers** — Constipation—17g PO qd for up to 2w
- **Contraindications**—hypersensitivity to drug or class, bowel obstruction
- **Caution**—elderly

■ **Maternal Considerations** — There is little if any systemic absorption of **polyethylene glycol**. There are no adequate reports or well-controlled studies in pregnant women. It is used successfully for the treatment of puerperal constipation.
Side effects include nausea, abdominal bloating, cramping, flatulence, diarrhea, urticaria, and electrolyte disorders.

■ **Fetal Considerations** — There are no adequate reports or well-controlled studies in human fetuses. It is unknown whether **polyethylene glycol** crosses the human placenta. However, it is unlikely a clinically significant quantity of **polyethylene glycol** is absorbed systemically. Rodent teratogenicity studies have not been performed.

■ **Breastfeeding Safety** — There are no adequate reports or well-controlled studies in nursing women. It is unknown whether **polyethylene glycol** enters human breast milk. Considering the lack of systemic absorption, **polyethylene glycol** is unlikely to achieve clinically relevant levels in breast milk.

■ **References** — Nardulli G, Limongi F, Sue G, et al. GEN 1995; 49:224-6.

■ **Summary** .... • **Pregnancy Category C**
• **Lactation Category S**
• **Polyethylene glycol** should be used during pregnancy
  and lactation only if the benefit justifies the potential
  perinatal risk.
• There are alternative agents for which there is more
  experience during pregnancy and lactation.

Polymyxin B/trimethoprim ophthalmic
(Polytrim)

■ **Class** .... *Antibacterial, antibiotic, combination*

■ **Indications** .... Ophthalmic infection

■ **Mechanism** .... Bacteriostatic, bactericidal—see individual drugs

■ **Dosage with Qualifiers** .... Ophthalmic infection—1 gtt each eye q3h ×7d; max
6 doses/d
• **Contraindications**—hypersensitivity to drug or class
• **Caution**—none

■ **Maternal Considerations** .... There are no adequate reports or well-controlled studies
in pregnant women. See individual drugs.
Side effects include superinfection, increased perspiration,
burning, stinging, itching, circumocular rash, and eyelid
edema.

■ **Fetal Considerations** .... There are no adequate reports or well-controlled studies
in human fetuses. Considering the dose and route, it is
unlikely the maternal systemic concentrations will reach
clinically relevant levels. See individual drugs.

■ **Breastfeeding Safety** .... There are no adequate reports or well-controlled studies
in nursing women. It is unknown whether **polymyxin B/
trimethoprim ophthalmic** enters human breast milk.
However, considering the indication, route, and dosing,
polymyxin B/trimethoprim use is unlikely to pose a
clinically significant risk to the breast-feeding neonate.
See individual drugs.

■ **References** .... There are no current relevant references.

■ **Summary** .... • **Pregnancy Category C**
• **Lactation Category S**
• **Polymyxin B/trimethoprim ophthalmic** should be used
  during pregnancy and lactation only if the benefit
  justifies the potential perinatal risk.

Polythiazide/prazosin (Minizide)

- **Class** — Antihypertensive, diuretic, combination

- **Indications** — Hypertension

- **Mechanism** — See individual drugs

- **Dosage with Qualifiers** — Hypertension—1 tab PO bid/tid, beginning in the evening
  - **Contraindications**—hypersensitivity to drug or class, anuria, hypersensitivity to sulfonamides
  - **Caution**—unknown

- **Maternal Considerations** — There are no adequate reports or well-controlled studies in pregnant women. See individual drugs.
  Side effects include first dose hypotension and/or syncope, orthostatic hypotension, dizziness, headache, somnolence, weakness, palpitations, nausea, paresthesias, tinnitus, abdominal pain, arthralgia, myalgia, and pruritus.

- **Fetal Considerations** — There are no adequate reports or well-controlled studies in human fetuses. See individual drugs.

- **Breastfeeding Safety** — There are no adequate reports or well-controlled studies in nursing women. It is unknown whether **polythiazide/prazosin** enters human breast milk. See individual drugs.

- **References** — There is no published experience in pregnancy or during lactation.

- **Summary**
  - **Pregnancy Category C**
  - **Lactation Category S**
  - **Polythiazide/prazosin** should be used during pregnancy and lactation only if the benefit justifies the potential perinatal risk.
  - There are alternative agents for which there is more experience during pregnancy and lactation.

Potassium chloride (Cena-K; Chloropotassuril; Durules; K Tab; K-10; K-Care; K-Dur; K-Lease; K-Lor; K-Lyte Cl; K-Norm; K-Sol; Kadalex; Kaochlor; Kaon Cl; Kay Ciel; Klor-Con; Klorvess; Klotrix; Kolyum; Micro-K; Rum-K; Slow-K; Ten-K; Ultra-K-Chlor)

■ **Class** — Electrolytes, minerals

■ **Indications** — Hypokalemia, treatment and prophylaxis

■ **Mechanism** — Electrolyte replacement

■ **Dosage with Qualifiers** — Hypokalemia, treatment—400mEq/d PO if K<2mEq/L; 10-20mEq/h PO if ECG changes
Hypokalemia, prophylaxis—begin 20mEq PO qd, adjust as needed
- **Contraindications**—hypersensitivity to drug or class, untreated Addison's disease, hyperkalemia, renal failure
- **Caution**—renal dysfunction, cardiovascular disease

■ **Maternal Considerations** — There are no adequate reports or well-controlled studies in pregnant women. The most common cause of hypokalemia during pregnancy is the administration of betamimetic agents for the treatment of preterm labor (see **terbutaline**, **ritodrine**). However, the decreased serum potassium does not reflect total body depletion, but rather an increase in intracellular potassium. Routine treatment is not necessary.
Side effects include arrhythmia, dyspepsia, nausea, vomiting, diarrhea, rash, and bleeding.

■ **Fetal Considerations** — There are no adequate reports or well-controlled studies in human fetuses. Potassium readily crosses the human placenta. It is unlikely that potassium supplementation would have an adverse effect on the fetus without maternal toxicity. Rodent reproduction studies have not been performed.

■ **Breastfeeding Safety** — There are no adequate reports or well-controlled studies in nursing women. **Potassium chloride** enters human breast milk; supplementation is generally considered compatible with breastfeeding.

■ **References** — There are no current relevant references.

■ **Summary** —
- **Pregnancy Category C**
- **Lactation Category S**
- **Potassium chloride** should be used during pregnancy and lactation only if the benefit justifies the potential perinatal risk.

Potassium iodide (SSKI)

■ **Class** .... *Thyroid, mineral, electrolyte replacement*

■ **Indications** .... Thyrotoxicosis, preoperative thyroidectomy, expectorant; radiation exposure

■ **Mechanism** .... Inhibits thyroid hormone synthesis

■ **Dosage with Qualifiers** .... Thyrotoxicosis—50-250mg PO tid
Preoperative thyroidectomy—50-250mg PO tid beginning 10-14d before surgery
Expectorant—50-250mg PO tid; max 500mg/dose
Radiation exposure—130mg/d if expected exposure >5cGy; continue until risk of expousre has passed
- **Contraindications**—hypersensitivity to drug or class, hyperkalemia, severe volume depletion, Addison's disease, hypothyroidism, acute bronchitis, tuberculosis
- **Caution**—renal dysfunction, cardiovascular disease, cystic fibrosis

■ **Maternal Considerations** .... **Potassium iodide** effectively reduces thyroid uptake of radioactive iodide and is an adjunct for women with hyperthyroidism associated with Graves' disease. There are no adequate reports or well-controlled studies in pregnant women. **Potassium iodide** replacement is effective during pregnancy for the treatment of mild to moderate iodine deficiency.
Side effects include arrhythmia, GI bleeding, angioedema, parotitis, goiter, thyroid adenoma, metallic taste, dyspepsia, urticaria, headache, acne, fever, rhinitis, lymphadenopathy, arthralgia, eosinophilia, confusion, numbness, and paresthesia.

■ **Fetal Considerations** .... There are no adequate reports or well-controlled studies in human fetuses. **Potassium iodide** crosses the human placenta, and an excess can cause fetal goiter and hypothyroidism. The limited rodent studies are reassuring.

■ **Breastfeeding Safety** .... There are no adequate reports or well-controlled studies in nursing women. Supplementation with **potassium iodide** has little effect on the iodine concentration of human breast milk. It is probably compatible with breastfeeding.

■ **References** .... Glinoer D, De Nayer P, Delange F, et al. J Clin Endocrinol Metab 1995; 80:258-69.
Reinhardt W, Kohl S, Hollmann D, et al. Eur J Med Res 1998; 3:203-10.
Vicens-Calvet E, Potau N, Carreras E, et al. J Pediatr 1998; 133:147-8.
Morales de Villalobos LM, Campos G, Ryder E. Enzyme 1986; 35:96-101.
Chierici R, Saccomandi D, Vigi V. Acta Paediatr Suppl 1999; 88:7-13.

■ **Summary**
- **Pregnancy Category D**
- **Lactation Category S**
- **Potassium iodide** should be used during pregnancy and lactation only if the benefit justifies the potential perinatal risk.

Pralidoxime (Protopam)

■ **Class**

Antidote; toxicology

■ **Indications**

Organophosphate poisoning, anticholinesterase overdose

■ **Mechanism**

Reactivates cholinesterase

■ **Dosage with Qualifiers**

Organophosphate poisoning—1-2g IV over 15-30min; may repeat in 1h if clinically indicated
Anticholinesterase overdose—1-2g IV over 15-30min
- **Contraindications**—hypersensitivity to drug or class
- **Caution**—myasthenia gravis, renal dysfunction

■ **Maternal Considerations**

There are no adequate reports or well-controlled studies in pregnant women. The published experience is limited to case reports.
Side effects include transient neuromuscular blockade, laryngospasm, muscle rigidity, blurred vision, diplopia, dizziness, headache, nausea, vomiting, hypertension, tachycardia, maculopapular rash, and elevated LFTs.

■ **Fetal Considerations**

There are no adequate reports or well-controlled studies in human fetuses. It is not known whether **pralidoxime** crosses the human placenta. Rodent teratogenicity studies have not been conducted.

■ **Breastfeeding Safety**

There is no published experience in nursing women. It is unknown whether **pralidoxime** enters human breast milk. However, considering the indication and dosing, one-time **pralidoxime** use is unlikely to pose a clinically significant risk to the breast-feeding neonate.

■ **References**

Bailey B. Ann Emerg Med 1997; 29:299.

■ **Summary**
- **Pregnancy Category C**
- **Lactation Category U**
- **Pralidoxime** should be used during pregnancy and lactation only if the benefit justifies the potential perinatal risk.

Pramipexole (Mirapex; Sifrol)

- **Class** — *Antiparkinsonian, dopaminergic*

- **Indications** — Parkinsonism

- **Mechanism** — Nonergot dopamine receptor agonist

- **Dosage with Qualifiers** — Parkinsonism—begin 0.125mg PO tid; increase by 0.25mg/d q7d for 7w
  NOTE—renal dosing
  - **Contraindications**—hypersensitivity to drug or class
  - **Caution**—renal dysfunction

- **Maternal Considerations** — **Pramipexole** clearance is 30% lower in women than men; most of this difference reflects body weight. There is no published experience with **pramipexole** during pregnancy.
  Side effects include hallucinations, orthostatic hypotension, dyskinesia, asthenia, dizziness, insomnia, somnolence, peripheral edema, dry mouth, headache, anorexia, and visual abnormalities.

- **Fetal Considerations** — There are no adequate reports or well-controlled studies in human fetuses. It is unknown whether **pramipexole** crosses the human placenta. **Pramipexole** in rodents reduces implantation and is embryotoxic. Teratogenicity studies have not been performed.

- **Breastfeeding Safety** — There is no published experience in nursing women. It is unknown whether **pramipexole** enters human breast milk. **Pramipexole** is concentrated in rodent milk.

- **References** — There is no published experience in pregnancy.

- **Summary** —
  - **Pregnancy Category C**
  - **Lactation Category U**
  - **Pramipexole** should be used during pregnancy and lactation only if the benefit justifies the potential perinatal risk.

Pravastatin (Pravachol)

■ **Class** — Antihyperlipidemic; HMG-CoA reductase inhibitor

■ **Indications** — Hypercholesterolemia

■ **Mechanism** — Inhibits HMG-CoA reductase

■ **Dosage with Qualifiers** — Hypercholesterolemia—begin 40mg/d; max 80mg/d
NOTE—renal and hepatic dosing; monitor hepatic transaminases at baseline and either q3mo or prior to increasing dose
- **Contraindications**—hypersensitivity to drug or class, active liver disease
- **Caution**—alcohol abuse, hepatic or renal dysfunction

■ **Maternal Considerations** — **Pravastatin** lowers lipids in two ways. First, it modestly reduces the intracellular pool of cholesterol by the reversible inhibition of HMG-CoA reductase, increasing the number of LDL-receptors on cell surfaces and enhancing receptor-mediated catabolism and clearance of circulating LDL. Second, **pravastatin** inhibits LDL production by inhibiting hepatic synthesis of VLDL, the LDL precursor. There are no adequate reports or well-controlled studies in pregnant women. Atherosclerosis is a chronic process; discontinuation of **pravastatin** during pregnancy should have little impact on long-term outcome.
Side effects include rhabdomyolysis, hepatotoxicity, cholelithiasis, dyspepsia, abdominal pain, flatulence, constipation, rash, myalgia, asthenia, and elevated CPK or transaminases.

■ **Fetal Considerations** — There are no adequate reports or well-controlled studies in human fetuses. It is unknown whether **pravastatin** crosses the human placenta. Cholesterol and other products of cholesterol biosynthesis are essential components for fetal development. Because HMG-CoA reductase inhibitors such as **pravastatin** decrease cholesterol synthesis and potentially other biologically active substances derived from cholesterol, they are considered contraindicated during pregnancy by the FDA.

■ **Breastfeeding Safety** — There are no adequate reports or well-controlled studies in nursing women. It is unknown whether **pravastatin** enters human breast milk. Certainly cholesterol and its by-products are important components of breast milk. In the absence of further study, **pravastatin** should be considered incompatible with breastfeeding.

■ **References** — There is no published experience in pregnancy or during lactation.

- **Summary** ....
  - **Pregnancy Category X**
  - **Lactation Category NS?**
  - Cholesterol and other products of cholesterol biosynthesis are essential components for fetal development.
  - **Pravastatin** decreases cholesterol synthesis and potentially other biologically active substances derived from cholesterol.
  - It should be considered contraindicated during pregnancy and lactation until additional study.
  - Atherosclerosis is a chronic process; discontinuation of **pravastatin** during pregnancy should have little impact on long-term outcome.

Praziquantel (Biltricide)

- **Class** .... *Antiparasitic, anthelminthic*

- **Indications** .... Schistosomiasis, tapeworms, liver flukes

- **Mechanism** .... Enhances cell membrane permeability

- **Dosage with Qualifiers** ....
  Schistosomiasis—20mg/kg PO q4-6h ×1d
  Tapeworms—5-25mg/kg PO ×1
  Liver flukes—25mg/kg PO q4-6h ×1d
  - **Contraindications**—hypersensitivity to drug or class, ocular schistosomiasis or cysticercosis
  - **Caution**—hepatic dysfunction

- **Maternal Considerations** ....
  There are no adequate reports or well-controlled studies in pregnant women. The main complication of helminth infection during pregnancy is anemia. Neurocysticercosis is a cause of first-time convulsions in pregnant patients, and there are several case reports of its successful treatment with **praziquantel** during pregnancy.
  Praziquantel has also been used during the puerperium to successfully treat hypersplenism secondary to chronic hepatosplenic schistosomiasis.
  Side effects include CSF reaction syndrome, malaise, headache, dizziness, abdominal pain, nausea, fever, urticaria, bitter taste, drowsiness, anorexia, sweating, and fever.

- **Fetal Considerations** ....
  There are no adequate reports or well-controlled studies in human fetuses. It is not known whether **praziquantel** crosses the human placenta. Congenital helminthic infection in humans is exceedingly rare. Rodent studies are reassuring, revealing no evidence of teratogenicity or IUGR despite the use of doses higher than those used

clinically. However, some studies report **praziquantel** is embryotoxic and may be genotoxic.

■ **Breastfeeding Safety**

There are no adequate reports or well-controlled studies in nursing women. **Praziquantel** enters human breast milk with an M:P ratio approximating 0.25 or a peak milk concentration of 0.5mg/ml. However, the mean excretion with the milk in 24h approximates 0.0008% of the given dose. Thus, the unsupplemented neonate of a woman treated for tapeworm would ingest less than 1mg of drug given to its mother.

■ **References**

Kurl R, Montella KR. Am J Perinatol 1994; 11:409-11.
Kopelman JN, Miyazawa K. Am J Perinatol 1990; 7:380-3.
Frohberg H. Arzneimittelforschung 1984; 34:1137-44.
Montero R, Ostrosky P. Mutat Res 1997; 387:123-39.
Putter J, Held F. Eur J Drug Metab Pharmacokinet 1979; 4:193-8.

■ **Summary**

- **Pregnancy Category B**
- **Lactation Category S?**
- **Praziquantel** should be used during pregnancy and lactation only if the benefit justifies the potential perinatal risk.

Prazosin (Lopres; Minipress)

■ **Class**

Antihypertensive, α-adrenergic antagonist

■ **Indications**

Hypertension

■ **Mechanism**

Unknown; peripheral α-1 adrenergic antagonist

■ **Dosage with Qualifiers**

Hypertension—begin 1mg PO bid; usual dose 3-20mg/d
- **Contraindications**—hypersensitivity to drug or class
- **Caution**—hepatic or renal dysfunction

■ **Maternal Considerations**

Unlike many other antihypertensive drugs, the effect of **prazosin** is closely related to its plasma concentration. The time to peak concentration is increased and its elimination half-life prolonged during pregnancy. **Prazosin** is a secondary agent for the treatment of preeclamptic hypertension. While as effective as **nifedipine,** the associated fetal death rate is higher. *Side effects* include syncope after the 1st dose, postural hypotension, dizziness, palpitations, edema, nausea, vomiting, diarrhea, headache, paresthesias, blurred vision, drowsiness, malaise, dry mouth, arthralgia, fever, and pruritus.

- **Fetal Considerations** — There are no adequate reports or well-controlled studies in human fetuses. **Prazosin** crosses the human placenta achieving an F:M ratio of 0.20. Rodent studies are reassuring, revealing no evidence of teratogenicity or IUGR despite the use of doses higher than those used clinically. Some decrease in litter size occurs at doses >200 times the MRHD. There is no apparent explanation for the increased perinatal mortality rate when used to treat preeclamptic hypertension.

- **Breastfeeding Safety** — There are no adequate reports or well-controlled studies in nursing women. Small quantities of **prazosin** enter human breast milk; however, it is generally considered compatible with breastfeeding.

- **References** — Rubin PC, Butters L, Low RA, Reid JL. Br J Clin Pharmacol 1983; 16:543-7.
Lowe SA, Rubin PC. J Hypertens 1992; 10:201-7.
Hall DR, Odendaal HJ, Steyn DW, Smith M. BJOG 2000; 107:759-65.
Bourget P, Fernandez H, Edouard D, et al. Eur J Drug Metab Pharmacokinet 1995; 20:233-41.

- **Summary** —
  - **Pregnancy Category C**
  - **Lactation Category S**
  - **Prazosin** is one of many second-line alternatives for the treatment of preeclamptic and chronic hypertension during pregnancy.
  - **Prazosin** should be used during pregnancy and lactation only if the benefit justifies the potential perinatal risk.

Prednicarbate topical (Dermatop)

- **Class** — Corticosteroid, dermatosis

- **Indications** — Steroid-responsive dermatitis

- **Mechanism** — Unknown

- **Dosage with Qualifiers** — Steroid-responsive dermatitis—apply bid
  - **Contraindications**—hypersensitivity to drug or class
  - **Caution**—avoid prolonged use on face, groin, axilla, or skin creases

- **Maternal Considerations** — **Prednicarbate** (0.1%) does not suppress the HPA-axis if used at 30g/d for 1w. There are no published studies in pregnant women.
Side effects include pruritus, skin atrophy, and acne.

- **Fetal Considerations** .... There are no published studies in human fetuses. It is unknown whether **prednicarbate** crosses the human placenta. Considering the dose and route, it is unlikely the maternal systemic concentration will reach a clinically relevant level. In some rodent studies, **prednicarbate** is teratogenic and embryotoxic if given SC at doses 45 times the recommended topical human dose, assuming a percutaneous absorption of approximately 3%.

- **Breastfeeding Safety** .... There is no published experience in nursing women. It is unknown whether **prednicarbate** enters human breast milk. Some systemically administered corticosteroids are excreted in breast milk. However, considering the route and concentration, limited **prednicarbate** use is unlikely to pose a clinically significant risk to the breast-feeding neonate.

- **References** .... There is no published experience in pregnancy or during lactation.

- **Summary** ....
  - **Pregnancy Category C**
  - **Lactation Category S?**
  - **Prednicarbate** should be used during pregnancy and lactation only if the benefit justifies the potential perinatal risk.

Prednisolone (Adnisolone; Cortalone; Delta-Cortef; Orapred; Prelone; Ultracortenol)

- **Class** .... Corticosteroid

- **Indications** .... Inflammatory disorders, multiple sclerosis, asthma (acute or persistent severe), adrenal insufficiency

- **Mechanism** .... Unknown

- **Dosage with Qualifiers** .... Inflammatory disorders—5-60mg/d PO/IV/IM, may give in divided doses
  Relapsing multiple sclerosis—begin 200mg PO qd ×1w, then 80mg PO qod ×1m
  Asthma (acute)—begin 120-180mg/d PO/IV/IM in 3-4 divided doses, then 60-80mg/d PO/IV/IM for severe exacerbations
  Asthma (persistent severe)—7.5-80mg PO qd-qod, taper slowly
  Adrenal insufficiency—4-5mg/m^2 PO qd
  NOTE—available in various tablet, syrup, parenteral and ophthalmic preparations

- **Contraindications**—hypersensitivity to drug or class, systemic fungal infection
- **Caution**—seizure disorder, diabetes mellitus, hypertension, tuberculosis, osteoporosis, hepatic dysfunction

■ **Maternal Considerations**

Prednisolone is a metabolite of **prednisone**. It provides effective relief (10mg PO tid) of severe hyperemesis unresponsive to primary therapy and characterized by at least a 10% weight loss. Dermatologic and ophthalmic applications have been used for decades during pregnancy without apparent sequelae. **Prednisolone** is used widely for the treatment of inflammatory/autoimmune disorders that are common in reproductive-age women. Once used for the treatment antiphospholipid syndrome, several trials document a higher loss rate with **prednisolone** and **aspirin** than **heparin** and **aspirin**.
Side effects include adrenal insufficiency, steroid psychosis, immunosuppression, peptic ulcer, CHF, osteoporosis, pseudotumor cerebri, nausea, vomiting, dyspepsia, edema, headache, dizziness, mood swings, insomnia, anxiety, menstrual irregularities, ecchymosis, acne, skin atrophy, impaired wound healing, hypertension, hypokalemia, and hyperglycemia.

■ **Fetal Considerations**

There are no adequate reports or well-controlled studies in human fetuses. The human placenta metabolizes **prednisone** reducing fetal exposure to perhaps 10% of the maternal level. Some authors suggest emotional stress during organogenesis could cause congenital malformations by increasing the level of glucocorticoids. Older, epidemiologic studies examined the association of oral clefting with corticosteroids exposure and concluded prenatal exposure carried 6-fold increase in risk for cleft lip with or without cleft palate. IUGR, shortening of the head and mandible were also suggested as sequelae. However, the Collaborative Perinatal Project followed women treated during the 1st trimester. While the number of exposures was limited, no increase in congenital malformations was detected. More recent studies also dismiss the risk of teratogenicity for all malformations except clefting. There is no increase in risk of anomalies when exposure occurs after organogenesis. Women exposed to topical **prednisone**-like compounds during pregnancy have no significantly increased risk of delivering a child with birth defects. In sum, the evidence that corticosteroids are human teratogens is weak, and confined only to cleft lip. Female rats exposed to **cortisone** *in utero* exhibit premature vaginal opening. **Cortisone** accelerates fetal rat intestinal maturation, perhaps explaining why corticosteroids decrease the incidence of NEC.

■ **Breastfeeding Safety**

There are no adequate reports or well-controlled studies in nursing women. It is unknown whether **prednisolone** enters human breast milk. However, long clinical experience suggests **prednisolone** therapy is compatible with breastfeeding.

■ **References** .... Moran P, Taylor R. QJM 2002; 95:153-8.
Guillonneau M, Jacqz-Aigrain E. J Gynecol Obstet Biol Reprod (Paris) 1996; 25:160-7.
Park-Wyllie L, Mazzotta P, Pastuszak A, et al. Teratology 2000; 62:385-92.
Rodriguez-Pinnilla E, Martinez-Frias ML. Teratology 1998; 58:2-5.

■ **Summary** ....
- **Pregnancy Category B**
- **Lactation Category S?**
- **Prednisolone** should be used during pregnancy and lactation only if the benefit justifies the potential perinatal risk.

Prednisone (Adasone; Cartancyl; Colisone; Cordrol; Cortan; Dacortin; Deltasone; Orasone; Paracort; Prednicot; Sterapred; Sterapred DS)

■ **Class** .... Corticosteroid

■ **Indications** .... Inflammatory disorders, multiple sclerosis, pneumocystic pneumonia, adrenal insufficiency

■ **Mechanism** .... Unknown

■ **Dosage with Qualifiers** .... Inflammatory disorders—5-60mg PO qd
Relapsing multiple sclerosis—begin 200mg PO qd ×1w, then 80mg PO qod ×1m
Pneumocystic pneumonia—begin 40mg PO bid x5d, then 40mg qd ×5d, then 20mg qd
Adrenal insufficiency—4-5mg/m^2 PO qd
- **Contraindications**—hypersensitivity to drug or class, systemic fungal infection
- **Caution**—seizure disorder, diabetes mellitus, hypertension, tuberculosis, osteoporosis, hepatic dysfunction

■ **Maternal Considerations** .... There are no adequate reports or well-controlled studies in pregnant women. Previously used for the treatment antiphospholipid syndrome, several trials report the loss rate is higher with **prednisolone** and **aspirin** versus **heparin** and **aspirin**.
Side effects include adrenal insufficiency, steroid psychosis, immunosuppression, peptic ulcer, CHF, osteoporosis, pseudotumor cerebri, nausea, vomiting, dyspepsia, edema, headache, dizziness, mood swings, insomnia, anxiety, menstrual irregularities, ecchymosis, acne, skin atrophy, impaired wound healing, hypertension, hypokalemia, and hyperglycemia.

■ **Fetal Considerations** ⋯⋯⋯ There are no adequate reports or well-controlled studies in human fetuses. The human placenta metabolizes **prednisone** reducing fetal exposure to perhaps 10% of the maternal level. Some authors suggest emotional stress during organogenesis could cause congenital malformations by increasing the level of glucocorticoids. Older, epidemiologic studies examined the association of oral clefting with corticosteroids exposure and concluded prenatal exposure carry a 6-fold increase in risk for cleft lip with or without cleft palate. IUGR, shortening of the head and mandible were also suggested as sequelae. However, the Collaborative Perinatal Project followed women treated during the 1st trimester. While the number of exposures was limited, no increase in congenital malformations was detected. More recent studies also dismiss the risk of teratogenicity for all malformations except clefting. There is no increase in risk of anomalies when exposure occurs after organogenesis. Women exposed to topical **prednisone**-like compounds during pregnancy have no significantly increased risk of delivering a child with birth defects. In sum, the evidence that **corticosteroids** are human teratogens is weak, and confined only to cleft lip. Female rats exposed to **cortisone** *in utero* exhibit premature vaginal opening. **Cortisone** accelerates fetal rat intestinal maturation, perhaps explaining why corticosteroids decrease the incidence of NEC.

■ **Breastfeeding Safety** ⋯⋯⋯ There are no adequate reports or well-controlled studies in nursing women. It is unknown whether **prednisone** enters human breast milk. However, long clinical experience suggests **prednisone** is compatible with breastfeeding.

■ **References** ⋯⋯⋯ Empson M, Lassere M, Craig JC, Scott JR. Obstet Gynecol 2002; 99:135-44.
Rotmensch S, Liberati M, Celentano C, et al. Acta Obstet Gynecol Scand 1999; 78:768-73.
Park-Wyllie L, Mazzotta P, Pastuszak A, et al. Teratology 2000; 62:385-92.
Rodriguez-Pinnilla E, Martinez-Frias ML. Teratology 1998; 58:2-5.

■ **Summary** ⋯⋯⋯
- **Pregnancy Category B**
- **Lactation Category S**
- **Prednisone** should be used during pregnancy and lactation only if the benefit justifies the potential perinatal risk.

Prilocaine hydrochloride (Citanest)

■ **Class** — Anesthetic, local

■ **Indications** — Dental nerve block

■ **Mechanism** — Inhibits propagation of nerve impulse by inhibiting trans-neuronal membrance ionic flux

■ **Dosage with Qualifiers** — Dental nerve block—1-2ml infiltrated in the anatomically correct zone; max 600mg per 24h
NOTE—1% and 4% solution; avoid IV administration; onset 2-3min, duration 2-3h
- **Contraindications**—hypersensitivity to drug or class, congenital or idiopathic methemoglobinemia
- **Caution**—severe hepatic dysfunction

■ **Maternal Considerations** — There are no adequate reports or well-controlled studies in pregnant women. **Prilocaine** is used in some locales for pudendal nerve block at delivery. **Prilocaine** causes vascular smooth muscle contraction in *in vitro* studies, suggesting injection in the region of the uterine artery for a paracervical block may be a risk.
Side effects include lightheadedness, nervousness, apprehension, euphoria, confusion, dizziness, drowsiness, tinnitus, blurred or double vision, vomiting, sensations of heat, cold or numbness, twitching, tremors, convulsions, unconsciousness, respiratory depression or arrest, and vasovagal reaction.

■ **Fetal Considerations** — There are no adequate reports or well-controlled studies in human fetuses. **Prilocaine** crosses the human placenta, and after pudendal nerve block achieves a F:M ratio near unity. There are several reports of neonatal methemoglobinemia after **prilocaine**. Rodent studies are reassuring, revealing no evidence of teratogenicity or IUGR despite the use of doses higher than those used clinically.

■ **Breastfeeding Safety** — There are no adequate reports or well-controlled studies in nursing women. It is unknown whether **prilocaine** enters human breast milk. However, considering the indication and dosing, one-time **prilocaine** use is unlikely to pose a clinically significant risk to the breast-feeding neonate.

■ **References** — Tuvemo T, Willdeck-Lund G. Acta Anaesthesiol Scand 1982; 26:104-7.
Shnider SM, Gildea J. Am J Obstet Gynecol 1973; 116:320-5.
Nau H. Dev Pharmacol Ther 1985; 8:149-81.

■ **Summary** .... • **Pregnancy Category B**
- **Lactation Category S**
- **Prilocaine** should be used during pregnancy and lactation only if the benefit justifies the potential perinatal risk.
- There are superior alternatives for labor analgesia.

Primaquine (Primaquine)

■ **Class** .... Antiprotozoal; antimalarial

■ **Indications** .... Malaria, Pneumocystis carinii pneumonia

■ **Mechanism** .... Unknown

■ **Dosage with Qualifiers** .... Malaria—1 tab (15mg) PO qd ×14d
Pneumocystis carinii pneumonia—1-2 tabs (15-30mg) PO qd in combination with clindamycin
- **Contraindications**—hypersensitivity to drug or class, bone marrow suppression, rheumatoid arthritis, SLE, recent quinacrine use
- **Caution**—G6PD deficiency, favism

■ **Maternal Considerations** .... There are no adequate reports or well-controlled studies in pregnant women.
Side effects include hemolytic anemia, methemoglobinemia, leukopenia, retinopathy, nausea, vomiting, abdominal pain, headache, pruritus, and vision disturbances.

■ **Fetal Considerations** .... There are no adequate reports or well-controlled studies in human fetuses. It is unknown whether **primaquine** crosses the human placenta. Except for the tetracyclines, there is no evidence that at recommended doses any of the antimalarial drugs are teratogenic. **Primaquine** is generally not recommended because of its theoretic potential to cause fetal hemolytic anemia. Rodent teratogenicity studies have not apparently been performed.

■ **Breastfeeding Safety** .... There are no adequate reports or well-controlled studies in nursing women. It is unknown whether **primaquine** enters human breast milk.

■ **References** .... Phillips-Howard PA, Wood D. Drug Saf 1996; 14:131-45.

■ **Summary** .... • **Pregnancy Category C**
- **Lactation Category U**
- **Primaquine** should be used during pregnancy and lactation only if the benefit justifies the potential perinatal risk.

Primidone (Midone; Mylepsin; Mysoline; PMS Primidone; Prysoline)

■ **Class** ⸺ *Anticonvulsant*

■ **Indications** ⸺ Seizure disorder, essential tremor

■ **Mechanism** ⸺ Unknown

■ **Dosage with Qualifiers** ⸺ Seizure disorder—begin 100-125mg PO qhs ×3d, 100-125mg PO bid ×3d, then 250mg PO tid-qid; max 2g/d
Essential tremor—begin 12.5-25mg PO qhs, increase 12.5-25mg/d qw; max 750mg/d
NOTE—renal dosing
- **Contraindications**—hypersensitivity to drug or class, porphyria
- **Caution**—unknown

■ **Maternal Considerations** ⸺ **Primidone** is metabolized to **phenobarbital** and phenylethylmalonamide (PEMA). PEMA potentiates the effect of **phenobarbital**. There are no adequate reports or well-controlled studies in pregnant women.
Side effects include dyspnea, megaloblastic anemia, thrombocytopenia, ataxia, vertigo, nausea, vomiting, anorexia, fatigue, irritability, diplopia, nystagmus, drowsiness, rash, and osteopenia.

■ **Fetal Considerations** ⸺ There are no adequate reports or well-controlled studies in human fetuses. **Phenobarbital** and PEMA readily crosses the human placenta, and are distributed throughout fetus. The highest concentrations are found in the placenta, fetal liver, and brain. Withdrawal symptoms may occur in infants exposed to barbiturates throughout the 3rd trimester. Reports suggesting an increased rate of birth defects (oral clefting and cardiac malformations) in children of drug-treated epileptic women are not adequate to prove a cause-and-effect relationship. The majority of mothers on anticonvulsant medication deliver normal infants. Anticonvulsant drugs should <u>not</u> be discontinued in patients in whom the drug is administered to prevent major seizures because of the strong possibility of precipitating status epilepticus with attendant hypoxia and threat to life. As for most psychotropic drugs, monotherapy and the lowest effective quantity given in divided doses to minimize the peaks can minimize the fetal risks. It is controversial whether enzyme-inducing drugs like **primidone** increase the risk of neonatal bleeding. And though the most recent studies indicate no, the administration of 1mg vitamin K IM at birth is common.

■ **Breastfeeding Safety** ⸺ There is no published experience in nursing women. **Primidone** and its metabolites are excreted into human breast milk and have been associated with neonatal sedation. If breastfeeding continues, the infant should be monitored for possible adverse effects, the drug given at the lowest effective dose, and breastfeeding avoided at times of peak drug levels.

■ **References**

Bruno MK; Harden CL. Curr Treat Options Neurol 2002; 4:31-40.

Kaaja E, Kaaja R, Matila R, Hiilesmaa V. Neurology 2002; 58:549-53.

Hagg S, Spigset O. Drug Saf 2000; 22:425-40.

Dessens AB, Cohen-Kettenis PT, Mellenbergh GJ, et al. Teratology 2001; 64:181-8.

Arpino C, Brescianini S, Robert E, et al. Epilepsia 2000; 41:1436-43.

Shankaran S, Papile LA, Wright LL, et al. Am J Obstet Gynecol 2002; 187:171-7.

Crowther CA, Henderson-Smart DJ. Cochrane Database Syst Rev 2001; (2):CD000164.

Kuhnz W, Koch S, Helge H, Nau H. Dev Pharmacol Ther 1988; 11:147-54.

■ **Summary**

- **Pregnancy Category B**
- **Lactation Category NS?**
- **Primidone** should be used during pregnancy and lactation only if the benefit justifies the potential perinatal risk.
- There are alternative agents for which there is more experience during pregnancy and lactation.

Probenecid (Benemid; Panuric; Probalan; Solpurin; Urocid)

■ **Class**

Antigout, *uricosuric*

■ **Indications**

Adjunct to penicillin, gout

■ **Mechanism**

Inhibits penicillin secretion and urate resorption by the renal tubules

■ **Dosage with Qualifiers**

Adjunct to penicillin therapy—500mg PO qid
Gout—begin 250mg PO bid ×7d; max 2-3g/d
- **Contraindications**—hypersensitivity to drug or class, CrCl<50ml/h, urate stones, acute gout
- **Caution**—hypersensitivity to sulfa drugs, peptic ulcer disease, renal dysfunction

■ **Maternal Considerations**

Probenecid is used during pregnancy with a penicillin almost exclusively for the treatment of STDs.
Side effects include hemolytic anemia, aplastic anemia, hepatic necrosis, headache, dizziness, anorexia, nausea,

823

vomiting, sore gums, nephrotic syndrome, renal colic, dermatitis, pruritus, flushing, fever, and exacerbation of gout.

■ **Fetal Considerations** — There are no adequate reports or well-controlled studies in human fetuses. **Probenecid** crosses the human placenta, but is not associated with adverse fetal affects. Rodent studies are reassuring, revealing no evidence of teratogenicity or IUGR despite the use of doses higher than those used clinically.

■ **Breastfeeding Safety** — There is no published experience in nursing women. It is unknown whether **probenecid** enters human breast milk. However, considering the indication and dosing, the typically one-time use of **probenecid** is unlikely to pose a clinically significant risk to the breastfeeding neonate.

■ **References** — There are no current relevant references.

■ **Summary** —
- **Pregnancy Category B**
- **Lactation Category S**
- **Probenecid** should be used during pregnancy and lactation only if the benefit justifies the potential perinatal risk.

Probucol (Bifenabid; Lesterol; Lorelco; Lurselle; Panesclerina; Sinlestal)

■ **Class** — Antihyperlipidemic

■ **Indications** — Hyperlipidemia

■ **Mechanism** — Increases the fractional rate of LDL catabolism; inhibits early stages of cholesterol biosynthesis

■ **Dosage with Qualifiers** — Hyperlipidemia—500mg PO bid
NOTE—do not begin if QT interval exceeds rate dependent guideline; any hypomagnesemia, hypokalemia, or severe bradycardia should be resolved before initiating
- **Contraindications**—hypersensitivity to drug or class, recent or progressive myocardial damage, prolonged QT interval syndrome, ventricular arrhythmia
- **Caution**—unknown

■ **Maternal Considerations** — There is no published experience with **probucol** during pregnancy. Atherosclerosis is a chronic process; discontinuation of **probucol** during pregnancy should have little impact on the long-term outcome of the disease process.

Side effects include prolongation of the QT interval, syncope, ventricular arrhythmia, sudden death, diarrhea, abdominal pain, nausea, vomiting, dyspepsia, GI bleeding, headache, dizziness, paresthesia, insomnia, tinnitus, peripheral neuritis, rash, pruritus, ecchymosis, petechiae, eosinophilia, anemia, and thrombocytopenia.

- **Fetal Considerations** There are no adequate reports or well-controlled studies in human fetuses. It is unknown whether **probucol** crosses the human placenta. Rodent studies are reassuring, revealing no evidence of teratogenicity or IUGR despite the use of doses higher than those used clinically.

- **Breastfeeding Safety** There is no published experience in nursing women. It is unknown whether **probucol** enters human breast milk. Certainly cholesterol and its by-products are important components of breast milk. In the absence of further study, **probucol** should be considered incompatible with breastfeeding.

- **References** There is no published experience in pregnancy or during lactation.

- **Summary**
  - **Pregnancy Category B**
  - **Lactation Category NS?**
  - **Probucol** should be used during pregnancy and lactation only if the benefit justifies the potential perinatal risk.
  - Cholesterol and other products of cholesterol biosynthesis are essential components for fetal development.
  - Atherosclerosis is a chronic process; discontinuation of probucol during pregnancy should have little impact on long-term outcome.

Procainamide (Biocoryl; Procan SR; Procanbid; Promine; Pronestyl; Ritmocam)

- **Class** Antiarrhythmic, class IA

- **Indications** Atrial or ventricular arrhythmia

- **Mechanism** Stabilizes membrane potential, depressing the phase 0 action potential

- **Dosage with Qualifiers** Atrial or ventricular arrhythmia—100mg IV over 5min, repeat up to 500mg then wait ≥ 10min before restarting infusion; alternatively, 15-17mg/kg IV over 30-60min until either QRS widens 50% or abnormality resolves, then 1-6mg/min IV; max 1.5g load, 9g/d maintenance

NOTE—renal dosing; therapeutic levels = 4-10mcg/ml, or 10-30mcg/ml **procainamide** + NAPA
- **Contraindications**—hypersensitivity to drug or class, 2nd or 3rd degree AV block, myasthenia gravis, SLE, torsades de pointes
- **Caution**—bone marrow depression, CHF, renal dysfunction

■ **Maternal Considerations** ⋯⋯ There are no adequate reports or well-controlled studies in pregnant women. **Procainamide** is well tolerated, and is a first-line agent for the treatment of acute, undiagnosed, wide-complex tachycardia. It may be used alone or in combination with **digoxin**. All IA agents should be administered in the hospital under continuous cardiac monitoring due to the potential risk of ventricular arrhythmia.
Side effects include asystole, ventricular fibrillation, seizures, lupus-like syndrome, hemolytic anemia, neutropena, thrombocytopenia, agranulocytosis, hypotension, bradycardia, flushing, urticaria, pruritus, angioedema, rash, fever, nausea, vomiting, bitter taste, hallucinations, confusion, depression, diarrhea, dizziness, and elevated LFTs.

■ **Fetal Considerations** ⋯⋯ There are no adequate reports or well-controlled studies in human fetuses. **Procainamide** crosses the human placenta and is not bound by the placenta. There are numerous case reports of its use as a transplacental agent to treat fetal arrhythmia. *In vitro*, it produces dose-dependent relaxation of the placental vasculature. Rodent teratogenicity studies have not been performed.

■ **Breastfeeding Safety** ⋯⋯ There are no adequate reports or well-controlled studies in nursing women. Both **procainamide** and its main metabolite, NAPA are excreted into human breast milk and absorbed by the nursing neonate. Yet, the circulating level is low and **procainamide** is considered compatible with breastfeeding.

■ **References** ⋯⋯ Joglar JA, Page RL. Drug Saf 1999; 20:85-94.
Bailey DN. Ann Clin Lab Sci 1999; 29:209-12.
Dumesic DA, Silverman NH, Tobias S, Golbus MS. N Engl J Med 1982; 307:1128-31.
Weiner CP, Thompson MI. Am J Obstet Gynecol 1988; 158:570-3.
Ito S, Magee L, Smallhorn J. Clin Perinatol 1994; 21:543-72.
Omar HA, Rhodes LA, Ramirez R, et al. J Cardiovasc Electrophysiol 1996; 7:1197-203.
Pittard WB 3rd, Glazier H. J Pediatr 1983; 102:631-3.

■ **Summary** ⋯⋯
- **Pregnancy Category C**
- **Lactation Category S**
- **Procainamide** should be used during pregnancy and lactation only if the benefit justifies the potential perinatal risk.

Procaine (Novocain)

- **Class** — *Local anesthetic*

- **Indications** — Local and regional anesthesia

- **Mechanism** — Inhibits propagation of nerve impulse by inhibition of trans-neuronal membrane ion flux.

- **Dosage with Qualifiers** — Local and regional anesthesia—dose varies; max 10mg/kg
  NOTE—typical onset 2-5min, duration 30-90min
  - **Contraindications**—hypersensitivity to drug or class, infection at site
  - **Caution**—heart block, hypotension, cholinesterase deficiency, sulfite allergy, renal disease, impaired cardiovascular function

- **Maternal Considerations** — There are no adequate reports or well-controlled studies in pregnant women. Procaine has been used for decades during labor to create spinal, nerve block, or infiltration anesthesia.
  Side effects include CNS toxicity, myocardial depression, cardiac arrest, convulsions, RDS, unconsciousness, heart block, hypotension, arrhythmia, drowsiness, nervousness, blurred vision, tremors, nausea, vomiting, pupil constriction, tinnitus, chills, and pruritus.

- **Fetal Considerations** — There are no adequate reports or well-controlled studies in human fetuses. Local anesthetics rapidly cross the placenta. The long clinical experience is reassuring. Rodent teratogenicity studies have not been performed.

- **Breastfeeding Safety** — There is no published experience in nursing women. It is unknown whether **procaine** enters human breast milk. However, considering the indication and dosing, one time **procaine** use is unlikely to pose a clinically significant risk to the breast-feeding neonate.

- **References** — There are no current relevant references.

- **Summary** —
  - **Pregnancy Category C**
  - **Lactation Category S?**
  - **Procaine** should be used during pregnancy and lactation only if the benefit justifies the potential perinatal risk.

Procarbazine (Matulane)

- **Class** — Antineoplastic

- **Indications** — Lymphomas, brain and lung cancers

- **Mechanism** — Unknown

- **Dosage with Qualifiers** — Lymphomas, brain and lung cancers—dosing protocols vary
  - **Contraindications**—hypersensitivity to drug or class, bone marrow depression
  - **Caution**—hepatic or renal dysfunction

- **Maternal Considerations** — There are no adequate reports or well-controlled studies in pregnant women. Procarbazine is usually combined with other potent, antineoplastic agents. Yet the outcomes for most treated pregnancies and the 2nd generation children are normal.
  Side effects include seizures, coma, thrombocytopenia, bleeding, leukopenia, anemia, hemolytic anemia, pleural effusion, nausea, vomiting, hallucinations, nervousness, dermatitis, anorexia, dry mouth, tachycardia, and neuropathy.

- **Fetal Considerations** — There are no adequate reports or well-controlled studies in human fetuses. While it is unknown whether **procarbazine** crosses the human placenta, there are case reports of malformations in the offspring of women exposed to **procarbazine** in combination with other antineoplastic agents. Rodent studies performed at multiples of the MRHD reveal a spectrum of malformations including a dose-dependent increase in microcephaly.

- **Breastfeeding Safety** — There is no published experience in nursing women. It is unknown whether **procarbazine** enters human breast milk.

- **References** — Aviles A, Neri N. Clin Lymphoma 2001; 2:173-7.
  Lishner M, Zemlickis D, Degendorfer P, et al. Br J Cancer 1992; 65:114-7.
  Johnson JM, Thompson DJ, Haggerty GC, et al. Teratology 1985; 32:203-12.

- **Summary** —
  - **Pregnancy Category D**
  - **Lactation Category U**
  - **Procarbazine** should be used during pregnancy and lactation only if the benefit justifies the potential perinatal risk.
  - Though the risks of chemotherapy to the fetus are real, most pregnancies end without complication.

Prochlorperazine (Buccastem; Compa-Z; Compazine; Cotranzine; Nautisol; Novomit; Prochlorperazine Edisylate; Prochlorperazine Maleate; Steremal; Tementil; Ultrazine-10; Vertigon)

■ **Class** —————————————— *Antiemetic/antivertigo, antipsychotic; phenothiazine*

■ **Indications** ——————————— Nausea, vomiting, anxiety, psychosis

■ **Mechanism** ———————————— Unknown

■ **Dosage with Qualifiers** ————— Nausea, vomiting—5-10mg PO/IM tid-qid, or 25mg PR bid, or 5-10mg IV over 2min; max 40mg/d
Psychosis—5-10mg PO tid/qid; max 150mg/d
- **Contraindications**—hypersensitivity to drug or class, CNS depression, adrenergic blockade, phenothiazine blood dyscrasia
- **Caution**—glaucoma, epilepsy, cardiovascular disease, bone marrow depression

■ **Maternal Considerations** ———— There are no adequate reports or well-controlled studies in pregnant women. Long clinical experience indicates efficacy for the treatment of hyperemesis when combined with hydration and rest. **Prochlorperazine** (10mg IV) is superior to **meclopramide** (10mg IV) for the relief of acute migraine headache.
Side effects include agranulocytosis, thrombocytopenia, hemolytic anemia, ECG abnormalities, exfoliative dermatitis, tardive dyskinesia, neuroleptic malignant syndrome, hepatotoxicity, leukopenia, drowsiness, amenorrhea, blurred vision, rash, orthstatic hypotension, jaundice, dry mouth, constipation, photosensitivity, anxiety, oculogyric crisis, and extrapyramidal effects.

■ **Fetal Considerations** —————— There are no adequate reports or well-controlled studies in human fetuses. It is unknown whether **prochlorperazine** crosses the human placenta. The extensive clinical experience during pregnancy is reassuring without any substantial evidence of teratogenicity. Rodent teratogenicity studies have not been performed.

■ **Breastfeeding Safety** ————— There are no adequate reports or well-controlled studies in nursing women. **Prochlorperazine** enters human breast milk, but the kinetics remain to be elucidated.

■ **References** ————————————— Mazotta P, Magee LA. Drugs 2000; 59:781-800.
Coppola M, Yealy DM, Leibold RA. Ann Emerg Med 1995; 26:541-6.

■ **Summary**

- **Pregnancy Category C**
- **Lactation Category U**
- **Prochloperazine** is a commonly used agent for the treatment of nausea during pregnancy.
- It should be used during pregnancy and lactation only if the benefit justifies the potential perinatal risk.

Procyclidine (Apricolin; Kemadren; Kemadrin; Osnervan)

■ **Class** — *Anticholinergic; antiparkinsonian*

■ **Indications** — Parkinson's disease

■ **Mechanism** — Anticholinergic

■ **Dosage with Qualifiers** — Parkinson's disease—2.5mg PO tid; increase slowly to 5mg PO tid
- **Contraindications**—hypersensitivity to drug or class, angle-closure glaucoma
- **Caution**—none

■ **Maternal Considerations** — There is no published experience in pregnancy. *Side effects* include dryness of the mouth, mydriasis, blurring of vision, giddiness, lightheadedness and GI disturbances such as nausea, vomiting, epigastric distress, and constipation.

■ **Fetal Considerations** — There are no adequate reports or well-controlled studies in human fetuses. It is unknown whether **procyclidine** crosses the human placenta. Rodent teratogenicity studies have not been performed.

■ **Breastfeeding Safety** — There is no published experience in nursing women. It is unknown whether **procyclidine** enters human breast milk.

■ **References** — There is no published experience in pregnancy or during lactation.

■ **Summary**
- **Pregnancy Category C**
- **Lactation Category U**
- **Procyclidine** should be used during pregnancy and lactation only if the benefit justifies the potential perinatal risk.

Progesterone (Gesterol 50; Lutolin-S; Progestaject-50; Prometrium; Crinone)

■ **Class** ······ *Hormone replacement, contraceptive, uterine hemorrhage*

■ **Indications** ······ Amenorrhea, secondary amenorrhea, hormone replacement, infertility

■ **Mechanism** ······ Inhibits GnRH, transforms proliferative into secretory endometrium

■ **Dosage with Qualifiers** ······ Amenorrhea—400mg PO qd ×10d
Hormone replacement—200mg PO given each day with estrogen
Infertility, progesterone deficiency—1 applicator 8% PV qd; continue through 10-12w of pregnancy
Infertility, ovarian failure—1 applicator 8% PV bid
Secondary amenorrhea—1 applicator 4% PV qod
NOTE—available in tablet, parenteral or vaginal cream (Crinone, 4% = 45mg/applicator) forms
- **Contraindications**—hypersensitivity to drug or class, peanut allergy, pregnancy, thromboembolism, breast cancer, undiagnosed vaginal bleeding, missed abortion
- **Caution**—CHF, hepatic dysfunction, lactation

■ **Maternal Considerations** ······ **Progesterone** is central for reproduction. This section applies only to native hormone and not synthetic compounds, which may differ significantly depending upon their receptor profile. Please see the individual progestogens. **Progesterone** is used throughout the 1st trimester to provide luteal phase support for women undergoing ovulation induction and IVF. Other than those, there are no proved indications for its use during pregnancy. **Progesterone** administration does not prevent pregnancy loss in women with spontaneous, clinically recognized conceptions greater than 7w when the placenta is hormonally functional and the pregnancy no longer corpus luteum dependent. The evidence that **progesterone** is an effective treatment for supposed luteal phase defects is weak. It is controversial whether **progesterone** can delay delivery in women with idiopathic preterm labor. Recent study suggests it may be beneficial in women at high risk.
Side effects include menstrual irregularities, amenorrhea, breast tenderness, weight gain, stroke, thromboembolism, MI, breast cancer, gallbladder disease, cholestatic jaundice, hypertension, headache, fluid retention, depression, rash, pruritus, libido changes, acne, hirsutism, galactorrhea, and alopecia.

■ **Fetal Considerations** ······ There are no adequate reports or well-controlled studies in human fetuses. Progestogens differ in their hormonal effects. Masculinization of the female fetus is attributed to some progestogens. The evidence that natural **progesterone** is a teratogen is weak.

■ **Breastfeeding Safety** — There are no adequate reports or well-controlled studies in nursing women. Exogenous **progesterone** enters human breast milk. The quantity of milk produced correlates with the antenatal progesterone level.

■ **References** — da Fonseca EB, Bittar RE, Carvalho MH, Zugaib M. Am J Obstet Gynecol 2003; 188:419-24.
Carp H, Torchinsky A, Fein A, Toder V. Gynecol Endocrinol 2001; 15:472-83.
Norwitz ER, Schust DJ, Fisher SJ. N Engl J Med 2001; 345:1400-8.
Dawood MY. Curr Opin Obstet Gynecol 1994; 6:121-7.
Ingram JC, Woolridge MW, Greenwood RJ, McGrath L. Acta Paediatr 1999; 88:493-9.

■ **Summary** —
- **Pregnancy Category D**
- **Lactation Category S**
- **Progesterone** should be used during pregnancy only for luteal phase support after ovulation induction.
- Its potential to reduce the incidence of preterm delivery in at-risk women remains under investigation.

Promazine (Liranol; Prazine; Primazine; Protactyl; Prozine-50; Savamine; Sparine; Talofen)

■ **Class** — *Antipsychotic, phenothiazine*

■ **Indications** — Psychotic disorders

■ **Mechanism** — Unknown

■ **Dosage with Qualifiers** — Psychotic disorders—begin 50-150mg IM; up to 300mg additional may be given after 30min to achieve desired effect; thereafter, 10-200mg PO q4-6h
NOTE—dose and route dictated by severity of the condition; IM preferred
- **Contraindications**—hypersensitivity to drug or class, drug-induced CNS depression, intra-arterial injection, bone marrow suppression
- **Caution**—atherosclerosis, severe hypotension, abrupt cessation

■ **Maternal Considerations** — **Promazine** is a prototype phenothiazine used with variable success for the treatment of depressive neurosis, alcohol withdrawal, nausea and vomiting, symptoms of dementia, Tourette's syndrome, Huntington's chorea, and

Reye's syndrome. Though **promazine** has been used in obstetrics for almost 3 decades, there are no adequate reports or well-controlled studies in pregnant women. *Side effects* include tardive dyskinesia, drowsiness, jaundice, agranulocytosis, eosinophilia, leukopenia, hemolytic anemia, thrombocytopenic purpura, fever, decreased appetite, paradoxical exacerbation of psychotic symptoms, seizures, cerebral edema, amenorrhea, galactorrhea, and dry mouth.

■ **Fetal Considerations**

There are no adequate reports or well-controlled studies in human fetuses. It is unknown whether **promazine** crosses the human placenta. However, it undergoes placental peroxidation, and the free radicals produced may be one source of fetal toxicity. Older reports suggest a relationship between antenatal **promazine** and neonatal hyperbilirubinemia. In one study, **promazine** had no effect on fetal cardiovascular function of sheep. But in a second study performed using a higher dose, **promazine** caused fetal hypotension and tachycardia, and exacerbated the effect of umbilical cord compression. Rodent teratogenicity studies have not been performed.

■ **Breastfeeding Safety**

There are no adequate reports or well-controlled studies in nursing women. It is unknown whether **promazine** enters human breast milk.

■ **References**

Yang X, Kulkkarni AP. Terat Carcinog Mutagen 1997; 17:139-51.
Ayromlooi J. Dev Pharmacol Ther 1985; 8:302-10.
Cottle MK, Van Patten GR, van Muyden P. Am J Obstet Gynecol 1983; 146:686-92.

■ **Summary**

- **Pregnancy Category C**
- **Lactation Category U**
- **Promazine** should be used during pregnancy and lactation only if the benefit justifies the potential perinatal risk.

Promethazine (Anergan; Antiallersin; Camergan; Fargan; Metaryl; Pentazine; Phenergan; Phenerzine; Promethacon; Prozine; Sayomol; Xepagan)

■ **Class**
Antiemetic, antihistamine, phenothiazine

■ **Indications**
Nausea, vomiting, motion sickness, sedation, allergic rhinitis

■ **Mechanism**
Antagonizes central and peripheral H_1 receptors

- **Dosage with Qualifiers** ⋯⋯ <u>Nausea, vomiting</u>—12.5-25mg PO/PR/IM q4-6h prn
<u>Motion sickness</u>—25mg PO bid
<u>Sedation</u>—25-50mg PO/PR/IM q4-6h prn
<u>Allergic rhinitis</u>—12.5-25mg PO q6h, or 25mg PO qhs
NOTE—may be combined with **codeine**
  - **Contraindications**—hypersensitivity to drug or class, narrow-angle glaucoma
  - **Caution**—seizure disorder, asthma, hepatic dysfunction, bone marrow suppression

- **Maternal Considerations** ⋯⋯ **Promethazine** has been used for decades in obstetrics to treat nausea and vomiting, as a sedative, and to relieve apprehension during the latent phase of labor. It is often combined with a narcotic such as **meperidine**. **Promethazine** (25mg tid x 3w) is similar to **ondansetron** but inferior to a short course (3d) of **methylprednisolone** for the relief of nausea and vomiting of pregnancy. **Promethazine** was a frequent component of lytic cocktails used in preeclamptic women to prevent seizures. These cocktails have been abandoned in favor of **magnesium sulfate**. Initial hopes that **promethazine** would ameliorate severe Rh alloimmunization have not been substantiated but remain poorly studied. It is not effective for the relief of nausea following after **thiopentone** anesthesia for abortion. Controlled trials do not support the use of **promethazine** as an adjuvant to reduce postoperative adhesions.
Side effects include tardive dyskinesia, extrapyramidal effects, respiratory depression, hypotension, bradycardia, tachycardia, agranulocytosis, thrombocytopenia, dry mouth, sedation, drowsiness, nausea, vomiting, rash, tachycardia, rash, and thickened bronchial secretions.

- **Fetal Considerations** ⋯⋯ There are no adequate reports or well-controlled studies in human fetuses. It is unknown whether **promethazine** crosses the human placenta. The combination of **promethazine** and **meperidine** during labor reduces fetal heart rate reactivity. There was no effect on somatic development in one study. Transport across the mouse placenta is limited. Rodent studies are reassuring, revealing no evidence of teratogenicity or IUGR despite the use of doses higher than those used clinically.

- **Breastfeeding Safety** ⋯⋯ There is no published experience in nursing women. It is unknown whether **promethazine** enters human breast milk.

- **References** ⋯⋯ Safari HR, Fassett MJ, Souter IC, et al. Am J Obstet Gynecol 1998; 179:921-4.
Sullivan CA, Johnson CA, Roach H, et al. Am J Obstet Gynecol 1996; 174:1565-8.
Duley L, Gulmezoglu AM. Cochrane Database Syst Rev 2001; (1):CD002960.
Sandhya Yaddanapudi LN. Singapore Med J 1994; 35:271-3.
Jonkman JH, Westenberg HG, Rijntjes NV, van der Kleijn E, Lindeboom SF. Arzneimittelforschung 1983; 33:223-8.

Gibble JW, Ness PM. Clin Lab Med 1992; 12:553-76.
Watson A, Vanderkerckhove P, Lilford R. Hum Fertil 1999; 2:149-57.
Solt I, Ganadry S, Weiner Z. Isr Med Assoc J 2002; 4:178-80.
Czeizel AE, Szegal BA, Joffe JM, Racz J. Neurotoxicol 1999; 21:157-67.

■ **Summary**
- **Pregnancy Category C**
- **Lactation Category U**
- **Promethazine** is effective as an antiemetic under certain circumstances.

Propafenone (Arythmol; Norfenon; Normorytmin; Rythmol; Rytmonorm)

■ **Class** — *Antiarrhythmic, class 1c*

■ **Indications** — Ventricular arrhythmia

■ **Mechanism** — Stabilizes membrane potential; depresses the phase 0 action potential

■ **Dosage with Qualifiers** — <u>Ventricular arrhythmia</u>—150mg PO q8h; may increase over 3-4d to a max of 900mg/d
- **Contraindications**—hypersensitivity to drug or class, CHF, bradycardia, SA or AV conduction defects, severe, hypotension, bronchospasm, electrolyte imbalances
- **Caution**—unknown

■ **Maternal Considerations** — There are no adequate reports or well-controlled studies in pregnant women. The published experience is confined to case reports.
Side effects include CHF, ventricular arrhythmia, nausea, vomiting, dizziness, constipation, taste change, dyspnea, fatigue, headache, blurred vision, palpitations, rash, angina, dry mouth, and syncope.

■ **Fetal Considerations** — There are no adequate reports or well-controlled studies in human fetuses. **Propafenone** crosses the human placenta, though the kinetics remain to be elucidated. Rodent studies reveal embryotoxicity but no evidence of teratogenicity. Embryotoxicity occurs increasingly with escalating doses.

■ **Breastfeeding Safety** — There are no adequate reports or well-controlled studies in nursing women. Limited study suggests low quantities of **propafenone** enter human breast milk.

■ **References** .... Braverman AC, Bromley BS, Rutherford JD. Int J Cardiol 1991; 33:409-12.
Grand A. Rev Fr Gynecol Obstet 1993; 88:297-312.
Libardoni M, Piovan D, Busato E, Padrini R. Br J Clin Pharmacol 1991; 32:527-81.

■ **Summary** ....
- **Pregnancy Category C**
- **Lactation Category U**
- **Propafenone** should be used during pregnancy and lactation only if the benefit justifies the potential perinatal risk.
- There are alternative agents for which there is more experience during pregnancy and lactation.

Propantheline (Bropantil; Corrigast; Ercoril; Norproban; Pantheline; Pro-Banthine)

■ **Class** .... *Antiulcer, antispasmotic*

■ **Indications** .... Peptic ulcer

■ **Mechanism** .... Cholinergic antagonist

■ **Dosage with Qualifiers** .... Peptic ulcer—begin 15mg PO qac, 30mg qhs; max 60mg PO qid
- **Contraindications**—hypersensitivity to drug or class, bowel obstruction, myasthenia gravis, angle closure glaucoma, bleeding, reflux esophagitis
- **Caution**—CAD, ulcerative colitis

■ **Maternal Considerations** .... There is no published experience in pregnancy.
Side effects include dry mouth, blurred vision, confusion, palpitations, headache, orthostatic hypotension, insomnia, somnolence, tachycardia, mydriasis, cycloplegia, constipation, nausea, bloating, urticaria, anhidrosis, and respiratory distress.

■ **Fetal Considerations** .... There are no adequate reports or well-controlled studies in human fetuses. It is unknown whether **propantheline** crosses the human placenta. Rodent teratogenicity studies have apparently not been performed.

■ **Breastfeeding Safety** .... There is no published experience during lactation. It is unknown whether **propantheline** enters human breast milk.

■ **References** .... There are no current relevant references.

■ **Summary**
- **Pregnancy Category C**
- **Lactation Category U**
- **Propantheline** should be used during pregnancy and lactation only if the benefit justifies the potential perinatal risk.
- There are alternative agents for which there is more experience during pregnancy and lactation.

Propofol (Diprivan)

■ **Class**
Anesthesia, induction/maintenance

■ **Indications**
Anesthesia induction and maintenance, sedation for ventilated patients

■ **Mechanism**
Unknown; positively modulates inhibitory function of GABA

■ **Dosage with Qualifiers**
Anesthesia induction—dose varies widely depending on patient health; typically 2-2.5mg/kg IV administered as 40mg q10sec until desired effect
Anesthesia maintenance—dose varies widely depending on patient health; typically 0.1-0.4mg/kg/min IV depending on use of inhalation or other intravenous anesthetics
Sedation for ventilated patients—begin 5mcg/kg/min IV, then increase by 5-10mcg/kg/min q5-10min until desired effect
- **Contraindications**—hypersensitivity to drug or class, allergy to either soybean, egg lecithin, or glycerol
- **Caution**—lipid metabolism disorder, increased ICP

■ **Maternal Considerations**
Propofol is popular for a variety of procedures including oocyte retrieval and suction curettage. Its administration (1.0mg/kg/h) after cord clamping at cesarean delivery performed under general anesthesia reduces postoperative nausea and vomiting. Its clearance, as reflected in the dose required to produce unconsciousness, is unaltered during early pregnancy. It has a direct inhibitory effect on uterine contractions, caused at least in part by interfering with calcium transport. In small series of patients whose anesthesia for cesarean delivery was induced and maintained with **propofol**, there were no differences in neonatal outcome as compared to more commonly administered anesthetic agents.
Side effects include pancreatitis, opisthotonus, apnea, bradycardia, hypotension, involuntary movement, nausea, vomiting, and injection site reactions.

- **Fetal Considerations** .... There are no adequate reports or well-controlled studies in human fetuses. **Propofol** crosses the human placenta in a time dependent manner, at a rate dependent on uterine and umbilical blood flows. The maternal albumen level also impacts on the extent of transfer. Reports of F:M ratio range widely from 0.35-1.0. **Propofol** infusions adequate for conscious sedation during cesarean section seem to have no adverse neonatal effects. While rodent studies are reassuring, revealing no evidence of teratogenicity, breast-fed pups of treated mothers have a higher mortality rate. **Propofol** transiently blocks NMDA receptors that lead to an increase in neuronal apoptosis in rodent.

- **Breastfeeding Safety** .... There are no adequate reports or well-controlled studies in nursing women. A small amount of **propofol** is excreted in human breast milk. However, considering the indications, prior exposure to **propofol** is not likely to pose a significant risk to the breastfeeding neonate.

- **References** .... He YL, Seno H, Sasaki K, Tashiro C. Anesth Analg 2002; 94:1312-4.
Tsujiguchi N, Yamakage M, Namika A. Anesthesiology 2001; 95:1245-55.
Higuchi H, Adachi Y, Arimura S, et al. Anesth Analg 2001; 93:1565-9.
Gaynot JS, Wertz EM, Alvis M, Turner AS. J Vet Pharmacol Ther 1998; 21:69-73.
He YL, Seno H, Tsujimoto S, Tashiro C. Anesth Analg 2001; 93:151-6.
Sanchez-Alcaraz A, Quintana MB, Laguarda M. J Clin Pharm Ther 1998; 23:19-23.
Ikonomidou C, Bittigau P, Koch C, et al. Biochem Pharmacol 2001; 62:401-5.

- **Summary** ....
  - **Pregnancy Category B**
  - **Lactation Category S?**
  - **Propofol** is an excellent anesthetic agent during pregnancy and lactation for a variety of indications.

Propoxyphene (Abalgin; Darvon; Deprancol; Develin; Dolotard; Dolpoxene; Margesic; Parvon)

- **Class** .... *Narcotic, analgesic*

- **Indications** .... Mild to moderate pain

- **Mechanism** .... Binds to opioid receptors

- **Dosage with Qualifiers** .... Mild to moderate pain—65mg PO q4h prn; max 390mg/d
  NOTE—often combined with one of several analgesic and
  antihistaminic compounds
  - **Contraindications**—hypersensitivity to drug or class
  - **Caution**—history of substance abuse, depression,
    suicidal ideation, hepatic or renal dysfunction

- **Maternal Considerations** .... **Propoxyphene** is a narcotic, and its combination with
  other CNS depressants such as alcohol has an additive
  effect. There are no adequate reports or well-controlled
  studies in pregnant women. **Propoxyphene** combinations
  offer no clinical advantage over NSAIDs for the treatment
  of episiotomy pain.
  Side effects include respiratory depression, dependency,
  somnolence, dizziness, hallucinations, dysphoria,
  constipation, hepatic dysfunction, and painful myopathy.

- **Fetal Considerations** .... There are no adequate reports or well-controlled studies
  in human fetuses. Both **propoxyphene** and its principal
  active metabolite, norporpoxyphene, cross the human
  placenta, and neonatal addiction/withdrawal occur.
  Though there are scattered case reports of miscellaneous
  birth defects, but no pattern has emerged.

- **Breastfeeding Safety** .... There are no adequate reports or well-controlled studies
  in nursing women. While low levels of **propoxyphene** are
  excreted into human breast milk, its use as directed is
  generally considered compatible with breastfeeding.

- **References** .... Gruber CM Jr, Bauer RO, Bettigole JB, et al. J Med 1979;
  10:65-98.
  Bloomfield SS, Barden TP, Mitchell J. Clin Pharmacol
  Ther 1980; 27:502-7.
  Golden NL, King KC, Sokol RJ. Clin Pediatr 1982; 21:752-4.
  Kunka RL, Venkataramanan R, Stern RM, Ladik CF. Clin
  Pharmacol Ther 1984; 35:675-80.

- **Summary** ....
  - **Pregnancy Category C**
  - **Lactation Category S**
  - **Propoxyphene** should be used during pregnancy and
    lactation only if the benefit justifies the potential
    perinatal risk.
  - There are non-narcotic alternatives that provide similar
    or superior analgesia for most indications.

Propranolol (Inderal)

■ **Class** .... Antiadrenergic, β-blocker, antiarrhythmic class II

■ **Indications** .... Hypertension, migraine headache prophylaxis, SVT, angina

■ **Mechanism** .... Nonselective β antagonist

■ **Dosage with Qualifiers** .... Hypertension—begin 40mg PO bid, increasing q3-7d; max 640mg/d
Migraine headache prophylaxis—begin 20mg PO qd; increase gradually to 40-60mg PO qid
SVT—begin 1-3mg IV at 1mg/min; may repeat 2min later; if control, then 10-30mg PO tid/qid beginning 4h later
Angina—80-120mg PO bid; may increase q7-10d
- **Contraindications**—hypersensitivity to drug or class, asthma, CHF, cardiogenic shock, 2nd or 3rd degree heart block, severe sinus bradycardia
- **Caution**—diabetes mellitus, hepatic or renal dysfunction

■ **Maternal Considerations** .... **Propranolol** is used extensively during pregnancy for the treatment of maternal hypertension, arrhythmia and migraine headache, and is generally considered safe. It is also used acutely to provide symptomatic relief of symptoms from thyrotoxicosis and pheochromocytoma. Several studies suggest the administration of **propranolol** (2mg IV) to nulliparas who require oxytocin augmentation for dysfunctional labor reduces the likelihood of a cesarean delivery by almost half. The studies of **propranolol** as an oral hypotensive are small. It appears as effective as **alpha methyldopa,** and is often coupled with other hypotensive agents such as **hydralazine**.
Side effects include CHF, arrhythmia, bronchospasm, bradycardia, dizziness, insomnia, weakness, fatigue, hallucinations, nausea, vomiting, abdominal pain, diarrhea, constipation, pharyngitis, rash, alopecia, and agranulocytosis.

■ **Fetal Considerations** .... There are no adequate reports or well-controlled studies in human fetuses. **Propranolol** crosses the human placenta, but has no effect on either uterine or umbilical Doppler determined resistances in chronically hypertensive women. There are case reports of its use, usually with **digoxin,** for the treatment of supraventricular tachycardia, though there are superior agents. The impact of **propranolol** on the fetus of women with chronic hypertension is unclear. Frequently combined with another agent, the risk of IUGR is reportedly increased. However, IUGR is more common when the maternal pressure is suboptimally controlled and in need of higher doses. The most recent information suggests the increased risk of IUGR reflects excessive maternal β blockade adequate to decrease maternal cardiac output. Other neonatal sequelae reported include bradycardia and hypoglycemia.

■ **Breastfeeding Safety** — Less than 1% of the maternal dose of **propranolol** enters human breast milk; it should not pose a risk to the breast-fed neonate.

■ **References** — Aube M. Neurology 1999; 53:S26-8.
Sanchez-Ramos L, Quillen MJ, Kaunitz AM. Obstet Gynecol 1996; 88:517-20.
Chow T, Galvin J, McGovern B. Am J Cardiol 1998; 82:581-62l.
Easterling TR, Carr DB, Brateng D, et al. Obstet Gynecol 2001; 98:427-33.
Livingstone I, Craswell PW, Bevan EB, et al. Clin Exp Hypertens B 1983; 2:341-50.
Smith MT, Livingstone I, Hooper WD, et al. Ther Drug Monit 1983; 5:87-93.
Oudijk MA, Ruskamp JM, Ambachtsheer BE, et al. Paediatr Drugs 2002; 4:49-63.
Meizner I, Paran E, Katz M, et al. J Clin Ultrasound 1992; 20:115-9.

■ **Summary** — • **Pregnancy Category C**
• **Lactation Category S**
• **Propranolol** should be used during pregnancy only if the benefit justifies the potential perinatal risk.

Propylthiouracil (PTU)

■ **Class** — Antithyroid; *hormone/hormone modifier*

■ **Indications** — Hyperthyroidism

■ **Mechanism** — Inhibits thyroid synthesis

■ **Dosage with Qualifiers** — Hyperthyroidism (Graves' disease)—begin 100-125mg PO tid; 200-300mg PO qid if thyroid storm
NOTE—renal dosing
• **Contraindications**—hypersensitivity to drug or class
• **Caution**—pregnancy, renal dysfunction, concurrent hepatotoxic or agranulocytosis agents, bone marrow suppression

■ **Maternal Considerations** — **Propylthiouracil** is the agent of choice for Graves' disease during pregnancy. It is generally recommended that the minimum dose necessary to control the maternal thyroid be used. Women with a history of Graves' disease in the past should be screened for the continued presence of thyroid-stimulating immunoglobulin even if she previously received definitive treatment, since fetal hyperthyroidism is still likely when positive. Fetal treatment may be necessary and the patient should be appropriately evaluated in a fetal care unit. There are no adequate reports or well-controlled studies in pregnant women.

Side effects include agranulocytosis, leukopenia, thrombocytopenia, aplastic anemia, hepatotoxicity, exfoliative dermatitis, urticaria, vasculitis, interstitial pneumonitis, nausea, vomiting, rash, drowsiness, dizziness, headache, arthralgia, lymphadenopathy, paresthesias, hyperpigmentation, jaundice, alopecia, and neuritis.

■ Fetal Considerations

There are no adequate reports or well-controlled studies in human fetuses. **Propylthiouracil** crosses the human placenta. Maternal treatment is most often associated with fetal hypothyroidism and fetal evaluation is mandatory. Aplasia cutis is a rare complication of maternal therapy.

■ Breastfeeding Safety

There are no adequate reports or well-controlled studies in nursing women. Small quantities of **propylthiouracil** are excreted into human breast milk, but thyroid function of breast-fed neonates is unaffected.

■ References

Polak M, Leger J, Luton D, et al. Ann Endocrinol 1997; 58:338-42.
Wenstrom KD, Weiner CP, Williamson RA, Grant SS. Obstet Gynecol 1990; 76:513-17.
Brunner JP, Dellinger EH. Fetal Diagn Ther 1997; 12:200-4.
Momotani N, Yamashita R, Makino F, et al. Clin Endocrinol 2000; 53:177-81.
Lee A, Moretti ME, Collantes A, et al. Pediatrics 2000; 106:27-30.
Kampmann JP, Johansen K, Hansen JM, Helweg J. Lancet 1980; i:736-7.

■ Summary

- **Pregnancy Category D**
- **Lactation Category S**
- **Propylthiouracil** should be used during pregnancy only if the benefit justifies the potential perinatal risk.

Protamine

■ **Class** — *Bleeding disorders, toxicology*

■ **Indications** — Heparin reversal

■ **Mechanism** — Binds heparin

■ **Dosage with Qualifiers** — Heparin reversal—1-1.5mg IV per 100U heparin estimated to remain in the body; if 0-30min from last dose, give 1-1.5mg/100U, if 30-60min give 0.5-0.75mg/100U, if >2h, give 0.25-0.375mg/100U
NOTE—monitor BP, ECG, and aPTT during reversal
- **Contraindications**—hypersensitivity to drug or class
- **Caution**—fish allergy or prior exposure to various protamine insulins

■ **Maternal Considerations** — There are no adequate reports or well-controlled studies in pregnant women. Case reports note acute hypotension, bradycardia and anaphylactic reactions. **Protamine** does not reverse anticoagulation secondary to the low molecular weight heparins.
Side effects include anaphylaxis, bronchospasm, fatigue, angioedema, circulatory collapse (due to sudden pulmonary hypertension, right ventricular then biventricular failure followed by circulatory collapse) bradycardia, bleeding, paradoxical hemorrhage, leukopenia, thrombocytopenia, dyspnea, flushing, urticaria, nausea, and vomiting.

■ **Fetal Considerations** — There are no adequate reports or well-controlled studies in human fetuses. It is unknown whether **protamine** crosses the human placenta. Rodent teratogenicity studies have not been conducted. However, insulin coupled to **protamine** has a long safety record.

■ **Breastfeeding Safety** — There is no published experience in nursing women. It is unknown whether **protamine sulfate** enters human breast milk. However, insulin coupled to **protamine** has a long safety record.

■ **References** — There are no current relevant references.

■ **Summary** —
- **Pregnancy Category C**
- **Lactation Category S?**
- **Protamine** sulfate should be used during pregnancy and lactation only if the benefit justifies the potential perinatal risk.

Protriptyline (Concordin; Triptil; Vivactil)

- **Class** — Antidepressant, tricyclic

- **Indications** — Depression

- **Mechanism** — Unknown; inhibits norepinephrine and serotonin reuptake

- **Dosage with Qualifiers** — Depression—5-10mg PO tid/qid; max 60mg/d
  - **Contraindications**—hypersensitivity to drug or class, SSRI use
  - **Caution**—hyperthyroidism, epilepsy, coronary artery disease

- **Maternal Considerations** — There are no published reports in pregnancy
  Side effects include MI, AV block, arrhythmia, stroke, seizures, fever, agranulocytosis, leukopenia, jaundice, agitation, anxiety, tachcardia, palpitations, hypotension, nausea, vomiting, blurred vision, dry mouth, mydriasis, photosensitivity, hallucinations, ataxia, peripheral neuropathy, SIADH, itching, rash, and black tongue.

- **Fetal Considerations** — There are no adequate reports or well-controlled studies in human fetuses. It is unknown whether **protriptyline** crosses the human placenta. There is no evidence after 5 years that either tricyclic antidepressants or **fluoxetine** adversely affect cognition and language development. In contrast, maternal depression is associated with lower language and cognitive achievement. Rodent studies are reassuring, revealing no evidence of teratogenicity or IUGR despite the use of doses higher than those used clinically.

- **Breastfeeding Safety** — There are no published reports in nursing women. It is unknown whether **protriptyline** enters human breast milk.

- **References** — Nulman I, Rovet J, Stewart DE, et al. Am J Psychiatry 2002; 159:1889-1895.

- **Summary** —
  - **Pregnancy Category C**
  - **Lactation Category S**
  - **Protriptyline** should be used during pregnancy and lactation only if the benefit justifies the potential perinatal risk.
  - There are alternative agents for which there is more experience during pregnancy and lactation.

Pseudoephedrine (Bronalin; Cenafed; Chlordrine; Novafed; Sufedrin)

■ **Class** ⋯⋯⋯⋯⋯⋯⋯⋯⋯⋯⋯⋯ *Decongestant, nasal; sympathomimetic*

■ **Indications** ⋯⋯⋯⋯⋯⋯⋯⋯⋯⋯ Nasal decongestion

■ **Mechanism** ⋯⋯⋯⋯⋯⋯⋯⋯⋯⋯ α agonist

■ **Dosage with Qualifiers** ⋯⋯⋯ Nasal decongestion—30-60mg PO q4-6h prn; max 240mg/d
NOTE—available in a sustained-release form, and in combination with either the antihistamine **triprolidine** (Actifed) or **codeine**
- **Contraindications**—hypersensitivity to drug or class, MAO use <14d, narrow-angle glaucoma, severe hypertension, severe CAD
- **Caution**—hypertension, diabetes mellitus, mild/moderate CAD, hyperthyroidism, renal dysfunction, PKU

■ **Maternal Considerations** ⋯⋯ **Pseudoephedrine** is second-line therapy behind 1st and 2nd generation antihistamines. There are no adequate reports or well-controlled studies in pregnant women. *Side effects* include hypertension, arrhythmia, nausea, vomiting, headache, dizziness, nervousness, excitability, agitation, anxiety, palpitations, weakness, and tremor.

■ **Fetal Considerations** ⋯⋯⋯⋯ There are no adequate reports or well-controlled studies in human fetuses. The chemical structure of **pseudoephedrine** indicates it crosses the human placenta. Epidemiological study suggests exposed fetuses are at increased risk of gastroschisis and small intestinal atresias. There is a single case report suggesting a relationship with fetal tachycardia. Rodent teratogenicity studies have not been conducted.

■ **Breastfeeding Safety** ⋯⋯⋯⋯ There are no adequate reports or well-controlled studies in nursing women. Less than 1% of the maternal dose of **pseudoephedrine** is excreted into human breast milk. It is generally considered compatible with breastfeeding.

■ **References** ⋯⋯⋯⋯⋯⋯⋯⋯⋯ Werler MM, Sheehnan JE, Mitchell AA. Am J Epidemiol 2002; 155:26-31.
Anastasio GD, Harston PR. J Am Board Fam Prac 1992; 5:527-8.
Mitchell JL. J Hum Lact 1999; 15:347-9.
Findlay JW, Butz RF, Sailstad JM, et al. Br J Pharmacol 1984; 18:901-6.

■ **Summary**

• **Pregnancy Category C**
• **Lactation Category S**
• **Pseudoephedrine** should be used during pregnancy and lactation only if the benefit justifies the potential perinatal risk.
• Avoid use in 1st trimester.
• Antihistamines are the drugs of choice for the treatment of nasal congestion during pregnancy.

Psyllium (Metamucil)

■ **Class** — Laxative

■ **Indications** — Constipation

■ **Mechanism** — Increases stool bulk

■ **Dosage with Qualifiers** — Constipation—1-2tsp PO dissolved in water or juice qd/tid
• **Contraindications**—hypersensitivity to drug or class, suspected appendicitis, intestinal obstruction
• **Caution**—unknown

■ **Maternal Considerations** — There are no adequate reports or well-controlled studies in pregnant women. **Psyllium** is not absorbed systemically. *Side effects* include esophageal obstruction, bowel obstruction, constipation, diarrhea, abdominal cramps, bronchospasm, rhinitis, and conjunctivitis.

■ **Fetal Considerations** — There are no adequate reports or well-controlled studies in human fetuses. **Psyllium** is not absorbed systemically and poses no direct threat to the fetus.

■ **Breastfeeding Safety** — There is no published experience in nursing women. As **psyllium** is not absorbed systemically, it is unlikely to be excreted into human breast milk.

■ **References** — There is no published experience in pregnancy or during lactation.

■ **Summary**

• **Pregnancy Category C**
• **Lactation Category S**
• **Psyllium** is not absorbed systemically. It should pose no additional risk during pregnancy and lactation.

Pyrantel pamoate (Antiminth)

- **Class** — Antiparasitic

- **Indications** — Pinworm, roundworm, hookworm, whipworm

- **Mechanism** — Depolarizing agent causing worm paralysis

- **Dosage with Qualifiers** — Pinworm—11mg/kg PO qd ×1d; may take with milk or juice, treat all family members
  Roundworm—11mg/kg PO qd ×1d; may take with milk or juice
  Hookworm—11mg/kg PO qd ×3d; may take with milk or juice
  Whipworm—11mg/kg PO qd ×1d; may take with milk or juice
  - **Contraindications**—hypersensitivity to drug or class
  - **Caution**—hepatic dysfunction, malnutrition

- **Maternal Considerations** — There are no published reports in pregnancy.
  Side effects include anorexia, nausea, vomiting, abdominal cramps, diarrhea, dizziness, drowsiness, insomnia, tenesmus, rash, weakness, and elevated hepatic transaminases.

- **Fetal Considerations** — There are no adequate reports or well-controlled studies in human fetuses. It is unknown whether **pyrantel pamoate** crosses the human placenta. Rodent teratogenicity studies have not been conducted.

- **Breastfeeding Safety** — There is no published experience in nursing women. It is unknown whether **pyrantel pamoate** enters human breast milk.

- **References** — There is no published experience in pregnancy or during lactation.

- **Summary** —
  - **Pregnancy Category C**
  - **Lactation Category S**
  - **Pyrantel** pamoate should be used during pregnancy and lactation only if the benefit justifies the potential perinatal risk.

Pyrazinamide

- **Class** — Antimycobacterial

- **Indications** — Tuberculosis, adjuvant

- **Mechanism** — Unknown

- **Dosage with Qualifiers** — Tuberculosis, adjuvant—15-30mg/kg PO qd given as part of a multidrug regimen; max 3g/d
  - **Contraindications**—hypersensitivity to drug or class, severe hepatic dysfunction
  - **Caution**—renal dysfunction, diabetes mellitus, gout

- **Maternal Considerations** — **Pyrazinamide** should only be given with other antituberculosis agents. It has an excellent safety record during pregnancy. However, there are no adequate reports or well-controlled studies in pregnant women. Most publications consist of case reports or limited series. *Side effects* include interstitial nephritis, hepatotoxicity, thrombocytopenia, elevated LFTs, hyperuricemia, anorexia, urticaria, rash, nausea, vomiting, arthralgia, malaise, photosensitivity, and gout.

- **Fetal Considerations** — There are no adequate reports or well-controlled studies in human fetuses. It is unknown whether **pyrazinamide** crosses the human placenta. Rodent teratogenicity studies have not been conducted.

- **Breastfeeding Safety** — There are no reports in nursing women. It is unknown whether **pyrazinamide** enters human breast milk.

- **References** — Bothamley G. Drug Saf 2001; 24:553-65.

- **Summary** —
  - **Pregnancy Category C**
  - **Lactation Category U**
  - **Pyrazinamide** should be used during pregnancy and lactation only if the benefit justifies the potential perinatal risk.

Pyridostigmine (Mestinon)

- **Class** — Cholinesterase inhibitor; musculoskeletal agent

- **Indications** — Myasthenia gravis

- **Mechanism** — Cholinesterase inhibitor

- **Dosage with Qualifiers** ········· <u>Myasthenia gravis</u>—begin 60mg PO q8h, individualizing to response and side effects; max 1500mg/d
  - **Contraindications**—hypersensitivity to drug or class, mechanical GI obstruction
  - **Caution**—asthma, peptic ulcer disease, arrhythmia, bradycardia, seizures, renal dysfunction

- **Maternal Considerations** ········· There are no adequate reports or well-controlled studies in pregnant women. The published literature consists of small series and case reports.
  Side effects include bronchospasm, bradycardia, hypertension, cholinergic crisis, paralysis, AV block, arrhythmia, cardiac or respiratory arrest, nausea, vomiting, diarrhea, dyspepsia, abdominal pain, weakness, rash, muscle cramps, increased bronchial secretions or salivation, miosis, and tearing.

- **Fetal Considerations** ········· There are no adequate reports or well-controlled studies in human fetuses. It is unknown whether **pyridostigmine** crosses the human placenta. Several case reports suggest a relationship between **pyridostigmine** and several neurologic abnormalities including arthrogryposis multiplex and microcephaly. Rodent teratogenicity studies have not been conducted.

- **Breastfeeding Safety** ········· There are no adequate reports or well-controlled studies in nursing women. **Pyridostigmine** is excreted into human breast milk at low concentration.

- **References** ········· Pijinenborg JM, Hansen EC, Brolmann HA, et al. Gynecol Obstet Invest 2000; 50:142-3.
  Garcia SA, Ogata AJ, Patriota RG, et al. Rev Paul Med 1989; 107:144-8.
  Niesen CE, Shah NS. Neurology 2000; 54:1873-4.
  Hardell LI, Lindstrom B, Lonnerholm G, Osterman PO. Br J Clin Pharmacol 1982; 14:565-7.

- **Summary** ·········
  - **Pregnancy Category C**
  - **Lactation Category U**
  - **Pyridostigmine** should be used during pregnancy and lactation only if the benefit justifies the potential perinatal risk.

Pyridoxine (Beesix; Hexa-Betalin; Rodex; Vitamin B$_6$)

- **Class** ········· *Vitamin*

- **Indications** ········· Pyridoxine deficiency or supplementation, PMS, INH adjunct

- **Mechanism** ········· Replacement

■ **Dosage with Qualifiers** ⋯⋯⋯⋯ Pyridoxine deficiency—10-20mg PO/IM/IV qd ×3w, then
2-5mg/d PO
Pyridoxine supplementation—2-5mg PO qd
PMS—40-500mg PO qd
Isoniazid adjunct—25-50mg PO qd to prevent associated
neuropathy
NOTE—available in some areas combined with
doxylamine (Diclectin); antagonizes **levodopa**
● **Contraindications**—hypersensitivity to drug or class,
levodopa therapy
● **Caution**—unknown

■ **Maternal Considerations** ⋯⋯⋯ **Pyridoxine** is a coenzyme for several amino acid
decarboxylases and transaminases. It reduces nausea and
vomiting of pregnancy, but does not reduce the side
effects associated with oral contraceptive use. **Pyridoxine**
is used in combination with antituberculosis therapy to
reduce the risk of neuropathy.
Side effects include numbness, unsteady gait, and
paresthesias.

■ **Fetal Considerations** ⋯⋯⋯⋯⋯ **Pyridoxine** crosses the human placenta and is not
teratogenic. **Pyridoxine** supplementation during
pregnancy increases neonatal stores in a dose-dependent
manner.

■ **Breastfeeding Safety** ⋯⋯⋯⋯ **Pyridoxine** requirements are thought to increase during
lactation. Maternal supplementation increases human
breast milk content in a dose-dependent manner.

■ **References** ⋯⋯⋯⋯⋯⋯⋯⋯⋯⋯
Jewell D, Young G. Cochrane Database Syst Rev 2002;
(1):CD000145.
Magee LA, Mazzotta P, Koren G. Am J Obstet Gynecol
2002; 185:S256-61.
Sahakian V, Rouse D, Sipes S, et al. Obstet Gynecol 1991;
78:33-6.
Vutyavanich T, Wongtrangan S, Ruangsri R. Am J Obstet
Gynecol 1995; 173:881-4.
Chang SJ. J Nutr Sci Vitaminol 1999; 45:449-58.
Chang SJ, Kirksey A. J Nutr Sci Vitaminol 2002; 48:10-17.

■ **Summary** ⋯⋯⋯⋯⋯⋯⋯⋯⋯⋯
● **Pregnancy Category A**
● **Lactation Category S**
● **Pyridoxine** reduces the severity of morning sickness.
● Routine supplementation during pregnancy and
lactation is recommended.

Pyrimethamine (Daraprim; Eraprelina; Malocide)

■ **Class** — *Antiprotozoal*

■ **Indications** — Malaria treatment and prophylaxis, toxoplasmosis, isosporiasis

■ **Mechanism** — Inhibits plasmodium dihydrofolate reductase

■ **Dosage with Qualifiers** — Malaria treatment—50mg PO qd ×2w in combination with **sulfadiazine** and **quinine**; use in **chloroquine**-resistant areas
Malaria prophylaxis—25mg PO qw for 10w after exposure; use in **chloroquine** resistant areas
Toxoplasmosis—begin 50-75mg PO qd ×1-3w, then 25-50mg PO qd ×4-5w in combination with **sulfadoxine** and **folinic acid**
Toxoplasmosis with HIV—begin 200mg PO ×1, then 50-100mg PO qd ×4-8w, then maintenance
Isosporiasis—50-75mg PO qd
NOTE—may be combined with **sulfadoxine** (Fansidar)
● **Contraindications**—hypersensitivity to drug or class, folate deficiency
● **Caution**—hepatic or renal dysfunction, G6PD deficiency

■ **Maternal Considerations** — Severe anemia is a cause of maternal morbidity in endemic areas and treatment leads to resolution. HIV infection during pregnancy is associated with an increased risk of malaria. **Pyrimethamine** has a long history of use during pregnancy, especially for the treatment of primary toxoplasmosis and malaria.
Side effects include aplastic anemia, pancytopenia, thrombocytopenia, Stevens-Johnson syndrome, agranulocytosis, megaloblastic anemia, seizures, pulmonary eosinophilia, erythema multiforme, nausea, vomiting, abdominal pain, dizziness, malaise, diarrhea, rash, fever, dry mouth, and increased skin pigmentation.

■ **Fetal Considerations** — **Pyrimethamine** crosses the human placenta with about 30% efficiency. While it has been long used for the treatment of toxoplasmosis during pregnancy, several recent studies conclude that antenatal therapy does not alter outcome, perhaps because fetal infection has already occurred. Other studies suggest **pyrimethamine** does not reduce transmission, but rather the sequelae of infection. Further research is required to define the role of prenatal screening and therapy. In contrast, the treatment of pregnant women (in combination with **sulfadoxine**) in malaria-endemic areas is cost-effective, reducing the risk of prematurity and IUGR secondary to placental malaria. In rodents, **pyrimethamine** is associated with embryotoxicity and IUGR. **Pyrimethamine** was associated with an increased risk of cleft palate, micrognathia, and clubfoot in pigs.

■ **Breastfeeding Safety** ⋯⋯⋯⋯ There are no adequate reports or well-controlled studies in nursing women. **Pyrimethamine** is excreted into human breast milk in low concentrations. It is estimated the breast-fed neonate would ingest less than 10% of the maternal dose over 48h.

■ **References** ⋯⋯⋯⋯⋯⋯⋯⋯

Shulman CE, Dorman EK, Cutts F, et al. Lancet 1999; 353:632-6.
Verhoeff FH, Brabin BJ, Hart CA, et al. Trop Med Int Health 1999; 4:5-12.
Shulman CE. Ann Trop Med Parasitol 1999; 93:S59-66.
Foulon W, Villena I, Stray-Pedersen B, et al. Am J Obstet Gynecol 1999; 180:410-5.
Peytavin G, Leng JJ, Forestier F, et al. 2000; 78:83-5.
Wallon M, Liou C, Garner F, Peyron F. BMJ 1999; 318:1511-4.
Gras L, Gilbert RE, Ades AE, Dunn DT. Int J Epidemiol 2001; 30:1309-13.
Gilbert RE, Gras L, Wallon M, et al. Int J Epidemiol 2001; 30:1303-8.
Wolfe EB, Parise ME, Haddix AC, et al. Am J Trop Med Hyg 2001; 64:178-86.

■ **Summary** ⋯⋯⋯⋯⋯⋯⋯⋯⋯

- **Pregnancy Category C**
- **Lactation Category S**
- **Pyrimethamine** should be used during pregnancy and lactation only if the benefit justifies the potential perinatal risk.

Quetiapine (Seroquel)

■ **Class** — Antipsychotic

■ **Indications** — Psychosis

■ **Mechanism** — Unknown; antagonizes multiple neurotransmitter receptors

■ **Dosage with Qualifiers** — Psychosis—begin 25mg PO bid, increase by 25-50mg/dose q1-2d; max 800mg/d
NOTE—hepatic dosing
- **Contraindications**—hypersensitivity to drug or class
- **Caution**—hepatic dysfunction, cardiac disease, CVD, seizures, hypotension, hypovolemia

■ **Maternal Considerations** — **Quetiapine** is a dibenzothiazepine derivative. The published experience during pregnancy is limited to case reports.
Side effects include hypotension, tardive dyskinesia, menstrual irregularities, hyperprolactinemia, hypothyroidism, diabetes mellitus, neuroleptic malignant syndrome, leukopenia, headache, somnolence, dizziness, constipation, tachycardia, dry mouth, asthenia, rash, hypercholesterolemia, hypertriglyceridemia, elevated LFTs, dyspepsia, abdominal pain, rhinitis, weight gain, and fever.

■ **Fetal Considerations** — There are no adequate reports or well-controlled studies in human fetuses. It is unknown whether **quetiapine** crosses the human placenta. Rodent studies are mostly reassuring, revealing no evidence of teratogenicity despite the use of doses higher than those used clinically. Embryotoxicity and IUGR were noted at the highest doses.

■ **Breastfeeding Safety** — There are no adequate reports or well-controlled studies in nursing women. **Quetiapine** is excreted into human breast milk, but detailed kinetic studies have not been published.

■ **References** — Taylor TM, O'Toole MS, Ohlsen RI, Walters J, Pilowsky LS. Am J Psychiatry 2003; 160:588-9.
Tenyi T, Trixler M, Keresztes Z. Am J Psychiatry 2002; 159:674.

■ **Summary**
- **Pregnancy Category C**
- **Lactation Category U**
- **Quetiapine** should be used during pregnancy and lactation only if the benefit justifies the potential perinatal risk.
- There are alternative agents for which there is more experience during pregnancy and lactation.

Quinapril (Accupril)

- **Class** — Antihypertensive, ACE-1/A2R-antagonist

- **Indications** — Hypertension, CHF

- **Mechanism** — ACE inhibitor

- **Dosage with Qualifiers** — Hypertension—begin 10mg PO qd, adjust for effect q2w moving to bid if necessary; max 80mg/d
  CHF—begin 5mg PO qd, adjust weekly for effect, moving to bid; max 40mg/d
  NOTE—renal dosing
  - **Contraindications**—hypersensitivity to drug or class, angioedema
  - **Caution**—renal dysfunction, renal artery stenosis, collagen vascular disease, hyponatremia, hypovolemia

- **Maternal Considerations** — There are no adequate reports or well-controlled studies in pregnant women. In general, ACE inhibitors should be avoided during pregnancy. The lowest effective dose should be used when **quinapril** is required for pressure control during pregnancy.
  Side effects include angioedema, hypotension, renal failure, cough, dizziness, fatigue, nausea, vomiting, URI symptoms, myalgia, arthralgia, hyperkalemia, neutropenia, agranulocytosis, and elevated BUN/Cr.

- **Fetal Considerations** — There is no published experience in human fetuses. **Quinapril** likely crosses the human placenta like other ACE inhibitors. As a group, no adverse fetal effects are reported from 1st trimester exposure to ACE inhibitors. Later exposure is associated with cranial hypoplasia, anuria, reversible or irreversible renal failure, death, oligohydramnios, prematurity, IUGR, and patent ductus arteriosus. The mechanism of renal dysfunction is likely related to fetal hypotension and prolonged decreased glomerular filtration. There is inadequate study to determine whether the response to **quinapril** is typical of this group. The one published rodent study is reassuring. If oligohydramnios is detected, **quinapril** should be discontinued unless lifesaving for the mother. Antenatal surveillance should be initiated (e.g., BPP) if the fetus is potentially viable. Oligohydramnios may not appear until after the fetus has irreversible injury. Neonates exposed *in utero* to ACE inhibitors should be observed closely for hypotension, oliguria, and hyperkalemia. If oliguria occurs despite adequate pressure and renal perfusion, exchange transfusion or peritoneal dialysis may be required.

- **Breastfeeding Safety** — There are no adequate reports or well-controlled studies in nursing women. **Quinapril** enters human breast milk with an M/P ratio of 0.12. No drug is detected more than 4h after maternal ingestion. It is unlikely the breast-fed neonate would ingest clinically relevant amounts.

■ **References** ·········· Dostal LA, Kim SN, Schardein JL, Anderson JA. Fundam Appl Toxicol 1991; 17:684-95.
Begg EJ, Robson RA, Gardiner SJ, et al. Br J Clin Pharmacol 2001; 51:478-81.

■ **Summary** ··········
- **Pregnancy Category C (1st trimester), D (2nd and 3rd trimesters)**
- **Lactation Category S?**
- **Quinapril** and other ACE inhibitors should be avoided during pregnancy if possible.
- When mother's disease requires treatment with **quinapril**, the lowest doses should be used followed by close monitoring of the fetus.

Quinidine gluconate/sulfate
(Quinaglute Dura-Tabs; Quinidex Extentabs; Quinora)

■ **Class** ·········· *Antiarrhythmic, class 1a, antiprotozoal*

■ **Indications** ·········· Atrial fibrillation, ventricular arrhythmia, SVT, malaria

■ **Mechanism** ·········· Depresses phase 0 action potential; intraerythrocytic schizonticide

■ **Dosage with Qualifiers** ·········· Atrial fibrillation—324-648mg PO q8-12h (gluconate), 200-300mg PO q4-6h (sulfate); adjust to therapeutic level of 2-6mcg/ml
Ventricular arrhythmia—324-648mg PO q8-12h (gluconate), 200-300mg PO q4-6h (sulfate); adjust to therapeutic level of 2-6mcg/ml
SVT—324-648mg PO q8-12h (gluconate), 200-300mg PO q4-6h (sulfate); adjust to therapeutic level of 2-6mcg/ml
Life-threatening malaria—15mg/kg (sulfate) (or 24mg/kg gluconate) in 250ml 0.9 NS over 4h, then 7.5mg/kg (sulfate) (12mg/kg gluconate) 8h after the load given over 4h q8h ×7d
- **Contraindications**—hypersensitivity to drug or class, myasthenia gravis, intraventricular conduction defects, complete AV block, history of TTP associated with **quinidine** or **quinine**
- **Caution**—**succinylcholine**, incomplete AV block, sick sinus syndrome, digoxin toxicity, QT interval prolongation, CHF, hypomagnesemia, hypokalemia, G6PD deficiency, and hepatic or renal dysfunction

■ **Maternal Considerations** ···· There are no adequate reports or well-controlled studies of **quinidine** in pregnant women. All IA agents should be administered with continuous cardiac monitoring in the hospital because of the risk of ventricular arrhythmia (torsades de pointes). **Quinidine** has a long record of safety during pregnancy, and is generally well tolerated. The clearance of **quinidine** is apparently unaffected by pregnancy. In women with severe P. *falciparum* malaria and hyperparasitemia, IV **quinidine** is often coupled with exchange transfusion, resulting in the clearing of the parasitemia and high survival rates. Therapeutic levels of **quinidine** inhibit pseudocholinesterase activity in pregnant women by 60-70%, necessitating caution if **succinylcholine** is to be used intraoperatively.

Side effects include QT interval prolongation, torsades de pointes, AV block, cardiac arrest, respiratory arrest, ventricular arrhythmia, syncope, hypotension, hemolytic anemia, thrombocytopenia, thrombocytopenic purpura, agranulocytosis, SLE-like syndrome, optic neuritis, nausea, vomiting, diarrhea, abdominal pain, dyspepsia, headache, fatigue, chest pain, blurred vision, rash, abnormal ECG, insomnia, tremor, and tinnitus.

■ **Fetal Considerations** ···· There are no adequate reports or well-controlled studies in human fetuses. **Quinidine** crosses the human placenta reaching an F:M ratio approaching unity over time. It causes *in vitro* significant dose-dependent relaxation of placental arteries and veins. **Quinidine** has been used successfully to correct fetal SVT and reverse hydrops. Elimination of maternal parasitemia does not necessarily mean elimination from the placenta. Rodent teratogenicity studies have not been performed.

■ **Breastfeeding Safety** ···· There are no adequate reports or well-controlled studies in nursing women. **Quinidine** is excreted into human milk with an M:P ratio near unity. Neonatal kinetics have not been studied.

■ **References** ···· Joglar JA, Page RL. Drug Saf 1999; 20:85-94.
Procop GW, Jessen R, Hyde SR, Scheck DN. J Perinatol 2001; 21:128-30.
Kambam JR, Franks JJ, Smith BE. Am J Obstet Gynecol 1987; 157:897-9.
Omar HA, Rhodes LA, Ramirez R, et al. J Cardiovasc Electrophysiol 1996; 7:1197-203.
Spinnato JA, Shaver DC, Flinn GS, et al. Obstet Gynecol 1984; 64:730-5.
Hill LM, Malkasian GD Jr. Obstet Gynecol 1979; 54:366-8.

■ **Summary** ···· • **Pregnancy Category C**
• **Lactation Category U**
• **Quinidine** should be used during pregnancy and lactation only if the benefit justifies the potential perinatal risk.

Quinine (Qm-260; Quin-Amino; Quinaminoph; Quinamm; Quinasul; Quindan; Quinite; Quiphile)

- ■ **Class** — Antiprotozoal, antimalarial

- ■ **Indications** — Malaria

- ■ **Mechanism** — Unknown; schizontocidal

- ■ **Dosage with Qualifiers** — Malaria—650mg PO q8h ×3-7d
  NOTE—use with other antimalarial agents
  - **Contraindications**—hypersensitivity to drug, class or **mefloquine** or **quinidine**, G6PD deficiency, optic neuritis, tinnitus, thrombocytopenic purpura, hypoglycemia, myasthenia gravis
  - **Caution**—arrhythmias

- ■ **Maternal Considerations** — Malaria is a major cause of maternal/perinatal morbidity and death in regions of the world. Treatment dramatically reduces those risks. **Quinine** is used extensively in developing countries for the treatment of malaria during pregnancy. It is one of a limited number of drugs used where multidrug resistant *Plasmodium falciparum* is endemic. However, **quinine** has a higher treatment failure rate than **chloroquine**. **Quinine** toxicity is associated with abortion.
  Side effects include cinchonism, hemolysis, prolonged QT interval, edema, hypoglycemia, thrombocytopenia, agranulocytosis, optic nerve damage, nausea, vomiting, diarrhea, headache, confusion, hypotension, altered color perception, photosensitivity, rash, pruritus, delirium, tinnitus, and mydriasis.

- ■ **Fetal Considerations** — There are no adequate reports or well-controlled studies in human fetuses. **Quinine** crosses the placenta achieving an F:M ratio of 0.32 ± 0.14. The risks of pregnancy loss, IUGR or malformation are unchanged after 1st trimester exposure for malaria treatment. Congenital malformations reported in the human were associated with large doses (up to 30g) taken to trigger abortion. In about half of these reports, the abnormality was deafness related to auditory nerve hypoplasia. Other abnormalities reported included limb anomalies, visceral defects, and visual changes. Teratogenic effects are observed in rabbits and guinea pigs but not mice, rats, dogs, and monkeys. Congenital malaria is rare, but elimination of the maternal parasitemia does not guarantee elimination from the placenta. **Quinine** is used for the treatment of neonatal malaria. Considering the kinetics of placental transport, fetal toxicity seems a low probability at recommended doses.

■ **Breastfeeding Safety** ⋯⋯⋯⋯ There are no adequate reports or well-controlled studies in nursing women. **Quinine** enters human breast milk achieving an M:P ratio of 0.31 (range 0.11-0.53). There are no reports of toxicity in breast-fed newborns.

■ **References** ⋯⋯⋯⋯⋯⋯⋯⋯⋯ McCready R, Thwai KL, Cho T, et al. Trans R Soc Trop Med Hyg 2002; 96:180-4.
Phillips RE, Looareesuwan S, White NJ, et al. Br J Clin Pharmacol 1986; 21:677-83.
Moran NF, Couper ID. S Afr Med J 1999; 89:943-6.
Zucker JR, Lackritz EM, Ruebush TK 2nd, et al. Am J Trop Med Hyg 1996; 55:655-60.
Phillips-Howard PA, Wood D. Drug Saf 1996; 14:131-45.

■ **Summary** ⋯⋯⋯⋯⋯⋯⋯⋯⋯⋯
- **Pregnancy Category X**
- **Lactation Category S?**
- Malaria is a major cause of maternal/perinatal illness.
- **Quinine** is an effective agent for the treatment of malaria.
- Except for the tetracyclines, there is no evidence that any of the antimalarial drugs in use are teratogenic at the recommended doses.
- **Quinine** should be used during pregnancy and lactation only if the benefit justifies the potential perinatal risk.

Rabeprazole (Aciphex)

- **Class** — Antiulcer, *proton pump inhibitor*

- **Indications** — GERD, esophagitis, duodenal ulcer, hypersecretory conditions, stress ulcer, ulcer prophylaxis

- **Mechanism** — Hydrogen-potassium ATP-ase inhibitor

- **Dosage with Qualifiers** — Gastroesophageal reflex disease—20mg PO qd/bid ×4-8w; may repeat for an additional 8w if needed
  Erosive esophagitis—20mg PO qd/bid ×4-8w; may repeat for an additional 8w if needed
  Duodenal ulcer—20mg PO qd/bid ×4w; may repeat for an additional 4w if needed
  Hypersecretory conditions—60mg PO qd
  NOTE—do not crush or chew
  - **Contraindications**—hypersensitivity to drug or class
  - **Caution**—hepatic dysfunction, long-term use

- **Maternal Considerations** — GERD and/or heartburn occur in 45-85% of women during pregnancy. The effect of estrogen and **progesterone** on lower esophageal sphincter tone is a recognized factor. The treatment for GERD is the reduction of gastric acidity. There is no published experience with **rabeprazole** during pregnancy. Other proton pump inhibitors are generally considered effective treatment for GERD during pregnancy. There are no reported adverse effects. Proton pump inhibitors are first-line agents for the prevention of "aspiration syndrome" during general anesthesia.
  Side effects include hepatic failure, blood dyscrasias, headache, and diarrhea.

- **Fetal Considerations** — There are no adequate reports or well-controlled studies in human fetuses. It is unknown whether **rabeprazole** crosses the human placenta. Rodent studies are reassuring, revealing no evidence of teratogenicity or IUGR despite the use of doses higher than those used clinically.

- **Breastfeeding Safety** — There is no published experience in nursing women. It is unknown whether **rabeprazole** enters human breast milk. It is concentrated in rodent breast milk.

- **References** — There is no published experience in pregnancy or during lactation.

- **Summary** —
  - **Pregnancy Category B**
  - **Lactation Category U**
  - **Rabeprazole** should be used during pregnancy and lactation only if the benefit justifies the potential perinatal risk.

- Proton pump inhibitors are agents of choice for the treatment of GERD in nonpregnant patients.
- Safety data are limited to animal studies and case reports. As a result, proton pump inhibitors are recommended during pregnancy only for the treatment of severe, intractable GERD.
- There are alternative agents for which there is more experience during pregnancy and lactation.

Rabies immune globulin, human
(BayRab; Hyperab; Imogam rabies)

■ **Class** — *Immune globulin, antiviral*

■ **Indications** — Rabies exposure

■ **Mechanism** — Passive immunization

■ **Dosage with Qualifiers** — Rabies exposure—20IU/kg (0.133ml/kg) concurrent with the 1st vaccine dose; if feasible, up to 1/2 the dose should be thoroughly infiltrated in the area of the wound and the rest IM in the gluteus
NOTE—may also be given up to day 7 after 1st vaccine dose; never give in the same syringe or site as vaccine
- **Contraindications**—none known
- **Caution**—hypersensitivity to drug or class, asthma

■ **Maternal Considerations** — Over 50% of the rabies cases among Americans result from exposure to dogs outside the U.S. Prevention is key. Rabies is almost universally fatal once it occurs. **Rabies immune globulin** is prepared from the plasma of donors hyperimmunized with **rabies vaccine**. The product is standardized to an average potency of 150IU/ml. **Rabies vaccine** and **rabies immune globulin** should be given to all suspected of rabies exposure unless previously immunized with **rabies vaccine** and with confirmed adequate antirabies titers. It has been used successfully during pregnancy. The reported adverse reaction rate is similar in pregnant and nonpregnant women.
Side effects include injection site reaction and mild fever.

■ **Fetal Considerations** — There are no adequate reports or well-controlled studies in human fetuses. Antirabies IgG likely crosses the human placenta. Fetal infection with rabies is reported. It is not known whether transfer provides any level of protection to the perinate. Animal reproduction studies have not been performed.

■ **Breastfeeding Safety** ⋯⋯⋯ There is no published experience in pregnancy. It is unknown whether **rabies immune globulin** enters human breast milk. However, other IgG antibodies are excreted into breast milk.

■ **References** ⋯⋯⋯⋯⋯⋯⋯ Chutivongse S, Wilde H, Benjavongkulchai M, et al. Clin Infect Dis 1995; 20:818-20.
Chabala S, Williams M, Amenta R, Ognjan AF. Am J Med 1991; 91:423-4.
Sipahioglu U, Alpaut S. Mikrobiyol Bul 1985; 19:95-9.

■ **Summary** ⋯⋯⋯⋯⋯⋯⋯⋯
- **Pregnancy Category C**
- **Lactation Category S?**
- Rabies remains a problem in many locales; it is almost uniformly fatal once manifest.
- Post-exposure prophylaxis with both immune globulin and vaccine reduces the risk of disease.
- Pregnant women respond to **rabies immune globulin**.

Rabies vaccine (Imovax Rabies; RabAvert)

■ **Class** ⋯⋯⋯⋯⋯⋯⋯⋯⋯⋯⋯ *Vaccine*

■ **Indications** ⋯⋯⋯⋯⋯⋯⋯⋯ Rabies exposure

■ **Mechanism** ⋯⋯⋯⋯⋯⋯⋯ Active immunization

■ **Dosage with Qualifiers** ⋯⋯ Rabies exposure, booster immunization—1ml IM on days 0, 7, 21 and 28 after exposure
Rabies exposure, immunization—1ml IM booster
NOTE—for IM use only
- **Contraindications**—none
- **Caution**—hypersensitivity to bovine gelatin, chicken protein, **neomycin**, **chlortetracycline**, **amphotericin B**

■ **Maternal Considerations** ⋯⋯ Over 50% of the rabies cases among Americans result from exposure to dogs outside the U.S. It is almost universally fatal once manifest. **Rabies vaccine** is an inactivated vaccine grown in chicken fibroblasts. **Rabies vaccine** and **rabies immune globulin** should be given to all suspected of rabies exposure unless previously immunized with **rabies vaccine** producing confirmed adequate antirabies titers. There is no data on the interchangeable use of different rabies vaccines in a single pre- or postexposure series. Thus, vaccine from a single manufacturer should be used for the complete series if possible. The vaccine has been used successfully during pregnancy, and pregnant women respond immunologically at least as well as nonpregnant women. The reported adverse reaction rate is similar in pregnant and nonpregnant women.

Side effects include anaphylaxis, paralysis, and muscular sclerosis.

■ **Fetal Considerations**

There are no adequate reports or well-controlled studies in human fetuses. Fetal rabies is reported. It is likely the IgG antibody produced in response to the vaccine crosses the placenta. It is not known whether transfer provides any level of perinatal protection. In one trial, intrauterine growth and pregnancy outcome were normal in women vaccinated for post-exposure prophylaxis.

■ **Breastfeeding Safety**

There is no published experience in nursing women. It is unknown whether **rabies vaccine** enters human breast milk. It is likely the antibodies produced in response to the vaccine are excreted into the milk.

■ **References**

Sudarshan MK, Madhusudana SN, Mahendra BJ, et al. Indian J Publ Health 1999; 43:76-8.
Chutivongse S, Wilde H, Benjavongkulchai M, et al. Clin Infect Dis 1995; 20:818-20.
Chabala S, Williams M, Amenta R, Ognjan AF. Am J Med 1991; 91:423-4.
Sipahioglu U, Alpaut S. Mikrobiyol Bul 1985; 19:95-9.
Sudarshan MK, Madhusudana SN, Mahendra BJ. J Commun Dis 1999; 31:229-36.

■ **Summary**

- **Pregnancy Category X**
- **Lactation Category U**
- Rabies remains a problem in many locales; it is almost uniformly fatal.
- Post-exposure prophylaxis with both immune globulin and vaccine reduces the risk of disease.
- Pregnant women respond to **rabies vaccine** at least as well as matched nonpregnant women.
- There is no evidence of fetal jeopardy from vaccination.

Raloxifene (Evista)

■ **Class**

SERM, *calcium metabolism*

■ **Indications**

Postmenopausal osteoporosis, prophylaxis and treatment

■ **Mechanism**

Estrogen-receptor modulator inhibiting bone resorption and turnover

- **Dosage with Qualifiers** ⋯⋯ Postmenopausal osteoporosis—60mg PO qd
  NOTE—take with **vitamin D** (400U qd) and **calcium**
  - **Contraindications**—hypersensitivity to drug or class,
    pregnancy, DVT, HRT or OCP use
  - **Caution**—unknown

- **Maternal Considerations** ⋯⋯ The decline in estrogen after oophorectomy and
  menopause enhances bone resorption and accelerates
  bone loss. Selective estrogen receptor modulators
  (SERMs) are a new family of drugs for the management of
  estrogen-related pathology. **Raloxifene** decreases
  resorption of bone and reduces biochemical markers of
  bone turnover to the premenopausal range. There is no
  published experience during pregnancy. **Raloxifene** does
  not stimulate the endometrium and may reduce the risk of
  ovarian cancer. Long-term effects are under study.
  Side effects include PE, DVT, hot flashes, arthralgia, flu-like
  symptoms, sinusitis, nausea, weight gain, pharyngitis,
  depression, cough, leg cramps, insomnia, and dyspepsia.

- **Fetal Considerations** ⋯⋯ There are no adequate reports or well-controlled studies
  in human fetuses. It is not known whether **raloxifene**
  crosses the human placenta. Studies in rodents reveal an
  increase in several types of defects including heart, brain,
  and skeleton. Different from estrogen, **raloxifene** does not
  alter the organization of the neuronal system related to
  sexual receptivity in rodents.

- **Breastfeeding Safety** ⋯⋯ There is no published experience in nursing women. It is
  unknown whether **raloxifene** enters human breast milk.

- **References** ⋯⋯ Pinilla L, Barreiro ML, Tena-Sempere M, Aguilar E.
  Neurosci Lett 2002; 329:285-8.

- **Summary** ⋯⋯
  - **Pregnancy Category X**
  - **Lactation Category U**
  - There are no indications for **raloxifene** during pregnancy.

Ramipril (Altace)

- **Class** ⋯⋯ ACE-I/A2R-*antagonist*

- **Indications** ⋯⋯ Hypertension, post-MI CHF, CV risk reduction

- **Mechanism** ⋯⋯ ACE inhibitor

- **Dosage with Qualifiers** ⋯⋯ Hypertension—begin 2.5mg PO qd; max 20mg PO qd
  Post-MI CHF—begin 2.5mg PO bid ×7d, then 5mg PO bid

CV risk reduction—begin 2.5mg PO qd ×7d, then 10mg PO qd; indicated for patients >55y with either CAD, CVA, PVD or with diabetes mellitus and at least 1 other risk factor
NOTE—renal dosing
- **Contraindications**—hypersensitivity to drug or class, angioedema
- **Caution**—severe CHF, renal dysfunction, renal artery stenosis, collagen vascular disease, hyponatremia and volume depletion

■ **Maternal Considerations** ⋯⋯ Some ACE inhibitors decrease proteinuria and preserve renal function in patients with hypertension and diabetes mellitus to a greater extent than other antihypertensive agents. More recently, they were shown to decrease the progression of nephropathy in normotensive patients with type II diabetes mellitus. There are no adequate reports or well-controlled studies in pregnant women. In general, ACE inhibitors are avoided during pregnancy because of fetal risks. The lowest effective dose should be used if **ramipril** is required for pressure control during pregnancy. *Side effects* include angioedema, severe hypotension, hyperkalemia, hepatotoxicity, pancreatitis, agranulocytosis, neutropenia, cough, dizziness, fatigue, nausea, vomiting, myalgias, arthralgias, and URI symptoms.

■ **Fetal Considerations** ⋯⋯ There is no published experience in human fetuses. **Ramipril** likely crosses the human placenta as similar agents do. Transfer was described as low in one rodent study. As a drug group, no adverse fetal effects are reported after 1st trimester exposure to ACE inhibitors. Later exposure is associated with cranial hypoplasia, anuria, reversible or irreversible renal failure, death, oligohydramnios, prematurity, IUGR, and patent ductus arteriosus. The mechanism of renal dysfunction is likely related to fetal hypotension associated with prolonged decreased glomerular filtration. There is inadequate study to decide whether **ramipril** is typical of ACE inhibitors. However, the one published rodent study is reassuring. If oligohydramnios is detected, **ramipril** should be discontinued unless lifesaving for the mother. Antenatal surveillance should be initiated (e.g., BPP) if the fetus is potentially viable. Oligohydramnios may not appear until after the fetus has irreversible injury. Neonates exposed *in utero* to ACE inhibitors should be observed closely for hypotension, oliguria, and hyperkalemia. If oliguria occurs despite adequate pressure and renal perfusion, exchange transfusion or peritoneal dialysis may be required.

■ **Breastfeeding Safety** ⋯⋯ There is no published experience in nursing women. It is unknown whether **ramipril** enters human breast milk. It is described as low in rodents.

■ **Reference** ⋯⋯ Eckert HG, Badian MJ, Gantz D, et al. Arzneimittelforschung 1984; 34:1435-47.

■ **Summary** ⋯⋯⋯⋯⋯⋯⋯⋯⋯⋯⋯⋯⋯
- **Pregnancy Category C (1st trimester), D (2nd and 3rd trimesters)**
- **Lactation Category U?**
- **Ramipril** and other ACE inhibitors should be avoided during pregnancy if possible.
- Neonatal skull hypoplasia and reversible or irreversible renal failure are the most frequent fetal consequences of ACE inhibitors during late pregnancy; 1st trimester exposure is probably safe.
- When the mother's disease requires treatment with **ramipril**, the lowest doses should be used followed by close monitoring of the fetus.

Ranitidine (Ranitiget; Zantac)

■ **Class** ⋯⋯⋯⋯⋯⋯⋯⋯⋯⋯⋯⋯⋯⋯⋯⋯⋯ Antiulcer

■ **Indications** ⋯⋯⋯⋯⋯⋯⋯⋯⋯⋯⋯⋯⋯ Duodenal or gastric ulcer, erosive esophagitis, GERD, dyspepsia

■ **Mechanism** ⋯⋯⋯⋯⋯⋯⋯⋯⋯⋯⋯⋯⋯ H_2 antagonist

■ **Dosage with Qualifiers** ⋯⋯⋯⋯⋯
Duodenal or gastric ulcer—150mg PO bid
Erosive esophagitis—150mg PO qid
GERD—150mg PO bid
Dyspepsia—75mg PO qd/bid
NOTE—renal dosing; may be combined with **bismuth** (Tritec)
- **Contraindications**—hypersensitivity to drug or class, porphyria
- **Caution**—hepatic or renal dysfunction

■ **Maternal Considerations** ⋯⋯⋯
Pregnant women with symptomatic GERD should be managed aggressively with lifestyle and dietary modification. Antacids are first-line therapy. Should they fail, **ranitidine** or **cimetidine** are second-line options effective during pregnancy. It has also been used successfully during pregnancy for the treatment of Zollinger-Ellison syndrome.
Side effects include hepatotoxicity, thrombocytopenia, myalgia, headache, nausea, vomiting, diarrhea, constipation, vertigo, dizziness, malaise, dry skin, rash and confusion.

■ **Fetal Considerations** ⋯⋯⋯⋯⋯⋯
There are no adequate reports or well-controlled studies in human fetuses. It is unknown whether **ranitidine** crosses the human placenta. Epidemiological study reveals no increased prevalence of adverse fetal outcomes following 1st trimester exposure. Rodent studies are reassuring,

noting no evidence of teratogenicity or IUGR despite the use of doses higher than those used clinically. **Ranitidine** reduces fetal gastric pH when administered to pregnant rabbits, thus suggesting placental transfer.

■ **Breastfeeding Safety** There is no published experience in nursing women. While **ranitidine** is concentrated in human breast milk, no adverse effects are reported. **Ranitidine** is approved for use in pediatric practice.

■ **References** Larson JD, Patatanian E, Miner PB Jr, et al. Obstet Gynecol 1997; 90:83-7.
Stewart CA, Termanini B, Sutliff VE, et al. Am J Obstet Gynecol 1997; 176:224-33.
Ruigomez A, Garcia Rodriguez LA, Cattaruzzi C, et al. Am J Epidemiol 1999; 150:476-81.
Aslan A, Karaguzel G, Uysal N, et al. Am J Perinetal 1999; 16:209-15.
Hagemann TM. J Hum Lact 1998; 14:259-62.
Kearns GL, McConnell RF Jr, Trang JM, Kluza RB. Clin Pharm 1985; 4:322-4.

■ **Summary**
- **Pregnancy Category B**
- **Lactation Category S?**
- **Ranitidine** should be used during pregnancy and lactation only if the benefit justifies the potential perinatal risk.
- Medications used for treating GERD are not routinely tested in randomized, controlled trials in pregnant women.

Remifentanil (Ultiva)

■ **Class** Narcotic

■ **Indications** Anesthesia

■ **Mechanism** Binds opiate receptors

■ **Dosage with Qualifiers** Anesthesia:
Induction—0.5-1mcg/kg/min; anesthesia induced when given with hypnotic and a muscle relaxant to avoid chest rigidity
Maintenance—0.05-2mcg/kg/min IV; usually given along with inhaled anesthetic or intravenous anesthetic agent
Postoperative—0.025-0.2mcg/kg/min IV
Sedation—0.025-0.2mcg/kg/min IV usually given with sedative/hypnotic (e.g., **propofol**)
NOTE—onset <1min, duration 5-10min, peak 1-5min

- **Contraindications**—hypersensitivity to drug or class, epidural or intrathecal use
- **Caution**—respiratory depression

■ **Maternal Considerations** ⋯⋯ Unlike other opioids, **remifentanil** undergoes rapid hydrolysis by nonspecific blood and tissue esterases. This characteristic suggested a potential for use in obstetrics. In a pilot study, **remifentanil** provided superior pain relief to laboring women when given by PCA compared to IM **meperidine**. However, **remifentanil** is difficult to titer in clinical practice, and produces high levels of sedation and excess rates of maternal oxygen desaturation.
Side effects include apnea, chest wall rigidity, ventricular arrhythmia, bradycardia, hypotension, dependency, seizures, nausea, vomiting, shivering, fever, dizziness, constipation, headache, blurred vision, pruritus, oliguria, confusion, tachycardia, agitation, anxiety, and biliary spasm.

■ **Fetal Considerations** ⋯⋯ There are no adequate reports or well-controlled studies in human fetuses. **Remifentanil** crosses the human placenta achieving an F:M ratio approximating 0.5. Neonatal sedation is reported. Rodent studies are reassuring, revealing no evidence of teratogenicity or IUGR despite the use of doses higher than those used clinically.

■ **Breastfeeding Safety** ⋯⋯ There is no published experience in nursing women. It is unknown whether **remifentanil** enters human breast milk. It is excreted into rodent breast milk. Considering the indication and half-life, one-time **remifentanil** use is unlikely to pose a clinically significant risk to the breast-feeding neonate.

■ **References** ⋯⋯ Thurlow JA, Laxton CH, Dick A, et al. Br J Anaesth 2002; 88:374-8.
Volmanen P, Akural EI, Raudaskoski T, Alahuhta S. Anesth Analg 2002; 94:913-7.

■ **Summary** ⋯⋯
- **Pregnancy Category C**
- **Lactation Category S?**
- There are alternative agents with a higher safety profile for which there is more experience during pregnancy and lactation.

Repaglinide (Prandin)

- **Class** — *Diabetes mellitus*

- **Indications** — Diabetes mellitus type 2

- **Mechanism** — ATP-dependent K channel antagonist that stimulates islet cell insulin release in a glucose-dependent manner

- **Dosage with Qualifiers** — Diabetes mellitus type 2—0.5-4mg PO 5-30min qAC; max 16mg/d
  NOTE—titer to glucose profile
  - **Contraindications**—hypersensitivity to drug or class, IDDM, ketoacidosis
  - **Caution**—severe renal disease

- **Maternal Considerations** — There is no published experience with **repaglinide** in pregnant women. Its clearance is lower in women than in men. **Insulin** remains the standard agent for the treatment of hyperglycemia during pregnancy. However, a growing body of research indicates that some oral hypoglycemic agents may be equally effective and safe, while more convenient.
  Side effects include hypoglycemia, pancreatitis, Stevens-Johnson syndrome, hemolytic anemia, hepatic dysfunction, headache, URI symptoms, nausea, vomiting, constipation, diarrhea, dyspepsia, myalgias, and chest pain.

- **Fetal Considerations** — There are no adequate reports or well-controlled studies in human fetuses. It is unknown whether **repaglinide** crosses the human placenta. Rodent studies are reassuring, revealing no evidence of teratogenicity. However, an increased risk of IUGR may be secondary to chronic maternal hypoglycemia.

- **Breastfeeding Safety** — There is no published experience in nursing women. It is unknown whether **repaglinide** enters human breast milk. It does enter rat milk and is associated with skeletal deformities in the feeding pups.

- **References** — Viertel B, Guttner J. Arzneimittelforschung 2000; 50:425-40.

- **Summary** —
  - **Pregnancy Category C**
  - **Lactation Category U**
  - **Repaglinide** should be avoided during pregnancy and lactation until additional research supports its use.

Reserpine (Reserpaneed; Serpalan; Serpasil; Serpatabs; Serpate; Serpivite)

- **Class** — *Antihypertensive, antiadrenergic*

- **Indications** — Hypertension, adjunct for psychosis

- **Mechanism** — Depletes catecholamine and 5-HT stores

- **Dosage with Qualifiers** — Hypertension—begin 0.5mg PO qd x1-2w, then 0.1-0.25mg PO qd
  Psychiatric disorders—begin 0.5mg PO qd
  NOTE—discontinue with first signs of depression
  - **Contraindications**—hypersensitivity to drug or class, depression (especially with suicidal tendencies), active peptic ulcer, active ulcerative colitis, electroconvulsive therapy
  - **Caution**—history of either peptic ulcer or ulcerative colitis, gallstones, renal insufficiency, anesthesia, use of **digoxin** or **quinidine**, or other antihypertensives

- **Maternal Considerations** — **Reserpine** is a pure crystalline alkaloid of rauwolfia. It is a second-line agent for the treatment of hypertension. **Reserpine** is also used for the treatment of cerebral vasospasm, migraines, Raynaud's syndrome, refractory depression, tardive dyskinesia, and thyrotoxic crisis. There is only limited study during pregnancy.
  Side effects include nausea, vomiting, diarrhea, anorexia, dryness of mouth, hypersecretion, arrhythmias, syncope, angina-like symptoms, bradycardia, edema, dyspnea, epistaxis, nasal congestion, dizziness, headache, paradoxical anxiety, depression, nervousness, nightmares, drowsiness, myalgias, weight gain, deafness and pruritus.

- **Fetal Considerations** — There are no adequate reports or well-controlled studies in human fetuses. **Reserpine** crosses the human placenta. It can increase neonatal respiratory tract secretions, and cause nasal congestion, cyanosis, and anorexia. While it is unclear whether **reserpine** is a human teratogen, rodent studies reveal evidence of teratogenicity and embryotoxicity. It is also tumorigenic.

- **Breastfeeding Safety** — **Reserpine** is excreted in human breast milk. Increased respiratory tract secretions, nasal congestion, cyanosis, and anorexia can occur in breast-fed infants.

- **References** — Southern African Hypertension Society Executive Committee 2000. S Afr Med J 2001; 91:163-72.
  Mirmiran M, Swaab DF. Neurotoxicology 1986; 7:95-102.

■ **Summary**
• **Pregnancy Category C**
• **Lactation Category NS**
• **Reserpine** should probably be avoided during pregnancy and lactation unless there is no other option.
• There are alternative agents for which there is more experience during pregnancy and lactation.

Reteplase (Rapilysin; Retavase)

■ **Class** — Anticoagulant

■ **Indications** — Acute MI

■ **Mechanism** — Promotes fibrinolysis by converting plasminogen to plasmin

■ **Dosage with Qualifiers** — Acute MI—10U IV over 2min; repeat 2nd dose 30min later if no complications
• **Contraindications**—hypersensitivity to drug or class, history of stroke or recent surgery or trauma, active bleeding, intracranial mass, AVM, aneurysm, severe hypertension
• **Caution**—unknown

■ **Maternal Considerations** — **Reteplase** is recombinant plasminogen activator. There are no adequate reports or well-controlled studies of **reteplase** in pregnant women. The published experience is limited to two case reports associated with life-threatening thrombosis. There were no reported adverse effects. There is a real risk of uterine hemorrhage if administered in the puerperium.
Side effects include intracranial hemorrhage, ventricular arrhythmia, pulmonary edema, cholesterol embolization, anemia, GI and GU bleeding, nausea and vomiting.

■ **Fetal Considerations** — There are no adequate reports or well-controlled studies in human fetuses. It is unknown whether **reteplase** crosses the human placenta. Rodent studies showed no evidence of teratogenicity, but there was an increased risk of genital hemorrhage and abortion.

■ **Breastfeeding Safety** — There is no published experience in nursing women. It is unknown whether **reteplase** enters human breast milk. However, considering the indication and dosing, one time **reteplase** use is unlikely to pose a clinically significant risk to the breast-feeding neonate.

■ **References** — Yap LB, Alp NJ, Forfar JC. Int J Cardiol 2002; 82:193-4.
Rinaldi JP, Yassine M, Aboujaoude F, et al. Arch Mal Coeur Vaiss 1999; 92:427-30.

Rh$_o$(D) immune globulin (Gamulin Rh;
HypRho-D; Mini-Gamulin Rh; Rhesonativ; WinRho SDF)

■ **Class** .... *Immune globulin*

■ **Indications** .... Risk for D alloimmunization

■ **Mechanism** .... Passive immunization

■ **Dosage with Qualifiers** .... Delivery >12w gestation—300mcg IM within 72h covers
transplacental hemorrhage up to 15ml PRBC
Pregnancy termination (spontaneous or iatrogenic)
≤12w—120-150mcg IM
Antenatal prophylaxis at 28w or after placental bleeding or
instrumentation—300mcg IM; repeat for each bleeding
episode >72h apart
Transfusion accident—Multiply the volume (in ml) of Rh-
positive whole blood administered by the hematocrit of
the donor unit. This equals the volume of packed red
blood cells transfused. Divide the volume (in ml) of
packed red blood cells by 15 to obtain the number of vials
or syringes of Rh IgG to be administered.
NOTE—available as a pooled plasma or engineered
product, in "indication specific" doses
• **Contraindications**—hypersensitivity to drug or class,
Rh$^+$
• **Caution**—unknown

■ **Maternal Considerations** .... Rh alloimmunization remains a perinatal health problem
even in countries with a developed program of
prophylaxis. Patient or medical error is the most common
cause of failed prophylaxis. Anti-D human
immunoglobulin has been in clinical use for more than 30
years. Its assessment is based more on experience than
on well-designed comparative trials. A meta-analysis of 6
trials involving more than 10,000 women demonstrated
efficacy of prophylaxis after delivery of a Rh$_o$(D) positive
infant to a Rh$_o$(D) negative woman reducing sensitization
from 10% to 1.5%. The addition of antenatal prophylaxis
reduces the rate of sensitization further, down to <0.5%.
However, the optimal dose regimen and route of

administration remain unclear. Some data favor the use of **Rh$_o$(D) immune globulin** after abortion, as it appears to reduce immunization rates from about 3-4% to 0.4%. **Rh$_o$(D) immune globulin** is also likely effective antenatally in circumstances or procedures carrying a risk of maternal exposure to fetal red blood cells, although this has not been proved in comparative trials. Criteria for an Rh-incompatible pregnancy requiring treatment includes: mother Rh$_o$(D) negative, not previously sensitized to the Rh$_o$(D) factor, and the neonate Rh$_o$(D) positive and direct antiglobulin negative. **Rh$_o$(D) immune globulin** should be administered to all nonsensitized Rh-negative women after spontaneous or induced abortion, after ruptured tubal pregnancy, chorion villus sampling, amniocentesis, abdominal trauma, or any occurrence of transplacental hemorrhage unless the fetus is known to be Rh$_o$(D) negative. If **Rh$_o$(D) immune globulin** is given antenatally, it is essential the mother receive another dose after delivery of a Rh$_o$(D) positive infant. If the father is known and Rh$_o$(D) negative, **Rh$_o$(D) immune globulin** is unnecessary. **Rh$_o$(D) immune globulin** should be given within 72h of delivery or abortion (spontaneous or iatrogenic). Passively acquired anti-Rh$_o$(D) may be detected after delivery following antenatal treatment; however, she should be treated again post partum if the neonate is Rh$_o$(D) positive. One vial or syringe of 300mcg is sufficient to prevent maternal sensitization if the transferred fetal PRBC volume is <15ml (30ml whole blood). More than one vial or syringe of **Rh$_o$(D) immune globulin** must be given when the fetomaternal hemorrhage >15ml PRBCs or 30ml whole blood. The number of vials required is calculated by taking the volume of packed fetal red blood cells determined by an approved laboratory assay, divided by 2 to get the volume of packed fetal red blood cells in the maternal blood, and dividing that number by 15 to get the number of syringes or vials. *Side effects* include injection site reaction and fever.

■ **Fetal Considerations**

There is no evidence of fetal harm after extensive clinical experience. Babies born of women given Rh immune globulin antepartum may have a weakly positive antiglobulin test at birth.

■ **Breastfeeding Safety**

There are no adequate reports or well-controlled studies in nursing women. **Rh$_o$(D) immune globulin** is excreted into human breast milk, but the amount of intact antibody detectable in the neonate is too low to cause clinically relevant hemolysis.

■ **References**

Crowther C, Middleton P. Cochrane Database Syst Rev 2000; (2): CD000021.
Bowman J.M., Chown B. Can Med J 1968; 99:385-388.
Bowman J.M., Pollock J.M. Can Med J 1978; 118:627-630.
Grimes DA, Ross WC, Hatcher RA. Obstet Gynecol 1977; 50:261-263.

Weinberg L. Emerg Med J 2001; 18:444-7.
Maayan-Metzger A, Schwartz T, Sulkes J, Merlob P. Arch
Dis Child Fetal Neonatal Ed 2001; 84:F60-2.

■ **Summary**

- **Pregnancy Category C**
- **Lactation Category S**
- **Rh$_o$(D) immune globulin** is safe and likely effective for each of the listed indications.
- Antenatal and postnatal prophylaxis is cost-effective in most developed countries.

Ribavirin (Rebetol; Viramid; Virazid; Virazole)

■ **Class**

Antiviral

■ **Indications**

Chronic hepatitis C

■ **Mechanism**

Unknown

■ **Dosage with Qualifiers**

Chronic hepatitis C—400mg PO qAM and 600mg qPM if <75kg; 600mg PO bid if >74.9kg
NOTE—may be combined with **interferon alfa-2b** (Rebetron)

- **Contraindications**—hypersensitivity to drug or class, male partners of pregnant women, significant cardiac disease, autoimmune hepatitis, hemoglobinopathy, CrCl<50ml/min
- **Caution**—psychiatric disorder, myelosuppression, pulmonary or cardiac disease, diabetes mellitus

■ **Maternal Considerations**

Hepatitis C is a growing problem worldwide. Perhaps a third of patients with HIV also have hepatitis C. Liver disease due to chronic HCV infection is now the 2nd leading cause of death in some HIV-infected populations. The published experience with **ribavirin** during pregnancy is limited to case reports. No adverse effects are reported. Considering the risk of viral transmission to the perinate is increased by coexistent infection, it seems likely future trials will address treatment of hepatitis C in HIV-infected pregnant women. The CDC does not recommend **ribavirin** for post exposure prophylaxis. Patients with chronic hepatitis whose therapy can be delayed should not be treated until controlled studies are available. However, women exposed to **ribavirin** inadvertently during pregnancy may be encouraged to continue pregnancy. In patients with acute hepatitis C during pregnancy, the use of **ribavirin** therapy should be considered with close monitoring.
Side effects include hemolytic anemia, thrombocytopenia, neutropenia, marrow suppression, MI, suicidal ideation, nausea, vomiting, autoimmune disorders, pulmonary

toxicity, pancreatitis, diabetes mellitus, headache, fatigue, myalgia, arthralgia, fever, insomnia, depression, alopecia, irritability, anorexia, rash, pruritus, dyspnea, dyspepsia, and loss of concentration.

■ **Fetal Considerations** — There are no adequate reports or well-controlled studies in human fetuses. It is unknown whether **ribavirin** crosses the human placenta. Rodent studies reveal an increased prevalence of limb, eye, and brain defects. The incidence and severity was proportional to drug dose. Teratogenicity was not seen at doses approximating the recommended human dose. **Ribavirin** is often used in the pediatric population for the treatment of RSV. The prevalence of hepatitis C in children is between 0.05% and 0.4%. The major mode of acquisition has shifted from parenteral to maternal-infant transmission. And while the actual rate of maternal-infant transmission is low, HIV increases the rate of transmission. Cesarean section reduces the transmission rate of both viruses.

■ **Breastfeeding Safety** — There is no published experience in nursing women. It is unknown whether **ribavirin** enters human breast milk. **Ribavirin** is toxic to lactating rats and their offspring.

■ **References** — Hegenbarth K, Maurer U, Kroisel PM, et al. Am J Gastroenterol 2001; 96:2286-7.
U.S. Public Health Service. MMWR Recomm Rep 2001; 50(RR-11):1-52.
Ferm VH, Willhite C, Kilham L. Teratology 1978; 17:93-101.
Prows CA, Shortridge L, Kenner C, Lemasters G. J Pediatr Nurs 1993; 8:370-5.

■ **Summary**
- **Pregnancy Category X**
- **Lactation Category U**
- **Ribavirin** is a teratogen in rodents.
- There is inadequate experience to conclude it is or is not a teratogen in humans. It is used clinically for the treatment of small children.
- Ribavirin should be used during pregnancy and lactation only if the benefit justifies the potential risk.
- Physicians are encouraged to register pregnant women with the Antiretroviral Pregnancy Registry (1-800-258-4263) for a better follow-up of the outcome while under treatment with ribavirin.

Riboflavin

■ Class .... *Vitamin*

■ Indications .... Replacement, supplementation

■ Mechanism ....

■ Dosage with Qualifiers .... Replacement—5-25mg PO qd
Supplementation—1.7mg PO qd (MDR)
- **Contraindications**—hypersensitivity to drug or class
- **Caution**—unknown

■ Maternal Considerations .... **Riboflavin** is an important nutrient contained in virtually all multivitamin supplements. Contrary to conventional wisdom, the maternal concentration of **riboflavin** does not decline during normal, unsupplemented pregnancy. However, maternal supplementation does generate supraphysiologic levels. Epidemiologic studies suggest multivitamin supplementation during the pregnancy of HIV-infected women improves maternal weight gain. *Side effects* include bright yellow urine.

■ Fetal Considerations .... There are no adequate reports or well-controlled studies in human fetuses. Observational studies note a positive relationship between maternal **riboflavin** levels and fetal size. This finding also applies to women who abuse tobacco. There is no substantative evidence **riboflavin** is a teratogen. In some animal models, **riboflavin** supplementation reduces the incidence of neural tube defects.

■ Breastfeeding Safety .... **Riboflavin** is excreted into human breast milk, and the concentration is proportional to the maternal concentration.

■ References .... Cikot RJ, Steegers-Theunissen RP, Thomas CM, et al. Br J Nutr 2001; 85:49-58.
Villamor E, Msamanga G, Spiegelman D, et al. Am J Clin Nutr 2002; 76:1082-90.
Baker H, DeAngelis B, Holland B, et al. J Am Coll Nutr 2002; 21:33-7.
Seller MJ. Ciba Found Symp 1994; 181:161-73; discussion 173-9.
Badart-Smook A, van Houwelingen AC, Al MD, et al. J Am Diet Assoc 1997; 97:867-70.
Faron G, Drouin R, Pedneault L, et al. Teratology 2001; 63:161-3.
Ortega RM, Quintas ME, Martinez RM, et al. J Am Coll Nutr 1999; 18:324-9.

■ **Summary**
- **Pregnancy Category A**
- **Lactation Category S**
- The maternal concentration of **riboflavin** does not change during normal pregnancy.
- Prenatal multivitamin supplements successfully increase the maternal concentration.

Rifabutin (Ansamycin; Mycobutin)

■ **Class**
Antimycobacterial

■ **Indications**
Prevention of disseminated *Mycobacterium avium* complex (MAC) disease in women with advanced HIV infection

■ **Mechanism**
Unknown; inhibits bacterial DNA-dependent RNA polymerase

■ **Dosage with Qualifiers**
MAC prevention—300mg PO qd
NOTE—renal dosing
- **Contraindications**—hypersensitivity to drug or class, active TB
- **Caution**—neutropenia, thrombocytopenia

■ **Maternal Considerations**
Rifabutin is an alternative to **rifampin** for the treatment of *Mycobacterium* tuberculosis in HIV-infected women taking certain antiretroviral agents concomitantly. It is also recommended by the U.S. Public Health Service/Infectious Diseases Society of America Prevention of Opportunistic Infections in Persons Infected with HIV Working Group as an alternative agent to **rifampin** for chemoprophylaxis of tuberculosis. There is no experience with **rifabutin** during pregnancy. In healthy nonpregnant women, **rifabutin** and **rifampin** significantly increase the clearance of **ethinyl estradiol**, suggesting women who use low-dose oral contraceptives should either switch to a higher dose, or use a back-up contraceptive method while taking **rifabutin.**
Side effects include thrombocytopenia, neutropenia, leukopenia, uveitis, rash, nausea, vomiting, abdominal pain, headache, dyspepsia, diarrhea, belching, discolored urine, taste changes, fever, anorexia, myalgias, asthenia, flatus, chest pain, and insomnia.

■ **Fetal Considerations**
There are no adequate reports or well-controlled studies in human fetuses. It is unknown whether **rifabutin** crosses the human placenta. Rodent studies are reassuring, revealing no evidence of teratogenicity or IUGR despite the use of doses higher than those used clinically.

- ■ **Breastfeeding Safety** ⋯ There are no adequate reports or well-controlled studies in nursing women. It is unknown whether **rifabutin** enters human breast milk. Breastfeeding is contraindicated in HIV-infected nursing women where formula is available to reduce the risk of neonatal transmission.

- ■ **References** ⋯ LeBel M, Masson E, Guilbert E, et al. J Clin Pharmacol 1998; 38:1042-50.

- ■ **Summary** ⋯
  - Pregnancy Category B
  - Lactation Category U
  - **Rifabutin** should be used during pregnancy and lactation only if the benefit justifies the potential perinatal risk.

Rifampin (Abrifam; Aptecin; Corifam; Fenampicin; Rifadin; Rifamate; Rifamed; Rifampicin; Rifamycin; Rifarad; Rifocina; Rifumycin; Rimactane; Rimpacin; Syntaxil; Syntoren; Tibirim; Visedan)

- ■ **Class** ⋯ Antimycobacterial

- ■ **Indications** ⋯ Tuberculosis, meningococcal prophylaxis

- ■ **Mechanism** ⋯ Bactericidal; inhibits DNA-dependent RNA polymerase

- ■ **Dosage with Qualifiers** ⋯ Tuberculosis—10-20mg/kg PO qd on an empty stomach (not to exceed 600mg/d)
  Meningococcal prophylaxis (not treatment)—600mg PO bid ×2d
  NOTE—may be combined with **isoniazid** +/– **pyrazinamide** and **ethambutol** or **streptomycin**
  - **Contraindications**—hypersensitivity to drug or class
  - **Caution**—hepatic dysfunction or use of a hepatic enzyme inducer

- ■ **Maternal Considerations** ⋯ Untreated TB poses a significant threat to the mother, fetus, and family. A 3-drug regimen of **rifampin**, **isoniazid**, and **pyrazinamide** is recommended for the initial 2mo treatment phase. All pregnant women taking **isoniazid** should also take **pyridoxine** to reduce the chance of hepatitis. The CDC recommends that either **streptomycin** or **ethambutol** be added during the initial treatment unless the likelihood of INH resistance is low. However, **streptomycin** is contraindicated in pregnancy. **Ciprofloxacin** has the best safety profile of second-line drugs for the treatment of drug-resistant TB. After the initial phase, treatment is continued with **rifampin** and

isoniazid for 4mo, or longer if the sputum or culture is positive, resistant organisms are present, or if patient is HIV positive. There are no adequate reports or well-controlled studies of **rifampin** in pregnant women. A long clinical experience suggests pregnancy does not increase the risk of an adverse effect. **Rifampin** may cause hemorrhage in the mother and neonate when administered during the 3rd trimester. Treatment with **vitamin K** may be indicated. **Rifampin** impairs the effectiveness of OCs. Women using a low-dose oral contraceptive should consider a higher dose preparation or a back-up method of contraception.
Side effects include renal failure, shock, hepatotoxicity, hemolytic anemia, thrombocytopenia, leukopenia, elevated LFTs, interstitial nephritis, nausea, vomiting, diarrhea, anorexia, headache, fatigue, dizziness, abdominal pain, pruritus, rash, dyspnea, ataxia, visual changes, and urticaria.

■ **Fetal Considerations**

There are no adequate reports or well-controlled studies in human fetuses. It is unknown whether **rifampin** crosses the human placenta. There is no substantive evidence of teratogenicity in humans. **Rifampin** does cross the rodent placenta, and it is teratogenic at oral doses 15-25 times the MRHD, affecting bone, spine, and palate, depending upon the species. Congenital TB does occur on occasion, especially in association with miliary TB. **Rifampin** is used to treat children in the first few months of life.

■ **Breastfeeding Safety**

There are no adequate reports or well-controlled studies in nursing women. Only trace amounts of **rifampin** are excreted into human breast milk.

■ **References**

From the Centers for Disease Control and Prevention. JAMA 1993; 270:694-8.
Bothamley G. Drug Saf 2001; 24:553-65.
Dickinson BD, Altman RD, Nielsen NH, Sterling ML. Obstet Gynecol 2001; 98:853-60.
Pillet P, Grill J, Rakotonirina G, et al. Arch Pediatr 1999; 6:635-9.
Holdiness MR. Early Hum Dev 1987; 15:61-74.
Tran JH, Montakantikul P. J Hum Lact 1998; 14:337-40.

■ **Summary**

- **Pregnancy Category C**
- **Lactation Category S**
- **Rifampin** and the core group of antituberculosis drugs appear safe and effective during pregnancy when given as recommended.

Rifapentine (Priftin)

- **Class** — *Antimycobacterial*

- **Indications** — Tuberculosis

- **Mechanism** — Bactericidal; inhibits DNA-dependent RNA polymerase

- **Dosage with Qualifiers** — Tuberculosis—begin 600mg PO with food 2x/w ×2mo; then 600mg PO qw × 2mo
  NOTE—not for monotherapy; take with meals to improve bioavailability
  - **Contraindications**—hypersensitivity to drug or class
  - **Caution**—hepatic dysfunction, nephrotoxic drug use

- **Maternal Considerations** — **Rifapentine** is similar to **rifampin**, but has a more convenient dosing protocol. It must be taken in tandem with at least one other antituberculosis drug to which the isolate is susceptible. There are no adequate reports or well-controlled studies of **rifapentine** in pregnant women. The published experience is limited to isolated case reports.
  Side effects include thrombocytopenia, neutropenia, leukopenia, elevated LFTs, hyperbilirubinemia, proteinuria, hematuria, pancreatitis, pseudomembranous colitis, interstitial nephritis, hepatotoxicity, urinary casts, rash, pruritus, acne, anorexia, arthralgia, pain, nausea, and vomiting.

- **Fetal Considerations** — There are no adequate reports or well-controlled studies in human fetuses. **Rifapentine** is teratogenic in rodents when given at doses similar to humans, affecting bone, heart, spine and palate (species-dependent). There is also evidence of embryotoxicity.

- **Breastfeeding Safety** — There is no published experience in nursing women. It is unknown whether **rifapentine** enters human breast milk.

- **References** — Temple ME, Nahata MC. Ann Pharmacother 1999; 33:1203-10.

- **Summary** —
  - **Pregnancy Category C**
  - **Lactation Category U**
  - **Rifapentine** has no significant clinical advantage over **rifampin** that would justify its use during pregnancy and lactation.

Riluzole (Rilutek)

■ **Class** — *Other neurologic, neuroprotective*

■ **Indications** — Amyotrophic lateral sclerosis

■ **Mechanism** — Unknown

■ **Dosage with Qualifiers** — ALS—50mg PO q12h taken on an empty stomach
- **Contraindications**—hypersensitivity to drug or class
- **Caution**—hepatic or renal dysfunction, hypertension, history of neutropenia

■ **Maternal Considerations** — Amyotrophic lateral sclerosis (ALS) is the most common, progressive motor neuron disease, but is rare in the obstetric population. There are no published reports of **riluzole** use during pregnancy.
Side effects include hepatotoxicity, asthenia, nausea, vomiting, diarrhea, rhinitis, headache, abdominal pain, weight loss, tachycardia, worsening of spasticity, insomnia, cough, paresthesias, edema, and depression.

■ **Fetal Considerations** — There are no adequate reports or well-controlled studies in human fetuses. It is unknown whether **riluzole** crosses the human placenta. Rodent studies are reassuring, revealing no evidence of teratogenicity or IUGR despite the use of doses higher than those used clinically. Maternal and embryo toxicity were seen.

■ **Breastfeeding Safety** — There are no adequate reports or well-controlled studies in nursing women. It is unknown whether **riluzole** enters human breast milk.

■ **References** — There are no current relevant references.

■ **Summary** —
- **Pregnancy Category C**
- **Lactation Category U**
- **Riluzole** should be used during pregnancy and lactation only if the benefit justifies the potential perinatal risk.

Rimantadine (Flumadine)

- **Class** — *Antiviral*

- **Indications** — Influenza A treatment and prophylaxis

- **Mechanism** — Unknown

- **Dosage with Qualifiers** — Influenza A treatment—100mg PO bid ×7d
  Influenza prophylaxis—100mg PO bid
  NOTE—renal dosing
  - **Contraindications**—hypersensitivity to drug or class
  - **Caution**—hepatic or renal dysfunction

- **Maternal Considerations** — Pregnant women suffered a higher mortality rate during the influenza pandemics of the last century and should be vaccinated prior to each influenza season. Prophylaxis is not a substitute for vaccination, although it is an important adjunct. **Rimantadine** is 70-90% effective in preventing influenza A. When used for prophylaxis, these antiviral agents can prevent illness while permitting subclinical infection and the genesis of protective antibodies. **Rimantadine** reduces the duration of the illness if administered within 2d of symptom onset should an unprotected woman contract influenza A. To reduce the emergence of antiviral drug-resistant viruses, **rimantadine** therapy is discontinued as soon as clinically warranted, typically after 3-5 days, or within 24-48h from resolution of signs and symptoms. There is no published experience with **rimantadine** in pregnant women.
  Side effects include CHF, AV block, bronchospasm, seizures, nausea, vomiting, insomnia, dizziness, anorexia, dry mouth, abdominal pain, nervousness, and fatigue.

- **Fetal Considerations** — There are no adequate reports or well-controlled studies in human fetuses. It is unknown whether **rimantadine** crosses the human placenta. It crosses the rodent placenta and is initially concentrated in the fetal liver. The elimination half-life is less than 3h. Rodent studies are generally reassuring, revealing no evidence of teratogenicity or IUGR despite the use of doses higher than those used clinically. Embryo and maternal toxicity occur at the highest doses. There is also an increase in pup death during the first 2-4d post partum, and decreased fertility of the F_1 generation. **Rimantadine** has not been tested in children under a year.

- **Breastfeeding Safety** — There is no published experience in nursing women. It is unknown whether **rimantadine** enters human breast milk. **Rimantadine** is concentrated in rat milk in a dose-dependent fashion, achieving twice plasma levels 2-3h after dosing. Until further study, breast-feeding women who choose to take **rimantadine** should probably stop feeding and pump until 48h after discontinuing the drug.

■ **References** Pravdina NF, Shobukhov VM, Petrova IG, et al. Biull Eksp Biol Med 1985; 99:74-6.

■ **Summary**
- **Pregnancy Category C**
- **Lactation Category U**
- **Rimantadine** should be used during pregnancy only if the benefit justifies the potential perinatal risk.

Risedronate (Actonel)

■ **Class** — Biphosphonate, calcium metabolism

■ **Indications** — Postmenopausal osteoporosis, steroid-induced osteoporosis, Paget's disease

■ **Mechanism** — Inhibits osteoclast bone resorption

■ **Dosage with Qualifiers** — Postmenopausal osteoporosis—5mg PO with water qd
Steroid-induced osteoporosis—5mg PO qd with water for women on **prednisone** 7.5mg/d or more
Paget's disease—30mg PO qd with water before breakfast ×2mo; supplement calcium and vitamin D
- **Contraindications**—hypersensitivity to drug or class
- **Caution**—unknown

■ **Maternal Considerations** — There is no published experience with **risedronate** during pregnancy.
Side effects include headache, irritability, nervousness, menstrual irregularities, sweating, increased bowel motility, shock, insomnia, tremor, tachycardia, arrhythmia, weight loss, heat intolerance, and diaphoresis.

■ **Fetal Considerations** — There are no adequate reports or well-controlled studies in human fetuses. It is unknown whether **risedronate** crosses the human placenta. In one study, placental transport was not confirmed in the mouse. Rodent studies are generally reassuring, revealing no clear evidence of teratogenicity or IUGR despite the use of doses higher than those used clinically. Pregnancy wastage was increased with maternal toxicity.

■ **Breastfeeding Safety** — There is no published experience in nursing women. It is unknown whether **risedronate** enters human breast milk. Small amounts are excreted into rodent milk.

■ **Reference** — Richardson AC, Tinling SP, Chole RA. Otolaryngol Head Neck Surg 1993; 109:623-33.

■ **Summary** ....
- **Pregnancy Category C**
- **Lactation Category U**
- **Risedronate** should be used during pregnancy and lactation only if the benefit justifies the potential perinatal risk.

Risperidone (Risperdal)

■ **Class** .... *Antipsychotic, type 4, atypical*

■ **Indications** .... Psychosis

■ **Mechanism** .... Unknown; antagonizes D_2 and 5-HT$_2$ receptors

■ **Dosage with Qualifiers** .... <u>Psychosis</u>—begin 1mg PO bid; increase by 1-2mg/d qw
NOTE—hepatic and renal dosing; avoid caffeine-containing products such as colas and tea
- **Contraindications**—hypersensitivity to drug or class, prolonged QT interval
- **Caution**—hepatic or renal dysfunction, seizures, cardiac or cerebrovascular disease, hypotension, hypovolemia, dehydration, agents that prolong the QT interval, aspiration pneumonia risk

■ **Maternal Considerations** .... There are no adequate reports or well-controlled studies of **risperidone** in pregnant women. The published experience is limited to two case reports.
Side effects include neuroleptic malignant syndrome, menstrual irregularities, hypotension, extrapyramidal signs, tardive dyskinesia, hyperglycemia, diabetes mellitus, seizures, QT interval prolongation, insomnia, agitation, headache, anxiety, rhinitis, constipation, nausea, vomiting, diarrhea, dyspepsia, dizziness, tachycardia, somnolence, increased REM sleep, and hyperprolactinemia.

■ **Fetal Considerations** .... There are no adequate reports or well-controlled studies in human fetuses. It is unknown whether **risperidone** crosses the human placenta. It does cross the rodent placenta. Rodent studies are generally reassuring, revealing no evidence of teratogenicity or IUGR despite the use of doses higher than those used clinically. The observed increased neonatal mortality may relate to either the drug or maternal toxicity.

■ **Breastfeeding Safety** .... There are no adequate reports or well-controlled studies in nursing women. It is unknown whether **risperidone** enters human breast milk. There are case reports of its use in breast-feeding women without apparent adverse effect.

■ **References** ················· Ratnayake T, Libretto SE. J Clin Psychiatry 2002; 63:76-7.
Hill RC, McIvor RJ, Wojnar-Horton RE, et al. J Clin
Psychopharmacol 2000; 20:285-6.

■ **Summary** ··················
- **Pregnancy Category C**
- **Lactation Category U**
- **Risperidone** should be used during pregnancy and
lactation only if the benefit justifies the potential risk.

Ritodrine (Yutopar)

■ **Class** ······························· *Tocolytic; adrenergic, betamimetic*

■ **Indications** ··················· Preterm labor

■ **Mechanism** ················· β-2 agonist

■ **Dosage with Qualifiers** ·········· Preterm labor—begin 0.05mg/min, increase by
0.05mg/min q10min (unless maternal heart rate>130bpm)
until contractions stop; continue that dose for 12h after
contractions end; max 0.35mg/min
- **Contraindications**—hypersensitivity to drug or class,
sulfite allergy, indication for delivery (e.g.,
chorioamnionitis, severe preeclampsia), fetal demise,
pulmonary hypertension, maternal hyperthyroidism,
uncontrolled diabetes mellitus
- **Caution**—diabetes mellitus, maternal infection, CAD

■ **Maternal Considerations** ·········· Preterm delivery is the leading cause of perinatal
morbidity and death. There is no tocolytic agent known to
change pregnancy outcome short of allowing
corticosteroid administration. **Ritodrine** decreases the
intensity and frequency of uterine contractions, but does
not alter in a clinically relevant fashion the gestational
age at delivery compared to placebo. It is inferior to
nifedipine both in terms of delivery delay and maternal
morbidity. **Ritodrine** produces an immediate dose-related
elevation of heart rate with maximum mean increase of
19-40bpm. The pulse pressure widens, the average systolic
pressure increases 4.0mmHg, and the average diastolic
pressure decreases 12.3mmHg. IV infusion transiently
elevates glucose, insulin, and free fatty acids, while serum
potassium declines. Maternal pulse rate and blood
pressure and fetal heart rate should be closely monitored.
Maternal signs and symptoms of pulmonary edema
should be sought constantly. A persistent tachycardia
(over 140bpm) may be a sign of impending pulmonary
edema. Occult cardiac disease may be unmasked by

ritodrine. If the patient complains of chest pain or tightness of chest, the drug should be temporarily discontinued. A baseline ECG is not cost-effective. Oral dosing after parenteral treatment is of no clinical benefit. **Ritodrine** has also been used to facilitate external version of a breech fetus.

Side effects include pulmonary edema, agranulocytosis, hypotension, palpitations, tachycardia, nausea, vomiting, paradoxical hypertension, flushing, hyperglycemia, tremor, headache, nervousness, and chest pain.

■ **Fetal Considerations** — **Ritodrine** crosses the human placenta. There is no evidence of teratogenicity in humans. Rodent studies are reassuring. It has been suggested that **ritodrine** and other betamimetics might promote fetal growth. This hypothesis cannot be confirmed. **Ritodrine** increases the fetal heart rate and left cardiac output, and has been used to treat fetal complete heart block.

■ **Breastfeeding Safety** — There is no published experience in pregnancy. However, considering the indication and clearance, it is unlikely the breast-fed neonate would ingest clinically relevant amounts of **ritodrine**.

■ **References** — Papatsonis DN, Van Geijn HP, Ader HJ, et al. Obstet Gynecol 1997; 90:230-4.
Sanchez-Ramos L, Kaunitz AM, Gaudier FL, Delke I. Am J Obstet Gynecol 1999; 181:484-90.
Ezra Y, Elram T, Plotkin V, Elchalal U. Eur J Obstet Gynecol Reprod Biol 2000; 90:63-6.
Weiner CP, Renk K, Klugman M. Am J Obstet Gynecol 1988; 159:216-22.
Chung T, Neale E, Lau TK, Rogers M. Acta Obstet Gynecol Scand 1996; 75:720-4.
Gulmezoglu AM, Hofmeyr GJ. Cochrane Database Syst Rev 2001; 4:CD000036.
Matsushita H, Higashino M, Sekizuka N, et al. Arch Gynecol Obstet 2002; 267(1):51-3.

■ **Summary** —
- **Pregnancy Category B**
- **Lactation Category S**
- **Ritodrine** should be used during pregnancy only if the benefit justifies the potential perinatal risk.
- The primary clinical goal of **ritodrine** administration is to delay delivery until there is maximal effect of corticosteroids; thereafter, its continued use provides risk but no benefit.
- The diagnosis of preterm labor requires cervical change and should not be based solely on the uterine contractions.
- **Ritodrine** and other betamimetics have not changed pregnancy outcome. There are superior alternative agents.

Ritonavir (Norvir)

- ■ **Class** — Antiviral, *protease inhibitor*

- ■ **Indications** — HIV

- ■ **Mechanism** — Binds to active site of HIV protease

- ■ **Dosage with Qualifiers** — HIV—begin 300mg PO bid ×1d, then 400mg PO bid ×2d, then 500mg PO bid ×1d, then 600mg PO bid
  NOTE—multiple drug interactions including antiarrhythmics, antihistamines, ergot derivatives, GI mobility agents, neuroleptics, and hypnotics; check before prescribing
  - **Contraindications**—hypersensitivity to drug or class, use of a potent CYP3A4 inhibitor
  - **Caution**—hepatic dysfunction

- ■ **Maternal Considerations** — There are no adequate reports or well-controlled studies of **ritonavir** in pregnant women. Published cohort studies and case reports do not suggest an increased risk of an adverse outcome during pregnancy. Many commonly used drugs alter the clearance of **ritonavir**. The patient should be questioned closely about concurrent drug use before prescribing.
  Side effects include seizures, diabetes mellitus, thrombocytopenia, neutropenia, hyperlipidemia, elevated LFTs, nausea, vomiting, diarrhea, asthenia, taste changes, paresthesias, vasodilation, anxiety, anorexia, pharyngitis, abdominal pain, myalgias, neuralgias and rash.

- ■ **Fetal Considerations** — There are no adequate reports or well-controlled studies in human fetuses. Placental transport of **ritonavir** is very low; most umbilical cord samples studied are below the level of detection. Limited transfer for most protease inhibitors reflects both their high degree of plasma protein binding and their backward transport by the P-glycoprotein expressed on placenta. Rodent studies are generally reassuring, revealing no evidence of teratogenicity or IUGR despite the use of doses higher than those used clinically. Maternal toxicity from high doses leads to embryo toxicity.

- ■ **Breastfeeding Safety** — There are no adequate reports or well-controlled studies in nursing women. It is unknown whether **ritonavir** enters human breast milk. Breastfeeding is contraindicated in HIV-infected nursing women where formula is available to reduce the risk of neonatal transmission.

- ■ **References** — Pinelli JM, Symington AJ, Cunningham KA, Paes BA. Am J Obstet Gynecol. 2002; 187:245-9.
  Mirochnick M, Dorenbaum A, Holland D, et al. Pediatr Infect Dis J 2002; 21:835-8.

Casey BM, Bawdon RE. Am J Obstet Gynecol 1998;
179:758-61.
Marzolini C, Rudin C, Decosterd LA, et al. AIDS 2002;
16:889-93.

■ **Summary**

- **Pregnancy Category B**
- **Lactation Category NS**
- **Ritonavir** is a protease inhibitor widely used during pregnancy as part of several treatment "cocktails."
- Breastfeeding is contraindicated in HIV-infected nursing women where formula is available to reduce the risk of neonatal transmission.
- Physicians are encouraged to register pregnant women under the Antiretroviral Pregnancy Registry (1-800-258-4263) for a better follow-up of the outcome while under treatment with **ritonavir**.

Rizatriptan (Maxalt; Rizalt)

■ **Class** — Migraine; serotonin receptor agonist

■ **Indications** — Migraine headache

■ **Mechanism** — 5-HT$_1$ agonist

■ **Dosage with Qualifiers** — Migraine headache—5-10mg PO ×1, may repeat in 2h; max 24mg/d
NOTE—max 5mg/dose, 3 doses/24h if taking **propranolol**

- **Contraindications**—hypersensitivity to drug or class, CAD, MI, uncontrolled hypertension, 5-HT$_1$ agonist <24h, MAO inhibitor <14d, ergot derivative <24h, basilar migraine, hemiplegic migraine
- **Caution**—peripheral or cerebrovascular disease, cardiac risk factors, hepatic dysfunction

■ **Maternal Considerations** — There is no published experience with **rizatriptan** during pregnancy. Clearance is slower in nonpregnant women compared to men.
Side effects include acute MI, arrhythmia, coronary spasm, palpitations, hypertensive crisis, cerebral hemorrhage, stroke, bowel or peripheral vascular ischemia, angioedema, somnolence, chest pain, neck tightness, dizziness, paresthesias, flushing, nausea, vomiting, diarrhea, dyspnea, decreased mental acuity, tremor, and euphoria.

■ **Fetal Considerations** — There are no adequate reports or well-controlled studies in human fetuses. It is unknown whether **rizatriptan** crosses the human placenta. Rodent studies are generally reassuring, revealing no evidence of teratogenicity. However, embryo toxicity and IUGR were noted unrelated to maternal toxicity.

■ **Breastfeeding Safety** ⋯⋯⋯⋯ There is no published experience in nursing women. It is unknown whether **rizatriptan** enters human breast milk.

■ **References** ⋯⋯⋯⋯⋯⋯⋯⋯ There is no published experience in pregnancy or during lactation.

■ **Summary** ⋯⋯⋯⋯⋯⋯⋯⋯⋯
- **Pregnancy Category C**
- **Lactation Category U**
- **Rizatriptan** should be used during pregnancy and lactation only if the benefit justifies the potential perinatal risk.
- There are alternative agents for which there is more experience during pregnancy and lactation.
- Health care workers are urged to report prenatal exposures to **rizatriptan** to the manufacturer's Pregnancy Registry: 1-800-986-8999.

Rocuronium (Zemuron)

■ **Class** ⋯⋯⋯⋯⋯⋯⋯⋯⋯⋯⋯ *Neuromuscular blocker, nondepolarizing*

■ **Indications** ⋯⋯⋯⋯⋯⋯⋯⋯ Anesthetic paralysis

■ **Mechanism** ⋯⋯⋯⋯⋯⋯⋯⋯ Nondepolarizing neuromuscular blocker

■ **Dosage with Qualifiers** ⋯⋯ Anesthetic, neuromuscular paralysis—0.6-1.2mg/kg IV for induction, 0.1-0.2mg/kg IV q12min based on train-of-four response to peripheral nerve stimulation
NOTE—onset 1min, duration 30min
- **Contraindications**—hypersensitivity to drug or class
- **Caution**—obesity, respiratory or hepatic dysfunction

■ **Maternal Considerations** ⋯⋯ There are no adequate reports or well-controlled studies of **rocuronium** in pregnant women, though it has been used for cesarean delivery as part of rapid-sequence general anesthesia in patients who have a contraindication to **succinylcholine** (e.g., suspected malignant hyperthermia, upper-motor neuron lesion). The manufacturer notes that tracheal intubation can be problematic 60sec after administration, and does not recommend its use (i.e., replacing **succinylcholine**) for rapid-sequence induction of general anesthesia for cesarean delivery. **Rocuronium** neuromuscular blockade may be prolonged by **magnesium sulfate** infusion or in the postpartum period if dosing is based on total rather than lean body weight.

Side effects include arrhythmia, bronchospasm, hypotension, hypertension, and injection site pain.

■ **Fetal Considerations** .... There are no adequate reports or well-controlled studies in human fetuses. **Rocuronium** crosses the human placenta. In women undergoing rapid-sequence induction of general anesthesia, the F:M ratio approximates 0.18 at delivery. No clinical sequelae are noted. Rodent studies are reassuring, revealing no evidence of teratogenicity or IUGR despite the use of doses higher than those used clinically assuming the mother was properly oxygenated.

■ **Breastfeeding Safety** .... There is no published experience in nursing women. However, considering the indication and dosing, limited use of **rocuronium** is unlikely to pose a clinically significant risk to the breast-feeding neonate.

■ **References** .... Gin T, Chan MT, Chan KL, Yuen PM. Anesth Analg 2002; 94:686-9.
Puhringer FK, Sparr HJ, Mitterschiffthaler G, et al. Anesth Analg 1997; 84:352-4.
Gaiser RR, Seem EH. Br J Anesth 1996; 77:669-71.

■ **Summary** .... • **Pregnancy Category C**
• **Lactation Category S**
• **Rocuronium** should be used during pregnancy and lactation only if the potential benefit justifies the perinatal risk.
• There are alternative agents for which there is more experience during pregnancy and lactation.

Rofecoxib (Vioxx)

■ **Class** .... *Analgesic*, NSAID; COX-2 *inhibitor*

■ **Indications** .... Dysmenorrhea, rheumatoid and osteoarthritis, mild to moderate pain

■ **Mechanism** .... Specific COX-2 inhibitor

■ **Dosage with Qualifiers** .... Dysmenorrhea—50mg PO qd for a max of 5d
Rheumatoid arthritis—begin 12.5mg PO qd; max 25mg/d
Osteoarthritis—25mg/d; max 25mg/d
Mild to moderate pain—50mg PO qd for a max of 5d
NOTE—hepatic dosing
• **Contraindications**—hypersensitivity to drug or class, NSAID asthma or urticaria, hepatic failure, severe renal dysfunction, aspirin triad

- **Caution**—GI bleeding, nasal polyps, hepatic or renal dysfunction, CHF, hypertension, ischemic heart disease, hypovolemia, asthma

■ **Maternal Considerations** .... **Rofecoxib** is a COX-2 inhibitor that has analgesic, anti-inflammatory and antipyretic properties. It is no more effective than **diclofenac** and **ibuprofen** for the relief of mild to moderate pain when used at maximal doses. Further, it only modestly reduces the risk of GI reactions (1.3% vs. 1.8% after a year of treatment). There are no adequate reports or well-controlled studies of **rofecoxib** in pregnant women. It has no effect on either the onset or duration of labor in rodents. **Rofecoxib** inhibits spontaneous contractions of isolated rat myometrium at lower concentrations than **indomethacin**.
Side effects include GI bleeding or ulcer, esophagitis, bronchospasm, hypertension, CHF, MI, hepatotoxicity, renal failure, renal papillary necrosis, anemia, blood dyscrasias, epigastric pain, nausea, vomiting, edema, dyspepsia, fatigue, and dizziness.

■ **Fetal Considerations** .... There are no adequate reports or well-controlled studies in human fetuses. **Rofecoxib** crosses the human placenta. Similar to other NSAIDs, **rofecoxib** is associated with oligohydramnios and constriction of the ductus arteriosus. The latter reverses with cessation, and the long-term impact of in utero ductal constriction on the otherwise healthy fetus is currently unknown. Rodent studies are generally reassuring, revealing no evidence of teratogenicity or IUGR despite the use of doses higher than those used clinically. Embryo toxicity was noted at higher doses.

■ **Breastfeeding Safety** .... There are no adequate reports or well-controlled studies in nursing women. It is unknown whether **rofecoxib** enters human breast milk. It is excreted into rodent milk and is associated with decreased pup growth and increased pup death.

■ **References** .... Editorial. Prescrire Int 2000; 9:166-7.
Dore M, Mellier G, Benchaib M, et al. BJOG 2002; 109:983-8.

■ **Summary** ....
- **Pregnancy Category C**
- **Lactation Category U**
- **Rofecoxib** should be used during pregnancy and lactation only if the benefit justifies the potential perinatal risk.
- There are alternative agents for which there is more experience during pregnancy and lactation.
- Health care practitioners are urged to report any prenatal exposure to **rofecoxib** by calling the manufacturer's Pregnancy Registry: 1-800-986-8999.

Ropinirole (Requip)

- **Class** — *Antiparkinsonian; dopaminergic*

- **Indications** — Parkinson's disease

- **Mechanism** — Dopamine agonist

- **Dosage with Qualifiers** — Parkinson's disease—begin 0.25mg PO tid; increase 0.25mg PO tid/w; max 24mg/d
  - **Contraindications**—hypersensitivity to drug or class
  - **Caution**—none

- **Maternal Considerations** — There is no published experience with **ropinirole** during pregnancy.
  Side effects include somnolence, atrial fibrillation, syncope, hypotension, nausea, vomiting, hallucinations, dizziness, fatigue, dyspepsia, malaise, edema, chest or abdominal pain, sweating, pharyngitis, anorexia, and visual changes.

- **Fetal Considerations** — There are no adequate reports or well-controlled studies in human fetuses. It is unknown whether **ropinirole** crosses the human placenta. Rodent teratogenicity studies reveal IUGR and digit abnormalities at doses that are multiples of the MRHD.

- **Breastfeeding Safety** — There is no published experience in nursing women. It is unknown whether **ropinirole** enters human breast milk. **Ropinirole** inhibits prolactin secretion in humans and could interfere with establishment of the milk reflex.

- **References** — There is no published experience in pregnancy or during lactation.

- **Summary** —
  - **Pregnancy Category C**
  - **Lactation Category U**
  - **Ropinirole** should be used during pregnancy and lactation only if the benefit justifies the potential perinatal risk.

Rosiglitazone (Avandia)

- **Class** — *Antidiabetic, thiazolidinediones*

- **Indications** — Diabetes mellitus, type 2

- **Mechanism** — Increases insulin sensitivity

- **Dosage with Qualifiers** ⸺ Diabetes mellitus, type 2—begin 4PO qd; max 8mg/d, adjust for glucose control
  NOTE—check AST/ALT at baseline and then q2mo × 12mo
  - **Contraindications**—hypersensitivity to drug or class, type 1 diabetes mellitus, diabetic ketoacidosis, concurrent insulin use, CHF (NYHA Class III and IV)
  - **Caution**—CHF (NYHA Class I and II), hypertension, hepatic dysfunction, edema

- **Maternal Considerations** ⸺ **Rosiglitazone** may be used alone or in combination with **metformin** or a sulfonylurea. The improved glucose control may lead to ovulation in premenopausal, anovulatory women and increase the risk of an unplanned pregnancy. Paradoxically, it may interfere with ovulation in spontaneously cycling women. There is no published experience with **rosiglitazone** during pregnancy, and **insulin** monotherapy is the current gold standard for the treatment of hyperglycemia during pregnancy.
  Side effects include hepatotoxicity, hepatitis, elevated LFTs, anemia, CHF, URI, fluid retention, edema, headache, weight gain, and hypoglycemia.

- **Fetal Considerations** ⸺ There are no adequate reports or well-controlled studies in human fetuses. It is unknown whether **rosiglitazone** crosses the human placenta. Rodent studies are generally reassuring, revealing no evidence of teratogenicity despite the use of doses higher than those used clinically. High doses were associated with fetal losses and IUGR, possibly reflecting sustained hypoglycemia.

- **Breastfeeding Safety** ⸺ There is no published experience in nursing women. It is unknown whether **rosiglitazone** enters human breast milk. It is excreted into rat milk.

- **References** ⸺ Cataldo NA, Abbasi F, McLaughlin TL, et al. Fertil Steril 2001; 76:1057-9.

- **Summary** ⸺
  - **Pregnancy Category C**
  - **Lactation Category U**
  - **Rosiglitazone** should be used during pregnancy and lactation only if the benefit justifies the potential perinatal risk.
  - Insulin is the drug of choice for the treatment of diabetes during pregnancy.

Rubella virus vaccine, live (Meruvax II)

- **Class** .... *Vaccine*

- **Indications** .... Rubella susceptibility

- **Mechanism** .... Active immunization

- **Dosage with Qualifiers** .... Susceptible women of childbearing age—0.5ml SC
  - **Contraindications**—hypersensitivity to drug or class, allergy to **neomycin**, any active febrile infection, untreated TB, immunosuppressive therapy (except replacement corticosteroids), blood dyscrasias, lymphoma, primary or acquired immune deficiency (including AIDS)
  - **Caution**—do not give with immunoglobulin

- **Maternal Considerations** .... The **rubella virus vaccine** produces a modified, noncommunicable rubella infection in susceptible persons. Vaccine-induced immunity persists for at least 10 years without significant decline. Vaccinating susceptible women confers individual protection against rubella during a subsequent pregnancy, thus preventing congenital rubella. Yet, only about half the world's countries vaccinate for rubella. Outbreaks continue to occur in countries with national immunization programs, typically involving women born in other countries. Perhaps the most convenient time to vaccinate is immediately post partum while the patient is still hospitalized. In that instance, conception should be delayed a month. Unfortunately, the opportunity is often missed because of physician/hospital oversight. Rubella susceptibility should be confirmed serologically before vaccinating.
  Side effects include injection site reaction, mild regional lymphadenopathy, urticaria, rash, malaise, sore throat, fever, headache, nausea, vomiting, diarrhea, polyneuritis, syncope, and thrombocytopenia.

- **Fetal Considerations** .... Rubella vaccine virus has been found in the products of conception in women undergoing termination and in the offspring of vaccinated women. Similar to natural viral infections, newborns may shed virus for an extended time. The manufacturer reports that in over 700 women inadvertently vaccinated within 3mo before or after conception, no newborn had stigmas of congenital rubella syndrome. Pregnancy termination is not recommended solely because of inadvertent vaccination.

- **Breastfeeding Safety** .... Rubella vaccine virus is excreted into human breast milk, and neonatal infection is reported.

■ **References** .... MMWR Morb Mortal Wkly Rep 2001; 50:1117.
Bath SK, Singleton JA, Strikas RA, et al. Am J Infect 2000;
28:327-32.
Hofmann J, Kortung M, Pustowoit B, et al. J Med Virol
2000; 61:155-8.

■ **Summary** ....
- **Pregnancy Category C**
- **Lactation Category U**
- **Rubella virus vaccine** prevents congenital rubella.
- Inadvertent vaccination during pregnancy is not associated with an adverse outcome.
- The immediate postpartum period is an excellent opportunity to vaccinate susceptible women, an opportunity overlooked too often.

Salmeterol xinafoate inhaled (Serevent; Serevent Diskus)

- **Class** — *Adrenergic agonist; bronchodilator*

- **Indications** — Asthma prophylaxis, exercise-induced asthma, COPD

- **Mechanism** — Selective β-2 adrenergic agonist

- **Dosage with Qualifiers** — Asthma prophylaxis—2 puffs INH q12h
  Exercise-induced asthma—2 puffs INH ×1
  COPD—2 puffs INH q12h
  NOTE—21mcg/spray MDI
  - **Contraindications**—hypersensitivity to drug or class, acute asthma, arrhythmia
  - **Caution**—hypertension, cardiovascular disease, diabetes mellitus, seizures, hyperthyroidism, hypokalemia

- **Maternal Considerations** — **Salmeterol** is a long-acting β-adrenergic agonist. It also is a potent inhibitor of mast cell release of histamine, leukotrienes, and prostaglandin D_2. Systemic levels of **salmeterol** are low or undetectable after inhalation. There is no published experience during pregnancy.
  Side effects include angioedema, paradoxical bronchospasm, laryngospasm, arrhythmia, hypertension, headache, nasal congestion, rhinitis, pharyngitis, urticaria, palpitations, tachycardia, tremor and nervousness.

- **Fetal Considerations** — There are no adequate reports or well-controlled studies in human fetuses. It is unknown whether **salmeterol inhaled** crosses the human placenta. Transfer across the rat placenta is low. Considering the low systemic levels achieved and the poor placental transport, it is unlikely the fetus is exposed to a clinically relevant concentration. When given orally at doses 50-100 times greater than those inhaled, **salmeterol** is associated with cleft palate and abnormal ossification. These studies do not seem relevant to clinical practice.

- **Breastfeeding Safety** — There is no published experience in breast-feeding women. However, considering the dose and route, it is unlikely the breast-fed neonate would ingest clinically relevant amounts. The transfer into rodent milk is limited.

- **References** — Manchee GR, Barrow A, Kulkarni S, et al. Drug Metab Dispos 1993; 21:1022-8.

- **Summary** —
  - **Pregnancy Category C**
  - **Lactation Category S**
  - **Salmeterol** should be used during pregnancy and lactation only if the benefit justifies the potential perinatal risk.
  - It seems unlikely that it poses any significant risk to fetus or neonate when used as directed.

Salsalate (Amigesic; Anaflex 750; Artha-G; Carsalate; Diagen; Disalcid; Marthritic; Mono-Gesic; Nobegyl; Ro-Salcid; Salflex; Salgesic; Salicylsalicylic acid; Salsitab)

■ **Class** — *Analgesic, salicylate*

■ **Indications** — Arthritis

■ **Mechanism** — Unknown; prostaglandin synthesis inhibitor

■ **Dosage with Qualifiers** — Arthritis—1000mg PO tid
- **Contraindications**—hypersensitivity to drug or class, NSAID/ASA-induced asthma hx, flu-like symptoms or varicella, peptic ulcer disease
- **Caution**—renal dysfunction

■ **Maternal Considerations** — **Salsalate** is a dimer of salicylic acid and absorbed in the intestine. Unlike **aspirin**, **salsalate** does not inhibit platelet aggregation, and there is no increase in GI bleeding over placebo. There is no published experience during pregnancy.
Side effects include hepatic or nephrotoxicity, Reye's syndrome, nausea, vomiting, epigastric pain, fatigue, rash, and dizziness.

■ **Fetal Considerations** — There is no published experience in human fetuses. It is unknown whether **salsalate** crosses the human placenta. **Salsalate** and salicylic acid are teratogenic and embryocidal in rats when given in doses 4-5 times the usual human dose; teratogenicity is not seen when given at twice the usual human dose.

■ **Breastfeeding Safety** — There is no published experience in nursing women. It is unknown whether **salsalate** enters human breast milk. Salicylic acid, the primary metabolite reaches an M:P ratio approximating unity. Caution is advised.

■ **References** — There is no published experience in pregnancy or during lactation.

■ **Summary** —
- **Pregnancy Category C**
- **Lactation Category S?**
- **Salsalate** should be used during pregnancy and lactation only if the benefit justifies the potential perinatal risk.
- There are alternative agents for which there is more experience during pregnancy and lactation.

Saquinavir (Fortovase; Invirase)

- **Class** — Antiviral, *protease inhibitor*

- **Indications** — HIV adjunct treatment

- **Mechanism** — HIV protease inhibitor

- **Dosage with Qualifiers** — HIV adjunct treatment—600mg PO tid (Invirase) or 1200mg tid PO (Fortovase) within 2h of eating
  - **Contraindications**—hypersensitivity to drug or class, **terfenadine**, **cisapride**, **astemizole**, **triazolam**, **midazolam** or ergot use
  - **Caution**—hepatic dysfunction, use of **lovastatin** or **simvastatin**

- **Maternal Considerations** — **Saquinavir** is well tolerated during pregnancy and is part of several treatment regimens. Its clearance is increased by pregnancy, and the usually recommended dose may be inadequate. **Ritonavir** significantly increases **saquinavir** concentration, and the combination during pregnancy may have some advantage.
  Side effects include nausea, vomiting, diarrhea, diabetes mellitus, hyperglycemia, peripheral neuropathy, headache, buccal ulceration, rash, dyspepsia, abdominal pain, and eczema.

- **Fetal Considerations** — There are no adequate reports or well-controlled studies in human fetuses. **Saquinavir**, like many protease inhibitors, does not significantly cross the human placenta probably because of reverse placental P glycoprotein transport. It is unlikely to pose a significant risk to the fetus. Rodent studies are reassuring, revealing no evidence of teratogenicity or IUGR.

- **Breastfeeding Safety** — There is no published experience in nursing women. It is unknown whether **saquinavir** enters human breast milk. Breastfeeding is contraindicated in HIV-infected nursing women where formula is available to reduce the risk of neonatal transmission.

- **References** — Acosta EP, Zorrilla C, Van Dyke R, et al. HIV Clin Trials 2001; 2:460-5.
  Huisman MT, Smit JW, Wiltshire HR, et al. Mol Pharmacol 2001; 59:806-13.
  Mirochnick M, Dorenbaum A, Holland D, et al. Pediatr Infect Dis J 2002; 21:835-8.
  Vithayasai V, Moyle GJ, Supajatura V, et al. J Acquir Immune Defic Syndr 2002; 30:410-2.

■ **Summary**
- **Pregnancy Category B**
- **Lactation Category NS**
- **Saquinavir** is an effective protease inhibitor when used in conjunction with other retroviral agents.
- It should be used during pregnancy and lactation only if the benefit justifies the potential perinatal risk.
- Breastfeeding is contraindicated in HIV-infected nursing women where formula is available to reduce the risk of neonatal transmission.
- Physicians are encouraged to register pregnant women under the Antiretroviral Pregnancy Registry (1-800-258-4263) for a better follow-up of the outcome while under treatment with **saquinavir**.

Sargramostim (GM-CSF; Granulocyte Macrophage-Colony Stimulating Factor; Leukine; Prokine)

■ **Class**
Hematopoietic agents

■ **Indications**
Neutropenia post bone marrow transplant, post-AML chemotherapy, progenitor mobilization, bone marrow transplant failure

■ **Mechanism**
Stimulates granulocyte and macrophage proliferation and differentiation

■ **Dosage with Qualifiers**
Neutropenia post bone marrow transplant—250mcg/m^2 IV qd over 2h beginning 2-4h after transplant and >24h post chemotherapy
Neuropenia post-AML chemotherapy—250mcg/m^2 IV qd over 4h beginning day 11 post chemotherapy; continue until ANC >1500 ×3d, max 42d
Progenitor mobilization—250mcg/m^2 IV qd over 24h
Bone marrow transplant failure—250mcg/m^2 IV qd over 2h ×14d; may repeat in 7d
- **Contraindications**—hypersensitivity to drug or class, leukemic myeloid blast cells >10%, current chemotherapy, current radiation therapy
- **Caution**—arrhythmia, CHF, pericardial effusion, pleural effusion

■ **Maternal Considerations**
Sargramostim is a recombinant human granulocyte-macrophage colony-stimulating factor. There is no published experience with **sargramostim** during pregnancy. *Side effects* include arrhythmias, anaphylaxis, pleural or pericardial effusion, capillary leak syndrome, RDS, fever, chills, headache, nausea, vomiting, diarrhea, myalgias, asthenia, bone pain, edema, rash, pruritus, dyspnea, flushing, hypotension, tachycardia, and syncope.

- **Fetal Considerations** .... There are no adequate reports or well-controlled studies in human fetuses. It is unknown whether **sargramostim** crosses the human placenta. Rodent teratogenicity studies have not been conducted.

- **Breastfeeding Safety** .... There is no reported experience in nursing women. It is unknown whether **sargramostim** enters human breast milk.

- **References** .... There is no published experience in pregnancy or during lactation.

- **Summary** ....
  - **Pregnancy Category C**
  - **Lactation Category U**
  - **Sargramostim** should be used during pregnancy and lactation only if the benefit justifies the potential perinatal risk.

Scopolamine (Isopto Hyoscine; Minims Hyoscine Hydrobromide; Scopoderm; Transderm Scop)

- **Class** .... *Vertigo/motion sickness, antiemetic, anticholinergic, preanesthetic*

- **Indications** .... Motion sickness, obstetric amnesia, preoperative sedation, intraoperative amnesia

- **Mechanism** .... Anticholinergic

- **Dosage with Qualifiers** .... Motion sickness—1 patch behind the ear 4h prior to need; may replace in 3d
  Obstetric amnesia or preoperative sedation—0.32-0.65 mg SC/IM
  Intraoperative amnesia—0.4mg IV
  - **Contraindications**—hypersensitivity to drug or class, narrow angle glaucoma
  - **Caution**—intestinal obstruction, history seizures or psychosis, impaired metabolic function, hepatic or renal dysfunction

- **Maternal Considerations** .... **Scopolamine** differs only quantitatively in antimuscarinic actions from **atropine**. It is ineffective for the prevention of postoperative nausea and vomiting. There are no adequate reports or well-controlled studies of **scopolamine** in pregnant women. At one time popular for "twilight sleep" during labor, **scopolamine** has appropriately fallen out of favor. It may reduce the post-cesarean section nausea and vomiting associated with epidural **morphine**.
  Scopolamine is rapidly cleared, but there is no significant relationship between heart rate changes, sedative and antisialogogue effects with serum concentration.

899

Side effects include narrow angle glaucoma, drowsiness, blurred vision, disorientation, dizziness, dilated pupils, hallucinations, confusion, psychosis, bronchospasm, respiratory depression, rash, muscle weakness, and red eyes.

■ **Fetal Considerations**

There are no adequate reports or well-controlled studies in human fetuses. **Scopolamine** rapidly crosses the human placenta and may cause tachycardia and decreased beat-to-beat and long-term variability. Rodent studies are reassuring, revealing no evidence of teratogenicity or IUGR despite the use of doses higher than those used clinically.

■ **Breastfeeding Safety**

There are no adequate reports or well-controlled studies in nursing women. **Scopolamine** enters human breast milk, but the kinetics remain to be elucidated. The long clinical experience is reassuring.

■ **References**

Koski EM, Mattila MA, Knapik D, et al. Br J Anaesth 1990; 64:16-20.
Kotelko DM, Rottman RL, Wright WC, et al. Anesthesiology 1989; 71:675-8.
Kanto J, Kentala E, Kaila T, Pihlajamaki K. Acta Anaesthesiol Scand 1989; 33:482-6.
Ayromlooi J, Tobias M, Berg P. J Reprod Med 1980; 25:323-6.

■ **Summary**

- **Pregnancy Category C**
- **Lactation Category S?**
- **Scopolamine** should be used during pregnancy and lactation only if the benefit justifies the potential perinatal risk.

Secobarbital (Immenoctal; Novosecobarb; Secanal; Seconal)

■ **Class**

Anxiolytic/hypnotic, barbiturate, preanesthetic

■ **Indications**

Short-term insomnia

■ **Mechanism**

Nonselective CNS depressant

■ **Dosage with Qualifiers**

Short-term insomnia—100mg PO qd
- **Contraindications**—hypersensitivity to drug or class, respiratory depression, porphyria
- **Caution**—unknown

■ **Maternal Considerations** ⋯⋯⋯ Barbiturates are dangerous drugs, with a narrow therapeutic index between that required for sedation and that causing coma and death. **Secobarbital** is used by patients to self-treat the unpleasant effects of illicit stimulants, to reduce anxiety, and to get "high." It is physiologically addicting if taken in high doses for a month or more, and the abstinence syndrome can be life-threatening. There are no adequate reports or well-controlled studies of **secobarbital** in pregnant women. As a short-acting agent, **secobarbital** was used for decades as a short-term sleeping aid for pregnant women. Unfortunately, the sleep produced is not restful, characterized by a low percentage of REM stage. Hypnotic doses of barbiturates do not impair uterine activity significantly during labor. Anesthetic doses of barbiturates decrease the force and frequency of uterine contractions. *Side effects* include respiratory depression, dependency, hepatotoxicity, Stevens-Johnson syndrome, angioedema, lethargy, and drowsiness.

■ **Fetal Considerations** ⋯⋯⋯ There are no adequate reports or well-controlled studies in human fetuses. It is likely **secobarbital** rapidly crosses the human placenta. There is no substantive evidence **secobarbital** is a human teratogen. Administration during labor may cause respiratory depression in the newborn. Premature infants are particularly susceptible to the depressant effects of barbiturates. Withdrawal symptoms occur in infants of women who receive **secobarbital** throughout the 3rd trimester.

■ **Breastfeeding Safety** ⋯⋯⋯ There is no published experience in nursing women. Small amounts of **secobarbital** are excreted into human breast milk, but its occasional use is generally considered compatible with breastfeeding.

■ **References** ⋯⋯⋯ No current relevant references.

■ **Summary** ⋯⋯⋯
- **Pregnancy Category D**
- **Lactation Category S**
- **Secobarbital** should be used during pregnancy and lactation only if the benefit justifies the potential perinatal risk.
- There are alternative agents with greater safety and efficacy for the same indications during pregnancy and lactation.

Selegiline (Alzene; Carbex; Deprenyl; Eldeprine; Eldepryl; Selgene)

■ **Class** — Antiparkinsonian

■ **Indications** — Parkinsonism

■ **Mechanism** — Selective MAO-B antagonist

■ **Dosage with Qualifiers** — Parkinsonism—5mg PO qam and qnoon
NOTE—death may occur if combined with **meperidine**
- **Contraindications**—hypersensitivity to drug or class, opiate use
- **Caution**—unknown

■ **Maternal Considerations** — **Selegiline** is a derivative of **phenethylamine**. It has also been used for the treatment of Alzheimer's dementia and narcolepsy. There are no adequate reports or well-controlled studies of **selegiline** in pregnant women. The literature consists of case reports involving 30-40 women with Parkinson's disease.
Side effects include ventricular arrhythmia, nausea, vomiting, diarrhea, dizziness, confusion, hallucinations, vivid dreams, headache, anxiety, anemia, hair loss, fatigue, and low back pain.

■ **Fetal Considerations** — There are no adequate reports or well-controlled studies in human fetuses. It is unknown whether **selegiline** crosses the human placenta. Monoamine neurotransmitters are important for the development of the immature brain. Their endogenous levels are highly regulated by monoamine oxidase (MAO), and any change in enzyme activity could have a profound effect on brain development. Some recommend discontinuing MAO inhibitors before conception. Unfortunately, there is little scientific information on which to base such decisions. Rodent studies are generally reassuring, revealing no evidence of teratogenicity at doses higher than those used clinically. There was evidence of embryotoxicity at high doses.

■ **Breastfeeding Safety** — There are no adequate reports or well-controlled studies in nursing women. It is unknown whether **selegiline** enters human breast milk.

■ **References** — Hagell P, Odin P, Vinge E. Mov Disord 1998; 13:34-8.
Golbe LI. Neurol Clin 1994; 12:497-508.

■ **Summary** —
- **Pregnancy Category C**
- **Lactation Category U**
- **Selegiline** should be used during pregnancy and lactation only if the benefit justifies the potential perinatal risk.

Selenium sulfide, topical (Abbottselsun; Exsel; Glo-Sel; Lenium; Micalon; Sebo-Lenium; Sel-Pen; Selsum; Selsun; Selukos; Versel)

■ **Class** — Other dermatologic, antifungal/dermatophyte

■ **Indications** — Dandruff, seborrhea, tinea versicolor

■ **Mechanism** — Reduces epidermal and follicular epithelial corneocyte production

■ **Dosage with Qualifiers** — Dandruff, seborrhea—massage 5-10ml to wet scalp 2×/w, rinse after 2-3min
Tinea versicolor—apply 2.5% lotion qd ×7d, then monthly ×3mo
NOTE—wash hands, avoid contact with jewelry
- **Contraindications**—hypersensitivity to drug or class, inflamed skin
- **Caution**—unknown

■ **Maternal Considerations** — There is no published experience with **selenium sulfide** during pregnancy. Systemic absorption is scant whether measured after shampooing or lotion application.
Side effects include skin irritation, hair loss, hair discoloration, and oily or dry scalp.

■ **Fetal Considerations** — There are no adequate reports or well-controlled studies in human fetuses. It is unknown whether **selenium sulfide** crosses the human placenta. Considering the dose and route, it is unlikely the maternal systemic concentration will reach a clinically relevant level.

■ **Breastfeeding Safety** — There is no published experience in nursing women. It is unknown whether **selenium sulfide** enters human breast milk. However, considering the indication and dosing, **selenium sulfide** use is unlikely to pose a clinically significant risk to the breast-feeding neonate.

■ **References** — There is no published experience in pregnancy or during lactation.

■ **Summary** —
- **Pregnancy Category C**
- **Lactation Category S?**
- **Selenium** sulfide is unlikely to pose a risk when used as indicated.

Senna (Ex-lax; Senna-Gen; Sennokot)

■ **Class** .... *Laxative*

■ **Indications** .... Constipation

■ **Mechanism** .... Cathartic; increases peristalsis

■ **Dosage with Qualifiers** .... Constipation—2-4 tabs PO qd/bid
- **Contraindications**—hypersensitivity to drug or class, bowel obstruction, undiagnosed abdominal pain
- **Caution**—unknown

■ **Maternal Considerations** .... Despite a long clinical experience, there are no adequate reports or well-controlled studies of **senna** in pregnant women. **Senna** is absorbed across the GI tract only to a limited degree. Some believe **senna** is the purgative of choice during pregnancy and lactation. It effectively relieves postpartum constipation. It does not affect the myometrial activity of the pregnant ewe.
Side effects include laxative abuse, nausea, bloating, cramps, flatulence, diarrhea, melanosis coli, and discolored urine.

■ **Fetal Considerations** .... There are no adequate reports or well-controlled studies in human fetuses. It is unknown whether it crosses the human placenta.

■ **Breastfeeding Safety** .... Less than 1% of the maternal dose of **senna** enters human breast milk. This amount is inadequate for a clinical effect.

■ **References** .... Pharmacology 1992; 44(Suppl 1):20-2.
Pharmacology 1992; 44(Suppl 1):23-5.
Shelton MG. S Afr Med J 1980; 57:78-80.
Garcia-Villar R. Pharmacology 1988; 36(Suppl 1):203-11.
Faber P, Strenge-Hesse A. Pharmacology 1988; 36 (Suppl 1):212-20.

■ **Summary** ....
- **Pregnancy Category C**
- **Lactation Category S**
- **Senna** should be used during pregnancy and lactation only if the benefit justifies the potential perinatal risk.
- Occasional use for the relief of constipation should be safe during pregnancy and lactation.

Sertraline (Lustral; Zoloft)

■ **Class** — *Antidepressant type 1, SSRIs*

■ **Indications** — Depression, obsessive-compulsive disorder, premenopausal dysphoric disorder, post-traumatic stress disorder, panic disorder

■ **Mechanism** — Selective serotonin reuptake inhibitor

■ **Dosage with Qualifiers** — Depression—begin 50mg PO qd; max 200mg PO qd
Obsessive-compulsive disorder—begin 50mg PO qd; max 200mg PO qd
Premenopausal dysphoric disorder—begin either 50mg PO qd or cycle days 15-28, may increase 50mg/d per cycle, max 150mg/d
Post-traumatic stress disorder—begin 25mg PO qd ×7d before increasing 25-50mg/d; max 200mg/d
Panic disorder—begin 25mg PO qd; max 200mg PO qd
NOTE—discontinue slowly
- **Contraindications**—hypersensitivity to drug or class, MAO inhibitor <14d
- **Caution**—renal dysfunction

■ **Maternal Considerations** — Depression is common during and after pregnancy, but typically goes unrecognized. Pregnancy is not a reason *apriori* to discontinue psychotropic drugs. There are no adequate reports or well-controlled studies of **sertraline** in pregnant women. In general, women taking SSRIs during pregnancy for depression require an increased dose to maintain euthymia.
Side effects include serotonin withdrawal syndrome, withdrawal syndrome, nausea, vomiting, diarrhea, insomnia, headache, dry mouth, somnolence, dizziness, fatigue, tremor, dyspepsia, constipation, decreased libido, sweating, anorexia, nervousness, agitation, anxiety, and visual disturbances.

■ **Fetal Considerations** — There are no adequate reports or well-controlled studies in human fetuses. **Sertraline** crosses the human placenta and enters the amniotic fluid; however, the kinetics remain to be elucidated. There is no evidence SSRIs are human teratogens at the doses used, but the experience with **sertraline** specifically is still limited. An increased prevalence of IUGR cannot be excluded. Newborns chronically exposed to SSRIs may have reduced responses to pain. Rodent studies are generally reassuring, though a delay in ossification was noted in rabbits. Further, the fetal loss rate is increased by late pregnancy exposure. The mechanism and significance are unclear. The exposure of mouse embryos in culture to **sertraline** at a high concentration (10μM) causes craniofacial malformations without evidence of general embryotoxicity, consistent with a direct action at 5HT uptake sites.

■ **Breastfeeding Safety** .... **Sertraline** and **desmethylsertraline** are present in human breast milk. The concentrations are affected by the fraction of milk sampled, the time after maternal dose (max 7-10h), and daily dose. The mean maximum calculated nursing infant dose of **sertraline**, 0.67mg/d, and **desmethylsertraline**, 1.44mg/d, represent 0.54% of the maternal daily dose. Neonatal serum concentration is usually below the detection limit of most commercial laboratories. If breast-fed, the infant should be monitored for possible adverse effects, the drug given at the lowest effective dose, and breastfeeding avoided at times of peak drug levels.

■ **References** .... Hendrick V, Smith LM, Suri R, et al. Am J Obstet Gynecol 2003; 188:812-5.

Hostetter A, Stowe ZN, Strader JR Jr, et al. Depress Anxiety 2000; 11:51-7.

Hostetter A, Ritchie JC, Stowe ZN. Biol Psychiatry 2000; 48:1032-4.

Oberlander TF, Eckstein Grunau R, et al. Pediatr Res 2002; 51:443-53.

Kulin NA, Pastuszak A, Sage SR, et al. JAMA 1998; 279:609-10.

Shuey DL, Sadler TW, Lauder JM. Teratology 1992; 46:367-78.

Stowe ZN, Owens MJ, Landry JC, et al. Am J Psychiatry 1997; 154:1255-60.

Stowe ZN, Hostetter AL, Owens MJ, et al. J Clin Psychiatry 2003; 64:73-80.

■ **Summary** ....
- **Pregnancy Category C**
- **Lactation Category S?**
- Depression is common during pregnancy and the puerperium and should not be ignored if treatment is otherwise indicated.
- **Sertraline** should be used during pregnancy and lactation only if the benefit justifies the potential perinatal risk.

Sevoflurane (Sevorane; Ultane)

■ **Class** .... *Anesthesia*

■ **Indications** .... Induction and maintenance of anesthesia

■ **Mechanism** .... Unknown

- **Dosage with Qualifiers** .... <u>Induction of anesthesia</u>—titrate inhalation to effect; a technique used mainly in children
<u>Maintenance of anesthesia</u>—titrate inhalation to anesthetic effect, typically inspired concentration of 0.5-3%
<u>NOTE</u>—consult anesthesia specialty text
  - **Contraindications**—hypersensitivity to drug or class, malignant hyperthermia
  - **Caution**—hepatitis, hepatic or renal dysfunction, aortic stenosis, mitral valve disease, head injury, myasthenia gravis, increased ICP

- **Maternal Considerations** .... There are no adequate reports or well-controlled studies of **sevoflurane** in pregnant women. It is popular for cesarean delivery when general anesthesia is elected, producing an intraoperative course and neonatal outcome similar to that of either **isoflurane** or a subarachnoid block. Like the other volatile anesthetics (**halothane** and **isoflurane**), **sevoflurane** reduces oxytocin-induced contraction of pregnant rat myometrium mediated, at least in part, by activation of Ca^{2+}-activated K^+ channels. A limited number of case reports in the 1st trimester do not report adverse outcomes.
Side effects include malignant hyperthermia, arrhythmias, hepatitis, increased intracranial pressure, nausea, vomiting, agitation, cough, hypotension, shivering, laryngospasm, breath holding, increased salivation, bradycardia, dizziness, tachycardia, hypertension, and apnea.

- **Fetal Considerations** .... **Sevoflurane** rapidly crosses the human placenta. It has been used for fetal anesthesia during the 'EXIT' procedure. Rodent studies are reassuring, revealing no evidence of teratogenicity or IUGR.

- **Breastfeeding Safety** .... There are no adequate reports or well-controlled studies in nursing women. It is unknown whether **sevoflurane** enters human breast milk. However, considering the indication and dosing, one-time **sevoflurane** use is unlikely to pose a clinically significant risk to the breast-feeding neonate.

- **References** .... Kanazawa M, Kinefuchi Y, Suzuki T, et al. Tokai J Exp Clin Med 1999; 24:53-5.
Yamakage M, Tsujiguchi N, Chen X, et al. Can J Anaesth 2002; 49:62-6.
Gambling DR, Sharma SK, White PF, et al. Anesth Analg 1995; 81:90-5.

- **Summary** ....
  - **Pregnancy Category B**
  - **Lactation Category S**
  - **Sevoflurane** should be used during pregnancy and lactation only if the benefit justifies the potential perinatal risk.

Sibutramine (Meridia)

- **Class** — *Anorexiant, stimulant*

- **Indications** — Obesity

- **Mechanism** — Inhibits norepinephrine, serotonin, and dopamine reuptake

- **Dosage with Qualifiers** — Obesity—begin 10mg PO qd, increase to 15mg PO qd after 4w; max 15mg/d
  - **Contraindications**—hypersensitivity to drug or class, MAO inhibitor <14d, CAD, CHF, arrhythmias, stroke, severe hepatic or renal dysfunction, anorexia nervosa
  - **Caution**—unknown

- **Maternal Considerations** — Obesity is a major epidemic in the industrialized countries. Observational studies confirm a relationship between obesity and cardiovascular disease, type 2 diabetes mellitus, certain forms of cancer, gallstones, certain respiratory disorders, and an increase in overall mortality rate. These studies suggest that weight loss, if maintained, may produce health benefits for patients with chronic obesity. **Sibutramine** leads to dose-dependent weight loss. Maintenance therapy enhances the likelihood of maintaining the loss. There is no published experience with **sibutramine** during pregnancy, and there are no apparent indications for its use during pregnancy. Clearance is modestly decreased in women.
  Side effects include menstrual irregularities, dysmenorrhea, tachycardia, severe hypertension, seizures, headache, dry mouth, insomnia, rhinitis, anorexia, constipation, increased appetite, dizziness, anxiety, dyspepsia, nausea, rash, and sinusitis.

- **Fetal Considerations** — There are no adequate reports or well-controlled studies in human fetuses. It is unknown whether **sibutramine** crosses the human placenta. Rodent studies are generally reassuring, with dysmorphology noted only at the highest doses concurrent with maternal toxicity and only in rabbits. Transport across the rodent placenta is limited.

- **Breastfeeding Safety** — There is no published experience in nursing women. It is unknown whether **sibutramine** enters human breast milk.

- **References** — There is no published experience in pregnancy or during lactation.

- **Summary** —
  - **Pregnancy Category C**
  - **Lactation Category U**
  - There are no indications for **sibutramine** during pregnancy and lactation.

Sildenafil (Viagra)

■ **Class** .... PDE *inhibitor*

■ **Indications** .... Erectile dysfunction

■ **Mechanism** .... Phosphodiesterase V inhibitor

■ **Dosage with Qualifiers** .... No FDA approved indications for women
- **Contraindications**—hypersensitivity to drug or class, nitrate use
- **Caution**—CAD, hepatic dysfunction, severe renal disease, hypotension

■ **Maternal Considerations** .... **Sildenafil** is suggested as a treatment for sexual arousal disorder in premenopausal women. Though there are no adequate reports or well-controlled studies of **sildenafil** in pregnant women, it is a potentially attractive agent as it increases the half-life of nitric oxide. **Sildenafil** has also been tested as an agent to increase uterine blood flow and endometrial development in women undergoing IVF. *Side effects* include severe hypotension, MI, ventricular arrhythmia, sudden death, stroke, TIA, increased intraocular pressure, headache, flushing, dyspepsia, nasal congestion, UTI, blurred or blue-tinted vision, diarrhea, dizziness, rash, and photophobia.

■ **Fetal Considerations** .... There are no adequate reports or well-controlled studies in human fetuses. It is unknown whether **sildenafil** crosses the human placenta. Rodent studies are reassuring, revealing no evidence of teratogenicity or IUGR despite the use of doses higher than those used clinically.

■ **Breastfeeding Safety** .... There is no published experience in pregnancy. It is unknown whether **sildenafil** enters human breast milk.

■ **Reference** .... Sher G, Fisch JD. Hum Reprod 2000; 15:806-9.

■ **Summary** ....
- **Pregnancy Category B**
- **Lactation Category U**
- There are currently no indications for **sildenafil** during pregnancy or lactation.

Silver nitrate

- **Class** — *Antibacterial, ophthalmic*

- **Indications** — Prevention of gonorrheal ophthalmia neonatorum

- **Mechanism** — Precipitates bacterial proteins

- **Dosage with Qualifiers** — Prevention of gonorrheal ophthalmia neonatorum—apply 2 gtt 1% solution each eye shortly after birth
  - **Contraindications**—hypersensitivity to drug or class
  - **Caution**—unknown

- **Maternal Considerations** — **Silver nitrate** has been used for decades to prevent neonatal gonorrheal conjunctivitis. Unfortunately, it does not prevent chlamydial conjunctivitis and has been largely replaced with **erythromycin** ointment.
  Side effects include chemical conjunctivitis.

- **Fetal Considerations** — Not relevant

- **Breastfeeding Safety** — Not relevant

- **References** — Schaller UC, Klauss V. Bull World Health Organ 2001; 79:262-3.
  de Toledo AR, Chandler JW. Infect Dis Clin North Am 1992; 6:807-13.

- **Summary** —
  - **Pregnancy Category B**
  - **Lactation Category S**
  - **Silver nitrate** provides effective prophylaxis for gonorrheal conjunctivitis, but does not well treat the more prevalent chlamydia.

Silver sulfadiazine topical (Canflame; Dermazin; Flamazine; Flammazine; Geben; Sildimac; Silvadene; SSD; Silvazine; Silverderma; Silverol; Silvirin; Sofargen; Thermazene)

- **Class** — *Dermatologic, antibacterial*

- **Indications** — 2nd or 3rd degree burns

- **Mechanism** — Bacteriostatic; inhibits dihydropteroate

- **Dosage with Qualifiers** — 2nd or 3rd degree burns—apply to debrided wound qd/bid
  NOTE—1% cream

910

- **Contraindications**—hypersensitivity to drug or class
- **Caution**—unknown

■ **Maternal Considerations** ⋯⋯ While burn injuries to pregnant women are not rare, the literature is indeed sparse. There are no adequate reports or well-controlled studies of **silver sulfadiazine** in pregnant women. Absorption of **silver sulfadiazine** varies depending upon the percent of body surface area and the extent of the tissue damage.
Side effects include neutropenia, leukopenia, erythema multiforme, burning, pain, pruritus, skin necrosis, and rash.

■ **Fetal Considerations** ⋯⋯ There are no adequate reports or well-controlled studies in human fetuses. It is unknown whether **silver sulfadiazine** crosses the human placenta. Considering the route and concentration, it is unlikely the maternal systemic concentration will reach a clinically relevant level. Rodent studies are reassuring, revealing no evidence of teratogenicity or IUGR despite the use of doses higher than those used clinically.

■ **Breastfeeding Safety** ⋯⋯ There are no adequate reports or well-controlled studies in nursing women. It is unknown whether **silver sulfadiazine** enters human breast milk. Considering the route and concentration, it is unlikely the breast-fed neonate will ingest a clinically relevant amount.

■ **References** ⋯⋯ Prasanna M, Singh K. Burns 1996; 22:234-7.
Gang RK, Bajec J, Tahboub M. Burns 1992; 18:317-20.

■ **Summary** ⋯⋯
- **Pregnancy Category B**
- **Lactation Category S?**
- **Silver sulfadiazine** should be used during pregnancy and lactation only if the benefit justifies the potential perinatal risk.

Simethicone (Mylicon)

■ **Class** ⋯⋯ *Gastrointestinal*

■ **Indications** ⋯⋯ Flatulence

■ **Mechanism** ⋯⋯ Alters gas surface tension

■ **Dosage with Qualifiers** ⋯⋯ Flatulence—80-120mg PO qid (pc and hs) prn; max 480mg/d
- **Contraindications**—hypersensitivity to drug or class, intestinal perforation, GI obstruction
- **Caution**—unknown

- **Maternal Considerations** .... **Simethicone** significantly reduces vomiting, stomach discomfort, and abdominal pain post-cesarean section. Bowel function appears to return more rapidly. *Side effects* include nausea and diarrhea.

- **Fetal Considerations** .... There are no adequate reports or well-controlled studies in human fetuses. And while it is unknown whether **simethicone** crosses the human placenta, it is unlikely the maternal systemic concentration reaches a clinically relevant level. Rodent teratogenicity studies have not been conducted.

- **Breastfeeding Safety** .... There are no adequate reports or well-controlled studies in nursing women. While it is unknown whether **simethicone** enters human breast milk, it is unlikely the maternal systemic concentration reaches a clinically relevant level. It is generally considered compatible with breastfeeding.

- **Reference** .... Avramovic D, Sulovic V, Lazarevic B, et al. Jugosl Ginekol Obstet 1979; 19:307-11.

- **Summary** ....
  - **Pregnancy Category C**
  - **Lactation Category S**
  - **Simethicone** is effective for the relief of flatulence and post-cesarean section abdominal discomfort.

Simvastatin (Zocor)

- **Class** .... *Antihyperlipidemic, HMG CoA reductase inhibitor*

- **Indications** .... Hypercholesterolemia, hypertriglyceridemia, dysbetalipoproteinemia, familial hypercholesterolemia, secondary prevention of cardiovascular events

- **Mechanism** .... HMG CoA reductase inhibitor

- **Dosage with Qualifiers** .... Hypercholesterolemia—begin 20mg PO qd; max 80mg/d
  Hypertriglyceridemia—begin 20mg PO qd; max 80mg/d
  Dysbetalipoproteinemia—begin 20mg PO qd; max 80mg/d
  Familial hypercholesterolemia—40mg PO qpm; max 80mg/d
  Secondary prevention of cardiovascular events—begin 20mg PO qd (40mg PO qd if goal >45% reduction LDL); max 80mg/d
  NOTE—multiple drug interactions alter dosing (e.g., **verapamil**, **amiodarone**, other fibrates or **cyclosporine**)

- **Contraindications**—hypersensitivity to drug or class, active hepatic disease, unexplained elevated LFTs
- **Caution**—hepatic dysfunction, alcohol abuse, severe renal disease

■ **Maternal Considerations**

Simvastatin is a synthetic statin that reduces the overall lipid level and the risk of adverse cardiovascular events. It may modestly increase the risk of cholelithiasis. **Simvastatin** does not affect gonadotropin function in premenopausal women. There are no adequate reports or well-controlled studies of **simvastatin** in pregnant women. Post-marketing studies do not suggest an increase in adverse outcomes. However, atherosclerosis is a chronic process. Discontinuation during pregnancy should have little impact on the long-term therapeutic outcome of primary hypercholesterolemia.
Side effects include rhabdomyolysis, hepatotoxicity, constipation, diarrhea, flatus, dyspepsia, nausea, gallstones, asthenia, myalgias, elevated CPK, elevated LFTs, and rash.

■ **Fetal Considerations**

There are no adequate reports or well-controlled studies in human fetuses. It is unknown whether **simvastatin** crosses the human placenta. Post-marketing studies are reassuring, as are rodent studies, which reveal no evidence of teratogenicity despite doses that were multiples of the MRHD. However, cholesterol and other products of the cholesterol biosynthesis pathway are essential components for fetal development, including synthesis of steroids and cell membranes, and it is generally considered the potential fetal risk outweighs the benefit to the mother. Inadvertent exposure is not an indication for pregnancy termination.

■ **Breastfeeding Safety**

There are no adequate reports or well-controlled studies in nursing women. It is unknown whether **simvastatin** enters human breast milk.

■ **References**

Plotkin D, Miller S, Nakajima S, et al. J Clin Endocrinol Metab 2002; 87:3155-61.
Caroli-Bosc FX, Le Gall P, Pugliese P, et al. Dig Dis Sci 2001; 46:540-4.
Manson JM, Freyssinges C, Ducrocq MB, Stephenson WP. Reprod Toxicol 1996; 10:439-446.

■ **Summary**

- **Pregnancy Category X**
- **Lactation Category NS**
- **Simvastatin** should be avoided during pregnancy and lactation.
- Inadvertent exposure is not an indication for pregnancy termination.

Sirolimus

- **Class** — *Immunosuppressive*

- **Indications** — Adjunct, renal transplant

- **Mechanism** — Inhibits T cell activation/proliferation in response to antigenic and IL-2, IL-4, and IL-15 stimulation

- **Dosage with Qualifiers** — Adjunct, renal transplant—2mg PO qd combined with **cyclosporine** and corticosteroids; alternative 15mg PO initially, then 5mg PO qd
  NOTE—hepatic dosing; monitor renal function, antimicrobial and CMV prophylaxis suggested; complete drug history essential because of interactions with commonly used agents
  - **Contraindications**—hypersensitivity to drug or class, acute infection
  - **Caution**—sun exposure

- **Maternal Considerations** — A growing number of obstetric patients have benefited from organ transplant. Pregnancy is considered safe if the patient is 2 years after transplantation, has good renal function without proteinuria, no uncontrolled arterial hypertension, and no evidence of ongoing rejection. The clearance of **sirolimus** is modestly increased in women. There are no adequate reports or well-controlled studies of **sirolimus** in pregnant women. It is generally avoided in favor of **tacrolimus**, **azathioprine** with or without steroids. *Side effects* include hyperlipidemia, hypercholesterolemia, increased BUN/Cr, opportunistic infection, epistaxis, lymphocele, insomnia, hemolytic-uremic syndrome, herpes zoster, malaise, skin ulcer, increased LDH, hypotension, diabetes mellitus, tinnitus, deafness, facial edema, atrial fibrillation, CHF, hemorrhage, hypervolemia, palpitation, peripheral vascular disorder, syncope, tachycardia, thrombophlebitis, thrombosis, vasodilatation, anorexia, dysphagia, eructation, esophagitis, flatulence, gastritis, gastroenteritis, gingivitis, ileus, abnormal LFTs, mouth ulceration, oral moniliasis, stomatitis, skin cancer, and lymphoma.

- **Fetal Considerations** — There are no adequate reports or well-controlled studies in human fetuses. It is unknown whether **sirolimus** crosses the human placenta. **Sirolimus** is embryotoxic in rodents. In *vitro*, it inhibits the growth of fetal myocardial cells.

- **Breastfeeding Safety** — There are no adequate reports or well-controlled studies in nursing women. It is unknown whether **sirolimus** enters human breast milk. Trace amounts are found in rat milk, and in *vitro*, **sirolimus** inhibited milk production.

■ **References** .... Nephrol Dial Transplant 2002; 17(Suppl 4):50-5.
Burton PB, Yacoub MH, Barton PJ. Pediatr Cardiol 1998;
19:468-70.
Hang J, Rillema JA. Biochim Biophys Acta 1997; 1358:209-14.

■ **Summary** ....
- **Pregnancy Category C**
- **Lactation Category U**
- **Sirolimus** should be used during pregnancy and lactation only if the benefit justifies the potential perinatal risk.
- There are alternative agents for which there is more experience during pregnancy and lactation.

Sodium bicarbonate (Baros granules; Neut)

■ **Class** .... *Electrolyte replacement, alkalinizing agents*

■ **Indications** .... Metabolic acidemia

■ **Mechanism** .... Increases serum bicarbonate

■ **Dosage with Qualifiers** .... Metabolic acidemia—1mEq/kg IV; adjust dose based on ABG and clinical scenario
- **Contraindications**—hypersensitivity to drug or class, hypochloridemia, hypocalcemia
- **Caution**—CHF

■ **Maternal Considerations** .... There are no adequate reports or well-controlled studies of **sodium bicarbonate** in pregnant women. There is no reason to expect pregnancy alters the risk of its use. It is most often used during pregnancy in association with the treatment of diabetic ketoacidosis.
Side effects include metabolic alkalosis, extravasation cellulitis, edema, and hyponatremia.

■ **Fetal Considerations** .... There are no adequate reports or well-controlled studies in human fetuses. Bicarbonate ions do equilibrate across the human placenta. There is no physiologic reason to expect a gradual correction of a metabolic acidosis would threaten the fetus. It is used during RBC transfusion of the profoundly anemic fetus to prevent severe acidemia and to resuscitate during fetal surgery. Rodent teratogenicity studies have not been conducted.

■ **Breastfeeding Safety** .... There are no adequate reports or well-controlled studies in nursing women. It is unknown whether infused **sodium bicarbonate** enters human breast milk and increases milk concentration.

■ References .... Jennings RW, Adzick NS, Longaker MT, et al. J Pediatr Surg 1992; 27:1329-33.
Weiner CP, Williamson RA, Wenstrom KD, et al. Am J Obstet Gynecol 1991; 165:1302-7.

■ Summary .... • **Pregnancy Category C**
• **Lactation Category S**
• **Sodium bicarbonate** should be used during pregnancy and lactation when medically indicated.

Sodium ferric gluconate (Ferrlecit)

■ **Class** .... *Minerals; replacement*

■ **Indications** .... Iron deficiency in hemodialysed patients

■ **Mechanism** .... Essential component for erythropoiesis

■ **Dosage with Qualifiers** .... Iron deficiency in hemodialysed patients—25mg IV test dose over 60min followed by 100mg IV over 1h
• **Contraindications**—hypersensitivity to drug or class, non-iron deficient anemia, iron overload
• **Caution**—unknown

■ **Maternal Considerations** .... There is no adequate published experience with **sodium ferric gluconate** complex during pregnancy.
Side effects include anaphylaxis, iron toxicity, hypotension, flushing, headache, nausea, vomiting, diarrhea, weakness, fatigue, injection site reactions, pain, fever, dyspnea, itching, and rash.

■ **Fetal Considerations** .... There are no adequate reports or well-controlled studies in human fetuses. It is unknown whether **sodium ferric gluconate** complex crosses the human placenta. Iron is transported across. There is no physiologic reason to expect an adverse effect if maternal iron content is in the normal range.

■ **Breastfeeding Safety** .... There is no published experience in nursing women. It is unknown whether **sodium ferric gluconate** complex enters human breast milk. However, iron is a normal component of breast milk and other iron supplements increase the milk concentration.

■ **References** .... There is no published experience in pregnancy or during lactation.

- **Pregnancy Category B**
- **Lactation Category S**
- **Sodium ferric gluconate** complex should be used during pregnancy and lactation only if the benefit justifies the potential perinatal risk.

Sodium polystyrene (Kayexalate; Resonium; SPS)

■ **Class** — *Electrolytes*

■ **Indications** — Hyperkalemia

■ **Mechanism** — Exchanges sodium for potassium in the large bowel

■ **Dosage with Qualifiers** — Hyperkalemia—15mg mixed in water or sorbitol PO qd/qid
- **Contraindications**—hypersensitivity to drug or class, hypokalemia
- **Caution**—severe CHF, severe hypertension, marked hypernatremia

■ **Maternal Considerations** — There is no published experience with **sodium polystyrene** during pregnancy.
Side effects include hypokalemia, alkalosis, gastric irritation, anorexia, nausea, vomiting, diarrhea, constipation, intestinal obstruction, fecal impaction, and hypocalcemia.

■ **Fetal Considerations** — There are no adequate reports or well-controlled studies in human fetuses. **Sodium polystyrene** is not absorbed systemically and should pose no direct risk to the fetus. Rodent teratogenicity studies have not been performed.

■ **Breastfeeding Safety** — There is no published experience in nursing women. However, the low maternal systemic concentration precludes a direct effect.

■ **References** — There is no published experience in pregnancy or during lactation.

■ **Summary** —
- **Pregnancy Category C**
- **Lactation Category S**
- **Sodium polystyrene** should be used during pregnancy and lactation when medically indicated.

Sotalol (Betapace; Sorine)

■ **Class** — *Antiarrhythmic class* III; *antiadrenergic, β-blocker*

■ **Indications** — Ventricular arrhythmia

■ **Mechanism** — Nonspecific β-blocker

■ **Dosage with Qualifiers** — Ventricular arrhythmia—begin 80mg PO q12h, titrate dose in hospital with continuous monitoring for at least 3d; max 640mg for refractory cases
NOTE—renal dosing; monitor ECG, QT interval and CrCl, avoid abrupt withdrawal
- **Contraindications**—hypersensitivity to drug or class, sinus bradycardia, 2nd and 3rd degree AV block, prolonged QT interval syndrome, cardiogenic shock, uncontrolled CHF, asthma, hypokalemia, hypomagnesemia
- **Caution**—renal dysfunction, sick sinus syndrome, compensated CHF, diabetes mellitus, diuretics, electrolyte abnormalities

■ **Maternal Considerations** — There are no adequate reports or well-controlled studies of **sotalol** in pregnant women. **Sotalol** reduces blood pressure in hypertensive women, but its reported use during pregnancy is restricted to its properties as an antiarrhythmic agent.
Side effects include torsades de pointes, ventricular arrhythmia, CHF, prolonged QT interval, severe bradycardia, dyspnea, fatigue, dizziness, bradycardia, chest pain, palpitations, asthenia, hypotension, headache, nausea, vomiting, diarrhea, edema, sweating, and dyspepsia.

■ **Fetal Considerations** — There are no adequate reports or well-controlled studies in human fetuses. **Sotalol** crosses the human placenta reaching an F:M ratio approximating unity and is found in amniotic fluid. It has been used to treat fetal tachyarrhythmia. Rodent studies are reassuring, revealing no evidence of teratogenicity or IUGR despite the use of doses higher than those used clinically. In rabbits, high doses are associated with embryonic death most likely secondary to embryonic arrhythmia.

■ **Breastfeeding Safety** — There are no adequate reports or well-controlled studies in nursing women. **Sotalol** enters human breast milk. And though the kinetics remain to be detailed, a mean M:P ratio of 5.4 was reported in one mother, raising the possibility of pharmacological effect in the newborn infant. It is highly protein bound. The nursing neonate should be observed closely for evidence of β-blockade.

■ **References** ⋯⋯⋯⋯⋯⋯⋯⋯⋯⋯ O'Hare MF, Murnaghan GA, Russell CJ, et al. Br J Obstet Gynaecol 1980; 87:814-20.
Oudijk MA, Ruskamp JM, Ambachtsheer BE, et al. Paediatr Drugs 2002; 4(1):49-63.
Skold AC, Danielsson BR. Pharmacol Toxicol 2001; 88:34-9.
Shannon ME, Malecha SE, Cha AJ. J Hum Lact 2000; 16:240-5.

■ **Summary** ⋯⋯⋯⋯⋯⋯⋯⋯⋯⋯
- **Pregnancy Category B**
- **Lactation Category U**
- **Sotalol** should be used during pregnancy and lactation only if the benefit justifies the potential perinatal risk.

Spectinomycin (Trobicin)

■ **Class** ⋯⋯⋯⋯⋯⋯⋯⋯⋯⋯⋯⋯⋯ *Antibiotic, aminoglycoside*

■ **Indications** ⋯⋯⋯⋯⋯⋯⋯⋯⋯ Gonorrhea

■ **Mechanism** ⋯⋯⋯⋯⋯⋯⋯⋯ Bactericidal; inhibits protein synthesis by binding the bacterial 30S ribosomal subunit

■ **Dosage with Qualifiers** ⋯⋯ Gonorrhea, uncomplicated—2g IM (gluteus) ×1; increase to 4g if resistance (2g per injection)
Gonorrhea, disseminated—2g IM (gluteus) ×3-7d
- **Contraindications**—hypersensitivity to drug or class
- **Caution**—unknown

■ **Maternal Considerations** ⋯⋯ **Spectinomycin** is not effective for the treatment of syphilis, and may in fact mask or delay the symptoms of incubating syphilis. All patients with gonorrhea should be serologically tested for syphilis at diagnosis, and again 3mo later. There are no adequate reports or well-controlled studies of **spectinomycin** in pregnant women. Failure to achieve "microbiologic cure" is similar for common antibiotic regimens: **amoxicillin** plus **probenecid** compared with **spectinomycin** (odds ratio (OR) 2.40, 95% confidence interval (CI) 0.71-8.12), **amoxicillin** plus **probenecid** compared with **ceftriaxone** (OR 2.40, 95% CI 0.71-8.12) and **ceftriaxone** compared with **cefixime** (OR 1.22, 95% CI 0.16-9.04). Thus, the selection is based on sensitivities in the geographic locale, price, and the prevalence of syphilis. Sex partners should be tested and treated when possible.
Side effects include urticaria, dizziness, nausea, chills, fever, injection site pain, insomnia, anemia, elevated BUN, and elevated LFTs.

- **Fetal Considerations** ⋯⋯ There are no adequate reports or well-controlled studies in human fetuses. It is unknown whether **spectinomycin** crosses the human placenta. Rodent studies are reassuring, revealing no evidence of teratogenicity or IUGR despite the use of doses higher than those used clinically.

- **Breastfeeding Safety** ⋯⋯ There is no published experience in nursing women. It is unknown whether **spectinomycin** enters human breast milk. Considering the likely dosage and that other aminoglycosides are generally considered safe for breastfeeding, the same should be true for **spectinomycin**.

- **References** ⋯⋯ Brocklehurst P. Cochrane Database Syst Rev 2002; (2):CD000098.

- **Summary** ⋯⋯
  - **Pregnancy Category B**
  - **Lactation Category S?**
  - **Spectinomycin** is one of several available effective agents for the treatment of gonorrhea during pregnancy and lactation.

Spironolactone (Aldactone; Diatensec; Flumach; Osiren)

- **Class** ⋯⋯ *Diuretic*

- **Indications** ⋯⋯ Edema, CHF, diuretic-induced hypokalemia, hyperaldosteronism test, hypertension

- **Mechanism** ⋯⋯ Aldosterone receptor antagonist active in the distal convoluted tubule

- **Dosage with Qualifiers** ⋯⋯ Edema—25-50mg PO qd/bid
  CHF—25mg PO qd
  Diuretic-induced hypokalemia—25-100mg PO qd (only if oral potassium not appropriate)
  Hyperaldosteronism test—400mg PO qd ×4-28d (until hypokalemia corrects)
  Hypertension—25-50mg PO qd/bid
  NOTE—renal dosing
  - **Contraindications**—hypersensitivity to drug or class, anuria, renal insufficiency, hyperkalemia
  - **Caution**—hepatic or renal dysfunction, hyponatremia, diabetes mellitus

- **Maternal Considerations** ⋯⋯ **Spironolactone** increases sodium and water excretion while retaining potassium. There are no adequate reports or well-controlled studies of **spironolactone** in pregnant women. Diuretics should not be used to treat the physiologic edema of pregnancy and do not prevent preeclampsia. There are superior agents for such off label indications as hirsutism. It has been used for the treatment of maternal Bartter's syndrome during pregnancy with success.

Side effects include renal failure, hepatotoxicity, menstrual irregularities, agranulocytosis, anaphylaxis, nausea, vomiting, diarrhea, abdominal pain, headache, confusion, hirsutism, fever, rash, hyperkalemia, and metabolic acidosis.

- **Fetal Considerations**

There are no adequate reports or well-controlled studies in human fetuses. It is unknown whether **spironolactone** crosses the human placenta. **Spironolactone** is an antiandrogen and can feminize male rats. However, there is at least one case report of an appropriately developed male newborn after high-dose treatment for maternal Bartter's syndrome.

- **Breastfeeding Safety**

While **spironolactone** and its major active metabolite enter human breast milk, it is estimated that the breast-feeding neonate would ingest <0.5% of the daily maternal dose.

- **References**

Groves TD, Corenblum B. Am J Obstet Gynecol 1995; 172:1655-6.
Rigo J Jr, Glaz E, Papp Z. Am J Obstet Gynecol 1996; 174:297.
Phelps DL, Karim Z. J Pharm Sci 1977; 66:1203.

- **Summary**

- **Pregnancy Category D**
- **Lactation Category S**
- **Spironolactone** should be used during pregnancy and lactation only if the benefit justifies the potential perinatal risk.

Stavudine (d4T; Zerit)

- **Class** — Antiviral

- **Indications** — HIV

- **Mechanism** — Reverse transcriptase inhibitor

- **Dosage with Qualifiers** — HIV—40mg PO q12h; hold if peripheral neuropathy develops
NOTE—renal dosing
  - **Contraindications**—hypersensitivity to drug or class, lactic acidosis, lactation

- **Caution**—hepatic or renal dysfunction, peripheral neuropathy, neurotoxic agents, AIDS, history of pancreatitis, bone marrow depression

■ **Maternal Considerations**

Stavudine is a synthetic thymidine nucleoside analog. There are no adequate reports or well-controlled studies of **stavudine** in pregnant women. Pregnancy increases the risk of potentially fatal lactic acidosis/hepatic steatosis when combined with **didanosine** and other antiretroviral agents.

Side effects include hepatotoxicity, pancreatitis, lactic acidosis, peripheral neuropathy, severe motor weakness, leukopenia, thrombocytopenia, headache, nausea, vomiting, diarrhea, abdominal pain, rash, fever, chills, anorexia, myalgia, insomnia, anemia, elevated LFTs and elevated amylase/lipase.

■ **Fetal Considerations**

There are no adequate reports or well-controlled studies in human fetuses. It is unknown whether **stavudine** crosses the human placenta. Rodent studies are generally reassuring, revealing only minor skeletal abnormalities when the dose approximated 400 times the MRHD. **Stavudine** readily crosses the rhesus macaque placenta and is present as parent compound and inactive metabolites. However, no active metabolites are found.

■ **Breastfeeding Safety**

There is no published experience in nursing women. It is unknown whether **stavudine** enters human breast milk. It is excreted into rodent milk. Breastfeeding is contraindicated in HIV-infected nursing women when formula is available to reduce the risk of neonatal transmission.

■ **References**

AIDS Treat News 2001; 358:8.
Sarner L, Fakoya A. Sex Transm Infect 2002; 78:58-9.
Patterson TA, Binienda ZK, Newport GD, et al. Teratology 2000; 62:93-9.

■ **Summary**

- **Pregnancy Category C**
- **Lactation Category U**
- **Stavudine** should be used during pregnancy and lactation only if the benefit justifies the potential perinatal risk.
- It may provide little HIV protection to the perinate despite placental transfer of the parent drug.
- Physicians are encouraged to register pregnant women under the Antiretroviral Pregnancy Registry (1-800-258-4263) for a better follow-up of the outcome while under treatment with **stavudine**.

Streptokinase (Kabikinase; K-Nase; Streptase; Zykinase)

■ **Class** — Thrombolytic

■ **Indications** — MI, PE/DVT, AV cannula occlusion

■ **Mechanism** — Converts plasminogen to plasmin

■ **Dosage with Qualifiers** — MI—1.5millionU IV over 60min
PE/DVT—begin 250,000U IV over 30min, then 100,000U/h for either 72h (DVT) or 24h (PE); begin within 7-10d of occlusion
AV cannula occlusion—100,000-250,000U IV over 30min
- **Contraindications**—hypersensitivity to drug or class, recent stroke, active internal bleeding, recent trauma, intracranial tumor, ulcerative colitis, severe hypertension, rheumatic valvular disease, <10d since a diagnostic arterial procedure
- **Caution**—recent delivery, recent GI bleeding, left-sided heart thrombosis, hypertension, diabetic retinopathy, subacute bacterial endocarditis

■ **Maternal Considerations** — **Streptokinase** is a purified bacterial protein produced by group C β-hemolytic streptococci. There is no residual thrombotic material in 60-75% of patients treated with **streptokinase** vs. only 10% of those treated with **heparin**. Therapy preserves venous valve function in most cases, avoiding the pathologic changes that cause postphlebitic syndrome, which follows in 90% of the DVT patients treated with heparin alone. There are no adequate reports or well-controlled studies of **streptokinase** in pregnant women, though numerous case reports suggest relative safety compared to therapeutic alternatives. Of note is its success with thrombotic mechanical mitral valves. Hemorrhage complicates <10%. Because of the increased likelihood of resistance due to antistreptokinase antibody, **streptokinase** may be ineffective within a year of prior administration, or a streptococcal infection, such as streptococcal pharyngitis, acute rheumatic fever, or acute glomerulonephritis secondary to a streptococcal infection. *Side effects* include anaphylaxis, cholesterol embolism, arrhythmia, severe bleeding, stroke, hypotension, fever, and bronchospasm.

■ **Fetal Considerations** — There are no adequate reports or well-controlled studies in human fetuses. It is unknown whether **streptokinase** crosses the human placenta. The published case reports provide some reassurance. Rodent teratogenicity studies have not been conducted.

■ **Breastfeeding Safety** — There is no published experience in nursing women. It is unknown whether **streptokinase** enters human breast milk.

■ **References** ⋯⋯⋯⋯⋯⋯⋯⋯⋯⋯⋯⋯⋯ Arneson H, Heilo A, Jakobsen E, et al. Acta Med Scand
1978; 203:457-463.
Anbarasan C, Kumar VS, Latchumanadhas K, Mullasari AS.
J Heart Valve Dis 2001; 10:393-5.
Henrich W, Schmider A, Henrich M, Dudenhausen JW.
J Perinat Med 2001; 29:155-7.
Turrentine MA, Braems G, Ramirez MM. Obstet Gynecol
Surv 1995; 50:534-41.

■ **Summary** ⋯⋯⋯⋯⋯⋯⋯⋯⋯⋯⋯⋯ • **Pregnancy Category C**
• **Lactation Category U**
• **Streptokinase** should be used during pregnancy and
lactation only if the benefit justifies the potential
perinatal risk.

Succinylcholine (Anectine; Celocurin; Quelicin; Sucostrin; Sux-Cert; Suxamethonium)

■ **Class** ⋯⋯⋯⋯⋯⋯⋯⋯⋯⋯⋯⋯⋯⋯⋯ *Neuromuscular blocker, depolarizing; musculoskeletal agents*

■ **Indications** ⋯⋯⋯⋯⋯⋯⋯⋯⋯⋯⋯⋯ Paralysis; anesthesia

■ **Mechanism** ⋯⋯⋯⋯⋯⋯⋯⋯⋯⋯⋯ Stimulates acetylcholine motor endplates

■ **Dosage with Qualifiers** ⋯⋯⋯⋯ <u>Paralysis, anesthesia, short term</u>—0.6-1.5mg/kg IV over
10-30sec; max 150mg
<u>Paralysis, long term</u>—0.5-10mg/min continuous IV
NOTE—onset 30-60sec, duration 6-10min
• **Contraindications**—hypersensitivity to drug or class,
pseudocholinesterase deficiency, narrow-angle
glaucoma, penetrating eye injury, history malignant
hyperthermia, bradycardia, severe burns, hyperkalemia,
neuromuscular disorders, history rhabdomyolysis
• **Caution**—stroke, severe hepatic disease, myasthenia
gravis

■ **Maternal Considerations** ⋯⋯⋯ There are no adequate reports or well-controlled studies
of **succinylcholine** in pregnant women. It is the drug
routinely used in rapid-sequence induction of general
anesthesia to facilitate tracheal intubation for cesarean
delivery. The large clinical experience is reassuring.
Plasma cholinesterase levels decrease by 1/4 during
pregnancy and for several days post-partum. Thus, a
higher proportion of patients may experience prolonged
apnea to **succinylcholine** when pregnant compared to
nonpregnant.
Side effects include arrhythmias, bradycardia, tachycardia,
respiratory depression, cardiovascular collapse, malignant
hyperthermia, apnea, hyperkalemia, rhabdomyolysis,

myoglobinemia, muscle twitching, postoperative myalgia and stiffness, excess salivation, and increased intraocular pressure.

■ **Fetal Considerations** There are no adequate reports or well-controlled studies in human fetuses. Small amounts of **succinylcholine** are known to cross the placenta, but under normal conditions the amount of drug does not endanger the fetus. But because the amount that crosses depends on the M:F concentration gradient, apnea and flaccidity can occur in the neonate after repeated high doses, or in the presence of atypical maternal plasma cholinesterase. Rodent teratogenicity studies have not been conducted.

■ **Breastfeeding Safety** There are no adequate reports or well-controlled studies in nursing women. It is unknown whether **succinylcholine** enters human breast milk. However, considering the indication and dosing, one-time **succinylcholine** use is unlikely to pose a clinically significant risk to the breast-feeding neonate.

■ **References** Guay J, Grenier Y, Varin F. Clin Pharmacokinet 1998; 34:483.
van der Kleijn E, Drabkova J, Crul JF. Br J Anaesth 1973; 45:1169-77.

■ **Summary**
- **Pregnancy Category C**
- **Lactation Category S**
- There is extensive clinical experience with succinylcholine during pregnancy that is reassuring.
- **Succinylcholine** should be used during pregnancy and lactation only if the benefit justifies the potential perinatal risk.

Sucralfate (Calmidan; Carafate; Scrat; Sucafate; Sucrace; Ulcona; Ulcumaag; Ulsidex; Yuwan-S)

■ **Class** *Cytoprotective, antiulcer*

■ **Indications** Duodenal ulcer

■ **Mechanism** Coats the ulcer with proteinaceous exudate

■ **Dosage with Qualifiers** Duodenal ulcer—1g PO qid (treatment) or bid (maintenance)
- **Contraindications**—hypersensitivity to drug or class, dysphagia, GI obstruction
- **Caution**—renal dysfunction

- **Maternal Considerations** .... GERD poses a special challenge in pregnancy. Lifestyle and dietary modifications, change in sleeping posture, and antacid medications are the first lines of therapy. When these interventions are unsuccessful, **sucralfate** should be considered next. Therapy with H$_2$ receptor antagonists or proton pump inhibitors are generally reserved for women with refractory symptoms. There are no adequate reports or well-controlled studies of **sucralfate** in pregnant women.
Side effects include diarrhea, nausea, vomiting, flatulence, constipation, rash, dizziness, insomnia, and bezoar formation.

- **Fetal Considerations** .... There are no adequate reports or well-controlled studies in human fetuses. It is only minimally absorbed across the GI tract, and thus should pose no risk to the fetus. Rodent studies are reassuring.

- **Breastfeeding Safety** .... There are no adequate reports or well-controlled studies in nursing women. While it is unknown whether **sucralfate** enters human breast milk, it is only minimally absorbed across the GI tract and should pose no risk to the breast-feeding neonate.

- **References** .... Charan M, Katz PO. Curr Treat Options Gastroenterol 2001; 4:73-81.
Broussard CN, Richter JE. Drug Saf 1998; 19:325-37.

- **Summary** ....
  - **Pregnancy Category B**
  - **Lactation Category S**
  - **Sucralfate** is a first-line agent for the treatment of GERD during pregnancy and lactation.

Sufentanil (Sufenta)

- **Class** .... *Anesthesia, opioid*

- **Indications** .... General anesthesia, neuraxial anesthesia

- **Mechanism** .... Binds to multiple opiate receptors

- **Dosage with Qualifiers** .... General anesthesia—begin 2-8mcg/kg IV when used with inhalational anesthetics; up to 30mcg/kg when used with amnestic and oxygen alone: titrate additional smaller doses to desired effect
Epidural during labor—several regimens including 10-15mcg **sufentanil** plus 10ml 0.125% **bupivacaine**
Intrathecal during labor—several regimens including 5-7.5mcg with or without **bupivacaine**

- **Contraindications**—hypersensitivity to drug or class
- **Caution**—respiratory depression, hepatic or renal dysfunction

■ **Maternal Considerations**

Sufentanil is a potent opioid. When used in balanced general anesthesia, **sufentanil** has as much as 10 times the potency as **fentanyl**. It is popular combined with a local anesthetic for a variety of neuraxial anesthetic techniques during labor. However, when choosing between **fentanyl** and **sufentanil**, **sufentanil** costs more and has a greater risk of dosing error because of its higher potency.

Side effects include laryngospasm, respiratory depression, chest stiffness, ventricular arrhythmia, bronchospasm, hypotension, bradycardia, pruritus, nausea, vomiting, chills, postoperative confusion, biliary spasm, constipation, ureteral colic, and blurred vision.

■ **Fetal Considerations**

There are no adequate reports or well-controlled studies in human fetuses. **Sufentanil** crosses the human placenta achieving an F:M ratio of unity. Because of its low initial umbilical vein concentration, **sufentanil** may be the opioid of choice when delivery is imminent (<45 min). Fetal acidosis increases placental transfer. It is used for fetal analgesia during a variety of procedures. Rodent studies are generally reassuring, revealing no evidence of teratogenicity or IUGR despite the use of doses higher than those used clinically. Embryotoxicity does occur at doses twice the recommended human dose.

■ **Breastfeeding Safety**

There are no adequate reports or well-controlled studies in nursing women. However, considering the indication and dosing, one-time **sufentanil** use is unlikely to pose a clinically significant risk to the breast-feeding neonate.

■ **References**

Clement HJ, Caruso L, Lopez F, et al. Br J Anaesth 2002; 88:809-13.
De Eccher L, Martino C, Bacchilega I, et al. Minerva Anestesiol 2002; 68:83-7.
Nelson KE, Rauch T, Terebuh V, D'Angelo R. Anesthesiology 2002; 96:1070-3.
Senat MV, Fischer C, Ville Y. Prenat Diagn 2002; 22:354-6.
Krishna BR, Zakowski MI, Grant GJ. Can J Anaesth 1997; 44:996-1001.

■ **Summary**

- **Pregnancy Category C**
- **Lactation Category S**
- **Sufentanil** should be used during pregnancy and lactation only if the benefit justifies the potential perinatal risk.
- It is a useful adjunct for labor epidural analgesia allowing for a decreased quantity of local anesthetic, which helps preserve motor function.

Sulconazole nitrate topical (Exelderm; Sulcosyn)

■ **Class** — *Dermatologic, antifungal*

■ **Indications** — Tinea pedis, tinea cruris, tinea corporis, tinea versicolor

■ **Mechanism** — Imidazole that inhibits cell membrane ergosterol synthesis

■ **Dosage with Qualifiers** —
<u>Tinea pedis</u>—apply bid ×4w
<u>Tinea cruris</u>—apply qd/bid ×3w
<u>Tinea corporis</u>—apply qd/bid ×3w
<u>Tinea versicolor</u>—apply qd/bid ×3w
NOTE—available in 1% cream or solution
- **Contraindications**—hypersensitivity to drug or class
- **Caution**—unknown

■ **Maternal Considerations** — There is no published experience with **sulconazole** during pregnancy.
Side effects include pruritus, burning and erythema.

■ **Fetal Considerations** — There are no adequate reports or well-controlled studies in human fetuses. It is unknown whether **sulconazole** crosses the human placenta. Considering the dose and route, it is unlikely the maternal systemic concentration will reach a clinically relevant level. Rodent studies are reassuring, revealing no evidence of teratogenicity or IUGR despite the use of doses higher than those used clinically. Embryotoxicity was noted at doses 100 times the MRHD.

■ **Breastfeeding Safety** — There is no published experience in nursing women. However, considering the dose and route, it is unlikely the breast-fed neonate would ingest clinically relevant amounts.

■ **References** — There are no current relevant references.

■ **Summary** —
- **Pregnancy Category C**
- **Lactation Category S?**
- **Sulconazole** should be used during pregnancy and lactation only if the benefit justifies the potential perinatal risk.

Sulfadiazine (Microsulfon)

- **Class** — Antibiotic, sulfonamide

- **Indications** — Toxoplasmosis

- **Mechanism** — Bacteriostatic; inhibits dihydropteroate synthesis

- **Dosage with Qualifiers** — Toxoplasmosis—2-8g PO qd in 3-4 divided doses ×4w plus **pyrimethamine** 25mg/d
  NOTE—if AIDS, give 6mo or longer
  - **Contraindications**—hypersensitivity to drug or class, porphyria
  - **Caution**—hepatic or renal dysfunction, G6PD deficiency, hypovolemia

- **Maternal Considerations** — Toxoplasmosis is one of the most common parasitic infections in humans. There are no adequate reports or well-controlled studies of **sulfadiazine** in pregnant women for maternal disease.
  Side effects include hemolytic anemia, Stevens-Johnson syndrome, thrombocytopenia, leukopenia, hepatitis, acute renal failure, kernicterus in the newborn, fever, dizziness, headache, nausea, vomiting, diarrhea, photosensitivity, rash, and hematuria.

- **Fetal Considerations** — There are no adequate reports or well-controlled studies in human fetuses. **Sulfadiazine** crosses the human placenta and is used as a treatment for fetal toxoplasmosis in combination with **pyrimethamine**. Controversy continues as to how effective it is in preventing disease transmission. Since it is effective in the rhesus monkey model, treatment delay may explain the controversy. Rodent teratogenicity studies have not been performed. Other sulfonamides given at multiples of the MRHD are associated with cleft palate and bony abnormalities. The extensive human experience associated with congenital toxoplasmosis is reassuring. There is no published experience to suggest any increase in the risk of kernicterus.

- **Breastfeeding Safety** — There is no published experience in nursing women. While it is unknown whether **sulfadiazine** enters human breast milk, it is excreted into cows' milk. There are no adverse effects published in breast-fed children.

- **References** — Gilbert RE, Gras L, Wallon M, et al. Int J Epidemiol 2001; 30:1303-8.
  Schoondermark-van de Ven EM, Melchers WJ, Galama JM, et al. Eur J Obstet Gynecol Reprod Biol 1997; 74:183-8.
  Couvreur J, Thulliez P, Daffos F, et al. Fetal Diagn Ther 1993; 8:45-50.

Sulfamethoxazole (Gamazole; Gantanol; Sinomin; Urobak)

■ **Class** ———————————— *Antibiotic, sulfonamide*

■ **Indications** ———————————— Bacterial infection, e.g., pyelonephritis, cystitis,
meningitis, otitis media

■ **Mechanism** ———————————— Bacteriostatic; inhibits dihydropteroate synthesis

■ **Dosage with Qualifiers** ———— <u>Bacterial infection</u>—begin 2g PO ×1, then 1g PO bid
NOTE—may be combined with **trimethoprim** (Septra)
• **Contraindications**—hypersensitivity to drug or class
• **Caution**—G6PD deficiency

■ **Maternal Considerations** ———— There are no adequate reports or well-controlled studies
of **sulfamethoxazole** in pregnant women. When combined
with **trimethoprim**, it is effective for the treatment of Q
fever and for the treatment/prophylaxis of *Pneumocystis
carinii* pneumonia. **Trimethoprim/sulfamethoxazole** is
an alternative to high-dose **penicillin** for the treatment
of listeriosis.
Side effects include agranulocytosis, aplastic anemia,
hemolytic anemia, seizures, erythema multiforme,
hypoglycemia, exfoliative dermatitis, rash, hepatocellular
necrosis, and various allergic reactions.

■ **Fetal Considerations** ———— There are no adequate reports or well-controlled studies
in human fetuses. **Sulfamethoxazole** readily crosses the
human placenta. One study noted a small increase in the
rate of cardiovascular malformations after treatment with
trimethoprim/sulfamethoxazole in the 2nd and 3rd
trimesters. The causative agent was unclear. There is no
published evidence to suggest it is associated with
bilirubin toxicity, as is **sulfisoxazole**. Rodent studies
performed at high multiples of the MRHD revealed an
increased prevalence of cleft palate.

■ **Breastfeeding Safety** ———— There are no adequate reports or well-controlled
studies in nursing women. It is unknown whether
sulfamethoxazole enters human breast milk.

■ **References** .... Raoult D, Fenollar F, Stein A. Arch Intern Med 2002; 162:701-4.
Ahmad H, Mehta NJ, Manikal VM, et al. Chest 2001; 120:666-71.
Silver HM. Obstet Gynecol Surv 1998; 53:737-40.
Bawdon RE, Maberry MC, Fortunato SJ, et al. Gynecol Obstet Invest 1991; 31:240-2.
Czeizel AE, Rockenbauer M, Sorensen HT, Olsen J. Reprod Toxicol 2001; 15:637-46.
Hernandez-Diaz S, Werler MM, Walker AM, Mitchell AA. N Engl J Med 2000; 343:1608-14.

■ **Summary** .... • **Pregnancy Category C**
• **Lactation Category U**
• **Sulfamethoxazole** should be used during pregnancy and lactation only if the benefit justifies the potential perinatal risk.

Sulfasalazine (Azaline; Azaline EC; Azulfidine)

■ **Class** .... *Inflammatory bowel, salicylate*

■ **Indications** .... Ulcerative colitis, rheumatoid arthritis, Crohn's disease

■ **Mechanism** .... Unknown

■ **Dosage with Qualifiers** .... Ulcerative colitis—begin 500mg PO qd after meals for several days of improvement, then 500mg PO qid after meals
Rheumatoid arthritis—begin 500mg PO qd after meals for several days, then 500mg PO qid after meals
Crohn's disease—begin 500mg PO qd after meals for several days, then 500mg PO qid after meals
NOTE—obtain a CBC biweekly for the first 3mo of treatment; monitor renal function periodically
• **Contraindications**—hypersensitivity to drug or class, hypersensitivity to salicylates, hepatic or renal dysfunction, porphyria, intestinal or urinary obstruction
• **Caution**—G6PD deficiency

■ **Maternal Considerations** .... Bacteria in the gut metabolize **sulfasalazine** to 5-aminosalicylic acid and **sulfapyridine** in a fashion unaffected by gender. There are no adequate reports or well-controlled studies of **sulfasalazine** in pregnant women.
Side effects include Stevens-Johnson syndrome, epidermal necrolysis, exfoliative dermatitis, agranulocytosis, hepatitis, peripheral neuropathy, hemolytic anemia, headache, depression, urticaria, rash, pruritus, nausea, vomiting, diarrhea, abdominal pain, anorexia, hematuria, leukopenia, jaundice, and fever.

- **Fetal Considerations** .... There are no adequate reports or well-controlled studies in human fetuses. **Sulfasalazine** and **sulfapyridine** cross the placenta with the M:F concentration ratios reaching unity. Large epidemiologic studies identify no evidence for human teratogenicity. Rodent studies are also reassuring, revealing no evidence of teratogenicity or IUGR despite the use of doses higher than those used clinically.

- **Breastfeeding Safety** .... There are no adequate reports or well-controlled studies in nursing women. Insignificant amounts of uncleaved **sulfasalazine** and 5-aminosalicylic acid are found in human milk; **sulfapyridine** levels are 30-60% of maternal serum. **Sulfapyridine** has poor bilirubin-displacing capacity.

- **References** .... Norgard B, Czeizel AE, Rockenbauer M, et al. Aliment Pharmacol Ther 2001; 15:483-6.
Esbjorner E, Jarnerot G, Wranne L. Acta Paediatr Scand 1987; 76:137-42.
Ambrosius Christensen L, Rasmussen SN, Hansen SH, et al. Acta Obstet Gynecol Scand 1987; 66:433-5.
Connell W, Miller A. Drug Saf 1999; 21:311-23.

- **Summary** ....
  - **Pregnancy Category B**
  - **Lactation Category S**
  - **Sulfasalazine** is first-line therapy for the treatment of inflammatory bowel disease during pregnancy and lactation.

Sulfisoxazole (Gantrisin; Gulfasin; Isoxazine; Lipo Gantrisin; Novosoxazole; Oxazole; Sosol; Soxa; Sulfalar; Sulfazin; Sulfazole; Sulphafurazole; Sulsoxin; Thiasin; Truxazole; Urazole)

- **Class** .... *Antibiotic, sulfonamide*

- **Indications** .... Bacterial infection, e.g., acute, recurrent or chronic urinary tract infections, meningococcal meningitis, otitis media

- **Mechanism** .... Bacteriostatic; inhibits dihydropteroate synthesis

- **Dosage with Qualifiers** .... Bacterial infection—500-1000mg PO q6h ×10-21d
NOTE—renal dosing
  - **Contraindications**—hypersensitivity to drug or class, porphyria
  - **Caution**—hepatic or renal dysfunction

- **Maternal Considerations** .... There are no adequate reports or well-controlled studies of **sulfisoxazole** in pregnant women. **Sulfisoxazole** is an alternative to **ampicillin**, which some feel should no longer be used in the treatment of asymptomatic bacteriuria because of high rates of resistance. It has been used as an alternative for the treatment of chlamydia in **erythromycin**-allergic women.

Side effects include Stevens-Johnson syndrome, jaundice, aplastic anemia, agranulocytosis, leukopenia, thrombocytopenia, pseudomembranous colitis, stomatitis, hepatitis, vasculitis, photosensitivity, anorexia, nausea, vomiting, rash, headache, and dizziness.

■ **Fetal Considerations** — There are no adequate reports or well-controlled studies in human fetuses. It is unknown whether **sulfisoxazole** crosses the human placenta. A large human experience is reassuring as there are no reports suggesting teratogenicity. Rodent studies performed at multiples of the MRHD were associated with cleft palate and bony abnormalities.

■ **Breastfeeding Safety** — There are no adequate reports or well-controlled studies in nursing women. Only small amounts of **sulfisoxazole** enter human breast milk, and it is generally considered compatible with breastfeeding.

■ **References** — McNeeley SG Jr, Ryan GM Jr, Baselski V. Sex Transm Dis 1989; 16:60-2.
Kauffman RE, O'Brien C, Gilford P. J Pediatr 1980; 97:839-41.

■ **Summary** —
- **Pregnancy Category C**
- **Lactation Category S**
- **Sulfisoxazole** should be used during pregnancy and lactation only if the benefit justifies the potential perinatal risk.
- A long clinical experience is reassuring.

Sulindac (Antribid; Arthridex; Biflace; Clinoril; Clisundac; Daclin; Imbaral; Lindak; Lyndak; Reumofil; Sudac)

■ **Class** — *Analgesic, non-narcotic*; NSAIDs

■ **Indications** — Osteoarthritis or rheumatoid arthritis, anti-inflammatory, ankylosing spondylitis, acute gout

■ **Mechanism** — Unknown; inhibits prostaglandin synthesis

■ **Dosage with Qualifiers** — Osteoarthritis or rheumatoid arthritis—150-200mg PO bid; max 400mg/d
Anti-inflammatory—200mg PO bid ×7-14d; max 400 mg/d
Ankylosing spondylitis—150-200mg PO bid; max 400mg/d
Acute gout—150-200mg PO bid; max 400mg/d

- **Contraindications**—hypersensitivity to drug or class, NSAID- or aspirin-induced asthma
- **Caution**—CHF, GI bleeding, hypertension

■ **Maternal Considerations** ⋯⋯⋯ **Sulindac** is a nonsteroidal anti-inflammatory drug, also possessing analgesic and antipyretic activities. It inhibits certain transcription factors such as NF-κβ and AP-1, as does **ibuprofen** but not **indomethacin**. There are no adequate reports or well-controlled studies of **sulindac** in pregnant women. Very limited study suggests it is equally effective as **indomethacin** for the prolongation of pregnancy in women with preterm labor. The use of **sulindac** until 34w after successful tocolysis fails to reduce the incidence of readmission for preterm labor or prolong the gestational age at delivery.
Side effects include GI bleeding, acute renal failure, bronchospasm, thrombocytopenia, Stevens-Johnson syndrome, interstitial nephritis, hepatotoxicity, agranulocytosis, nausea, vomiting, abdominal pain, dyspepsia, constipation, headache, dizziness, rash, drowsiness, urticaria, elevated LFTs, and tinnitus.

■ **Fetal Considerations** ⋯⋯⋯⋯⋯ There are no adequate reports or well-controlled studies in human fetuses. **Sulindac** crosses the human placenta producing F:M ratios approximating 0.4. Like other NSAIDs, **sulindac** causes dose-dependent and reversible ductal constriction and oligohydramnios. Rodent studies reveal an increased incidence of cleft palate (not seen with **indomethacin**), and there is an increased risk of IUGR and fetal death.

■ **Breastfeeding Safety** ⋯⋯⋯⋯ There are no adequate reports or well-controlled studies in nursing women. It is unknown whether **sulindac** enters human breast milk; it does enter rat milk.

■ **References** ⋯⋯⋯⋯⋯⋯⋯⋯⋯ Carlan SJ, O'Brien WF, O'Leary TD, Mastrogiannis D. Obstet Gynecol 1992; 79:223-8.
Humphrey RG, Bartfield MC, Carlan SJ, et al. Obstet Gynecol 2001; 98:555-62.
Kramer WB, Saade GR, Belfort M, et al. Am J Obstet Gynecol 1999; 180:396-401.
Lampela ES, Nuutinen LH, Ala-Kokko TI, et al. Am J Obstet Gynecol 1999; 180:174-80.
Tegeder I, Pfeilschifter J, Geisslinger G. FASEB J 2001; 15:2057-72.
Montenegro MA, Palomino H. J Craniofac Genet Dev Biol 1990; 10:83-94.

■ **Summary** ⋯⋯⋯⋯⋯⋯⋯⋯⋯⋯
- **Pregnancy Category C**
- **Lactation Category U**
- Though NSAIDs share certain characteristic effects on pregnant women and their fetus, they are not interchangeable.
- **Sulindac** should be used during pregnancy and lactation only if the benefit justifies the potential perinatal risk.

Sumatriptan (Imigran; Imitrex)

- **Class** — Migraine; serotonin receptor agonist

- **Indications** — Migraine headache

- **Mechanism** — 5HT-1 agonist

- **Dosage with Qualifiers** — Migraine headache—6mg SC ×1, may repeat in 1h; max 12mg/d, or 25-100mg PO ×1, may repeat after 2h, max 200mg/d, or 1 spray per nostril (20mg/spray)
  NOTE—available in oral, parenteral and nasal spray forms
  - **Contraindications**—hypersensitivity to drug or class, uncontrolled hypertension, CAD, basilar or hemiplegic migraine, MAO inhibitor <14d
  - **Caution**—peripheral or cerebrovascular disease, hepatic dysfunction, 5HT-1 or ergot derivative agonist <24h, cardiac risk factors

- **Maternal Considerations** — There are no adequate reports or well-controlled studies of **sumatriptan** in pregnant women.
  Side effects include coronary vasospasm, acute MI, ventricular tachycardia, ventricular arrhythmia, death, hypertensive crisis, stroke, bowel or peripheral vascular ischemia, asthenia, chest pain, neck tightness, dizziness, flushing, paresthesias, rhinitis (spray), rash, taste changes (spray), pruritus, urticaria, tinnitus (spray), myalgias, palpitations, somnolence, and sweating.

- **Fetal Considerations** — There are no adequate reports or well-controlled studies in human fetuses. Only a small amount of **sumatriptan** (<5%) crosses the human placenta by passive transport, and should pose minimal risk to the fetus. Metabolites do not cross. Epidemiologic studies are reassuring. Rodent studies conducted at doses at least 6 times the MRHD revealed embryotoxicity and vascular and skeletal abnormalities. No adverse effects were noted at lower doses.

- **Breastfeeding Safety** — There are no adequate reports or well-controlled studies in nursing women. A small amount of **sumatriptan** enters human breast milk, but the quantity absorbed by the neonate will be negligible.

- **References** —
Loder E. CNS Drugs 2003; 17:1-7.
Schenker S, Yang Y, Perez A, et al. Proc Soc Exp Biol Med 1995; 210:213-20.
Shuhaiber S, Pastuszak A, Schick B, et al. Neurology 1998; 51:581-3.
Fox AW, Chambers CD, Anderson PO, et al. Headache 2002; 42:8-15.
Wojnar-Horton RE, Hackett LP, Yapp P, et al. Br J Clin Pharmacol 1996; 41:217-21.

■ Summary ·······························

- **Pregnancy Category C**
- **Lactation Category S?**
- **Sumatriptan** should be used during pregnancy and lactation only if the benefit justifies the potential perinatal risk.
- A fairly large body of clinical experience is reassuring.

Tacrine (Cognex; THA)

- **Class** — *Alzheimer's*

- **Indications** — Alzheimer's dementia

- **Mechanism** — Reversible cholinesterase inhibitor

- **Dosage with Qualifiers** — Alzheimer's dementia—begin 10mg PO qid ×4w; increase by 10mg qid q4w based on response
  - **Contraindications**—hypersensitivity to drug or class, **tacrine** hepatotoxicity, hepatic dysfunction, cardiac conduction defects
  - **Caution**—unknown

- **Maternal Considerations** — **Tacrine** acts presumably to elevate acetylcholine in the cerebral cortex by slowing the degradation of acetylcholine released by still intact cholinergic neurons. There is no evidence it alters the underlying dementia process. Plasma concentrations are 50% higher in women than men. There are no adequate reports or well-controlled studies of **tacrine** in pregnant women. The published literature is limited to two case reports 3 decades ago when it was used as a general anesthetic adjunct during cesarean delivery.
  Side effects include hepatotoxicity, bradycardia, seizures, nausea, vomiting, diarrhea, constipation, flatulence, abdominal pain, dyspnea, anorexia, weight loss, rash, agitation, insomnia, ataxia, and confusion.

- **Fetal Considerations** — There are no adequate reports or well-controlled studies in human fetuses. It is unknown whether **tacrine** crosses the human placenta. Rodent teratogenicity studies have not been conducted.

- **Breastfeeding Safety** — There is no published experience in nursing women. It is unknown whether **tacrine** enters human breast milk.

- **References** — No current relevant references

- **Summary** —
  - **Pregnancy Category C**
  - **Lactation Category U**
  - **Tacrine** should be used during pregnancy and lactation only if the benefit justifies the potential perinatal risk.

Tacrolimus (FK 506; Prograf)

■ **Class** — Transplant, immunosuppressant

■ **Indications** — Prophylaxis against liver or kidney transplant rejection

■ **Mechanism** — Inhibits T-cell activation

■ **Dosage with Qualifiers** — Transplant rejection prophylaxis—0.1-0.2mg/kg/d PO in 2 divided doses; alternatively, 0.03-0.05mg/kg/d as continuous IV infusion
  - **Contraindications**—hypersensitivity to drug or class
  - **Caution**—hepatic or renal dysfunction

■ **Maternal Considerations** — A growing number of obstetric patients have benefited from organ transplant. Pregnancy is considered safe if the patient is 2 years after transplantation, has good renal function without proteinuria, no uncontrolled arterial hypertension, and no evidence of ongoing rejection. There are no adequate reports or well-controlled studies of **tacrolimus** in pregnant women. It has been used widely during pregnancy without obvious adverse effect. Clearance is not significantly altered.
Side effects include thrombocytopenia, nephrotoxicity, hypertension, hyperkalemia, seizures, diabetes mellitus, immunosuppression, malignancy, nausea, diarrhea, headache, insomnia, abdominal pain, tremor, weakness, fever, hyperglycemia, anemia, itching, elevated LFTs, anorexia, and renal dysfunction.

■ **Fetal Considerations** — There are no adequate reports or well-controlled studies in human fetuses, and little animal experience. It is unknown whether **tacrolimus** crosses the placenta. Human studies do not reveal obvious evidence of teratogenicity. Immunosuppression is a theoretic concern.

■ **Breastfeeding Safety** — There are no adequate reports or well-controlled studies in nursing women. It is unknown whether **tacrolimus** enters human breast milk.

■ **References** — Kainz A, Harabacz I, Cowlrick IS, et al. Transplantation 2000; 70:1718-21.
Armenti VT, Moritz MJ, Davison JM. Drug Saf 1998; 19:219-32.
Farley DE, Shelby J, Alexander D, Scott JR. Transplantation 1991; 52:106-10.

■ **Summary** —
  - **Pregnancy Category C**
  - **Lactation Category U**
  - Widely used in transplant patients, there is limited information on its reproductive effects.
  - Current experience suggests the benefits of **tacrolimus** far exceed its theoretic risks to the pregnancy and newborn.

Tamoxifen (Dignotamoxi; Nolvadex; Valodex)

- **Class** — *Hormonal oncologic*, SERM, *antineoplastic*

- **Indications** — Breast cancer, mastalgia, ovulation induction

- **Mechanism** — Partial estrogen receptor antagonist/agonist

- **Dosage with Qualifiers** — Breast cancer, metastatic—10-20mg PO qd/bid
  Breast cancer, adjuvant—10mg PO bid ×5y
  Breast cancer, ductal *in situ*—10mg PO bid ×5y after surgery and radiation therapy
  Breast cancer, prophylaxis—10mg PO bid ×5y for high-risk women begun during menses after a negative hCG test
  Mastalgia—10mg PO qd ×4mo
  Ovulation induction—5-40mg PO bid ×4d
  - **Contraindications**—hypersensitivity to drug or class, undiagnosed genital bleeding, history of thromboembolism, **coumarin** anticoagulation
  - **Caution**—bone metastases, thrombocytopenia, leukopenia

- **Maternal Considerations** — **Tamoxifen** is one of four <u>s</u>elective <u>e</u>strogen <u>r</u>eceptor <u>m</u>odulators (SERMs) marketed in the U.S. The effect of SERMs on the estrogen receptor is tissue-dependent. It is an antagonist in the breast. The potential role of **tamoxifen** in the prevention of breast cancer is unclear and the subject of several large ongoing trials. It appears to reduce the incidence of ER+ invasive and noninvasive cancer. Until the completion of these trials, prophylaxis should probably be confined to women at high risk. **Tamoxifen** is an agonist in the uterus, increasing the risk of endometrial cancer and sarcoma. It is associated with an increased risk of thromboembolic disease. **Tamoxifen** does not cause infertility. Rather, it appears equal to **clomiphene** for ovulation induction in anovulatory women. There are no adequate reports or well-controlled studies of **tamoxifen** in pregnant women. The addition of **tamoxifen** to a regimen of **misoprostol** for medical abortion is unnecessary. The published literature includes numerous cases of breast cancer diagnosis during pregnancy, surgery followed by **tamoxifen** therapy usually after the 1st trimester. There were no obvious drug related complications.
  Side effects include thromboembolism, CVA, endometrial cancer, endometrial hyperplasia, hot flashes, vaginal discharge, irregular menses, increased bone or tumor pain, hypercalcemia, thrombocytopenia, leukopenia, pancytopenia, leiomyomas, ovarian cysts, retinopathy, cataracts, dizziness, peripheral edema, fatigue, headache, visual changes, vulvar pruritus, hair loss, anorexia, and elevated LFTs.

■ **Fetal Considerations** .... There are no adequate reports or well-controlled studies in human fetuses. It is unknown whether **tamoxifen** crosses the human placenta. **Tamoxifen** has similar effects on genital tract development as estrogen does. In rodents, **tamoxifen** inhibits uteroplacental artery dilation, decreases placental and fetal weights, and as a consequence increases the risk of fetal death.

■ **Breastfeeding Safety** .... There are no adequate reports or well-controlled studies in nursing women. It is unknown whether **tamoxifen** enters human breast milk. It is generally recommended women not breastfeed while taking **tamoxifen**.

■ **References** .... No authors. Obstet Gynecol 2002; 100:835-43.
Boostanfar R, Jain JK, Mishell DR Jr, Paulson RJ. Fertil Steril 2001; 75:1024-6.
Boostanfar R, Jain JK, Park M, Mishell DR Jr. Contraception 1999; 60:353-6.
Issacs RJ, Hunter W, Clark K. Gynecol Oncol 2001; 80:405-8.
Woo JC, Yu T, Hurd TC. Arch Surg 2003; 138:91-8.
Sadek S, Bell SC. Br J Obstet Gynaecol 1996; 103:630-41.
Nakai M, Uchida K, Teuscher C. J Androl 1999; 20:626-34.
Tewari K, Bonebrake RG, Asrat T, Shanberg AM. Lancet 1997; 350:183.
Helewa M, Levesque P, Provencher D, et al. J Obstet Gynaecol Can 2002; 24:164-80.

■ **Summary** .... • **Pregnancy Category D**
• **Lactation Category U**
• **Tamoxifen** should be avoided during pregnancy and lactation unless maternal survival requires it.

Tazarotene topical (Tazorac)

■ **Class** .... *Dermatologic, retinoid*

■ **Indications** .... Psoriasis, acne vulgaris

■ **Mechanism** .... Unknown; retinoid

■ **Dosage with Qualifiers** .... Psoriasis—apply to affected area qhs
Acne vulgaris—apply to affected area qhs
NOTE—obtain pregnancy test before initiating therapy; available in cream (.05%) and gel (0.05 and 0.1%) formats
• **Contraindications**—hypersensitivity to drug or class, pregnancy
• **Caution**—avoid sun

■ **Maternal Considerations** ⋯⋯⋯ There is no published experience with **tazarotene** during pregnancy. The maternal systemic concentration is reportedly low.
Side effects include birth defects, pruritus, burning, erythema, and irritation.

■ **Fetal Considerations** ⋯⋯⋯ There are no adequate reports or well-controlled studies in human fetuses. It is unknown whether **tazarotene** crosses the human placenta. The maternal systemic concentration is reportedly low, and unpublished rodent teratogenicity studies reputedly are reassuring. Other drugs in this group are potent teratogens in mammals. Rodents treated topically with doses approximating 20% of the surface area have a greater risk of embryo loss and fetal malformation including neural tube and cardiac anomalies.

■ **Breastfeeding Safety** ⋯⋯⋯ There is no published experience in nursing women. It is unknown whether **tazarotene** enters human breast milk. It is excreted into rodent milk. However, considering the dose and route, it is unlikely the breast-fed neonate would ingest clinically relevant amounts.

■ **References** ⋯⋯⋯ Duvic M. Cutis 1998; 61:22-6.

■ **Summary** ⋯⋯⋯
- **Pregnancy Category X**
- **Lactation Category U**
- **Tazarotene** is a known teratogen in rodents even at levels below the MRHD, and should probably be avoided during pregnancy and lactation pending the availability of additional study confirming safety.

Technetium Tc⁹⁹ᵐ (Cardiolite; Cardiotec; Cardiotech; Ceretec; Miraluma; Neurolite; NeoTect; RBC-Scan; Ultratag)

■ **Class** ⋯⋯⋯ *Diagnostic radiopharmaceutical*

■ **Indications** ⋯⋯⋯ Diagnostic imaging

■ **Mechanism** ⋯⋯⋯ Radioactive label attached to a variety of peptides with assorted binding profiles

■ **Dosage with Qualifiers** ⋯⋯⋯ Available in multiple formats bound to a variety of peptides for imaging of structures such as the heart, brain and biliary system, localization of malignancy and bleeding
- **Contraindications**—hypersensitivity to drug or class
- **Caution**—unknown

■ **Maternal Considerations** ---- **Technetium Tc[99m]** decays by isomeric transition with a half-life of 6h. Its clearance is reduced in women. There are no adequate reports or well-controlled studies of **technetium** in pregnant women. There is a long clinical experience, which supports its use during pregnancy when medically indicated. A diagnostically indicated test should not be withheld because of pregnancy.
Side effects include metallic taste, burning at the injection site, facial swelling, numbness of hand/arm, hypotension and nausea.

■ **Fetal Considerations** ---- There are no adequate reports or well-controlled studies in human fetuses. **Technetium** crosses the human placenta, but delivers a maximal total fetal dose of <5mGy, far below the 50mGy considered the threshold for concern. Rodent teratogenicity studies have not been performed.

■ **Breastfeeding Safety** ---- There are no adequate reports or well-controlled studies in nursing women. **Technetium Tc[99m]** is excreted in human milk during lactation for about 24h after administration. Formula feedings for at least 24h after testing seem prudent.

■ **References** ---- Romney BM, Nickoloff EL, Esser PD, Alderson PO. Radiology 1986; 160:549-54.
Adelstein SJ. Teratology 1999; 59:236-9.
Owunwanne A, Omu A, Patel M, et al. J Nucl Med 1998; 39:1810-3.

■ **Summary** ----
- **Pregnancy Category C**
- **Lactation Category S?**
- **Technetium** should be used during pregnancy and lactation only if the benefit justifies the potential perinatal risk.
- Pregnancy is not a valid reason to withhold a diagnostically indicated test.

Tegaserod (Zelnorm)

■ **Class** ---- *Gastrointestinal; serotonin receptor agonist*

■ **Indications** ---- Irritable bowel syndrome in women characterized by constipation

■ **Mechanism** ---- 5-HT4 agonist stimulating peristalsis while decreasing visceral sensitivity

■ **Dosage with Qualifiers** ---- Irritable bowel syndrome—6mg PO 30-60min before meals bid ×4-6w; may repeat ×1

- **Contraindications**—hypersensitivity to drug or class, severe renal dysfunction, moderate to severe hepatic disease, history bowel obstruction, abdominal adhesions, sphincter Oddi dysfunction, symptomatic gallbladder disease, diarrhea
- **Caution**—mild hepatic dysfunction

■ **Maternal Considerations** ·········· There are no published reports of **tegaserod** during pregnancy.
Side effects include cholecystitis, headache, nausea, abdominal pain, flatulence, diarrhea, and dizziness.

■ **Fetal Considerations** ············ There are no adequate reports or well-controlled studies in human fetuses. It is unknown whether **tegaserod** crosses the human placenta. Rodent studies are reassuring, revealing no evidence of teratogenicity or IUGR despite the use of doses higher than those used clinically.

■ **Breastfeeding Safety** ············ There is no published experience in nursing women. **Tegaserod** enters human breast milk with a high M:P ratio. Its impact on the neonate is unknown.

■ **References** ·········· There is no published experience in pregnancy or during lactation.

■ **Summary** ··········
- **Pregnancy Category B**
- **Lactation Category U**
- **Tegaserod** should be used during pregnancy and lactation only if the benefit justifies the potential perinatal risk.
- There are alternative agents for which there is more experience during pregnancy and lactation that may suffice in the short term.

Telmisartan (Micardis)

■ **Class** ·········· ACE-I/A2R-*antagonist*

■ **Indications** ·········· Hypertension

■ **Mechanism** ·········· AT1 antagonist

■ **Dosage with Qualifiers** ·········· Hypertension—begin 40mg PO qd if monotherapy; max 80mg/d
- **Contraindications**—hypersensitivity to drug or class, pregnancy
- **Caution**—history of ACE-I angioedema, renal artery stenosis, hepatic or renal dysfunction, CHF, hyponatremia

- **Maternal Considerations** ········ The plasma concentration of **telmisartan** is 2-3 times higher in females than in males. There is no published experience with **telmisartan** during pregnancy. Inhibitors of the renin angiotensin system should be avoided during pregnancy for fetal indications. The lowest dose effective should be used when **telmisartan** is required during pregnancy for pressure control.

  Side effects include angioedema, hypotension, dizziness, URI symptoms, back pain, diarrhea, fatigue, dyspepsia, neutropenia, leukopenia, and hyperkalemia.

- **Fetal Considerations** ········ There are no adequate reports or well-controlled studies in human fetuses. It is unknown whether **telmisartan** crosses the human placenta. Inhibitors of the renin angiotensin system are considered contraindicated during pregnancy. No adverse fetal effects are reported from 1st trimester exposure to AT1 antagonists. However, later exposure is associated with cranial hypoplasia, anuria, reversible or irreversible renal failure, death, oligohydramnios, prematurity, IUGR, and patent ductus arteriosus. If oligohydramnios is observed, **telmisartan** should be discontinued unless considered lifesaving. Antenatal surveillance may be appropriate, depending upon gestational age. Oligohydramnios may not appear until after irreversible injury. Neonates exposed should be closely observed for hypotension, oliguria, and hyperkalemia. Rodent studies are reassuring, revealing no evidence of teratogenicity or IUGR despite the use of doses higher than those used clinically.

- **Breastfeeding Safety** ········ There is no published experience in nursing women. It is unknown whether **telmisartan** enters human breast milk. It is excreted into rodent milk.

- **References** ········ There is no published experience in pregnancy or during lactation.

- **Summary** ········
  - **Pregnancy Category C (1st trimester), D (2nd and 3rd trimesters)**
  - **Lactation Category U**
  - **Telmisartan** should be used during pregnancy and lactation only if the benefit justifies the potential perinatal risk.
  - The lowest dose effective should be used when **telmisartan** is required during pregnancy for pressure control.
  - There are numerous alternative agents with a superior safety profile for which there is more experience during pregnancy and lactation.

Temazepam (Euhypnos; Levanxol; Normison; Planum; Restoril)

- **Class** — *Benzodiazepine 2, sedative/hypnotic*

- **Indications** — Insomnia

- **Mechanism** — Benzodiazepine and possibly GABA receptor agonist

- **Dosage with Qualifiers** — Insomnia, short-term—7.5-30mg PO qhs
  - **Contraindications**—hypersensitivity to drug or class
  - **Caution**—azole antifungal

- **Maternal Considerations** — Residual medication effects ("hangover") are essentially absent, and early morning awakening, a particular problem for the geriatric patient, is significantly reduced compared to similar agents. REM sleep is unchanged. There are no adequate reports or well-controlled studies of **temazepam** in pregnant women. One case report suggested an association with a fetal demise.
  Side effects include respiratory depression, seizures, coma, drowsiness, headache, fatigue, nervousness, lethargy, dizziness, nausea, vomiting, anxiety, depression, dry mouth, diarrhea, abdominal pain, euphoria, weakness, blurred vision, nightmares, and vertigo.

- **Fetal Considerations** — There are no adequate reports or well-controlled studies in human fetuses. **Temazepam** crosses the second trimester human placenta achieving an F:M ratio approximating 0.38 1h after 10mg IV. The ratio was stabile between 60-120min, but rose with advancing gestation age. Third trimester studies are unavailable. Several studies suggest an increased prevalence of fetal malformation after **diazepam** use during the 1st trimester. Decreased fetal movement frequently follows IV **diazepam** administration, and prolonged CNS depression may occur in neonates due to their inability to metabolize. It is unknown whether the effect of **temazepam** is similar. The shortest course and the lowest dose should be used if indicated during pregnancy. Rodent teratogenicity studies reveal an increased prevalence of skeletal abnormalities and embryo loss.

- **Breastfeeding Safety** — There is no published experience in nursing women. It is unknown whether **temazepam** enters human breast milk. Benzodiazepines in general, and **diazepam** specifically enter human breast milk and may cause lethargy, sedation, and weight loss in infants. Some newborns exposed antenatally to **diazepam** exhibit either the floppy infant syndrome, or marked neonatal withdrawal symptoms.

■ References .... Cooper J, Jauniaux E, Gulbis B, Bromley L. Reprod Biomed Online 2001; 2:165-171.

■ Summary ....
• **Pregnancy Category X**
• **Lactation Category NS?**
• **Temazepam** should be used during pregnancy and lactation only if the benefit justifies the potential perinatal risk.
• There are alternative agents for which there is more experience during pregnancy and lactation.
• While it is unlikely a one-time use would cause harm, continuous use should be avoided during pregnancy and lactation.

Temozolomide (Temodar; Temoxol)

■ **Class** .... *Antineoplastic, alkylating agent*

■ **Indications** .... Astrocytoma, refractory

■ **Mechanism** .... Alkylates guanine

■ **Dosage with Qualifiers** .... <u>Astrocytoma, refractory</u>—multiple dosing regimens based on response and side effects
• **Contraindications**—hypersensitivity to drug or class, hypersensitivity to DTIC
• **Caution**—hepatic or renal dysfunction

■ **Maternal Considerations** .... There is no published experience with **temozolomide** during pregnancy.
Side effects include myelosuppression, nausea, vomiting, abdominal pain, constipation, diarrhea, headache, fever, convulsions, hemiparesis, amnesia, insomnia, and viral infection.

■ **Fetal Considerations** .... There are no adequate reports or well-controlled studies in human fetuses. It is unknown whether **temozolomide** crosses the human placenta. Rodent teratogenicity studies reveal an increased prevalence of multiple malformations.

■ **Breastfeeding Safety** .... There is no published experience in nursing women. It is unknown whether **temozolomide** enters human breast milk.

■ **References** .... There is no published experience in pregnancy or during lactation.

■ **Summary** .... • **Pregnancy Category D**
• **Lactation Category U**
• **Temozolomide** should be used during pregnancy and lactation only if the benefit justifies the potential perinatal risk; it is reserved for life-threatening circumstances.

Tenecteplase (THKase)

■ **Class** .... *Anticoagulant, thrombolytic*

■ **Indications** .... Myocardial infarction

■ **Mechanism** .... Tissue plasminogen activator

■ **Dosage with Qualifiers** .... Myocardial infarction, acute—30-50mg IV ×1, weight dependent; max 50mg
• **Contraindications**—hypersensitivity to drug or class, active internal bleeding, stroke, aneurysm, intracranial/spinal surgery or trauma, bleeding diathesis, uncontrolled hypertension
• **Caution**—severe hepatic disease, hypertension, recent surgery or trauma, CVD, GPIIb/IIIa use, endocarditis, acute pericarditis, LV thrombus,

■ **Maternal Considerations** .... There is no published experience with **tenecteplase** during pregnancy.
Side effects include intracranial hemorrhage, stroke, severe bleeding, arrhythmia, and angioedema.

■ **Fetal Considerations** .... There are no adequate reports or well-controlled studies in human fetuses. It is unknown whether **tenecteplase** crosses the human placenta. Rodent studies are reassuring, revealing no evidence of teratogenicity or IUGR despite the use of doses higher than those used clinically. Embryotoxicity occurs with high doses.

■ **Breastfeeding Safety** .... There is no published experience in nursing women. It is unknown whether **tenecteplase** enters human breast milk.

■ **References** .... There is no published experience in pregnancy or during lactation.

■ **Summary** .... • **Pregnancy Category C**
• **Lactation Category U**
• **Tenecteplase** should be used during pregnancy and lactation only if the benefit justifies the potential perinatal risk.

Tenofovir (Viread)

- **Class** — Antiviral; *reverse transcriptase inhibitor*

- **Indications** — HIV infection

- **Mechanism** — Nucleotide reverse transcriptase inhibitor

- **Dosage with Qualifiers** — HIV infection—300mg PO qd in combination with other retrovirals
  - **Contraindications**—hypersensitivity to drug or class, CrCl <60ml/min, lactic acidosis
  - **Caution**—alcoholism, hepatic dysfunction

- **Maternal Considerations** — There is no published experience with **tenofovir** during pregnancy.
  Side effects include lactic acidosis, hepatomegaly with steatosis, nausea, vomiting, diarrhea, anorexia, and flatulence.

- **Fetal Considerations** — There are no adequate reports or well-controlled studies in human fetuses. It is unknown whether **tenofovir** crosses the human placenta. **Tenofovir** crosses the rhesus monkey placenta sufficiently well to lower the fetal viral load. In doing so, there is a transient delay in bone growth that may be IGF-I mediated. Rodent studies are reassuring, revealing no evidence of teratogenicity or IUGR despite the use of doses higher than those used clinically.

- **Breastfeeding Safety** — There is no published experience in nursing women. It is unknown whether **tenofovir** enters human breast milk. It is excreted into rodent milk. Breastfeeding is contraindicated in HIV-infected nursing women where formula is available to reduce the risk of neonatal transmission.

- **References** — Tarantal AF, Castillo A, Ekert JE, et al. J Acquir Immune Defic Syndr 2002; 29:207-20.

- **Summary** —
  - **Pregnancy Category B**
  - **Lactation Category NS**
  - **Tenofovir** should be used during pregnancy and lactation only if the benefit justifies the potential perinatal risk.
  - There are alternative agents for which there is more experience during pregnancy and lactation.
  - Breastfeeding is contraindicated in HIV-infected nursing women where formula is available to reduce the risk of neonatal transmission.
  - Physicians are encouraged to register pregnant women under the Antiretroviral Pregnancy Registry (1-800-258-4263) for a better follow-up of the outcome while under treatment with **tenofovir**.

Terazosin (Hytrin)

- **Class** — Antiadrenergic, α blocker

- **Indications** — Hypertension

- **Mechanism** — Peripheral α-1 antagonist

- **Dosage with Qualifiers** — Hypertension—begin 1mg PO qhs; max 20mg/d
  - **Contraindications**—hypersensitivity to drug or class
  - **Caution**—unknown

- **Maternal Considerations** — There is no published experience with **terazosin** during pregnancy.
  Side effects include hypotension after the first dose, dizziness, vertigo, headache, palpitations, atrial fibrillation, thrombocytopenia, asthenia, nasal congestion, peripheral edema, pain, paresthesias, polyuria, nervousness, and blurred vision.

- **Fetal Considerations** — There are no adequate reports or well-controlled studies in human fetuses. It is unknown whether **terazosin** crosses the human placenta. While rodent studies are generally reassuring, revealing no evidence of teratogenicity, embryotoxicity and IUGR were noted after doses higher than those used clinically.

- **Breastfeeding Safety** — There are no adequate reports or well-controlled studies in nursing women. It is unknown whether **terazosin** enters human breast milk.

- **References** — There is no published experience in pregnancy or during lactation.

- **Summary** —
  - **Pregnancy Category C**
  - **Lactation Category U**
  - **Terazosin** should be used during pregnancy and lactation only if the benefit justifies the potential perinatal risk.
  - There are alternative agents for which there is more experience during pregnancy and lactation.

Terbinafine (Lamisil)

■ Class — Antifungal

■ Indications — Onychomycosis, tinea

■ Mechanism — Inhibits squalene epoxidase, reducing cell membrane ergosterol synthesis

■ Dosage with Qualifiers — Onychomycosis—250mg PO qd ×6w (fingernails) or 12w (toenails)
Tinea—250mg PO qd ×2w
NOTE—check LFTs at baseline; CBC count if >6w
- **Contraindications**—hypersensitivity to drug or class
- **Caution**—hepatic or renal dysfunction

■ Maternal Considerations — There is no published experience with **terbinafine** during pregnancy.
Side effects include hepatic failure, hepatotoxicity, Stevens-Johnson syndrome, erythema multiforme, toxic epidermal necrolysis, rash, pruritus, neutropenia, headache, diarrhea, dyspepsia, nausea, abdominal pain, constipation, flatulence, and urticaria.

■ Fetal Considerations — There are no adequate reports or well-controlled studies in human fetuses. It is unknown whether **terbinafine** crosses the human placenta. Rodent studies are reassuring, revealing no evidence of teratogenicity or IUGR despite the use of doses higher than those used clinically.

■ Breastfeeding Safety — There is no published experience in nursing women. Reportedly, **terbinafine** achieves an M:P ratio of 7:1 after oral administration. Until data to the contrary, breastfeeding should be avoided.

■ References — There is no published experience in pregnancy or during lactation.

■ Summary
- **Pregnancy Category B**
- **Lactation Category NS**
- **Terbinafine** should be used during pregnancy only if the benefit justifies the potential perinatal risk.
- **Terbinafine** should probably be avoided during breastfeeding.
- There are alternative agents for which there is more experience during pregnancy and lactation.

Terbutaline (Brethaire; Brethancer; Brethine; Bricanyl; Monovent; Syntovent)

- **Class** .... *Adrenergic, β agonist; bronchodilator*

- **Indications** .... Asthma, tocolysis

- **Mechanism** .... β-2 agonist

- **Dosage with Qualifiers** .... Asthma—5mg PO q6h prn; max 15mg/d; or, 2 puffs INH q4-6h; or 0.25mg SC q15-30min ×2
  Tocolysis—0.25mg SC q30min; max 1mg/4h; or, 2.5-10mcg/min IV, max 30mcg/min
  NOTE—available in oral, inhaler, or parenteral forms
  - **Contraindications**—hypersensitivity to drug or class
  - **Caution**—diabetes mellitus, infection (with tocolysis), hypertension, hyperthyroidism, arrhythmia, seizures, hypokalemia

- **Maternal Considerations** .... **Terbutaline** is a popular and effective agent for the treatment of asthma during pregnancy. While generally considered a selective β-2 agonist based on *in vitro* study, its clinical profile is less specific. As with all other betamimetics and most tocolytic agents, **terbutaline** is associated with approximately a 48h delay in delivery compared to placebo in women with preterm labor. Pregnancy outcome is altered only when coupled with antenatal steroid administration. As it is for all other currently available drugs, the use of either oral or continuous SC treatment is ineffective preterm labor prophylaxis. Maternal side effects are common and often lead to discontinuation of therapy. Serious adverse reactions include pulmonary edema and maternal death has been reported with **terbutaline**. Several large meta-analyses conclude that of the currently available agents, **nifedipine** is the tocolytic of choice.
  Side effects include pulmonary edema, hypotension, tachycardia, palpitations, arrhythmia, nervousness, tremor, headache, nausea, vomiting, drowsiness, sweating, muscle cramps, and hyperglycemia.

- **Fetal Considerations** .... There are no adequate reports or well-controlled studies in human fetuses. **Terbutaline** crosses the human placenta, achieving an F:M ratio between 0.11-0.48 after a single IV dose immediately prior to elective cesarean delivery. Multiple case reports suggest it is chronotropic in fetuses with complete heart block. The effect, if any, is often transient perhaps because β-adrenergic innervation is still relatively immature even at birth. Paradoxically, there is no receptor desensitization demonstrable in the fetal rat heart exposed chronically to **terbutaline**. Rodent studies are reassuring showing no evidence of teratogenicity or IUGR despite the use of doses higher than those used clinically. **Terbutaline** increases the frequency of fetal breathing. Chronic **terbutaline** exposure increases cardiac size and the heart rate in fetal guinea pigs. Overall, it appears long-term **terbutaline** use has measurable fetal affects.

■ **Breastfeeding Safety** ⋯ There are no adequate reports or well-controlled studies in nursing women. **Terbutaline** is excreted into human breast milk reaching M:P ratios in excess of 2. Yet, the amount ingested is less than 1% of the maternal dose, and the neonatal level undetectable.

■ **References** ⋯
Ann Allergy Asthma Immunol 2000; 84:475-80.
Goldenberg RL. Obstet Gynecol 2002; 100:1020-37.
Wenstrom KD, Weiner CP, Merrill D, Niebyl J. Am J Perinatol 1997; 14:87-91.
Guinn DA, Goepfert AR, Owen J, et al. Am J Obstet Gynecol 1998; 179:874-8.
Tsatsaris V, Papatsonis D, Goffinet F, et al. Obstet Gynecol 2001; 97:840-7.
Robinson BV, Ettedgui JA, Sherman FS. Cardiol Young 2001; 11:683-6.
Auman JT, Seidler FJ, Slotkin TA. Am J Physiol Regul Integr Comp Physiol 2001; 281:R1079-89.
Petersen R, Carter LS, Chescheir NC, et al. Am J Obstet Gynecol 1989; 161:509-12.
Hallak M, Moise K Jr, Lira N, et al. Am J Obstet Gynecol 1992; 167:1059-63.
Lindberg C, Boreus LO, de Chateau P, et al. Eur J Respir Dis (Suppl)1984; 134:87-91.

■ **Summary** ⋯
- **Pregnancy Category B**
- **Lactation Category S**
- **Terbutaline** is a first-line treatment of asthma during pregnancy and lactation.
- There are alternative agents for tocolysis such as **nifedipine** that are more effective and with a superior safety profile.

Terconazole (Terazol)

■ **Class** ⋯ *Vaginal antifungal, dermatologic*

■ **Indications** ⋯ Vulvovaginal candidiasis

■ **Mechanism** ⋯ Unknown

■ **Dosage with Qualifiers** ⋯ Vulvovaginal candidiasis—1 applicator 4% qhs ×7d, or 8% ×3d, or 1 suppository PV qhs ×3d

NOTE—available in cream (0.4%, 0.8%) and suppository (80mg)
- **Contraindications**—hypersensitivity to drug or class
- **Caution**—unknown

■ **Maternal Considerations** .... **Terconazole** is a member of a series of imidazoles whose effectiveness appears similar. There are no adequate reports or well-controlled studies of **terconazole** in pregnant women. Topical imidazole appears to be more effective than **nystatin** for treating symptomatic vaginal candidiasis in pregnancy. Treatment periods of 7d may be necessary during pregnancy rather than the shorter courses typically recommended.
Side effects include irritation, headache, and pruritus.

■ **Fetal Considerations** .... There are no adequate reports or well-controlled studies in human fetuses. It is unknown whether **terconazole** crosses the human placenta. Rodent studies are generally reassuring, revealing no evidence of teratogenicity or IUGR until the dose exceeds 20 times the MRHD when skeletal abnormalities and embryotoxicity are noted. The no-effect oral dose (10 mg/kg/d) produces a mean peak plasma level in pregnant rats 44 times the mean peak plasma levels seen after intravaginal administration.

■ **Breastfeeding Safety** .... There is no published experience in nursing women. It is unknown whether **terconazole** enters human breast milk.

■ **Reference** .... Young GL, Jewell D. Cochrane Database Syst Rev 2001; (4):CD000225

■ **Summary** ....
- **Pregnancy Category C**
- **Lactation Category U**
- **Terconazole** should be used during pregnancy and lactation only if the benefit justifies the potential perinatal risk.
- There are alternative agents for which there is more experience during pregnancy and lactation.

Tetanus immune globulin (Hyper-Tet; Hypertet)

■ **Class** .... *Immune globulin*

■ **Indications** .... Tetanus prophylaxis following injury with unknown/uncertain vaccination history, active tetanus

■ **Mechanism** .... Passive immunity

- **Dosage with Qualifiers** ········· Tetanus prophylaxis following injury with unknown/uncertain vaccination history—250IU deep IM; administer in different extremities and with separate syringes, **tetanus** and **diphtheria toxoids**
Active tetanus—dose depends on severity; see package insert
  - **Contraindications**—hypersensitivity to drug or class
  - **Caution**—thrombocytopenia, bleeding disorder

- **Maternal Considerations** ······· **Tetanus immune globulin** creates passive immunity to the toxin of *Clostridium tetani*. Naturally acquired immunity to tetanus toxin is rare in the U.S. Universal primary vaccination, with subsequent timed boosters to maintain adequate antitoxin levels, is required for all age groups. There are no adequate reports or well-controlled studies of **tetanus immune globulin** in pregnant women. Tetanus is a highly lethal disease and a significant cause of maternal death in some locales. It appears the antibodies produced in response to **tetanus toxoid** during pregnancy have low protective capacity, strengthening the importance of **tetanus immune globulin** prophylaxis during pregnancy. The long clinical experience suggests safety. *Side effects* include injection site soreness, fever, angioneurotic edema, and nephrotic syndrome.

- **Fetal Considerations** ················ There are no adequate reports or well-controlled studies in human fetuses. **Tetanus immune globulin** crosses the human placenta and provides at least partial coverage for the neonate. Maternal immunization does not interfere with neonatal response to the DPT series. The degree of IgG transfer is lower in the preterm compared to the term neonate, and there appears a maximal transfer rate. Rodent teratogenicity studies have not been performed, but there is no reason to hypothesize the antibody may damage the fetus.

- **Breastfeeding Safety** ············· There are no adequate reports or well-controlled studies in nursing women. It is unknown whether **tetanus immune globulin** enters human breast milk. However, the long clinical experience in humans is reassuring. It does enter the colostrum of horses and actually can reduce the foal's response to vaccination.

- **References** ······························· Pasetti MF, Dokmetjian J, Brero ML, et al. Am J Reprod Immunol 1997; 37:250-6.
Okoko BJ, Wesuperuma LH, Ota MO, et al. J Health Popul Nutr 2001; 19:59-65.
Kutukculer N, Kurugol Z, Egemen A, et al. J Trop Pediatr 1996; 42:308-9.
Morell A, Sidiropoulos D, Herrmann U, et al. Pediatr Res 1986; 20:933-6.
Wesumperuma HL, Perera AJ, Pharoah PO, Hart CA. Ann Trop Med Parasitol 1999; 93:169-77.
Wilson WD, Mihalyi JE, Hussey S, Lunn DP. Equine Vet J 2001; 33:644-50.

■ **Summary** • **Pregnancy Category C**
 • **Lactation Category S**
 • **Tetanus immune globulin** is considered safe and
    effective during pregnancy and lactation.

Tetanus toxoid (Tetanus toxoid adsorbed)

■ **Class** — *Vaccine*

■ **Indications** — Tetanus susceptibility

■ **Mechanism** — Active immunization

■ **Dosage with Qualifiers** — Tetanus susceptibility—primary immunization, 0.5ml IM
q4-8w ×2, then 0.5ml IM 6-12m after the 2nd trimester;
booster, 0.5ml IM q10y
 • **Contraindications**—hypersensitivity to drug or class,
    acute respiratory infection or other active infection
    (unless emergency), immunosuppressive agents
 • **Caution**—unknown

■ **Maternal Considerations** — Serologic tests demonstrate naturally acquired immunity
to tetanus toxin is rare in the U.S. Universal primary
vaccination, with subsequent timed boosters to maintain
adequate antitoxin levels are required for the protection
all age groups. Tetanus is a highly lethal disease and a
significant cause of maternal death in some locales.
Tetanus toxoid is a highly effective antigen; a completed
primary series generally induces protection that persists
≥10 years. Increasing the interval between primary
immunizing doses for 6mo or longer does not interfere
with the final immunity. Any dose of **tetanus toxoid**
received, even a decade earlier, is counted as the first
immunizing injection. There are no adequate reports or
well-controlled studies of **tetanus toxoid** in pregnant
women. Pregnant women do respond. In many geographic
locales, a cogent argument can be made for routine
immunization with at least one dose during pregnancy to
protect both mother and newborn.
Side effects include injection site soreness, fever, malaise,
lymphadenopathy, generalized aches, hypotension, and
pruritus.

■ **Fetal Considerations** — There are no adequate reports or well-controlled studies
in human fetuses. The antibodies generated in response
to **tetanus toxoid** appear to cross the human placenta,
and are capable of stimulating active immunity in the
term fetus. The long clinical experience with immunization
during pregnancy is reassuring. Maternal immunization

protects against neonatal tetanus and should be public policy in many geographic locales.

■ **Breastfeeding Safety** ⋯⋯⋯ There are no adequate reports or well-controlled studies in nursing women. It is unknown whether **tetanus toxoid** enters human breast milk.

■ **References** ⋯⋯⋯⋯⋯

Rochat R, Akhter HH. Lancet 1999; 354:565.
Maral mI, Cirak M, Aksakal FN, et al. Eur J Epidemiol 2001; 17:661-5.
Gupta SD, Keyl PM. Pediatr Infect Dis J 1998; 17:316-21.
Vanderbeeken Y, Sarfati M, Bose R, Delespesse G. Am J Reprod Immunol Microbiol 1985; 8:39-42.
Czeizel AE, Rockenbauer M. In J Gynaecol Obstet 1999; 64:254-8.

■ **Summary** ⋯⋯⋯⋯⋯
- **Pregnancy Category C**
- **Lactation Category S**
- **Tetanus toxoid** is considered safe and effective during pregnancy and lactation.

Tetracaine (Ak-T-Caine; Dermacaine; Pontocaine; Tetocain)

■ **Class** ⋯⋯⋯⋯⋯ *Anesthetic, spinal/local*

■ **Indications** ⋯⋯⋯⋯⋯ Spinal anesthetic

■ **Mechanism** ⋯⋯⋯⋯⋯ Blocks Na/K channels, inhibiting nerve impulse transmission

■ **Dosage with Qualifiers** ⋯⋯⋯ Spinal anesthesia—5-15mg intraspinal between L2-L4
NOTE—volume load to minimize the risk of hypotension
- **Contraindications**—hypersensitivity to drug or class, associated conditions which increase the risks of spinal anesthesia, including generalized septicemia (relative), injection site infection (absolute), increased ICP (absolute), uncontrolled hypotension (absolute)
- **Caution**—arrhythmia, hypotension, hypovolemia, shock

■ **Maternal Considerations** ⋯⋯⋯ **Tetracaine** produces 2-3h of surgical anesthesia depending on the site of surgery (i.e., intra-abdominal vs lower limb/perineal). The extent and degree of anesthesia depend on dose, specific gravity of the anesthetic solution, volume used, and the position of the patient during and immediately after injection. There are no adequate reports or well-controlled studies of **tetracaine** in pregnant women. Although once routinely used (mixed with either 10% glucose or 10% procaine) for spinal anesthesia for cesarean delivery, **tetracaine** has been supplanted by **bupivacaine** as the spinal agent of choice for cesarean delivery.

Side effects of spinal anesthesia include those related to systemic hypotension-associated medullary/pontine hypoperfusion (e.g., unconsciousness, respiratory/cardiac arrest, nausea, vomiting) as well as those related to post dural puncture headache (e.g., tinnitus, blurry vision, occipitofrontal cephalgia).

■ **Fetal Considerations**

There are no adequate reports or well-controlled studies in human fetuses. It is unknown whether **tetracaine** crosses the human placenta. Considering the dose and route, it is unlikely the maternal systemic concentration will reach clinically relevant level. Rodent teratogenicity studies have not been performed.

■ **Breastfeeding Safety**

There is no published experience in nursing women. It is unknown whether **tetracaine** enters human breast milk. Other local anesthetics are excreted. Considering the indication and dosing, one-time **tetracaine** use is unlikely to pose a clinically significant risk to the breast-feeding neonate.

■ **Reference**

Pan PM, Lin ZF, Lim J, et al. Ma Zui Xue Za Zhi 1989; 27:349-52.

■ **Summary**

- **Pregnancy Category C**
- **Lactation Category S**
- Although supplanted by **bupivacaine** for cesarean delivery, **tetracaine** is still a popular agent for spinal anesthesia for longer surgical procedures.

Tetracycline (Achromycin; Acrimicina; Actisite; Ala-Tet; Alphacycline; Ambramycin; Austramycin; Bekatetracyn; Biocycline; Bristacycline; Brodspec; Cofarcilina; Cyclopar; Emtet-500; Hydracycline; Maviciclina; Nelmicyn; Nor-Tet; Panmycin; Polfamycine; Robitet; Sarocycline; Sumycin; Supramycin; Tega-Cycline; Teline; Telmycin; Tetocyn; Tetracap; Tetrachel; Tetraciclina; Tetracitro-S; Tetracon; Tetracyn; Tetralan; Tetram; Tetramed; Topicycline; Upcyclin; Wesmycin; Wintellin; Wintrex; Xepacycline)

■ **Class**   *Antibiotic, tetracycline*

■ **Indications**   Bacterial infection, *Chlamydia* infection, acne vulgaris

- **Mechanism** — Bacteriostatic; inhibits protein synthesis

- **Dosage with Qualifiers** — Bacterial infection—1-2g qd divided bid or qid at least 1h before or 2h after meals
Chlamydia infection—500mg PO qid at least 1h before or 2h after meals ×7d
Acne vulgaris—250-500mg PO qid at least 1h before or 2h after meals
NOTE—renal dosing; available in oral, ointment (3%) and parenteral formats
  - **Contraindications**—hypersensitivity to drug or class, pregnancy
  - **Caution**—hepatic or renal dysfunction

- **Maternal Considerations** — **Tetracycline** is a broad-spectrum antibiotic prepared from certain *Streptomyces* species. When **penicillin** is contraindicated, tetracycline class agents are alternatives for the treatment of gonorrhea (1.5g PO, then 0.5g qid for a total of 9.0g), syphilis and yaws, *Listeria monocytogenes*, *Clostridium* species, *Bacillus anthracis*, *Fusobacterium fusiforme* (Vincent's infection), and *Actinomyces* species. There are no adequate reports or well-controlled studies of **tetracycline** in pregnant women. It is generally avoided during pregnancy because of fetal considerations.
Side effects include pseudotumor cerebri, hepatotoxicity, Jarisch-Herxheimer reaction, pseudomembranous colitis, pericarditis, tooth discoloration in progeny, nausea, vomiting, dyspepsia, anorexia, diarrhea, photosensitivity, stomatitis, oral and or vulvovaginal candidiasis, urticaria, lightheadedness, dizziness, ataxia, tinnitus, headache, blurred vision, neutropenia, thrombocytopenia and increased BUN.

- **Fetal Considerations** — There are no adequate reports or well-controlled studies in human fetuses. **Tetracycline** crosses the human placenta and may cause a yellow-gray-brown tooth discoloration in adults after fetal/childhood exposure. It is unlikely topically applied **tetracycline** achieves a clinically relevant systemic level. Another tetracycline, **oxytetracycline** (but not **doxycycline**) is associated with an increased risk of NTDs, cleft palate and cardiovascular defects. There are no similar studies for **tetracycline**. Rodent studies are otherwise generally reassuring, revealing no evidence of teratogenicity, but some embryotoxicity at high doses.

- **Breastfeeding Safety** — There are no adequate reports or well-controlled studies in nursing women. **Tetracycline** enters human breast milk, though the kinetics remain to be elucidated. Clinical experience suggests that maternal oral ingestion is compatible with breastfeeding.

- **References** — Czeizel AE, Rockenbauer M. Eur J Obstet Gynecol Reprod Biol 2000; 88:27-33.

■ **Summary**
- **Pregnancy Category D**
- **Lactation Category S**
- Parenteral and oral **tetracycline** should be avoided during pregnancy whenever possible.

Thalidomide (Thalomid)

■ **Class**
Other dermatologic, immunomodulator

■ **Indications**
Erythema nodosum leprosum, HIV wasting, aphthous ulcer

■ **Mechanism**
Unknown

■ **Dosage with Qualifiers**
Restricted access in U.S.—call 1-888-423-5436 for information.
Erythema nodosum leprosum—begin 100-300mg PO ×2w or until symptoms improve, then decrease by 50mg/d q2-4w
HIV wasting—100-300mg PO qhs
Aphthous ulcer—200mg PO qd
NOTE—effective contraception obligatory 1mo before, during, and until 1mo after therapy; document negative hCG test 24h prior to initiating
- **Contraindications**—hypersensitivity to drug or class, pregnancy, moderate /severe neuritis
- **Caution**—seizure disorder, reproductive age, cardiovascular disease

■ **Maternal Considerations**
Thalidomide is a known human teratogen and contraindicated during pregnancy. It is also excreted in semen and treated males should wear a condom during coitus. Initially banned in the U.S., it has proven a superb drug for the treatment of several formerly resistant diseases. Its potential indications are growing, increasing the likelihood of an inadvertent pregnancy. There are no adequate and well-controlled studies of **thalidomide** in pregnant women.
Side effects include severe birth defects, peripheral neuropathy, toxic epidermal necrolysis, seizures, bradycardia, hypertension, orthostatic hypotension, headache, Stevens-Johnson syndrome, drowsiness, dizziness, rash, diarrhea, fever, chills, increased appetite, weight gain, confusion, amnesia, mood changes, photosensitivity, neutropenia, and increased HIV viral load.

■ **Fetal Considerations**
There are no adequate reports or well-controlled studies in human fetuses. **Thalidomide** crosses the human placenta and is a potent human (but not rodent) teratogen causing limb abnormalities after 1st trimester

exposure. Even a single 50mg dose can cause defects. If pregnancy occurs, the drug should be discontinued and the patient referred to a fetal medicine expert for evaluation and counseling. Any suspected fetal exposure to **thalidomide** must be reported to the FDA via the MedWatch program at 1-800-FDA-1088 and also to the Celgene Corporation.

■ **Breastfeeding Safety** — There is no published experience in nursing women. It is unknown whether **thalidomide** enters human breast milk.

■ **References** — Kane S, Stone LJ, Ehrenpreis E. J Clin Gastroenterol 2002; 35:149-50.
Ances BM. Obstet Gynecol 2002; 99:125-8.
Fieldston E. Princet J Bioeth 1998; 1:83-93.
Teo SK, Harden JL, Burke AB, et al. Drug Metab Dispos 2001; 29:1355-7.

■ **Summary** —
- **Pregnancy Category X**
- **Lactation Category U**
- **Thalidomide** is a known and potent human teratogen. It should be avoided during pregnancy and pregnancy termination considered after inadvertent exposure.
- Any suspected fetal exposure to **thalidomide** must be reported to the FDA via the MedWatch program at 1-800-FDA-1088 and also to Celgene Corporation.

Theophylline (Accurbron; Aerolate; Aloefilina; Aminomal; Aquaphyllin; Asmalix; Asperal; Bilordyl; Bronkodyl; Bykofilin; Constant-T; Elixicon; Elixomin; Elixophyllin; Hydro-Spec; Labid; Lanophyllin; Lixolin; Neulin-SA; Phyllocontin; Provent; Pulmo; Respbid; Slo-Bid; Slo-Phyllin; Solu-Phyllin; Somophyllin; Sustaire; T-Phyl; Talofren; Teofilina; Teophyllin; Theo-24; Theo-Dur; Theo-Time; Theobid; Theochron; Theoclear; Theocontin; Theocot; Theolair; Theomar; Theophyl; Theophylline Anhydrous; Theosol-80; Theospan Sr; Theostat 80; Theovent; Theox; Truxophyllin; Uni-Dur; Unifyl; Uniphyl)

■ **Class** — *Bronchodilator; xanthine derivative*

■ **Indications** — Chronic asthma, COPD (maintenance)

■ **Mechanism** — PDE inhibitor increasing cAMP; adenosine receptor antagonist

■ **Dosage with Qualifiers** ⸳⸳⸳⸳ <u>Chronic asthma</u>—begin 300mg PO qd in divided doses bid/tid ×3d, then 400mg/d ×3d, then 600mg/d if tolerated
<u>COPD (maintenance)</u>—begin 300mg PO qd in divided doses bid/tid ×3d, then 400mg/d ×3d, then 600mg/d if tolerated
NOTE—therapeutic level 10-20mcg/ml; exists in multiple formats with varying release rates. Dosing quoted for **theophylline** only.
- **Contraindications**—hypersensitivity to drug or class, arrhythmia, seizures, peptic ulcer disease
- **Caution**—hepatic or renal dysfunction, hypothyroidism

■ **Maternal Considerations** ⸳⸳⸳⸳ **Theophylline** has two distinct actions on the airways of women with reversible airway obstruction: bronchodilation and nonbronchodilator prophylactic effects. Although 1% of pregnant women have asthma, it is often under-recognized and suboptimally treated. Severe, uncontrolled asthma increases the likelihood of maternal and fetal morbidity and death. Pharmacologic therapy is often necessary during pregnancy. Women with well-controlled asthma during pregnancy have outcomes as good as those of their nonasthmatic peers. There are no adequate reports or well-controlled studies of **theophylline** in pregnant women. Its clearance is altered little during either the 1st and 2nd trimesters, but significantly decreased in the 3rd trimester and puerperium. Benefit-risk considerations suggest inhaled asthma medications such as betamimetics and corticosteroids are first-line agents, with **theophylline** a second-line agent for the treatment of asthma during pregnancy. The risk of exacerbation is high immediately post partum, but overall severity usually reverts to preconception levels postpartum. Asthma tends to follow a similar course in subsequent pregnancies.
Side effects include arrhythmia, seizures, respiratory arrest, nausea, vomiting, headache, insomnia, rash, alopecia, flushing, fever, nervousness, agitation, tremor, tachycardia, and palpitations.

■ **Fetal Considerations** ⸳⸳⸳⸳ There are no adequate reports or well-controlled studies in human fetuses. **Theophylline** crosses the human placenta reaching an F:M ratio of unity in a brief time. It dilates *in vitro* constricted placental arteries. While the limited rat teratogen studies are reassuring, **theophylline** producing more than 5 times the recommended human therapeutic concentration causes fetal toxicity, cleft palate, and skeletal malformations in rabbits. In the chick (a poor model for humans), **theophylline** is associated with an increased prevalence of cardiovascular malformations.

■ **Breastfeeding Safety** ⸳⸳⸳⸳ There are no adequate reports or well-controlled studies in nursing women. **Theophylline** enters human breast milk, achieving an M:P ratio between 0.6 and 0.9. It can cause irritability in the nursing newborn, presumably because of the long neonatal half-life. Neonatal toxicity is unlikely. Women who choose to breastfeed should monitor their children's behavior closely.

■ **References** .... Dombrowski MP. Obstet Gynecol Clin North Am 1997; 24:559-74.

Schatz M. Semin Perinatol 2001; 25:145-52.

Shibata M, Wachi M, Kawaguchi M, et al. Methods Find Exp Clin Pharmacol 2000; 22:101-7.

Omarini D, Barzago MM, Bortolotti A, et al. Eur J Drug Metab Pharmacokinet 1993; 18:369-74.

Walters WA, Boura AL. Reprod Fertil Dev 1991; 3:475-81.

Gardner MJ, Schatz M, Cousins L, et al. Eur J Clin Pharmacol 1987; 32:289-95.

Reinhardt D, Richter O, Brandenburg G. Monatsschr Kinderheilkd 1983; 131:66-70.

■ **Summary** ....
- **Pregnancy Category C**
- **Lactation Category S?**
- **Theophylline** should be used during pregnancy and lactation only if the benefit justifies the potential perinatal risk.
- Though the long clinical experience is reassuring, **theophylline** cannot be excluded as a weak human teratogen at high doses.

Thiabendazole (Mintezol; Tiabendazole; Triasox)

■ **Class** .... *Antiparasitic*

■ **Indications** .... Helminthic infection, cutaneous larva migrans, visceral larva migrans, trichinosis, dracunculosis

■ **Mechanism** .... Unknown

■ **Dosage with Qualifiers** .... Helminthic (systemic pinworm, whipworm, roundworm, threadworm) infection—1.5g PO q12h ×2d; max 3g/d
Cutaneous larva migrans—25mg/kg PO q12h ×5-7d; max 3g/d
Visceral larva migrans—25mg/kg PO q12h ×5-7d; max 3g/d
Trichinosis—25mg/kg PO q12h ×5-7d; max 3g/d
Dracunculosis—25-37.5mg/kg PO q12h ×3d; max 3g/d
NOTE—take after meals with fruit juice; chew tablets before swallowing
- **Contraindications**—hypersensitivity to drug or class, pinworm prophylaxis
- **Caution**—hepatic or renal dysfunction, anemia, volume depletion, malnutrition

■ **Maternal Considerations** .... **Thiabendazole** is usually a second-line therapy for pinworm behind **piperazine**. However, when enterobiasis occurs, additional therapy is not required for most patients. **Thiabendazole** should be used for the following only when more specific therapy is unavailable or cannot be used or when further therapy with a second agent is desirable: uncinariasis (hookworm: *Necator americanus* and *Ancylostoma duodenale*); trichuriasis (whipworm); ascariasis (large roundworm). There are no adequate reports or well-controlled studies of **thiabendazole** in pregnant women. *Side effects* include hepatic dysfunction, jaundice, Stevens-Johnson syndrome, erythema multiforme, seizures, hallucinations, nausea, vomiting, diarrhea, malodorous urine, nephrotoxicity, leukopenia, headache, numbness, tinnitus, yellow or blurred vision, dry mouth, rash, pruritus, dizziness, somnolence, and altered mental state.

■ **Fetal Considerations**

There are no adequate reports or well-controlled studies in human fetuses. It is unknown whether **thiabendazole** crosses the human placenta. It crosses the rodent placenta, though the kinetics remain to be elucidated. Rodent teratogen studies are inconsistent, revealing skeletal and cleft palate abnormalities at 10 times the MRHD in only some investigations. These adverse effects are now thought likely the product of maternal toxicity.

■ **Breastfeeding Safety**

There are no adequate reports or well-controlled studies in nursing women. It is unknown whether **thiabendazole** enters human breast milk.

■ **References**

Lankas GR, Nakatsuka T, Ban Y, et al. Food Chem Toxicol 2001; 39:367-74.
Yoneyama M, Ogata A, Fujii T, Hiraga K. Food Chem Toxicol 1984; 22:731-5.

■ **Summary**

- **Pregnancy Category C**
- **Lactation Category U**
- **Thiabendazole** should be used during pregnancy and lactation only if the benefit justifies the potential perinatal risk.
- Though probably not a significant human teratogen, it should be used only as a second-line agent.

Thiamine (Actamin; Alivio; Anacrodyne; Benerva; Beneuril; Beneuron; Betabion; Betalin S; Betamin; Betatabs; Betaxin; Bevitine; Bewon; Biamine; Dumovit; Invite; Metabolin; Oryzanin; Ottovit; Tiamina; Vitamin B₁; Vitanon; Vitantial)

■ **Class**

Vitamin, nutritional

■ **Indications**

Dietary supplement, Wernicke's encephalopathy, beriberi, wet beriberi with CHF

■ **Mechanism** ⋯⋯⋯⋯⋯⋯⋯⋯⋯ Replacement

■ **Dosage with Qualifiers** ⋯⋯⋯ <u>Dietary supplement</u>—1.1mg PO qd
<u>Wernicke's encephalopathy</u>—100mg IV ×1, then 50-100mg
IM/IV qd
<u>Beriberi</u>—10-20mg IM tid ×2w
<u>Wet beriberi with CHF</u>—10-30mg IV tid
- **Contraindications**—hypersensitivity to drug or class,
- **Caution**—unknown

■ **Maternal Considerations** ⋯⋯⋯ Pure **thiamine** deficiency is rare. Multiple vitamin
deficiencies should be suspected in any case of dietary
inadequacy. There are no adequate reports or well-controlled
studies of **thiamine** in pregnant women. Despite its
inclusion in prenatal vitamins, **thiamine** deficiency is not
uncommon during pregnancy. Wernicke's encephalopathy is
reported, often in association with hyperemesis. When given
as part of a multivitamin prenatal supplement, **thiamine**
improves weight gain among HIV-infected women.
Side effects include cyanosis, angioedema, pruritus,
urticaria, warmth, and injection site reaction.

■ **Fetal Considerations** ⋯⋯⋯⋯ There are no adequate reports or well-controlled studies
in human fetuses. **Thiamine** is actively transported across
the human placenta, reaching an F:M ratio of 10. Thus,
maternal supplementation is unlikely to alter the fetal
thiamine to any clinically relevant extent.

■ **Breastfeeding Safety** ⋯⋯⋯⋯ There are no adequate reports or well-controlled studies
in nursing women. **Thiamine** enters human breast milk,
and maternal supplementation increases milk content.
The **thiamine** content in milk from unsupplemented
women is considered inadequate for requirements of the
neonate.

■ **References** ⋯⋯⋯⋯⋯⋯⋯⋯⋯ Villamor E, Msamanga G, Spiegelman D, et al. Am J Clin
Nutr 2002; 76:1082-90.
Baker H, DeAngelis B, Holland B, et al. J Am Coll Nutr
2002; 21:33-7.
Zempleni J, Link G, Kubler W. Int J Vitam Nutr Res 1992;
62:165-72.
Link G, Zempleni J, Bitsch I. Int J Vitam Nutr Res 1998;
68:242-8.
Nail PA, Thomas MR, Eakin R. Am J Clin Nutr 1980;
33:198-204.

■ **Summary** ⋯⋯⋯⋯⋯⋯⋯⋯⋯⋯ - **Pregnancy Category A**
- **Lactation Category S**
- **Thiamine** is a standard component of prenatal vitamins.
  Yet, thiamine deficiency is not rare.
- Attention to **thiamine** replacement is important in
  women with presumed hyperemesis.

Thioguanine (Tabloid)

■ Class — *Antineoplastic, antimetabolite*

■ Indications — Acute nonlymphocytic leukemia

■ Mechanism — Purine analog that interfere with nucleic acid biosynthesis

■ Dosage with Qualifiers — <u>Acute nonlymphocytic leukemia</u>—multiple dosing regimens, typically as part of a multidrug protocol
- **Contraindications**—hypersensitivity to drug or class
- **Caution**—unknown

■ Maternal Considerations — There are no adequate reports or well-controlled studies of **thioguanine** in pregnant women. The published literature includes only case reports.
Side effects include bone marrow suppression, hyperuricemia, nausea, vomiting, anorexia, stomatitis, intestinal necrosis and perforation, jaundice and hepatomegaly.

■ Fetal Considerations — There are no adequate reports or well-controlled studies in human fetuses. It is unknown whether **thioguanine** crosses the human placenta. Though many of the reported cases end with a normal outcome, few women receive monotherapy. It seems likely **thioguanine** is at least a modest teratogen in humans. **Thioguanine** is teratogenic in rats at 5 times the MRHD, causing embryotoxicity and an increased prevalence of cranial defects, general skeletal hypoplasia, hydrocephalus, ventral hernia, situs inversus, incomplete limb development, and IUGR.

■ Breastfeeding Safety — There is no published experience in nursing women. It is unknown whether **thioguanine** enters human breast milk.

■ References — Requena A, Velasco JG, Pinilla J, Gonzalez-Gonzalez A.Eur J Obstet Gynecol Reprod Biol 1995; 63:139-41.
De Souza JJ, Bezwoda WR, Jetham D, Sonnendecker EW. S Afr Med J 1982; 62:295-6.
Schafer AI. Arch Intern Med 1981; 141:514-5.

■ Summary
- **Pregnancy Category D**
- **Lactation Category U**
- **Thioguanine** may be used in life-threatening scenarios during pregnancy and lactation where maternal benefit takes precedence.
- **Thioguanine** is likely at least a modest human teratogen.

Thiopental (Pentothal)

■ **Class** — *Barbiturate, anesthesia induction/maintenance*

■ **Indications** — Induction and maintenance of anesthesia, increased intracranial pressure

■ **Mechanism** — CNS depressant

■ **Dosage with Qualifiers** — Induction and maintenance of anesthesia—induction, 4-6mg/kg IV; maintenance 50-100mg IV; repeat as necessary for short surgical procedures
Increased intracranial pressure (ICP)—1.5-3.5mg/kg IV in patients being mechanically hyperventilated; repeat as necessary before continuous IV infusion or substitution with **pentobarbital**
- **Contraindications**—hypersensitivity to drug or class, porphyria
- **Caution**—hepatic or renal dysfunction, severe cardiovascular disease, hypotension, increased ICP, myasthenia gravis, status asthmaticus

■ **Maternal Considerations** — **Thiopental** is an ultra short-acting CNS depressant in use for more than 60 years. It induces hypnosis and anesthesia, but not analgesia. Recovery after a small dose is rapid, with some somnolence and retrograde amnesia. Repeated IV doses lead to prolonged anesthesia because fatty tissues act as a reservoir. There are no adequate reports or well-controlled studies of **thiopental** in pregnant women. It remains a popular agent for rapid sequence induction of general anesthesia for cesarean section. Hypotension and awareness are more common when it is used for induction than when **ketamine** is used. *Side effects* include habituation, respiratory depression, cardiovascular collapse, arrhythmia, hypotension, tachycardia, thrombophlebitis, bradycardia, and dyspnea.

■ **Fetal Considerations** — There are no adequate reports or well-controlled studies in human fetuses. **Thiopental** rapidly crosses the human placenta achieving an F:M ratio approximating 0.8 within 5min of maternal IV administration. However, the long clinical history of use in pregnant women is reassuring. Peak levels occur in the fetal rat in 10min. In the fetal sheep, **thiopental** reduces cerebral blood flow and oxygen delivery, suggesting it should be avoided during a delivery for fetal distress. Rodent teratogen studies have not been performed. **Thiopental** is a teratogen in the chick embryo, increasing the prevalence of CNS malformations.

■ **Breastfeeding Safety** — There are no adequate reports or well-controlled studies in nursing women. **Thiopental** enters human breast milk, but the concentrations are negligible by 36h postoperatively.

- **References** .... Krissel J, Dick WF, Leyser KH, et al. Eur J Anaesthesiol 1994; 11:115-22.
  Esener Z, Sarihasasan B, Guven H, Ustun E. Br J Anaesth 1992; 69:586-8.
  Pickering BG, Palahniuk RJ, Cote J, et al. Can Anaesth Soc J 1982; 29:463-7.
  Morgan DJ, Blackman GL, Paull JD, Wolf LJ. Anesthesiology 1981; 54:474-80.
  Novitt AD, Gilani SH. J Clin Pharmacol 1979; 19:697-700.
  Andersen LW, Qvist T, Hertz J, Mogensen F. Acta Anaesthesiol Scand 1987; 31:30-2.

- **Summary** ....
  - **Pregnancy Category C**
  - **Lactation Category S**
  - **Thiopental** has been used as an adjunct for general anesthesia for decades without obvious pregnancy-specific risk.

Thioridazine (Dazine; Meleretten; Mellaril; Mellaril-S; Novoridazine; Sonapex; Thinin; Winleril)

- **Class** .... *Antipsychotic, phenothiazine*

- **Indications** .... Refractory schizophrenia

- **Mechanism** .... Unknown; D_2 antagonist

- **Dosage with Qualifiers** .... Refractory schizophrenia—begin 50-100mg PO qd after baseline ECG and potassium; max 800mg/d
  - **Contraindications**—hypersensitivity to drug or class, severe hypertension, hypotension, prolonged QT interval, arrhythmia, CNS depression, coma, narrow-angle glaucoma, electrolyte imbalance, paralytic ileus, GI obstruction, bone marrow depression, decreased CY P450 2D6 levels
  - **Caution**—hepatic dysfunction, cardiovascular disease, CNS depressants, seizures, Parkinson's disease

- **Maternal Considerations** .... There are no adequate reports or well-controlled studies of **thioridazine** in pregnant women. The published literature is confined to case reports.
  Side effects include paralytic ileus, neuroleptic malignant syndrome, tardive dyskinesia, torsade de pointes, arrhythmia, menstrual irregularities, cholestatic jaundice, blood dyscrasias, seizures, QT interval prolongation, drowsiness, dry mouth, constipation, nausea, blurred vision, akathisia, tremor, weight gain, edema, galactorrhea, agranulocytosis, and skin or ocular pigmentation.

- **Fetal Considerations** — There are no adequate reports or well-controlled studies in human fetuses. It is unknown whether **thioridazine** crosses the human placenta.

- **Breastfeeding Safety** — There is no published experience in nursing women. It is unknown whether **thioridazine** enters human breast milk.

- **References** — Scanlan FJ. Med J Aust 1972; 1:1271-2.

- **Summary** —
  - **Pregnancy Category C**
  - **Lactation Category U**
  - **Thioridazine** should be used during pregnancy and lactation only if the benefit justifies the potential perinatal risk.

Thiothixene (Navane)

- **Class** — *Antipsychotic; psychosis 3*

- **Indications** — Schizophrenia

- **Mechanism** — Unknown; selective D_2 antagonist

- **Dosage with Qualifiers** — Schizophrenia—begin 2-5mg PO tid; max 60mg/d
  - **Contraindications**—hypersensitivity to drug or class, coma, CNS depression, blood dyscrasias
  - **Caution**—seizures, glaucoma, alcohol withdrawal, CAD

- **Maternal Considerations** — There are no adequate reports or well-controlled studies of **thiothixene** in pregnant women. The published literature consists of a single case report.
  Side effects include neuroleptic malignant syndrome, seizures, tardive dyskinesia, agranulocytosis, drowsiness, restlessness, agitation, insomnia, tardive dyskinesia, hypotension, blurred vision, dry mouth, acute withdrawal syndrome, tachycardia, photosensitivity, and elevated LFTs.

- **Fetal Considerations** — There are no adequate reports or well-controlled studies in human fetuses. It is unknown whether **thiothixene** crosses the human placenta. Rodent studies are reassuring, revealing no evidence of teratogenicity or IUGR despite the use of doses higher than those used clinically.

- **Breastfeeding Safety** — There is no published experience in nursing women. It is unknown whether **thiothixene** enters human breast milk.

■ **Reference** ···················· Milhovilovic M. Neuropsihijatrija 1970; 18:261-3.

■ **Summary** ·····················
- **Pregnancy Category C**
- **Lactation Category U**
- **Thiothixene** should be used during pregnancy and lactation only if the benefit justifies the potential perinatal risk.

Tiagabine (Gabitril)

■ **Class** ·················· Anticonvulsant

■ **Indications** ·················· Partial complex seizures

■ **Mechanism** ·················· Unknown

■ **Dosage with Qualifiers** ·················· <u>Partial complex seizures</u>—begin 4mg PO qd, increase prn to 56mg/d in divided doses with food
NOTE—taper slowly to avoid withdrawal seizures
- **Contraindications**—hypersensitivity to drug or class
- **Caution**—hepatic dysfunction, EEG spike/wave

■ **Maternal Considerations** ·················· **Tiagabine** is a 2nd generation anticonvulsant frequently employed as adjunct therapy. It is not an enzyme inducer, and there is no interaction between **tiagabine** and oral contraceptive agents. There are no adequate reports or well-controlled studies of **tiagabine** in pregnant women. *Side effects* include CNS depression, withdrawal seizures, dizziness, asthenia, somnolence, nausea, vomiting, impaired memory, and nervousness.

■ **Fetal Considerations** ·················· There are no adequate reports or well-controlled studies in human fetuses. It is unknown whether **tiagabine** crosses the human placenta. **Tiagabine** is a rodent teratogen, increasing the prevalence of craniofacial, appendicular, and visceral defects in addition to IUGR.

■ **Breastfeeding Safety** ·················· There is no published experience in nursing women. It is unknown whether **tiagabine** enters human breast milk. It is excreted in rodent milk.

■ **Reference** ·················· Crawford P. CNS Drugs 2002; 16:263-72.

■ **Summary** ··················
- **Pregnancy Category C**
- **Lactation Category U**
- **Tiagabine** should probably be avoided during pregnancy and lactation unless there is no other option.

Ticarcillin (Ticar; Timentin)

■ **Class** ⋯⋯⋯⋯⋯⋯⋯⋯⋯⋯⋯⋯⋯ *Antibiotic, penicillin*

■ **Indications** ⋯⋯⋯⋯⋯⋯⋯⋯⋯ Bacterial infection including septicemia, skin and soft tissue, and acute and chronic respiratory infection

■ **Mechanism** ⋯⋯⋯⋯⋯⋯⋯⋯⋯ Bactericidal; inhibits cell wall mucopeptide synthesis

■ **Dosage with Qualifiers** ⋯⋯ <u>Bacterial infection</u>—3-4g IV/IM q4-6h, or 200-300mg/kg IV div q4-6h; max 24g/d
NOTE—renal dosing; may be combined with **clavulanate** (Timentin) to extend bacterial coverage
● **Contraindications**—hypersensitivity to drug or class
● **Caution**—cephalosporin allergy, renal dysfunction, seizures, sodium restriction, bleeding disorder

■ **Maternal Considerations** ⋯⋯ **Ticarcillin** is an extended spectrum **penicillin**. It is primarily indicated for gram-negative infections and is often combined with an aminoglycoside. **Clavulanic acid** is a β-lactam that inactivates a wide range of β-lactamase enzymes commonly found in microorganisms resistant to penicillins and cephalosporins. The combination of **ticarcillin/clavulanate** has a microbiologic spectrum similar to **gentamicin** and **clindamycin**. There are no adequate reports or well-controlled studies of **ticarcillin** in pregnant women. Like other antibiotics, it reduces the risk of postpartum endomyometritis in women with PPROM, but may increase the proportion of neonates with sepsis secondary to **ampicillin**-resistant organisms. *Side effects* include seizures, thrombocytopenia, Stevens-Johnson syndrome, neutropenia, rash, urticaria, prolonged bleeding time, bleeding, headache, dizziness, hypokalemia, hypernatremia, fatigue, fever, pseudomembranous colitis, flatulence, phlebitis, and elevated LFTs.

■ **Fetal Considerations** ⋯⋯⋯⋯ There are no adequate reports or well-controlled studies in human fetuses. Transfer of **ticarcillin** across the human placenta is slow, but it does accumulate in the fetal compartment over time. Rodent studies are reassuring, revealing no evidence of teratogenicity or IUGR despite the use of doses higher than those used clinically.

■ **Breastfeeding Safety** ⋯⋯⋯⋯ There are no adequate reports or well-controlled studies in nursing women. **Ticarcillin** enters human breast milk. However, the quantity (2-2.5mg/L) is too low to have clinical relevance.

■ **References** ⋯⋯⋯⋯⋯⋯⋯⋯⋯ Edwards RK, Locksmith GJ, Duff P. Obstet Gynecol 2000; 96:60-4.
Fortunato SJ, Bawdon RE, Swan KF, et al. Am J Obstet Gynecol 1992; 167:1595-9.
Von Kobyletzki D, Dalhoff A, Lindemeyer H, Primavesi CA. Infection 1983; 11:144-9.

■ **Summary** ⸺ • **Pregnancy Category B**
• **Lactation Category S**
• **Ticarcillin** is generally considered safe during pregnancy and lactation for the indicated uses.

Ticlopidine (Ticlid)

■ **Class** ⸺ *Platelet inhibitor*

■ **Indications** ⸺ Thrombotic stroke prophylaxis

■ **Mechanism** ⸺ Inhibits ADP-induced platelet fibrinogen binding

■ **Dosage with Qualifiers** ⸺ Thrombotic stroke prophylaxis—250mg PO bid with meals
• **Contraindications**—hypersensitivity to drug or class, severe hepatic dysfunction, active bleeding, blood dyscrasias
• **Caution**—mild to moderate hepatic dysfunction

■ **Maternal Considerations** ⸺ **Ticlopidine** potentiates the effect of **aspirin** or other NSAIDs on platelet aggregation. There are no adequate reports or well-controlled studies of **ticlopidine** in pregnant women. The published experience is limited to case reports. *Side effects* include pancytopenia, agranulocytosis, thrombocytopenia, intracranial hemorrhage, nephrotic syndrome, allergic pneumonitis, TTP, serum sickness, nausea, vomiting, diarrhea, rash, hyponatremia, purpura, and neutropenia.

■ **Fetal Considerations** ⸺ There are no adequate reports or well-controlled studies in human fetuses. It is unknown whether **ticlopidine** crosses the human placenta. Rodent studies are reassuring, revealing no evidence of teratogenicity or IUGR despite the use of doses higher than those used clinically.

■ **Breastfeeding Safety** ⸺ There is no published experience in nursing women. It is unknown whether **ticlopidine** enters human breast milk. It is excreted into rodent milk.

■ **References** ⸺ Ueno M, Masuda H, Nakamura K, Sakata R. Surg Today 2001; 31:1002-4.
Rezig K, Diar N, Walcker JL. Ann Fr Anesth Reanim 2000; 19:544-8.

■ **Summary** ⸺ • **Pregnancy Category B**
• **Lactation Category U**
• **Ticlopidine** is rarely indicated during pregnancy, but does not appear to require any unique considerations.
• There are alternative agents for which there is more experience during pregnancy and lactation.

Timolol (Aquanil; Blocadren; Cusimolol; Dispatim; Equiton; Glauco-Opu; Glucolol; Glucomol; Nyolol; Ocupres; Optimol; Tiloptic; Timoptic; Timoptic-Xe; Timoptol; Timpotic)

■ **Class** — Antiadrenergic, *β-blocker*

■ **Indications** — Hypertension, angina, acute MI, migraine prophylaxis, glaucoma

■ **Mechanism** — Nonselective β-blocker

■ **Dosage with Qualifiers** — Hypertension—begin 10mg PO bid; max 60mg/d
Angina—5-15mg PO tid
Acute MI—10mg PO bid within 4w of MI
Migraine prophylaxis—10mg PO bid
Elevated intraocular pressure—1 gtt qd/bid
- **Contraindications**—hypersensitivity to drug or class, CHF, bradycardia, 2nd or 3rd degree heart block, asthma, cardiogenic shock
- **Caution**—hepatic or renal dysfunction, diabetes mellitus

■ **Maternal Considerations** — There are no adequate reports or well-controlled studies of **timolol** in pregnant women. **Timolol** is superior to α **methyldopa** for the treatment of puerperal hypertension. It is unclear whether **timolol** offers any therapeutic advantage over another β-blocker.
Side effects include CHF, bradycardia, hypotension, bronchospasm, fatigue, dizziness, headache, dyspnea, pruritus, nightmares, and Raynaud's syndrome.

■ **Fetal Considerations** — There are no adequate reports or well-controlled studies in human fetuses. **Timolol** crosses the isolated perfused human placenta, though the *in vivo* kinetics remain to be elucidated. It decreases the fetal heart rate after administration to the ewe. Rodent studies are reassuring, revealing no evidence of teratogenicity or IUGR despite the use of doses higher than those used clinically.

■ **Breastfeeding Safety** — There are no adequate reports or well-controlled studies in nursing women. **Timolol** is excreted into human milk, achieving an M:P ratio of 0.8 in one study, but higher in another. However, the amount ingested by the neonate is likely clinically insignificant.

■ **References** — Schneider H, Proegler M. Am J Obstet Gynecol 1988; 159:42-7.
Fidler J, Smith V, De Swiet M. Br J Obstet Gynaecol 1983; 90:961-5.

■ Summary
• **Pregnancy Category C**
• **Lactation Category S?**
• **Timolol** should be used during pregnancy and lactation only if the benefit justifies the potential perinatal risk.
• There are alternative agents for which there is more experience during pregnancy and lactation.

Tinzaparin (Innohep)

■ **Class** — Anticoagulant, antithrombotic

■ **Indications** — DVT

■ **Mechanism** — Binds ATIII, accelerating its anti-Xa activity

■ **Dosage with Qualifiers** — DVT—175 anti-Xa IU/kg sc qd at least 6d in hospitalized patients; overlap with **warfarin** until therapeutic INR
NOTE—renal dosing
• **Contraindications**—hypersensitivity to drug or class, hypersensitivity to pork products, active or recent bleeding, conduction anesthesia, thrombocytopenia, history of heparin-induced thrombocytopenia
• **Caution**—bleeding tendency, recent major surgery, bacterial endocarditis, uncontrolled hypertension, diabetic retinopathy, platelet inhibitors, renal dysfunction

■ **Maternal Considerations** — Thromboembolic disease remains a major cause of pregnancy morbidity and death. **Tinzaparin** is a low-molecular-weight heparin (LMWH) extracted from pig. It is at least as effective as unfractionated **heparin** for the treatment and prevention of thromboembolic disease. There are no adequate reports or well-controlled studies of **tinzaparin** in pregnant women. Post-cesarean section, it reduces thrombin antithrombin (TAT) complex concentration more effectively than **enoxaparin**. It is unknown whether that enhancement means improved prophylaxis. Most anesthesiologists prefer to wait 24h after the last dose of **tinzaparin** (even if given once a day 175U/kg) before induction of neuraxial anesthesia.
Side effects include hemorrhage, hematoma, skin necrosis, Stevens-Johnson syndrome, injection site reaction, and elevated LFTs.

■ **Fetal Considerations** — There are no adequate reports or well-controlled studies in human fetuses. **Tinzaparin** does not cross the human placenta. Rodent studies are reassuring, revealing no evidence of teratogenicity or IUGR despite the use of doses higher than those used clinically.

Breastfeeding Safety	There are no adequate reports or well-controlled studies in nursing women. It is unknown whether **tinzaparin** enters human breast milk.

References	Ellison J, Thomson AJ, Conkie JA, et al. Thromb Haemoat 2001; 86:1374-8. Samama MM, Gerotziafas GT. Semin Thromb Hemost 2000; 26(Suppl 1): 31-8.

Summary	• **Pregnancy Category B** • **Lactation Category U** • **Tinzaparin** is an alternative to heparin and other LMWHs during pregnancy, but has no clear advantage.

Tobramycin (Aktob; Tobrex; Trazil; Nebcin; Tobradistin; Tobrasix; Toround)

■ **Class**	*Antibiotic, aminoglycoside*

■ **Indications**	Bacterial infection, endocarditis prophylaxis, cystic fibrosis, ocular infection

■ **Mechanism**	Bactericidal; binds 30S ribosomal subunit inhibiting protein synthesis

■ **Dosage with Qualifiers**	Bacterial infections—3-5mg/kg/d in divided doses Endocarditis prophylaxis—1.5mg/kg IV 30-60min pre-procedure Cystic fibrosis—300mg NEB q12h following 28d on/off cycles Ocular infection—1-2 gtt OS/OD q4-6h NOTE—peak 4-12mcg/ml, trough 0.5-2mcg/ml after parenteral use • **Contraindications**—hypersensitivity to drug or class • **Caution**—myasthenia gravis, vestibular/cochlear implant, nephrotoxic agents, renal dysfunction

■ **Maternal Considerations**	There are no adequate reports or well-controlled studies of **tobramycin** in pregnant women. The clearance of **tobramycin** during pregnancy and the puerperium is increased, requiring 3mg/kg or more to obtain adequate peak and trough levels. *Side effects* include nephrotoxicity, ototoxicity, neurotoxicity, pseudotumor cerebri, enterocolitis, diarrhea, nausea, vomiting, pruritus, rash, weakness, tremor, muscle cramps, anorexia, headache, edema, increased salivation, tinnitus, vertigo, agranulocytosis, thrombocytopenia, elevated BUN/Cr, and muscle weakness.

- **Fetal Considerations** ···· There are no adequate reports or well-controlled studies in human fetuses. It is unknown whether **tobramycin** crosses the human placenta. Other aminoglycoside antibiotics do cross, and there are reports of total, irreversible, bilateral congenital deafness after **streptomycin**. Serious side effects to mother, fetus, or newborn are not reported after the treatment with other aminoglycosides. **Tobramycin** likely poses no greater risk than **gentamicin** to the fetus. Systemic levels are much lower after nebulizer or ophthalmic administration compared to parenteral route. In the rat, **tobramycin** accumulates in the placenta. Rodent studies are reassuring, revealing no evidence of teratogenicity or IUGR despite the use of doses higher than those used clinically. The highest doses caused excess maternal toxicity with increased fetal wastage.

- **Breastfeeding Safety** ···· There is no published experience in nursing women. It is unknown whether **tobramycin** enters human breast milk.

- **References** ···· Ferrini AM, Aureli P, Ricciardi C, et al. Pharmacol Res 1992; 26:277-84.

- **Summary** ····
  - **Pregnancy Category D (B for ophthalmic applications)**
  - **Lactation Category U**
  - **Tobramycin** should be used during pregnancy and lactation only if the benefit justifies the potential perinatal risk.
  - There are alternative agents for which there is more experience during pregnancy and lactation.

Tocainide (Tonocard)

- **Class** ···· *Antiarrhythmic* 1B

- **Indications** ···· Ventricular arrhythmia

- **Mechanism** ···· Depresses phase 0 action, potential, stabilizing the membrane

- **Dosage with Qualifiers** ···· Ventricular arrhythmia—begin 400mg PO q8h; max 2g/d; alternate 7.5-11.3mg/kg IV over 15min
  - **Contraindications**—hypersensitivity to drug or class, CHF, 2nd or 3rd degree heart block, hepatic or renal dysfunction
  - **Caution**—unknown

- **Maternal Considerations** ……… **Tocainide** is similar to **lidocaine**. There is no published experience with **tocainide** during pregnancy.
Side effects include blood dyscrasias, pulmonary fibrosis, CHF, ventricular arrhythmia, respiratory arrest, pulmonary edema, pneumonitis, dizziness, nausea, vomiting, diarrhea, rash, nervousness, tremor, confusion, anorexia, mood changes, ataxia, blurred vision, paresthesias, arthritis, tachycardia, and hypotension.

- **Fetal Considerations** ……… There are no adequate reports or well-controlled studies in human fetuses. It is unknown whether **tocainide** crosses the human placenta. Rodent studies are reassuring, revealing no evidence of teratogenicity or IUGR despite the use of doses higher than those used clinically. Embryotoxicity occurs at high doses with maternal toxicity.

- **Breastfeeding Safety** ……… There are no adequate reports or well-controlled studies in nursing women. **Tocainide** enters human breast milk, though the kinetics remain to be elucidated.

- **References** ……… Wilson JH. J Cardiovasc Pharmacol 1988; 12:497.

- **Summary** ………
  - **Pregnancy Category C**
  - **Lactation Category U**
  - **Tocainide** should be used during pregnancy and lactation only if the benefit justifies the potential perinatal risk.
  - There are alternative agents for which there is more experience during pregnancy and lactation.

Tolazamide (Diabewas; Tolinase; Tolisan)

- **Class** ……… *Hypoglycemic, sulfonylurea, 1st generation*

- **Indications** ……… Diabetes mellitus type 2

- **Mechanism** ……… Stimulates islet cell insulin release

- **Dosage with Qualifiers** ……… Diabetes mellitus type 2—100-250mg PO qd; max 1g/d
  - **Contraindications**—hypersensitivity to drug or class, hypersensitivity to sulfonamides
  - **Caution**—unknown

- **Maternal Considerations** ……… Diet remains the first-line treatment of diabetes mellitus type 2. Caloric restriction and weight loss are essential in the obese diabetic patient, and may alone be effective controlling blood glucose and symptoms. The importance of regular physical activity should be stressed, and cardiovascular risk factors identified and corrected if possible. When this approach fails, oral hypoglycemic agents may be indicated. **Tolazamide** is a first-generation sulfonylurea. Sulfonylureas may be associated with an excess of cardiovascular death. There are no adequate reports or well-controlled studies of **tolazamide** in pregnant women. Additional study is necessary. **Insulin** remains the hypoglycemic agent of choice during pregnancy.

Side effects include hypoglycemia, nausea, epigastric fullness, heartburn, leukopenia, agranulocytosis, thrombocytopenia, hemolytic anemia, aplastic anemia, pancytopenia, pruritus, erythema, urticaria, and morbilliform or maculopapular eruptions.

■ **Fetal Considerations** ···········
There are no adequate reports or well-controlled studies in human fetuses. It is unknown whether **tolazamide** crosses the human placenta. Prolonged, severe hypoglycemia (4-10d) has been reported in neonates delivered to women receiving a sulfonylurea at delivery. This is most common with agents with prolonged half-lives. **Tolazamide** should be discontinued at least 2w before the EDC. Rodent studies are reassuring, revealing no evidence of teratogenicity or IUGR despite the use of doses higher than those used clinically. Only with the highest doses (>100 times the MRHD) was embryotoxicity noted.

■ **Breastfeeding Safety** ···········
There are no adequate reports or well-controlled studies in nursing women. It is unknown whether **tolazamide** enters human breast milk. Other sulfonylurea drugs are excreted into breast milk.

■ **References** ···········
There are no current relevant references.

■ **Summary** ···········
- **Pregnancy Category C**
- **Lactation Category U**
- **Insulin** remains the hypoglycemic agent of choice during pregnancy.
- Though some oral hypoglycemic agents may have a role in the treatment of type 2 diabetes mellitus during pregnancy, there are alternative agents for which there is more experience during pregnancy and lactation.

Tolbutamide (Aglicem; Aglycid; Ansulin; Diabecid-R; Dolipol; Fordex; Glucosulfa; Guabeta; Mobenol; Noglucor; Novobutamide; Orabet; Orinase; Orinase Diagnostic; Raston; Tolbusal; Tolbutamida Valdecases)

■ **Class** — *Hypoglycemic, sulfonylurea*

■ **Indications** — Diabetes mellitus type 2

■ **Mechanism** — Stimulates islet cell insulin release

■ **Dosage with Qualifiers** — <u>Diabetes mellitus type 2</u>—1-2g PO qd in divided doses; max 3g/d
  - **Contraindications**—hypersensitivity to drug or class, IDDM sole therapy, DKA
  - **Caution**—hypersensitivity to sulfonamides

■ **Maternal Considerations** — Diet remains the first-line treatment of diabetes mellitus type 2. Caloric restriction and weight loss are essential in the treatment of the obese diabetic patient, and may alone be effective in controlling blood glucose and symptoms. The importance of regular physical activity must also be stressed and cardiovascular risk factors identified and corrected where possible. When this approach fails, oral hypoglycemic agents may be indicated. There are no adequate reports or well-controlled studies of **tolbutamide** in pregnant women. **Insulin** remains the standard hypoglycemic agent of choice during pregnancy.
Side effects include aplastic anemia, thrombocytopenia, bone marrow suppression, hypoglycemia, jaundice, leukopenia, SIADH, **disulfiram**-like reaction, headache, constipation, diarrhea, dyspepsia, anorexia, dizziness, rash, and photosensitivity.

■ **Fetal Considerations** — There are no adequate reports or well-controlled studies in human fetuses. **Tolbutamide** crosses the human placenta relatively efficiently compared to **glyburide**. The fetal pancreas is responsive. Prolonged and severe hypoglycemia (4-10d) is reported in neonates born to mothers receiving a sulfonylurea at the time of delivery. This is reported more frequently with the use of agents having prolonged half-lives. If **tolbutamide** is used during pregnancy, it should be discontinued at least 2w before the expected delivery date. **Tolbutamide** is teratogenic in rats associated with an increased prevalence of ocular and bony abnormalities at doses 25-100 times the human dose. Similar studies in rabbits were negative.

■ **Breastfeeding Safety** — There are no adequate reports or well-controlled studies in nursing women. **Tolbutamide** enters human breast milk, but the kinetics remain to be elucidated.

■ **References** ⋯⋯⋯⋯⋯⋯⋯⋯ Elliott BD, Schenker S, Langer O, et al. Am J Obstet Gynecol 1994; 171:653-60.
Philipps AF, Dubin JW, Raye JR. Pediatr Res 1979;13:1375-8.
Jensen DM, Sorensen B, Feilberg-Jorgensen N, et al. Diabet Med 2000; 17:281-6.
Christesen HB, Melander A. Eur J Endocrinol 1998; 138:698-701.
Moiel RH, Ryan JR. Clin Pediatr (Phila) 1967; 6:480.

■ **Summary** ⋯⋯⋯⋯⋯⋯⋯⋯⋯
- **Pregnancy Category C**
- **Lactation Category S**
- **Insulin** remains the hypoglycemic agent of choice for the treatment of diabetes mellitus during pregnancy and lactation.

Tolmetin (Donison; Midocil; Reutol; Safitex; Tolectin)

■ **Class** ⋯⋯⋯⋯⋯⋯⋯⋯⋯⋯⋯ *Analgesic, non-narcotic*; NSAID

■ **Indications** ⋯⋯⋯⋯⋯⋯⋯⋯ Osteo and rheumatoid arthritis

■ **Mechanism** ⋯⋯⋯⋯⋯⋯⋯⋯ Unknown; inhibits cyclooxygenase and lipoxygenase reducing prostaglandin synthesis

■ **Dosage with Qualifiers** ⋯⋯ Osteoarthritis—200-600mg PO with food tid; max 1800mg/d
Rheumatoid arthritis—200-600mg PO with food tid; max 1800mg/d
- **Contraindications**—hypersensitivity to drug or class, ASA/NSAID-induced asthma
- **Caution**—nasal polyps, GI bleeding, hypertension, CHF

■ **Maternal Considerations** ⋯ There are no adequate reports or well-controlled studies of **tolmetin** in pregnant women.
Side effects include GI bleeding, acute renal failure, bronchospasm, Stevens-Johnson syndrome, interstitial nephritis, hepatotoxicity, dyspepsia, nausea, vomiting, abdominal pain, headache, dizziness, rash, urticaria, drowsiness, tinnitus, agranulocytosis, thrombocytopenia, elevated LFTs, and fluid retention.

■ **Fetal Considerations** ⋯⋯⋯ There are no adequate reports or well-controlled studies in human fetuses. It is unknown whether **tolmetin** crosses the human placenta. Rodent studies performed up to 1.5 times the MRHD were reassuring, revealing no evidence of teratogenicity. However, other drugs in this class are known to cause constriction of the ductus arteriosus *in utero*.

- **Breastfeeding Safety** ⋯⋯⋯ There are no adequate reports or well-controlled studies in nursing women. **Tolmetin** enters human breast milk, though the kinetics remain to be elucidated.

- **Reference** ⋯⋯⋯ Sagraves R, Waller ES, Goehrs HR. Drug Intell Clin Pharm 1985; 19:55-6.

- **Summary** ⋯⋯⋯
  - **Pregnancy Category C**
  - **Lactation Category U**
  - **Tolmetin** should be used during pregnancy and lactation only if the benefit justifies the potential perinatal risk.
  - There are many alternative agents for which there is more experience during pregnancy and lactation.

Tolterodine (Detrol)

- **Class** ⋯⋯⋯ *Antispasmodic*

- **Indications** ⋯⋯⋯ Overactive bladder

- **Mechanism** ⋯⋯⋯ Cholinergic receptor antagonist

- **Dosage with Qualifiers** ⋯⋯⋯ Overactive bladder—2mg PO bid
  NOTE—hepatic dosing
  - **Contraindications**—hypersensitivity to drug or class, narrow-angle glaucoma, gastric obstruction
  - **Caution**—hepatic or renal dysfunction

- **Maternal Considerations** ⋯⋯⋯ There is no published experience with **tolterodine** during pregnancy.
  Side effects include anticholinergic psychosis, dry mouth, headache, dyspepsia, constipation, dry eyes, dizziness, blurred vision, somnolence, chest pain, cough, tachycardia, and peripheral edema.

- **Fetal Considerations** ⋯⋯⋯ There are no adequate reports or well-controlled studies in human fetuses. It is unknown whether **tolterodine** crosses the human placenta. It crosses the rodent placenta concentrating in the placenta and fetal liver, brain, and spinal cord. Rodent studies conducted at does 20-25 times the MRHD revealed embryotoxicity, IUGR, and birth defects including cleft palate and skeletal malformations. In guinea pigs, maternal treatment decreases acetylcholine-mediated relation of isolated aorta.

- **Breastfeeding Safety** ⋯⋯⋯ There is no published experience in nursing women. It is unknown whether **tolterodine** enters human breast milk. It is excreted at low levels into rodent milk with neonates ingesting <0.5% of the dose.

■ **References** .... Pahlman I, d'Argy R, Nilvebrant L. Arzneimittelforschung 2001; 51:125-33.

■ **Summary** ....
- **Pregnancy Category C**
- **Lactation Category U**
- **Tolterodine** should be used during pregnancy and lactation only if the benefit justifies the potential perinatal risk.
- Considering that the indication is not life-threatening, **tolterodine** should be avoided during pregnancy.

Topiramate (Topamax)

■ **Class** .... *Anticonvulsant*

■ **Indications** .... Tonic clonic seizures, adjunct therapy

■ **Mechanism** .... Unknown

■ **Dosage with Qualifiers** .... Seizures, adjunct therapy—25-50mg PO qd, increase 25-50mg/wk; usual dose 400mg/d in divided doses
NOTE—renal dosing
- **Contraindications**—hypersensitivity to drug or class, hepatic dysfunction
- **Caution**—unknown

■ **Maternal Considerations** .... **Topiramate** increases the metabolism of **ethinylestradiol** and progestogens. If a women wishes to take the oral contraceptive pill, the preparation should contain at least 50mcg of **ethinylestradiol**. **Levonorgestrel** implants are contraindicated because of the increased risk of contraceptive failure. Further, it is recommended that **medroxyprogesterone** injections be given q10w rather than q12w. There are no adequate reports or well-controlled studies of **topiramate** in pregnant women. **Folate** supplementation preconception is prudent. As for most psychotropic drugs, monotherapy and the lowest effective quantity given in divided doses to minimize the peaks may minimize the risks. Many recommend vitamin K, 10mg PO qd be given the last 4w of pregnancy for women taking hepatic enzyme-inducing anticonvulsants like **topiramate**. The scientific support for this practice is weak.
Side effects include nephrolithiasis, acute myopia, secondary angle closure glaucoma, dizziness, somnolence, fatigue, language problems, memory difficulty, psychomotor slowing, nervousness, ataxia, nystagmus, depression, diplopia, mood disturbances, paresthesias, tremor, weight loss, confusion, abdominal pain, agitation, and URI.

- **Fetal Considerations** .... There are no adequate reports or well-controlled studies in human fetuses. **Topiramate** readily crosses the human placenta reaching F:M ratios approaching unity. There is too little human experience to make any judgment on fetal risks. **Topiramate** is a teratogen in rodents. There is a dose-dependent increase in the prevalence of craniofacial and limb malformations, and IUGR, even at doses a fraction of the recommended human dose.

- **Breastfeeding Safety** .... There are no adequate reports or well-controlled studies in nursing women. **Topiramate** enters human breast milk at low concentrations; breast-feeding neonates have levels around the lower limit of detection.

- **References** .... Ohman I, Vitols S, Luef G, et al. Epilepsia 2002; 43:1157-60.

- **Summary** ....
  - **Pregnancy Category C**
  - **Lactation Category S**
  - **Topiramate** should be used during pregnancy only if alternative therapy fails to provide adequate seizure control.
  - As for most psychotropic drugs, using monotherapy and the lowest effective quantity given in divided doses to minimize the peaks can minimize the risks.
  - **Topiramate** appears a good choice for breast-feeding women.
  - There are alternative agents for which there is more experience during pregnancy.

Torsemide (Demadex; Presaril)

- **Class** .... Diuretic, loop

- **Indications** .... Hypertension, diuresis for CHF, renal failure, hepatic failure

- **Mechanism** .... Inhibits Na/K/Cl carriers in ascending loop of Henle

- **Dosage with Qualifiers** .... Hypertension—5mg PO qd
  Diuresis for CHF—10-20mg PO/IV qd, double until desired response; max 200mg/d
  Diuresis for renal failure—20mg PO/IV qd, double until desired response; max 200mg/d
  Diuresis for hepatic failure—5-10mg PO/IV qd, double until desired response; max 40mg/d
  - **Contraindications**—hypersensitivity to drug or class, hypersensitivity to sulfonylureas
  - **Caution**—hypersensitivity to sulfonamides, hepatic or renal dysfunction

- ■ **Maternal Considerations** — There is no published experience with **torsemide** during pregnancy. Diuretics should not be used for the treatment of physiologic edema of pregnancy.
  Side effects include ototoxicity, GI bleeding, arrhythmia, ECG abnormalities, dizziness, headache, frequency, nausea, vomiting, diarrhea, dyspepsia, weakness, rhinitis, cough, arthralgia, hyperglycemia, hyperuricemia, hypokalemia, and insomnia.

- ■ **Fetal Considerations** — There are no adequate reports or well-controlled studies in human fetuses. It is unknown whether **torsemide** crosses the human placenta. Rodent studies are reassuring, revealing no evidence of teratogenicity or IUGR despite the use of doses higher than those used clinically.

- ■ **Breastfeeding Safety** — There are no adequate reports or well-controlled studies in nursing women. It is unknown whether **torsemide** enters human breast milk.

- ■ **References** — There is no published experience in pregnancy or during lactation.

- ■ **Summary** —
  - **Pregnancy Category B**
  - **Lactation Category U**
  - **Torsemide** should be used during pregnancy and lactation only if the benefit justifies the potential perinatal risk.
  - There are alternative agents for which there is more experience during pregnancy and lactation.

Tramadol (Adamon; Ultram)

- ■ **Class** — *Other analgesic, narcotic-like*

- ■ **Indications** — Moderate to severe pain

- ■ **Mechanism** — Unknown

- ■ **Dosage with Qualifiers** — Moderate to severe pain—50-100mg PO q4-6h prn
  NOTE—renal and hepatic dosing
  - **Contraindications**—hypersensitivity to drug or class, alcohol or drug use
  - **Caution**—history substance abuse, CNS depressant use, respiratory depressant use, respiratory depression, seizures, head injury, increase ICP, acute abdomen, hepatic or renal dysfunction

- ■ **Maternal Considerations** — **Tramadol** is a centrally acting analgesic. There are no adequate reports or well-controlled studies of **tramadol** in pregnant women. A single study comparing **tramadol** with

meperidine for labor analgesia concluded it created less maternal sedation and fetal respiratory depression. **Tramadol** reduces post-anesthetic shivering with a lower frequency of somnolence than **meperidine**. There is no evidence of a difference between **meperidine** and **tramadol** in terms of pain relief, interval to delivery, or instrumental or operative delivery. It is an excellent oral agent for the relief of significant postoperative pain. *Side effects* include dependency, seizures, angioedema, bronchospasm, respiratory depression, Stevens-Johnson syndrome, toxic epidermal necrolysis, orthostatic hypotension, serotonin syndrome, hallucinations, suicidal ideation, dizziness, nausea, vomiting, somnolence, pruritus, nervousness, anxiety, agitation, euphoria, tremor, spasticity, visual disturbances, incoordination, anorexia, rash, and vasodilatation.

■ **Fetal Considerations**

There are no adequate reports or well-controlled studies in human fetuses. **Tramadol** crosses the human placenta, achieving an F:M ratio of 0.83. Chronic use during pregnancy may lead to physical dependence and postpartum withdrawal symptoms in the newborn. Rodent studies are generally reassuring, revealing only embryo and maternal toxicity at high concentrations, and no teratogenicity or IUGR.

■ **Breastfeeding Safety**

There is no published experience in nursing women. A small amount of **tramadol** enters human breast milk, but the kinetics remain to be elucidated.

■ **References**

Fieni S, Angeri F, Kaihura CT, et al. Acta Biomed Ateneo Parmense 2000; 71(Suppl 1):397-400.
Tsai YC, Chu KS. Anesth Analg 2001; 93:1288-92.
Elbourne D, Wiseman RA. Cochrane Database Syst Rev 2000; (2):CD001237.
Siddik-Sayyid S, Aouad-Maroun M, Sleiman D, et al. Can J Anaesth 1999; 46:731-5.

■ **Summary**

- **Pregnancy Category C**
- **Lactation Category S?**
- **Tramadol** should be used during pregnancy and lactation only if the benefit justifies the potential perinatal risk.
- It is a reasonable oral agent for the management of postoperative pain.

Trandolapril (Mavik)

- **Class** — ACE-I/A2R-*antagonist*

- **Indications** — Hypertension, CHF

- **Mechanism** — ACE inhibitor

- **Dosage with Qualifiers** — Hypertension—begin 1-2mg PO qd; max 8mg/d
  CHF—begin 0.5mg PO qd; max 4mg/d
  NOTE—renal and hepatic dosing; may be combined with **verapamil** (Tarka, 1 tab PO qd/bid) for the treatment of hypertension
  - **Contraindications**—hypersensitivity to drug or class, history of ACE-I angioedema, hereditary angioedema, idiopathic angioedema
  - **Caution**—severe CHF, renal artery stenosis, collagen vascular disease, renal dysfunction, volume depletion, hyponatremia

- **Maternal Considerations** — There is no published experience with **trandolapril** during pregnancy. Agents that inhibit the renin angiotensin system should be avoided during pregnancy for fetal indications.
  Side effects include angioedema, hypotension, acute renal failure, hyperkalemia, hepatotoxicity, neutropenia, agranulocytosis, pancreatitis, cough, hypotension, dizziness, fatigue, hyperkalemia, nausea, vomiting, URI symptoms, musculoskeletal pain, and elevated BUN/Cr levels.

- **Fetal Considerations** — There are no adequate reports or well-controlled studies in human fetuses. It is unknown whether **trandolapril** crosses the human placenta. Other drugs of this class do cross the placenta. No adverse fetal effects are reported from drugs that inhibit the renin angiotensin system given in the 1st trimester exposure. Later exposure is associated with cranial hypoplasia, anuria, reversible or irreversible renal failure, death, oligohydramnios, prematurity, IUGR, and patent ductus arteriosus. If oligohydramnios is observed, **trandolapril** should be discontinued unless considered lifesaving. Antenatal surveillance may be appropriate, depending upon the week of pregnancy. Oligohydramnios may not appear until after the fetus has sustained irreversible injury. Neonates exposed *in utero* should be closely observed for hypotension, oliguria, and hyperkalemia. Rodent and primate studies are reassuring, revealing no evidence of teratogenicity or IUGR despite the use of doses higher than those used clinically.

- **Breastfeeding Safety** — There is no published experience in nursing women. It is unknown whether **trandolapril** enters human breast milk. It is excreted into rodent milk.

- **Reference** ———————————— Matsuura T, Kurio W, Maeda H, et al. J Toxicol Sci 1993; 18(Suppl 1):107-32.

- **Summary** —————————
  - **Pregnancy Category C (1st trimester), D (2nd and 3rd trimesters)**
  - **Lactation Category U**
  - **Trandolapril** should not be used during pregnancy and breastfeeding unless there is no alternative for the control of severe maternal hypertension.
  - There are alternative agents for which there is more experience during pregnancy and lactation.

Tranylcypromine (Parnate)

- **Class** ———————————— Antidepressant 3, MAO inhibitor

- **Indications** ———————— Depression

- **Mechanism** ——————— MAO inhibitor, prostacyclin (PGI2) synthetase inhibitor

- **Dosage with Qualifiers** ——— Depression—30mg PO qd, increase by 10mg/d q1-3w; max 60mg/d
  NOTE—withdraw slowly
  - **Contraindications**—hypersensitivity to drug or class, alcoholism, CHF, severe hepatic or renal dysfunction, pheochromocytoma, narcotic use, alcohol use, ingestion of cheese or other foods with a high tyramine content, excessive caffeine intake
  - **Caution**—unknown

- **Maternal Considerations** ——— Depression is common during and after pregnancy, but typically goes unrecognized. Pregnancy is not a reason *apriori* to discontinue psychotropic drugs.
  Tranylcypromine is best suited for patients who have failed to respond to drugs more commonly used for depression. There is no published experience with **tranylcypromine** during pregnancy. Its inhibition of PGI2 synthetase raises theoretic concerns.
  Side effects include hypertensive crisis, blurred vision, orthostatic hypotension, hepatitis, thrombocytopenia, agranulocytosis, CNS stimulation, increased sweating, shakiness, and weakness.

- **Fetal Considerations** ———— There are no adequate reports or well-controlled studies in human fetuses. It is unknown whether **tranylcypromine** crosses the human placenta. It does cross the rat placenta, but rodent teratogen studies have not been performed.

- **Breastfeeding Safety** — There is no published experience in nursing women. It is unknown whether **tranylcypromine** enters human breast milk. It is excreted into rodent milk. As for most psychotropic drugs, monotherapy and the lowest effective quantity given in divided doses to minimize the peaks may minimize the risks.

- **References** — There is no published experience in pregnancy or during lactation.

- **Summary**
  - **Pregnancy Category C**
  - **Lactation Category U**
  - **Tranylcypromine** should be used during pregnancy and lactation only if the benefit justifies the potential perinatal risk.
  - There are alternative agents for which there is more experience during pregnancy and lactation.
  - As for most psychotropic drugs, using monotherapy and the lowest effective quantity given in divided doses to minimize the peaks can minimize the risks.

Trazodone (Desyrel; Sideril; Trazalon; Trazonil)

- **Class** — *Depression 4*

- **Indications** — Depression

- **Mechanism** — Unknown; serotonin reuptake inhibitor

- **Dosage with Qualifiers** — Depression—begin 150mg PO with meals qd or in divided doses, and increase by 50mg q3d until desired effect; max 400mg/d
  - **Contraindications**—hypersensitivity to drug or class, recent acute MI
  - **Caution**—suicidal risk, CNS depressants, antihypertensive use, electroconvulsive therapy, arrhythmia

- **Maternal Considerations** — Depression is common in reproductive-age women and frequently overlooked or minimized by their care provider. There is no reason *apriori* to deny indicated treatment during pregnancy. The published experience with **trazodone** during pregnancy is limited but reassuring. *Side effects* include hypotension, syncope, drowsiness, bitter taste, dry mouth, nausea, vomiting, headache, blurred vision, fatigue, arthralgia, incoordination, and tremor.

- **Fetal Considerations** — There are no adequate reports or well-controlled studies in human fetuses. It is unknown whether **trazodone** crosses the human placenta. Cohort studies are reassuring, revealing no increase in the prevalence of adverse outcomes. **Trazodone** crosses the rat placenta, and rodent teratogenicity studies reveal an increased risk of embryo absorption and malformations (rabbit) at doses that are multiples of the MRHD.

■ **Breastfeeding Safety** ·············· **Trazodone** enters human breast milk, but the amount ingested by the neonate is not clinically relevant.

■ **References** ············· Einarson A, Bonari L, Voyer-Lavigne S, et al. Can J Psychiatry 2003; 48:106-10.
DeVane CL, Boulton DW, Miller LF, Miller RL. Int J Neuropsychopharmcol 1999; 2:17-23.
Verbeeck RK, Ross SG, McKenna EA. Br J Clin Pharmacol 1986; 22:367-70.

■ **Summary** ·············· • **Pregnancy Category C**
• **Lactation Category S**
• **Trazodone** should be used during pregnancy only if the benefit justifies the potential perinatal risk.
• There are alternative agents for which there is more experience during pregnancy.
• As for most psychotropic drugs, monotherapy and the lowest effective quantity given in divided doses to minimize the peaks may minimize the risks.

Treprostinil (Remodulin)

■ **Class** ·············· *Platelet inhibitor; prostaglandin; vasodilator*

■ **Indications** ·············· Pulmonary hypertension, NYHA class II-IV symptoms

■ **Mechanism** ·············· Unknown; inhibits platelet aggregation, dilates systemic and pulmonary vasculature

■ **Dosage with Qualifiers** ·········· Pulmonary hypertension—begin 1.25ng/kg/min continuous SC infusion, increased in increments no more than 1.25ng/kg/min/w for first 4w, then no more than 2.5ng/kg/min/w for remaining duration depending on clinical response.
NOTE—hepatic dosing
• **Contraindications**—hypersensitivity to drug or class
• **Caution**—abrupt withdrawal, hepatic or renal dysfunction

■ **Maternal Considerations** ·········· Significant pulmonary hypertension is associated with a high maternal mortality rate during the peripartum. There is no published experience with **treprostinil** during pregnancy.

Side effects include rebound pulmonary hypertension, infusion site reaction, headache, diarrhea, nausea, rash, vasodilatation, jaw pain, dizziness, edema, pruritus, and hypotension.

■ **Fetal Considerations** ⋯⋯⋯⋯ There are no adequate reports or well-controlled studies in human fetuses. It is unknown whether **treprostinil** crosses the human placenta. Rodent studies are reassuring, revealing no evidence of teratogenicity or IUGR despite the use of doses higher than those used clinically.

■ **Breastfeeding Safety** ⋯⋯⋯⋯ There is no published experience in nursing women. It is unknown whether **treprostinil** enters human breast milk.

■ **References** ⋯⋯⋯⋯ There is no published experience in pregnancy or during lactation.

■ **Summary** ⋯⋯⋯⋯
- **Pregnancy Category B**
- **Lactation Category U**
- **Treprostinil** should be used during pregnancy and lactation only if the benefit justifies the potential perinatal risk.

Tretinoin (Acnavit; Avita; Avitoin; Cordes-Vas; Dermojuventus; Kerlocal; Relief; Renova; Retin-A; Retin-A Micro; Retinoic Acid; SteiVAA; Vesanoid)

■ **Class** ⋯⋯⋯⋯ *Antineoplastic; acne, retinoid; dermatologic, topical*

■ **Indications** ⋯⋯⋯⋯ Acne vulgaris, acute promyelocytic leukemia

■ **Mechanism** ⋯⋯⋯⋯ Unknown

■ **Dosage with Qualifiers** ⋯⋯⋯ <u>Acne vulgaris</u>—apply qhs 30min after washing and drying skin
<u>Acute promyelocytic leukemia</u>—45 mg/m^2/d PO given in evenly divided doses bid until complete remission; discontinue 30d after remission or after 90d of treatment; continue effective contraception during and 1mo after completion of therapy
- **Contraindications**—hypersensitivity to drug or class
- **Caution**—unknown

■ **Maternal Considerations** ⋯⋯⋯ Some retinoid agents can be highly toxic to the fetus. Within 7d of tretinoin therapy, a blood or urine pregnancy test with a sensitivity of at least 50 mIU/L should be performed. When possible, **tretinoin** should be delayed until a negative result from this test is obtained. When a delay is

989

not possible, the patient should be placed on two reliable forms of contraception. Pregnancy testing and contraception counseling should be repeated monthly throughout the period of tretinoin treatment. **Tretinoin** inhibits *in vitro* decidualization of endometrial stroma. There are no adequate reports or well-controlled studies of **tretinoin** in pregnant women. The published experience consists of case reports of acute promyelocytic leukemia. *Side effects* include peeling, erythema, and blistering after topical therapy; retinoic acid-APL syndrome, hypercholesterolemia and/or hypertriglyceridemia, pseudotumor cerebri, and elevated LFTs after oral therapy.

■ **Fetal Considerations**

There are no adequate reports or well-controlled studies in human fetuses. **Tretinoin** crosses the human placenta. Fewer than 10 neonates have been born to women treated with **tretinoin** during pregnancy (virtually all after the 1st trimester) for acute promyelocytic leukemia. All infants have shown normal growth without any complications. **Tretinoin** is a teratogen in rodents and primates when given orally. Reported defects in these species include abnormalities of the CNS, musculoskeletal system, ear, eye, thymus, great vessels, facial dysmorphia, cleft palate, and parathyroid hormone deficiency. The offspring of diabetic mice are more prone to develop caudal regression after **tretinoin** exposure. The teratogenic effect of topically applied drug is less clear and is likely low if used as directed.

■ **Breastfeeding Safety**

There is no published experience in nursing women. It is unknown whether **tretinoin** enters human breast milk.

■ **References**

Nau H. J Am Acad Dermatol 2001; 45:S183-7.
Brar AK, Kessler CA, Meyer AJ, et al. Mol Hum Reprod 1996; 2:185-93.
Maeda M, Tyugu H, Okubo T, et al. Rinsho Ketsueki 1997; 38:770-5.
Chan BW, Chan KS, Koide T, et al. Diabetes 2002; 51:2811-6.

■ **Summary**

- **Pregnancy Category D (oral), C (topical)**
- **Lactation Category U**
- **Tretinoin** should be avoided during pregnancy and lactation unless maternal risk dictates it and there are no alternatives.
- The fetal risk remains unclear.

Triamcinolone (Aristcort; Aristo-Pak; Aristocort; Extracort; Kenacort; Oricort; Triaminoral; Acetocot; Aricin; Aristocort Topical; Aristogel; Azmacort; Cenocort A-40; Cinalog; Cinolar; Cinonide 40; Delta-Tritex; Flutex; Kena-Plex 40; Kenac; Kenaject-40; Kenalog; Kenalog-10; Kenalone; Kenonel; Nasacort; Oracort; Oralone; Sholog K; Tac; Tramacort 40; Tri-Kort; Triacet; Triacort; Triam-A; Triamcinair; Triamcot; Triamonide 40; Trianide; Triatex; Triderm; Trilog; Trylone A; Trymex; Amcort; Aristocort Forte; Aristocort Suspension; Articulose-L.A.; Cenocort Forte; Kenacort; Sholog A; Tramacort-D; Tri-Med; Triam-Forte; Triamcot; Triamolone 40; Trilone; Tristo-Plex; Tristoject; Trylone D; U-Tri-Lone; Aristospan Intralesional; Aristospan Parenteral)

■ **Class** — Corticosteroid

■ **Indications** — Adrenal insufficiency, inflammatory disorders, chronic asthma, allergic rhinitis, steroid-responsive dermatitis

■ **Mechanism** — Unknown anti-inflammatory; replacement

■ **Dosage with Qualifiers** —
Adrenal insufficiency—4-12mg PO qd
Inflammatory disorders—4-48mg PO in divided doses qd
Chronic asthma—2 puffs INH tid/qid, rinse mouth after use; max 16 puffs qd
Allergic rhinitis—1-2 sprays/nostril qd; max 2 sprays/nostril qd; discontinue after 3w if no improvement
Steroid-responsive dermatitis—apply sparingly to affected area bid/qid
NOTE—available in oral, topical, inhalational forms
● **Contraindications**—hypersensitivity to drug or class, systemic fungal infection
● **Caution**—CHF, seizures, diabetes mellitus, hypertension, tuberculosis, osteoporosis, hepatic dysfunction, respiratory infection (inhalation), nasal surgery, herpes infection (nasal)

■ **Maternal Considerations** — **Triamcinolone** is a fluorinated glucocorticoid. There are no adequate and well-controlled studies of **triamcinolone** in pregnant women. **Triamcinolone** appears to be at least as efficacious for the treatment of asthma during pregnancy as is **beclomethasone**. The suggestion that chronic topical application might lead to IUGR has yet to be confirmed by others. It is less likely the maternal systemic concentration will reach a clinically relevant level after either topical or inhalational use. In one study, PO **triamcinolone** caused a loss of circadian rhythms of **cortisol**, ACTH, **estradiol** and unconjugated estriol, and modified the ultradian and circadian patterns of FHR. No differences in hormonal and biophysical parameters were found after the end of treatment, suggesting the inhibition of fetal and maternal adrenal glands modifies FHR patterns.

Side effects vary by route of use and include adrenal insufficiency (long-term therapy, LT), steroid psychosis (LT), immunosuppression (LT), menstrual irregularities, peptic ulcer, CHF, osteoporosis (LT), cataracts, nausea, vomiting, dyspepsia, appetite change, edema, headache, dizziness, mood swings, insomnia, anxiety, sinusitis, hypertension, pharyngitis, oral candidiasis, eczema, hyperglycemia, hypokalemia, ecchymoses, acne, folliculitis, dry skin, skin atrophy, and impaired wound healing.

■ **Fetal Considerations** ⋯⋯⋯⋯ There are no adequate reports or well-controlled studies in human fetuses. It is unknown whether **triamcinolone** crosses the human placenta. However, it does cross the nonhuman primate placenta and is relatively resistant to placental metabolism. The resulting F:M ratio approximates 0.6. Further, its administration to nonhuman primates at doses 5-60 times (10mg/kg) the MRHD increases the prevalence of IUGR and craniofacial defects. The extensive fetoplacental metabolism of **cortisol** to inactive metabolites and the resistance of **triamcinolone** to metabolic conversion result in greater **triamcinolone** than **cortisol** exposure. **Triamcinolone** also crosses the rodent placenta, and its fetal half-life is significantly prolonged compared to **cortisol**. In several rodent models, **triamcinolone** causes cleft lip and palate, whereas **cortisol** does not. While there is no epidemiologic evidence suggesting PO **triamcinolone** is a teratogen in humans, prescribing caution especially during the 1st trimester seems prudent. It is less likely the maternal systemic concentration will reach a clinically relevant level after either topical or inhalational use.

■ **Breastfeeding Safety** ⋯⋯⋯ There is no published experience in nursing women. It is unknown whether **triamcinolone** enters human breast milk. Topically applied drug likely poses little risk to the nursing newborn.

■ **References** ⋯⋯⋯⋯⋯⋯⋯⋯

Dombrowski MP, Brown CL, Berry SM. J Matern Fetal Med 1996; 5:310-3.
Katz VL, Thorp JM Jr, Bowes WA Jr. Am J Obstet Gynecol 1990; 162:396-7.
Arduini D, Rizzo G, Parlati E, et al. Prenat Diagn 1986; 6:409-17.
Tarara RP, Wheeldon EB, Hendrickx AG. Teratology 1988; 38:259-70.
Parker RM, Hendrickx AG. Teratology 1983; 28:35-44.
Czeizel AE, Rockenbauer M. Teratology 1997; 56:335-40.
Rowland JM, Althaus ZR, Slikker W Jr, et al. Teratology 1983; 27:333-41.
Slikker W Jr, Althaus ZR, Rowland JM, et al. J Pharmacol Exp Ther 1982; 223:368-74.
Rowland JM, Hendrickx AG. Teratog Carcinog Mutagen 1983; 3:313-9.

■ **Summary**
- **Pregnancy Category C**
- **Lactation Category U**
- **Triamcinolone** should be used during pregnancy and lactation only if the benefit justifies the potential perinatal risk.
- While there is no epidemiologic evidence suggesting PO **triamcinolone** is a human teratogen, prescribing caution seems prudent especially during the 1st trimester.
- It is less likely the maternal systemic concentration will reach a clinically relevant level after either topical or inhalational use.

Triamterene (Dyrenium)

■ **Class** — Diuretic 3, potassium sparing

■ **Indications** — Peripheral edema associated with CHF, cirrhosis, nephrotic syndrome or idiopathic

■ **Mechanism** — Inhibits aldosterone-induced Na^+ resorption in the distal tubule (K^+ sparing)

■ **Dosage with Qualifiers** — Peripheral edema—100mg PO bid after meals
- **Contraindications**—hypersensitivity to drug or class, hyperkalemia, other potassium-sparing agents
- **Caution**—hepatic or renal dysfunction, diabetes mellitus

■ **Maternal Considerations** — **Triamterene** has a unique mode of action. In addition to its diuretic effect, **triamterene** is also a folate antagonist. There are no adequate reports or well-controlled studies of **triamterene** in pregnant women.
Side effects include hyperkalemia, ventricular arrhythmia, nausea, vomiting, fatigue, photosensitivity, rash, dizziness, diarrhea, headache, muscle cramps, dry mouth, weakness and azotemia.

■ **Fetal Considerations** — There are no adequate reports or well-controlled studies in human fetuses. **Triamterene** rapidly crosses the human placenta reaching F:M levels approaching unity. Epidemiologic studies suggest that folate antagonists, including **triamterene**, may increase the risk of not only NTDs, but also of cardiovascular defects, oral clefts, and urinary tract defects. It crosses the rodent placenta. Rodent studies are reassuring, revealing no evidence of teratogenicity or IUGR despite the use of doses higher than those used clinically.

- **Breastfeeding Safety** ⸻ There is no published experience in nursing women. It is unknown whether **triamterene** enters human breast milk. It is excreted into rodent milk.

- **References** ⸻ Hernandez-Diaz S, Werler MM, Walker AM, Mitchell AA. N Engl J Med 2000; 343:1608-14.
Ching MS, Czuba MA, Mihaly GW, et al. J Pharmacol Exp Ther 1988; 246:1093-7.

- **Summary** ⸻
  - **Pregnancy Category B**
  - **Lactation Category U**
  - **Triamterene** should be used during pregnancy and lactation only if the benefit justifies the potential perinatal risk.
  - Epidemiologic studies suggest that folate antagonists, including **triamterene** may increase the risk not only of NTDs, but also of cardiovascular defects, oral clefts, and urinary tract defects.
  - There are alternative agents for which there is more experience during pregnancy and lactation.

Triazolam (Halcion; Somniton; Tialam; Trizam)

- **Class** ⸻ *Benzodiazepine, short-acting; sedative/hypnotic*

- **Indications** ⸻ Insomnia, short-term

- **Mechanism** ⸻ Benzodiazepine receptor agonist

- **Dosage with Qualifiers** ⸻ Insomnia, short term—0.25mg PO qhs
NOTE—hepatic dosing
  - **Contraindications**—hypersensitivity to drug or class
  - **Caution**—hepatic dysfunction, CNS depression, substance abuse

- **Maternal Considerations** ⸻ There are no adequate reports or well-controlled studies of **triazolam** in pregnant women. The published literature consists of scattered case reports.
Side effects include dependency, rebound insomnia, behavioral abnormalities, drowsiness, headache, anxiety, lightheadedness, dizziness, confusion, nervousness, ataxia, dry mouth, constipation, diarrhea, tachycardia, chest pain, dermatitis, and blurred vision.

- **Fetal Considerations** ⸻ There are no adequate reports or well-controlled studies in human fetuses. It is unknown whether **triazolam** crosses the human placenta. However, neonatal CNS depression has followed its use in the immediate antepartal period. Other benzodiazepines do cross the placenta, and in some rodent models, **diazepam** and **chlordiazepoxide** are associated with cleft lip and palate. Rodent teratogen studies have not been conducted.

■ **Breastfeeding Safety** — There is no published experience in nursing women. It is unknown whether **triazolam** enters human breast milk. It is excreted in rodent milk.

■ **References** — Attallah A, Seilanian M, Bavoux F, Choisy H. Rev Fr Gynecol Obstet 1989; 84:47-51.
Sakai T, Matsuda H, Watanabe N. Eur J Pediatr 1996; 155:1065-6.

■ **Summary** —
- **Pregnancy Category X**
- **Lactation Category U**
- **Triazolam** is poorly studied during pregnancy and lactation.
- There are alternative agents for which there is more experience during pregnancy and lactation.

Trifluoperazine (Calmazine; Flupazine; Novoflurazine; Stelazine; Suprazine; TFP)

■ **Class** — Antipsychotic, phenothiazine

■ **Indications** — Schizophrenia, anxiety

■ **Mechanism** — Unknown; selective D_2 antagonist

■ **Dosage with Qualifiers** — Schizophrenia—begin 1-2mg PO bid; typical dose 2.5mg PO bid; max 40mg/d
Anxiety—1-2mg PO bid; max 6mg/d ×3mo
- **Contraindications**—hypersensitivity to drug or class, coma, CNS depression, hepatic disease, bone marrow depression
- **Caution**—unknown

■ **Maternal Considerations** — **Trifluoperazine** has a number of effects, including the inhibition of calmodulin. There are no adequate reports or well-controlled studies of **trifluoperazine** in pregnant women. **Trifluoperazine** also has antiemetic properties similar to other phenothiazines. The published literature consists of scattered, typically uninformative case reports. *Side effects* include neuroleptic malignant syndrome, dry mouth, constipation, orthostatic hypotension, extrapyramidal effects, dizziness, blurred vision, tardive dyskinesia, photosensitivity, rash, nausea, tachycardia, fatigue, headache, weight gain, agranulocytosis, and jaundice.

■ **Fetal Considerations** ⋯⋯⋯ There are no adequate reports or well-controlled studies in human fetuses. **Trifluoperazine** apparently crosses the human placenta, but the kinetics remain to be elucidated. It is oxidized by human placental peroxidase. Calmodulin inhibition has the potential to adversely affect multiple developmentally important pathways. Rodent studies are generally reassuring, revealing no evidence of teratogenicity or IUGR despite the use of doses higher than those used clinically.

■ **Breastfeeding Safety** ⋯⋯⋯ There are no adequate reports or well-controlled studies in nursing women. **Trifluoperazine** enters human breast milk, but apparently at lower concentrations than **haloperidol** and **chlorpromazine**. As for most psychotropic drugs, monotherapy and the lowest effective quantity given in divided doses to minimize the peaks may minimize the risks.

■ **References** ⋯⋯⋯ Boiko SS, Smol'nikova NM. Farmakol Toksikol 1975; 38:701-3.
Yang X, Kulkarni AP. Teratog Carcinog Mutagen 1997; 17:139-51.
Yoshida K, Smith B, Craggs M, Kumar R. Psychol Med 1998; 28:81-91.

■ **Summary** ⋯⋯⋯
- **Pregnancy Category C**
- **Lactation Category S?**
- **Trifluoperazine** should be used during pregnancy and lactation only if the benefit justifies the potential perinatal risk.
- As for most psychotropic drugs, using monotherapy and the lowest effective quantity given in divided doses to minimize the peaks can minimize the risks.
- There are alternative agents for which there is more experience during pregnancy and lactation.

Trimethobenzamide (Anaus; Arrestin; Benzacot; Bio-Gan; Ibikin; Navogan; Stemetic; T-Gen; Tebamide; Tegamide; Ti-Plex; Ticon; Tigan; Tiject-20; Triban; Tribenzagan; Trimazide)

■ **Class** ⋯⋯⋯ *Anticholinergic; antiemetic/antivertgo*

■ **Indications** ⋯⋯⋯ Nausea/vomiting

■ **Mechanism** ⋯⋯⋯ Unknown

■ **Dosage with Qualifiers** ⋯⋯⋯ Nausea/vomiting—300mg PO tid/qid, or 200mg PR/IM tid/qid

- **Contraindications**—hypersensitivity to drug or class
- **Caution**—unknown

■ **Maternal Considerations** ········ There are no adequate reports or well-controlled studies of **trimethobenzamide** in pregnant women. It has been used for the treatment of morning sickness.

Side effects include coma, seizures, diarrhea, disorientation, dizziness, drowsiness, and muscle cramps.

■ **Fetal Considerations** ·············· There are no adequate reports or well-controlled studies in human fetuses. It is unknown whether **trimethobenzamide** crosses the human placenta. One epidemiologic study several decades old suggested an increased prevalence of major malformations. This observation has not been supported by subsequent study. Rodent studies are reassuring, revealing no evidence of teratogenicity or IUGR despite the use of doses higher than those used clinically. Embryotoxicity occurred in several animals treated at 50-60 times the human dose.

■ **Breastfeeding Safety** ·············· There is no published experience in nursing women. It is unknown whether **trimethobenzamide** enters human breast milk.

■ **References** ··························· Kousen M. Am Fam Physician 1993; 48:1279-84.
Miklovich L, van den Berg BJ. Am J Obstet Gynecol 1976; 125:244-8.

■ **Summary** ···························
- **Pregnancy Category C**
- **Lactation Category U**
- **Trimethobenzamide** should be used during pregnancy and lactation only if the benefit justifies the potential perinatal risk. It is a second-line agent.
- There are alternative agents for which there is more experience during pregnancy and lactation.

Trimethoprim (Abaprim; Alprim; Bactin; Idotrim; Ipral; Lidaprim; Methoprim; Monotrim; Primosept; Primsol; Proloprim; Syraprim; TMP-Ratiopharm; Tiempe; Trimexazole; Trimopan; Trimpex; Triprim; Unitrim; Wellcoprim)

■ **Class** ······························· *Antibiotic, folate antagonist*

■ **Indications** ························· UTI, UTI prophylaxis, traveler's diarrhea, P*neumocystis carinii* pneumonia treatment

■ **Mechanism** ························· Inhibits bacterial dihydrofolate reductase

- **Dosage with Qualifiers** ⋯⋯⋯ <u>UTI</u>—100mg PO q12h ×10d
<u>UTI prophylaxis</u>—100mg PO qhs ×6-24w
<u>Traveler's diarrhea</u>—200mg PO bid ×5d
<u>*Pneumocystis carinii* pneumonia treatment</u>—20mg/kg/d PO
in divided doses
NOTE—renal dosing; often combined with sulfamethoxazole
- **Contraindications**—hypersensitivity to drug or class, megaloblastic anemia
- **Caution**—hepatic or renal dysfunction, bone marrow depression, folate deficiency

- **Maternal Considerations** ⋯⋯⋯ Bacteriuria, with or without clinical symptoms, is common during pregnancy. If left untreated, 20-30% develop acute pyelonephritis, which increases the risk of preterm labor and low-birth-weight infants. Established first-line drugs such as **ampicillin, amoxicillin**, and **trimethoprim/sulfamethoxazole** are associated with a high degree of resistance in E. *coli*, the most common pathogen in the urinary tract. **Nitrofurantoin** or a β-lactam agent are also first-line agents for the treatment of asymptomatic bacteriuria. There are no adequate reports or well-controlled studies of **trimethoprim** in pregnant women. A growing number of women are being treated with **trimethoprim** in combination of an array of antivirals for HIV-related complications. The impacts of these combinations are poorly studied. **Trimethoprim/sulfamethoxazole** is used for the treatment of Q fever during pregnancy. Women who develop Q fever should be treated for the duration of pregnancy, specifically if infected during the 1st trimester. *Side effects* include thrombocytopenia, leukopenia, megaloblastic anemia, methemoglobinemia, exfoliative dermatitis, Stevens-Johnson syndrome, fever, aseptic meningitis, toxic epidermal necrolysis, rash, erythema multiforme, pruritus, nausea, vomiting, epigastric pain, glossitis, taste changes, hyperkalemia, hyponatremia, eosinophilia, elevated LFTs, elevated BUN/Cr, and photosensitivity.

- **Fetal Considerations** ⋯⋯⋯ There are no adequate reports or well-controlled studies in human fetuses. Transfer of **trimethoprim** across the human placenta is limited. The combination of **trimethoprim/sulfamethoxazole** has been associated with an increased risk of cardiovascular, NTD and urinary tract malformations. And while there is no solid evidence solo therapy with **trimethoprim** is a human teratogen, the possibility it is a weak human teratogen cannot be excluded. **Trimethoprim** is teratogenic in the rat if given at doses 40 times the MRHD.

- **Breastfeeding Safety** ⋯⋯⋯ There are no adequate reports or well-controlled studies in nursing women. **Trimethoprim** enters human breast milk, but the kinetics remain to be elucidated. Breastfeeding is contraindicated in HIV-infected nursing women where formula is available to reduce the risk of neonatal transmission.

■ **References** .... Raoult D, Fenollar F, Stein A. Arch Intern Med 2002; 162:701-4.

Bawdon RE, Maberry MC, Fortunato SJ, et al. Gynecol Obstet Invest 1991; 31:240-2.

Shepard TH, Brent RL, Friedman JM, et al. Teratology 2002; 65:153-61.

Hernandez-Diaz S, Werler MM, Walker AM, Mitchell AA. Am J Epidemiol 2001; 153:961-8.

■ **Summary** ....
- **Pregnancy Category C**
- **Lactation Category U**
- **Trimethoprim** should be used during pregnancy and lactation only if the benefit justifies the potential perinatal risk.
- Avoid 1st trimester administration.

Trimethoprim/sulfamethoxazole (Bactrim DS/SS; Cotrim DS/SS; SeptraDS/SS/IV)

■ **Class** .... *Sulfonamide, folate antagonist*

■ **Indications** .... Bacterial infection, *Pneumocystis carinii* pneumonia treatment and prophylaxis, acute otitis media, shigellosis

■ **Mechanism** .... See individual drugs

■ **Dosage with Qualifiers** .... Bacterial infection—2 tab (SS) or 1 tab (DS) PO bid, or 4-5mg/kg **trimethoprim** IV q12h, max 960mg/d
Pneumocystis carinii pneumonia treatment—15-20mg/kg **trimethoprim** PO qd divided qid; or 4-5mg/kg **trimethoprim** IV q6h
Pneumocystis carinii pneumonia prophylaxis—2 tab (SS) or 1 tab (DS) PO qd
Acute otitis media—4-5mg/kg **trimethoprim** IV q12h; max 960mg/d
Shigellosis—4-5mg/kg **trimethoprim** IV q12h; max 960mg/d
NOTE—**SS** consists of 80mg **trimethoprim** and 400mg **sulfamethoxazole** and **DS** means double the concentration; renal dosing
- **Contraindications**—hypersensitivity to drug or class, hypersensitivity to sulfonamides, megaloblastic anemia, folate deficiency, G6PD deficiency
- **Caution**—bone marrow suppression, hepatic or renal dysfunction

■ **Maternal Considerations** .... Bacteriuria, with or without clinical symptoms, is common during pregnancy. If left untreated, 20-30% develop acute pyelonephritis, which increases the risk of preterm labor and low-birth-weight infants. Established first-line drugs such as **ampicillin**, **amoxicillin**, and **trimethoprim/ sulfamethoxazole** are associated with a high degree of resistance in E. *coli*, the most common pathogen in the urinary tract. **Nitrofurantoin** or a β-lactam agent are also first-line agents for the treatment of asymptomatic bacteriuria. There are no adequate and well-controlled studies of **trimethoprim/sulfamethoxazole** in pregnant women. See the entries for the individual drugs. A growing number of women are being treated with **trimethoprim** in combination of an array of antivirals for HIV-related complications. The impacts of these combinations are poorly studied. **Trimethoprim/sulfamethoxazole** is also used for the treatment of Q fever during pregnancy. Women who develop Q fever should be treated for the duration of pregnancy, specifically if infected during the 1st trimester. *Side effects* include aplastic anemia, agranulocytosis, blood dyscrasias, Stevens-Johnson syndrome, toxic epidermal necrolysis, fulminate hepatic necrosis, hepatitis, hepatotoxicity, interstitial nephritis, nephrotoxicity, pseudomembranous colitis, aseptic meningitis, bone marrow suppression, methemoglobinemia, hyperkalemia, goiter, SLE, nausea, vomiting, diarrhea, rash, urticaria, photosensitivity, dizziness, GI upset, headache and lethargy.

■ **Fetal Considerations**

There are no adequate reports or well-controlled studies in human fetuses. Transfer of **trimethoprim** across the human placenta is limited. And while there is no solid evidence of teratogenicity in humans, the possibility it is a weak human teratogen cannot be excluded. In contrast, **sulfamethoxazole** readily crosses reaching an F:M ratio approximating unity even in the 1st trimester. See the entries for the individual drugs. The combination has been associated with an increased risk of cardiovascular and urinary tract malformations.

■ **Breastfeeding Safety**

There are no adequate reports or well-controlled studies in nursing women. **Trimethoprim** enters human breast milk, but the kinetics remain to be elucidated. It is unknown whether **sulfamethoxazole** enters human breast milk. Breastfeeding is contraindicated in HIV-infected nursing women where formula is available to reduce the risk of neonatal transmission.

■ **References**

Bawdon RE, Maberry MC, Fortunato SJ, et al. Gynecol Obstet Invest 1991; 31:240-2.
Prokopczyk J, Raczynski A, Troszynski M, et al. Probl Med Wieku Rozwoj 1979; 9:132-3.
Czeizel AE, Rockenbauer M, Sorensen HT, Olsen J. Reprod Toxicol 2001; 15:637-46.

■ **Summary**

- **Pregnancy Category C**
- **Lactation Category U**
- **Trimethoprim/sulfamethoxazole** should be used during pregnancy and lactation only if the benefit justifies the potential perinatal risk.
- Avoid 1st trimester administration.

Trimetrexate (Neutrexin)

■ **Class** .... *Antibiotic, folate antagonist; antiprotozoal*

■ **Indications** .... Pneumocystis carinii pneumonia treatment

■ **Mechanism** .... Inhibits protozoal dihydrofolate reductase

■ **Dosage with Qualifiers** .... *Pneumocystis carinii pneumonia treatment*—45mg/m^2 IV qd
×21d given with **leucovorin**
- **Contraindications**—hypersensitivity to drug or class
- **Caution**—bone marrow depression, hepatic or renal dysfunction

■ **Maternal Considerations** .... **Trimetrexate** with **leucovorin** may have lower toxicity than **trimethoprim/sulfamethoxazole**. There is no published experience with **trimetrexate** during pregnancy. *Side effects* include neutropenia, thrombocytopenia, anemia, nausea, vomiting, confusion, GI pain, hepatic dysfunction, peripheral neuropathy and rash.

■ **Fetal Considerations** .... There are no adequate reports or well-controlled studies in human fetuses. It is unknown whether **trimetrexate** crosses the human placenta. **Trimetrexate** (without **leucovorin**) is teratogenic in rodents with increased risks of skeletal, visceral, ocular, and cardiovascular abnormalities.

■ **Breastfeeding Safety** .... There is no published experience in nursing women. It is unknown whether **trimetrexate** enters human breast milk. Breastfeeding is contraindicated in HIV-infected nursing women where formula is available to reduce the risk of neonatal transmission.

■ **References** .... There is no published experience in pregnancy or during lactation.

■ **Summary** ....
- **Pregnancy Category D**
- **Lactation Category U**
- **Trimetrexate** should be used during pregnancy and lactation only if the benefit justifies the potential perinatal risk.
- There are alternative agents for which there is more experience during pregnancy and lactation.

Trimipramine (Surmontil)

- **Class** — *Antidepressant, tricyclic*

- **Indications** — Depression

- **Mechanism** — Unknown; inhibits serotonin and norepinephrine reuptake

- **Dosage with Qualifiers** — Depression—begin 50-75mg PO qd; max 300mg/d
  NOTE—taper slowly; do not switch rapidly to and from SSRIs
  - **Contraindications**—hypersensitivity to drug or class, acute MI, MAO inhibitor <14d
  - **Caution**—seizures, hepatic dysfunction, glaucoma

- **Maternal Considerations** — Depression is common during and after pregnancy, but typically goes unrecognized. Pregnancy is not a reason *apriori* to discontinue psychotropic drugs. There is no published experience with **trimipramine** during pregnancy.
  Side effects include seizures, ventricular arrhythmia, MI, complete AV heart block, stroke, drowsiness, dizziness, orthostatic hypotension, dry mouth, blurred vision, constipation and diaphoresis.

- **Fetal Considerations** — There are no adequate reports or well-controlled studies in human fetuses. It is unknown whether **trimipramine** crosses the human placenta. Rodent studies are generally reassuring, revealing no evidence of teratogenicity, though embryotoxicity was noted at the highest doses.

- **Breastfeeding Safety** — There is no published experience in nursing women. It is unknown whether **trimipramine** enters human breast milk.

- **References** — There is no published experience in pregnancy or during lactation.

- **Summary** —
  - **Pregnancy Category C**
  - **Lactation Category U**
  - **Trimipramine** should be used during pregnancy and lactation only if the benefit justifies the potential perinatal risk.
  - As for most psychotropic drugs, monotherapy and the lowest effective quantity given in divided doses to minimize the peaks may minimize the risks.
  - There are alternative agents for which there is more experience during pregnancy and lactation.

Tripelennamine (PBZ; PBZ-SR; Pelamine; Pyribenzamine; Triplen)

■ **Class** — Antihistamine

■ **Indications** — Allergy

■ **Mechanism** — Nonselective H antagonist

■ **Dosage with Qualifiers** — Allergy—100mg PO bid SR; alternative 25-50mg PO q4-6h immediate release
- **Contraindications**—hypersensitivity to drug or class, MAO <14d, narrow angle glaucoma, asthma, GI obstruction
- **Caution**—increased intraocular pressure, hyperthyroidism, cardiovascular disease, hypertension

■ **Maternal Considerations** — **Tripelennamine** is often paired illicitly with **pentazocine** to produce euphoria. Known as T's and Blues, users have a greater risk of adverse pregnancy outcome. There are no adequate reports or well-controlled studies of **tripelennamine** in pregnant women.
Side effects include drowsiness, dry mouth, nose, and throat, thickening of bronchial secretions, dizziness, disturbed coordination, epigastric distress, fatigue, chills, confusion, excitation, hysteria, nervousness, irritability, insomnia, anorexia, nausea, vomiting, diarrhea, constipation, hypotension, wheezing, blurred vision, vertigo, tinnitus, convulsions, headache, palpitations, and tachycardia.

■ **Fetal Considerations** — There are no adequate reports or well-controlled studies in human fetuses. It is unknown whether **tripelennamine** crosses the human placenta. However, fetuses of women who abuse T's and Blues have significantly reduced birthweight, length, and head circumference. Withdrawal occurs in about a third. Children of mothers who abused throughout pregnancy demonstrate interactive deficits and withdrawal similar to **methadone**-addicted newborns. The limited rodent studies are reassuring, revealing no evidence of teratogenicity or IUGR despite the use of doses higher than those used clinically.

■ **Breastfeeding Safety** — There is no published experience in nursing women. It is unknown whether **tripelennamine** enters human breast milk.

■ **References** — Little BB, Snell LM, Breckenridge JD, et al. Am J Perinatol 1990; 7:359-62.
von Almen WF 2nd, Miller JM Jr. J Reprod Med 1986; 31:236-9.
Chasnoff IJ, Hatcher R, Burns WJ, Schnoll SH. Dev Pharmacol Ther 1983; 6:162-9.

■ **Summary**
- **Pregnancy Category C**
- **Lactation Category U**
- **Tripelennamine** should be used during pregnancy and lactation only if the benefit justifies the potential perinatal risk.
- There are alternative agents for which there is more experience during pregnancy and lactation.

Trovafloxacin (Trovan)

■ **Class** — Antibiotic, quinolone

■ **Indications** — Bacterial infection due to wide range of gram-negative and gram-positive aerobic and anaerobic bacteria

■ **Mechanism** — Bactericidal; inhibits DNA gyrase and topoisomerase IV

■ **Dosage with Qualifiers** — Bacterial infection—begin 200-300mg IV qd ×1, then switch to 200mg PO qd ×7-14d
NOTE—hepatic dosing
- **Contraindications**—hypersensitivity to drug or class
- **Caution**—hepatic or renal dysfunction, seizures, CNS disorder, dehydration, diabetes mellitus, sun exposure

■ **Maternal Considerations** — There is no published experience with **trovafloxacin** during pregnancy.
Side effects include lethal hepatotoxicity, pseudomembranous colitis, superinfection, increased intracranial pressure, seizures, toxic psychosis, tendon rupture, pancreatitis, nausea, vomiting, diarrhea, abdominal pain, headache, dyspepsia, restlessness, lightheadedness, elevated LFTs, vaginitis, arthralgia, insomnia, pruritus, anxiety, rash, and photosensitivity.

■ **Fetal Considerations** — There are no adequate reports or well-controlled studies in human fetuses. **Trovafloxacin** crosses the human placenta by simple diffusion and is unlikely to reach toxic levels. Rodent studies conducted with more than 10 times the MRHD reveal fetal toxicity and an increased prevalence of skeletal malformations.

■ **Breastfeeding Safety** — There is no published experience in nursing women. **Trovafloxacin** is excreted into human breast milk, but the kinetics remain to be elucidated.

■ **References** — Casey B, Bawdon RE. Infect Dis Obstet Gynecol 2000; 8:228-9.

■ **Summary**

- **Pregnancy Category C**
- **Lactation Category U**
- **Trovafloxacin** should be used during pregnancy and lactation only if the benefit justifies the potential perinatal risk.
- There are alternative agents for which there is more experience during pregnancy and lactation.

Tubocurarine

■ **Class**

Musculoskeletal agent, neuromuscular blocker, nondepolarizing

■ **Indications**

Adjunct to general anesthesia, diagnosis of myasthenia gravis

■ **Mechanism**

Competitive cholinergic receptor blocker at the motor endplate interrupting nerve impulses transmission

■ **Dosage with Qualifiers**

Adjunct to general anesthesia—0.5mg/kg IV for abdominal relaxation or non-emergent tracheal intubation; may repeat 0.1mg/kg q40-60min as indicated by response to train-of-four peripheral nerve stimulation
Diagnosis of myasthenia gravis—0.02-0.04mg/kg IV followed by 2mg **neostigmine**

- **Contraindications**—hypersensitivity to drug or class
- **Caution**—renal or hepatic dysfunction, cardiovascular disease, hyperthyroidism

■ **Maternal Considerations**

Tubocurarine is the active ingredient of the curare-producing plant, *Chondodendron tomentosum*. Nondepolarizing relaxants are longer acting than depolarizing muscle relaxants. While there are no adequate reports or well-controlled studies of **tubocurarine** in pregnant women, there is a long clinical experience. **Magnesium sulfate** therapy prolongs the effect of **tubocurarine**. Long-acting agents like **tubocurarine** or **pancuronium** have generally been abandoned by anesthesiologists/intensivists in favor of synthetic short-to-intermediate-acting agents (e.g., **rocuronium**, **cisatracurium**, **vecuronium**) which have fewer side effects (e.g., histamine release, tachycardia) profiles
Side effects include histamine release characterized by erythema, edema, skin rash, flushing, tachycardia, arterial hypotension, bronchospasm, circulatory collapse, cardiac arrhythmias, bradycardia, and prolonged apnea.

■ **Fetal Considerations**

There are no adequate reports or well-controlled studies in human fetuses. Placental transfer of **tubocurarine** is greater than **atracurium,** with an F:M ratio of 0.09 for

atracurium and 0.12 for **tubocurarine** (p <0.05). However, it may be more rapidly cleared by the neonate. **Tubocurarine** is well tolerated by the neonate if used during cesarean delivery, provided the interval between drug and delivery is short (1-10min). One woman treated for tetanus at 10-12w with **tubocurarine** for 10d delivered a term infant with joint contractures. **Tubocurarine** is administered directly to the fetus (3 or 1.5mg/kg SEFW IM/IV) to facilitate fetal therapeutic efforts. It lowers HR and BP in comparison to **pancuronium**. The duration of action of **tubocurarine** is directly related to the relative sensitivities of the different muscle groups, which are ranked from most sensitive to least sensitive as extraocular muscles, nuchal muscle, and diaphragm. Rodent studies reveal an increase in deformations consistent with absent fetal muscle tone.

■ **Breastfeeding Safety**

There is no published experience in nursing women. It is unknown whether **tubocurarine** enters human breast milk. However, considering the indication and dosing, one time **tubocurarine** use is unlikely to pose a clinically significant risk to the breast-feeding neonate.

■ **References**

Perreault C, Guay J, Gaudreault P, et al. Can J Anaesth 1991; 38:587-91.
Chestnut DH, Weiner CP, Thompson CS, McLaughlin GL. Am J Obstet Gynecol 1989; 160:510-3.
Weiner CP, Wenstrom KD, Sipes SL, Williamson RA. Am J Obstet Gynecol 1991; 165:1020-5.
Moise KJ Jr, Carpenter RJ Jr, Deter RL, et al. Am J Obstet Gynecol 1987; 157:874-9.
Szeto HH, Hinman DJ. Am J Obstet Gynecol 1990; 163:202-9.

■ **Summary**

- **Pregnancy Category C**
- **Lactation Category S?**
- **Tubocurarine** has been used during pregnancy and lactation as an anesthetic adjunct during surgery for decades.
- Newer synthetic agents may have advantages in specific clinical settings.

Urea (Ureaphil)

■ **Class** — *Cerebral edema, hypertension*

■ **Indications** — Increased intracranial pressure, increased intraocular pressure, SIADH

■ **Mechanism** — Osmotic diuretic

■ **Dosage with Qualifiers** — Increased intracranial pressure—1-1.5g/kg IV over 1-3h; max 120g/d
Increased intraocular pressure—1-1.5g/kg IV over 1-3h; max 120g/d
SIADH—80g IV over 6h
- **Contraindications**—hypersensitivity to drug or class, dehydration, hepatic failure, intracranial hemorrhage, renal dysfunction, lower extremity infusion
- **Caution**—cardiovascular disease

■ **Maternal Considerations** — There are no adequate reports or well-controlled studies of **urea** in pregnant women. Intra-amniotic urea is a valuable adjunct for late pregnancy termination. There is no published experience in pregnant women for the remaining listed indications.
Side effects include headache, nausea, vomiting, syncope, disorientation, and injection site reaction.

■ **Fetal Considerations** — There are no adequate reports or well-controlled studies in human fetuses. **Urea** crosses the human placenta. Intra-amniotic injection of **urea** (80-120g) in combination with a prostaglandin is used for 2nd and 3rd trimester termination. The **urea** is typically lethal when given prior to skin keratinization. Rodent teratogenicity studies have not been conducted.

■ **Breastfeeding Safety** — There is no published experience in nursing women. **Urea** likely enters human breast milk, but the effect of its use for the above indications has not been studied. However, most of the **urea** ingested by the infant is not bioavailable. Thus any increase in milk urea from maternal treatment should be clinically irrelevant.

■ **References** — Haning RV Jr, Peckham BM. Am J Obstet Gynecol 1985; 151:92-6.
Hern WM, Zen C, Ferguson KA, et al. Obstet Gynecol 1993; 81:301-6.
Fomon SJ, Matthews DE, Bier DM, et al. J Pediatr 1987; 111:221-4.

■ **Summary** —
- **Pregnancy Category C**
- **Lactation Category S**
- **Urea** should be used during pregnancy and lactation only if the benefit justifies the potential perinatal risk.

- The published experience demonstrates that intra-amniotic urea is a valuable adjunct for the performance of midtrimester pregnancy termination.

Urokinase (Abbokinase)

■ **Class** — Anticoagulant, *thrombolytic*

■ **Indications** — Pulmonary embolus, coronary artery thrombosis

■ **Mechanism** — Converts plasminogen to plasmin

■ **Dosage with Qualifiers** — **Unavailable in the U.S.**
Pulmonary embolus—begin 4400IU/kg IV over 10min, then 4400IU/kg qh ×12h within 7d
Coronary artery thrombosis—load heparin 2500-10,000U IV, then 6000IU/min IV until lysis (up to 2h, average 500,000IU)
IV catheter clearance—5000IU contained in 1ml
- **Contraindications**—hypersensitivity to drug or class, stroke history, active bleeding, aneurysm, AV malformation, recent trauma, intracranial malignancy, ulcerative colitis, severe uncontrolled hypertension
- **Caution**—venipuncture, arterial puncture, IM injections, diabetic retinopathy, CVD, severe hepatic dysfunction, surgery or delivery <10d

■ **Maternal Considerations** — Urokinase is produced by the kidney and excreted in the urine. **Urokinase** treatment must be instituted as soon as possible after onset of pulmonary embolism, and no later than 7d. Any delay instituting lytic therapy, even to evaluate the effect of heparin, decreases the potential for optimal efficacy. The diagnosis of a thromboembolus should always be confirmed by objective testing. Therapy should be instituted within 6h of symptom onset if used to treat coronary artery thrombosis associated with an evolving transmural MI. Concurrent use of anticoagulants with IV administration of **urokinase** is not recommended except as noted. There are no adequate reports or well-controlled studies of **urokinase** in pregnant women. The published literature consists of case reports using **urokinase** to treat MI, pulmonary embolus and cerebral and ovarian vein thrombosis either during pregnancy or in the puerperium. There may be a substantial risk of hemorrhage in the puerperium.
Side effects include bleeding, reperfusion arrhythmia, rash, bronchospasm, and injection site phlebitis.

- ■ **Fetal Considerations** There are no adequate reports or well-controlled studies in human fetuses. It is unknown whether **urokinase** crosses the human placenta. Rodent studies are reassuring, revealing no evidence of teratogenicity or IUGR despite the use of doses higher than those used clinically.

- ■ **Breastfeeding Safety** There are no adequate reports or well-controlled studies in nursing women. It is unknown whether **urokinase** enters human breast milk. Plasminogen and plasminogen activator are normal components of breast milk. Considering the indication and dosing, one-time **urokinase** use is unlikely to pose a clinically significant risk to the breast-feeding neonate.

- ■ **References** Lee EH, Im CY, Kim JW. Ultrasound Obstet Gynecol 2001; 18:384-6.
  Wang S, Liang Y, Zhao F. Zhonghua Fu Chan Ke Za Zhi 1998; 33:412-4.
  Webber MD, Halligan RE, Schumacher JA. Cathet Cardiovasc Diagn 1997; 42:38-43.
  Heegaard CW, Larsen LB, Rasmussen LK, et al. Pediatr Gastroenterol Nutr 1997; 25:159-66.

- ■ **Summary**
  - ● **Pregnancy Category B**
  - ● **Lactation Category S?**
  - ● **Urokinase** should be used during pregnancy and lactation only if the benefit justifies the potential perinatal risk.

Ursodiol (Actigall; Ursacol; Ursodamor)

- ■ **Class** *Gallstone solubilizer, other gastrointestinal*

- ■ **Indications** Gallstone dissolution or prevention, primary biliary cirrhosis, primary sclerosing cholangitis, nonalcoholic steatohepatitis

- ■ **Mechanism** Decreases cholesterol synthesis, secretion, and absorption

- ■ **Dosage with Qualifiers** Gallstone dissolution—8-10mg/kg/d PO in divided doses; monitor response q6mo by ultrasound, and continue drug for 3mo after dissolution
  Gallstone prevention—300mg PO bid for obese women losing weight
  Primary biliary cirrhosis—13-15mg/kg/d PO in divided doses with food
  Primary sclerosing cholangitis—25-30mg/kg/d PO in divided doses with food
  Nonalcoholic steatohepatitis—10-15mg/kg/d PO in divided doses with food

- **Contraindications**—hypersensitivity to drug or class, hypersensitivity to bile acids, unremitting acute cholecystitis, acute cholangitis, biliary obstruction, gallstone pancreatitis, biliary-GI fistula, calcified/radiopaque/radiolucent gallstones
- **Caution**—unknown

■ **Maternal Considerations** ······· There are no adequate reports or well-controlled studies of **ursodiol** in pregnant women. Small series suggest it can be effective for the treatment of cholestasis of pregnancy (approximately 16mg/kg). One report chronicles a woman with primary biliary cirrhosis treated throughout pregnancy. The drug was effective, though a preterm cesarean delivery was required for uteroplacental dysfunction.

Side effects include nausea, vomiting, dyspepsia, abdominal pain, diarrhea, constipation, dizziness, alopecia, leukopenia, and URI symptoms.

■ **Fetal Considerations** ············ There are no adequate reports or well-controlled studies in human fetuses. **Ursodiol** apparently does not cross the human placenta.

■ **Breastfeeding Safety** ············ **Ursodiol** does not enter human breast milk.

■ **References** ·································· Paumgartner G, Beuers U. Hepatology 2002; 36:525-31.
Palma J, Reyes, H, Ribalta J, et al. J Hepatol 1997; 27:1022-6.
Mazzella G, Rizzo N, Azzaroli F, et al. Hepatology 2001; 33:504-8.
Rudi J, Schonig T, Stremmel W. Z Gastroenterol 1996; 34:188-91.

■ **Summary** ·································
- **Pregnancy Category B**
- **Lactation Category S**
- **Ursodiol** is a first-line agent for the treatment of intrahepatic cholestasis of pregnancy.

Valacyclovir (Valtrex)

- **Class** — Antiviral

- **Indications** — Genital herpes, herpes zoster

- **Mechanism** — Inhibits DNA polymerase

- **Dosage with Qualifiers** — Genital herpes—primary, 1000mg PO bid ×10d; recurrent, 500mg PO bid ×3d; prophylaxis, 1000mg PO qd
  Herpes zoster—1000mg PO tid ×7d
  NOTE—renal dosing
  - **Contraindications**—hypersensitivity to drug or class, immunocompromised
  - **Caution**—renal dysfunction

- **Maternal Considerations** — After ingestion, **valacyclovir** is metabolized to and actually enhances **acyclovir** bioavailability. It is effective and well tolerated for HSV suppression for up to 10 years of continuous use. Neonatal herpes affects 1/15,000 newborns. The vast majority of infected infants are born to women with a primary infection during pregnancy. While there are no adequate reports or well-controlled studies of **valacyclovir** in pregnant women, it is used extensively for the listed indications. If initiated prophylactically at 36w, **acyclovir** reduces both the risk of recurrence and the frequency of a positive cervical culture at delivery in women who either experience a primary infection or at least one secondary episode during pregnancy. As a result, prophylaxis reduces the need for cesarean delivery. *Side effects* include renal failure, dysmenorrhea, nausea, vomiting, headache, dizziness, arthralgia, depression, facial edema, hypertension, tachycardia, angioedema, rash, confusion, hallucinations, aplastic anemia, thrombocytopenia, anemia, leukopenia, and erythema multiforme.

- **Fetal Considerations** — There are no adequate reports or well-controlled studies in human fetuses. It is unknown whether **valacyclovir** crosses the human placenta. **Acyclovir** crosses the rodent placenta. Post-marketing surveys suggest no increased frequency of birth defects. Rodent studies are reassuring, revealing no evidence of teratogenicity or IUGR despite the use of doses higher than those used clinically.

- **Breastfeeding Safety** — **Valacyclovir** is converted to **acyclovir**, which enters human breast milk. However, the amount of **acyclovir** in breast milk during **valacyclovir** administration is <5% of the dose used to treat neonates.

- **References** — Watts DH, Brown ZA, Money D, et al. Am J Obstet Gynecol 2003; 188:836-43.
  Brown SD, Bartlett MG, White CA. Antimicrob Agents Chemother 2003; 47:991-6.

Tyring SK, Baker D, Snowden W. J Infect Dis 2002; 186(Suppl 1):S40-6.

Scott LL, Hollier LM, McIntire D, et al. Infect Dis Obstet Gynecol 2001; 9:75-80.

Braig S, Luton D, Sibony O, et al. Eur J Obstet Gynecol Reprod Biol 2001; 96:55-8.

Sheffield JS, Fish DN, Hollier LM, et al. Am J Obstet Gynecol 2002; 186:100-2.

■ **Summary**

- **Pregnancy Category B**
- **Lactation Category S**
- **Valacyclovir** should be used during pregnancy only if the benefit justifies the potential perinatal risk.
- **Valacyclovir** is a first-line agent for the treatment of genital herpes and herpes zoster during pregnancy and lactation.
- Herpes prophylaxis at 36w reduces the risk of recurrence, and as a result, the need for cesarean delivery for recurrence.
- Physicians are encouraged to register pregnant women under the Pregnancy Registry (1-800-336-2176) for a better follow-up of the outcome while under treatment with **valacyclovir.**

Valdecoxib (Bextra)

■ **Class**

Analgesic, non-narcotic; NSAID; *antiarthritic*

■ **Indications**

Osteoarthritis and rheumatoid arthritis, dysmenorrhea

■ **Mechanism**

Selective COX-2 antagonist

■ **Dosage with Qualifiers**

Osteoarthrits—10mg PO qd
Rheumatoid arthritis—10mg PO qd
Dysmenorrhea—20mg PO bid

- **Contraindications**—hypersensitivity to drug or class, hypersensitivity to ASA, NSAIDs, ASA/NSAID-induced asthma or urticaria, hepatic failure, severe renal dysfunction
- **Caution**—CHF, hypertension, nasal polyps, peptic ulcer disease, history of GI bleeding, hepatic or renal dysfunction, dehydration, asthma, fluid retention

■ **Maternal Considerations**

Valdecoxib is an NSAID with anti-inflammatory, analgesic, and antipyretic properties. In general, the COX-2 inhibitors are associated with a lower incidence of GI upset. **Valdecoxib** provides effective relief of dysmenorrhea, but does not appear to be more effective than alternative, nonselective NSAIDs. There is no published experience with **valdecoxib** during pregnancy. It has no effect on the timing of onset of rodent labor. *Side effects* include GI bleeding or ulceration, esophagitis, bronchospasm, hypertension, CHF, hepatotoxicity, renal papillary necrosis, anemia, blood dyscrasias, dyspepsia, abdominal pain, nausea, vomiting, diarrhea, dizziness, and peripheral edema.

- **Fetal Considerations** — There are no adequate reports or well-controlled studies in human fetuses. It is unknown whether **valdecoxib** crosses the human placenta. Other NSAIDs do cross and are associated with gastroschisis (1st trimester exposure), oligohydramnios, and ductal constriction. **Valdecoxib** increases the risk of skeletal malformations in some rodents when given at >70 times the MRHD. IUGR is noted with doses >5 times MRHD.

- **Breastfeeding Safety** — There is no published experience in nursing women. It is unknown whether **valdecoxib** enters human breast milk. It is found in rodent milk.

- **Reference** — Stichtenoth DO, Frolich JC. Drugs 2003; 63:33-45.

- **Summary** —
  - **Pregnancy Category C**
  - **Lactation Category U**
  - **Valdecoxib** should be used during pregnancy and lactation only if the benefit justifies the potential perinatal risk.
  - There are alternative agents for which there is more experience during pregnancy and lactation.

Valganciclovir (Valcyte)

- **Class** — Antiviral

- **Indications** — CMV retinitis associated with AIDS

- **Mechanism** — Inhibits DNA polymerase

- **Dosage with Qualifiers** — CMV retinitis associated with AIDS—begin 900mg PO bid with food ×21d, then qd
  NOTE—renal dosing
  - **Contraindications**—hypersensitivity to drug or class, ANC <500/mcl, HB <8mg/dl, platelets <25,000/mcl
  - **Caution**—bone marrow suppression, concomitant radiation, renal dysfunction

- **Maternal Considerations** ---- **Valganciclovir** is metabolized to **ganciclovir**. There is no published experience with **valganciclovir** during pregnancy. (See **ganciclovir**.)
Side effects include leukopenia, neutropenia, thrombocytopenia, aplastic anemia, bone marrow suppression, infertility, nephrotoxicity, peripheral neuropathy, retinal detachment, seizures, psychosis, nausea, vomiting, diarrhea, fever, insomnia, abdominal pain, confusion, agitation, and increased creatinine.

- **Fetal Considerations** ---- There are no adequate reports or well-controlled studies in human fetuses. **Valganciclovir** crosses the isolated human placenta by passive diffusion. **Ganciclovir** is embryotoxic and teratogenic in various rodent models. Birth defects include cleft palate, craniofacial abnormalities, and pancreas and renal agenesis.

- **Breastfeeding Safety** ---- There is no published experience in nursing women. It is unknown whether **valganciclovir** enters human breast milk. Breastfeeding is contraindicated in HIV-infected nursing women where formula is available to reduce the risk of neonatal transmission. (See **ganciclovir**.)

- **References** ---- There is no published experience in pregnancy or during lactation.

- **Summary** ----
  - **Pregnancy Category C**
  - **Lactation Category U**
  - **Valganciclovir** should be used during pregnancy and lactation only if the benefit justifies the potential perinatal risk.
  - See **ganciclovir**.
  - Physicians are encouraged to register pregnant women under the Pregnancy Registry (1-800-336-2176) for a better follow-up of the outcome while under treatment with **valganciclovir**.

Valproate (Depacon; Epival)

- **Class** ---- Anticonvulsant

- **Indications** ---- Seizures

- **Mechanism** ---- Unknown

- **Dosage with Qualifiers** ---- Seizures—10-15mg/kg/d IV in divided doses qd/tid, increase by 5-10mg/kg/d q7d to achieve therapeutic trough of 50-100mcg/ml; max 60mg/kg/d
NOTE—switch to PO when feasible

- **Contraindications**—hypersensitivity to drug or class, hepatic disease or dysfunction
- **Caution**—renal dysfunction, bone marrow suppression, bleeding tendencies, congenital metabolic disorders, anticonvulsant use

■ **Maternal Considerations**

Valproate is the sodium salt of **valproic acid**. There are no adequate reports or well-controlled studies of **valproate** in pregnant women. There is a long clinical experience with **valproate**. It does not alter the efficacy of hormonal contraception. Patients planning pregnancy should be counseled on the risks and the importance of periconceptual folate supplementation.

Side effects include potentially fatal hepatotoxicity, pancreatitis, bone marrow suppression, pancytopenia, aplastic anemia, thrombocytopenia, bleeding, hyponatremia, hyperammonemia, erythema multiforme, Stevens-Johnson syndrome, nausea, vomiting, appetite and weight changes, dyspepsia, abdominal pain, diarrhea, asthenia, somnolence, tremor, alopecia, rash, peripheral edema, petechiae, blurred vision, nystagmus, tinnitus, SIADH, psychosis, and respiratory disorders.

■ **Fetal Considerations**

Valproate is a recognized human teratogen, increasing the relative risk by a factor of 4. The risk is compounded by a low serum folate. **Valproate** is rapidly and actively transported across the human placenta reaching an F:M ratio exceeding 2. For unknown reasons, **valproate** accumulates in the fetal plasma. A distinct facial appearance, coupled with a cluster of minor and major anomalies and CNS dysfunction characterize the *fetal valproate syndrome*. The likelihood of an affected offspring is dose dependent. Ten percent die in infancy, and 1 of 4 survivors have either developmental deficits or mental retardation. A fetal medicine specialist should evaluate women taking **valproate** during pregnancy. Affected fetuses may have an increased nuchal translucency measurement. As for most psychotropic drugs, monotherapy and the lowest effective quantity given in divided doses to minimize the peaks can theoretically minimize the risks.

■ **Breastfeeding Safety**

Valproate sodium enters human breast milk, but the neonatal concentration is less than 10% of the maternal.

■ **References**

Kaaja E, Kaaja R, Hiilesmaa V. Neurology 2003; 60:575-9.
Crawford P. CNF Drugs 2002; 16:263-72.
Mawer G, Clayton-Smith J, Coyle H, Kini U. Seizure 2002; 11:512-8.
Samren EB, van Duijn CM, Koch S, et al. Epilepsia 1997; 38:981-90.
Kozma C. Am J Med Genet 2001; 98:168-75.
Witters I, Van Assche F, Fryns JP. Prenat Diagn 2002; 22:834-5.
Nakamura H, Ushigome F, Koyabu N, et al. Pharm Res 2002; 19:154-61.

ten Berg K, Lindhout D. Clin Dysmorphol 2002; 11:227-8.
Nau H, Kuhnz W, Egger HJ, et al. Clin Pharmacokinet 1982; 7:508-43.
Chaudron LH, Jefferson JW. J Clin Psychiatry 222; 61:79-90.
Tsuru N, Maeda T, Tsuruoka M. Jpn J Psychiatry 1988; 42:89-96.
Philbert A, Pedersen B, Dam M. Acta Neurol Scand 1985; 72:460-3.

■ Summary	
	• **Pregnancy Category D**
	• **Lactation Category S**
	• **Valproate** is a recognized human teratogen.
	• The risk of a defect is compounded by folate deficiency.
	• **Valproate** should be used during pregnancy only if the benefit justifies the potential perinatal risk.
	• As for most psychotropic drugs, monotherapy and the lowest effective quantity given in divided doses to minimize the peaks may minimize the risks.

Valproic acid (Depakene; Myproic acid)

■ Class	Anticonvulsant, migraine, mania, bipolar
■ **Indications**	Seizures, mania, migraine prophylaxis
■ **Mechanism**	Unknown
■ **Dosage with Qualifiers**	Seizures—10-15mg/kg/d PO with meals in divided doses qd/tid, increase by 5-10mg/kg/d q7d to achieve therapeutic trough of 50-100mcg/ml; max 60mg/kg/d Mania—10-15mg/kg/d PO with meals in divided doses qd/tid, increase by 5-10mg/kg/d q7d to achieve therapeutic trough of 50-100mcg/ml; max 60mg/kg/d Migraine prophylaxis—250-500mg PO with meals bid • **Contraindications**—hypersensitivity to drug or class, hepatic disease or dysfunction • **Caution**—renal dysfunction, bone marrow suppression, bleeding tendencies, congenital metabolic disorders, anticonvulsant use
■ **Maternal Considerations**	There is a long clinical experience with **valproic acid**. It does not alter the efficacy of hormonal contraception. Patients planning pregnancy should be counseled on the risks and the importance of periconceptual folate supplementation. *Side effects* include potentially fatal hepatotoxicity, pancreatitis, SIADH, thrombocytopenia, pancytopenia, aplastic anemia, bone marrow suppression, bleeding, hyponatremia, hyperammonemia, erythema multiforme,

Stevens-Johnson syndrome, psychosis, nausea, vomiting, appetite and weight change, dyspepsia, diarrhea, abdominal pain, asthenia, somnolence, tremor, alopecia, rash, peripheral edema, petechiae, blurred vision, nystagmus, tinnitus, and respiratory disorders.

■ **Fetal Considerations**

Valproic acid is a recognized human teratogen, increasing the relative risk by a factor of 4. The risk is compounded by a low serum folate. **Valproic acid** is rapidly and actively transported across the human placenta reaching an F:M ratio exceeding 2. For unknown reasons, **valproic acid** accumulates in the fetal plasma. A distinct facial appearance, coupled with a cluster of minor and major anomalies and CNS dysfunction characterize the *fetal valproate syndrome*. The likelihood of an affected offspring is dose-dependent. Ten percent die in infancy, and 1 of 4 survivors have either developmental deficits or mental retardation. A fetal medicine specialist should evaluate women taking **valproic acid** during pregnancy. Affected fetuses may have an increased nuchal translucency measurement. As for most psychotropic drugs, monotherapy and the lowest effective quantity given in divided doses to minimize the peaks can theoretically minimize the risks.

■ **Breastfeeding Safety**

Valproic acid enters human breast milk, but the neonatal concentration is less than 10% of the maternal.

■ **References**

Kaaja E, Kaaja R, Hiilesmaa V. Neurology 2003; 60:575-9.
Crawford P. CNF Drugs 2002; 16:263-72.
Mawer G, Clayton-Smith J, Coyle H, Kini U. Seizure 2002; 11:512-8.
Samren EB, van Duijn CM, Koch S, et al. Epilepsia 1997; 38:981-90.
Kozma C. Am J Med Genet 2001; 98:168-75.
Witters I, Van Assche F, Fryns JP. Prenat Diagn 2002; 22:834-5.
Nakamura H, Ushigome F, Koyabu N, et al. Pharm Res 2002; 19:154-61.
ten Berg K, Lindhout D. Clin Dysmorphol 2002; 11:227-8.
Nau H, Kuhnz W, Egger HJ, et al. Clin Pharmacokinet 1982; 7:508-43.
Chaudron LH, Jefferson JW. J Clin Psychiatry 61:79-90.
Tsuru N, Maeda T, Tsuruoka M. Jpn J Psychiatry 1988; 42:89-96.
Philbert A, Pedersen B, Dam M. Acta Neurol Scand 1985; 72:460-3.

■ **Summary**

- **Pregnancy Category D**
- **Lactation Category S**
- **Valproic acid** is a recognized human teratogen.
- The risk of a defect is compounded by folate deficiency.
- **Valproic acid** should be used during pregnancy only if the benefit justifies the potential perinatal risk.
- As for most psychotropic drugs, monotherapy and the lowest effective quantity given in divided doses to minimize the peaks may minimize the risks.

Valsartan (Diovan)

■ **Class** ACE-I/A2R-*antagonist*

■ **Indications** .... Hypertension

■ **Mechanism** .... Selective AT-1 antagonist

■ **Dosage with Qualifiers** .... Hypertension—begin 80-160mg PO qd if monotherapy; max 320mg/d
  - **Contraindications**—hypersensitivity to drug or class
  - **Caution**—CHF, history ACE inhibitor angioedema, renal artery stenosis, hepatic or renal dysfunction, volume depletion, hyponatremia

■ **Maternal Considerations** ...... **Valsartan** has no significant advantages over similar agents in its class for which there is more experience. Nor has it been demonstrated to reduce the complications of arterial hypertension. There are no adequate reports or well-controlled studies of **valsartan** in pregnant women. There are only 4 pregnancy exposures reported. Inhibitors of the renin angiotensin system should be avoided during pregnancy because of their fetal implications.
Side effects include angioedema, severe hypotension, hyperkalemia, URI symptoms, dizziness, fatigue, dyspepsia, back pain, and diarrhea.

■ **Fetal Considerations** .... There are no adequate reports or well-controlled studies in human fetuses. Drugs that act directly on the renin-angiotensin system can cause perinatal morbidity and death. Adverse outcomes similar to other drugs in this class are reported for **valsartan** suggesting it crosses the human placenta. Adverse effects are not likely if exposure is limited to the 1st trimester; 2nd and 3rd trimester morbidity includes hypotension, neonatal skull hypoplasia, anuria, and reversible or irreversible renal failure. Oligohydramnios may be associated with limb contractures, craniofacial deformation, and hypoplastic lung development. Rarely, an alternative drug is not available. In these cases, the women should be counseled on the hazards, and serial ultrasound examinations should be performed to assess the intra-amniotic environment. If oligohydramnios is observed, the **valsartan** should be discontinued unless lifesaving for the mother. Antenatal surveillance may be appropriate depending upon gestation. Oligohydramnios may not appear until after the fetus has sustained irreversible injury.

■ **Breastfeeding Safety** .... There is no published experience in nursing women. It is unknown whether **valsartan** enters human breast milk.

- **References** .... Biswas PN, Wilton LV, Shakir SW. J Hum Hypertens 2002; 16:795-803.
  Briggs GG, Nageotte MP. Ann Pharmacother 2001; 35:859-61.

- **Summary** .... • **Pregnancy Category C (1st trimester), D (2nd and 3rd trimesters)**
  - **Lactation Category U**
  - **Valsartan** should be used during pregnancy and lactation only if the benefit justifies the potential perinatal risk.
  - Women should be counseled on the risks and switched to a different class of antihypertensives prior to conception or during the 1st trimester.
  - There are alternative agents for which there is more experience during pregnancy and lactation.

Vancomycin (Balcorin; Edicin; Ledervan; Lyphocin; Vancocin; Vancoled; Vancor)

- **Class** .... Antibiotic, glycopeptide

- **Indications** .... Bacterial infections, endocarditis prophylaxis

- **Mechanism** .... Bactericidal; inhibits cell wall and RNA synthesis

- **Dosage with Qualifiers** .... Bacterial infections—500mg IV q6h; peak 25-40mcg/ml, trough 5-10mcg/ml
  Endocarditis prophylaxis—1g slow IV over 1h
  NOTE—renal dosing
  - **Contraindications**—hypersensitivity to drug or class
  - **Caution**—hepatic or renal dysfunction, hearing loss, nephrotoxic agents

- **Maternal Considerations** .... **Vancomycin** is most commonly used for the treatment of **methicillin**-resistant Staphylococcus aureus infections. There are no adequate reports or well-controlled studies of **vancomycin** in pregnant women. It is used as a second-line agent for the treatment of postpartum endomyometritis, and as a first-line agent and alternative to **metronidazole** for the treatment of Clostridium difficile diarrhea. Other applications during pregnancy include listeriosis and bacterial endocarditis in IV drug users. *Side effects* include neutropenia, Stevens-Johnson syndrome, thrombocytopenia, toxic epidermal necrolysis, nephrotoxicity, ototoxicity, chills, fever, nausea, tinnitus, superinfection, urticaria, rash, red-man syndrome, and phlebitis.

- **Fetal Considerations** ⋯⋯⋯ There are no adequate reports or well-controlled studies in human fetuses. **Vancomycin** crosses the human placenta, though the kinetics remain to be elucidated. Concern that **vancomycin** exposure might cause ototoxicity has not been substantiated. Rodent studies are reassuring, revealing no evidence of teratogenicity or IUGR despite the use of doses higher than those used clinically.

- **Breastfeeding Safety** ⋯⋯⋯ There are no adequate reports or well-controlled studies in nursing women. **Vancomycin** enters human breast milk, but the kinetics remain to be elucidated. Considering the poor oral absorption, it is unlikely the breast-fed neonate would ingest a clinically relevant amount.

- **References** ⋯⋯⋯ James AH, Katz VL, Dotters DJ, Rogers RG. South Med J 1997; 90:889-92.
  Bonacorsi S, Doit C, Aujard Y, et al. Clin Infect Dis 1993; 17:139-40.
  Bourget P, Fernandez H, Delouis C, Ribou F. Obstet Gynecol 1991; 78:908-11.
  Reyes MP, Ostrea EM Jr, Cabinian AE, et al. Am J Obstet Gynecol 1989; 161:977-81.

- **Summary** ⋯⋯⋯
  - **Pregnancy Category B**
  - **Lactation Category S**
  - **Vancomycin** should be used during pregnancy only if the benefit justifies the potential perinatal risk.
  - It should probably be reserved for antibiotic-resistant bacterial infections.

Varicella vaccine (Varivax)

- **Class** ⋯⋯⋯ Vaccine

- **Indications** ⋯⋯⋯ Varicella susceptibility

- **Mechanism** ⋯⋯⋯ Active immunity

- **Dosage with Qualifiers** ⋯⋯⋯ Varicella susceptibility—0.5ml SC and a second 0.5ml SC 4-8w
  - **Contraindications**—hypersensitivity to drug or class, blood dyscrasias, leukemia, lymphomas, or other malignant neoplasms affecting the bone marrow or lymphatic systems, immune suppression or compromise (acquired or congenital), febrile illness, active tuberculosis
  - **Caution**—acute lymphocytic leukemia in remission

■ **Maternal Considerations** ········· Varicella is a cause of significant maternal and fetal morbidity and mortality. The attack rate of natural varicella after household exposure among healthy susceptible people approaches 90%. **Varicella vaccine** is a live attenuated preparation, and as such is usually contraindicated during pregnancy. Most adverse events associated with varicella vaccine are minor, and serious complications rare. If vaccine virus transmission occurs, it does so at a very low rate and possibly without recognizable clinical disease. Most complications are instead associated with wild-type virus. Seventy percent of women in North America who do not remember having childhood varicella are actually immune. It is wise to test women of reproductive age planning pregnancy, and selectively immunize preconception if indicated. It is estimated that selective serologic screening of pregnant women with postpartum vaccination of susceptible women is cost-effective and would prevent half the cases of congenital varicella. There are no adequate reports or well-controlled studies of **varicella vaccine** in pregnant women. Inadvertent administration during pregnancy produces maternal immunity. There are reports of its erroneous administration when **varicella zoster immune globulin** was ordered.

Side effects include fever, injection site reactions, vesicular lesions, upper respiratory illness, headache, fatigue, cough, myalgia, disturbed sleep, nausea, malaise, diarrhea, stiff neck, irritability/nervousness, lymphadenopathy, chills, eye complaints, abdominal pain, loss of appetite, arthralgia, otitis, itching, vomiting, other rashes, constipation, lower respiratory illness, and allergic reactions.

■ **Fetal Considerations** ·············· Varicella is a human teratogen. Abnormalities are usually related to CNS and peripheral nerve infection. They include skin lesions in dermatomal distribution, neurologic disease and skeletal anomalies. The frequency of the syndrome is low (0.4-1.2% of infected cases) and gestational age related. There are no adequate reports or well-controlled studies in human fetuses. It is unknown whether the attenuated virus comprising the **varicella vaccine** crosses the human placenta. Wild-type virus does cross. Inadvertent immunization during pregnancy is unassociated with fetal pathology and is not *apriori* an indication for pregnancy termination. A voluntary Pregnancy Registry established by the manufacturer, Merck & Co., recorded 92 women inadvertently vaccinated during the 1st trimester between 1995-2000, of which there were 56 live births. Five infants had a variety of abnormalities not associated with congenital varicella syndrome. Longitudinal study demonstrates the fetal immunologic response to congenital varicella may not be sustained. Molecular testing is recommended. Rodent teratogenicity studies have not been performed.

- **Breastfeeding Safety** ⸱⸱⸱⸱⸱⸱⸱⸱⸱⸱⸱ There is no published experience in nursing women. It is unknown whether the attenuated virus comprising **varicella vaccine** enters human breast milk. However, wild-type virus is excreted into human breast milk and can cause neonatal infection.

- **References** ⸱⸱⸱⸱⸱⸱⸱⸱⸱⸱⸱⸱⸱⸱⸱⸱⸱⸱⸱⸱⸱⸱ Wise RP, Salive ME, Braum MM, et al. JAMA 2000; 284:3129.
  Wise RP, Braum MM, Seward JF, et al. Pharmacoepidemiol Drug Saf 2002; 11:651-4.
  Salzman MB, Sharrar RG, Steinberg S, LaRussa P. J Pediatr 1997; 131:151-4.
  Smith WJ, Jackson LA, Watts, DH, Koepsell TD. Obstet Gynecol 1998; 92:535-45.
  Shields KE, Galil K, Seward RG, et al. Obstet Gynecol 2001; 98:14-9.
  Harger JH, Ernest JM, Thurnau GR, et al. Obstet Gynecol 2002; 100:260-5.
  Yoshida M, Yamagami N, Tezuka T, Hondo R. J Med Virol 1992; 38:108-10.

- **Summary** ⸱⸱⸱⸱⸱⸱⸱⸱⸱⸱⸱⸱⸱⸱⸱⸱⸱⸱⸱⸱⸱⸱
  - **Pregnancy Category C**
  - **Lactation Category NS?**
  - **Varicella** vaccine administration is contraindicated during pregnancy.
  - A cogent societal cost-benefit argument can be made for selective serologic screening during pregnancy and postpartum vaccination of susceptible women.
  - Inadvertent immunization during pregnancy is not associated with fetal pathology and is not *apriori* an indication for pregnancy termination.

Varicella zoster immune globulin
(VZIG; Varitect)

- **Class** ⸱⸱⸱⸱⸱⸱⸱⸱⸱⸱⸱⸱⸱⸱⸱⸱⸱⸱⸱⸱⸱⸱⸱⸱⸱⸱⸱ *Immunoglobulin*

- **Indications** ⸱⸱⸱⸱⸱⸱⸱⸱⸱⸱⸱⸱⸱⸱⸱⸱⸱⸱⸱⸱ Varicella susceptibility and exposure

- **Mechanism** ⸱⸱⸱⸱⸱⸱⸱⸱⸱⸱⸱⸱⸱⸱⸱⸱⸱⸱⸱⸱⸱ Passive immunization

- **Dosage with Qualifiers** ⸱⸱⸱⸱⸱ Varicella-susceptibility and exposure—625U IM ×1
  - **Contraindications**—hypersensitivity to drug or class, severe thrombocytopenia if IM
  - **Caution**—avoid intravascular injection

- **Maternal Considerations** ⸱⸱⸱⸱⸱ Varicella is a cause of significant maternal and fetal morbidity and mortality. Varicella pneumonia is perhaps the most serious maternal complication with mortality rates in excess of 10%. Current smokers and women with more than 100 lesions are at particularly high risk. There are no adequate reports or well-controlled studies of **varicella zoster immune globulin** in pregnant women. There is no evidence that VZIG administration to a susceptible, pregnant woman prevents viremia, fetal infection or congenital varicella syndrome. The goal is to reduce the maternal sequelae of varicella rather than to prevent intrauterine infection. Women with no history of varicella and an unknown immune status should be tested as soon as the exposure is recognized. Seventy percent of women with no history of childhood varicella are immune. **Varicella zoster immune globulin** administered within 24h of exposure may reduce the severity of maternal disease and is typically coupled with a course of **acyclovir**. The newer IV form achieves higher initial anti-varicella antibodies than the IM format. Though the effectiveness of this practice is unclear, case series indicate improved outcomes. Neonatal studies suggest the combination of immune globulin and **acyclovir** is more effective than monotherapy.

Side effects include pain, redness, or swelling at the injection site, GI symptoms, malaise, headache, rash, respiratory symptoms, and angioneurotic edema.

■ **Fetal Considerations**

There are no adequate reports or well-controlled studies in human fetuses. It is likely **varicella zoster immune globulin** (VZIG) crosses the human placenta, but it is unknown whether such transfer conveys a level of passive immunity. Newborns of women who develop varicella 7d before or up to 28d after delivery should be given **varicella zoster immune giobulin** and possibly **acyclovir**.

■ **Breastfeeding Safety**

There are no adequate reports or well-controlled studies in nursing women. It is unknown whether **varicella zoster immune globulin** enters human breast milk. Other IgG immunoglobulins do, and breastfeeding is encouraged as a potential source of neonatal passive immunization.

■ **References**

Gregorakos L, Myrianthefs, Markou N, et al. Respiration 2002; 69:330-4.
Harger JH, Ernest JM, Thurnau GR, et al. J Infect Dis 2002; 185:422-7.
Wise RP, Braun MM, Seward JF, et al. Pharmacoepidemiol Drug Saf 2002; 11:651-4.
Koren G, Money D, Boucher M, et al. J Clin Pharmacol 2002; 42:267-74.
Heuchan AM, Issacs D. Med J Aust 2001; 174:288-92.

■ **Summary**

- **Pregnancy Category C**
- **Lactation Category S**
- Varicella is a cause of significant maternal and fetal morbidity and death.
- **Varicella zoster immune globulin** should be used during pregnancy only if the benefit justifies the potential perinatal risk.

- 70% of pregnant women who do not recall childhood varicella are immune.
- Susceptible women may benefit from **varicella immune globulin** and **acyclovir** given within 24-48h of exposure.

Vasopressin (Pitressin)

- **Class** — *Antidiuretic, hormone*

- **Indications** — Diabetes insipidus, abdominal distention, abdominal radiographs, renal biopsy, GI hemorrhage, ACLS, VF/pulseless V tachycardia

- **Mechanism** — Smooth muscle V1 agonist

- **Dosage with Qualifiers** — Diabetes insipidus—5-10U IM/SC bid/qid; max 60U/d
  Abdominal distension—5-10U IM q3-4h prn
  Abdominal radiographs—5-15U IM/IV 2h and 30min preoperatively
  Renal biopsy—5-15U IM/IV 2h and 30min preoperatively
  GI hemorrhage—0.2-0.4U/min IV
  ACLS, VF/pulseless V tachycardia—40U IV ×1
  - **Contraindications**—hypersensitivity to drug or class
  - **Caution**—CHF, coronary artery disease, severe hepatic disease, renal dysfunction, asthma, migraine

- **Maternal Considerations** — V1 receptors are widely distributed in smooth muscle including the myometrium. Women with dysmenorrhea have higher vasopressin levels. There are no adequate reports or well-controlled studies of **vasopressin** in pregnant women. Doses of **vasopressin** sufficient for an antidiuretic effect are unlikely to produce tonic uterine contractions deleterious to the fetus or threaten the continuation of the pregnancy. **Deamino-arginine-vasopressin (DDAVP)** is now the 1st choice for the treatment of diabetes insipidus and von Willebrand's disease.
  Side effects include MI, water intoxication, arrhythmia, bradycardia, angina, hypertension, headache, uterine cramping, bronchospasm, angioedema, venous thrombosis, nausea, vomiting, abdominal pain, flatulence, diarrhea, sweating, tremor, pallor, vertigo, rash, fever, and urticaria.

- **Fetal Considerations** — There are no adequate reports or well-controlled studies in human fetuses. It is unknown whether **vasopressin** crosses the human placenta. Rodent teratogenicity studies have not been performed.

■ **Breastfeeding Safety** ⋯⋯⋯ There are no adequate reports or well-controlled studies in nursing women. Little **vasopressin** enters human breast milk and does not pose a significant risk to the breast-feeding neonate.

■ **References** ⋯⋯⋯ Burrow GN, Wassenaar W, Robertson GL, Sehl H. Acta Endocrinol 1981; 97:23-5.
Silcox J, Schultz P, Horbay GL, Wassenaar W. Obstet Gynecol 1993; 82:456-9.

■ **Summary** ⋯⋯⋯
- **Pregnancy Category C**
- **Lactation Category S**
- **Vasopressin** should be used during pregnancy only if the benefit justifies the potential perinatal risk.
- Pregnancy should not preclude its use for diagnostic or lifesaving procedures.

Vecuronium (Musculax; Norcuron)

■ **Class** ⋯⋯⋯ *Neuromuscular blocker, nondepolarizing; adjunct anesthesia, skeletal muscle relaxant*

■ **Indications** ⋯⋯⋯ Paralysis

■ **Mechanism** ⋯⋯⋯ Competitive acetylcholine motor endplate antagonist

■ **Dosage with Qualifiers** ⋯⋯⋯ Paralysis—begin 0.08-0.1mg/kg IV, then 25-45min after load, 0.01-0.015mg/kg IV q15-30min as indicated by train-of-four peripheral nerve stimulation
- **Contraindications**—hypersensitivity to drug or class, bronchogenic carcinoma
- **Caution**—hepatic dysfunction, hypovolemia

■ **Maternal Considerations** ⋯⋯⋯ **Vecuronium** is a nondepolarizing neuromuscular blocker. There are no adequate reports or well-controlled studies of **vecuronium** in pregnant women. Popular during cesarean delivery as an adjunct to general anesthesia, its effect may be prolonged by the concurrent administration of **magnesium sulfate** and possibly **clindamycin**.
Side effects include arrhythmia, tachycardia, bradycardia, hypotension, bronchospasm, and flushing.

■ **Fetal Considerations** ⋯⋯⋯ There are no adequate reports or well-controlled studies in human fetuses. A limited amount of **vecuronium** crosses the human placenta within 5min, achieving a fetal concentration of 79ng/ml and an F:M ratio <0.07. It is administered directly to the fetus as an alternative to **pancuronium** during fetal procedures. In contrast to **pancuronium**, **vecuronium** has no effect on the fetal heart rate tracing. This is an advantage for many procedures, but a potential drawback when used with fetal intravascular transfusion. Fetal paralysis modestly reduces oxygen consumption. Rodent teratogenicity studies have not been performed.

■ **Breastfeeding Safety** — There is no published experience in nursing women. It is unknown whether **vecuronium** enters human breast milk. Though similar to **pancuronium**, **vercuronium**'s clearance is faster and half-life shorter. Considering the indication and dosing, limited **vecuronium** use is unlikely to pose a clinically significant risk to the breast-feeding neonate.

■ **References** — Sloan PA, Rasul M. Anesth Analg 2002; 94:123-4.
Kaneko T, Iwama H, Tobishima S, et al. Masui 1997; 46:750-4.
Watson WJ, Atchison SR, Harlass FE. JU Matern Fetal Med 1996; 5:151-4.
Weiner CP, Anderson TL. Obstet Gynecol 1989; 73:219-24.

■ **Summary** —
- **Pregnancy Category C**
- **Lactation Category S**
- **Vecuronium** is a useful adjunct to general anesthesia during pregnancy and lactation and for fetal procedures.
- **Vecuronium** should be used during pregnancy and lactation only if the benefit justifies the potential perinatal risk.

Venlafaxine (Effexor; Trewilor)

■ **Class** — *Antidepressant, miscellaneous*

■ **Indications** — Depression

■ **Mechanism** — Inhibits norepinephrine, serotonin, and dopamine reuptake

■ **Dosage with Qualifiers** — Depression—begin 37.5mg PO with meals bid and increase q4h as needed; max 375mg/d
NOTE—hepatic and renal dosing; taper over 2w
- **Contraindications**—hypersensitivity to drug or class, MAO inhibitor <14d
- **Caution**—hepatic or renal dysfunction, seizures, history of mania, suicide risk

■ **Maternal Considerations** — Depression is common during and after pregnancy, but typically goes unrecognized. Pregnancy is not a reason *apriori* to discontinue psychotropic drugs. There are no adequate reports or well-controlled studies of **venlafaxine** in pregnant women. **Venlafaxine** may be effective for the treatment of other disorders including obsessive compulsive disorder, panic disorder, eating disorders, substance abuse, headaches, hot flashes, and chronic pain (including neuropathic pain).

Side effects include seizures, headache, nausea, vomiting, diarrhea, somnolence, anorexia, weight loss, constipation, anxiety, blurred vision, dizziness, dry mouth, insomnia, hypertension, and sweating.

■ **Fetal Considerations**

There are no adequate reports or well-controlled studies in human fetuses. **Venlafaxine** and its active metabolites cross the human placenta and enter the amniotic fluid, though the kinetics remain to be elucidated. Case control study suggests it is unassociated with an increased prevalence of fetal malformations. Rodent studies are generally reassuring, revealing no evidence of teratogenicity despite the use of doses higher than those used clinically. IUGR is seen in some models.

■ **Breastfeeding Safety**

Venlafaxine enters human breast milk achieving an M:P ratio approximating 2.5, and 2.7 for its active metabolite. Yet, the mean total drug exposure of the breast-fed infants is only 6.4%. Though this level of exposure should be safe, the breast-fed neonate should be monitored closely, since low but detectable levels are found in about half.

■ **References**

Hostetter A, Ritchie JC, Stowe ZN. Biol Psychiatry 2000; 48:1032-4.
Einarson A, Fatoye B, Sarkar M, et al. Am J Psychiatry 2001; 158:1728-30.
Ilett KF, Kristensen JH, Hackett LP, et al. Br J Clin Pharmacol 2002; 53:17-22.

■ **Summary**

- **Pregnancy Category C**
- **Lactation Category U**
- **Venlafaxine** should be used during pregnancy and lactation only if the benefit justifies the potential perinatal risk.
- As for most psychotropic drugs, monotherapy and the lowest effective quantity given in divided doses to minimize the peaks can minimize the risks.

Verapamil (Calan; Calan SR; Cardiabeltin; Covera-HS; Isoptin; Isoptin SR; Verelan; Verpal)

■ **Class** ··· *Antiarrhythmic, antihypertensive, calcium-channel blocker*

■ **Indications** ·· Angina, hypertension, supraventricular arrhythmia, atrial flutter/fibrillation, migraine prophylaxis

■ **Mechanism** ··· Inhibits Ca^{2+} influx into muscle

■ **Dosage with Qualifiers** ··············· Angina—80-480mg PO tid; max 480mg/d
Hypertension—begin 80mg PO tid; max 480mg/d
Supraventricular arrhythmia—80-120mg PO tid; max 480mg/d; alternative for paroxysmal SVT 2.5-5mg IVP, may repeat as dictated by response
Atrial flutter/fibrillation—80-120mg PO tid/qid; max 480mg/d
Migraine prophylaxis—80mg PO tid; adjust dose based effect
NOTE—renal dosing
- **Contraindications**—hypersensitivity to drug or class, severe hypotension, cardiogenic shock, severe LV dysfunction, 2nd or 3rd degree AV block, atrial fibrillation/flutter with bypass tract, sick sinus syndrome
- **Caution**—bradycardia, CHF, hepatic or renal dysfunction, muscular dystrophy, myasthenia gravis, GERD

■ **Maternal Considerations** ··········· In addition to the listed indications, **verapamil** is used in some locales for the treatment of bipolar disorder and for tocolysis in women with preterm labor. There are no adequate reports or well-controlled studies of **verapamil** in pregnant women. There is no randomized or case control study using **verapamil** as the primary tocolytic, and the practice of combining it with a β-blocker has been appropriately abandoned. Isolated case reports describe its successful use to treat maternal SVT. There are also rare reports of its use to treat preeclamptic hypertension, though there is no suggestion it offers advantages over other, more commonly used antihypertensives. Clearance is not altered in the rabbit pregnancy.
Side effects include CHF, severe hypotension. AV block, severe bradycardia, constipation, dizziness, nausea, headache, edema, and fatigue.

■ **Fetal Considerations** ················ There are no adequate reports or well-controlled studies in human fetuses. **Verapamil** readily crosses the human placenta, achieving an F:M ratio of 0.7. Similar levels are found in the amniotic fluid. Relaxation of precontracted placental arteries by **verapamil** is reduced in placentas obtained from preeclamptic women. Doppler-determined fetal blood flow resistances in preeclamptic women are unaltered by **verapamil**. **Verapamil** has been used as transplacental therapy for fetal SVT with unclear efficacy. **Flecainide** remains the drug of choice for SVT and fetal hydrops. Direct fetal administration has been reported with success. **Verapamil** crosses the rabbit placenta, though the kinetics remain to be elucidated. Rodent studies are generally reassuring, revealing no teratogenicity despite the use of doses higher than those used clinically. However, IUGR and embryotoxicity occur.

■ **Breastfeeding Safety** — There are no adequate reports or well-controlled studies in nursing women. **Verapamil** enters human breast milk, but the amount excreted is <0.05% and does not result in measurable levels in the nursing newborn.

■ **References** —
Wisner KL, Peindl KS, Perel JM, et al. Biol Psychiatry 2002; 51:745-52.
Solans C, Bregante MA, Aramayona JJ, et al. Xenobiotica 2000; 30:93-102.
Byerly WG, Hartmann A, Foster DE, Tannenbaum AK. Ann Emerg Med 1991; 20:552-4.
Szymanski W, Skublicki S, Jankowski A, Kotzbach R. Ginekol Pol 1992; 63:166-71.
Belfort MA, Anthony J, Buccimazza A, Davey DA. Obstet Gynecol 1990; 75:970-4.
Simpson JM, Sharland GK. Heart 1998; 79:576-81.Kook H, Yoon YD, Baik YH. J Korean Med Sci 1996; 11:250-7.
Belfort M, Akovic K, Anthony J, et al. J Clin Ultrasound 1994; 22:317-25.
Gembruch U, Hansmann M, Redel DA, Bald R. J Perinat Med 1988; 16:39-44.
Anderson P, Bondesson U, Mattiasson I, Johansson BW. Eur J Clin Pharmacol 1987; 31:625-7.

■ **Summary** —
- **Pregnancy Category C**
- **Lactation Category S**
- **Verapamil** should be used during pregnancy only if the benefit justifies the potential perinatal risk.
- There are alternative agents for which there is more experience during pregnancy and lactation.

Vidarabine (Vira-A)

■ **Class** — *Antiviral, ophthalmologic, encephalitis*

■ **Indications** — HSV keratoconjunctivitis, HSV epithelial keratitis

■ **Mechanism** — Inhibits DNA synthesis

■ **Dosage with Qualifiers** HSV epithelial keratitis—apply 0.5in ribbon OS/OD 5×/d
HSV keratoconjunctivitis—apply 0.5in ribbon OS/OD 5×/d
HSV encephalitis—15mg/kg/d ×10d (IV preparation no
longer released in the U.S.)
- **Contraindications**—hypersensitivity to drug or class,
  sterile trophic ulcers
- **Caution**—unknown

■ **Maternal Considerations** **Vidarabine** is a purine nucleoside obtained from
fermentation cultures of Streptomyces antibioticus. There
is no published experience with **vidarabine** for the above
indications during pregnancy. Treatment for encephalitis
should be discontinued when the brain biopsy is negative
for herpes simplex virus in cell culture.
Side effects include tearing, foreign body sensation, burning,
photophobia, and superficial punctuate keratitis.

■ **Fetal Considerations** There are no adequate reports or well-controlled studies
in human fetuses. It is unknown whether **vidarabine**
crosses the human placenta. **Vidarabine** is teratogenic in
rodents after parenteral administration. And though this
concern remains for topical administration, it is unlikely
the maternal systemic concentration will reach clinically
relevant level. **Vidarabine** is used for neonatal treatment.

■ **Breastfeeding Safety** There is no published experience in nursing women. It is
unknown whether **vidarabine** enters human breast milk.
It is unlikely to pose a clinically significant risk to the
breast-feeding neonate after topical use.

■ **References** There are no current relevant references.

■ **Summary**
- **Pregnancy Category C**
- **Lactation Category S? (topical), U (IV)**
- **Vidarabine** should be used during pregnancy and
  lactation only if the benefit justifies the potential
  perinatal risk.

Vinblastine (Velban; Velsar)

■ **Class** *Mitosis inhibitor*

■ **Indications** Ovarian or breast cancer, choriocarcinoma, Hodgkin's
disease, lymphoma, Kaposi's sarcoma, mycosis fungoides

■ **Mechanism** Arrests mitosis in metaphase by inhibiting microtubule
formation

- **Dosage with Qualifiers** ⋯⋯ <u>Chemotherapy</u>—dosing protocols vary; usually combined with other agents
  - **Contraindications**—hypersensitivity to drug or class, bacterial infection, granulocytopenia, intrathecal use, intestinal obstruction, paralytic ileus
  - **Caution**—bone marrow depression, neuropathy, neuromuscular disease, neurotoxic agents, ototoxic agents, pulmonary disease, hepatic dysfunction, cytochrome P3A4 interactions

- **Maternal Considerations** ⋯⋯ **Vinblastine** is a vinca alkaloid. Fertility is retained when **vinblastine** is used for either gestational trophoblastic disease or ovarian cancer after ovary-sparing surgery. There are no adequate reports or well-controlled studies of **vinblastine** in pregnant women. The literature consists of isolated case reports of its use for the treatment of lymphoma.
  Side effects include myelosuppression, peripheral neuropathy, paralytic ileus, intestinal obstruction, intestinal necrosis, hemorrhagic enterocolitis, loss of DTRs, severe neuromuscular impairment, bronchospasm, infertility, SIADH, extravasation necrosis, leukopenia, anorexia, nausea, vomiting, alopecia, constipation, paresthesias, stomatitis, anemia, malaise, headache, diarrhea, dizziness, bone pain, injection site reaction, thrombophlebitis, decreased DTRs, and blood pressure changes.

- **Fetal Considerations** ⋯⋯ There are no adequate reports or well-controlled studies in human fetuses. It is unknown whether **vinblastine** crosses the human placenta. *In vitro*, its transfer involves P-glycoprotein, whose back transfer of **vinblastine** may help protect the fetus. Most fetuses exposed deliver without apparent adverse effects. The risk of birth defects in pregnant women previously treated is similar to the background rate. **Vinblastine** is teratogenic and embryotoxic in rodents. Exposed fetuses should be evaluated in a fetal medicine unit.

- **Breastfeeding Safety** ⋯⋯ There is no published experience in nursing women. It is unknown whether vinblastine enters human breast milk.

- **References** ⋯⋯ Yoshinaka A, Fukasawa I, Sakamoto T, et al. Arch Gynecol Obstet 2000; 264:124-7.
  Ross GT. Cancer 1976; 37:1043-7.
  Ushigome F, Takanaga H, Matsuo H, et al. Eur J Pharmacol 2000; 408:1-10.
  Nisce LZ, Tome MA, He S, et al. Am J Clin Oncol 1986; 9:146-51.

- **Summary** ⋯⋯
  - **Pregnancy Category D**
  - **Lactation Category U**
  - **Vinblastine** should be used during pregnancy and lactation only if the benefit justifies the potential perinatal risk.
  - *In utero* exposure appears for the most part well tolerated, and is not *apriori* an indication for pregnancy termination.

Vincristine (Citomid; Oncovin; Vincasar PFS; Vincrex)

■ **Class** — Mitosis inhibitor

■ **Indications** — Trophoblastic disease, Hodgkin's disease, leukemia, non-Hodgkin's lymphoma, neuroblastoma, rhabdomyosarcoma, Wilms' tumor, etc

■ **Mechanism** — Arrests mitosis in metaphase by inhibiting microtubule formation

■ **Dosage with Qualifiers** — Chemotherapy—multiple protocols; typically 1.4mg/m²; max 2mg/dose usually combined with other agents
   • **Contraindications**—hypersensitivity to drug or class, acute bacterial infection, intestinal obstruction, paralytic ileus, demyelinating Charcot-Marie-Tooth syndrome
   • **Caution**—bone marrow suppression, neuromuscular disease, neurotoxic agents, ototoxic agents, pulmonary disease, hepatic dysfunction, cytochrome P3A4 interactions

■ **Maternal Considerations** — **Vincristine** is a vinca alkaloid. There are no adequate reports or well-controlled studies of **vincristine** in pregnant women. The literature consists of isolated case reports and series of women treated during pregnancy for leukemia or lymphoma.
   Side effects include myelosuppression, peripheral neuropathy, paralytic ileus, intestinal necrosis, cranial nerve palsy, decreased DTRs, severe neuromuscular impairment, seizures, bronchospasm, MI, SIADH, infertility, extravasation necrosis, tumor lysis syndrome, uric acid nephropathy, alopecia, nausea, anorexia, vomiting, constipation, diarrhea, fatigue, paresthesias, peripheral neuropathy, dizziness, nystagmus, thrombophlebitis, ataxia, blood pressure changes, weakness, and electrolyte abnormalities.

■ **Fetal Considerations** — There are no adequate reports or well-controlled studies in human fetuses. It is unknown whether **vincristine** crosses the human placenta. In vitro, its transfer involves P-glycoprotein, whose back transfer may help protect the fetus. Most fetuses exposed deliver without apparent adverse effects. **Vincristine** is teratogenic and embryotoxic in rodents, and in limited study teratogenic in a subhuman primate. Exposed fetuses should be evaluated in a fetal medicine unit.

■ **Breastfeeding Safety** — There is no published experience in nursing women. It is unknown whether **vincristine** enters human breast milk. It inhibits goat milk production in a dose-dependent manner.

- **References** ·········· Ushigome F, Takanaga H, Matsuo H, et al. Eur J Pharmacol 2000; 408:1-10.
  Fassas A, Kartalis G, Klearchou N, et al. Nouv Rev Fr Hematol 1984; 26:19-24.
  Aviles N, Neri N. Clin Lymphoma 2001; 2:173:7.
  Henderson AJ, Faulkner A. Q J Exp Physiol 1985; 70:15-22.

- **Summary** ··········
  - **Pregnancy Category D**
  - **Lactation Category U**
  - **Vincristine** should be used during pregnancy and lactation only if the benefit justifies the potential perinatal risk.
  - *In utero* exposure appears for the most part well tolerated, and is not *apriori* an indication for pregnancy termination.

Vinorelbine (Navelbine)

- **Class** ·········· *Mitosis inhibitor*

- **Indications** ·········· Breast, cervical, and non-small cell lung cancers, Kaposi's sarcoma

- **Mechanism** ·········· Inhibits microtubule formation in metaphase arresting mitosis

- **Dosage with Qualifiers** ·········· Chemotherapy—multiple protocols alone or in combination with **cisplatin**
  - **Contraindications**—hypersensitivity to drug or class, acute bacterial infection, granulocytopenia, intrathecal administration, GI obstruction, paralytic ileus
  - **Caution**—bone marrow depression, neuropathy, neuromuscular disease, neurotoxic agents, pulmonary disease, hepatic dysfunction, cytochrome P3A4 interactions

- **Maternal Considerations** ·········· **Vinorelbine** is a vinca alkaloid. There are no adequate reports or well-controlled studies of **vinorelbine** in pregnant women. The literature consists of multiple case reports of women treated during pregnancy.
  Side effects include myelosuppression, peripheral neuropathy, paralytic ileus, intestinal necrosis, radiation recall reaction, severe neuromuscular impairment, interstitial pulmonary disease, dyspnea, MI, SIADH, infertility, extravasation necrosis, leukopenia, granulocytopenia, anemia, increased LFTs, infusion site reactions, constipation, anorexia, alopecia, peripheral neuropathy, diarrhea, dizziness, nausea, vomiting, nystagmus, thrombophlebitis, and thrombocytopenia.

- **Fetal Considerations** ...... There are no adequate reports or well-controlled studies in human fetuses. It is unknown whether **vinorelbine** crosses the human placenta. The case reports of its use during pregnancy usually note no adverse effects attributable to treatment on the perinate.

- **Breastfeeding Safety** ...... There is no published experience in nursing women. It is unknown whether **vinorelbine** enters human breast milk.

- **References** ...... Janne PA, Rodriguez-Thompson D, Metcalf DR, et al. Oncology 2001; 61:175-83.
Cuvier C, Espie M, Extra JM, Marty M. Eur J Cancer 1997; 33:168-9.

- **Summary** ......
  - **Pregnancy Category D**
  - **Lactation Category U**
  - **Vinorelbine** should be used during pregnancy and lactation only if the benefit justifies the potential perinatal risk.

Voriconazole (Vfend)

- **Class** ...... Antifungal

- **Indications** ...... Invasive aspergillosis, severe fungal infections

- **Mechanism** ...... Inhibits sterol C-14 α demethylation and cytochrome p450

- **Dosage with Qualifiers** ...... Invasive aspergillosis—begin 6mg/kg IV q12h, then 4mg/kg IV q12h or convert to PO
Severe fungal infections—begin 6mg/kg IV q12h, then 4mg/kg IV q12h or convert to PO
NOTE—renal and hepatic dosing
NOTE—check LFTs at baseline and periodically during treatment; monitor visual fields if >28d treatment
  - **Contraindications**—hypersensitivity to drug or class, use of either **terfenadine, astemizole, cisapride, quinidine, pimozide, sirolimus, rifampin, carbamazepine, rifabutin**, or long-acting barbiturates, galactose intolerance
  - **Caution**—hepatic or renal dysfunction, hematologic malignancy, prolonged use

- **Maternal Considerations** ...... There are no adequate reports or well-controlled studies of **voriconazole** in pregnant women.
Side effects include cholecystitis, hepatitis, fulminant hepatic necrosis, acute renal failure, Stevens-Johnson syndrome, photosensitivity, and angioedema,

blood dyscrasias, fever, nausea, vomiting, rash, chills, headache, increased LFTs, hallucinations, visual changes, blurred vision, and photophobia.

■ **Fetal Considerations** .... There are no adequate reports or well-controlled studies in human fetuses. It is unknown whether **voriconazole** crosses the human placenta.

■ **Breastfeeding Safety** .... There is no published experience in nursing women. It is unknown whether **voriconazole** enters human breast milk.

■ **References** .... There is no published experience in pregnancy or during lactation.

■ **Summary** ....
- **Pregnancy Category D**
- **Lactation Category U**
- **Voriconazole** should be used during pregnancy and lactation only if the benefit justifies the potential perinatal risk

Warfarin (Coumadin)

■ **Class** .... Anticoagulant, thrombolytic

■ **Indications** .... Anticoagulation, therapeutic and prophylactic

■ **Mechanism** .... Inhibits vitamin K-dependent clotting factor synthesis (II, VII, IX, X, proteins C and S)

■ **Dosage with Qualifiers** .... Chronic treatment of thrombophilia—5-10mg PO qd, keep INR >3
Acute therapy of thromboembolic disease—begin 2.5mg, increase gradual over 2-4d to achieve desired INR
Prosthetic cardiac valves or atrial fibrillation—2.5-10mg PO qd, INR should be maintained between 2.5-3.0 depending on the valve type
- **Contraindications**—hypersensitivity to drug or class, active bleeding, recent surgery, esophageal varices, thrombocytopenia, vitamin K deficiency, concurrent thrombolytics, recent lumbar puncture, congenital clotting defect
- **Caution**—congenital clotting defects, thrombocytopenia, concurrent thrombolytics, lumbar puncture

■ **Maternal Considerations** .... Thromboembolic disease remains a major cause of maternal morbidity and mortality. There are no adequate reports or well-controlled studies in pregnant women. It is most likely that a woman with a prior thromboembolic event unrelated to a permanent risk factor does not require prophylaxis during a subsequent pregnancy. The risk of a bleeding complication during pregnancy approximates 18% with **warfarin**. An INR of 3.0 is sufficient for either prophylaxis or treatment of venous thromboembolism, thus minimizing the risk of hemorrhage associated with higher INRs. Women on **warfarin** planning pregnancy should switch to a heparinoid agent prior to conception if possible. However, therapeutic **heparin** is not effective prophylaxis in women with a prosthetic heart valve. In this instance, it is best to continue **warfarin**, though some recommend replacement with **heparin** between 6-12w. A daily dose >5mg is associated with a greater risk of an adverse outcome. If the mother's condition requires anticoagulation with **warfarin**, it should be substituted with **heparin** at 36w to decrease the risk to the fetus. Neuraxial anesthesia is contraindicated because of the risk of puncture-associated bleeding. **Warfarin** treatment is resumed postpartum.
Side effects include hemorrhage, skin necrosis, rash, major hemorrhage, diarrhea, nausea, abdominal pain, hepatitis, dermatitis, and blue toe syndrome.

■ **Fetal Considerations** ········· **Warfarin** is a known teratogen. While there are no adequate reports or well-controlled studies in human fetuses, exposure from 6-10w gestation is associated with an embryopathy, and exposure subsequently with a fetopathy. The *fetal* **warfarin** *syndrome* includes nasal hypoplasia (failure of nasal septum development), micropthalmia, hypoplasia of the extremities, IUGR, heart disease, scoliosis, deafness, and mental retardation. While the embryopathy appears secondary to a fetal vitamin K deficiency, the fetopathy results from microhemorrhages. The most common CNS malformations include agenesis of the corpus callosum, Dandy-Walker malformation, and optic atrophy. In a large series of women treated the duration of pregnancy for a prosthetic valve, the overall incidence of fetal **warfarin** syndrome was 5.6%. The pregnancy loss rate was 32% and the stillbirth rate 10% of pregnancies achieving at least 20w. School-age children exposed *in utero* have an increased frequency of mild neurologic dysfunction and an IQ <80.

■ **Breastfeeding Safety** ········· **Warfarin** does not enter human breast milk and is compatible with breastfeeding.

■ **References** ·········

Wesseling J, Van Driel D, Heymans HS, et al. Thromb Haemost 2001; 85:609-130.
Cotrufo M, De Feo M, De Santo LS, et al. Obstet Gynecol 2002; 99:35-40.
Brill-Edwards P, Ginsberg JS, Gent M, et al. N Engl Med 2000; 343:1439-44.
Clark SL, Porter TF, West FG. Obstet Gynecol 2000; 95:938-40.
Wesseling J, Van Driel D, Smrkovsky M, et al. Early Hum Dev 2001; 63:83-95.
Suri V, Sawhney H, Vasishta K, et al. Int J Gynaecol Obstet 1999; 64:239-46.
Rosove MH, Brewer PM. Ann Intern Med 1992; 117:303-8.
Cotrufo M, de Luca TS, Calabro R, et al. Eur J Cardiothorac Surg 1991; 5:300-4.

■ **Summary** ·········

- **Pregnancy Category X**
- **Lactation Category S**
- **Warfarin** may cause an embryopathy in the 1st trimester, and a fetopathy in the 2nd and 3rd trimesters
- Heparinoids are the preferred substitutes for most anticoagulant needs during pregnancy except when the prophylaxis is for a mechanical heart valve.
- **Warfarin** should be used during pregnancy only if the benefit justifies the potential perinatal risk.

Zafirlukast (Accolate)

- **Class** — *Leukotriene antagonist, asthma*

- **Indications** — Asthma prophylaxis

- **Mechanism** — Leukotriene D4 and E4 receptor antagonist

- **Dosage with Qualifiers** — Asthma prophylaxis—20mg PO 1h before or 2h after meals bid
  NOTE—hepatic dosing
  - **Contraindications**—hypersensitivity to drug or class, acute asthma
  - **Caution**—hepatic dysfunction, systemic corticosteroid taper

- **Maternal Considerations** — There is no published experience with **zafirlukast** during pregnancy.
  Side effects include Churg-Strauss syndrome, headache, rhinitis, nausea, diarrhea, pain, asthenia, abdominal pain, dizziness, myalgia, fever, back pain, vomiting, increased hepatic transaminases, and dyspepsia.

- **Fetal Considerations** — There are no adequate reports or well-controlled studies in human fetuses. It is unknown whether **zafirlukast** crosses the human placenta. Rodent and primate studies are reassuring, revealing no evidence of teratogenicity or IUGR (unless there was maternal toxicity) despite the use of doses higher than those used clinically.

- **Breastfeeding Safety** — There is no published experience in nursing women. **Zafirlukast** is excreted into human breast milk with an M:P ratio of 0.2.

- **References** — Spector SL. Ann Allergy Asthma Immunol 2001; 86:18-23.

- **Summary** —
  - **Pregnancy Category B**
  - **Lactation Category S?**
  - **Zafirlukast** should be used during pregnancy and lactation only if the benefit justifies the potential perinatal risk.
  - There are alternative agents for which there is more experience during pregnancy and lactation.

Zalcitabine (DDC; ddC; Dideoxycytidine; Hivid)

■ **Class** — *Antiviral*, HIV

■ **Indications** — Advanced HIV

■ **Mechanism** — Nucleoside reverse transcriptase inhibitor

■ **Dosage with Qualifiers** — <u>Advanced HIV</u>—0.75mg PO q8h
- **Contraindications**—hypersensitivity to drug or class
- **Caution**—hepatic or renal dysfunction, peripheral neuropathy, CHF, history pancreatitis

■ **Maternal Considerations** — There are no adequate reports or well-controlled studies of **zalcitabine** in pregnant women. The treatment of HIV during pregnancy significantly reduces the risk of mother-to-child transmission. Triple therapy (**zidovudine, lamivudine, nevirapine**) remains the standard of care for management of HIV infection in adults. The U.S. FDA has approved only 4 nucleoside analog reverse transcriptase inhibitors: **zidovudine**, **zalcitabine**, **didanosine**, and **stavudine**. **Zalcitabine** is a 2nd selection should the patient not respond to **zidovudine**.
Side effects include seizures, lactic acidosis, thrombocytopenia, leukopenia, anemia, eosinophilia, peripheral neuropathy, hepatic dysfunction, fatigue, nausea, abdominal pain, vomiting, diarrhea, constipation, rash, pruritus, urticaria, oral lesions, depression, headache, fever, cough, and rhinitis.

■ **Fetal Considerations** — There are no adequate reports or well-controlled studies in human fetuses. It is unknown whether **zalcitabine** crosses the human placenta. It does cross the primate (*Macaca nemestrina*) placenta. Rodent studies revealed evidence of teratogenicity at doses >1000 times the MRHD.

■ **Breastfeeding Safety** — There are no adequate reports or well-controlled studies in nursing women. It is unknown whether **zalcitabine** enters human breast milk. However, breastfeeding is contraindicated in HIV-infected nursing women where formula is available to reduce the risk of neonatal transmission.

■ **References** — Temesgen Z, Wright AJ. Mayo Clin Proc 1999; 74:1284-301.
Tuntland T, Nosbisch C, Baughman WL, et al. Am J Obstet Gynecol 1996; 174:856-63.
Spector SA. AIDS 1994; 8(Suppl 3):S15-8.
Matthews SJ, Cersosimo RJ, Spivack ML. Pharmacotherapy 1991; 11:419-48.

■ **Summary**
- **Pregnancy Category C**
- **Lactation Category NS**

- Combination therapy with of **zidovudine**, **lamivudine**, and **nevirapine** significantly reduces the risk of mother-to-child transmission and remains the standard of care for management of HIV infection in adults.
- **Zalcitabine** is an alternative reverse transcriptase inhibitor in patients unresponsive to **zidovudine**.
- Physicians are encouraged to register pregnant women under the Antiretroviral Pregnancy Registry (1-800-258-4263) for a better follow-up of the outcome while under treatment with **zalcitabine**.

Zaleplon (Sonata)

■ **Class** — *Hypnotic, anxiolytic*

■ **Indications** — Short-term treatment of insomnia

■ **Mechanism** — Interacts with GABA/benzodiazepine receptor complex

■ **Dosage with Qualifiers** — Short-term treatment of insomnia—5-10mg PO qhs prn; onset 60min, duration <5h
- **Contraindications**—hypersensitivity to drug or class
- **Caution**—hepatic dysfunction, history of substance abuse, pulmonary disease

■ **Maternal Considerations** — There is no published experience with **zaleplon** during pregnancy.
Side effects include dependency, drowsiness, amnesia, paresthesias, abnormal vision, dizziness, headache, hangover, rebound insomnia, and confusion.

■ **Fetal Considerations** — There are no adequate reports or well-controlled studies in human fetuses. It is unknown whether **zaleplon** crosses the human placenta.

■ **Breastfeeding Safety** — Small quantities of **zaleplon** are excreted into human breast milk. It is calculated that the breast-feeding neonate would ingest approximately 0.015% of the maternal dose. This quantity is unlikely to result in a clinically relevant level.

■ **References** — Darwish M, Martin PT, Cevallos WH, et al. J Clin Pharmacol 1999; 39:670-4.

■ **Summary** —
- **Pregnancy Category C**
- **Lactation Category S**

Zanamivir (Relenza)

■ **Class** — Antiviral, other

■ **Indications** — Uncomplicated influenza

■ **Mechanism** — Inhibits influenza neuraminidase

■ **Dosage with Qualifiers** — Uncomplicated influenza—begin within 48h of symptoms, 10mg INH q2-4h ×2, then 12h ×5d
  - **Contraindications**—hypersensitivity to drug or class, COPD, asthma, unable to use inhaler
  - **Caution**—unknown

■ **Maternal Considerations** — There is no published experience with **zanamivir** during pregnancy. Pregnant women should consider vaccination prior to influenza season.
Side effects include bronchospasm, nausea, dizziness, headache, bronchitis, cough, nasal symptoms, and ENT infection.

■ **Fetal Considerations** — There are no adequate reports or well-controlled studies in human fetuses. It is unknown whether **zanamivir** crosses the human placenta. It does cross the rodent placenta. Rodent studies are for the most part reassuring, with only minor skeletal abnormalities occurring in one strain of rat when the dose exceeded 1000 times the MRHD.

■ **Breastfeeding Safety** — There is no published experience in nursing women. It is unknown whether **zanamivir** enters human breast milk. It is excreted into rodent milk.

■ **References** — There is no published experience in pregnancy or during lactation.

■ **Summary** —
  - **Pregnancy Category C**
  - **Lactation Category U**
  - **Zanamivir** should be used during pregnancy and lactation only if the benefit justifies the potential perinatal risk.

Zidovudine (Aviral; AZT; Retrovir; Retrovis)

■ **Class** .... *Antiviral*, HIV

■ **Indications** .... HIV

■ **Mechanism** .... Nucleoside reverse transcriptase inhibitor

■ **Dosage with Qualifiers** .... <u>HIV during pregnancy</u>—begin 100mg PO 5×/d after 14w until onset of labor; in intrapartum period: 2mg/kg IV over 1h, then 1mg/kg/h until cord clamping
<u>HIV in nonpregnant women</u>—300mg PO q12h, or 1mg/kg IV q4h
- **Contraindications**—hypersensitivity to drug or class, severe bone marrow suppression
- **Caution**—hepatic or renal dysfunction

■ **Maternal Considerations** .... The treatment of HIV infection during pregnancy significantly reduces the risk of mother-child transmission. Combination therapy (**zidovudine, lamivudine, nevirapine**) remains the standard of care for management of HIV infection in adults due to its high efficacy. The Pediatric AIDS Clinical Trials Group (protocol 076) documented that **zidovudine** chemoprophylaxis reduced perinatal HIV-1 transmission by nearly 70%. Since then, multiple randomized studies confirm **zidovudine** monotherapy is extremely effective in preventing vertical transmission of the virus. Shorter regimens reduced the risk of transmission by 50% in a non-breastfeeding population, and by about 37% in breastfeeding populations. When **zidovudine** is combined with other antiretroviral drugs (protease inhibitors), the effectiveness is almost 90%. The addition of **nevirapine** to the standard IV **zidovudine** labor regimen further reduces perinatal HIV transmission in women not already receiving antenatal antiretroviral therapy. The addition of **nevirapine** is not beneficial when the patient has been using "triple therapy" prenatally. It is possible in developed countries to lower the transmission rate below 4% using combinations of available medications and for the selective patient, elective cesarean section before labor. Thus, it is important to encourage women to undergo testing for HIV during pregnancy, maximizing opportunities for offering antiretroviral therapy. Unfortunately, adherence to **zidovudine** therapy may be relatively low during the last 3w of gestation and during the first 3w postpartum. **Zidovudine** prophylaxis is not associated with the development of resistance. Women should be monitored closely for hepatotoxicity after initiation of **zidovudine**. *Side effects* include agranulocytosis, thrombocytopenia, bone marrow suppression, seizures, anemia, pancreatitis, myopathy, lactic acidosis, granulocytopenia, hepatotoxicity, nausea, vomiting, abdominal pain, diarrhea, headache, asthenia, rash, fever, anorexia, somnolence, myalgia, malaise, dyspepsia, diaphoresis, dyspnea, taste changes, pigmented nails, and paresthesias.

■ **Fetal Considerations** .... **Zidovudine** rapidly crosses the human placenta achieving concentrations that approach unity. Maternal antiretroviral drug therapy during pregnancy and labor, followed by 6w of neonatal **zidovudine**, significantly reduces the risk of vertical transmission. Additional antiretroviral drugs may be needed in some high-risk newborns. Asymptomatic women with HIV who lack a social support network are more likely not to comply with the recommended neonatal prophylactic regimen of antiretroviral therapy. Elective cesarean section prior to the onset of labor also reduces the rate of vertical transmission if there is a detectable maternal viral load. Mitochondrial disorders are described in children exposed to **zidovudine** *in utero*. Fetuses exposed to triple therapy may be at increased risk for malformations.

■ **Breastfeeding Safety** .... There is no published experience in nursing women. It is unknown whether **zidovudine** enters human breast milk. It is excreted into rodent milk. However, breastfeeding is contraindicated in HIV-infected nursing women where formula is available to reduce the risk of neonatal transmission.

■ **References** ....
Mofenson LM. MMWR Recomm Rep 2002; 51(RR-18):1-38.
No authors. Arch Pediatr Adolesc Med 2002; 156:915-21.
Demas PA, Webber MP, Schoenbaum EE, et al. Pediatrics 2002; 110:e35.
Simon T, Funke AM, Hero B, Reiser-Hartwig S, Fuhrmann U. Zentralbl Gynakol 2002; 124:413-7.
Ickovics JR, Wilson TE, Royce RA, et al. J Acquir Immune Defic Syndr 2002; 30:311-5.
Bhana N, Ormrod D, Perry CM, et al. Paediatr Drugs 2002; 4:515-53.
Dorenbaum A, Cunningham CK, Gelber RD, et al. JAMA 2002; 288:189-98.
Sperling RS, Roboz J, Dische R, et al. Am J Perinatol 1992; 9:247-9.
Brocklehurst P, Volmink J. Cochrane Database Syst Rev 2002; CD003510.
Nolan M, Fowler MG, Mofenson LM. J Acquir Immune Defic Syndr 2002; 30:216-29.
Cooper ER, Charurat M, Mofenson L, et al. J Acquir Immune Defic Syndr 2002; 29:484-94.
Lancet 2002; 359:1178-86.
Ekpini RA, Nkengasong JN, Sibailly T, et al. AIDS 2002; 16:625-30.
Brocklehurst P, Volmink J. Cochrane Database Syst Rev 2002; CD003510.
Hill JB, Sheffield JS, Zeeman GG, Wendel GD Jr. Obstet Gynecol 2001; 98:909-11.
Lansky A, Jones JL, Frey RL, Lindegren ML. Am J Public Health 2001; 91:1291-3.

Rovira MT, Antorn MT, Paya A, et al. Eur J Obstet
Gynecol Reprod Biol 2001; 97:46-9.
Rutstein RM. Curr Opin Pediatr 2001; 13:408-16.

■ **Summary**

- **Pregnancy Category C**
- **Lactation Category NS**
- "Triple therapy" consisting of **zidovudine**, **lamivudine**, and **nevirapine** significantly reduces the risk of mother-child transmission; it is the standard of care for HIV infection in adults.
- A short course of **zidovudine** or a single-dose of **nevirapine** is an effective therapy to reduce mother-child transmission of HIV.
- Breastfeeding is not recommended.
- Physicians are encouraged to register pregnant women under the Antiretroviral Pregnancy Registry (1-800-258-4263) for a better follow-up of the outcome while under treatment with **zidovudine**.

Zileuton (Zyflo)

■ **Class** — Asthma; *leukotriene antagonist*

■ **Indications** — Asthma

■ **Mechanism** — 5-lipoxygenase inhibitor reducing leukotrienes

■ **Dosage with Qualifiers** — Asthma—600mg PO qid; max 2400mg/d
NOTE—check LFTs baseline, qmo ×3mo, then q3mo ×1y
- **Contraindications**—hypersensitivity to drug or class, acute asthma, hepatotoxicity
- **Caution**—alcohol abuse, hepatic dysfunction

■ **Maternal Considerations** — There is no published experience with **zileuton** during pregnancy.
Side effects include hepatotoxicity, insomnia, headache, dizziness, nausea, dyspepsia, abdominal pain, neutropenia, and elevated LFTs.

■ **Fetal Considerations** — There are no adequate reports or or well-controlled studies in human fetuses. It is unknown whether **zileuton** crosses the human placenta. Rodent studies revealed evidence for an increased prevalence of IUGR, skeletal abnormalities and cleft palate.

■ **Breastfeeding Safety** — There is no published experience in nursing women. It is unknown whether **zileuton** enters human breast milk. It is excreted into rodent milk.

- **References** ⸺ Spector SL. Ann Allergy Asthma Immunol 2001; 86:18-23.
  No authors. Ann Allergy Asthma Immunol 2000; 84:475-80.

- **Summary** ⸺
  - **Pregnancy Category C**
  - **Lactation Category U**
  - **Zileuton** should be used during pregnancy and lactation only if the benefit justifies the potential perinatal risk.
  - There are alternative agents for which there is more experience during pregnancy and lactation.

Ziprasidone (Aygestin; Milligynon; Norcolut; Nordron; Geodon; Norlutate; Shiton)

- **Class** ⸺ *Antipsychotic*

- **Indications** ⸺ Schizophrenia

- **Mechanism** ⸺ Unknown; antagonizes D2 and 5-HT2 receptors

- **Dosage with Qualifiers** ⸺ Schizophrenia—begin 20mg PO with meals bid, adjust to response; max 160mg/d
  - **Contraindications**—hypersensitivity to drug or class, prolonged QT interval, recent MI, uncompensated CHF, hypokalemia, hypomagnesemia, history of arrhythmia
  - **Caution**—hepatic dysfunction, seizures, cerebrovascular disease, cardiovascular disease, hypotension, hypovolemia, dehydration, agents that prolong the QT interval, risk aspiration pneumonia

- **Maternal Considerations** ⸺ There is no published experience with **ziprasidone** during pregnancy.
  Side effects include neuroleptic malignant syndrome, tardive dyskinesia, hypertension, QT interval prolongation, syncope, extrapyramidal symptoms, irregular menses, somnolence, nausea, constipation, dyspepsia, akathisia, dizziness, respiratory disorders, asthenia, diarrhea, weight gain, rash, urticaria, visual disturbances, tachycardia, hyperglycemia, and hyperprolactinemia.

- **Fetal Considerations** ⸺ There are no adequate reports or well-controlled studies in human fetuses. It is unknown whether **ziprasidone** crosses the human placenta. Rodent studies reveal evidence of embryotoxicity, IUGR and an increased prevalence of malformation (cardiac, renal, and skeletal depending upon species and model) at doses similar to the recommended human dose.

- **Breastfeeding Safety** — There is no published experience in nursing women. It is unknown whether **ziprasidone** enters human breast milk.

- **References** — There is no published experience in pregnancy or during lactation.

- **Summary**
  - **Pregnancy Category C**
  - **Lactation Category U**
  - **Ziprasidone** should be used during pregnancy and lactation only if the benefit justifies the potential perinatal risk.
  - There are alternative agents for which there is more experience in pregnancy and lactation.

Zolmitriptan (Zomig; Zomigoro)

- **Class** — Migraine; serotonin agonist

- **Indications** — Migraine headache

- **Mechanism** — Selective 5HT-1 receptor agonist

- **Dosage with Qualifiers** — Migraine headache—1.25-2.5mg PO ×1, may repeat after 2h prn; max 10mg/24h
  - **Contraindications**—hypersensitivity to drug or class, CAD, coronary vasospasm, history MI, uncontrolled hypertension, 5-HT1 agonist <24h, MAO inhibitor <14d, ergot <24h, basilar migraine, hemiplegic migraine, WPW with symptoms
  - **Caution**—cardiac risk factors, hepatic dysfunction, severe renal disease, PVD, CVD

- **Maternal Considerations** — Pregnancy has a beneficial effect on migraine in 55-90% of women and mainly during the 2nd and 3rd trimesters. A higher percentage of women with menstrual migraine compared to other migraines improve during pregnancy. There is no published experience with **zolmitriptan** during pregnancy. Mean plasma concentrations of **zolmitriptan** are up to 1.5-fold higher in females than males. It is not known whether pregnancy alters clearance.
  Side effects include acute MI, arrhythmias, coronary vasospasm, cerebral hemorrhage, stroke, hypertensive crisis, peripheral vascular ischemia, bowel ischemia, asthenia, nausea, vomiting, dizziness, chest pain, neck and jaw tightness, somnolence, sweating, palpitations, and myalgia.

- **Fetal Considerations** — There are no adequate reports or well-controlled studies in human fetuses. It is unknown whether **zolmitriptan** crosses the human placenta. Rodent studies revealed embryotoxicity and skeletal abnormalities at doses more than 500 times the MRHD.

■ **Breastfeeding Safety** There is no published experience in nursing women. It is unknown whether **zolmitriptan** enters human breast milk. It is excreted into rodent milk. However, considering the indication and dosing, one-time or occasional **zolmitriptan** use is unlikely to pose a clinically significant risk to the breast-feeding neonate. If desired, the patient may pump her breasts for 24h and then resume breastfeeding.

■ **References** Diener HC, Limmroth V. Expert Opin Investig Drugs 2001; 10:1831-45.
Pfaffenrath V, Rehm M. Drug Saf 1998; 19:383-8.

■ **Summary**
- **Pregnancy Category C**
- **Lactation Category U**
- **Zolmitriptan** should be used during pregnancy and lactation only if the benefit justifies the potential perinatal risk.
- There are alternative agents for which there is more experience during pregnancy and lactation.

Zolpidem (Ambien)

■ **Class** *Hypnotic, anxiolytic*

■ **Indications** Short-term treatment of insomnia

■ **Mechanism** Interacts with GABA/benzodiazepine receptor complex

■ **Dosage with Qualifiers** Short-term treatment of insomnia—5-10mg PO qhs prn
- **Contraindications**—hypersensitivity to drug or class
- **Caution**—depression, substance abuse, impaired respiratory function

■ **Maternal Considerations** There are no adequate reports or well-controlled studies of **zolpidem** in pregnant women. **Zolpidem** significantly inhibits smooth muscle contractility *in vitro*.
Side effects include ataxia, hallucinations, headache, drowsiness, lethargy, depression, dizziness, URI, sinusitis, pharyngitis, dry mouth, nausea, dyspepsia, diarrhea, constipation, palpitations, arthralgia, back pain, and myalgias.

■ **Fetal Considerations** There are no adequate reports or well-controlled studies in human fetuses. It is unknown whether **zolpidem** crosses the human placenta. Rodent studies are reassuring, revealing no evidence of teratogenicity or IUGR despite the use of doses higher than those used clinically. Prenatal exposure to **diazepam** and **alprazolam**, but not to **zolpidem**, affects behavioral stress reactivity in adult male rats.

■ **Breastfeeding Safety** Less than 0.02% of the total administered maternal dose is excreted into milk, but the effect of **zolpidem** on the infant is unknown. It seems unlikely the occasional use of **zolpidem** would pose a clinically insignificant risk to the breast-feeding neonate. If desired, the patient may pump her breasts for 8h and then resume breastfeeding.

■ **References** Alvarez de Sotomayor M, Herrera MD, et al. Z Naturforsch 1997; 52:687-93.
Cannizzaro C, Martire M, Steardo L, et al. Brain Res 2002; 953:170-80.

■ **Summary**
- **Pregnancy Category B**
- **Lactation Category S**
- **Zolpidem** should be used during pregnancy and lactation only if the benefit justifies the potential perinatal risk.

Zonisamide (Zonegran)

■ **Class** *Anticonvulsant*

■ **Indications** Partial seizures

■ **Mechanism** Unknown

■ **Dosage with Qualifiers** Partial seizures—begin 100mg PO qd, increasing q2w or greater for control; max dose 600mg/d in divided doses if necessary
- **Contraindications**—hypersensitivity to drug or class, hypersensitivity to sulfonamides
- **Caution**—hepatic or renal dysfunction, hot weather, history of nephrolithiasis

■ **Maternal Considerations** There are no interactions between **zonisamide** and the combined oral contraceptive pill, progesterone-only pill, **medroxyprogesterone** injections, or **levonorgestrel** implants. There are no adequate reports or well-controlled studies of **zonisamide** in pregnant women.
Side effects include Stevens-Johnson syndrome, toxic epidermal necrolysis, agranulocytosis, heat stroke, withdrawal seizures, aplastic anemia, somnolence, fatigue, anorexia, dizziness, headache, irritability, agitation,

impaired concentration, speech disturbance, impaired memory, mental slowing, confusion, depression, insomnia, diplopia, tremor, and incoordination.

■ **Fetal Considerations** ⋯⋯⋯ There are no adequate reports or well-controlled studies in human fetuses. **Zonisamide** crosses the human placenta achieving F:M ratios of 0.92. The current data do not indicate an increased risk of teratogenicity in humans. However, studies in rodents, dogs and nonhuman primates reveal embryotoxicity and an increased prevalence of malformations when **zonisamide** is given at doses within the human range during organogenesis.

■ **Breastfeeding Safety** ⋯⋯⋯ There are no adequate reports or well-controlled studies in nursing women. **Zonisamide** enters human milk, achieving in one report an M:P ratio less than 0.6.

■ **References** ⋯⋯⋯⋯⋯⋯⋯⋯⋯ Kawada K, Itoh S, Kusaka T, et al. Brain Dev 2002; 24:95-7.
Kondo T, Kaneko S, Amano Y, Egawa I. Epilepsia 1996; 37:1242-4.

■ **Summary** ⋯⋯⋯⋯⋯⋯⋯⋯⋯⋯⋯
- **Pregnancy Category C**
- **Lactation Category U**
- **Zonisamide** should be used during pregnancy and lactation only if the benefit justifies the potential perinatal risk.

(reprinted from http://www.fda.gov/womens/registries/registries.html)

Pregnancy Registries Enrolling Pregnant Women for Specific Medical Conditions (as of Aug. 23, 2002)

Medicine(s) Being Studied	Condition Treated by the Medicine(s)	Registry/Study Name	Contact Information
Antipsychotic Medicines Eight antipsychotic medicines are included in the Registry. List.	Acute and chronic psychoses, psychotic disorders	Antipsychotic Medicines during Pregnancy	Motherisk Program The Hospital for Sick Children, Toronto, Canada Phone: 416-813-8298 http://www.motherisk.org/
Antiretroviral Medicines All antiretroviral medicines are included in the Registry. Examples	HIV infection	Antiretroviral Pregnancy Registry	PharmaResearch Corporation * *North America:* Phone: 1-800-258-4263 (toll-free) Fax: 1-800-800-1052 *Outside North America:* Phone: 910-256-0238 (call collect) Fax: 910-256-0637 http://www.apregistry.com/
Asthma Medicines All asthma medicines (including inhaled or systemic steroids) are included in the Registry. Examples	Asthma	Asthma Medications and Pregnancy Project	Organization of Teratology Information Services (OTIS) Phone: 1-888-523-4847 (toll-free) Fax: 619-543-2066 http://www.otispregnancy.org
Cancer Medicines All chemotherapeutic agents are included in the registry. Examples	Cancer diagnosed during pregnancy	Cancer and Childbirth Registry	Thomas Jefferson University Hospital Phone: 215-955-9202 Fax: 215-955-5041 http://www.tju.edu/obgyn/info/cp.cfm
Epilepsy Medicines All epilepsy medicines are included in the Registry. Examples	Epilepsy	AED (antiepileptic drug) Pregnancy Registry	Genetics and Teratology Unit Massachusetts General Hospital Phone: 1-888-233-2334 (toll-free) Fax: 617-724-8307 http://www.massgeneral.org/aed/

| Rheumatoid Arthritis Medicines All rheumatoid arthritis medicines are included in the Registry. Examples | Rheumatoid arthritis | Rheumatoid Arthritis and Pregnancy Study | Organization of Teratology Information Services (OTIS) Phone: 1-866-626-6847 (toll-free) http://www.otispregnancy.org |

*The Antiretroviral Pregnancy Registry is a collaboration of product manufacturers managed by PharmaResearch Corporation.
http://www.pharmaresearch.com/aregistries.htm

Pregnancy Registries Enrolling Pregnant Women for Specific Medicines (as of July 5, 2002)

Medicine(s) Being Studied	Condition Treated by the Medicine(s)	Registry/Study Name	Contact Information
Aldara (imiquimod)	external genital and perianal warts (condyloma)	Aldara Pregnancy Health Line	Motherisk Program The Hospital for Sick Children, Toronto, Canada Phone: 1-800-670-6126 (toll-free) Phone: 416-813-8490 http://www.motherisk.org/
Amerge (naratriptan) Imitrex (sumatriptan)	migraine attacks	Sumatriptan and Naratriptan Pregnancy Registry	*North America:* PharmaResearch Corporation for GlaxoSmithKline Phone: 1-800-336-2176 (toll-free) Phone: 910-256-0549 (call collect) Fax: 1-800-800-1052 *Outside North America:* Contact local GlaxoSmithKline company or use numbers below: Phone: 910-256-0549 (call collect) Fax: 910-256-0637 http://pregnancyregistry.gsk.com/ naratriptan.html
Lamictal (lamotrigine)	partial seizure in adults with epilepsy	Lamotrigine Pregnancy Registry	*North America:* *Health-care providers and pregnant women should contact:* PharmaResearch Corporation for GlaxoSmithKline Phone: 1-800-336-2176 (toll-free) Phone: 910-256-0549 (call collect) *Pregnant women may contact:* North American AED Registry Phone: 1-888-233-2334 (toll-free) *Outside North America:* Contact local GlaxoSmithKline company or use numbers below: Phone: 910-256-0549 (call collect) Fax: 910-256-0637 http://pregnancyregistry.gsk.com/ lamotrigene.html

Medicine(s) Being Studied	Condition Treated by the Medicine(s)	Registry/Study Name	Contact Information
Maxalt (rizatriptan)	migraine attacks	Merck Pregnancy Registry Program	Merck & Company, Inc. Merck National Service Center Phone: 1-800-986-8999 (toll-free) Fax: 484-344-2328 http://www.merckpregnancyregistries.com/maxalt.html
Singulair (montelukast)	asthma	Merck Pregnancy Registry Program	Merck & Company, Inc. Merck National Service Center Phone: 1-800-986-8999 (toll-free) Fax: 484-344-2328 http://www.merckpregnancyregistries.com/singulair.html
Varivax (varicella virus vaccine): exposure anytime from 3 months before pregnancy through the end of pregnancy	prevention of chickenpox	Merck Pregnancy Registry Program	Merck & Company, Inc. Merck National Service Center Phone: 1-800-986-8999 (toll-free) Fax: 484-344-2328 http://www.merckpregnancyregistries.com/varivax.html
Vioxx (rofecoxib)	osteoarthritis, pain in adults, pain from menstrual cramps	Merck Pregnancy Registry Program	Merck & Company, Inc. Merck National Service Center Phone: 1-800-986-8999 (toll-free) Fax: 484-344-2328 http://www.merckpregnancyregistries.com/vioxx.html
Wellbutrin, Wellbutrin SR, and Zyban (bupropion)	depression	Bupropion Pregnancy Registry	*North America*: PharmaResearch Corporation for GlaxoSmithKline Phone: 1-800-336-2176 (toll-free) Fax: 1-800-800-1052 *Outside North America*: Contact local GlaxoSmithKline company or use numbers below: Phone: 910-256-0549 (call collect) Fax: 910-256-0637 http://pregnancyregistry.gsk.com/bupropion.html
Zofran (ondansetron)	nausea and vomiting	Zofran Use for the Treatment of Nausea and Vomiting During Pregnancy	Motherisk Program The Hospital for Sick Children, Toronto, Canada Phone: 1-800-436-8477 (toll-free) http://www.motherisk.org/

Pregnancy Registries Enrolling New Mothers (as of Nov. 1, 2002)

Medicine(s) Being Studied	Condition Treated by the Medicine(s)	Registry/Study Name	Contact Information
Cancer Medicines All chemotherapeutic agents are included in the registry <u>Examples</u>	Cancer diagnosed during pregnancy	Cancer and Childbirth Registry	Thomas Jefferson University Hospital Phone: 215-955-9202 Fax: 215-955-5041 http://www.tju.edu/obgyn/info/cp.cfm
Immunosuppressant Medicines All types of immunosuppression and other related medications and conditions such as high blood pressure and diabetes <u>Examples</u>	Any solid organ recipient (e.g., kidney, pancreas/kidney, liver, heart, heart/lung, lung, small bowel) who has had a pregnancy after transplant	National Transplantation Pregnancy Registry (NTPR)	National Transplantation Pregnancy Registry (NTPR) Thomas Jefferson University * Phone: 215-955-2840 *or* 877-955-6877 (toll-free) Fax: 215-923-1420 http://www.tju.edu/ntpr/

* Grant support for the National Transplantation Pregnancy Registry has been provided by Novartis Pharmaceuticals Corporation,
Fujisawa Healthcare, Inc., Roche Laboratories Inc., and Wyeth-Ayerst Pharmaceuticals, Inc.

Appendix 2 AHA Guidelines: Bacterial Endocarditis Prophylaxis

Reference: Dajani AS et al. Prevention of bacterial endocarditis: Recommendations by the American Heart Association. JAMA, 277(22): 1794-1801, June 11, 1997.

Table 1: Cardiac Conditions Associated with Endocarditis

Endocarditis prophylaxis recommended	Endocarditis prophylaxis NOT recommended: Negligible-risk category (no greater risk than the general population)
High-risk category *Prosthetic cardiac valves, including bioprosthetic and homograft valves *Previous bacterial endocarditis *Complex cyanotic congenital heart disease (eg, single ventricle states, transposition of the great arteries, tetralogy of Fallot) *Surgically constructed systemic pulmonary shunts or conduits **Moderate-risk category** *Most other congenital cardiac malformations (other than above and below) *Acquired valvar dysfunction (eg, rheumatic heart disease) *Hypertrophic cardiomyopathy *Mitral valve prolapse with valvar regurgitation and/or thickened leaflets	*Isolated secundum atrial septal defect Surgical repair of atrial septal defect, ventricular septal defect, or patent ductus arteriosus (without residua beyond 6mo) *Previous coronary artery bypass graft surgery *Mitral valve prolapse without valvar regurgitation *Physiologic, functional, or innocent heart murmurs *Previous Kawasaki disease without valvar dysfunction *Previous rheumatic fever without valvar dysfunction *Cardiac pacemakers (intravascular and epicardial) and implanted defibrillators

Table 2: Dental Procedures and Endocarditis Prophylaxis

Endocarditis prophylaxis recommended[1]	Endocarditis prophylaxis NOT recommended
*Dental extractions *Periodontal procedures including surgery, scaling and root planing, probing, and recall maintenance *Dental implant placement and reimplantation of avulsed teeth *Endodontic (root canal) instrumentation or surgery only beyond the apex *Subgingival placement of antibiotic fibers or strips *Initial placement of orthodontic bands but not brackets *Intraligamentary local anesthetic injections *Prophylactic cleaning of teeth or implants where bleeding is anticipated	*Restorative dentistry[2] (operative and prosthodontic) with or without retraction cord[3] *Local anesthetic injections (nonintraligamentary) *Intracanal endodontic treatment; post placement and buildup *Placement of rubber dams *Postoperative suture removal *Placement of removable prosthodontic or orthodontic appliances *Taking of oral impressions *Fluoride treatments *Taking of oral radiographs *Orthodontic appliance adjustment *Shedding of primary teeth

[1] Prophylaxis is recommended for patients with high- and moderate-risk cardiac conditions.
[2] This includes restoration of decayed teeth (filling cavities) and replacement of missing teeth.
[3] Clinical judgment may indicate antibiotic use in selected circumstances that may create significant bleeding.

Table 3: Other Procedures and Endocarditis Prophylaxis

Endocarditis prophylaxis recommended	Endocarditis prophylaxis NOT recommended
Respiratory tract: *Tonsillectomy and/or adenoidectomy *Surgical operations that involve respiratory mucosa *Bronchoscopy with a rigid bronchoscope	**Respiratory tract:** *Endotracheal intubation *Bronchoscopy with a flexible bronchoscope, with or without biopsy *Tympanostomy tube insertion
Gastrointestinal tract[1]: *Sclerotherapy for esophageal varices *Esophageal stricture dilation *Endoscopic retrograde cholangiography with biliary obstruction *Biliary tract surgery *Surgical operations that involve intestinal mucosa	**Gastrointestinal tract:** *Transesophageal echocardiography *Endoscopy with or without gastrointestinal biopsy
Genitourinary tract: *Cystoscopy *Urethral dilation	**Genitourinary tract:** *Vaginal hysterectomy[2] *Vaginal delivery[3] *Cesarean section -In uninfected tissue: *Urethral catheterization *Uterine dilatation and curettage *Therapeutic abortion *Sterilization procedures *Insertion or removal of intrauterine devices
	Other: *Cardiac catheterization, including balloon angioplasty *Implanted cardiac pacemakers, implanted defibrillators, and coronary stents *Incision or biopsy of surgically scrubbed skin

[1] Prophylaxis is recommended for high-risk patients; it is optional for medium-risk patients.
[2] Prophylaxis is optional for high-risk patients.
[3] Prophylaxis is optional for high-risk patients.

Table 4: Prophylactic Regimens for Dental, Oral, Respiratory Tract, or Esophageal Procedures

Situation	Agent	Regimen[1]
Standard general prophylaxis	Amoxicillin	Adults: 2.0g;
Unable to take oral medications	Ampicillin	Adults: 2.0g IM or IV;
Allergic to penicillin	Clindamycin or Cephalexin[1] or cefadroxil or Azithromycin or clarithromycin	Adults: 600mg; Adults: 2.0g; Adults: 500mg;
Allergic to penicillin and unable to take oral medications	Clindamycin or Cefazolin[1]	Adults: 600mg; Adults: 1.0g;

[1] Cephalosporins should not be used in individuals with immediate-type hypersensitivity reaction (urticaria, angioedema, or anaphylaxis) to penicillins

Table 5: Prophylactic Regimens for Genitourinary/Gastrointestinal (Excluding Esophageal) Procedures

Situation	Agents	Regimen[1]
High-risk patients	Ampicillin plus gentamicin	Adults: ampicillin 2.0g IM or IV plus gentamicin 1.5mg/kg (not to exceed 120 mg) within 30 min of starting procedure; 6 h later, ampicillin 1 g IM/IV or amoxicillin 1 g orally
High-risk patients allergic to ampicillin/amoxicillin	Vancomycin plus gentamicin	Adults: vancomycin 1.0 g IV over 1-2 h plus gentamicin 1.5 mg/kg IV/IM (not to exceed 120 mg); complete injection/infusion within 30 min of starting procedure
Moderate-risk patients	Amoxicillin or ampicillin	Adults: amoxicillin 2.0 g orally 1 h before procedure, or ampicillin 2.0 g IM/IV within 30 min of starting procedure
Moderate-risk patients allergic to ampicillin/ amoxicillin	Vancomycin	Adults: vancomycin 1.0 g IV over 1-2 h complete infusion within 30 min of starting procedure

[1] No second dose of vancomycin or gentamicin is recommended.

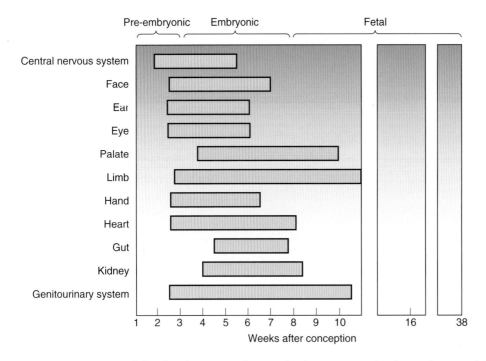

Figure 1. Timing of the development of major body structures in the embryo and fetus. Reproduced with permission from Hanretty KP and Whittle MJ. Identifying abnormalities *in* Rubin PC (ed): Prescribing in pregnancy, 2nd ed. pp. 8-21. London: British Medical Journal Publishing, 1995.

Examples of Known or Likely Teratogens or Fetal Toxins

Radiation
Radioiodine
Infections

      Cytomegalovirus
      Herpes simplex virus I and II
      Parvovirus B-19 (Erythema infectiosum)
      Rubella virus
      Syphilis
      Toxoplasmosis
      Varicella virus
      Venezuelan equine encephalitis virus

Maternal & Metabolic Imbalance

      Alcoholism
      Amniocentesis, early
        (before day 70 post conception)
      Chorionic villus sampling
        (before day 60 post conception)
      Cretinism, endemic
      Diabetes mellitus
      Folic acid deficiency
      Hyperthermia
      Phenylketonuria
      Rheumatic disease
      Sjögren's syndrome
      Virilizing tumors

Drugs and Environmental Chemicals

      ACE inhibitors (benazepril, captopril, enalapril, fosinopril, lisinopril, moexipril, quinapril, ramipril, trandolapril)
      Aminopterin
      Androgenic hormones
      Busulfan
      Chlorobiphenyls
      Cocaine
      Coumarin anticoagulants
      Cyclophosphamide
      Diethylstilbestrol
      Etretinate
      Fluconazole (high doses)
      Iodides
      Isotretinoin
      Indomethacin and related NSAIDs
      Lithium
      Mercury, organic
      Methimazole
      Methotrexate
      Methylene blue (after intraamniotic injection)
      Misoprostol
      Penicillamine
      Phenobarbital
      Phenytoin

Tetracyclines and its derivatives
Thalidomide
Toluene (abuse)
Trimethadione
Valproic acid

Possible Teratogens or Fetal Toxins

Binge drinking
Carbamazepine
Cigarette smoking
Colchicine
Disulfiram
Ergotamine
Lead
Primidone
Quinine (suicidal doses)
Streptomycin
Vitamin A (high doses)
Zinc deficiency

Unlikely Teratogens

Agent Orange
Anesthetics
Aspartame
Aspirin
Bendectin ® (antinauseant)
Hydroxyprogesterone
LSD
Marijuana
Medroxyprogesterone
Metronidazole
Oral contraceptives
Progesterone
Rubella vaccine
Spermicides
Video display terminals & electromagnetic waves
Ultrasound

Category A Controlled studies in women fail to demonstrate a risk to the fetus in the first trimester (and there is no evidence of a risk in later trimesters), and the possibility of fetal harm appears remote.

Category B Either animal-reproduction studies have not demonstrated a fetal risk but there are no controlled studies in pregnant women, or animal-reproduction studies.have shown an adverse effect (other than a decrease in fertility) that was not confirmed in controlled studies in women in the first trimester (and there is no evidence of a risk in later trimesters).

Category C Either study in animals has revealed adverse effects on the fetus (teratogenic or embryocidal or other) and there are no controlled studies in women, or studies in women and animals are not available. Drugs should be given only if the potential benefit justifies the potential risk to the fetus.

Category D There is positive evidence of human fetal risk, but the benefits from use in pregnant women may be acceptable despite the risk (e.g., if the drug is needed in a life-threatening situation or for a serious disease for which safer drugs cannot be used or are ineffective).

Category X Studies in animals or human beings have demonstrated fetal abnormalities, or there is evidence of fetal risk based on human experience or both, and the risk of the use of the drug in pregnant women clearly outweighs any possible benefit. The drug is contraindicated in women who are or may become pregnant.

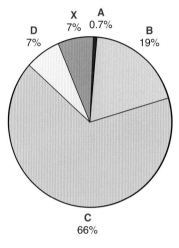

Abbreviations

ABG	arterial blood gases
ac	before meals
ACE	angiotensin–converting enzyme
ACEI	angiotensin–converting enzyme inhibitor
ACh	acetylcholine
ACLS	advanced cardiac life support
ACOG	American College of Obstetricians and Gynecologists
ACTH	adrenocorticotropic hormone
ADD	attention deficit disorder
ADHD	attention deficit hyperactivity disorder
ADP	adenosine diphosphate
AF	amniotic fluid
AF:M ratio	amniotic fluid:maternal plasma ratio
AGA	average for gestational age
AIDS	acquired immunodeficiency syndrome
Al	aluminum
ALS	amyotrophic lateral sclerosis
ALT	alanine aminotransferase
AML	acute myelogenous leukemia
ANC	absolute neutrophil count
APL	antiphospholipid (syndrome)
aPTT	activated partial thromboplastin time
A2R-antagonist	angiotensin 2 receptor antagonist
ARDS	adult respiratory distress syndrome
ASA	acetylsalicylic acid (aspirin)
ASAP	as soon as possible
AST	aspartate aminotransferase
ATI	angiotensin I
ATIII	antithrombin III
ATP	adenosine triphosphate
ATPase	adenosine triphosphatase
AV	atrioventricular
AVM	arteriovenous malformation
AZT	3′-azido-3′-deoxythymidine zidovudine (azidothymidine)
B.	*Bacillus*
	Bacteroides
beta-hCG	beta–human chorionic gonadotropin
bid	twice a day
BNP	B-type natriuretic peptide
BP	blood pressure
bpm	beats per minute
BPP	biophysical profile
BUN	blood urea nitrogen
BV	bacterial vaginosis
BZD	benzodiazepine
C.	*Candida*
	Clostridium
CA	cancer
Ca	calcium

CAD	coronary artery disease
cAMP	cyclic adenosine monophosphate
CBC	complete blood count
CD_4	type of white blood cell
CDC	Centers for Disease Control
cGMP	cyclic guanosine monophosphate
CHB	congenital heart block
chemo	chemotherapy
CHF	congestive heart failure
CI	confidence interval
CK	creatine kinase
Cl	chloride
cm	centimeter
cm^2	square centimeter
CML	chronic myelocytic leukemia
cml	cubic milliliter
CMV	cytomegalovirus
CN^-	cyanide anion
CNS	central nervous system
CO_2	carbon dioxide
COPD	chronic obstructive pulmonary disease
COX-2	cyclooxygenase-2
CPD	cephalopelvic disproportion
CPK	creatine phosphokinase
Cr	creatinine
CrCl	creatinine clearance
CSF	cerebrospinal fluid
CV	cardiovascular
CVA	cerebrovascular accident
CVD	cerebrovascular disease
CVS	chorionic villus sampling
cyp	cyproheptadine

d	day
DDAVP	1-deamino(8-D-arginine) vasopressin
DES	diethylstilbestrol
DIC	disseminated intravascular coagulation
DKA	diabetic ketoacidosis
dl	deciliter
DNA	deoxyribonucleic acid
DPT	diphtheria, pertussis, and tetanus
DS	double strength
DSM-IV	4th edition; Diagnostic and Statistical Manual of Mental Disorders
D5W	5% dextrose in water
DTIC	dimethyltriazenoimidazole carboxamide (dacarbazine)
DTR	deep tendon reflex
DVT	deep vein thrombosis

E.	*Escherichia*
EBV	Epstein-Barr virus
ECG	electrocardiogram
EDC	estimated date of confinement
EEG	electroencephalogram
ER+	estrogen receptor-positive
ET	endotracheal, also endothelin

| FDA | Food and Drug Administration |

FDP	fibrin degradation products
Fe	iron
FEV	forced expiratory volume
FFP	fresh frozen plasma
FHR	fetal heart rate
F:M ratio	fetal:maternal ratio
FSH	follicle–stimulating hormone
g	gram
G6PD	glucose-6-phosphate dehydrogenase
GABA	gamma-aminobutyric acid
GBS	group B streptococcus
GERD	gastroesophageal reflux disease
GFR	glomerular filtration rate
GH	growth hormone
GI	gastrointestinal
GIFT	gamete intrafallopian transfer
gm	gram
GnRH	gonadotropin-releasing hormone
GPIIb/IIIa	glycoprotein IIb/glycoprotein IIIa
GTD	gestational trophoblastic disease
gtt	drops
GU	genitourinary
h	hour
H.	*Haemophilus*
	Helicobacter
HB	hepatitis B
Hb	hemoglobin
HCG	human chorionic gonadotropin
HCV	hepatitis C virus
HDL	high-density lipoprotein
HELLP	hemolysis, elevated liver enzymes, and low platelets
HIV	human immunodeficiency virus
HIV-1	human immunodeficiency virus type 1
HMG CoA	3-hydroxy-3-methylglutaryl coenzyme A
HPA	hypothalamic–pituitary–adrenal
HR	heart rate
HRT	hormone replacement therapy
hs	at bedtime
HSV	herpes simplex virus
5-HT	5-hydroxytryptamine
hx	history
ICP	intracranial pressure
ICU	intensive care unit
IDDM	insulin-dependent diabetes mellitus
Ig	immunoglobulin
IgA	immunoglobulin A
IGF-I	insulin-like growth factor-I
IgG	immunoglobulin G
IHSS	idiopathic hypertrophic subaortic stenosis
IKr	inward delayed rectified potassium channel
IL-2	interleukin-2
IL-4	interleukin-4
IL-11	interleukin-11
IL-15	interleukin-15
IM	intramuscular

IN	intranasal
INH	inhalation
	isoniazid
INR	International Normalized Ratio
IQ	intelligence quotient
ITP	immune thrombocytopenic purpura
IU	International Unit
IUD	intrauterine device
IUGR	intrauterine growth restriction
IUI	intrauterine insemination
IV; iv	intravenous
IVF	in vitro fertilization
IVH	intraventricular hemorrhage
IVP	intravenous pyelogram
K	potassium
kg	kilogram
L	liter
L2	second lumbar vertebra
L4	fourth lumbar vertebra
lb	pound(s)
LDL	low-density lipoprotein
LDL-C	low-density lipoprotein cholesterol
LFTs	liver function tests
LH	luteinizing hormone
LMP	last menstrual period
LMWH	low molecular weight heparin
L:S ratio	lecithin/sphingomyelin ratio
LT	long-term therapy
LV	left ventricle
M.	*Microsporum*
m²	square meter [body surface]
MAC	*Mycobacterium avium* complex
MAO	monoamine oxidase
MAP	mean arterial pressure
max	maximum
mcg	microgram
MDI	metered-dose inhaler
MDR	minimum daily requirement
mEq	milliequivalent
meth	methamphetamine
Mg	magnesium
mg	milligram(s)
mGy	milligray
MI	myocardial infarction
MIC	minimal inhibitory concentration
min	minute
mIU	milli–International unit
ml	milliliter(s)
mm³	cubic millimeter
mmHg	millimeter(s) of mercury
mmol	millimole
MMP	metalloprotease
mo	month(s)
M:P	milk:maternal plasma ratio

MRHD	maximal recommended human dose
MRI	magnetic resonance imaging
MS	multiple sclerosis
msec	millisecond
MSRA	methicillin-resistant S. *aureus*
MSSA	methicillin-sensitive S. *aureus*
MTHFR	5,10 methylene tetrahydrofolate reductase
MW	molecular weight
N.	*Neisseria*
Na	sodium
NaCl	sodium chloride
NAPA	N-acetyl-procainamide
NAS	nasal
NE	norepinephrine
NEB	nebulizer spray
NEC	necrotizing enterocolitis
NG	nasogastric
ng	nanogram
NICU	neonatal intensive care unit
NMDA	N-methyl-D-aspartate
NNRTI	non–nucleoside reverse transcriptase inhibitor
NO	nitric oxide
NRT	nicotine replacement therapy
NSAID	nonsteroid anti-inflammatory drug
NST	nonstress test
NTD	neural tube defect
N/V	nausea and vomiting
NYHA	New York Heart Association
OCD	obsessive–compulsive disorder
OCP	oral contraceptive pill
OCs	oral contraceptives
OCT	oxytocin challenge test
OD	right eye
OR	odds ratio
OS	left eye
p	probability value
P.	*Pasteurella*
	Plasmodium
	Proteus
PaO$_2$	partial pressure of oxygen in arterial blood
pc	after meals
PCA	patient-controlled analgesia
PCEA	patient-controlled epidural analgesia
PCOS	polycystic ovary syndrome
PCP	pneumocystis carinii pneumonia
PDE	phosphodiesterase
PE	pulmonary embolism
PEMA	phenylethylmalonamide
PGI$_2$	prostacyclin
PGE	prostaglandin E
PGF	prostaglandin F
PGHS-II	prostaglandin H synthase
pH	hydrogen ion concentration
PID	pelvic inflammatory disease

PKU	phenylketonuria
PLT	platelet
PMS	premenstrual syndrome
PO	by mouth
post-op	postoperative
PPAR	peroxisome proliferator activated receptor
ppd	packs per day
PPH	primary pulmonary hypertension
PPROM	prolonged premature rupture of membranes
PR	by way of the rectum
PRBC	packed red blood cells
prn	as required
PROM	premature rupture of membranes
PTH	parathyroid hormone
PTT	partial thromboplastin time
PTU	propylthiouracil
PV	through the vagina
PVC	premature ventricular contraction
PVD	peripheral vascular disease
q	every
qac	before every meal
qam	every morning
qd	every day
qhs	every hour of sleep
qid	four times daily
qmo	every month
qnoon	every noon
qod	every other day
qpm	every night
QT	the Q-T interval on an electrocardiogram
qw	every week
RA-APL	retinoic acid–acute promyelocytic leukemia
RBC	red blood cell(s)
RDA	recommended daily allowance
RDS	respiratory distress syndrome
REM	rapid eye movement
Rh factor	Rhesus factor
RNA	ribonucleic acid
ROM	rupture of membranes
RSV	respiratory syncytial virus
S.	*Staphylococcus*
	Streptococcus
SA	sinoatrial
SC	subcutaneous
S/D	systolic/diastolic
sec	second(s)
SEFW	sonographic estimate of fetal weight
SERM	selective estrogen receptor modulators
SGA	small for gestational age
SIADH	syndrome of inappropriate antidiuretic hormone
sib	sibling
SIDS	sudden infant death syndrome
SL	sublingual
SLE	systemic lupus erythematosus
SOB	shortness of breath

SR	slow release
SSRI	selective serotonin reuptake inhibitor
STD	sexually transmitted disease
SVT	supraventricular tachycardia
T.	*Treponema*
	Trichomonas
	Trichophyton
T₃	triiodothyronine
T₄	thyroxine
tab(s)	tablet(s)
TAT	thrombin antithrombin
TB	tuberculosis
tbsp	tablespoon
TCA	tricyclic antidepressants
TIA	transient ischemic attack
tid	three times a day
TNF	tumor necrosis factor
T's and Blues	tripelennamine and pentazocine
TSH	thyroid-stimulating hormone
tsp	teaspoon
TT	thrombin time
TTP	thrombotic thrombocytopenic purpura
U	unit
mg; mcg	microgram
URI	upper respiratory infection
USP	United States Pharmacopeia
usu.	usually
UTI	urinary tract infection
UV	ultraviolet
UVA	ultraviolet A
V	ventricular
V.	*Vibrio*
VACTERL	vertebral, anal, cardiac, tracheoesophageal, renal, limb malformations
VATER	vertebral defects, imperforate anus, tracheoesophageal fistula, and radial and renal dysplasia
VBAC	vaginal birth after cesarean section
VF	ventricular fibrillation
VIP	vasoactive intestinal polypeptide
VLDL	very low–density lipoprotein
VSD	ventricular septal defect
VTE	venous thromboembolism
vWD	von Willebrand's disease
VZIG	varicella zoster immune globulin
VZV	varicella-zoster virus
w	week(s)
WBC	white blood count
x	times
Xa	activated Factor X
XR	extended release
y	year(s)

Index

Ansulin, 978–979
Antabuse, 280–281
Antadict, 280–281
Antcucs, 795–796
Antepar, 795–796
Anthraderm, 45–46
Anthra-Derm, 45–46
Anthraforte, 45–46
anthralin, 45–46
Anthra-Tex, 45–46
Anthrax
    ciprofloxacin, 178–180
    doxycycline, 293–294
    penicillin G aqueous, 755
Antiallersin, 833–835
Anticholinesterase
        overdose
    pralidoxime, 810
Anticoagulant overdose
    factor IX, 336
antihemophilic factor, 46
Antihistamine
    diphenhydramine as,
        275–276
Antilirium, 785–786
Antiminth, 847
Antipernicin, 211–212
Antiphospholipid
        syndrome
    heparin, 410–411
Antipres, 403
Antipyretic
    flurbiprofen, 364–365
Antispas, 257–258
antithrombin III
        concentrate, 47–48
Antitroide-GW, 587–589
Antitussive
    codeine, 203–204
Antivert, 545–546
Antizol, 370–371
Antribid, 933–934
Anusol-Hc, 420–422
Anxiety
    buspirone, 94–95
    chloral hydrate, 157
    chlordiazepoxide,
        160–161
    clonazepam, 194–195
    clorazepate, 197–198
    diazepam, 250–252
    doxepin, 291
    hydroxyzine, 427–428
    lorazepam, 525–527
    mephobarbital, 562–563
    meprobamate, 563–564
    mesoridazine, 570
    oxazepam, 726–727
    paroxetine, 746–748
    prochlorperazine,
        829–830
    trifluoperazine, 995–996
Anzemet, 287–288
Apacet, 3–4
APAP, 3–4
Apatef, 136–137
Aphthous ulcer
    thalidomide, 959–960
Aphtiria, 512–513

Apitart, 35–36
Aplacassee, 525–527
Apnea, prematurity
    caffeine, 101–102
Apo-Alpraz, 18–19
Apoterin, 190–191
Appecon, 772–773
Appendicitis
    meropenem, 567–568
Apresoline, 416–417
Apresrex, 416–417
Apricolin, 830
Aprovel, 463–464
Aptecin, 877–878
Aptide, 218–219
Apurol, 16–17
Aquabid-Dm, 246–247
Aquachloral, 157
Aqua-Mephyton,
    786–787
Aquanil, 972–973
Aquaphyllin, 960–962
Aquatensen, 599
Aquazide H, 418–419
Aragest, 547–549
Aralen, 162–163
Aralen Injection, 162–163
Aramine, 574–575
Arava, 493–494
arbutamine, 48
Archifen, 159–160
ardeparin sodium, 49
Aredia, 739–740
Arestin, 632–633
argatroban, 50
Aricin, 991–993
Aristocort, 991–993
Aristocort Suspension,
    991–993
Aristocort Topical,
    991–993
Aristogel, 991–993
Aristo-Pak, 991–993
Aristospan Intralesional,
    991–993
Aristospan Parenteral,
    991–993
Arixtra, 371–372
Arm-A-Med, 572–573
Arodoc, 168–170
Aromasin, 335
Aromycetin, 159–160
Arrestin, 996–997
Arret, 522–523
Arrhythmia. See also specific
        types of arrhythmia,
        e.g., Bradycardia.
    atrial
        flecainide, 349–350
        procainamide,
            825–826
    isoproterenol, 469–470
    mexiletine, 620–621
    nadolol, 652–653
    supraventricular
        verapamil, 1028–1029
    ventricular. See
        Ventricular
        arrhythmia.

Arteoptik, 118–119
Artha-G, 896
Arthridex, 933–934
Arthritis
    betamethasone, 78–79
    fenoprofen, 343–344
    osteoarthritis. See
        Osteoarthritis.
    rheumatoid. See
        Rheumatoid arthritis.
    salsalate, 896
Articulose-L.A., 991–993
Artomin, 167–168
Artril, 430–431
Arumil, 24–25
Aruzilina, 62–63
Arythmol, 835–836
Asacol, 568–569
Ascalix, 795–796
Ascaris lumbricoides
        (Roundworm) infection
    mebendazole, 541–542
    piperazine, 795–796
    pyrantel pamoate, 847
Ascaryl, 500–501
Asconale, 547–549
Asendin, 34
Asidon, 3–4
Asiplatin, 181–183
Asmalin, 12–13
Asmalix, 960–962
Asmanil, 12–13
Asmavent, 12–13
A-Spas, 257–258
A-Spas S L, 428–429
Aspenil, 35–36
Asperal, 960–962
Aspergillosis
    voriconazole, 1034–1035
aspirin, 51–52
Asthma
    beclomethasone, 69–70
    budesonide, 90–91
    cromolyn, 209–210
    epinephrine, 308–309
    exercise-induced
        albuterol, 12–13
        cromolyn, 209–210
        formoterol, inhaled,
            372–373
        salmeterol xinafoate
            inhaled, 895
    flunisolide, 355–356
    fluticasone, 365–366
    formoterol, inhaled,
        372–373
    metaproterenol, 572–573
    nedocromil, 667–668
    oxtriphylline, 729–730
    prednisolone, 816–818
    salmeterol xinafoate
        inhaled, 895
    terbutaline, 951–952
    theophylline, 960–962
    triamcinolone, 991–993
    zafirlukast, 1038
    zileuton, 1044–1045
Astrocytoma, refractory
    temozolomide, 946–947

Atacand, 107–108
Atacin, 563–564
Atarax, 427–428
Atazina, 427–428
atenolol, 53–54
Ativan, 525–527
ATnativ, 47–48
Atolmin, 53–54
Atopic dermatitis
    pimecrolimus, topical,
        788–789
atorvastatin calcium, 54–55
atovaquone, 55–56
Atp, 11–12
atracurium, 56–57
Atretol, 111–112
Atrial arrhythmia
    flecainide, 349–350
    procainamide, 825–826
Atrial fibrillation
    digitoxin, 264–265
    digoxin, 266–268
    diltiazem, 270–272
    dofetilide, 286–287
    ibutilide, 431–432
    quinidine
        gluconate/sulfate,
            855–856
    verapamil, 1028–1029
Atrial flutter
    digitoxin, 264–265
    digoxin, 266–268
    diltiazem, 270–272
    dofetilide, 286–287
    ibutilide, 431–432
    verapamil, 1028–1029
Atrial tachycardia,
        paroxysmal
    digoxin, 266–268
Atrioventricular cannula
        occlusion
    streptokinase, 923–924
Atromid-S, 190–191
Atro Ofteno, 57–58
Atropair, 57–58
Atropen, 57–58
Atrophic vaginitis
    chlorotrianisene,
        165–166
    dienestrol, 260
    estradiol, 319–321
atropine, 57–58
Atropine Sulfate, 70–71
Atropinol, 57–58
Atrovent, 462–463
A/T/S, 315–316
attapulgite, 58–59
Attention deficit disorder
        (ADD)
    dexmethylphenidate, 244
    methamphetamine,
        581–583
Attention deficit
        hyperactivity disorder
        (ADHD)
    dextroamphetamine,
        245–246
    methylphenidate,
        607–608

Hypercholesterolemia
(*Continued*)
colestipol, 207
dextrothyroxine, 247–248
familial
simvastatin, 912–913
fluvastatin, 366–367
gemfibrozil, 387–388
lovastatin, 527–528
niacin, 678–679
pravastatin, 812–813
simvastatin, 912–913
Hyperex, 416–417
Hyperhep, 413–414
Hyperkalemia
sodium polystyrene, 917
Hyperlipidemia
fenofibrate, 341–342
probucol, 824–825
Hypermagnesemia
calcium chloride,
105–106
Hypermet, 601–603
Hyperparathyroidism
paricalcitol, 745
Hyperpigmentation
hydroquinone topical,
423–424
Hyperprolactinemia
cabergoline, 99–100
Hypersecretory conditions
lansoprazole, 491–492
pantoprazole, 742
rabeprazole, 859–860
Hyperstat, 252–253
Hypertension
acebutolol, 2–3
benazepril, 71–72
bendroflumethiazide,
72–74
betaxolol, 80–81
bisoprolol fumarate, 83
candesartan, 107–108
captopril, 108–109
carteolol, 118–119
carvedilol, 119–120
chlorothiazide, 164–165
chlorthalidone, 170–171
clonidine, 195–196
diazoxide, 252–253
doxazosin, 290
enalapril, 300–301
eprosartan mesylate,
311–312
esmolol, 316–317
ethacrynic acid, 324–325
felodipine, 340–341
fenoldopam, 342–343
fosinopril, 375–376
furosemide, 379–381
guanabenz acetate, 401
guanadrel sulfate, 402
guanethidine
monosulfate, 403
guanfacine
hydrochloride, 404
hydralazine, 416–417
hydrochlorothiazide,
418–419

Hypertension (*Continued*)
indapamide, 437–438
irbesartan, 463–464
isradipine, 474–475
labetalol, 484–486
lisinopril, 516–517
malignant
mecamylamine, 543
mecamylamine, 543
methyclothiazide, 599
methyldopa, 601–603
metolazone, 614–615
metoprolol, 615–617
minoxidil, 634–635
moexipril, 642–643
nadolol, 652–653
nicardipine, 679–682
nisoldipine, 690–691
nitroprusside, 697–699
olmesartan medoxomil,
714–715
penbutolol, 752
perindopril erbumine,
767
pindolol, 790–791
polythiazide/prazosin,
807
prazosin, 814–815
propranolol, 840–841
propylthiouracil, 841–842
pulmonary
epoprostenol, 310–311
treprostinil, 988–989
quinapril, 854–855
ramipril, 863–865
reserpine, 869–870
spironolactone, 920–921
telmisartan, 943–944
terazosin, 949
timolol, 972–973
torsemide, 982–983
trandolapril, 985–986
valsartan, 1018–1019
verapamil, 1028–1029
Hypertensive crisis
phentolamine, 779–780
Hypertet, 953–955
Hyper-Tet, 953–955
Hyperthyroidism
methimazole, 587–589
Hypertriglyceridemia
gemfibrozil, 387–388
niacin, 678–679
simvastatin, 912–913
Hypnorex, 518–520
Hypocalcemia
calcifediol, 102–103
calcitriol, 104–105
calcium chloride,
105–106
dihydrotachysterol,
269–270
Hypoglycemia
glucagon, 392–393
Hypogonadism
estropipate, 323–324
Hypokalemia
potassium chloride, 808
spironolactone, 920–921

Hypomagnesemia
magnesium chloride, 531
magnesium oxide, 533
magnesium sulfate,
534–538
Hyponrex, 518–520
Hypoparathyroidism
calcifediol, 102–103
calcitriol, 104–105
ergocalciferol, 312–313
Hypophosphatemia,
familial
ergocalciferol, 312–313
Hypoprothrombinemia
phytonadione, 786–787
Hypotension
mephentermine, 559–560
methoxamine, 594–595
midodrine, 626–627
Hypotension, postural
fludrocortisone, 353–354
Hypothyroidism
levothyroxine, 507–508
liotrix, 515–516
HypRho-D, 871–873
Hyrexin, 275–276
Hysterone, 360
Hytakerol, 269–270
Hytone, 420–422
Hytrin, 949
Hyzine, 427–428

I

Ibikin, 996–997
Ibren, 430–431
Ibugen, 430–431
ibuprofen, 430–431
Ibuprohm, 430–431
Ibu-Tab, 430–431
ibutilide, 431–432
I-Chlor, 159–160
Idamycin, 432–433
idarubicin, 432–433
Idenal, 96–97
Idotrim, 995–997
idoxuridine, 433–434
Ifen, 430–431
Iletin I, 448–449
Iletin II, 448–449
Iletin II Lente(Pork),
448–449
Iletin II Lente Pork,
448–449
Iletin II Nph(Pork),
448–449
Iletin II Nph Pork, 448–449
**Iletin II Protamine,
Zinc(Pork)**, 448–449
Iletin II Pzi Pork, 448–449
Iletin II Reg. Pork, 448–449
Iletin II Regular(Pork),
448–449
**Iletin II
Regular(Pork)Conc**,
448–449
Ilotycin, 315–316
Ilozyme, 740–741
Imavate, 433–434

Imbaral, 933–934
Imdur, 472–473
Imigran, 935–936
imipenem/cilastatin,
434–435
imipramine, 435–436
Imipramine HCL, 435–436
Imiprin, 435–436
imiquimod, 437
Imitrex, 935–936
Immenoctal, 900–901
Immuno, 336
Immunol, 500–501
Imode, 522–523
Imodium, 522–523
Imogam Rabies, 860–861
Imovax Rabies, 861–862
Imoxil, 35–36
Imtrate, 472–473
Imuran, 61–62
I-Naphline, 662–663
Inapsine, 295–296
Incontinence, urinary
midodrine, 626–627
indapamide, 437–438
Inderal, 840–841
indinavir, 438–439
Indocin, 440–442
indomethacin, 440–442
Infa-Chlor, 159–160
Infections. *See also specific
types of infections, e.g.,
Mycobacterium infection.*
bacterial. *See Bacterial
infections.*
Infectoflu, 21–22
Infergen, 456–457
Infertility
progesterone, 831–832
Inflammatory bowel disease
cromolyn, 209–210
Inflammatory disorders
betamethasone, 78–79
cortisone, 208–209
dexamethasone, 239–241
hydrocortisone, 420–422
methylprednisolone,
608–610
nabumetone, 651
naproxen, 663–664
prednisolone, 816–818
prednisone, 818–819
triamcinolone, 991–993
infliximab, 442–443
Influenza A
oseltamivir phosphate,
723
rimantadine, 881–882
Influenza B
oseltamivir phosphate,
723
Influenza, uncomplicated
zanamivir, 1041
influenza vaccine, 443–444
Ingadine, 403
INH, 468–469
Inidrase, 5–6
Innohep, 973–974
Inophyline, 27–28

Tri-Med, 991–993
trimethobenzamide, 996–997
trimethoprim, 997–999
trimethoprim/
   sulfamethoxazole,
   999–1000
trimetrexate, 1001
Trimexazole, 995–997
trimipramine, 1002
Trimopan, 995–997
Trimox, 35–36
Trimpex, 995–997
Tri-Onex Dm, 246–247
Triostat, 514–515
tripelennamine, 1003–1004
Tripid, 387–388
Triplen, 1001–1002
Triprim, 995–997
Triptil, 844
Tristoject, 991–993
Tristo-Plex, 991–993
Trizam, 994–995
Trobicin, 919–920
Trophoblastic disease
   chlorambucil, 158
   gestational
      cyclophosphamide,
      214–215
      dactinomycin, 223–224
      fluorouracil, 357–358
      methotrexate, 590–593
      vincristine, 1032–1033
   trovafloxacin, 1004–1005
Trovan, 1002–1003
Troymycetin, 159–160
Truphylline, 27–28
Truxadryl, 275–276
Truxazole, 932–933
Truxophyllin, 960–962
Trylone A, 991–993
Trylone D, 991–993
Trymex, 991–993
T-Stat, 315–316
Tuberculosis
   cycloserine, 215–216
   isoniazid, 468–469
   pyrazinamide, 848
   rifampin, 877–878
   rifapentine, 879
tubocurarine, 1005–1006
Tumor
   carcinoid
      octreotide acetate,
      710–711
   head and neck
      hydroxyurea, 426–427
   malignant. See Cancer.
   solid
      hydroxyurea, 426–427
   Wilms'
      dactinomycin, 223–224
      doxorubicin, 292–293
      vincristine, 1032–1033
Turimycin, 188–189
Tusnel, 246–247
Tusside, 246–247
Tussidin Dm, 246–247
Tussidin Dm Nr, 246–247
Tussigon, 419–420

Tussin, 400–401
Tussin Dm, 246–247
Tussi-Organidin DM,
   246–247
Tussi-Organidin DM NR,
   246–247
Tussi-Organidin DM-S NR,
   246–247
Tussi-R-Gen Dm, 246–247
Tusso-DM, 246–247
Tussol, 579–581
Tusstat, 275–276
Twicyl, 35–36
Tylenol, 3–4

U

Uad Dryl, 275–276
Ubacillin, 41–42
Ukapen, 40–41
Ulcer
   aphthous
      thalidomide, 959–960
   corneal
      ofloxacin, 712–713
   duodenal. See Duodenal
      ulcer.
   gastric
      famotidine, 338
      nizatidine, 700–701
      omeprazole, 717–718
      ranitidine, 865–866
   lansoprazole, 491–492
   peptic. See Peptic ulcer
      disease.
   stress
      lansoprazole, 491–492
      rabeprazole, 859–860
Ulcerative colitis
   balsalazide, 67–68
   hydrocortisone, 420–422
   mercaptopurine, 564–566
   mesalamine, 568–569
   olsalazine, 716–717
   sulfasalazine, 931–932
Ulcinfan, 176–177
Ulcona, 925–926
Ulcumaag, 925–926
Ulpax, 176–177
Ulsidex, 925–926
Ultane, 906–907
Ultiva, 866–867
Ultracef, 122
Ultracortenol, 816–818
Ultragris, 399–400
Ultra-K-Chlor, 808
Ultram, 983–984
Ultramicrosize
   Griseofulvin, 399–400
Ultrase, 740–741
Ultrase Mt, 740–741
Ultratag, 941–942
Ultravate, 407
Ultraxime, 128–130
Ultrazine-10, 829–830
Umi-Pex 30, 778–779
Unasyn, 41–42
Uni-Ace, 3–4
Unicillin, 35–36

Unicort, 78–79
Uni-Dur, 960–962
Unifyl, 960–962
Unipen, 653–654
Uniphyl, 960–962
Unitrim, 995–997
Univasc, 642–643
Unizuric, 16–17
Unstable angina
   dalteparin, 224–226
Upcyclin, 957–959
Urazole, 932–933
urea, 1007
Ureaphil, 1005
Urecholine, 81–82
Uricemil, 16–17
Uriconorm-E, 16–17
Urimor, 599
Urinary alkalinization
   acetazolamide, 5–6
Urinary incontinence
   midodrine, 626–627
Urinary retention
   neostigmine, 672–674
Urinary tract infection
   cinoxacin, 177–178
   ciprofloxacin, 178–180
   enoxacin, 303–304
   methenamine, 585–586
   nitrofurantoin, 691–693
   piperacillin, 792–794
   piperacillin/tazobactam,
      794–795
   sulfisoxazole, 932–933
   trimethoprim, 997–999
Urispas, 349
Uri-Tet, 734–736
Urobak, 930–931
Urocid, 823–824
Urodic, 656–657
Urodine, 771
Urodol, 771
urokinase, 1008–1009
Urolene Blue, 603–604
Urolin, 170–171
Uropyridine, 771
Urovist Cysto, 249–250
Urovist Cysto 100Ml in
   300Ml, 249–250
Urovist Cysto 300Ml in
   500Ml, 249–250
Urovist Cysto Pediatric,
   249–250
Urovist Meglumine,
   249–250
Urovist Meglumine
   DIU/CT, 249–250
Ursacol, 1007–1008
Ursodamor, 1007–1008
ursodiol, 1009–1010
Urticaria, 154–155
   cetirizine, 154–155
   clemastine fumarate, 187
   fexofenadine, 347
   loratadine, 524–525
Uterine atony
   carboprost
      tromethamine,
      115–116

Uterine bleeding
   dysfunctional
      medroxyprogesterone,
      547–549
      mestranol, 571–572
      norethindrone,
      701–702
      norgestrel, 704–705
   postpartum
      methylergonovine,
      605–606
      oxytocin, 736–737
Uterine carcinoma
   dactinomycin, 223–224
Uterine fibroids
   leuprolide, 498–499
U-Tri-Lone, 991–993

V

Vaginitis, atrophic
   chlorotrianisene,
      165–166
   dienestrol, 260
   estradiol, 319–321
   ethinyl estradiol,
      326–327
Vaginosis, bacterial
   clindamycin, 188–189
Vagistat, 708–709
valacyclovir, 1011–1012
Valcyte, 1011–1012
valdecoxib, 1012–1013
valganciclovir, 1013–1014
Valisone, 79–80
Valitran, 250–252
Valium, 250–252
Valmagen, 176–177
Valodex, 939–940
valproate, 1014–1016
valproic acid, 1016–1017
Valrelease, 250–252
valsartan, 1018–1019
Valtrex, 1009–1010
Valvulopathy
   dipyridamole, 276–277
Vanatrip, 30–31
Vanceril, 69–70
Vanceril DS, 69–70
Vancocin, 1017–1018
Vancoled, 1017–1018
vancomycin, 1019–1020
Vancor, 1017–1018
Vantin, 139–140
Vapine, 160–161
Vapo-Iso, 469–470
Vaqta, 412–413
Varicella pneumonia
   acyclovir, 8–9
varicella vaccine,
   1020–1022
varicella zoster immune
   globulin, 1022–1023
Varitect, 1020–1022
Varivax, 1018–1020
Vascor, 77
Vasocon, 662–663
Vasomotor symptoms
   chlorotrianisene, 165–166